Unlocking the Brain

Unlocking the Brain

VOLUME II: CONSCIOUSNESS

GEORG NORTHOFF

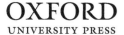

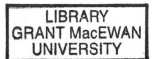

OXFORD
UNIVERSITY PRESS

Oxford University Press is a department of the University of Oxford.
It furthers the University's objective of excellence in research, scholarship,
and education by publishing worldwide.

Oxford   New York
Auckland   Cape Town   Dar es Salaam   Hong Kong   Karachi
Kuala Lumpur   Madrid   Melbourne   Mexico City   Nairobi
New Delhi   Shanghai   Taipei   Toronto

With offices in
Argentina   Austria   Brazil   Chile   Czech Republic   France   Greece
Guatemala   Hungary   Italy   Japan   Poland   Portugal   Singapore
South Korea   Switzerland   Thailand   Turkey   Ukraine   Vietnam

Oxford is a registered trademark of Oxford University Press
in the UK and certain other countries.

Published in the United States of America by
Oxford University Press
198 Madison Avenue, New York, NY 10016

Library of Congress Cataloging-in-Publication Data
Northoff, Georg.
Unlocking the brain / Georg Northoff.
   p. ; cm.
Includes bibliographical references and indexes.
ISBN 978-0-19-982698-8 (alk. paper)—ISBN 978-0-19-982699-5 (alk. paper)
I. Title.
[DNLM: 1. Brain—physiology.   2. Brain Mapping—psychology.   3. Cognition—physiology.   4. Neural
Pathways—physiology.   5. Neuropsychiatry. WL 335]
612.8—dc23
2012029357

9 8 7 6 5 4 3 2 1

Printed in the United States of America
on acid-free paper

CONTENTS OF VOLUME II

LIST OF FIGURES FOR VOLUME II

PREFACE

What is consciousness? Everybody experiences it daily. For instance, when reading this preface, you perceive these lines and subjectively experience them as the content of your perception. This is your consciousness. Everybody seems to know what consciousness is, since we experience it daily. Isn't that sufficient to answer the question?

Current philosophy, for instance, philosophy of mind, discusses different concepts of consciousness like "phenomenal and access consciousness." And it points out different phenomenal features like qualia, which describe the subjective and qualitative dimension of consciousness, the "what it is like"; such as what the experience of seeing blackness is like when experiencing the black cover of this book.

The philosophical discussion of consciousness is complemented on the neuroscientific side by the investigation of the neuronal states underlying the consciousness of contents. The search for these neural states has been described as the "neural correlates of consciousness" (NCC) that target the sufficient neural conditions for the constitution of consciousness and its contents by the brain's neuronal states. Various suggestions have been made recently for the NCC, and many will be discussed in this book.

What about the necessary neural conditions of consciousness, though? "Necessary conditions" are those without which any consciousness remains in principal impossible, even if it is not actually realized and manifested. At present, though, we do not know anything about the necessary neural conditions of consciousness. More specifically, we do not know how the brain's purely neuronal resting-state and stimulus-induced activity can possibly be associated with consciousness and its phenomenal features.

Let us describe the situation in more detail. We currently know a lot about the different regions and networks in the brain, including their different functions (e.g., sensorimotor, affective, cognitive, etc.) and how they process particular contents independently of whether they become conscious or not. In contrast, we do not know the neuronal mechanisms and processes that predispose the various contents and their respective stimulus-induced activities to become associated with consciousness.

What must the neuronal mechanisms look like that make possible and thus predispose consciousness? This leads us away from the current focus on particular regions and networks and their respective functions. And it also leads us away from the stimulus-induced and task-related activities we observe in the brain during our experimental manipulations. Instead, we may need to shift our focus to the very neuronal mechanisms and processes that occur prior to the distinction between different regions and networks as well as prior to the neuronal differentiation between different functions, that is, sensory, motor, affective, and cognitive to name just a few.

Where does such a shift away from both regions/networks and functions lead us? I argue that it will lead us back to the brain itself and its intrinsic features. Let me explain this briefly. We usually investigate the brain by applying specific stimuli and tasks to probe the brain's regions and functions in our experimental paradigms. This causes us to easily neglect what happens prior to the arrival of these stimuli in the brain itself. Rather than searching for what the brain does with extrinsic stimuli from body and environment, we have to look for what happens in the brain itself and its intrinsic features prior to the arrival of the extrinsic stimuli. This leads me back to Volume I, where I discussed two of the brain's intrinsic features in quite some detail, its resting-state activity and its neural code.

Why are the brain's intrinsic activity and its neural code so important? I showed in Volume I how the brain's resting state and its neural code, difference-based coding, shape and predispose stimulus-induced and task-related activity. Thereby, I presupposed a purely neuronal context, thus considering only how these two intrinsic features predispose and shape the brain's neural activity during both resting state and stimulus-induced activity independently of any kind of consciousness. This was the focus in Volume I.

What about Volume II? I now shift from the purely neuronal context of Volume I to a more phenomenal or better neurophenomenal context here in Volume II. This allows me to show the central relevance of both resting-state activity and difference-based coding for generating consciousness and its various phenomenal features. My aim is to develop specific neurophenomenal hypotheses that show how the brain's intrinsic features, that is, its resting-state activity and neural code, predispose the intrinsic features of consciousness and its phenomenal features in a necessary and unavoidable way and thus by default. In short, without resting-state activity and/or a different neural code, consciousness remains impossible. How will I structure this volume? The necessity of the brain's resting–state activity and its neural code will be shown for different phenomenal features, time and space in Chapters 13 to 17, unity in Chapters 18–22,

self and intentionality in Chapters 23 to 27, and finally qualia in Chapters 28 to 32. The reader may therefore select the chapters according to his primary interest and the contents predominating in his own consciousness.

Now that I have set up the general framework of this book and its relationship to Volume I, I want to turn to the more formal side of things. While working on these two volumes, I came across different and truly exciting studies in neuroscience. The field of neuroscience is booming with plenty of methods, hypotheses, and investigations. I could unfortunately only pick up a few while probably neglecting many others that would have also been relevant to both the neuronal hypotheses in Volume I and the neurophenomenal hypotheses in Volume II. The only thing I can do is to excuse myself to the many authors whose work I neglected. I hope they will make me aware of their findings in the future.

I want to thank several people. First and foremost, I want to thank Catharine Carlin and especially Joan Bossart from Oxford University Press, who supported me very much in all stages by giving excellent advice. A big thank-you to both of you for making such a complex project possible. The editorial assistants Jennifer Milton and Miles Osgaard should also be thanked at this stage.

Several anonymous reviewers also need to be thanked for providing very thoughtful comments, with one of them even suggesting to write these two volumes. My institution, the Institute of Mental Health Research in Ottawa/Canada and its head, Zul Merali, shall also be thanked for the freedom and mental space it provides me to tackle such a complex project. The Canadian funding agencies like the CIHR, the EJLB, National Science Foundation of China, and the Michael Smith Foundation as well as others like the HDRF/ISAN shall also be thanked for their generous support of my research and work.

My friend and dear colleague Jaak Panksepp should also be thanked. I cherish my discussions with him, his out-of-the-box thinking, and his excellent ideas and understanding. Thank you, Jaak. Thank you also to Todd Feinberg, Heinz Boeker, Eric Chen, Marina Farinelli,

Shinobura Kimura, Xuchu Weng, Mark Solms, Winnie Chu, and Shihui Han for stimulating discussions! A big thanks also goes to Timothy Lane, Nir Lipsman, Zirui Huang, Alexander Heinzel and Alexander Sartorius who provided extremely helpful comments in earlier stages. The members of research group also deserve a thank-you for inspiring discussions; hence, my thanks go to Dave Hayes, Niall Duncan, Takashi Nakao, Christine Wiebking, Zirui Huang (he offered excellent ideas for some of the figures in the introduction), Pedro Chaves, Nils-Frederic Wagner, Eyup Suzgun, and Pengmin Qin. Omar Han, Giles Holland, Samuel Kim, and Jonathan Hyslop should be thanked for putting the references together. For excellent support in some editorial work, my thanks go to Leslie Anglin. Finally, I need to give a big thank-you to my partner, John Sarkissian, who has to endure my often rather absent mind with its consciousness dwelling and musing in its mental states about the brain and its consciousness rather than focusing its own consciousness on the more physical and biological requirements of daily life.

INTRODUCTION I: THE BRAIN AND ITS INTRINSIC FEATURES

Do we really need yet another book about consciousness? "No," you are inclined to say, "since everybody knows what it is to be conscious." You are conscious while reading this book. Even worse, you cannot avoid becoming conscious of what is written here about consciousness: You perceive the black colors of the cover, you feel certain emotions like frustration about this seemingly banal beginning, and you think certain thoughts while reading. You may also become conscious of your own thoughts and cognitions tempting you to contradict the definition given here. Ultimately even your self, the one who reads these lines, enters consciousness yielding what is called "self-consciousness."

What is *consciousness*? Consciousness is such a basic phenomenon that any definition seems superfluous. However, if we want to understand how consciousness is generated, we need to at least somehow determine what it is we are searching for. Otherwise we remain blind in our search for the neural basis of consciousness. Let me give at least a tentative definition at this point.

Philosopher Thomas Nagel (1974) characterized consciousness as "what it is like." The concept of "what it is like" describes that experience and thus consciousness goes along with a particular quality, a phenomenal-qualitative feel that has been called *qualia*. You experience the book's black color in terms of this phenomenal-qualitative feel, you have a *quale* of the color black, the blackness of the book in your experience in first-person perspective. In contrast to your experience in the first-person perspective, the quale of the color black, that is, the blackness, remains absent during your observation of the book's cover in the third-person perspective. There is no experience of the book's blackness and thus a phenomenal-qualitative feel when you observe the book.

How is such phenomenal-qualitative feel possible? By answering that, Nagel argues, you need to take a particular "point of view." What is a "point of view"? Most generally, a point of view anchors us as humans in a particular position or stance compared to the rest of the physical and biological world. This distinguishes, for instance, the human's point of view from the ones of other species, like the bat: The bat's biophysical equipment allows it to perceive ultra-sonar frequencies that we humans, due to our brain's frequency range, are unable to capture. Due to their brain's biophysical properties, bats and humans are differently anchored and positioned within the same physical world (see Chapters 20 and 21 for more details on the concept of "point of view"). In short, your point of view is *species-specific*.

Things are even more complicated, though. The particular point of view you are taking while reading these lines is not only different from the ones of other species but also different from the ones of other human individuals. In other words, your point of view is not only species-specific, but also individually distinct, that is specific for a particular individual subject or person. And it is that individually specific point of view, your particular first-person perspective, from which you experience the world in terms of the qualitative-phenomenal feel; that is, qualia. Hence qualia are tied not only to a point of view of a particular species, but also to the perspective of an individual person, his first-person perspective.

Let us stop here. We already see that consciousness is not as simple as it seems to be. It can be characterized by different features of our subjective experience, like qualia, point of view, and first-person perspective (and many others, as we will see later). Since they concern our subjective experience, philosophers (see for instance van Gulick 2004) call them "phenomenal features" as distinguished from, say, physical features. Just like as in the case of physical features, our brief account already shows that there are different phenomenal features. There is thus phenomenal heterogeneity rather than phenomenal homogeneity.

Why is such phenomenal heterogeneity important for the neuroscientist? The different phenomenal features of consciousness may be related to different neuronal mechanisms in the brain. Rather than claiming that one particular neuronal mechanism underlies consciousness in general, as is often suggested these days (see later), we may do better to develop a specific neuronal hypothesis for each phenomenal feature, "neurophenomenal hypotheses," as I will call them later. Therefore, the main aim of this volume is to develop specific neurophenomenal hypotheses for the different phenomenal features of consciousness.

PRELUDE II: THE SUBJECTIVE NATURE OF CONSCIOUSNESS

Consciousness is characterized by different phenomenal features, including qualia, a point of view, and first-person perspective. Since all these phenomenal features are tied to a particular individual person rather than being shared between different individuals, philosophers characterize consciousness and its various

phenomenal features as "subjective." "Subjective" in this context means that it is specific to you, i.e., your individual person, implying that no other person can share your particular point of view and its associated experience. Consciousness is essentially subjective and therefore to be distinguished from the objective character of the physical world that is shared and similar across different individuals (rather than being specific for each particular individual person).

The subjective nature of consciousness presents a real puzzle to both neuroscientists and philosophers these days and (at least in the case of the philosophers) also some days ago: How is it possible that something as subjective as consciousness and its phenomenal features can arise within the objective physical world in general, and our seemingly purely physical brain in particular? This question touches upon what philosophers like David Chalmers (2000, 2010) describe as the "hard problem."

Put in an abbreviated way, this hard problem is the question of why there *is* and how it is possible that there is consciousness and thus subjectivity at all in the midst of an otherwise purely objective and completely non-conscious physical world. To address this question, the focus in this second volume shifts from the brain itself and its physical features, as dealt with in the first volume, to consciousness and its phenomenal features: How can the seemingly objective and purely physical brain (see Chapter 21 for details about the concepts of the "physical" and the "objective") possibly generate something as subjective and phenomenal as consciousness?

We remember that the first volume talked about the brain and how it generates and encodes its own neuronal activity. I proposed a particular theory of brain activity; namely, that neural activity in the brain is generated by the brain's application of a particular encoding strategy—difference-based coding as distinguished from stimulus-based coding. Therefore, the first volume was about the brain itself and its encoding of neural activity, thus remaining within a purely neuronal context.

The present volume goes one step further: from the brain's encoding of neural activity to how the brain, associates the phenomenal and subjective features of consciousness with its otherwise purely neuronal resting state and stimulus-induced activity. I propose that the brain's application of a particular encoding strategy, namely, difference-based coding, makes possible and thus predisposes the generation of the subjective nature of consciousness and its various phenomenal features. Accordingly, unlike the first volume, this volume is no longer about the brain itself and its encoding of neural activity. Instead, this second volume is about subjectivity and, more specifically, about how the subjective nature of consciousness and its phenomenal features are predisposed by the particular way the brain encodes its own neural activity.

PRELUDE III: CONSCIOUSNESS AND BRAIN DESIGN

How is consciousness related to the brain? At first glance you may be inclined to say that consciousness cannot be found in the brain and its neuronal activity as encoded by difference-based coding. Why? The brain is everything that consciousness is not. Let me be more specific. The brain and its neuronal activity do not seem to harbor the kind of phenomenal-qualitative feel that our experience and thus consciousness are associated with. All we can observe and measure in the brain are quantitative and neuronal changes in its spatiotemporal activity whereas nothing like the alleged qualia can be found. There is, for instance, no quale and thus no blackness visible in the brain and its neuronal states when you experience the black cover of this book in your consciousness. All you can observe amounts to nothing but mere changes in biochemical and electrical activity: you cannot detect any kind of phenomenal-qualitative feel like blackness in the brain. Even worse, nobody has ever observed a "point of view" in the brain and its neuronal activity. All we can observe are mere neuronal activities at different levels (cellular, population, regional, etc.), and those, importantly, can be accessed in an objective way, from a third-person perspective, rather than in a subjective way as experienced in first-person perspective. The very same neuronal activity can thus be observed not only by you, but also by others, your neuroscientific colleagues, for instance, in the very same way, that is intersubjectively. Since none of the above-mentioned phenomenal features characterizing consciousness can be observed in the brain's neuronal activity, you may be tempted to argue that consciousness cannot be associated with the brain at all. Localization of consciousness in the brain and its neuronal activity seems to be simply impossible. What shall we do? One could deny consciousness altogether, assuming that it does not exist. This amounts to the claim that there is no "subjective experience" at all. The phenomenal features of consciousness like qualia, point of view, and first-person perspective are then nothing but conceptual illusions that have no counterparts in the real world. The "real" world is here the purely objective and physical world, whereas the "subjective world of consciousness and its phenomenal features" is illusory rather than real (see, for instance, Metzinger 2003 with regard to the self). That is absurd, however, since it contradicts our daily experience—and your consciousness while reading these lines. Even if we do not want it to occur, consciousness is always already there; we can simply not avoid experiencing phenomenal features like a point of view, qualia, and a first-person perspective (and so forth). It is not up to us to decide and invoke the various phenomenal features and thus consciousness. Instead, consciousness, its subjective nature and its phenomenal features, come by default and are therefore necessary and thus unavoidable (as the philosophers would express it).

How is it possible that consciousness and its phenomenal features come by default and are thus necessary or unavoidable? Let us compare the situation to the heart. The heart is designed as a muscle that by its very nature contracts. Such contraction makes possible the pumping of blood throughout the whole organism; pumping blood is thus a necessary or unavoidable consequence of the heart's design as a muscle. In short, due to its muscle design, the heart cannot help but pump blood.

Analogous to the heart and pumping, one may now suggest that the brain generates consciousness by default; that is, by the very nature of its design that in turn makes the generation of the various phenomenal features necessary or unavoidable. While we know the design of the heart very well, we currently do not know the design of the brain and how and why it cannot avoid associating consciousness and its phenomenal features with its otherwise purely neuronal resting state and stimulus-induced activity. Therefore, the focus in this volume is on how the brain and its particular design make possible, that is, *predispose*, consciousness and its phenomenal features (see later for explanation of the term "predisposition").

PRELUDE IV: CONTENT AND LEVEL OF CONSCIOUSNESS

What shall we do with "consciousness"? Metaphorically speaking, consciousness seems to be like an obstinate child who refuses to obey on any terms. This is well reflected in the fact that none of the various neuronal mechanisms suggested to underlie consciousness have yet provided a satisfactory explanation of why consciousness occurs by default (in at least healthy subjects). That inclined many past and even current philosophers (and even neuroscientists) to postulate some kind of *mind* (as a mental entity) to underlie the subjective nature of consciousness and its phenomenal heterogeneity. Presupposing such a mind-based approach, consciousness has often been considered the domain of philosophy in general and philosophy of mind in particular, rather than science, including neuroscience.

Nowadays we claim to know better, however. Consciousness is brain-based rather than mind-based (or even "brain-reductive" as some philosophers like to say; see Churchland 2002; see, though, Appendix 3 in Volume I for the necessary distinction between brain-based and brain-reductive accounts). That is what we claim to know. We do not know, however, why and how consciousness is based on the brain. More specifically, we do not know why and how the brain can associate its own objective and physical neural activity with something as subjective and phenomenal as consciousness.

What about empirical evidence? Empirical evidence tells us indeed that consciousness must have something to do with the brain. Patients with selected lesions in particular regions of their brain, like the visual cortex, remain unable to experience specific contents in consciousness like visual contents. Accordingly, what is described as the "content of consciousness" (see second Introduction for more detail on the concept of the "content" of consciousness) must be somehow related to the brain and its neural activity in particular regions.

There are also disorders of consciousness like the vegetative state: patients in a vegetative state lose consciousness, meaning that they seem to no longer exhibit any phenomenal features like qualia, a point of view, or first-person perspective. These patients show a rather low degree of what is described as the "level or state of consciousness" that concerns mainly arousal as distinguished from the contents of consciousness. Most important, these patients show major changes in their brain in its various networks and their biochemical modulation (see Part VIII for details). The level or state of consciousness may thus be mediated by specific, yet unclear, neuronal mechanisms that differ from the ones underlying the contents of consciousness.

Finally, further support comes from neuropsychiatric disorders like schizophrenia and depression. While the qualia, that is, the phenomenal-qualitative feel, are basically preserved in these patients, their point of view and their first-person perspective are abnormally altered, leading to strange and bizarre symptoms like delusions, ego disorders, negative mood, increased self-focus, and hallucinations. These symptoms can be associated neither with the contents nor with the level or state of consciousness; they thus seem to hint at an "additional dimension" in consciousness.

PRELUDE V: FORM AND THE BRAIN'S INTRINSIC ACTIVITY

How can we describe this "additional dimension" in consciousness in further detail? We will characterize this additional dimension as the form, structure, or organization of consciousness in the second Introduction (see also Northoff 2012a and 2013). The psychiatric disorders of schizophrenia and depression seem to show major abnormalities in the brain's intrinsic activity (see Chapters 22 and 27 for details), its *resting-state activity* as it is often called these days. One may thus suppose that form as a possible third dimension of consciousness may be related to the brain's intrinsic activity.

We recall from Volume I that we described the brain's intrinsic activity by a particular virtual statistically-based spatiotemporal structure (see Chapters 4–6). Such a spatiotemporal structure is supposed to be based on neuronal measures like functional connectivity and low-frequency fluctuations that allow the intrinsic activity to span in a virtual and statistically based way across different discrete points in physical time and space. While we discussed the purely neuronal features of such spatiotemporal structure in Volume I (see Chapters 4–6), we now focus on how the brain's intrinsic activity and its particular spatiotemporal organization make possible and thus predispose consciousness and its various phenomenal features.

I propose that we can understand how the brain's neural activity generates consciousness by default only by considering form as its third dimension. For that, as I suggest, we need to go back to the brain's intrinsic activity and its spatiotemporal structure and how the latter provides the form (or structure or organization) for the various phenomenal features of consciousness. By relating the brain's intrinsic activity and its spatiotemporal structure to the form of consciousness, the brain and its intrinsic activity cannot avoid predisposing the possible association of its own neural activity with consciousness and its phenomenal features. Accordingly, the brain's intrinsic activity itself may hold the key to consciousness and its subjective nature.

I here postulate what I describe as a "resting state-based account of consciousness." The "resting state-based account of consciousness" claims that the brain's intrinsic activity predisposes and thus makes necessary and unavoidable the possible association of its otherwise purely neuronal resting state and stimulus-induced activity with consciousness and its phenomenal features (see later for more details on this resting state-based account of consciousness).

The central role of the brain's resting state activity distinguishes the "resting state-based account of consciousness" from a "stimulus-bound account of consciousness." A "stimulus-bound account of consciousness," as is often suggested these days by neuroscientists and philosophers alike, focuses on the extrinsic stimulus-induced (or task-related) activity in the brain and its associated neurosensory, neuromotor, neuroaffective, neurocognitive, or neurosocial functions in order to reveal the neural correlates of the contents of consciousness (see later for more details about the distinction between resting state-based and stimulus-bound accounts of consciousness).

Taking both phenomenal and empirical characterizations together, we see that consciousness is far from being homogenous. We need to distinguish among different empirical dimensions of consciousness like content, level, and form. And we also need to consider different phenomenal features of consciousness like qualia, point of view, first-person perspective, and many others, as will become clear in the course of this book. What does such empirical and phenomenal heterogeneity imply for a neuroscientific, or better, *neurophenomenal*, approach to consciousness? The different empirical dimensions and phenomenal features may be mediated by different neuronal mechanisms. Accordingly, rather than searching for one overarching unifying principle of brain function, as is often suggested these days to account for consciousness, we need to discuss different neuronal mechanisms.

BRAIN AND CONSCIOUSNESS IA: EXTRINSIC ACTIVITY- RE-ENTRANT LOOPS AND INFORMATION INTEGRATION

How can we search for the neuronal mechanisms underlying consciousness? Neuroscientists speak of what they describe as "neural correlates of consciousness" (NCC). The concept of NCC describes the neural mechanisms that are sufficient for the occurrence of consciousness (Crick and Koch 1998; Koch 2004; Chalmers 2000, 2010; Tononi and Koch 2008; and see a more detailed account of the concept of NCC and its distinction from neural predispositions, neural prerequisites, and neural consequences in the second Introduction; see also de Graaf et al. 2012; Aru et al. 2012; Northoff 2013). Several neuronal mechanisms have been discussed as possible candidate mechanisms for the NCC. In the following paragraph I briefly highlight some of the main and most popular suggestions, with these and others being discussed more extensively in subsequent parts of this volume (see also Appendix 1).

G. Edelman (2003, 2004) and Seth et al. (2006) consider cyclic processing and thus circularity within the brain's neural organization as central for constituting consciousness (see also Llinas 1998, 2002). Cyclic processing describes the re-entrance of neural activity in the same region after looping and circulating in other regions via so-called re-entrant (or feedback) circuits. This is, for instance, the case in primary visual cortex (V1): the initial neural activity in V1 is transferred to higher visual regions such as the inferotemporal cortex (IT) in feed-forward connections. From there it is conveyed to the thalamus, which relays the information back to V1 and the other cortical regions, implying thalamo-cortical re-entrant connections (see also Tononi and Koch 2008 as well as Lamme and Roelfsema 2000; Lamme 2006; van Gaal and Lamme 2011). Consciousness is postulated to be constituted on the basis of such feedback or re-entrant connections that allow for cyclic processing (see also Edelman and Tononi 2000).

What is the exact neuronal mechanism of the feedback or re-entrant circuits? Re-entrant circuits integrate information from different sources as associated with the neural activity in different regions and networks. This leads Guilio Tononi to emphasize the integration of information as the central neuronal mechanism in yielding consciousness. He consequently developed what he calls the "integrated information theory" (IIT; Tononi 2004; Tononi and Koch 2008). The IIT proposes the degree of information that is linked and integrated to be central for consciousness: if the degree of integrated information is low due to, for instance, disruption in functional connectivity between different regions, consciousness remains impossible. This is supported by experimental data that indeed show disruption of functional connectivity between different regions in various disorders of consciousness like vegetative state (Rosanova et al. 2012; see Chapter 29 for details), NREM sleep, and anesthesia (see Massimini et al. 2010; see Chapters 15 and 16 for details; see also Appendix 1 for more detailed discussion of the IIT).

To measure the degree of information integration across, for instance, different regions in the brain, Tononi and others (Seth et al. 2006, 2008, 2011) developed specific quantifiable measures as will be discussed later (see Chapters 15 and 16 and Chapter 29, as well as Appendix 1). Neurobiologically, Tononi postulates the integration of information to be particularly related to the thalamo-cortical re-entrant connections. These re-entrant connections process all kinds of stimuli from different sources and regions, thus remaining unspecific with regard to the selected content. Such integration of different contents from different sources and regions is proposed to make possible the generation of a particular quality on the phenomenal level of consciousness, that is, qualia (see earlier discussion and later discussion for exact determination of "qualia"), as a phenomenal hallmark of consciousness.

Linkage of these qualia to the contents, as they are processed via thalamo-cortical information integration, may then allow for the association of consciousness to the respective contents. This distinguishes the conscious contents from the unconscious contents that do not undergo such cyclic processing via the thalamus. The addition of the specific quality, the qualia, remains consequently impossible in the absence of cyclic re-entrant processing so that the contents remain unconscious (see Chapters 28–30 for the discussion of qualia).

BRAIN AND CONSCIOUSNESS IB: EXTRINSIC ACTIVITY—GLOBAL WORKSPACE

Another suggestion for the neural correlate of consciousness comes from B. Baars (Baars 2005; Baars and Franklin 2007) and others like S. Dehaene (Dehaene and Changeux 2005, 2011;

Dehaene et al. 2006 for excellent overviews). They postulate global distribution of neural activity across many brain regions in a so-called global workspace to be central for yielding consciousness. The information and its contents processed in the brain must be globally distributed across the whole brain in order for them to become associated with consciousness.

If, inversely, information is only processed locally within particular regions but no longer globally throughout the whole brain, it cannot be associated with consciousness anymore. The main distinction between unconsciousness and consciousness is then supposed to be manifest in the difference between local and global distribution of neural activity. Hence, the global distribution of neural activity is here considered a sufficient condition and thus neural correlate of consciousness.

Dehaene and Changeux (2005, 2011) take the assumption of a global workspace of consciousness as starting point and determine it in more neuronal detail when suggesting what they call the *global neuronal workspace* theory (GNW). They postulate that neural activity in the prefrontal-parietal cortical network is central for yielding consciousness. More specifically, the prefrontal-parietal cortical network has to be recruited by the single stimulus in order to link and recruit the different neural networks. That in turn makes possible the global distribution and processing of the stimulus, which is central for associating consciousness with the stimulus (see Chapter 24 and Appendix 1 for more details).

The global workspace theory must be distinguished from more cognitive theories of consciousness. Some accounts link attention closely to consciousness and its contents (see, for instance, Lamme and Roelfsema 2000; Lamme 2006; van Gaal and Lamme 2011; Prinz 2012). However, recent investigations have shed some doubt on attention being implicated in selecting the contents of consciousness (see van Boxtel et al. 2010a and b; Graziano and Kastner 2011; see also Chapters 14 and 25 for more detailed discussion of the phenomenal contents of consciousness). This is supported by recent analyses that demonstrated consciousness and attention

to occur independently of each other (see Koch and Tsuchiya 2012; van Boxtel et al. 2010a and b).

Other cognitive theories of consciousness emphasize the central role of higher-order cognitive functions like memory, executive functions, metacognition, metarepresentation, and so on, in constituting consciousness (see, for instance, Augustenborg 2010; Lau 2008). On the philosophical side, this is reflected in higher-order thought theories of consciousness such as, for instance, that advanced by David Rosenthal, that propose the meta-representation of contents as contents to generate consciousness.

This is the case if one becomes aware that one is reading these lines and its respective contents; consciousness is here determined not by the contents themselves, but rather by the awareness of those contents *as* contents (which amounts to access or reflective consciousness as it is called in philosophy; see Chapters 18 and 19 for details). Cognitive functions like attention or working memory are now proposed to be central in enabling such an awareness of contents as contents (see, for instance, Prinz 2012; as well as Appendix 1 for details). This amounts to a "cognitive-based account of consciousness" (as distinguished from both a resting state-based and a stimulus-bound account of consciousness; see earlier) as it is often favored especially among philosophers.

BRAIN AND CONSCIOUSNESS IC: EXTRINSIC ACTIVITY—NEURAL SYNCHRONIZATION

Neural synchronization is yet another neural candidate mechanism for consciousness. Neural synchronization describes the temporal coordination and integration of neural activity changes across different brain regions. For instance, rhythmic discharges in the gamma range (30–40 Hz) have been observed in conjunction with conscious states (Fries et al. 2006; Varela et al. 2001; Koch 2004; Tononi and Koch 2008; Tononi 2008; Bars 2007, 2009a and b; Singer 1999; Llinas 1998, 2002; Buzsaki 2006; John 2005). Such synchronous activity allows for binding together the neural activities of different neurons (and regions) across time so that they form a "neural coalition" (Crick and Koch 2003, 2005). This is called "binding by synchronization" (see Chapter 13 for more details, as well as Chapter 10).

Considered in a purely neuronal way, binding by synchronization makes possible the linkage, or so-called binding, of different stimuli into one particular content, that is, an object or event. Such an object or event can then become conscious, yielding a conscious percept and a corresponding experience (see Chapter 18 for more extensive discussion). Since "binding" and "binding by synchronization" may be central for consciousness, Crick and Koch consider the gamma oscillations as their underlying neuronal mechanisms to be sufficient conditions and thus neural correlates of consciousness (Crick 1994; Crick and Koch 2003, 2005).

Where does this leave us? There are currently various suggestions for neuronal mechanisms related to consciousness. Most of them seem to presuppose consciousness as a homogenous and unitary entity while not accounting separately for its distinct phenomenal (and conceptual) features. Moreover, they concern mainly the sufficient neural conditions of consciousness, the neural correlates, while leaving open its necessary neuronal conditions (see later for details). Finally, they seem to target predominantly the contents, the phenomenal contents, of consciousness, whereas the other dimensions of consciousness, level and form (see second Introduction for more details), are apparently not covered by these approaches.

There is yet another characteristic shared by the various suggestions for the NCC. They all focus on neural activity related to stimuli, i.e., stimulus-induced activity. The guiding question here is: how is a stimulus to be processed neuronally in order for it to become conscious? The answers consisted in re-entrant thalamo-cortical processing, globalized neuronal processing, and neuronal synchronization. One may thus speak of "stimulus-bound accounts of consciousness" that consider the brain's extrinsic activity, its stimulus-induced (or task-related) activity as a sufficient neural condition of consciousness, and thus as NCC.

BRAIN AND CONSCIOUSNESS IIA: INTRINSIC ACTIVITY—SLOW WAVES

The "stimulus-bound accounts of consciousness" must be distinguished from "resting state-based accounts of consciousness" that consider the brain's resting-state activity and thus its intrinsic activity (see below for conceptual definition) as the very basis for consciousness (see also earlier and later). Let us be more precise. Stimulus-induced activity is elicited by stimuli from the outside of the brain and can thus be characterized as *extrinsic activity*. How about the neural activity stemming from the inside of the brain, the brain's intrinsic activity? This shall be addressed in this and the next section.

The term "intrinsic activity" describes spontaneous activity generated inside the brain itself (see Volume I, Chapter 4, for details). Since the observation of spontaneous activity implies the absence of extrinsic stimuli and thus a mere resting state, the term "intrinsic activity" is often used interchangeably with "resting-state activity" as it is also done in the following (see Chapter 4 in Volume I for discussion of these issues; see also Logothetis 2009 for a discussion on the concept of the resting state). After having reviewed the proposals for the relationship of extrinsic stimulus-induced (or task-related) activity to consciousness, we now focus on whether the brain's intrinsic activity, its resting-state activity, may be a viable candidate for consciousness (see also Lundervold 2010 for a more technical overview).

One recent proposal suggests that the resting-state activity's slow wave fluctuations in the frequency ranges between 0.001 Hz and 4 Hz are central in yielding consciousness (He et al. 2008; He and Raichle 2009; Raichle 2009). Due to the long time windows of their ongoing cycles, that is, phase durations, the slow wave fluctuations may be particularly suited for integrating different information together. Such information integration may then allow for the respective content to become associated with consciousness (see Chapter 14 for a detailed discussion of this hypothesis).

The assumption of information integration is supported by the origin of the slow wave fluctuations: they are generated in cortical layers I and

II, where the afferences from many different cortical layers and regions converge onto each other. This predisposes the slow wave fluctuations to integrate the different information from the various afferences (see later for further details, as well as Fingelkurts et al. 2010 for the consideration of the resting state's functional connectivity and low-frequency fluctuations in the context of consciousness). Such integration of different information by the afferences meshes nicely with the assumption of the information integration theory (IIT) mentioned earlier. Moreover, the "slow wave" hypothesis can be regarded as complementary to the one on neuronal synchronization. Low-frequency fluctuations (0.001–4 Hz) are mainly observed in the resting state, while neuronal synchronization targets predominantly higher frequency fluctuation in the gamma range (30–40 Hz) during stimulus-induced activity.

This raises the question for the role of the resting state's low-frequency fluctuations (<0.1 Hz) in the synchronization of the higher frequency oscillations (around 30 Hz) during stimulus-induced activity: Do the resting state's low-frequency oscillations have a say in synchronizing higher-frequency oscillations during stimulus-induced activity? This question may be central not only for understanding how intrinsic and extrinsic neural activity, i.e., resting state and stimulus-induced activity, are linked, but also for how both forms of neural activity may need to interact in order to associate consciousness with the processed stimuli (see Chapters 18 and 19 for more detailed discussions).

BRAIN AND CONSCIOUSNESS IIB: INTRINSIC ACTIVITY—METABOLISM

Another suggestion for the relevance of the brain's resting-state activity in consciousness comes from Robert Shulman (see the recent excellent book by Shulman 2012). Shulman et al. (2003, 2004) and van Eijsden et al. (2009) propose the resting state's baseline metabolism and the brain's energy demand as necessary conditions of consciousness. Following him, a certain level of baseline metabolism and energetic activity is necessary to develop consciousness, more specifically a certain level or state of

consciousness. If, in contrast, the level of baseline metabolism and energy supply are too low, one glides into a non-conscious state as, for instance, in anesthesia.

This is empirically supported by the investigation of the brain's metabolism using positron emission tomography (PET; Shulman et al. 2003, 2004; van Eijsden et al. 2009). These data show highly reduced metabolism in anesthesia: the more reduced the brain metabolism and energy supply, the lower the level of consciousness, and the deeper the level of anesthesia. Most important, this did not concern reduction of metabolism in specific regions, but rather an overall global reduction throughout the whole brain. Metabolism and thus energy levels are uniformly globally reduced by about 40%–50% in anesthesia compared to the values in the awake state (during rest).

Shulman proposes this reduction of metabolism and energy to be central for the loss of consciousness in anesthesia. Based on his own investigations (see Parts V and VIII for details), about 80%–85% of the glucose and thus of the energy is used to maintain and sustain high neuronal activity even during the absence of specific stimulation, that is, the resting state (see Logothetis 2009). The high metabolic and energy demand of the brain may be used to maintain a continuously high level of resting-state activity, which seems to be essential for consciousness, while metabolic and energetic reduction seems to go along with a decrease in the level of consciousness and ultimately the loss of consciousness (as in anesthesia).

CONSCIOUSNESS AND THE BRAIN IIC: INTRINSIC ACTIVITY—SLEEP AND GATING

A third suggestion for the central role of the resting state in consciousness comes from Rudolfo Llinas (1998, 2002). He investigated subjects in the awake state and during sleep. Conducting MEG studies, he observed that 40 Hz oscillations are present in both awake and sleeping (REM sleep) states. Both states differed from each other, however, in that a sensory stimulus could reset (and thus modulate) the 40 Hz oscillations only in the awake state but not during REM sleep state (where we dream). Hence, the neural reactivity of the resting-state activity's 40 Hz oscillations to external stimuli seems to distinguish the awake state from REM sleep.

The same was observed in NREM sleep that showed a similar nonreactivity to external stimuli. In addition, NREM sleep also exhibited reduced amplitude in the 40 Hz oscillations themselves, which distinguished it from REM sleep. Hence, the amplitude in the 40 Hz oscillations in the resting state seems to distinguish REM and NREM sleep. This underlines the central importance of the resting state and especially of its interaction with stimuli, that is, rest–stimulus interaction (see also Freeman 2003, 2010; Northoff et al. 2010; as well as Chapter 11), in yielding consciousness.

A fourth suggestion for a central role of intrinsic activity in consciousness comes from Dehaene (Dehaene and Changeux 2005, 2011). Depending on the timing of the stimulus relative to the ongoing spontaneous phase fluctuations, the stimulus may or may not lead to the recruitment of the neurons and network in fronto-parietal cortex, which they consider to be central in allowing for global distribution of the stimulus and its subsequent association with consciousness. That, however, needs to be specified.

If, for instance, the spontaneous firing activity in the fronto-parietal network is too strong and continuous, it can block and thus prevent its ignition by the external stimulus. Since Dehaene and Changeux postulate the fronto-parietal network to be a global neuronal workspace that is necessary for consciousness, the stimulus may consequently be "denied" conscious access and remain unconscious, that is, preconscious (see later for conceptual details; see Chapter 19 for more extensive discussion of the global neuronal workspace theory). The level of the ongoing spontaneous activity in fronto-parietal cortex may thus set a threshold and thereby gate whether the stimulus can induce neural activity changes and thus consciousness.

Taken together, these hypotheses point out the central relevance of the brain's intrinsic activity, its resting-state activity (throughout

I use both terms interchangeably; see Chapter 4 in Volume I for their definition), for consciousness. One may thus want to characterize them as "resting state-based accounts of consciousness," which claim that the brain's intrinsic activity is somehow related to consciousness. The exact neuronal mechanisms by means of which the brain's intrinsic activity makes consciousness possible and (to put it even more strongly) necessary and unavoidable remain unclear, however.

CONSCIOUSNESS AND THE BRAIN IID: INTRINSIC ACTIVITY— "SUBJECTIVIZATION" OF NEURAL ACTIVITY

Where do the different proposals for the neural correlates of consciousness, including both the brain's intrinsic and extrinsic activity, leave us? We recall from the beginning of this introduction that we discussed the different phenomenal features of consciousness. How can these various phenomenal features of consciousness and its subjective nature be accounted for by the various extrinsic and intrinsic candidate mechanisms of the NCC as presented here?

Rather than suggesting different neuronal mechanisms to underlie the different phenomenal features, the various NCC candidate mechanisms seem to presuppose consciousness as homogenous unitary phenomenon. Qualia are often considered the phenomenal hallmark feature of consciousness in neuroscience (and philosophy). If we can account for qualia, we can explain consciousness. The presupposition of consciousness as homogenous unitary phenomenon is well reflected in the fact that neuroscientists often suggest one particular unitary neuronal mechanism to underlie qualia which they assume to account for consciousness. They thus seem to tacitly presuppose the phenomenal homogeneity of consciousness limiting it to qualia only. This, however, contradicts the phenomenal heterogeneity of consciousness as described at the beginning of this introduction.

Instead of focusing on one unitary neuronal mechanism only, we need to develop more specific hypotheses that link the various phenomenal features of consciousness to distinct neuronal mechanisms in the brain. We thus need to develop what I refer to as "neurophenomenal hypotheses." Tentatively defined, the concept of "neurophenomenal hypotheses" describes suggestions for how particular neuronal mechanisms of the brain are related to specific phenomenal features of consciousness. The aim of this book is to develop specific neurophenomenal hypotheses for the different phenomenal features of consciousness, like qualia, first-person perspective, intentionality, unity, and so on (see the second Introduction for the specification of the phenomenal features of consciousness).

Besides the phenomenal heterogeneity, we also need to account for the subjective nature of consciousness (see also earlier): How can the objective physical features of the brain generate something as subjective as consciousness and its phenomenal features? This is not addressed by the current neuroscientific theories of consciousness, which most often focus on the contents or level of consciousness but not on consciousness itself and its subjective nature. Most of the current neuroscientific accounts consider consciousness rather in an objective way and therefore defined in terms of its contents and level (see earlier). This, however, leaves out one, if not *the*, essential characteristic of consciousness—its subjective nature.

Accordingly, we need to understand the kind of neuronal mechanisms that make necessary or unavoidable the association of the brain's seemingly objective neuronal activity with a subjective state; that is, consciousness and its phenomenal features. For the answer to that, I propose, we need to go back to the brain's intrinsic activity and its spatiotemporal structure that provide the kind of form (or structure, or organization) that I postulate as the third dimension of consciousness. I postulate that the form (or structure or organization) of the brain's intrinsic activity makes possible the association of consciousness and its subjective nature with the otherwise purely objective neural activity of the brain.

Metaphorically speaking, one may be inclined to say that the brain's intrinsic activity "subjectivizes" its own neural activity. Such "subjectivization" makes possible and thus predisposes the association of stimulus-induced activity and

its respective contents with consciousness and its phenomenal features. How does the brain's intrinsic activity "subjectivize" its own neural activity? This is a hard nut to crack, which dents deeply into many of our empirical and conceptual preconceptions about the brain and consciousness. To better understand the suggested role of the brain's intrinsic activity, we will now make a little detour to another organ of the body, the pancreas.

NEUROMETAPHORICAL COMPARISON IA: INSULIN AND RESTING-STATE ACTIVITY

Despite all the efforts and impressive empirical data and conceptual accounts, we still have the feeling that something is lacking in our explanation of how brain and consciousness are related to each other. Let's compare the situation to insulin and its role in diabetes mellitus.

Imagine that we only know that the level of insulin is abnormally low in diabetes, but that we do not know why this goes along with the various symptoms typical of diabetes. We know, for instance, that insulin is produced by the pancreas, but we do not know how insulin is connected to the different symptoms across the various body organs (eyes, legs, etc.) we can observe in diabetes. We also know that insulin is somehow connected to diabetes since our recent scientific data show some kind of correlation between the level of insulin and the degree of diabetic symptoms. In contrast, we do not know anything about the underlying mechanisms and processes that make such a correlation possible (see Fig. I-1, left).

Physiologically, we thus do not know how insulin controls and modulates the level of glucose. The knowledge of glucose and its relationship to insulin, however, is central to understanding why and how the various kinds of symptoms are yielded in diabetes. In our thought experiment, glucose by itself may even be known, whereas it remains unknown how it is connected to both insulin and the diabetic symptoms. In other words, we may treat glucose as a different ballgame when compared to the one of insulin and diabetes in our thought experiment.

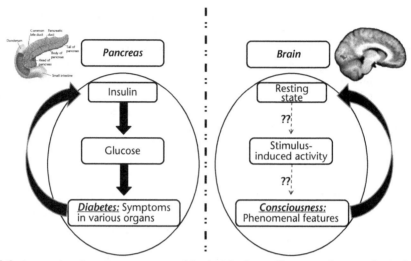

Figure I-1 Comparison between pancreas and brain. The figure illustrates the metaphorical comparison between pancreas and brain with regard to our current state of knowledge (I owe the basic design of this figure to Zirui Huang). *Left*: In the case of the pancreas we do know that insulin regulates and controls the level of glucose (upper). Abnormal levels of glucose can be traced back to insulin deficiency in the pancreas; while abnormal levels of glucose cause diabetes with various symptoms throughout the whole body (lower). To fully understand diabetes and its various symptoms, we thus have to go back to the pancreas itself and the insulin and its intrinsic features, i.e., how it impacts and controls glucose, as indicated by the big arrow. Imagine now if we know only about insulin, glucose, and the diabetes symptoms in a segregated way, while not being aware of their relationships as indicated by the arrows. That would be analogous to the current state of knowledge in the case of the brain, as indicated on the right. Note that the comparison with diabetes as disorder in no way indicates that consciousness is regarded as a pathological symptom of the brain; the illustration of the pancreas's function by diabetes makes it just clearer that we need to consider the pancreas's intrinsic functions, which, I claim, is also necessary in the case of the brain in order to understand consciousness. *Right*: In the case of the brain, we know some features about its resting-state activity; i.e., its intrinsic activity (upper), its stimulus-induced activity (middle), and the various phenomenal features of consciousness (lower). But we currently know neither how the resting state controls the stimulus-induced activity, nor how the latter brings forth and generates consciousness and its various phenomenal features. This is indicated by the dotted lines and the question marks. In order to understand consciousness, we may need to go back to the brain itself, the resting-state activity and its intrinsic features and how these predispose and modulate stimulus-induced activity. This is indicated by the big arrow on the side.

This is the situation we are currently facing in the neuroscience of consciousness. We know something about the brain's resting state (see later discussion and Chapters 4–6) that may be considered analogous to our knowledge of insulin in our thought experiment on diabetes. And at best we also know that there seems to be some kind of correlation between the level of the brain's resting state neuronal activity and the degree of consciousness, as especially suggested by the results from Shulman and the observations in anesthesia and vegetative state (see Chapters 28 and 29 for details).

In contrast, the underlying neuronal mechanisms and processes that yield this correlation remain unclear to us. We do not know how the neuronal activity in the brain yields the phenomenal-qualitative feel, the point of view, and the first-person perspective and thus the various phenomenal features of consciousness. Moreover, we have no knowledge about how the subjective nature of the phenomenal features is generated by the neuronal features of the brain. What we are missing are therefore the neuronal mechanisms and processes that allow the brain's seemingly objective intrinsic activity to yield something like subjective consciousness and its various phenomenal features. In other words, we are lacking the knowledge about the specific neuronal mechanisms that make necessary and thus unavoidable the generation of the various phenomenal features of consciousness (see Fig. I-1, right).

This is very much analogous to our imaginary scenario when we remain unable to causally connect insulin to glucose and the various symptoms of diabetes. In the same way we miss the link between insulin and the various diabetic symptoms in our imaginary scenario, we currently remain unable to account for the link between the brain's intrinsic activity and the various phenomenal features of consciousness.

NEUROMETAPHORICAL COMPARISON IB: GLUCOSE AND STIMULUS-INDUCED ACTIVITY

One may now want to argue that the analogy between our current knowledge of consciousness and the imaginary diabetes scenario does not hold. We do have plenty of knowledge of stimulus-induced activity, which may well correspond to the knowledge about glucose, while our knowledge of resting-state activity corresponds to the one about insulin. Accordingly, unlike in our thought experiment, we may have already plenty of knowledge of both insulin, that is resting-state activity, and glucose, that is stimulus-induced activity.

However, even if so, the analogy remains untouched by that. Why? In our "diabetic thought experiment" we lack the knowledge that the level of glucose is controlled and predisposed by insulin. Analogously, we currently lack the knowledge about the relationship between resting-state activity and stimulus-induced activity. More specifically, we do not know how the resting-state activity controls and thus predisposes subsequent stimulus-induced activity.

How, then, is the relationship between resting-state activity and stimulus-induced activity related to consciousness? Consciousness is usually associated with extrinsic stimuli and consequently with stimulus-induced activity in

the brain. Since we currently do not know how resting-state and stimulus-induced activity are related to each other, we also remain unable to directly link the brain and its intrinsic activity to consciousness as associated with the extrinsic stimuli and their stimulus-induced activity.

Lets briefly reconsider our "diabetic thought experiment" and more specifically see how we advanced our knowledge about diabetes. Once we were able to connect insulin to glucose, we could understand the common physiological mechanisms underlying the manifestation of the different diabetic symptoms in the various organs across the whole body. We then understood and knew how the level of insulin predisposes the various symptoms via its impact on glucose. The analogous scenario may now be suggested to hold true in the case of consciousness. I here aim to link resting-state activity and stimulus-induced activity. This may enable us to see how the brain's intrinsic activity predisposes the neuronal mechanisms that make necessary and thus unavoidable the constitution of the various phenomenal features of consciousness during stimulus-induced activity.

Analogous to insulin, the resting-state activity itself may then be supposed to provide the very basis, for example, or neural predisposition (see the second Introduction for details about the concept of neural predisposition), for the various phenomenal features of consciousness. In the same way as the level of insulin predisposes the level of glucose, the brain's intrinsic activity and its particular spatiotemporal organization may predispose the kind (and degree) of phenomenal features that characterize consciousness.

The analogy goes even further. Too little insulin will affect the glucose level and hence our general level of arousal. We may lose consciousness and slip into a coma: diabetic coma as it is called in the context of insulin. The same seems to hold on the side of the brain's resting-state activity. If the resting-state activity level is too low, we lose consciousness and end up in a vegetative state or, even worse, in a coma (a disorder of consciousness as it is called in the context of the brain; see Chapters 28 and 29). In short, both too little insulin and too little resting-state activity lead to coma.

NEUROMETAPHORICAL COMPARISON IC: DETOURS THROUGH INSULIN AND RESTING-STATE ACTIVITY

What does the figurative comparison with our "diabetic thought experiment" tell us? The detection of the intrinsic link of insulin to glucose revealed its central role in the control of both the glucose level and the various body functions (as visible in the symptoms of diabetes). Analogously, we may need to decipher the intrinsic link of the brain's resting-state activity to stimulus-induced activity in order to understand how the purely neuronal stimulus-induced activity can be associated with phenomenal features; that is, consciousness. More specifically, we need to understand how the brain's resting-state activity impacts and controls and thus predisposes the subsequent stimulus-induced activity (see also Chapters 11 and 12 in Volume I). This will not only shed some light on the neuronal mechanisms underlying stimulus-induced activity but, most important, on how the respective stimulus can be associated with the phenomenal features of consciousness.

How can we investigate consciousness? To reveal the neuronal mechanisms underlying consciousness, we must better understand stimulus-induced activity, that is analogous to the investigation of glucose in our "diabetic thought experiment." This is possible, however, only by going back to its predisposition by the resting-state activity that corresponds to the role of insulin in the case of diabetes. Most important, in the case of our research into diabetes, we had to make the detour via insulin and its intrinsic features to better understand the mechanisms of glucose itself and how and why it yields the various diabetic symptoms. Analogously, we have to make the detour via the brain's resting-state activity in order to better understand how and why the purely neuronal stimulus-induced activity can be associated with consciousness and its various phenomenal features.

Accordingly, the brain's intrinsic activity and how it predisposes consciousness may be central and will therefore be the main focus of my neurophenomenal hypotheses as developed in Parts V–VII. This, in turn, will make it easier for us to understand how the purely neuronal stimulus-induced activity can be associated with the various phenomenal features of consciousness as they will be discussed in the final part, Part VIII.

NEUROCONCEPTUAL REMARK IA: WHAT ARE NEURONAL MECHANISMS?

Let us go back to the brain and leave both insulin and diabetes behind. What kind of specific knowledge is missing in order to account for the neuronal mechanisms of consciousness? We have plenty of knowledge about the brain's neuronal states, including both resting-state and stimulus-induced activity. However, we lack an understanding of the neural mechanisms of how such objective and purely neuronal states can be associated with the subjective and phenomenal features of consciousness.

What do I mean by the term "mechanism"? In answering that, I briefly turn to philosopher M. Tye (2007, 26–27) and what he calls the "problem of mechanism." Following Tye, there must be some basic mechanism in the brain itself that operates in such way as to constitute consciousness: "The problem of mechanism, then, can be put as follows: How do objective, physical changes in the brain generate subjective feelings and experiences? What is the mechanism which is responsible for the production of the 'what it is like' aspects of our mental lives?" (Tye 2007, 27). Following Tye, we currently have no idea about the neuronal mechanisms underlying consciousness:

> What the above examples strongly suggest is that, in the natural world, the generation of higher-level states or processes or properties by what is going on at lower neurophysiological or chemical or microphysical levels is grounded in mechanisms which explain the generation of the higher-level items. So, if phenomenal consciousness is a natural phenomenon, a part of the physical world, there should be a mechanism that provides an explanatory link between the subjective and the objective. Given that there is such a mechanism, the place of phenomenally conscious states in the natural, physical domain is not threatened. But what could this mechanism

be? We currently have no idea. (Tye 2007, 27; see also Neisser 2011a and b and Hohwy 2012, for the discussion of "mechanisms" as distinguished from "correlates" of consciousness)

Where can we find such a mechanism? The mechanism must be predisposed by the brain itself and its intrinsic features. Intrinsic features of the brain are those that define the brain as brain (see later for more discussion). These intrinsic features predispose the brain to react in certain ways (rather than others) to extrinsic stimuli. We therefore need to understand the brain's intrinsic features and how they predispose the association of consciousness and its phenomenal features with the otherwise purely neuronal neural activity of the brain during either the resting state (as during dreams) or stimulus-induced activity of extrinsic stimuli. What are the brain's intrinsic features? We first need to briefly determine what exactly is meant by the term "intrinsic features," which is the focus of the next section.

NEUROCONCEPTUAL REMARK
IB: INTRINSIC FEATURES OF THE BRAIN

What are intrinsic features? Let's discuss an example Tye himself (2007, 27) gives when he speaks of *brittleness*:

> Like liquidity, brittleness is a predisposition. Brittle objects are supposed to shatter easily. This predisposition is produced in a thin glass sheet via the irregular alignment of crystals. Such an alignment results in there being weak forces between crystals holding them together. So, when a force is applied, the glass shatters. The generation of brittleness is now explained (Tye 2007, 27).

How can we compare the example of brittleness to our quest for the neuronal mechanisms underlying consciousness? Tye distinguishes here between intrinsic and extrinsic features: an intrinsic feature consists of the irregular alignment of crystals, whereas the external force is an extrinsic feature. How are intrinsic and extrinsic features related to each other? The intrinsic features, the irregular alignment of crystals, predispose the shattering of the brittle object during the application of the external force as extrinsic feature.

How does that stand in relation to consciousness? In the case of the brain, the intrinsic feature may consist in its intrinsic activity, its resting-state activity, whereas the stimuli from body and environment correspond to the external and thus extrinsic force applied to the brittle object. The resulting stimulus-induced activity and its associated phenomenal features may hence be considered the neural analogue to the shattering of the brittle object. The scattered broken and fragmented pieces on the side of the brittle object may then correspond to the scattering and the fragmentation of the brain's intrinsic activity and its spatiotemporal structure by the extrinsic stimuli.

Following Tye's example, the brain's intrinsic activity must somehow predispose the association of the stimulus and its stimulus-induced activity with consciousness. How is that possible? We do not know. Unlike in the case of the brittle object, we currently do not know the exact neuronal features of the brain's intrinsic activity. Hence, we lack the knowledge about the brain's analogue to the "irregular alignment of crystals" and thus of its intrinsic features (see Fig. I-2).

Moreover, we need to gain insight into how the brain's analogue to the "irregular alignment of crystals" predisposes the brain's reaction to extrinsic stimuli such as the latter can be associated with consciousness. To proceed, we therefore must better understand the brain's intrinsic features and what exactly is meant by the concept of "predisposition." Let me start with the former, the brain's intrinsic features, which will be discussed in the remainder of this introduction, while the latter, the concept of "predisposition," will be taken up in the second Introduction in more detail.

INTRINSIC FEATURES OF THE *BRAIN*
IA: SPATIOTEMPORAL STRUCTURE OF THE BRAIN'S RESTING-STATE ACTIVITY

After our little detour to the pancreas and the world of crystals, we can now finally return to the brain itself and more concrete to its neuronal mechanisms. More specifically, we may want to shed some light on the brain's intrinsic features. The brain's intrinsic features are the features that the brain itself provides to its own

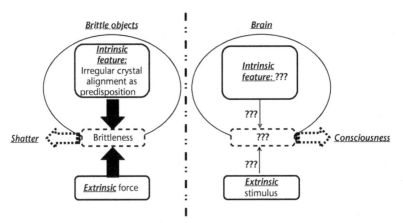

Figure I-2 Intrinsic features and predispositions. The figure shows the comparison between brittle objects (left part) and the brain (right) (I owe the basic design of this figure to Zirui Huang). *Left part*: In the case of brittle objects, we do know that an irregular alignment of crystals is an intrinsic feature of brittle objects that predisposes them to brittleness. If force as an extrinsic feature is applied, such brittleness lets the object shatter. *Right part*: In the case of the brain, we do know that extrinsic stimuli induce consciousness (lower part) and that that is somehow related to the brain. But we do not know the brain's intrinsic features that predispose it to generate consciousness in the presence of extrinsic stimuli. Hence we do not know the brain's neural analogue to the irregular crystal alignment, as indicated by the question marks. Nor do we know the neural mechanisms by means of which such an intrinsic feature could affect the brain's ability to generate consciousness as the neural analogue to the object's brittleness. This is indicated by the dotted line and the question marks. Hence, we know neither the brain's intrinsic features and thus its neural predispositions, nor the mechanisms by means of which these are related to consciousness. We consequently also lack the knowledge about the neural mechanisms by means of which the extrinsic stimulus can generate consciousness, as again indicated by question marks.

neural processing of extrinsic stimuli. They thus reflect the brain's active contribution, that is, its specific input, to its own neural processing of the intero- and exteroceptive inputs from body and environment.

Two such active contributions of the brain and thus intrinsic features were investigated in detail in Volume I: the spatiotemporal structure of the brain's intrinsic activity, and the neural code the brain applies to generate and encode its own neuronal activity. To understand how the brain predisposes consciousness, we thus have to better understand the resting state's spatiotemporal structure and the brain's encoding strategy. Let us start with the spatiotemporal structure of the brain's resting-state activity.

The resting-state activity can be characterized by both spatial and temporal dimensions. This is reflected in functional connectivity and low-frequency fluctuations. Functional connectivity describes the linkage between the neural activities of different regions across the space of the brain (see also Fingelkurts et al. 2004a and b, 2005 for the discussion of this issue), whereas low-frequency fluctuations concern the fluctuations in neural activity across time. As based on the encoding of temporal and spatial differences (see later), functional connectivity and low-frequency fluctuations reflect neural activity across different discrete points in physical time and space, rather than corresponding to different single discrete points in physical time and space.

The encoding of neural activity across different discrete points in physical time and space makes possible the constitution of a spatiotemporal structure. Such spatiotemporal structure must be considered "virtual" rather than "real." This is because the spatiotemporal structure is based on the encoding of temporal and spatial differences between different stimuli rather than on the stimuli themselves and their respective physical features.

The spatiotemporal structure is based on the encoding of the statistical frequency distribution of the stimuli across different discrete points in physical time and space, that is, the natural statistics of the encoded stimuli. Accordingly, the resting state's spatiotemporal structure is statistically based rather than physically based, which I postulate to be possible on the basis of difference-based coding as distinguished from stimulus-based coding (Fig. I-3a; see later).

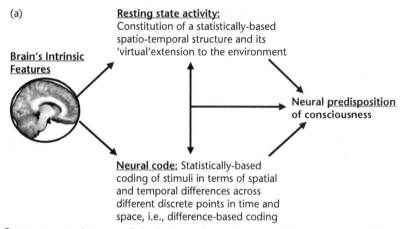

Figure I-3a-c Intrinsic features of the brain and consciousness. The figures show the relationship between the brain's intrinsic features and consciousness. (*a*) As illustrated on the left and the middle, the resting state and the neural code are intrinsic features of the brain. Thereby the brain's intrinsic activity is supposed to make possible the coding of neural activity changes in terms of spatial and temporal differences, which in turn leads to the constitution of a spatiotemporal structure during the resting state itself. This is indicated by the bilateral arrow between the brain's two intrinsic features, which both predispose the constitution of consciousness and can thus be considered neural predispositions of consciousness (NPC). (*b*) The figure depicts the relationship between the physical world (bottom), the brain and its resting state (middle circle), and consciousness (upper circle). The brain's resting state develops a statistically based virtual spatiotemporal structure (dotted lines within the circle symbolizing the brain) that aligns itself to the stimuli (simple non-dotted vertical lines), though not to all stimuli in the physical world and their statistically based occurrence across time and space (dotted lines between stimuli and brain). Taken together, both the statistically based neural alignment to the stimuli in the environment and the constitution of a statistically based spatiotemporal structure predispose (big vertical arrow) the subsequent constitution of consciousness (upper circle). Thereby, consciousness and its phenomenal features are supposed to show a spatiotemporal structure that can be traced back to the one of the resting state and its alignment to the environment. The big arrow on the left side indicates that we access, i.e., perceive, and cognize, the world through consciousness as the "medium of all our experience." (*c*) The figure illustrates where the linkage between the environment and the brain may be disrupted. It may be disrupted on the level of the intrinsic activity's neural alignment to the extrinsic stimuli. I suggest this to be central in schizophrenia (see Chapter 22 for details). The abnormal neural alignment is indicated by the absent lines and the abnormal arrows in the relationship between environment and brain. Alternatively, the resting state itself may not receive enough energy to encode a proper spatiotemporal structure, which is then simply no longer reactive to any kind of changes. The resting-state activity is quasi-frozen or,dormant: this is indicated by the absent lines in the brain's spatiotemporal structure. I suppose this to be the case in disorders of consciousness like the vegetative state, which will be explained in full detail in Chapters 28 and 29. Finally, the intrinsic activity's spatiotemporal structure may be abnormally altered by itself, as indicated by the thick abnormal lines in the brain itself. This may be the case in depression (see Chapters 17 and 22). All three—schizophrenia, depression, and vegetative state—lead to an abnormal spatiotemporal structure and to changes in consciousness of the environment, as indicated by the lines in the connecting arrows from consciousness to the environment.

(b)

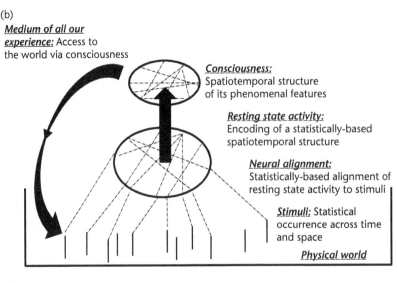

(c)

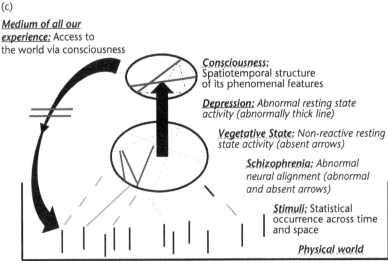

Figure I-3a-c (Continued)

INTRINSIC FEATURES OF THE BRAIN IB: STATISTICALLY VERSUS NON-PHYSICALLY BASED SPATIOTEMPORAL STRUCTURE

Philosophers and neuroscientists alike may now be concerned by the characterization of the spatiotemporal structure as not physically based. Does this mean that we have to propose some kind of nonphysical, mental property (like a "deep further fact" (Parfit, 1984) or a Cartesian ego) like a mind being located and inherent somewhere in the brain's resting state?

No, nothing is further from the truth. The resting state's spatiotemporal structure is not physically based because it does not reflect or correspond one to one to the stimuli's physical features at their specific discrete points in physical time and space. Instead, the resting state's spatiotemporal structure may rather correspond to the spatial and temporal differences in the occurrences of the different stimuli's physical features across their different discrete points in physical time and space. I consequently characterize the resting state's spatiotemporal structure as difference- and statistically based rather than stimulus- and physically based.

Do I henceforth propose nonphysical and thus mental properties to be prevalent in the brain and its resting state? The characterization of the resting state's spatiotemporal structure as not physically based does not imply that it is nonphysical. It is still physical but, and that is important, it is no longer based on the single stimuli and their respective physical features themselves. Instead, the spatiotemporal structure is based on the statistical frequency distribution of the stimuli across their physically discrete points in time and space. Hence, the statistically based characterization of the resting state's spatiotemporal structure does not introduce any nonphysical features like mental stimuli and properties (as it is, for instance, suggested by the term "cerebral mental field" by Libet [2006]).

The assumption of a spatiotemporal structure only considers the very same stimuli and their respective physical features in a different way, in a statistical way rather than a purely physical way. Instead of encoding each stimulus' single discrete point in physical time and space by itself into neural activity, i.e., stimulus-based coding, the resting state encodes the spatial and temporal differences between different stimuli and their different discrete points in physical time and space, e.g., difference-based coding. Accordingly, to confuse the statistically and difference-based nature of the resting state's spatiotemporal structure with mental properties would be to confuse two different ways of encoding one and the same stimuli, e.g., stimulus- and difference-based coding, with two different types of stimuli (i.e., physical and mental).

INTRINSIC FEATURES OF THE *BRAIN* IC: SPATIOTEMPORAL STRUCTURE AND "ENVIRONMENT–BRAIN UNITY"

How does the resting state's spatiotemporal structure predispose consciousness? For that, we have to go back to the spatiotemporal structure itself. One may now postulate that it may be

"located" within the brain itself. That is certainly true. But at the same time it extends toward the environment.

Recent investigations in both animals and humans (Lakatos et al. 2008; Stefanics et al. 2009) demonstrated that the resting state's low-frequency fluctuations (like delta oscillations in the range between 1 Hz and 4 Hz) can shift their phase onsets in order to align themselves to the onsets especially of rhythmic stimuli in the environment (see Chapters 19 and 20 for details). The brain's resting state may thus align itself to the environmental activity by encoding the latter's statistical frequency distribution into its neural activity; that is, the phase onsets (see Schroeder et al. 2008, 2010; Schroeder and Lakatos 2009a and b, 2012; Lakatos et al. 2005, 2007, 2008, 2009; and see Chapter 20 herein for details).

What does this imply for the resting state's spatiotemporal structure? Such neural alignment suggests the resting state's spatiotemporal structure to extend beyond the brain to the environment (including one's own body) in a statistically based and thus "virtual" way. There may thus be a statistically based spatiotemporal grid, matrix, or interface between environment and brain: the brain links us continuously to the environment by encoding its stimuli's statistical frequency distribution into its resting-state activity.

Metaphorically speaking, the resting state's spatiotemporal structure extends and spans its statistically based virtual net beyond the brain itself into the environment. I will therefore later speak of a statistically and spatiotemporally based virtual "environment–brain unity" (see Chapter 20).

INTRINSIC FEATURES OF THE *BRAIN* ID: "ENVIRONMENT–BRAIN UNITY" AND CONSCIOUSNESS

How is all that related to consciousness? Consciousness is our entrance door to the world (which is taken to be distinct from the concept of the environment; see Chapter 20 for details). We can access and thus perceive, act, feel, and so on the persons, objects and events in the world only via consciousness (and unconscious; see the second Introduction for conceptual clarification). Consciousness is the "medium of all our experience" (Merker 2007, 64).

How is that possible? Consciousness is the medium that always already anchors and embeds us in a very basic way in the world (and our own body). This, in turn, makes it possible for us to access the world and its persons, objects, and events in our perceptions, actions, emotions, cognitions, and so on, with these various functions thus presupposing (rather than causing) consciousness (see Appendix 1 and Chapter 24 for detailed discussion of this point, the relationship between the phenomenal functions of consciousness and the various other functions; that is, sensory, motor, affective, cognitive, and social).

Where does this basic relationship between consciousness and the environment come from? I suppose that it may ultimately be traced back to the above-described neural alignment of the brain's resting-state activity to its environment with the consequent constitution of a statistically and spatiotemporally based virtual net between environment and brain, the statistically and "spatiotemporally based virtual environment–brain unity" as I will call it later (see Chapters 20 and 21).

Only if brain and environment are to some degree aligned to each other via the statistically based spatiotemporal structure of our brain's resting state activity, we will we be able to develop consciousness (see Chapters 19, 24, 25, and 30 for more detailed discussion). I consequently propose the possibility of consciousness, i.e., possible consciousness (see second Introduction for conceptual clarification), to be necessarily dependent upon the statistically and spatiotemporally based virtual linkage of the brain's resting-state activity to the environment (and the body) (see Figure I-3b).

If, in contrast, there were no such statistically based virtual spatiotemporal structure between environment and brain, consciousness would remain impossible and could then no longer serve as "medium of all our experience" (see Chapter 20 for more discussion). This statistically and spatiotemporally based linkage between brain and environment may be disrupted at different stages. Either the intrinsic activity no longer aligns itself properly to the extrinsic stimuli, as may be the case in schizophrenia (see Chapter 22). Or, alternatively, the resting-state activity itself may be altered, no longer having (for instance) sufficient energy and metabolism to properly encode the stimuli from the environment; this may be the case in the vegetative state. The resting-state activity may then simply be no longer reactive to changes in the stimuli in the environment. Finally, the resting state may have sufficient energy, but it may be imbalanced leading to an abnormal spatiotemporal structure, which then also affects its relationship to the environment, as may be the case in depression (see Chapter 27; see Figure I-3c).

Accordingly, the resting-state activity's spatiotemporally and statistically based structure and its extension toward the environment may predispose and thus make possible the subsequent association of extrinsic stimuli and their purely neuronal stimulus-induced activity with the phenomenal features of consciousness. The resting-state activity's spatiotemporal structure and its neural alignment to the stimuli in the environment may be regarded as what I will call "neural predisposition of consciousness" (NPC), a necessary neural condition of the possibility of consciousness (see the second Introduction for conceptual clarification, as well as Northoff 2013).

INTRINSIC FEATURES OF THE *BRAIN* IIA: DIFFERENCE-BASED CODING AS THE BRAIN'S ENCODING STRATEGY

How is the resting state's spatiotemporal structure and its statistically based "virtual" extension toward the environment constituted? For that, I propose, we need to focus our attention on the second intrinsic feature of the brain, the neural code and thus the encoding strategy the brain applies to generate its own neural activity. That leads me back to Volume I, of which I give a short summary below.

In a nutshell, the brain's resting-state activity is highly dynamic, structured, and organized, yielding continuously ongoing rest–rest interactions (see Part II in Volume I). I postulated these rest–rest interactions (and subsequently also rest–stimulus and stimulus–rest interaction) to be encoded into neural activity in terms of spatial and temporal differences amounting to what I called "difference-based coding."

Before going into detail about difference-based coding itself, we need to briefly clarify the concept of *coding* itself as I use it. The term "code" was understood in a broad and general way as the most basic algorithm the brain applies to format and organize its neural activity, that is, any kind of neural activity during both resting-state and stimulus-induced activity (see the introduction in Volume I for more details). Coding in such a broad sense implies both encoding and decoding. As detailed in the Introduction of Volume I, encoding concerns the generation of neural activity during the exposure to intero- and exteroceptive stimuli (and spontaneous activity changes in the brain itself, its resting-state activity).

In contrast, decoding refers to the deciphering of the contents that are associated with and processed by the neural activity. Taken in this sense, decoding of the contents associated with neural activity presupposes that the very same neural activity has been generated and thus encoded. My focus in Volume I was on the encoding of neural activity rather than its decoding and the associated contents. I proposed a purely neuronal account of the brain's encoding strategy, which I determined as difference-based coding as distinguished from stimulus-based coding.

What do I exactly mean by difference-based coding? "Difference-based coding" refers to the brain's general encoding strategy and thus the formal measure or metric the brain applies to generate its own neural activity during both resting state and stimulus-induced activity. More specifically, "difference-based coding" describes that the neural activity in the brain encodes the spatial and temporal differences between the same and/or other stimuli across their different discrete points in physical time and space. What is encoded into neural activity is the statistical frequency distribution of stimuli, that is, their "natural statistics" (and also their "social, vegetative, and neuronal statistics"; see Chapters 8 and 9 as well as Chapter 20).

Such encoding of the stimuli's "natural statistics" (and social, vegetative, and neuronal statistics) must be distinguished from the encoding of the stimuli themselves and their discrete points in physical time and space. This would amount to stimulus-based coding as the brain's general encoding strategy, rather than difference-based coding. Since there is no empirical evidence for stimulus-based coding, as described in Volume I, one may consider difference-based coding as the general encoding strategy the brain applies to generate any kind of neural activity. Difference-based coding may consequently be considered an intrinsic feature of the brain that the brain applies by default and thus in a necessary and unavoidable way to encode its neural activity.

INTRINSIC FEATURES OF THE *BRAIN* IIB: DIFFERENCE-BASED CODING AND REST–STIMULUS AND STIMULUS–REST INTERACTION

Difference-based coding in this sense is proposed to apply to any stimulus being processed in the brain, including exteroceptive stimuli from the environment, interoceptive stimuli from the body, and "neural stimuli" describing the brain's intrinsic activity changes (see Chapter 4 for details). Accordingly, difference-based coding (rather than stimulus-based coding) is proposed to be the neural code the brain applies, as its intrinsic feature, to encode its own neural activity, including both resting-state activity and stimulus-induced activity.

The encoding of neural activity in terms of differences was supposed to constitute a fine-grained and well-organized, statistically based spatial and temporal structure in the brain's resting-state activity. Neuronally, the constitution of a spatial structure is proposed to be mediated by structural and functional connectivity that connects different regions' activities across the whole brain. While the constitution of a temporal structure is hypothesized to be realized by frequency fluctuations in neuronal activity especially in the lower-frequency ranges (0.001–0.1 Hz). Both functional connectivity and low-frequency fluctuations are postulated to organize and structure the brain's intrinsic activity in both spatial and temporal regard (see Volume I, Chapters 4–6).

What about the extrinsic stimuli and their effects? Taking the brain's intrinsic activity and its spatiotemporal structure as a departure point, the subsequent induction of stimulus-induced activity by extrinsic stimuli must be regarded as a mere modulation of the resting state's functional connectivity and low-frequency fluctuations. This is supposed to be manifest in what I described as rest–stimulus interaction (see Volume I, Part IV).

However, the interaction between resting-state and stimulus-induced activity is bilateral, being directed not only from the former to the latter, that is, rest–stimulus interaction, but also from the latter to the former, yielding what I call "stimulus–rest interaction" (see Volume I, Chapters 11 and 12). Both rest–stimulus and stimulus–rest interaction are possible only on the basis of encoding the extrinsic stimulus in relation to the brain's intrinsic activity; that is, in terms of their statistically based spatial and temporal differences, thus presupposing difference-based rather than stimulus-based coding.

Intrinsic Features of the *Brain* IIC—Difference-Based Coding and Other Neural Codes

How does difference-based coding stand in relation to other suggestions for neural coding? Another suggestion for the brain's neural code is sparse coding as discussed in Volume I, Part I. Briefly, sparse coding describes the encoding of the stimuli's statistical frequency distribution across different points in physical time and space, that is, its natural statistics, into the brain's neural activity. This has been demonstrated on the cellular and population level, especially in the sensory cortex (as, for instance, in the visual cortex) but also in other regions of the brain (Volume I, Part I). Based on recent evidence, I proposed such statistically based coding strategy and thus sparse coding to also hold on the regional level of the brain (see Chapter 3). The encoding of the stimuli's natural statistics implies that the

stimulus is encoded in a sparse way into the brain's neural activity, hence the name "sparse coding." This means that there is no one-to-one correspondence between stimuli and neurons/regions, but rather a many-to-one relationship with many stimuli leading to the activation of one neuron or region.

How is such sparse coding possible? The encoding of the stimuli's natural statistics is possible only by coding the differences between the same or different stimuli across their different discrete points in physical time and space. Sparse coding consequently presupposes difference-based coding, while it would remain impossible in the case of stimulus-based coding.

How about predictive coding? Predictive coding describes that the brain's neural activity yields an anticipation or prediction of a possible stimulus, the predicted input, which is then matched and compared with the actual input (see Part III in Volume I). The difference between the predicted input and the actual input yields what is called a "prediction error," whose degree determines the degree of stimulus-induced activity. This is possible, however, only if the difference between predicted and actual input is encoded into neural activity thus presupposing difference-based rather than stimulus-based coding (see also Mesulam 2008 for the possible role of predictive coding in consciousness).

Volume I demonstrated the brain's neural code to actively format and organize neural activity in terms of spatial and temporal differences by encoding its own neural activity in terms of difference- rather than stimulus-based coding. Such encoding of temporal and spatial differences into neural activity makes possible the constitution of a statistically based virtual spatiotemporal structure in the resting-state activity.

Neuronal Hypothesis of Consciousness IA: "Coding Hypothesis of Consciousness" (CHC)

Having reviewed two of the brain's intrinsic features, its intrinsic activity and its encoding strategy, we are now ready to propose a neuronal hypothesis that explains consciousness. This neuronal hypothesis aims to show why and how the brain's intrinsic features make necessary or unavoidable, and thus predispose, the association of consciousness and its phenomenal features with the otherwise purely neuronal resting state and stimulus-induced activity in the brain.

The hypothesis is purely neuronal in that it focuses exclusively on the neuronal mechanisms that are supposed to underlie consciousness. In contrast, our neuronal hypothesis does not yet refer specifically to any particular phenomenal feature of consciousness nor to its subjective nature. This requires the extension of our neuronal hypotheses to the neurophenomenal hypothesis which will be developed in the second introduction. Before making such a neurophenomenal extension, though, we first need to be clear about the neuronal mechanisms. This is the upcoming task of this section and the following sections herein.

How can the brain's resting-state activity make possible and thus predispose the constitution of the various phenomenal features of consciousness, including its essentially subjective nature? I claim that this requires a particular coding strategy that encodes any neural activity in the brain, that is, during rest–rest, rest–stimulus, and stimulus–rest interaction in a specific way. This particular encoding strategy, as I hypothesize in this book, is difference-based coding. By encoding its own neural activity during rest–rest, rest–stimulus, and stimulus–rest interaction in a difference-based rather than stimulus-based way, the brain predisposes the constitution of the various phenomenal features of consciousness.

If, in contrast, the encoding of the brain's neural activity were stimulus-based rather than difference-based, the phenomenal features of consciousness and their subjective nature could not be generated at all. The otherwise purely neuronal and objective features of the brain's resting state and stimulus-induced activity could then no longer be associated with possible consciousness including its phenomenal and subjective features (see Introduction II for the concept of "possible consciousness") by default; that is, in a necessary or unavoidable way.

This amounts to what I call the "coding hypothesis of consciousness" (CHC). The CHC claims that consciousness is predisposed and thus possible only on the basis of a particular coding strategy that is applied by the brain to encode and generate its own neural activity during both resting state and stimulus-induced activity (see Fig. I-4a).

NEURONAL HYPOTHESIS OF CONSCIOUSNESS IB: "ENCODING AND DIFFERENCE-BASED HYPOTHESIS OF CONSCIOUSNESS" (EHC, DHC)

I suggest that the CHC includes two subsets. The "first subset" of the CHC refers to the encoding of stimuli into neural activity as described by the "encoding hypothesis of consciousness" (EHC), while the "second subset" of the CHC concerns the coding of neural activity during rest–rest, rest–stimulus, and stimulus–rest interaction, which I subsume under the "difference-based coding hypothesis of consciousness" (DHC).

Let's go into more detail, and start with the EHC. The EHC describes the specific way stimuli are encoded into the brain's neural activity and thus the formal measure or metric the brain applies to generate any kind of neural activity (see the Introduction in Volume I for details). As pointed out earlier, the brain encodes the statistically based frequency distribution of the stimuli's physical features, for example, their natural statistics, rather than the stimuli's physical features themselves. This means that the EHC describes a statistically rather than physically based encoding strategy of the brain.

If, in contrast, the brain were encoding and thus generating its own neural activity in terms of a physically rather than statistically based encoding strategy, consciousness would remain impossible. I therefore deem a statistically based encoding strategy to be distinguished from a physically based encoding strategy as a necessary condition, that is, neural predisposition, for the generation of possible consciousness. Accordingly, the EHC is a neuronal hypothesis about the way or strategy the brain must use in encoding and thus generating its own neural activity in order to make possible consciousness and its various phenomenal features.

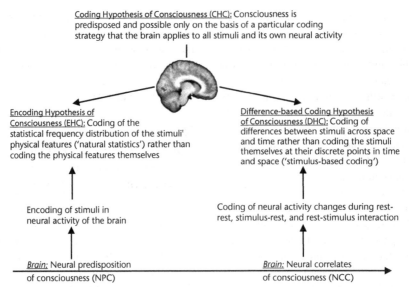

Figure I-4a Coding Hypothesis of Consciousness (CHC). The figure depicts the coding hypothesis of consciousness (CHC) and its two subsets, the encoding hypothesis of consciousness (EHC) (left), and the difference-based coding hypothesis of consciousness (DHC) (right). The EHC is related to the encoding of stimuli into neural activity on the basis of their spatial and temporal differences across the different discrete points in physical time and space, thus mirroring their statistical frequency distribution; i.e., natural statistics. That must be considered a neural predisposition of consciousness (NPC) (bottom). The DHC claims that neural activity changes during the various kinds of neural interactions in the brain, i.e., rest–rest, rest–stimulus, and stimulus–rest, are also coded in terms of differences. If the spatial and temporal differences encoded into neural activity are large enough, the respective neural differences will be associated with a phenomenal state, e.g., consciousness. The degree of the encoded neural difference may thus be regarded a neural correlate of consciousness (NCC) (bottom).

How about the DHC? The DHC describes the second specific subset of the CHC. The DHC refers to the kind of neural coding the brain applies to code its own neural activity during stimulus–rest, rest–rest, and rest–stimulus interaction. This pertains to difference-based coding as distinguished from stimulus-based coding. By encoding the spatial and temporal differences between both neural and intero- and exteroceptive stimuli rather than the isolated stimuli themselves, the brain makes possible the constitution of a statistically and spatiotemporally based virtual structure and its virtual extension to the environment (and the body). This results in what I earlier described as "statistically and spatiotemporally based virtual environment–brain unity" (see Chapters 20 and 21).

Since the statistically and spatiotemporally based virtual environment–brain unity predisposes consciousness, as described earlier, difference-based coding must be considered a neural predisposition of possible consciousness and its various phenomenal features. Accordingly, the DHC is a neuronal hypothesis about the way or strategy the brain must use in encoding extrinsic stimuli in relation to its own intrinsic activity (during rest–stimulus and stimulus–rest interaction) in order to make possible consciousness and its various phenomenal features.

NEURONAL HYPOTHESIS OF CONSCIOUSNESS IIA: *"CONTENT-VERSUS CODE-BASED HYPOTHESES"* OF CONSCIOUSNESS

How does the CHC stand in relation to the other neuroscientific theories of consciousness we sketched earlier? We will discuss in the various chapters and Appendix 1 the details of the relationship between the CHC and the other neuroscientific theories of consciousness. In order to put the CHC into the context of current neuroscientific and philosophical approaches to consciousness, I here sketch a broad and basic comparison that points out the radically different starting point and path the CHC takes compared to those of other approaches.

Most of the current neuroscientific theories focus on the neural mechanisms that underlie the contents or state/level of consciousness. Theories on extrinsic stimulus-induced or task-related activity like neuronal synchronization, re-entrant loops, global workspace, and information integration (see earlier) focus on the constitution of contents in consciousness rather than on consciousness itself; that is, the phenomenal features that are associated with the respective contents. These neuroscientific theories are thus what one may describe as "content-based hypotheses" of consciousness (see Fig. I-4b).

The CHC takes a radically different stance. Rather than focusing on how the contents of consciousness are processed and related to neural activity, the CHC is interested in the neural

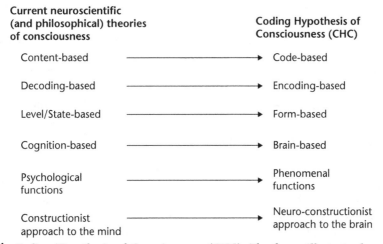

Figure I-4b Coding Hypothesis of Consciousness (CHC). The figure illustrates how the coding hypothesis of consciousness (CHC) differs from current neuroscientific and philosophical theories of consciousness. Rather than focusing on the contents of consciousness and their underlying neuronal mechanisms, the CHC aims to search for how the brain's encodes that very same neural activity that the other theories take for granted and as given when they associate it with the contents of consciousness. This implies that the CHC focuses on the encoding of neural activity rather than the decoding of contents from neural activity. The CHC is thus a "code-based hypothesis" and an "encoding-based hypothesis" rather than a "content-based hypothesis" and a "decoding-based hypothesis." Rather than on the level or state of consciousness itself, the CHC traces the level or state of consciousness back to the degree to which its form, the spatiotemporal structure of the brain's intrinsic activity, is recruited or activated during changes in neural activity. The CHC is thus a "form-based hypothesis" rather than a "level-based hypothesis" of consciousness. Finally, rather than being based on cognitive (or some other) function, the CHC claims a direct relationship between the brain's neural code and the phenomenal features of consciousness. This entails a "brain-based hypothesis" rather than a "cognition-based hypothesis" of consciousness. The focus on cognitive and, more generally, psychological functions is replaced by a focus on the brain's phenomenal functions. Finally, the constructionist approach to the mind in psychology is replaced by a neuro-constructionist approach to the brain's neural activity, where the processes of the encoding and structuring and organizing of the brain's neural activity, rather than the brain's psychological functions, are the main focus.

activity itself: how neural activity by itself is encoded and generated, and how that impacts the processing of any subsequent contents, as during rest–stimulus and rest–rest interaction. The CHC aims to reveal exactly what is usually taken for granted and tacitly presupposed in the current approaches; namely, how the brain encodes and generates its own neural activity during both resting state and stimulus-induced activity that in turn allow for the subsequent processing of contents.

Due to the shift from content to code, the CHC must be considered a "code-based hypothesis" of consciousness rather than a "content-based hypothesis" like most of the current neuroscientific and philosophical theories. As such, the CHC is a hypothesis about the brain's encoding of neural activity and how that predisposes consciousness, rather than a theory how the brain's neural activity processes contents.

Neuronal hypothesis of consciousness IIB: "*decoding*-based versus *encoding*-based hypotheses" of consciousness

Let us explicate this difference in further detail. Most neuroscientific and philosophical theories of consciousness take the brain's neural activity for granted and tacitly presuppose it as "given and ready-made." Rather than focusing on the neuronal mechanisms how the brain encodes and generates its own neural activity, they search for the kind of contents and the level or state of arousal that are processed by brain's neural activity once it is encoded and generated.

Most current neuroscientific (and philosophical) approaches aim to decipher and thus to decode the information about the content and level of consciousness that is "contained" in the neural activity of the brain. Since the focus is here on the decoding, one can characterize these approaches as "decoding-based hypotheses" of consciousness. The "decoding-based hypotheses" of consciousness aim to decipher and thus to decode the information about content and level of consciousness as it is supposedly contained (or represented as the philosophers say) in the brain's neural activity.

This is different in the CHC. The CHC does not presuppose the brain's neural activity as "given and ready-made." Instead, the CHC dents deeply into the neuronal mechanisms by which the brain encodes and generates its own neural activity. Accordingly, the CHC must be considered an "encoding-based hypothesis" of consciousness rather than a "decoding-based hypothesis."

As "encoding-based hypothesis," the CHC postulates that the brain's particular encoding strategy makes necessary or unavoidable and thus predisposes consciousness. If, for instance, the brain were encoding its own neural activity in terms of stimulus- rather than difference-based coding, consciousness, including both contents and level/state, would remain altogether impossible. Therefore, the CHC chooses a starting point that precedes the starting points of the current approaches. The brain must encode and generate its own neural activity before it can process and associate it with information about content and level of consciousness. The CHC can thus be considered more basic and fundamental than the current approaches.

How does my CHC stand in relation to the coding as discussed in Volume I? Volume I focused on the neuronal mechanisms underlying the brain's encoding of its neural activity. This purely neuronal account of the brain's neural activity is now extended to consciousness and its phenomenal features. The focus in this second volume is on how the brain's encoding of its own neural activity predisposes the various empirical dimensions (content, level, form) and phenomenal features (point of view, qualia, first-person perspective, etc.) of consciousness as mentioned at the beginning of this Introduction.

Neuronal hypothesis of consciousness IIC: "*level*-based versus *form*-based hypotheses" of consciousness

We have so far distinguished the CHC as "code- and encoding-based hypothesis" of consciousness from "content- and decoding-based hypotheses" of consciousness. This, however, left open how the CHC stands in relation to the hypotheses which focus on the level or state rather than on the contents of consciousness.

As discussed earlier, several neuroscientific theories suggest a central role for the brain's intrinsic activity and its metabolism and information integration in consciousness. Besides the contents of consciousness, this also concerns the level or state of consciousness as it is predominantly investigated in the disorders of consciousness like vegetative state, anesthesia, or NREM sleep (see above, as well as especially Chapters 14–16 and Chapters 28 and 29). Since they target the neuronal mechanisms underlying the level or state of consciousness, these approaches may be described as "level-based hypotheses" of consciousness.

How does the CHC compare with the "level-based hypotheses" of consciousness? We remember from Volume I that difference-based coding comes in different degrees as is manifested in the degree of spatial and temporal differences that are encoded into neural activity during both resting state and stimulus-induced activity (see Chapters 11 and 12 in Volume I). I now postulate that the degree of difference-based coding is directly proportional to the degree and thus the level or state of consciousness: the larger the spatial and temporal differences that are encoded into neural activity during, for instance, intero- or exteroceptive stimuli, the more likely it is that the purely neuronal stimulus-induced activity will be associated with a particular level or state of consciousness (see Chapter 29 for details).

Why, however, does the degree of difference-based coding entail the modulation of the level or state of consciousness? This is, I postulate, possible only on the basis of the brain's intrinsic activity and the spatiotemporal structure of its neural activity, its form (or structure or organization) as the third dimension of consciousness (see second Introduction for details, as well as Northoff 2013). The CHC can therefore be considered a "form-based hypothesis" of consciousness, rather than a "level-based hypothesis."

By encoding larger degrees of spatial and temporal differences into neural activity, the spatiotemporal structure of the brain's intrinsic activity will be activated, transferred, and carried over to the extrinsic stimulus and its stimulus-induced activity. Such a neuronal transfer of the intrinsic activity's spatiotemporal structures to the extrinsic stimulus-induced activity makes possible the association of the extrinsic (purely physical) stimulus with consciousness and its phenomenal features (see Chapter 29 and especially Chapter 30 for details).

NEURONAL HYPOTHESIS OF CONSCIOUSNESS IIIA: *"COGNITION*-BASED HYPOTHESES" OF CONSCIOUSNESS

The CHC does not focus on the brain's neural processing of contents but on the brain's neural code, its encoding strategy in particular. The focus on content in content-based hypotheses of consciousness is often linked to certain cognitive processes; namely, how the content is processed and which kind of processes and functions are involved. Therefore, many neuroscientific and philosophical theories target higher-order cognitive functions like memory, attention, or others. The various neurocognitive functions of the brain are thus supposed to be central for consciousness.

This has recently been complemented by a shift toward medium- or even lower-order functions like neurosensory, neuromotor, and neuroaffective functions (see earlier as well as Chapters 31 and 32, and Appendix 1). Despite the focus on different functions, the different hypotheses nevertheless share the assumption that the processing of stimuli in terms of some kind of function (whether sensory, motor, affective, cognitive, or social functions) and their underlying neuronal mechanisms can account for consciousness and its phenomenal features.

Since these approaches highlight the role of cognition (taken in a broad sense as "the processing of any kind of stimuli and their related contents"), one may describe them as neurocognitive or "cognition-based hypotheses" of consciousness. The "cognition-based hypotheses" of consciousness postulate that consciousness and its phenomenal features are dependent on the cognitive processes and their underlying neuronal mechanisms. This means that the link between brain and consciousness is here rather indirect via some mediating cognitive processes, the neurocognitive functions. This however leaves open how consciousness can be linked in a more direct way to the brain.

NEURONAL HYPOTHESIS OF CONSCIOUSNESS IIIB: "*COGNITION*-VERSUS *BRAIN*-BASED HYPOTHESES" OF CONSCIOUSNESS

I claim that the CHC provides a more direct link between consciousness and brain than the cognition-based approaches. The CHC postulates direct relationship between brain and consciousness without a third mediating variable like the cognitive processes (or some sensory, motor, affective, cognitive or social function). By focusing on the brain's encoding strategy and its intrinsic activity's spatiotemporal structure, the CHC targets the brain itself and more specifically its intrinsic features. These intrinsic features must be distinguished from the brain's extrinsic features, like the various functions and their related contents the brain processes in its neural activity that underlies its sensory, motor, affective, and cognitive functions.

The CHC postulates that the brain's intrinsic features themselves predispose, and thus make necessary or unavoidable, the generation of consciousness. If the brain were characterized by different intrinsic features, a different encoding strategy, and/or an intrinsic activity without a spatiotemporal structure, consciousness would be altogether impossible. There would no longer be any phenomenal features. Due to such direct dependence on the brain's intrinsic features, I characterize the CHC as a "brain-based hypothesis" of consciousness as distinguished from "cognition-based hypotheses."

I postulate, based on these considerations, a direct link between the brain's intrinsic features and its phenomenal functions that account for the phenomenal features of consciousness, a "neurophenomenal link" if one wants to say so. Such "neurophenomenal link" is direct rather than indirect and does therefore not require the mediation by any other function, including neurosensory, neuromotor, neuroaffective, or neurocognitive functions. This distinguishes my neurophenomenal approach from neurocognitive ones and the cognition-based hypotheses of consciousness that presuppose an indirect rather than direct link between brain and consciousness.

The focus in this volume will be on investigating the various "neurophenomenal links" between the brain's intrinsic features and the phenomenal features of consciousness. In contrast, I will not so much discuss the various neurosensory, neuromotor, neuroaffective, neurocognitive, and neurosocial functions of the brain and how they are related to consciousness. Despite the fact that my focus is not on the cognition-based hypotheses of consciousness, I will nevertheless discuss them in various places throughout this book to clarify the contrast to my neurophenomenal approach.

NEURONAL HYPOTHESIS OF CONSCIOUSNESS IIIC: "PRIORITY OF *PHENOMENAL* FUNCTION" VERSUS "PRIORITY OF *PSYCHOLOGICAL* FUNCTION" AND "THEORY OF BRAIN *ACTIVITY*" VERSUS "THEORY OF BRAIN *FUNCTION*"

How does such a "brain-based hypothesis" stand in relation to the "cognition-based hypotheses" of consciousness? Reversing the traditional relationship between cognitive and phenomenal functions, I here postulate that the brain's phenomenal functions are more basic and fundamental than the brain's processing of contents through its various psychological functions: cognitive, sensory, motor, social, or affective. To put it differently, I postulate that phenomenal functions precede psychological functions. This can be described as the "priority of phenomenal function." The concept of "priority of phenomenal function" describes that the phenomenal functions of the brain are more basic and fundamental than its psychological functions—the sensory, motor, affective, cognitive, and social functions. In short, phenomenology comes first, and psychology second.

This reverses the traditional relationship between psychological and phenomenal functions. Traditionally, the brain's psychological functions (sensory, motor, affective, cognitive, social) are considered the very basis and fundament of consciousness and its phenomenal features. This is well reflected in the cognition-based hypotheses of consciousness that seem to implicitly presuppose the "priority of psychological function" over phenomenal function. The concept of "priority of psychological function" describes that psychological functions are more basic and must therefore precede the phenomenal functions. In order to explain the phenomenal functions and thus consciousness, we must first understand the psychological functions. In short, psychology rather than phenomenology comes first.

What do both the "priority of phenomenal function" and the "priority of psychological function" imply for the relationship between brain and consciousness? The "priority of psychological function" considers consciousness and its phenomenal features to be dependent on the various psychological functions. When applied to the brain, the "priority of *psychological* function" presupposes a "theory of brain *function*" that investigates how the brain and its neural activity generate the various psychological functions (see Introduction in Volume I for details).

This is different in the "priority of *phenomenal* function." Rather than a "theory of brain function," the "priority of phenomenal function" presupposes a "theory of brain *activity*" that investigates the neuronal mechanisms of how the brain encodes and thus generates its own neural activity (see Introduction in first volume for details). Since neural activity must first and foremost be generated before it can process certain functions, a "theory of brain activity" must be considered more basic and fundamental than a "theory of brain function."

What does this imply for the relationship between phenomenal and psychological functions? Phenomenal functions presuppose a "theory of brain activity," while psychological functions require a "theory of brain function." Since a "theory of brain activity" must precede a "theory of brain function," phenomenal functions must also be considered more basic and fundamental than psychological functions. Therefore I opt for "priority of phenomenal

function" rather than "priority of psychological function."

Even more radically, I claim psychological functions to be based on phenomenal functions. Why? No psychological function can be generated without the prior encoding of neural activity, which, I postulate, is necessarily and unavoidably linked to consciousness and its phenomenal features. Therefore, psychological functions cannot avoid being based on the brain's encoding of neural activity and the related phenomenal functions. To put this in an abbreviated way, the generation of neural activity precedes the generation of function; code precedes content; and consciousness precedes cognition.

NEURONAL HYPOTHESIS OF CONSCIOUSNESS IIID: "FACULTY PSYCHOLOGY" VERSUS THE "CONSTRUCTIONIST APPROACH" TO THE *MIND*

How does the CHC stand in relation to psychology and its recent extension into cognitive neuroscience? In order to answer this question, let us briefly reflect how psychology considers mental functions like consciousness, attention, etc. One standard view in psychology often held (though contradicted early on by W. Wundt and W. James) is the assumption of certain mental categories or faculties that have a distinct, separate, and exclusively psychological basis. Such an approach to the mind in terms of mental categories or faculties has led to the term "faculty psychology" (see Lindquist and Barrett 2012 for an overview).

For instance, cognitive functions like working memory, attention, episodic memory, etc., have been suggested to be such different faculties. The same can be observed on the side of emotion, where different emotions like fear, happiness, disgust, or pleasure have been suggested to be different faculties or categories (see, for instance, Panksepp 1998). The introduction of brain imaging extended such faculty psychology to the brain and its different regions and networks. The different psychological faculties were assumed to be related to separate and distinct regions and networks in the brain.

That, however, turned out to be problematic, as the different functions or faculties show extensive overlapping in their respectively recruited regions and neural networks (see Chapters 4–5 as well as Bar et al. 2007, 2009a and b; Spreng et al. 2009, 2013; Oosterwijk et al. 2012; Lindquist and Barrett 2012, for recent overviews). This has led some researchers to postulate a different view of the mind. They claim that a "constructionist approach" to the mind should replace the old "faculty psychology" (see, for instance, Lindquist and Barrett 2012; Oosterwijk et al. 2012).

Rather than suggesting different faculties and the respective functions in the brain, this "constructionist approach" searches for some basic psychological processes, operations, and mechanisms that "construct" the different psychological functions. Psychological functions like perceptions, memories, attention, and emotions (including their various subdivisions) are then no longer considered "ready-made and given" categories or entities. Instead, they are supposed to result from constructing processes that involve some basic psychological operations.

Such construction of the various psychological functions presupposes some very basic ingredients, the sensation from the world, the sensations from the body, and the prior experiences. These basic ingredients are combined in various ways, which leads to the construction of the different psychological functions. Prior knowledge and associations are used here to assign meaning to the different contents—this is called "situated conceptualization" (see Lindquist and Barrett 2012).

NEURONAL HYPOTHESIS OF CONSCIOUSNESS IIIE: "CONSTRUCTIONIST APPROACH" TO THE *MIND'S PSYCHOLOGICAL FUNCTIONS* VERSUS "NEUROCONSTRUCTIONIST APPROACH" TO THE *BRAIN'S NEURAL ACTIVITY*

How is this constructionist approach to the mind in terms of basic psychological ingredients and mechanisms related to the CHC and its approach to the brain? The constructionist approach in psychology does not focus on the localization of psychological functions in the brain, the "where," but rather on their "how," that reflects the underlying psychological processes and ingredients.

This is more or less analogous to my approach to the brain. In the same way that the constructionist approach focuses on the construction of the mind's psychological functions, I target the construction of the brain's neural activity. How does the brain construct its own neural activity? I postulate that the brain constructs its own neural activity by applying a particular encoding strategy; namely, difference-based coding. Moreover, in the same way that the constructionist approach in psychology claims some basic ingredients, my approach argues as well that difference-based coding is based on three basic more or less analogous ingredients. The interoceptive stimuli from the body, the exteroceptive stimuli from the environment, and the brain's intrinsic or spontaneous activity are the three basic ingredients on the basis of which the brain constructs and thus encodes its own neural activity in a difference- rather than stimulus-based way (see Volume I for details).

Accordingly, I here pursue a constructionist approach to the brain and, more specifically, to its neural activity. Therefore I speak of a "neuroconstructionist approach." The concept of a "neuroconstructionist approach" means that I do not take the neural activity of the brain for "granted and as a given." Instead, the concept suggests that the neural activity as reflected in the term "neuro" must be generated and thus constructed, as indicated by the term "constructionist." The main claim of my "neuroconstructionist approach" is that the brain itself has a strong impact on the construction of its own neural activity by applying its particular neural code and its intrinsic activity.

How does my "neuroconstructionist approach" to the brain compare with the constructionist approach to the mind in psychology? While superficially being analogous, my "neuroconstructionist approach" must nevertheless be distinguished from the constructionist approach in psychology and its application to the brain: its proponents focus on the construction of psychological functions of the mind and the underlying neuronal mechanisms rather than on the brain's construction of its own neural activity prior to any function.

How do both the "constructionist approach" to the mind and the "neuroconstructionist approach" to the brain stand in relation to consciousness? The constructionist approach to psychology assumes that consciousness is constructed by some basic psychological ingredients and their underlying neuronal mechanisms. This is different in the neuroconstructionist approach to the brain. My neuroconstructionist approach suggests that consciousness and its phenomenal features directly result from the construction of the neural activity by the brain itself and its particular encoding strategy. The CHC requires consequently a "neuroconstructionist approach" to the brain and its neural activity, rather than a constructionist approach to the mind and its various psychological functions, as in current psychology and cognitive neuroscience.

CODA: THE "CODE-BASED HYPOTHESIS" OF CONSCIOUSNESS" AS "SOMETHING NEW"

Danish-Australian philosopher Jacob Hohwy (2009) points out that we need "something new" in our neuroscientific and philosophical theories to explain consciousness:

> It therefore appears likely that further progress in the search for the neural correlates of consciousness requires that *something new* be brought to the study of consciousness. Rather than merely conjoining the approaches, it may be that they must be integrated in a new type of experimental approach *that targets the presumably causal, mechanistic interplay between content processing and overall conscious state across different contents and across different types of conscious and unconscious states.* (Hohwy 2009, 435; *italics mine*)

I claim that the CHC does indeed provide *"something new"* by introducing the importance of the encoding, the EHC; and the coding, the DHC, of neural activity for consciousness. The CHC seems to fulfill the central criterion for the *"something new"*; namely, that it describe the brain's neural operation *"across different contents and across different types of conscious and unconscious states."* (as J.Hohwy says in his article, as quoted above).

By determining a particular encoding and coding strategy, namely, difference-based coding, the CHC targets the necessary neural conditions of possible consciousness including both contents and level or states. This amounts to what I refer to as the neural predispositions of consciousness (NPC) (see second Introduction for more details) that make possible and thus predispose both level/state and contents of consciousness. Metaphorically speaking, the NPC target the ground or the floor upon which most of the current neuroscientific and philosophical theories of consciousness stand when focusing on the sufficient rather than necessary neural conditions of actual rather than possible consciousness.

However, the here-targeted floor or ground was so far characterized only in purely neuronal terms, while not really touching the phenomenal features and the subjective nature of consciousness. We have not yet shown how the here-discussed neuronal mechanisms allow the brain to generate the various phenomenal features of consciousness, the phenomenal heterogeneity, and their essentially subjective nature. Therefore, we need to extend the here-postulated neuronal hypothesis of consciousness to the phenomenal realm of consciousness and develop specific neurophenomenal hypotheses. Since this requires some detouring into conceptual and phenomenal territories, we delegate that to the second Introduction, where the "code hypothesis of consciousness" (CHC) is extended into a truly neurophenomenal hypothesis.

INTRODUCTION II: CONSCIOUSNESS AND ITS INTRINSIC FEATURES

The reader may be rather surprised to see a second Introduction. Isn't one Introduction enough? While the first Introduction described the brain's intrinsic features in detail and a corresponding neuronal hypothesis how they could possibly be related to consciousness, I left open the exact determination of the phenomenal (and conceptual) features of consciousness. In other words, I covered the neuronal side of consciousness while neglecting the intrinsic features of consciousness itself.

How can we define the intrinsic features of consciousness? The intrinsic features of consciousness are the features that define consciousness *as* consciousness. Why, though, do we need to consider the intrinsic features of consciousness? I postulated in the first Introduction that the intrinsic features of the brain predispose consciousness. Consecutively the question is now what exactly do the brain's intrinsic features predispose on the side of consciousness.

I propose that the brain's intrinsic features predispose exactly those features that define consciousness as consciousness; that is, its intrinsic features. In order to extend our so far only neuronal hypothesis to the phenomenal realm of consciousness and to develop it into a truly neurophenomenal hypothesis, we need to understand the intrinsic features of consciousness. Which are the intrinsic features of consciousness? One may distinguish among empirical, conceptual, and phenomenal features, which shall be discussed briefly in the following section. This will allow us to formulate a truly neurophenomenal hypothesis of consciousness, which will be followed by an overview of the contents in this volume.

EMPIRICAL CHARACTERIZATION OF CONSCIOUSNESS IA: CONTENTS OF CONSCIOUSNESS

We are conscious of a book and its black color on the cover. The book is therefore the content of consciousness, the phenomenal content as philosophers say. Our consciousness is always about contents like events, persons, or objects in the environment. Or about some imaginary scene referring to imaginary persons, objects, or events as for instance during our dreams when we are asleep. Contents in this sense, that is, phenomenal contents, must be considered one central dimension of consciousness (see, for instance, Monaco et al. 2005; Cavanna et al. 2008, 2011, Laureys 2005a and b, Laureys et al. 2005 (see Fig. I-1a)).

Neuroscientific research on consciousness has focused mainly on the contents of consciousness, the phenomenal contents (as distinguished from unconscious, i.e., nonphenomenal contents). Neuronally, as discussed in the first introduction, phenomenal contents have been associated with various neuronal mechanisms, including cyclic thalamo-cortical reentrant processing (Edelman 2003, 2005), information integration

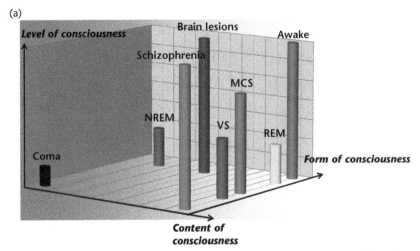

Figure II-1a-c Multidimensional view of consciousness. The figure illustrates the three dimensions of consciousness, content (x-axis), level (y-axis), and form (z-axis) and their involvement in different conditions (a), the interplay between extrinsic stimuli and intrinsic activity with the latter providing the form for the former (b), and the conceptual, neuronal, and pathological characterization of the three dimensions of consciousness (c). (a)The figure illustrates the three dimensions of consciousness—form, content, and level—in a three-dimensional view. The different cylinders reflect the changes of the three dimensions in different conditions: awake state in healthy subjects (awake); REM sleep in healthy subjects (REM: reduced level); NREM sleep in healthy subjects (NREM: reduced level and content); regional brain lesions (Brain lesions: reduced content); minimally conscious state (MCS: reduced level and form); vegetative state (VS: stronger reduced level form); coma (Coma: extremely reduced content, form, and level); and psychiatric disorders like schizophrenia (and depression, not shown) (Schizophrenia: reduced form).(b) The figure illustrates how the intrinsic activity and its spatiotemporal continuity provide the form for the extrinsic stimuli and their organization in consciousness. *Upper part*: The upper part of the figure shows the occurrence of different extrinsic stimuli (vertical lines) at different discrete points in physical time and space. *Middle part*: Independently of the extrinsic stimuli themselves, the intrinsic activity constitutes spatiotemporal continuity in its neural activity by linking different discrete points in time and space which by itself can be experienced in the gestalt of "inner time and space consciousness." The spatiotemporal continuity of the brain's intrinsic activity provides a grid, matrix, or template that is imposed upon and aligned to the extrinsic stimuli and their different discrete points in physical time and space. *Lower part*: This shows how the intrinsic activity's spatiotemporal continuity (light gray) is imposed upon the extrinsic stimuli and their discrete points in physical time and space (black) and how that yields contents (dark gray) in consciousness as part of the continuous flow of consciousness, the "stream or dynamic flow of consciousness." (c) The figure shows the three main dimensions of consciousness (left row), their role in consciousness (left middle row), their underlying neuronal mechanisms (right middle row), and their alterations in corresponding disorders (right row). The concept of *content* refers to the persons, objects and events in consciousness, the *phenomenal contents* as philosophers say. The contents are the main focus in the various neuroscientific suggestions for the neural correlates of consciousness (NCC). They imply stimulus-induced activity and are altered in patients with selective brain lesions. The concept of *level* refers to the different degrees of arousal and awakeness and thus to the state of consciousness. The level or state of consciousness is related to global metabolism and energy supply which are found to be impaired and highly reduced in disorders of consciousness like vegetative state and coma. Moreover, neural activity in brain stem and midbrain is supposed to play an essential role in maintaining arousal. This reflects what is described as "enabling conditions" or "neural prerequisites" of consciousness. The concept of *form* describes the spatiotemporal organization and structuring ("putting together") of the contents in consciousness. As such, form or organization and their underlying neuronal mechanisms signify the neural predisposition of consciousness (NPC) which I propose to be related to the resting state and the spatiotemporal continuity of its neuronal activity. The resting state itself and thus the neural predisposition of consciousness themselves seem to be abnormal in psychiatric disorders like depression or schizophrenia.

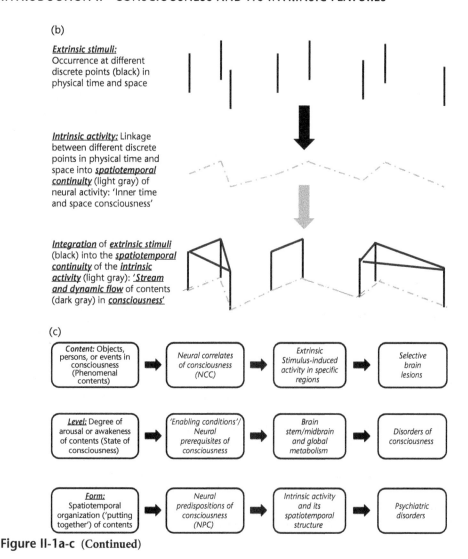

Figure II-1a-c (Continued)

(Tononi 2004; Tononi and Koch 2008; Seth et al. 2006, 2011), global neuronal workspace (Baars 2005; Dehaene and Changeux 2011; Dehaene et al. 2006), pre-stimulus resting-state activity (see Kleinschmidt et al. 2012), and neuronal synchronization (Fries et al. 2001; Fries 2005; Varela et al. 2001; Koch 2004; Singer 1999; Llinas et al. 1998; Llinas 2002; Buzsaki 2006; John 2005) (see first Introduction and subsequent parts for details).

In addition to healthy subjects, patients with selected regional lesions in the brain have been investigated extensively in order to reveal which brain region is "in charge" of which phenomenal content in consciousness (see Fig. I-1b; Haynes 2009; Seth et al. 2006, 2011;, Frith et al. 1999; Zeki 2003, 2008). For instance, patients with lesions in visual cortex show deficits in especially visual contents entering consciousness (see Zeki 2003, 2005). Why? Visual cortical regions process mainly visual stimuli related to visual objects, persons, or events; lesions in these regions go then along with deficits in visual contents such as that visual consciousness and more specifically visual content-based consciousness is impaired (see Figure I-1a).

EMPIRICAL CHARACTERIZATION OF CONSCIOUSNESS IB: LEVEL OF CONSCIOUSNESS

Beyond the contents entering consciousness, we may also need to consider another dimension of consciousness, the level or state of consciousness that is signified by arousal or awakeness. When you sleep, for instance, your degree of arousal or awakeness is rather low. And when you undergo surgery, you are in complete anesthesia so that your degree of consciousness is zero. This has been described as the state, or better level, of consciousness. The level of consciousness is thus proposed to be a second dimension of consciousness besides the contents (see, for instance, Monaco et al. 2005; Cavanna et al. 2008, 2011; Laureys 2005a and b; Laureys et al. 2005).

The level of consciousness is particularly relevant when discussing disorders of consciousness like coma, vegetative state, sleep, anesthesia (are sleep and anesthesia considered "disorders" of consciousness?), and epilepsy (see, for instance, Schiff 2010; Plum and Posner 1980; Danielson et al. 2011; Laureys 2005; Hohwy 2009; Laureys and Schiff 2012; Monaco et al. 2005; Cavanna et al. 2008, 2011; Cavanna and Monaco 2009). The level of consciousness is low in a minimally conscious state (Laureys 2005) and sleep (especially in what is described as non–rapid eye movement [NREM] sleep as distinguished from REM sleep; see, for instance, Nir and Tononi 2010). Further decrease in the level of consciousness can be observed in the vegetative state (although this has been doubted most recently; Laureys et al. 2005; Qin et al. 2010; Owen et al. 2006; Monti et al. 2010; Laureys and Schiff 2012) and comes to its lowest tending toward zero in anesthesia and coma (see Figure I-1a).

Neuronally, the focus has here been on especially subcortical regions like the brainstem/midbrain (see, for instance, Cavanna and Monaco 2009; Panksepp et al. 2007; and Parvizi and Damasio 2003) and the thalamus (see, for instance, Schiff 2010) that seem to be essential in constituting the level or state of consciousness. These regions seem to be affected in disorders of consciousness like vegetative state and coma (see Schiff and Laureys 2012 for review) as well as in anesthesia and NREM sleep (see Part VIII for details).

In addition to subcortical regions, the brain's global metabolism and energy supply seem to be closely related to the level of consciousness (see Hyder et al. 2006, 2013, van Eijsden et al. 2009; Laureys 2005a and b; Schiff and Laureys 2012). Low levels of global metabolism and energy supply with 40-50% deficit (when compared to healthy subjects) have been observed in both anesthesia and vegetative state (see part VIII for details). This suggests a central role for the global metabolism and the energy supply of the brain as a whole in constituting the level or state of consciousness.

EMPIRICAL CHARACTERIZATION OF CONSCIOUSNESS IIA: NEURAL CORRELATES OF CONSCIOUSNESS (NCC)

Current neuroscientific research aims to find the neural conditions underlying consciousness in both its content and its level. This has been subsumed under the concept of the neural correlates of consciousness: Following Francis Crick and Christoph Koch (1998) and Koch (2004), the aim is to identify what they call the "neural correlates of consciousness" (NCC). The NCC describe the search for those minimally neuronal conditions that are jointly sufficient for any one being specifically conscious, that is, the distinct phenomenal content that we can experience (see also Tononi and Koch 2008 for a recent review, as well as Chalmers 1996, 2002, 2010 for a more conceptual account). Several neuronal mechanisms have been discussed as possible candidate mechanisms for the NCC. The main contender have been mentioned earlier; these will be discussed in further detail throughout this book.

Following the distinction between contents and level of consciousness, one may want to distinguish between the neural correlates of the contents and the neural correlates of the level of consciousness. This has recently been put forward by Hohwy (2009). He distinguishes between the minimally sufficient neural conditions of the contents of consciousness, that is, "content-based NCC," and the minimally sufficient neural conditions of the level or state of consciousness,[1] that is, "level/state-based NCC" (see also Seth et al. 2006, 2008, as well as Monaco et al. 2005; and Cavanna et al. 2008; for discussing different measures of consciousness targeting the level/state and/or content of consciousness).

Such a distinction between "content-based NCC" and "level/state-based NCC" is further supported by the observation of a possible dissociation between level and content in consciousness in extreme states. While you are dreaming, you still experience contents, that is, phenomenal contents, even though your level of consciousness is rather low during sleep (see Chapter 26 for a detailed discussion about dreams). The same holds true for particular forms of epilepsy in which one can still perceive vivid phenomenal contents while the level of consciousness is decreased (see Monaco et al. 2005; Cavanna et al. 2008). The reverse scenario seems to occur in patients with lesions in specific regions of the brain as for instance, in subregions of the visual cortex (see earlier). In that case, specific phenomenal contents like visual motion are lost, that is, motion blindness occurs, while your level of consciousness is still intact (see Haynes 2009; Zeki 2005; Frith et al. 1999).

EMPIRICAL CHARACTERIZATION OF CONSCIOUSNESS IIB: FROM CONSCIOUSNESS TO UNCONSCIOUSNESS

In addition to the distinction between content- and level-based NCC, some authors describe yet another set of neural conditions of consciousness, the "enabling conditions" (Koch 2004; van Eijsden et al. 2009; Dehaene et al. 2006) or "neural prerequisites" (de Graaf et al. 2012; Aru et al. 2012; Northoff 2013) of consciousness. "Enabling conditions" or "neural prerequisites" are those neuronal mechanisms that are necessary to yield consciousness, while they remain unable to generate consciousness by themselves independent of some additional sufficient neural condition.

What exactly are the "enabling conditions" or neural prerequisites of consciousness? The "enabling conditions" are necessary prerequisites,

e.g., "neural prerequisites" for setting the sufficient neural conditions of consciousness, the neural correlate or neural substrate of consciousness, into motion. These in turn may then be followed by some neural events, the neural consequences of consciousness, that can occur only on the basis of the preceding neural substrate or neural correlate of consciousness (see Aru et al. 2012; Northoff 2013).

For instance, neural activity in brainstem and midbrain is often considered an enabling condition that needs to be met in order for thalamo-cortical connections to yield consciousness (see Koch 2004; de Graaf et al. 2012; Parvizi and Damasio 2003). However, in the absence of thalamo-cortical connections, neural activity in brainstem and midbrain will not be able to yield consciousness by itself. Whether such enabling conditions, or neural prerequisites, can be equated with the neural conditions underlying the level (rather than the content) of consciousness and thus the level-based NCC remains open at this point.

Both the NCC, whether they are content- or level-based, and the enabling conditions, the neural prerequisites, focus on the neuronal mechanisms that make possible the transition from unconscious to conscious states. The central question here is: How can an unconscious state be transformed into a conscious state? The main aim is here to find the neuronal mechanisms that allow to distinguish between unconscious and consciousness. This presupposes that the unconscious state can in principle be transformed into a conscious state. The unconscious state must thus contain certain features that in principle allow for such transformation into a conscious state in the presence of the NCC.

What are the neuronal mechanisms underlying these features that allow for the possible transformation of the unconscious into a conscious state? The question here no longer targets the NCC but rather some more basic neuronal mechanisms that, unlike the NCC, are already present in the unconscious state itself. Instead, the central question here is: What are the features of the unconscious state that in principle make possible its transformation into a conscious state? Hence rather than targeting the conscious state and its distinction from the unconscious state, as in the NCC, we are now targeting the unconscious state itself (and what it has in common with the conscious state with both being distinguished from a non-conscious state; see later).

EMPIRICAL CHARACTERIZATION OF CONSCIOUSNESS IIC: FROM NEURAL CORRELATES OF CONSCIOUSNESS (NCC) TO NEURAL PREDISPOSITION OF CONSCIOUSNESS (NPC)

The shift from consciousness to the unconscious (and its distinction from the non-conscious) implies a shift in the search for the neural conditions of consciousness. Rather than searching for the neural correlates and prerequisites of consciousness itself as distinguished from the unconscious, we are now targeting the neural conditions underlying those features of the unconscious itself that distinguishes it from the non-conscious and therefore make possible its transformation into a conscious state. Since these neural conditions predispose the principal (or possible) transformation of the unconscious into a conscious state, one may want to speak of neural predispositions of consciousness (NPC) (see Northoff 2013).

What do I mean by "neural predisposition of consciousness" (NPC)? The concept of the neural predispositions of consciousness (NPC) refers to those neural conditions that make it necessary or unavoidable for the unconscious to be possibly transformed into consciousness (in the "right" circumstances like in the presence of the "right" neuronal mechanisms). In contrast to the unconscious, the non-conscious can well avoid of being transformed into either unconscious or consciousness. How is that possible and what does the brain itself contributes to the difference between the non-conscious on the one hand and the unconscious and consciousness on the other? This is the focus of this volume that primarily targets the neural predispositions of consciousness (NPC) rather than its neural correlates (NCC).

EMPIRICAL CHARACTERIZATION OF CONSCIOUSNESS IIIA: FORM OF CONSCIOUSNESS—TEMPORAL CONTINUITY

How can we find the NPC, the neural conditions that make possible the association of the purely neuronal activity with the phenomenal features of consciousness? For that, we may need to introduce yet another dimension of consciousness complementing the content and level/state of consciousness. We so far discussed a bi-dimensional view of consciousness that characterizes consciousness by content and level. While this may open the door to investigate the NCC and the enabling conditions/neural prerequisites, it does not provide a key to the NPC. For that, one may need to introduce yet another dimension of consciousness, what I call the "form" or organization of consciousness (see also Northoff 2012a, 2013).

What do I mean by "form" of consciousness? The contents of consciousness have to be put together, ordered, structured, and ultimately organized in a certain way. Such "putting together" requires a certain form or organization (see later for a more extensive definition) which is well manifest on the level of subjective experience and thus on the phenomenal level. How is the form of consciousness manifest in our subjective experience and its particular phenomenal features? Experience of contents in consciousness presupposes a dynamic and continuous flow of time extending from the past over the present to the future all crystallized and condensed in the present moment. This is what William James (1890) described as "specious present" or "dynamic flow." How can we define the concept of the "dynamic flow"? The concept of the "dynamic flow" describes the organization of time as a continuum rather than as a discontinuum in consciousness. This leads to the experience of what James described as the "stream of consciousness," a continuous temporal flow analogous to the flow of water in a river as distinguished from a discontinuous time experience with gaps between different discrete points in time (and space) (see Chapter 13–15 for details).

Most important, any content we experience in consciousness is integrated and embedded within this "dynamic flow" of time and becomes thereby part of the ongoing stream of consciousness. Metaphorically speaking, consciousness of contents can be compared to a boat in a river: In very much the same way the boat cannot function as a boat without the flowing water of the river, the contents cannot become conscious without the underlying temporal flow, the dynamic flow as the "stream of consciousness" (see lower part in Fig. I-1b).

Lets consider the same point from a different angle, this time from the perspective of the contents. The contents themselves occur at specific discrete points in physical time. At most, they may last for some seconds, after which they disappear and are replaced by others. One content goes and the next one comes, each at its distinct and discrete point in physical time. Despite their occurrence at different discrete points in physical time, we nevertheless experience a temporal continuum, a transition, between the different contents. This temporal continuum in consciousness does not seem to obey the laws of physical time and its discrete points in time. Instead, there is a continuum between the different discrete points in physical time and thus what phenomenally is described as "dynamic flow" (James) or "phenomenal time" (E. Husserl) as distinguished from physical time (see Chapters 13–15 for details).

Where is this continuum of time that underlies our experience of contents in consciousness coming from? It must be constituted somewhere. I will later suggest that the brain's intrinsic activity has a major role in constituting such temporal continuity (see Chapter 13–15). However, before going into the neuronal mechanisms of time, we need to consider the other major dimension, namely space.

EMPIRICAL CHARACTERIZATION OF CONSCIOUSNESS IIIB: FORM OF CONSCIOUSNESS—SPATIAL CONTINUITY

While there has been much debate about time and consciousness (see Chapters 13–15 for details), there has been less discussion about

the experience of space in consciousness. Analogously to time, the contents in consciousness are not experienced at their different discrete points in physical space. Instead, they are embedded and integrated into a spatial continuum with multiple transitions between the different discrete points in physical space. As in the case of time, the contents are woven into a spatial grid or template that emphasizes continuity and transition over discontinuity and segregation (see Chapter 16 for details).

Taken together, consciousness may phenomenally be characterized by an underlying temporal and spatial template or grid into which the different contents are woven. This underlying spatiotemporal grid or template seems to provide continuity between the different discrete points in time and space at which the different contents (and their underlying stimuli) occur. The spatiotemporal grid or template can thus be characterized by spatiotemporal continuity in the phenomenal realm of consciousness as distinguished from the spatiotemporal discontinuity in the realm of physical time and space.

EMPIRICAL CHARACTERIZATION OF CONSCIOUSNESS IIIC: FORM OF CONSCIOUSNESS—"THIRD" DIMENSION

I demonstrated the presence of spatiotemporal continuity on the phenomenal level of consciousness. The contents we subjectively experience in consciousness are always already interwoven into an underlying spatiotemporal grid or template that provides some continuity between the different discrete points in physical time and space. Such spatiotemporal continuity can obviously not be equated with the contents, e.g., the phenomenal contents, themselves since the latter presuppose the former. Hence, the first dimension of consciousness, the dimension of content, cannot account for such spatiotemporal continuity.

Moreover, the spatiotemporal continuity cannot be accounted for by the second dimension of consciousness, the level or state, either. The level or state of consciousness describes the degree of arousal or awakeness that does not imply any reference to the spatiotemporal continuity itself. How then can we account for the spatiotemporal continuity in consciousness? The current bi-dimensional view with its distinction between content and level of consciousness seems to turn out insufficient in this regard. We may therefore need to introduce a third dimension, the form of consciousness (see Northoff 2013).

I propose that the spatiotemporal continuity structures and organizes the content in consciousness by putting their discrete points in physical time and space into a spatial and temporal continuum. Since this structures and organizes the contents in a novel way, one may want to speak of a "form" of consciousness. I thus advocate a tri-dimensional rather than a bi-dimensional view of consciousness that suggests to characterize consciousness by three dimensions, content, level, and form (see Northoff 2013).

What exactly do I mean by form as the third dimension of consciousness? The form as third dimension concerns the organization and structuring of the contents of consciousness in space and time and, more specifically, the integration of their different discrete points in physical time and space into a spatial and temporal continuum. Such underlying spatiotemporal continuum provides the form of consciousness which, as I postulate, is constructed by the brain's intrinsic activity itself and its spatiotemporal structure. This will be the focus in the next section.

EMPIRICAL CHARACTERIZATION OF CONSCIOUSNESS IIID: FORM OF CONSCIOUSNESS— PSYCHIATRIC DISORDERS

How can we empirically support our hypothesis of the brain's intrinsic activity as the designer of the spatiotemporal continuity of consciousness? One possible hint in this direction comes from patients with psychiatric disorders like schizophrenia or depression. These patients often experience abnormal time and space in their consciousness, that is, inner time and space consciousness (see Chapter 17 and 22 for details). This suggests an abnormal form

of consciousness which then also affects their experience of the various contents in consciousness as manifest in the sometimes rather bizarre symptoms.

How is the form of consciousness altered in psychiatric disorders? For instance, schizophrenic patients experience disruption and thus temporal discontinuity rather than a temporal continuum in their consciousness. This in turn affects their experience of the still somehow intact contents as manifest in delusions and hallucinations (see Chapter 17 and 22 for details). Unlike in schizophrenia, patients with depression still experience a temporal continuum in their consciousness, which though is abnormally shifted toward the past at the expense of the future (see Chapters 17 and 26 for details). Due to their preserved contents in their consciousness, the latter are abnormally associated with the past rather than present and future (see Fig. I-1a).

What is wrong in the brain of psychiatric patients? Recent investigations suggest the brain's intrinsic activity, its resting-state activity (Logothetis et al. 2009; see later for details), to be abnormal in psychiatric disorders like depression and schizophrenia (see Chapters 27 and 32 for details). They may consequently be regarded as "resting-state disorders" (see, for instance, Northoff et al. 2011a and b, Northoff 2013). Hence, in order to better understand the neural basis of the form of consciousness, we may need to investigate the brain's intrinsic activity in further detail.

More specifically, we need to understand how the brain's intrinsic activity can yield the aforementioned spatiotemporal continuity as the template or grid for the contents of consciousness. That may be possible if, for instance, the intrinsic activity itself constitutes a particular spatial and temporal structure on the basis of its own neural activity. This will then also open the door toward understanding the kind of neuronal features that predispose the unconscious to be converted into a conscious state. In other words, the brain's intrinsic activity may provide insight into what I describe as the neural predispositions of consciousness (NPC) (see Fig. I-1c).

EMPIRICAL CHARACTERIZATION OF CONSCIOUSNESS IIIE: FORM OF CONSCIOUSNESS—THE INTRINSIC ACTIVITY'S SPATIOTEMPORAL STRUCTURE PROVIDES THE FORM OF CONSCIOUSNESS

How can we characterize the brain's intrinsic activity in such a way as to link it to the form of consciousness and thus the spatiotemporal continuity? I so far discussed the empirical, e.g., neuronal features of the brain's intrinsic activity and its spatiotemporal structure in length in Volume I (see Chapter 4–6) and postulated that they predispose consciousness in the first introduction. This however left open what exactly the brain's intrinsic activity and its spatiotemporal structure predispose on the side of consciousness.

What kind of feature of consciousness is predisposed in what way by the brain's intrinsic activity and its spatiotemporal structure? This is the moment where the form as third dimension of consciousness becomes relevant. I postulate that the brain's intrinsic activity and its spatiotemporal structure predispose the form as third dimension of consciousness. The intrinsic activity's spatiotemporal structure may provide the spatiotemporal grid or template within which the various contents of contents are integrated, structured and organized (see middle part in Fig. I-1b).

Taken together, I here postulate a more refined empirical characterization of consciousness in terms of a threefold distinction between content, level, and form. All three can be distinguished from each other and may be related to different underlying neuronal mechanisms while at the same time being dependent and closely related to each other. How does such threefold empirical distinction of consciousness relate to consciousness including its phenomenal features and their essentially subjective nature? For that we need to go into more conceptual and phenomenal detail which will be the focus of the next sections. Before though we need to exemplify form as third dimension of consciousness in a more illustrative way.

NEUROMETAPHORICAL COMPARISON I: IS CONSCIOUSNESS THE LIVING ROOM OF THE BRAIN?

Let me illustrate the threefold distinction between content, level, and form of consciousness by a metaphorical comparison with the living room of your apartment. Your apartment is located at a certain level in the building as, for instance, the second or eighth floor. And obviously there is furniture inside the living room, which is set and organized spatiotemporally in a specific way, with the sofa, for instance, standing in the right-hand corner, the table in the middle, and so on.

How can we now compare the apartment to the here suggested threefold distinction within the realm of consciousness? The level or floor of your apartment corresponds to the level of consciousness; the furniture represents the contents of consciousness; and the way the furniture is set and organized in the rooms, e.g., space and time, of your apartment is analogous to what I described as form or organization of consciousness.

Where is the form or organization, the spatiotemporal continuity as the grid or template underlying the contents of consciousness coming from? In the case of the apartment it is easy. The designer organizes the furniture in particular ways and arranges it spatially and temporally. Who, however, is the designer in the case of consciousness? We currently do not know. One suspect, as it will turn out, is the brain itself and more specifically its intrinsic activity by means of which the brain itself may act as the designer of its own living room in which the extrinsic stimuli and their associated contents are processed. More concretely, it is the brain itself and its intrinsic activity that may constitute the spatiotemporal continuity as the form of consciousness.

After having clarified the brain itself and its neuronal features (see first introduction) and the empirical characterization of consciousness (see this introduction so far), we now need to tackle some conceptual issues. More specifically, we need to discuss what exactly we mean by the concept of consciousness and how it is related to concepts like unconscious and non-conscious. This will be the focus of the next sections.

NEUROCONCEPTUAL REMARK IA: INTRINSIC FEATURES OF THE BRAIN AND CONSCIOUSNESS

We remember from the first introduction the example of crystal and its brittleness which, relying on the philosopher Michael Tye, we invoked in order to distinguish between the brain's extrinsic and intrinsic features. In addition, Tye also emphasized that its intrinsic features may predispose the brain to associate consciousness with its own neural activity in the same way the crystal's intrinsic features predispose the crystal to brittleness. While focusing on the brain's intrinsic features in the first introduction, we left open what exactly is meant by the concept of "predisposition." After having discussed the empirical characterization of consciousness in a threefold way by content, level, and form, we are now in a good position to shed some more detailed light on the meaning of the concept of "predisposition" itself.

How does Tye's emphasis on mechanism and intrinsic features stand in relation to the various suggestions for the NCC as discussed in the first introduction? Suggestions like re-entrant circuits, information integration, and global workspace focus mainly on stimulus-induced activity. By starting from the stimulus and how it must affect the brain to elicit consciousness presupposes a focus on the brain's extrinsic features rather than its intrinsic features. Lets go back briefly to Tye and his example of the crystal and its brittleness. This scenario is comparable to a detailed investigation of the external and thus extrinsic force itself and how it affects the brittle object. That, however, leaves open the intrinsic features of the brittle object, its irregular alignment of crystals, without which the effects of the extrinsic force cannot be understood.

Coming back to the brain this yields the following question: What are the brain's intrinsic features themselves and how do they predispose the association of the extrinsic stimuli and their respective stimulus-induced activity with consciousness? The focus is thus no longer on the extrinsic stimuli themselves and their stimulus-induced activity. Instead, the brain's intrinsic activity, its resting-state activity, is regarded central for consciousness. The exact features of the brain's intrinsic activity that predispose it to associate the extrinsic stimuli and their purely neuronal and objective stimulus-induced activity with consciousness and its phenomenal and subjective features remain unclear, however. In the case of the brittle object, we know that its irregular alignment of crystals predisposes it to become shattered during the application of external force. What is the corresponding "irregular alignment of crystals" in the case of the brain's intrinsic activity? We currently do not know.

NEUROCONCEPTUAL REMARK IB: ACTUAL VERSUS POSSIBLE CONSCIOUSNESS

What does the NCC tell us? The NCC concerns the sufficient neural conditions of consciousness as it is manifest, that is, actual consciousness.[2] While the necessary neural conditions of actual consciousness may be touched upon with the concepts of "enabling conditions" (Koch 2004, 88; van Eijsden et al. 2009; Dehaene et al. 2006) and "neural prerequisite" (as distinguished from "neural substrates," "neural causes" and "neural consequences" (de Graaf et al. 2012; Neisser 2011a and b; Aru et al. 2012). As indicated earlier, these may, for instance, concern the involvement of subcortical structures like the brainstem that may remain insufficient by themselves to yield consciousness (see Chapter 31 for a discussion of subcortical regions and consciousness; see Koch 2004). Psychologically arousal or vigilance may be regarded an "enabling" and thus necessary nonsufficient condition of consciousness (see Deheaene et al. 2006).

We must, however, go one step further. Besides the necessary and sufficient (neural and psychological) conditions of actual or manifest consciousness, we may also need to distinguish those neural conditions that predispose consciousness. As mentioned above, we need to understand those features of the unconscious itself that predispose its possible conversion into a conscious state. In the same way, Tye considered the crystal itself to reveal its predispositions, we need to go back to the unconscious itself and ultimately to the brain itself and its intrinsic activity.

Lets starts with the crystal. The "irregular alignment of the crystal" makes possible the shattering of the brittle object during external force. However, the irregular alignment of the crystal does not by itself imply any shattering; which would require some external force. Therefore, the irregular alignment of the crystal concerns and predisposes only "possible shattering" rather than "actual shattering." Analogously, one may distinguish those conditions that predispose "*possible* consciousness" from those that are necessary and sufficient for "*actual* consciousness." We already discussed those necessary and sufficient neural conditions that are supposed to underlie *actual* consciousness, the NCC and its recent siblings, the neural prerequisites of consciousness. In contrast, we left open those neural conditions that account for *possible* consciousness. Therefore, I here propose that what I described as the neural predispositions of consciousness, the NPC, reflect the necessary neural conditions of possible consciousness and more specifically of those features of the unconscious that makes possible its principle transformation into consciousness. This needs to be detailed as it will be the focus of the next section.

NEUROCONCEPTUAL REMARK IC: FROM POSSIBLE CONSCIOUSNESS TO NEURAL PREDISPOSITIONS OF CONSCIOUSNESS (NPC)

One the basis of the distinction between actual and possible consciousness, I distinguish the following conditions. We have to reveal the necessary and sufficient neural conditions of *actual* consciousness. This concerns the manifestation of consciousness and thus actual consciousness in relation to extrinsic stimuli (and strong intrinsic activity changes, as in dreams; see Chapter 26) as it is usually targeted by the NCC.

The NCC needs to be complemented by considering the necessary and sufficient conditions of *possible* consciousness. This concerns the predisposition of consciousness by the brain itself and its intrinsic features. Since it refers to the predispositions rather than the correlates, one may speak of NPC as indicated earlier (see Fig. I-2) (see also Northoff 2013).[3]

Neuroscientists and philosophers alike may now be puzzled about such unnecessary conceptual inflation. All one needs are the NCC while the NPC seem to be superfluous. But this is not so. We are searching for the brain's analogue to the "irregular alignment of crystals" that predisposes the crystal's possible shattering of the brittle object. That is analogous to the predisposing role of the brain's intrinsic features for the possible association of stimuli and their purely neuronal stimulus-induced activity with consciousness and its phenomenal features.

Let us return one more time to the brittle object. The mechanisms underlying the brittle objects' "irregular alignment of crystals" must be distinguished from the ones underlying the application of external force with the consequent shattering. The latter corresponds to the correlate of shattering, while the former mirrors the predisposition of shattering. This can also be applied to the case of the brain: the neuronal mechanisms that predispose the brain to associate the extrinsic stimuli and their purely neuronal stimulus-induced activity with phenomenal features, that is consciousness, must be distinguished from the ones that underlie the actual consciousness itself. We therefore need to distinguish between the NCC and the NPC. Put differently, the NCC characterize consciousness as distinct from the unconscious. The central question here is: What are the neural conditions that transform an unconscious into a conscious state? This concerns what we above described as actual consciousness. That is to be distinguished from the NPC that concerns the unconscious as distinct from the non-conscious. The guiding question here is: What are the neural conditions that underlie the features of the unconscious (as distinct from the non-conscious) that make possible its distinction from the non-conscious and entail its possible transformation into a conscious state? The central target in this volume is no longer actual consciousness, as in the NCC (see Chapters 28–32), but rather

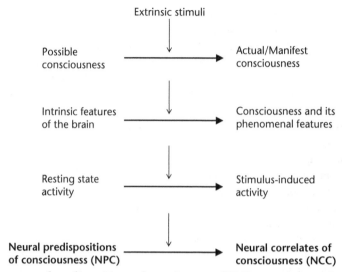

Figure II-2 From neural predispositions of consciousness (NPC) to neural correlates of consciousness (NCC). The figure shows the comparison between neural predispositions of consciousness (NPC) (left) and the neural correlates of consciousness (right). *Left part*: The intrinsic features (second from top) of the brain must make consciousness possible so that one can speak conceptually of "possible consciousness" (top). That must be related to the brain's intrinsic features and more specifically its intrinsic activity (or its resting-state activity) (second from top). The brain's intrinsic features predispose the possibility of consciousness, thus concerning the neural predispositions of consciousness (NPC) (bottom). *Right part*: During its encounter with the extrinsic stimuli (see middle part), the intrinsic predisposition generates consciousness and its phenomenal features (second from top) and thus what conceptually can be described as "actual consciousness" (top). That is neuronally related to stimulus-induced activity (second from top) concerning the neural correlates of consciousness (NCC) (bottom).

possible consciousness and thus the NPC (see Chapters 13–27).

NEUROCONCEPTUAL REMARK ID: FROM THE NEURAL PREDISPOSITIONS OF CONSCIOUSNESS (NPC) TO THE BRAIN'S INTRINSIC FEATURES

How and where can we search for the NPC? For that, we have to understand the intrinsic features of the brain independent of the extrinsic stimuli and their stimulus-induced activity. How can we define the intrinsic features of the brain? The brain's intrinsic features are those features that the brain itself provides; i.e., its own neural processing of extrinsic stimuli in the brain. They thus reflect the brain's active contribution, that is, its specific neuronal input, to its own neural processing of the intero- and exteroceptive inputs from body and environment.

Two such active contributions of the brain and its intrinsic features were identified in detail in Volume I and the first introduction in this volume: the spatiotemporal structure of the brain's intrinsic activity and the neural code the brain applies to encode and thus generate its neuronal activity. To understand how the brain predisposes consciousness, we thus have to better understand how the resting state's spatiotemporal structure and the brain's coding strategy are related to consciousness.

I therefore postulated in my first introduction that the resting state's spatiotemporal structure predisposes possible consciousness—the resting state's spatiotemporal structure can therefore be regarded as a neural predisposition of consciousness (NPC). While the brain's specific way of coding rest–stimulus and stimulus–rest interaction, more specifically the degree of difference-based coding, can be regarded as a sufficient neural condition of actual consciousness and thus as a neural correlate of consciousness (NCC) (see first introduction). Accordingly, what we empirically described as different intrinsic features of the brain, its spatiotemporal structure and coding strategy, can now be aligned with two different conceptual characterizations, NPC and NCC, in the search for the neuronal mechanisms underlying consciousness.

Now the neuro-conceptual ground is well cleared to go ahead with a more detailed conceptual and phenomenal characterization of consciousness itself as it shall be discussed in the following. More specifically, we first need to discuss which and what concept of consciousness we refer to when we postulate that the brain's intrinsic activity and its spatiotemporal structure predispose consciousness. This amounts to a conceptual clarification of the term consciousness which is the focus of the subsequent sections.

Conceptual characterization of consciousness Ia: Concept of unconsciousness—"preconscious" and "dynamic unconscious"

In the first introduction, I have discussed the brain's intrinsic features, the resting state's spatiotemporal structure and the brain's neural code, and how they predispose consciousness. While suggesting some specific neuronal mechanisms in the first introduction, I simply presupposed the concept of consciousness and took it for granted. That, however, is rather naive since different concepts of consciousness may need to be distinguished from each other.

While such a distinction is certainly important on the conceptual level, it also bears relevance for the empirical context: different concepts of consciousness may entail different neuronal mechanisms. Therefore, I here venture briefly and very superficially into the philosophical debate about different concepts of consciousness. The concept of consciousness needs to be distinguished first and foremost from the one of the unconscious. What is the unconscious? Notions of the unconscious can be traced back as far as Plato and Aristotle and have been

elaborated since then in philosophical and later in psychological thought.

Whatever frameworks have been presupposed, unconscious states have been characterized by hidden characteristics of a person's self (fate, temperament, soul, character) that need to be inferred and cannot be accessed directly. Such hidden characteristics were distinguished from those that were believed to be transparent, experienced directly, open to introspection, and thus accessible to consciousness (Uleman 2005; Northoff 2011, 2012a and b). Philosopher John R. Searle (2004, 165–172) distinguishes among different types of unconsciousness. He first speaks of the "preconscious," which refers to a state that is on the verge of becoming conscious though not yet conscious by itself; as such, it resembles what Sigmund Freud described as "system preconscious." Another concept of the unconscious concerns the "dynamic unconscious": "unconscious mental states function causally, even when unconscious" (Searle 2004, 167). Unlike in the case of the preconscious, the state is here not on the verge of becoming conscious but remains unconscious by itself. This corresponds to some degree to what Freud referred as "dynamic or repressed unconscious" where the contents are actively repressed in order to avoid their entrance into consciousness. Important, though, even the dynamically unconscious state has at least the potential or principal possibility of becoming conscious.

Searle's philosophical (and ultimately Freud's psychodynamic) distinction between the "dynamic unconscious" and the "preconscious" is mirrored in the more empirically and neuroscientifically based distinction between the "subliminal" and the "preconscious" by S. Dehaene (Dehaene et al. 2006; Kouider and Dehaene 2009; Dehaene and Changeux 2011): the "subliminal" is supposed to describe neural processing where the stimulus remains unconscious. In this case, the stimulus cannot enter consciousness because it is simply too weak to induce the "right" kind of neural processing, like the suggested "ignition" of neural activity in a large-scale fronto-parietal network (see first introduction and part VI for details). This is different in the case of the "preconscious," where the stimulus itself is strong enough while the fronto-parietal network is not ready because it is occupied with other stimuli (see Chapter 19 for extensive discussion of this "global neuronal workspace" theory [GNW] by Dehaene and Changeux, 2005, 2011; see Fig. I-3a).

CONCEPTUAL CHARACTERIZATION OF CONSCIOUSNESS IB: CONCEPT OF UNCONSCIOUSNESS— "DEEP UNCONSCIOUS" AND "NON-CONSCIOUS"

Let's return to philosopher John Searle and his different concepts of the unconscious. The third concept of the unconscious is what Searle describes as "deep unconscious." Here the unconscious mental state cannot only factually be brought into consciousness, as in the "dynamic unconscious," but even stronger it remains also principally impossible to do so. Following Searle, this is so because what is unconscious here is not "the sort of thing that can form the content of a conscious intentional state" (Searle 2004, 168).

Searle underlines this by the example of the computational rules that we follow unconsciously in acquiring language. While we can be preconscious or dynamically unconscious about the language and its letters, we remain deeply unconscious about the rules and principles of its universal grammar that guide our learning of the language. Hence, rules that guide the acquisition of language (or for instance our construction of perception in the retina and the visual cortex) are simply not the sort of things we can become conscious of at all.

Finally, there is what Searle describes as the "non-conscious." The concept of the non-conscious refers to neurobiological phenomena that remain non-conscious and cannot become instances of consciousness at all. This will be described in further detail in the next section.

> There are all sorts of things going on in the brain, many of which function crucially in controlling our mental lives but that are not cases of mental phenomena at all. So, for example, the secretion of serotonin at the synaptic cleft is simply not a mental phenomenon. Serotonin is important for several kinds of mental phenomena, and indeed some important drugs, such as Prozac, are used specifically to influence serotonin, but there is no mental reality to the behaviour of serotonin as such. Let us call these sorts of cases the "non-conscious."
>
> There are other examples of the non-conscious that are more problematic. So, for example, when I am totally unconscious, the medulla will still control my breathing. This is why I do not die when I am unconscious or in a sound sleep. But there is no mental reality to the events in the medulla that keep me breathing even when unconscious. I am not unconsciously following the rule "Keep breathing"; rather, the medulla is just functioning in a nonmental fashion, in the same way that the stomach functions in a nonmental fashion when I am digesting food. (Searle 2004, 168)

NEUROMETAPHORICAL COMPARISON IIA: UNCONSCIOUSNESS AS THE ENTRANCE GATE OF A CASTLE

How can we better illustrate Searle's four different concepts of unconsciousness? Let's invoke a thought experiment. Imagine you are standing in the entrance hallway of a castle waiting to enter the ballroom where the dance party is taking place. The guests inside are already dancing and enjoying themselves—obviously showing full-blown consciousness.

What about you who are standing outside? Now the main door to the hallway opens for a moment and you get a glimpse of what is going on inside. You consequently step forward and are on the verge of entering the ballroom—that is analogous to you being preconscious. But imagine an even earlier situation. You entered the castle through its main entrance door, the big door, and now you are standing in the hallway. Suddenly you notice that you forgot something important, the ticket you bought yesterday. What can you do? You have the principal option of entering the ballroom if you decide to return home and pick up the ticket—that compares to you being dynamically unconscious.

Let's imagine yet another scenario. By chance you pass by the castle and see all the people

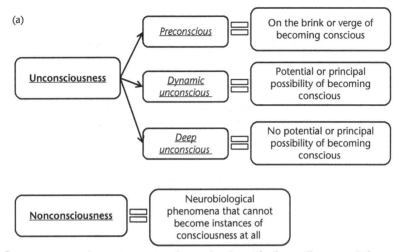

Figure II-3a-c Concepts of consciousness and neural coding. The figure illustrates different concepts of consciousness (*a, b*) and how they relate to the brain's neural coding (*c*). (*a*) The figure describes different concepts of unconsciousness (upper part) as distinguished from the concept of the non-consciousness (lower part) in orientation to the definitions suggested by the philosopher John R. Searle (see text). The concept of the *unconsciousness* includes the preconscious, the dynamic unconscious (corresponding more or less to the "subliminal" as a more empirically based concept as suggested by, for instance, S. Dehaene; see text), and the deep unconscious (middle part from top to bottom). The *preconscious* describes states that are on the verge of becoming conscious, while the *dynamic unconscious* refers to states that are not yet conscious but can in principle become so in the "right" circumstances. The *deep unconscious*, in contrast, does not show the potential or principal possibility of becoming conscious at all. Such a characterization distinguishes the concept of the unconscious from the concept of the non—consciousness, which refers to features (including neurobiological features like certain molecules) that have no access to consciousness and therefore cannot become conscious at all, hence the name *non-consciousness*. Searle raises the question of whether the deep unconscious and non-consciousness can be distinguished empirically from each other which he objects. While conceptually the concepts of the deep unconscious and non-consciousness differ from each other, they remain indistinguishable in empirical terms, as reflected in, for instance, their output or result that, in both cases, the respective states, i.e., deep unconscious and non-conscious, have in principle no access to consciousness at all, so that their respective contents can in principle never become conscious. (*b*) The figure depicts the distinction between the "principal consciousness" (upper part) and the "principal non-consciousness" (lower part). Both serve as umbrella terms to distinguish the potential or principal possibility of consciousness; i.e., "principal consciousness," from states lacking potential or principal impossibility of consciousness; i.e., principal non-consciousness." Hence, the concept of the "principal consciousness" includes both possible and actual consciousness referring to any state that can in principle be associated with consciousness. While this remains impossible in the case of the "principal non-consciousness," I propose that both "principal consciousness" and "principal non-consciousness" can be distinguished not only conceptually but also empirically by the kind of neural coding (right part): I propose "principal consciousness" to be possible on the basis of difference-based coding as the "right" kind of code for possible and actual consciousness; while stimulus-based coding is the "wrong" code for consciousness, thus being related to "principal non-consciousness" (see text for details). (*c*) The figure illustrates the relationship between the degree of difference-based coding (upper part, y-axis), the biophysical and physical spectrum (upper part, x-axis), unconsciousness and consciousness (lower middle part), and the concepts of the principal consciousness and the principal non-consciousness (lower part). *Upper part*: The world has a physical minimum and maximum in terms of physical properties the species living in the physical world can display; this is indicated by the outer ranges of the x-axis. Each species within that physical world has a species-dependent biophysical-computational range with an optimum and biophysical minima and maxima that define an inverted U-curve with regard to the degree of difference-based coding (as distinguished from stimulus-based coding). Highest degrees of difference-based coding are possible in the

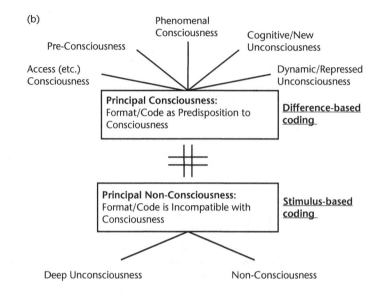

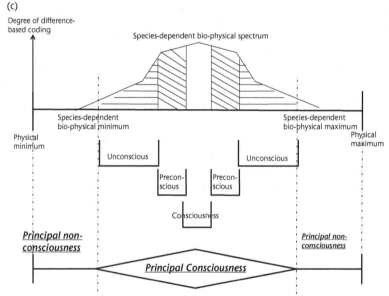

Figure II-3a-c (Continued)

middle, the optimal range, of the biophysical spectrum. *Middle and lower parts*: The higher degrees of difference-based coding in the middle of the species-specific biophysical-computational spectrum are related to higher degrees of consciousness, while the outer fringes of the biophysical-computational spectrum go along with lower degrees of difference-based coding and higher degrees of preconscious and unconsciousness (rather than consciousness). They remain, though, within the spectrum of what conceptually can be described as the "principal consciousness" (see below) as distinguished from the "principal non-consciousness." The "principal non-consciousness" is more related to the physical features that are part of the physical world but are not included in the biophysical-computational spectrum of the respective species. This is indicated by the difference between the inner and outer vertical dotted lines. One should be careful, though, in that some of the species' biophysical-computational features may also not be accessible to consciousness in which case they would need to be subsumed under *principal non-consciousness*; this is indicated here by the difference between the inner dotted vertical lines and the maximal and minimal ends of the inverted U-shape curve.

entering the main door to its entrance hall-way. They all have to show a ticket at the main entrance door, which provides them entrance. You are standing at the outside watching but cannot access the castle at all because you do not have a ticket; you did not know about the party at all and had thus not the chance of buying a ticket which by now are sold out completely. Hence, there is no way for you to pass through the entrance door and to enter the entrance hall-way, let alone the ballroom. This compares to you being deeply unconscious or non-conscious, as Searle would claim.

CONCEPTUAL CHARACTERIZATION OF CONSCIOUSNESS IIA: CONCEPT OF "PRINCIPAL NON-CONSCIOUSNESS"

Why does the "non-conscious" remain princi-pally inaccessible to consciousness? The format of these states may remain incompatible with the form of consciousness. This is, for instance, illustrated by the analogous example of the DNA by Revonsuo (2006, 63): "There is biologi-cal information coded in the DNA of our brain cells, but that type of information is in a totally non-conscious format and we will never be able to read it out just by reaching into our own minds and trying to retrieve it into consciousness. It is in a format unreadable at the phenomenal level."

The same holds in the case of the "deep unconscious." We cannot become conscious of the rules of language acquisition (or the retina's processing) (see earlier) because their format remains inaccessible to us. Our format in which we process data and stimuli is simply not com-patible with the one in which the rules of lan-guage acquisition (and the retina's processing) are coded. With the wrong code and wrong format, consciousness remains impossible. In other words, we remain deeply unconscious. In short, wrong code and wrong format make you non-conscious.

This implies, however, that the concept of the "deep unconscious" differs no longer, at least in its outcome, from the concept of the non-conscious. Everything that is deeply uncon-scious remains necessarily non-conscious. Hence, the concepts of the "non-conscious" and

the "deep unconscious" are intrinsically con-nected to each other in that they imply con-sciousness to be principally impossible. They thus presuppose what one may want to call "principal non-consciousness."

What do I mean by the concept of the "prin-cipal non-consciousness"? The concept of the "principal non-consciousness" describes that a particular state can in principle not become conscious at all because its intrinsic features like its format or code (principally) pre-vent its association with consciousness. The "principal non-consciousness" includes what Searle described as "deep unconscious" and "non-conscious" (see Fig. I-3b).

CONCEPTUAL CHARACTERIZATION OF CONSCIOUSNESS IIB: CONCEPT OF "PRINCIPAL CONSCIOUSNESS"

This is different in the other concepts of the uncon-scious, the "preconscious" and the "dynamic unconscious." While they do not describe actual or manifest consciousness itself, they at least carry the principal possibility in themselves (and thus the "right" intrinsic features) by means of which certain yet-unclear other features can in principle transform them into an actually con-scious state. The "preconscious" describes a state on the verge of becoming conscious, while the "dynamic unconscious" refers to states that can become in principle conscious even though they are actually not conscious.

Both "preconscious" and "dynamic uncon-scious" must share some intrinsic features like coding in the "right" format or code, which makes possible their principal transforma-tion into consciousness. Preconscious and the dynamic unconscious are thus "the kind of thing that could be a conscious mental state" (Searle 2004, 171; see also Revonsuo 2006, 63; Strawson 1994).

What does this imply for our concept of con-sciousness? Both preconscious and dynamic unconscious (or the "preconscious" and the "subliminal" in the more empirical sense of Dehaene and Changeux; see earlier, as well as Dehaene and Changeux 2011) are intrinsically linked to consciousness by sharing the same intrinsic features like the "right" format or code. There is thus some intrinsic connection between unconscious and consciousness, which Searle describes as the "connection principle": The connection principle states the logical connection between the concepts of the unconscious and the conscious. As such, it refers to some intrinsic feature like the "right" format or code that characterizes and commonly underlies both unconscious and consciousness.

Since the "connection principle" links both the unconscious and the conscious together by their principal possibility of becoming conscious, I here speak of "principal consciousness." The concept of the principal consciousness describes that a particular state can in principle become conscious because its intrinsic features like its format or code make principally possible its association with consciousness and its phenomenal features. Hence, the concept of the "principal consciousness" is based on the "right" kind of intrinsic features like the coding or formatting that therefore includes what we earlier described as *possible* and *actual* consciousness (see prior sections for this distinction). As such, the concept of the "principal consciousness" provides a wide umbrella term for the various forms of unconscious, that is, preconscious, dynamic unconscious, cognitive unconscious, as well as the different forms of consciousness like access consciousness, phenomenal consciousness, and so on (see Chapter 19 as well as Appendix 1).

CONCEPTUAL CHARACTERIZATION OF CONSCIOUSNESS IIC: "PRINCIPAL CONSCIOUSNESS" AND THE "RIGHT" CODE

My focus in this book will be on the "principal consciousness" as distinguished from the "principal non-consciousness." By searching for the neuronal mechanisms underlying "principal consciousness," I include both actual and possible consciousness as described earlier. This distinguishes my approach from most neuroscientific (and several philosophical) approaches that focus rather on how the brain's neuronal mechanisms allow to distinguish between actual and possible consciousness with the latter including

both "dynamic unconscious" and "preconscious." The investigation of the neuronal mechanisms of the "principal consciousness" and its distinction from the "principal non-consciousness" leads me to search for the consequent "right" kind of code or format.

More specifically, my aim is to investigate how the brain's neural activity needs to be encoded in order to associate its purely neuronal resting state and stimulus-induced activity with consciousness and its phenomenal features. Rather than comparing conscious and preconscious/dynamically unconscious contents as the current neuroscientific approaches. I compare different coding strategies in order to distinguish "right" and "wrong" codes or formats in the brain's encoding of its own neural activity. The search for the "right" code or format links the here presupposed concept of the "principal consciousness" to the "Coding Hypothesis of Consciousness" (CHC) as suggested in the first Introduction; this will be elaborated in the following sections. First, though, let us return once more to our castle to better illustrate the distinction between "principal consciousness" and "principal non-consciousness."

NEUROMETAPHORICAL COMPARISON IIB: "PRINCIPAL CONSCIOUSNESS" AND THE INSIDE OF THE CASTLE

How can we compare the concepts of the "principal consciousness" and "principal non-consciousness" to the metaphorical example of the dance party in the castle from the last section? The castle itself and its different rooms can be compared to the "principal consciousness." In the same way the castle has many rooms besides the big ballroom, the "principal consciousness" includes different forms of possible and actual consciousness as described earlier. And analogous to the rooms in the castle that are all somehow directly or indirectly connected with each other, the different forms of consciousness within the "principal consciousness" are connected to each other as described by the "connection principle."

How about the "principal non-consciousness"? The "principal non-consciousness" corresponds to everything that lies outside the castle. This is when you are standing outside in the rain watching all the people entering the castle while you have no access at all because you are lacking the ticket or, as one may say, the "right" kind of "entrance code."

Applied to our context, this means that your brain simply no longer provides you with the "right" kind of neural code or format to associate its own neural activity with consciousness. In the same way you remain principally unable to enter the castle and participate in the party of consciousness; the neuronal states of your brain have in principle no chance of ever making you conscious of, for instance, your exclusion from the party of consciousness. Lucky you, that you are no longer able to experience the rather miserable situation of your exclusion in your own consciousness? No, because, as we will see in Part VIII, you are then in a vegetative state or coma or, even worse, your brain may already be dead.

NEUROPHENOMENAL HYPOTHESIS OF CONSCIOUSNESS IA: "PRINCIPAL CONSCIOUSNESS" AND DIFFERENCE-BASED CODING

The first introduction focused on the neuronal mechanisms of consciousness without going into detail about its empirical, conceptual and phenomenal characterization. This was reflected in the assumption of a neuronal hypothesis about consciousness, the coding hypothesis of consciousness (CHC). The CHC postulated a particular neural code, difference-based coding (as distinguished from stimulus-based coding), to be central, e.g., necessary, in associating the brain's purely neuronal neural activity, e.g., resting state or stimulus-induced activity, with the phenomenal features of consciousness.

From there we moved on to the second introduction where I discussed so far the empirical and conceptual characterization of consciousness. This puts me now in the position to formulate not only a neuronal hypothesis of consciousness, as in the first introduction, but a truly neurophenomenal hypothesis of consciousness. Based on the conceptual considerations discussed here, I determine the conceptual range and scope of

the neuronal hypothesis by postulating a specific definition of consciousness as "principal consciousness."

The concept of "principal consciousness" is supposed to provide the conceptual ground and framework upon which any subsequent neurophenomenal hypotheses must be built. More specifically, I postulate particular neural mechanisms (see later) that make possible the "principal consciousness" and thus predispose the kind and range of the possible phenomenal features. This "locates" my first neurophenomenal hypothesis right at the border between empirical, e.g., neuronal, conceptual, and phenomenal domains.

What, then, is my first neurophenomenal hypothesis? I hypothesize the brain's particular coding strategy, difference-based coding, to provide the "right" kind of code and format that predisposes and makes possible the association of the brain's otherwise purely neuronal resting state and stimulus-induced activity with consciousness and its phenomenal features. Accordingly, I propose difference-based coding to provide the "right" code or format that allows it to distinguish the "principal consciousness" from the "principal non-consciousness."

NEUROPHENOMENAL HYPOTHESIS OF CONSCIOUSNESS IB: "PRINCIPAL NON-CONSCIOUSNESS" AND STIMULUS-BASED CODING

How can we further specify this first neurophenomenal hypothesis? Difference-based coding concerns the encoding of the spatial and temporal differences in the stimuli's statistical frequency distribution, e.g., their "natural statistics" (and "social, vegetative and neuronal statistics": see Chapters 8 and 9), into the brain's neural activity (see first Introduction and Volume I). This distinguishes difference-based coding from stimulus-based coding that encodes the single stimuli and their respective discrete points in physical time and space. Therefore, as detailed described in the first introduction, stimulus-based coding may be characterized as physically based, as distinguished from the more statistically based difference-based coding.

In contrast to difference-based coding, stimulus-based coding does not provide the "right" coding strategy or format to associate a stimulus and its stimulus-induced activity with consciousness. Why? Stimulus-based coding can be characterized as a format that is based on the stimuli themselves and their different discrete points in physical time and space; the format is thus stimulus- rather than difference-based and it is physically rather than statistically based.

I propose such stimulus- and physically based format to be simply the "wrong" format for associating the stimulus and its purely neuronal stimulus-induced activity with the phenomenal features of consciousness. Hence, I propose stimulus-based coding to predispose what Searle describes as "deep unconscious" and "non-consciousness" and thus the "principal non-consciousness" as distinguished from the "principal consciousness."

Taken together, I hypothesize difference-based coding and thus the CHC (and its two distinct subsets, the EHC and the DHC; see first introduction) to provide the "right" "format" or code that predisposes the constitution of the "principal consciousness." In contrast, stimulus-based coding would predispose the "principal non-consciousness" rather than the "principal consciousness." In short, I hypothesize difference-based coding to be a neural predisposition of "principal consciousness."

NEUROPHENOMENAL HYPOTHESIS OF CONSCIOUSNESS IC: DIFFERENCE-BASED CODING AND THE "BIOPHYSICAL-COMPUTATIONAL SPECTRUM" OF "PRINCIPAL CONSCIOUSNESS"

How does my first neurophenomenal hypothesis stand to the other neuroscientific hypotheses of consciousness as discussed earlier that target the neural correlates of consciousness (NCC) rather than neural predispositions of consciousness (NPC)? The current neuroscientific hypotheses (see earlier in this introduction and the first introduction) target consciousness as distinguished from unconsciousness and do

thus remain within the realm of the "principal consciousness" itself.

In contrast, I propose difference-based coding (as distinguished from stimulus-based coding) to allow for the distinction between the "principal consciousness" and the "principal non-consciousness." What about the distinction between consciousness and unconsciousness within the realm of the "principal consciousness"? I suggest the degree of the spatial and temporal differences encoded via difference-based coding to account for the difference between consciousness and unconsciousness within the realm of the "principal consciousness."

I hypothesize that the encoding of larger differences entails a higher probability of consciousness, while lower differences may favor unconsciousness (see Chapters 28 and 29 for details). I consequently propose the difference between consciousness and unconsciousness (within the realm of the "principal consciousness") to be, not a principal one, that is, all-or-nothing, but rather a continuous or gradual, that is, more-or-less, distinction (see Chapters 28 and 29). Consciousness and unconsciousness may thus be distinguished from each other by the degree of spatial and temporal differences that are encoded into neural activity on the basis of difference-based coding (see Fig. I-3c).

We may also want to set difference-based coding in relation to the brain's biophysical-computational equipment (see first Introduction). Difference-based coding can only operate within the available spectrum of the minimal and maximal bio-physical-computational limits of the respective organism: the more the organism's neural activity operates closer to either its minimal or maximal bio-physical-computational limits, the lower the degree of difference-based coding (and conversely higher degrees of stimulus-based coding),and the lower the subsequent probability of "principal consciousness" (with conversely higher probability of "principal non-consciousness") (see Chapters 28 and 29 for details on the relationship between consciousness and the biophysical-computational spectrum as well as Chapter 31, and Panksepp

2007; Edelman and Seth 2009; and Edelman et al. 2005 for the discussion of consciousness in non-human species).

This means that at the fringes of the organism's biophysical-computational spectrum, the degree of difference-based coding will decrease while the degree of stimulus-based coding may increase here. And that, as I propose, goes along with decreased probability of "principal consciousness" and increased probability of "principal non-consciousness" (see Chapters 28 and 29 for more details). Taken together, this amounts to what I will later describe as the "biophysical spectrum hypothesis of consciousness" (see Chapters 28 and 29).

NEUROPHENOMENAL HYPOTHESIS OF CONSCIOUSNESS ID: DIFFERENCE-BASED CODING AND THE "HARD PROBLEM" OF CONSCIOUSNESS

Finally, we may want to discuss yet another central point of distinction. My hypothesis of difference-based coding as neural predisposition of "possible consciousness" targets the following question: Why is there consciousness at all rather than non-consciousness? And how is consciousness possible? This addresses the "hard problem", as it is called in current philosophy of mind (see Chalmers 1996, 2000, 2010).

How about my answer to the "hard problem"? I provide both a conceptual and an empirical answer. In contrast, I will leave open the metaphysical problem of how to characterize the existence and reality of consciousness as distinguished from its conceptual definition and empirical mechanisms. I also leave open epistemological issues that concern the difference in our knowledge of brain and consciousness (which is often thematized in the explanatory gap argument in philosophy; see though chapter 30). Since such a metaphysical and epistemological discussion is the territory of philosophers, I leave it to them to discuss the implications of my empirical, conceptual, and phenomenal approach to consciousness.

How about my conceptual answer to the "hard problem"? My conceptual answer consists in the distinction between the concepts of the "principal consciousness" and the "principal unconsciousness." By subsuming both actual and possible consciousness under the umbrella of the "principal consciousness" and by distinguishing it from the "principal non-consciousness," we can provide a conceptual answer. Why is there consciousness rather than non-consciousness? Because our brain predisposes us to obtain "principal consciousness" rather than "principal non-consciousness."

How about my empirical answer to the "hard problem"? I propose that the "right" kind of code or format, namely, difference-based coding, provides an empirical answer to the "hard problem." (as it occurs in the natural world (as it is relevant for neurophilosophy) while my hypothesis leaves open the answer to the "hard problem" in the logical world as it is dealt with in philosophy). By generating and encoding its own neural activity in terms of statistically based spatial and temporal differences, that is difference-based coding, the brain predisposes the association of its otherwise purely neuronal and objective resting state and stimulus-induced activity with consciousness, including its various phenomenal features and their essentially subjective nature. Accordingly, the question of why and how there is consciousness rather than non-consciousness can be answered empirically by referring to difference-based coding as the "right" code or format for predisposing and thus making possible consciousness.

The direct reference to the "hard problem" distinguishes my coding hypothesis of consciousness (CHC) and its focus on difference-based coding from the many current neuroscientific suggestions for the NCC. As explicated above, they target the distinction between consciousness and unconscious rather than the one between consciousness/unconsciousness and non-consciousness. Therefore, these theories remain within the realm of the "principal consciousness" itself, rather than addressing the latter's distinction from the "principal non-consciousness." The current neuroscientific (and many philosophical) theories of consciousness remain consequently unable to provide an empirical (and conceptual) answer to the "hard problem," i.e., why there is consciousness rather than non-consciousness.

Phenomenal characterization of consciousness Ia: spatiotemporal continuity with "inner time and space consciousness"

So far, I have discussed how the brain's neural code, difference-based coding, predisposes consciousness as I postulated in the first introduction. This was specified in conceptual regard in the preceding section when postulating that difference-based coding predisposes "principal consciousness" as distinguished from "principal non-consciousness." I thus clarified my initial neuronal hypothesis from the first introduction in conceptual regard.

In contrast to the conceptual clarification, I left open the question of the phenomenal features of consciousness. More specifically, it remains unclear which phenomenal features of consciousness are predisposed in what way and how, by the brain's neuronal mechanisms in general and difference-based coding in particular. For the answer to that, we need to specify the phenomenal features of consciousness, which will then allow us to link the phenomenal features to specific neuronal mechanisms. We thus need phenomenal clarification and specification which is the focus of the present section.

Let us start with our experience of time. While reading these lines, you experience a continuous flow of time (and space)—there is a smooth and continuous transition from the past over the present to the future. It reminds you of previous books on consciousness you've read. You are also well able to link to and integrate that memory into your current reading of this book. And you also anticipate the next pages to come that you will read in the near future and, going even further in time, you may already envision another book on consciousness written by yourself.

This short description indicates that your experience of reading is embedded in a dynamic and continuous flow of time extending from the past over the present to the future all crystallized and condensed in the present moment. This is what William James (1890) described as "specious present" or "dynamic flow" and the philosopher E. Husserl as "phenomenal time": the dynamic flow describes the organization of time

as a continuum (rather than as a discontinuum) in consciousness. This was about our subjective experience of time. How about our consciousness of space? The same holds for space that is also homogenically and continually rather than heterogenically and discontinually organized and structured. One may consequently want to speak of a *spatiotemporal continuity* as central feature of our experience of time and space, that is, "inner time and space consciousness" (see earlier and part V for details).

Phenomenal characterization of consciousness Ib: qualia and unity

Another typical phenomenal feature of consciousness is the phenomenal-qualitative feel, as mentioned at the beginning of the first introduction. The phenomenal-qualitative character is the phenomenal hallmark feature of consciousness that is often described by the term *"qualia"* (see Part VIII for details): You have a certain feel, a "raw feel" when reading these lines. Your experience of reading this introduction is manifest in a certain qualitative character that comes with any experience, whether it is your experience of reading this book or your experience during the perception of, for instance, tomatoes.

This qualitative feel or qualia has been described by Thomas Nagel (1974) as the "what it is like" to have a certain perception. The "what it is like" captures the qualitative feel and associates it with a specific point of view. Based on their specific echo-locatory senses, bats, for instance, experience the world in a different way than humans—there is "something that it is like for the bat to experience the world." And that "something it is like" that signifies the qualitative character of experience is different between humans and bats (see Fig. I-4a).

Another important phenomenal feature of consciousness is *unity* (see part VI for details). You do not experience the pages of this introduction lying in front of you as principally diverse and segregated from the table, the floor, the room, and so on. Instead of such diversity, you rather experience the pages in continuity and thus relation to the table and the rest of the room, including yourself (see also Searle 2004

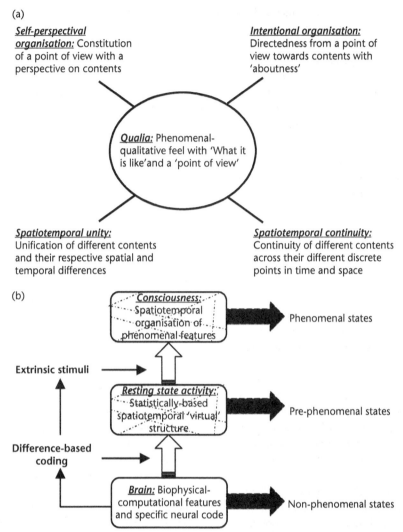

Figure II-4a and b Phenomenal features of consciousness and the brain. The figure illustrates the phenomenal features of consciousness and how they relate to the neuronal features of the brain (b). (*a*) The figure points out different phenomenal features of consciousness. The phenomenal hallmarks of consciousness are qualia as characterized by a phenomenal qualitative feel, "what it is like," and a point of view (see middle). Other phenomenal features that are closely related to qualia (and somehow resurface in them as will be pointed out in Parts V–VII) are self-perspectival organization (upper left), intentional organization (upper right), spatiotemporal unity (lower left), and spatiotemporal continuity (lower right). (*b*) The figure illustrates the relationship of consciousness and its phenomenal features (upper) to the resting state's spatiotemporal structure (middle) and the brain's basic biophysical-computational features (lower). I propose that the brain itself applies a particular encoding strategy as its neural code, namely, difference-based coding, in order to generate neuronal activity within the range of its underlying biophysical-computational spectrum (lower part). This makes possible the constitution of a statistically based "virtual" spatiotemporal structure in the resting state, as indicated by the dotted lines within the box (middle part). That in turn predisposes the constitution of consciousness, including the spatiotemporal organization of its phenomenal features (as indicated again by the dotted lines within the box) (upper part) during the encounter and difference-based coding of extrinsic stimuli (left part of the figure). The resting state's spatiotemporal structure can consequently be characterized as pre-phenomenal, as distinguished from both phenomenal and non-phenomenal states (see right part of the figure).

and Bayne 2010). There is a distinction between the pages of the book as the figure and the table as the background in your experience. However, you nevertheless experience them as unity, as a homogenous unified field of which both book and table are distinct aspects or parts. Hence, consciousness may be characterized by unity, which is to be distinguished from diversity.

PHENOMENAL CHARACTERIZATION OF CONSCIOUSNESS IC: INTENTIONAL ORGANIZATION AND THE SELF

There is more to consciousness than spatiotemporal continuity, qualia, and unity. When reading these lines, your experience is directed toward the book; your consciousness is about something, the book and its introduction. Perception is always perception of something else of, for instance, the book and that, in turn, structures and organizes your experience. Hence, consciousness seems to be almost always directed toward something outside itself that lies beyond consciousness itself by referring to something else in the world (or one's own body) as, for example, an object, person or event.

Most important, this holds even when the respective person, object or event remains absent in the real physical world as, for instance, during dreams (see Chapter 26 for dreams) or auditory hallucinations in schizophrenia (see Chapters 22 and 27 for details on schizophrenia). What is important here is not the physical presence but the presence of some kind of object, event, or person whether mentally or physically toward which the experience that is consciousness is directed and targeted. Such directedness toward or aboutness structures and organizes our consciousness which therefore can be characterized by intentionality, or *intentional organization* (see Part VII for details).

Consciousness, however, is not only about the book you experience while reading. It is also about your own self. You may experience the reading of this book completely different than your friend experiences the same book because your self is rather different from his. Consciousness is always already tied to the perspective of a particular self like your specific self

that provides the particular perspective, the perspectival point, from which you experience the reading of this book (see for instance van Gulick 2004; see Chapter 19 for details). The individual first-person perspective.

Some authors on the neuroscientific side like Panksepp (1998a and b; see also Northoff and Panksepp 2008) and Damasio (see Parvizi and Damasio 2001; Damasio 1999a and b, 2010) propose what they describe as "protoself," which cannot yet be experienced as such (thus remaining what I will describe later as prephenomenal; see Chapters 23 and 24). This "protoself" is supposed to be empirically associated with neural activity in subcortical regions (brainstem, midbrain) and, important in our context, considered necessary for the occurrence of consciousness. What exactly such a "protoself" looks like and how it is related to our self remains unclear however (see Chapter 24 and Appendix 4 for more extensive discussion).

PHENOMENAL CHARACTERIZATION OF CONSCIOUSNESS ID: SELF-PERSPECTIVAL ORGANIZATION

The "protoself" is often supposed to provide some kind of point of view or perspective from which experiences can be made. One can thus characterize the "protoself" as "perspectival point." You can experience the world only from the point of view of your own self (see also Dennett 2001 for the importance of the self in consciousness). In contrast, you remain unable to take the point of view of another person's self, let alone the one of another species, for instance, the bat when experiencing and perceiving this book. Your experience is thus centered around your point of view and the perspective associated with it. Such organization of consciousness as centered around your point of view and perspective has been described by what philosophers call *"self-perspectival organization"* (see Chapters 23 and 24 for details).

Besides these phenomenal features, others like subjectivity and first-person perspective have been described (van Gulick 2004). Consciousness implies a point of view and is therefore essentially subjective and must as such be distinguished from the brain, which has no point of view and is therefore objective. Thereby the objective character of the brain and its neuronal states is often linked to observation in third-person perspective. In contrast, the subjective character of consciousness is associated with the first-person perspective since it characterizes our experience, that is consciousness.

This makes it particularly difficult to link consciousness and brain: How can we link and relate something as subjective as consciousness and its point of view to the brain's neural activity that is by definition objective and shows no point of view? This also raises the question of how the subjective-objective distinction is related to the one between first- and third-person perspective, as the two distinctions are often associated with each other in the current discussion (see Chapter 21 for details on subjectivity).

NEUROPHENOMENAL HYPOTHESIS OF CONSCIOUSNESS IIA: WHAT ARE NEUROPHENOMENAL HYPOTHESES?

How are these phenomenal features of consciousness related to the brain and its neuronal states? In a recent review paper, the neuroscientist J. D. Haynes (2009) claims that future neuroscientific studies on consciousness not only need to explain the mere presence or absence of consciousness as, for instance, whether a stimulus has been seen, that is consciously experienced—they have to go beyond that, by accounting for the details of the participant's subjective experience and how they are related to the underlying neuronal state. In other words, we need to consider the different phenomenal features of consciousness and relate them to distinct neuronal mechanisms.

To put it even more strongly, we need to directly link the neuronal mechanisms of the brain to the phenomenal features of consciousness in a necessary and unavoidable way. This results in what I describe as "neurophenomenal hypotheses." The concept of neurophenomenal hypotheses describes particular neuronal mechanisms that, by virtue of their nature, make necessary and unavoidable the association of

consciousness and its phenomenal features to the otherwise purely neuronal resting state and/or stimulus-induced activity. The neurophenomenal hypotheses as understood here aim to reveal the neuronal mechanisms that predispose the otherwise purely neuronal resting state and stimulus-induced activity to become associated with consciousness and its various phenomenal features by default.

"Neurophenomenal hypotheses" in this sense refer to the brain's intrinsic features, its neural code, and particularly the encoding of its own neural activity as well as to the spatiotemporal structure of its intrinsic activity (see first Introduction and Volume I). The hypothesis is that the brain's intrinsic features necessarily and unavoidably imply the association of the brain's otherwise purely neuronal activity with consciousness and its phenomenal features. Accordingly, the neurophenomenal hypotheses claim for a direct link between neuronal and phenomenal features, the "neurophenomenal link" (see first Introduction).

The focus on the brain's intrinsic features and their neurophenomenal link distinguishes the neurophenomenal hypotheses from neurophenomenal hypotheses, as suggested in neurophenomenology (see Appendix 1 for details). Here the focus is mainly on sensorimotor functions and the body and how they are related to consciousness and more specifically to experience in the first-person perspective. Following the "priority hypothesis" of neurophenomenal function" (see first Introduction and Chapter 17), I claim that the neurophenomenal hypotheses are more basic and fundamental than the neurophenomenological hypotheses.

After having determined the concept of "neurophenomenal hypothesis" in more detail, we are now ready to formulate our second neurophenomenal hypothesis. We remember that the first neurophenomenal hypothesis concerned the predisposition of "principal consciousness" by difference-based coding as the "right" code (see earlier). While this specified the concept of consciousness by "principal consciousness," it left unresolved the different phenomenal features of consciousness. These are the target of my second neurophenomenal hypothesis.

NEUROPHENOMENAL HYPOTHESIS OF CONSCIOUSNESS IIB: SPATIOTEMPORAL STRUCTURE OF THE PHENOMENAL FEATURES OF CONSCIOUSNESS

We recall from Volume I and the first Introduction that I proposed the resting state to constitute a statistically based virtual spatiotemporal structure that spans between environment and brain. How is this statistically based spatiotemporal structure of the brain's resting-state activity related to the various phenomenal features of consciousness? Let me first go into more detail on the phenomenal side. More specifically, I will briefly show that the various phenomenal features of consciousness describe distinct ways of how the different contents in consciousness are organized and structured spatially and temporally (see Chapter 30 for more details).

How can we describe the different phenomenal features of consciousness in spatiotemporal terms? As explicated earlier, the different contents show, for instance, a dynamic flow following each other in a temporally and spatially continuous way as manifest in spatiotemporal continuity. And the contents seem to be closely related to the person's point of view, its particular stance within the world from which it experiences the world's various objects, persons, and events. This is subsumed under the umbrella term "self-perspectival organization," which describes the centeredness of the different spatial and temporal trajectories upon the own person (see earlier).

Though being related to your own self and its particular point of view, your consciousness is nevertheless directed toward specific objects, persons, or events in the outside world beyond your own self. Such directedness implies a special organization with a temporal and spatial distance between your own self, that is, its point of view, and the respective contents, that is, objects, persons, or events. This special organization is described as intentional organization, as we discussed earlier. Finally, qualia may also be intrinsically spatiotemporal since they allow for the convergence of the spatial and temporal differences between the various contents in one

spatiotemporally homogenous experience and its particular phenomenal-qualitative feel.

This brief discussion (see Chapter 30 for more details) already shows that the different phenomenal features of consciousness signify different forms of spatiotemporal organization. Therefore, it is important to note that such spatiotemporal organization does not refer to the notions of a purely physical and objective space and time, but rather to phenomenal and more subjective space and time; that is, the kind of time and space that provide the template or grid for our subjective experience. In short, the here suggested spatiotemporal organization implies the phenomenal rather than the physical level.

NEUROPHENOMENAL HYPOTHESIS OF CONSCIOUSNESS IIC: SPATIOTEMPORAL RELATIONSHIP BETWEEN INTRINSIC ACTIVITY AND PHENOMENAL FEATURES

How can we now relate these forms of spatiotemporal organization on the phenomenal level of consciousness to the brain's intrinsic activity and its spatiotemporal structure? This is where my second neurophenomenal hypothesis comes in.

I suggest that the various forms of spatiotemporal organization on the phenomenal level of consciousness are predisposed and thus made possible in a necessary and unavoidable way by the brain's intrinsic activity and its spatiotemporal structure. There is, as I claim, some kind of spatiotemporal relation or correspondence (see below for more discussion of the concept of "correspondence" which needs to be distinguished from mere "isomorphism") between the brain's intrinsic activity and the phenomenal features of consciousness. As pointed out, this correspondence is based on spatiotemporal features, with the spatiotemporal structure of the brain's intrinsic activity resurfacing in some way or another in the spatiotemporal structure of the phenomenal features of consciousness.

Let us specify this neurophenomenal hypothesis in empirical and thus neuronal terms. I propose that the spatial and temporal neuronal measures of the brain's intrinsic activity, like low-frequency fluctuations and functional connectivity, are structured and organized in such way that they cannot but predispose, e.g., necessarily and unavoidably, the organization of the subsequent extrinsic stimuli and their associated contents along the lines of the phenomenal features and their spatiotemporal structures (see Chapter 30 for details).

This means that the statistically based spatiotemporal virtual structure of the resting state's neural activity on the one hand, and the phenomenal features and their spatiotemporal structure on the other, may be structured and organized in a more or less related or corresponding way (see below for the discussion of whether this amounts to neuro-phenomenal isomorphism, as the philosophers may want to claim). That leads us back to the resting state's organizational and structural features of the spatiotemporal structure as constituted by its neural activity.

Neurophenomenal hypothesis of consciousness IID: Need for activity change as argument against "neurophenomenal isomorphism"

What exactly does the brain's resting state must provide in order to make possible consciousness? By means of its neuronal organization via low-frequency fluctuations and functional connectivity, the resting state's spatiotemporal structure may provide some kind of grid, template, or matrix for the organization of the extrinsic stimuli and their associated stimulus-induced activity. That by itself, however, is not yet sufficient to associate consciousness and its phenomenal features with the purely neuronal resting-state activity.

In addition to the resting-state activity's spatiotemporal structure as constituted by its low-frequency fluctuations and functional connectivity, the latter also need to undergo some kind of change to yield sufficiently large spatial and temporal differences in order to make possible their association with consciousness. Such a change is usually triggered by extrinsic stimuli from either body or environment that can yield sufficiently large differences in the resting state's neural activity (see Chapter 28 and especially Chapter 29). However, the resting-state activity

itself may undergo spontaneous activity changes that, as for example during dreams in sleep, may be large enough by themselves to associate consciousness and its phenomenal features to the otherwise purely neuronal resting-state activity (see Chapter 26 for dreams).

In sum, my second neurophenomenal hypothesis proposes some degree of relationship or correspondence between the spatiotemporal structures of the brain's intrinsic activity and that of the phenomenal features of consciousness. However, such spatiotemporal correspondence does not amount to one-to-one correspondence between neuronal and phenomenal features. The neuronal and phenomenal features thus do not need to map one-to-one onto each other. To suggest that would be to neglect the need to induce large enough spatial and temporal differences in the brain's intrinsic activity in order to assign its neural activity with phenomenal features, that is consciousness. One can thus not speak of what the philosophers may want to describe as a "spatiotemporal or neurophenomenal isomorphism" between the brain's intrinsic activity and the phenomenal features of consciousness (see Chapter 30 for details, as well as Roy and Llinas 2008, and Fingelkurts et al. 2010, for suggesting such a neurophenomenal isomorphism).

Neurophenomenal hypothesis of consciousness IIE: Resting-state activity is neither phenomenal nor nonphenomenal

How can we further characterize the resting state's spatiotemporal structure in both phenomenal and conceptual regards? The resting state's spatiotemporal grids or templates may not yet be ready by themselves to be associated with consciousness (except in dreams; see Chapter 25 and 26). They are not yet fully phenomenal by themselves since for that, usually (except in dreams) an extrinsic stimulus from either body or environment is needed that can induce the encoding of sufficiently large spatial and temporal differences into the resting state's neural activity.

Metaphorically speaking, the extrinsic stimuli may trigger sufficiently large changes in the resting-state activity to "wake up" its "dormant" spatiotemporal structure. Once "woken up," the intrinsic activity's spatiotemporal structure can integrate the extrinsic stimulus. This in turn makes possible the association of the stimulus and its purely neuronal stimulus-induced activity with consciousness and its phenomenal features (see Chapter 29 for details of such rest–stimulus interaction).

How can we now characterize the resting-state activity and its spatiotemporal structure by themselves in further conceptual detail? First and foremost, the resting state activity is purely neuronal. And second, the resting state activity is not phenomenal, since usually the resting-state activity is not associated with consciousness by itself (except in dreams; see Chapter 26). That is the easy part. Does this imply that the resting-state activity is nonphenomenal? This is the hard part.

If the concept of *nonphenomenal* implies the absence of any kind of relationship to the phenomenal features and thus to consciousness, the intrinsic activity cannot be characterized as nonphenomenal. There must be some kind of relationship between the brain's intrinsic activity and the phenomenal features of consciousness. Otherwise the brain's intrinsic activity could not predispose and thus make necessary and unavoidable consciousness in the case of sufficiently large neural activity changes. This means that, as said earlier, there must be some "dormant" feature in the neuronal activity of the resting-state activity itself that reacts to change in such a way that it makes possible the association of these activity changes with consciousness. Accordingly, to conceptually characterize the resting-state activity as nonphenomenal would mean to deny that it has any role in associating extrinsic stimuli and their stimulus-induced activity with consciousness and its phenomenal features.

NEUROPHENOMENAL HYPOTHESIS OF CONSCIOUSNESS IIF: RESTING-STATE ACTIVITY IS "PREPHENOMENAL" RATHER THAN "NONPHENOMENAL"

How can we conceptually characterize the brain's spatiotemporal structure if not as phenomenal or nonphenomenal? I propose that conceptually (and phenomenally), the brain's resting state

and its statistically based spatiotemporal structure need to be "positioned" right in between the full-blown phenomenal features of consciousness and the completely nonphenomenal features of purely physical states. Rather than being either full-blown phenomenal or purely physical, the resting state's spatiotemporal structure may be characterized as statistical-based by means of which it is able to predispose the phenomenal features of consciousness. Therefore, the resting state's spatiotemporal structure may be characterized as "prephenomenal" rather than either phenomenal or nonphenomenal.

What do I mean by the concept of "prephenomenal"? The concept of prephenomenal describes that the resting state's spatiotemporal structure makes possible, e.g., necessary and unavoidable, the association of the purely neuronal resting state or stimulus-induced activity, with consciousness and its phenomenal features. Let me be more specific.

The term "phenomenal" in the concept "prephenomenal" points out the analogous similarity between the phenomenal features of consciousness and the neuronal features in the resting state's spatiotemporal structure (see later for the definition of the term "pre"): I suggest that what is described as spatiotemporal continuity, unity, self-perspectival organization, and intentional organization on the phenomenal side of consciousness (see earlier) can be traced back to and is predisposed by the organization of different neuronal features (like functional connectivity and the low frequency fluctuations) in the resting state's spatiotemporal structure (see Fig. I-4b).

How about the prefix "pre-" in "prephenomenal"? The term "pre-" in "prephenomenal" refers to the actual absence of the phenomenal features of consciousness in the resting state itself. We will not be able to find (and experience) self-perspectival and intentional organization nor unity—let alone qualia—when considering the resting state itself, e.g. independent of and in isolation from extrinsic stimuli and their stimulus-induced activity (or independent of major neural activity changes in the resting state itself as in dreams; see Chapters 25 and 26).

How, then, can the resting state's activity prephenomenal features of its spatiotemporal structure be transformed into a full-blown phenomenal state that is consciousness? Something additional is required to associate the neural activity in the resting state and its spatiotemporal structure with consciousness. What is that something additional? I suppose that an extrinsic stimulus (or some large rest–rest interaction as in dreams or auditory hallucinations) must trigger sufficiently large enough neural activity changes in the resting-state activity itself to allow it to associate the newly resulting neural activity level with a full-blown consciousness and its phenomenal features.

NEUROMETAPHORICAL COMPARISON III: SLEEP AND BRAIN OR "THE DORMANT INTRINSIC ACTIVITY"

Metaphorically speaking, one may therefore want to characterize the resting-state activity's prephenomenal features of its spatiotemporal structure as "sleeping or dormant versions" of the phenomenal features of consciousness. In the same way, we often require some external signal like an alarm clock, to wake us up and come to full-blown awake consciousness, the resting-state activity apparently needs the extrinsic stimulus (or some major activity changes within the resting-state activity itself as during dreams) as external signal to associate its own purely neuronal neural activity with consciousness and its phenomenal features.

We transform our unconscious or non-conscious state during our night's sleep into a conscious awake state in the morning when the clock rings. Analogously, the brain's intrinsic activity is transformed by the extrinsic stimulus as its alarm clock that triggers it to associate phenomenal features and thus consciousness with its otherwise purely neuronal resting state and stimulus-induced activity. Accordingly, the waking up of both us and our brain is associated with one and the same state; namely, consciousness.

AIM AND OUTLOOK I: AIM OF THE BOOK

What is the aim of this book? The main and overarching aim of this book is to develop neurophenomenal hypotheses about the relationship between the brain's intrinsic features, that is, its resting-state activity and neural code, and the various phenomenal features of consciousness. My focus here is exclusively on the earlier-described phenomenal features of consciousness like qualia, "inner time and space consciousness," phenomenal unity, and self-perspectival and intentional organization. In contrast, I do not discuss the various cognitive features like awareness, attention, willful modulation, reporting, access, and volition that are often associated with consciousness (see Hohwy and Fox 2012 for a good overview of these). Accordingly, the approach taken here is strictly neurophenomenal rather than neurocognitive (or neuroaffective, neurosensory, neuromotor, or neurosocial).

Since I aim to directly link the different phenomenal features of consciousness to their neural predispositions in the brain's intrinsic activity without assuming any intermediating functions (sensory, motor, affective, cognitive, social, etc.), my approach can be described as a truly "neurophenomenal approach" (in the literal sense of the term). This distinguishes my approach from other approaches to consciousness that associate consciousness with particular sensory, motor, affective, cognitive, or social functions of the brain and their respective neuronal mechanisms (See end of the first introduction).

Let me be more specific. By referring to particular functions of the brain, most of the current neuroscientific (and philosophical) approaches to consciousness can be characterized as neuro-sensory, -motor, -affective, -cognitive, and -social theories of consciousness. Rather than targeting the various neuro-sensory, -motor, -affective, -cognitive, and -social functions of the brain, I here aim to search for what can be called the brain's "neurophenomenal functions." The concept of "neurophenomenal functions" refers to the neuronal mechanisms that are related to the various phenomenal features of consciousness, as described earlier.

How are these neurophenomenal functions related to the brain's neuro-sensory, -motor, -affective, -cognitive, and -social functions? While the latter are associated with mainly stimulus-induced or task-related activity as extrinsic activity in the brain, I suppose the neurophenomenal functions to be rather related to the brain's intrinsic activity and its spatiotemporal structure. This means that, in the same way as the brain's intrinsic activity provides the ground for the extrinsic stimulus-induced or task-related activity, I propose the brain's neurophenomenal functions to be more basic and fundamental than its neuro-sensory, -motor, -affective, -cognitive, and -social functions (see also the end of the first introduction for the discussion of this point). This is obviously a rather controversial thesis, which will be elaborated on and discussed throughout the course of this book, especially in Chapter 24 and Appendix 1.

Consciousness is such a wide field, covering many different domains and disciplines, that it is impossible to cover the whole field in one sweep. Hence, instead of a broad and general overview of consciousness that pays the price for lack of specificity on both sides, neuronal and phenomenal, I here focus on the development of specific neurophenomenal hypotheses. These neurophenomenal hypotheses aim to go into as much detail and specifics as possible about the linkage between neuronal mechanisms and phenomenal features. This may open the doors for both novel ways of future experimental testing (in neuroscience) and shifts in the focus of the conceptual discussions (in neurophilosophy and philosophy of mind).

AIM AND OUTLOOK
II: OVERVIEW OF THE BOOK

The book consists of four main parts, with each part containing five chapters. Each Part addresses a particular phenomenal feature of consciousness and how it is related to the brain's resting-state activity and its intrinsic features. This serves to develop specific neuronal and neurophenomenal hypotheses for each particular phenomenal feature of consciousness and how it is predisposed by particular neuronal mechanisms. I give a quick overview in what follows.

Part V focuses on spatiotemporal continuity in the neuronal activity of the resting state, while Part VI discusses how the phenomenal feature of unity is related to the neuronal mechanisms

of the resting state. This is followed by Part VII, which targets the self-perspectival organization and the intentional organization of consciousness and how these are related to the neuronal organization of the resting-state activity (Part VII). Finally, the fourth Part targets the phenomenal hallmark feature of consciousness, qualia, and how they are related to the interaction between resting-state activity and stimulus-induced activity (Part VIII; see also Fig. I-5).

Let me be a little more detailed. Part V, on spatiotemporal continuity, discusses neuronal mechanisms like neuronal oscillations in different frequency ranges and the baseline metabolism that allow for the constitution of spatiotemporal continuity in the brain's resting state. I suggest the constitution of spatiotemporal continuity in the brain's resting state to predispose the constitution of a "dynamic flow" and "stream of consciousness" as characterized by continuity of time and space in our subjective experience. That may be manifest on the phenomenal level of consciousness in what has been described as "inner time consciousness."

Part VI, on spatiotemporal unity, focuses on neuronal mechanism like entrainment of high-frequency neuronal oscillations by low-frequency ones including their implications for the encoding and coding strategies the brain applies to process and format stimuli. I hypothesize that these encoding and coding strategies yield spatiotemporal unity in the brain's resting state and its dynamic changes; that is, rest–rest interaction (see Chapters 18 and 19). This leads me to propose that the resting state's spatiotemporal unity may predispose the development of phenomenal unity in consciousness during subsequent rest–stimulus interaction.

Moreover, based on the statistically based encoding of environmental stimuli by the brain and its intrinsic activity, I propose the constitution of what I describe as statistically based "environment–brain unity" (see first Introduction and especially Chapter 20). Such statistically and spatiotemporally based "environment–brain unity" may correspond on the conceptual side to what Thomas Nagel described as "point of view" as a hallmark of the subjective nature of consciousness (see Chapter 22). This will be further

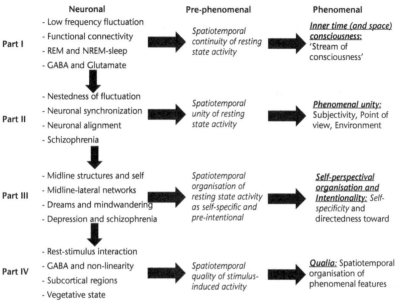

Figure II-5 Plan and overview of the book. The figure illustrates a schematic overview of the book. The book is divided into four main parts (left from top to bottom). Each part discusses different neuronal mechanisms (like low-frequency fluctuations) in the context of specific states of consciousness (like REM and N-REM sleep) and various disorders of consciousness (like schizophrenia or vegetative state) (second row from left). These neuronal mechanisms are proposed to lead to a particular way of neuronal organization in either the resting state (see Parts V–VII) or stimulus-induced activity (see Part VIII) (third row from the left). Since such neuronal organization is supposed to predispose the constitution of consciousness, it can be characterized as prephenomenal (third row from the left). That in turn makes possible consciousness and its phenomenal features that are based upon the pre-phenomenal organization of the neural activity (fourth row from the left at the very right). The relationship between neuronal, pre-phenomenal, and phenomenal states is indicated by horizontal arrows. In addition, I propose the different neuronal mechanisms and their respective pre-phenomenal and phenomenal states to build on each other as it is indicated by the vertical arrows within the row of the neuronal (second from the left). Finally, it should be noted that the book is concluded with an epilogue not indicated here. Furthermore, the book includes four appendices (not shown in the figure) about current neuroscientific theories of consciousness concerning time, unity, and self where my own neurophenomenal stance and position is directly compared to others' accounts and theories.

supported by the example of schizophrenia in both neuronal and phenomenal regards (see Chapter 32).

Part VII on spatiotemporal organization investigates the brain's resting-state activity and particularly rest–rest interaction and how it is affected by prior stimulus–rest interaction. Based on the neuroanatomical organization of the brain and its translation into functions, I propose the neuronal organization of the brain's resting state to be self-specific and intentional (see Chapters 23–25). This, in turn, predisposes the brain's resting-state activity to yield

the self-perspectival and intentional organizational features of consciousness during subsequent rest–stimulus interaction. I will support these neurophenomenal hypotheses by making excursions into the neuronal mechanisms of dreams and mind wandering as well as psychiatric disorders like depression and schizophrenia (see Chapters 26 and 27).

Finally, Part VIII, on spatiotemporal quality, focuses on rest–stimulus interaction and its relation to the constitution of phenomenal-qualitative properties, that is, qualia. I will demonstrate how the resting state's prephenomenal structures, as discussed in the first three parts, converges and resurfaces in the phenomenal feature during rest–stimulus interaction.

Thereby I will especially rely on the neuronal mechanisms underlying rest–stimulus interaction. Conceptually I here move from the neural predispositions (NPC), the necessary conditions of possible consciousness as hitherto discussed in Parts V–VII, to the neural correlates of consciousness (NCC), that is, the sufficient neural conditions of actual consciousness. The here-suggested neurophenomenal hypotheses of the NCC will be empirically supported and exemplified by extensive discussion of the recent imaging results from patients in vegetative state where qualia remain absent.

The book concludes with a short epilogue that provides a general summary about my approach to consciousness and a brief outlook into the future. Finally, I include four appendices that discuss some topics and other theories in more detail. Appendix 1 focuses on various neuroscientific theories of consciousness and how they stand in relation to my neurophenomenal approach. Appendix 2 complements part V by discussing others' theories and approaches to time. Appendix 3 focuses more on the unity of consciousness as discussed by the neuroscientist S. Zeki and the philosopher Immanuel Kant. Finally, Appendix 4 gives a short overview of different concepts of self and their relation to my own neurophenomenal hypotheses. However, the appendices can make up at best only partly for the neglected data, issues, and topics.

Notes

1. Thereby the characterization of consciousness by levels or states, that is, "state consciousness," may come close to the one of "creature consciousness" that is often used in philosophical debates to characterize species by wakefulness, sentience, or self-awareness, with both concepts being only more or less analogous, but not fully identical (see van Gulick 2004; Hohwy 2009). Their fine-grained conceptual differences, however, are not of importance here and are thus left for the philosophers to discuss.

2. The proponents of the NCC argue that it cannot be excluded that a device other than the brain and its neuronal mechanisms can have consciousness, such as a computer consisting of silicon chips rather than neurons. This is more of a philosophical issue that shall be touched upon only briefly. While it is certainly correct to exclude such cases and thus necessary conditions, it may hinder empirical progress. In addition to the sufficient neuronal conditions, one may also consider the necessary and non-sufficient neuronal conditions of consciousness. Once these are revealed, one may then discuss whether they are also necessary for the occurrence of consciousness in all possible worlds, that is, in a logical sense or only in our actual and thus natural world. In the first case, the necessary conditions would refer to logical conditions, while in the second instance they may only be natural conditions but not logical ones (see also Northoff 2004).

3. It should be noted that the NPC do still concern the very natural conditions of our brain rather than some purely logical conditions unrelated to the brain. Hence, the NPC remain fully within the boundaries of the natural world, for example, the brain, while not going beyond to some merely logically possible worlds as presupposed in philosophical discussion. One may, however, be inclined to argue that the NPC, due to their focus on the necessary predisposing conditions of possible (rather than actual) consciousness, may provide a bridge from the natural realm of neuroscience/science to the more logical realm of philosophy (see also Northoff 2004, 2011, for the relationship between natural and logical conditions and their respective realms). That is certainly so and may be exploited by philosophers in the future. The focus in this book is completely on the natural world and thus the natural conditions of our very human brain.

PART V
Spatiotemporal Continuity and Consciousness

I proposed in the first Introduction (to Volume I) to approach the neural basis of consciousness by investigating the brain's neural code when suggesting the "coding hypothesis of consciousness" (CHC). Coupled closely to a theory of brain activity, the CHC postulated that the brain needs to encode its own neural activity in a particular way in order to make possible—that is predispose—the association of its otherwise purely neuronal resting state and stimulus-induced activity with consciousness and its phenomenal features. In order to understand consciousness, we therefore need to explore how the brain encodes and thus generates its neural activity. For that, we briefly have to go back to Volume I.

In Volume I, I described the brain's neural code and suggested it was difference-based coding rather than stimulus-based coding. "Difference-based coding" means that spatial and temporal differences between the different stimuli's discrete points in physical time and space are encoded into neural activity. This must be distinguished from stimulus-based coding, where the single stimulus itself, including its single discrete point in physical time and space, is encoded into the brain's neural activity. Extending the principle of difference-based coding to any kind of neural activity in the brain made it clear that this mechanism also applies to the encoding of the resting-state activity itself, where its changes are encoded in terms of spatial

and temporal differences (see Chapters 4–6). Notably, when speaking of physical time and space, we here presume only a standard intuitive (Newtonian) conception of physical time and space; anything beyond that is likewise beyond our scope (see also Introduction in Volume I for more details on this point).

What does such difference-based coding imply for the characterization of the resting-state activity itself? The encoding of spatial and temporal differences amounts to the encoding of the statistical frequency distribution of the activity changes in the resting state. This leads, as I proposed, to the constitution of a virtual statistically based spatiotemporal structure by the resting-state activity itself (see Volume I, Part II). While I discussed the neuronal details of such spatiotemporal structure in Volume I, I left open its implications for consciousness and its various phenomenal features. This is the focus of the present volume.

How is such virtual statistically-based spatiotemporal structure related to consciousness? The resting-state activity's statistically based spatiotemporal structure is supposed to be essential in providing the very ground upon which stimuli and their purely neuronal stimulus-induced activity can possibly be associated with consciousness and its phenomenal features: Without such very "spatiotemporal ground" in the brain's resting-state activity, the stimulus will not be able to induce the kind of phenomenal features that

1

define consciousness, including its spatiotemporal features (see below). Therefore, I regard the resting state's statistically based spatiotemporal structure as a necessary condition and thus neural predisposition of possible consciousness (NPC); this distinguishes it from the sufficient neural conditions of actual consciousness, the neural correlates of consciousness (NCC).

We need to specify, however, the properties and features of the neural activity in the resting state itself and particularly its spatiotemporal structure. Since the resting state's spatiotemporal structure is necessary, though not sufficient, for consciousness to occur, it cannot yet be considered phenomenal by itself. But at the same it predisposes the phenomenal states of consciousness and must somehow related to them. I therefore characterize the resting state's statistically based spatiotemporal structure as prephenomenal rather than being either nonphenomenal or phenomenal (see also the second Introduction for the exact conceptual determination of the term "prephenomenal").

How must the resting-state activity's spatiotemporal structure operate in order to be prephenomenal and to consecutively predispose consciousness? Let us have a look at the very basics; how the brain itself and its neural activity deal with space and time. The brain and its neural activity operate in space and time and are thereby subject to physical space and time: time and space are here determined by different discrete points in time and space, which amounts to what we as outside observers generally describe as "physical time and space." This is, for instance, manifested temporally in the discrete time points of past, present, and future, while it is spatially manifested in the different points in space and thus the different locations of body and environment in space.

How does such a characterization of physical time and space stand in relation to the space and time we experience in consciousness? Consciousness provides us with a different experience of time and space. Instead of different discrete points in time and space amounting to spatial and temporal discontinuity, we rather experience spatial and temporal continuity.

For instance, we experience a temporal flow or stream—that is, temporal continuity—between the different discrete time points of past, present, and future. And we also experience spatial continuity across the different spatial discrete positions of body and environment, implying spatial continuity rather than discontinuity.

How are such temporal and spatial continuity generated by the brain and its neural activity? If the brain and its neuronal processes were strictly operating and encoding neural activity in orientation to physical time and space and its different discrete points in time and space, such a constitution of spatial and temporal continuity should remain impossible. The spatial and temporal discontinuity of the different discrete points in physical time and space of the purely physical (understood in a Newtonian sense) brain must thus be somehow transformed into the kind of spatial and temporal continuity we experience in consciousness.

How can the different discrete points in physical time and space of the physical brain be transformed into the kind of spatial and temporal continuity we experience in consciousness? This is the question of how the temporal and spatial discontinuity of physical processes can be transformed into the temporal and spatial continuity on the phenomenal level of consciousness.

I postulate that such a transformation may be predisposed by the brain and its resting state activity. More specifically, the brain's strategy of encoding spatial and temporal differences into its neural activity leads by default (i.e., necessarily and unavoidably) to the constitution of a statistically based virtual spatiotemporal structure. I now postulate that the resting-state activity's statistically based virtual spatiotemporal structure provides the kind of spatial and temporal continuity in its neural activity that predisposes temporal and spatial continuity on the phenomenal level of consciousness. The focus of this Part is to investigate the neuronal mechanisms that allow constituting temporal and spatial continuity in the neural activity of the resting-state activity, such that the latter can predispose its association with consciousness and its phenomenal features during changes in its activity level as during stimulus-induced activity.

GENERAL OVERVIEW:

Chapter 13 will focus on the intrinsic activity of the resting state itself and how it is related to the extension of time into the future and past in consciousness. We will see that the cortical midline regions in the brain are central for that. I propose that the midline regions' neural activity during both resting-state and stimulus-induced activity is central for constituting what on the phenomenal level of consciousness has been described as "dynamic flow" or "stream of consciousness." While many details may remain unclear here (and are provided in the subsequent chapters), this first chapter provides a general and sketchy overview of a first neurophenomenal hypothesis on the linkage between the brain's neural activity and the phenomenal experience of time in consciousness.

Chapter 14 focuses in more detail on the constitution of local temporal continuity of the neural activity across different discrete points in physical time as associated with the neural activity in particular regions of the brain. Based on recent findings, I here propose the slow cortical potentials to be essential in constituting continuity of neural activity across the limited time span of the neural activities in particular regions. Such "local temporal continuity" in the resting state's neural activity is supposed to be manifested on the phenomenal level of consciousness in what has been described as the "width of present," the extension of the single point in time beyond its discrete actual moment.

Chapter 15 proceeds from regions to the brain as a whole and investigates how low-frequency fluctuations in neural activity integrate and thus already entrain higher ones during the resting state itself. This leads to the integration of higher frequency fluctuations (like gamma) into the phases and time course of lower ones (like delta or even infraslow frequencies), which can

be described as "temporal nestedness." I suggest that such "temporal nestedness" is central in constituting what I describe as "global temporal continuity" of neural activity across the whole brain during the resting state. This may correspond on the phenomenal level of consciousness to what has been described as the "duration bloc," the extension of the present into both past and future in "inner time consciousness."

Chapter 16 focuses on the neuronal mechanisms underlying the constitution of space in consciousness. Based on recent results, I propose resting state functional connectivity between different regions' neural activities to be central in constituting what I describe as "global spatial continuity" of neural activity. Such "global spatial continuity" extends across different discrete points in physical space as associated with the different regions' neural activities. This may correspond on the phenomenal level of consciousness to what I describe as "dimension bloc," the extension of the single discrete points in space into a three-dimensional space.

Chapter 17 describes the biochemical mechanisms constituting "inner time consciousness." in particular I thereby focus on especially glutamate and GABA, which, as described in Volume I, have been shown to be central in constituting the resting state's spatiotemporal structure. Based on recent data, I propose GABA to disrupt the temporal continuity of neural activity, which, on the phenomenal level of consciousness, may be manifested in corresponding disruption of the duration bloc in inner time consciousness. In contrast, glutamate may rather abnormally shrink or extend the temporal continuity of the brain's neural activity, which may correspond on the phenomenal level to abnormal shifts of "inner time consciousness" into either past or future, as it is (for instance) observed in the psychiatric disorder of depression. This is further supported by corresponding neuronal findings and phenomenal observations in patients with neuropsychiatric disorders like depression and schizophrenia.

CHAPTER 13
Midline Regions and the "Stream of Consciousness"

Summary

William James spoke of a "stream of consciousness" that describes the continuously ongoing and changing nature of consciousness across the different discrete points in physical time. How is it possible that objects and events in the environment can be consciously experienced as part of a continuously ongoing "stream or flow" of time? Empirical findings show that the neuronal activity of especially the cortical midline structures is continuously changing, even in the resting state itself. The brain's intrinsic activity can thus be characterized by what I describe as "temporal flow." In addition to such continuous change leading to "temporal flow," the neural activity in especially the midline regions also shows strong low-frequency fluctuations. Low-frequency fluctuations are characterized by long time intervals, that is, phase durations, where the neural activity remains the same until either spontaneous neural activity change occurs or a stimulus interrupts the ongoing phase. I propose the degree of phase durations of the brain's high- and low-frequency fluctuations to constitute a certain degree of "temporal continuity" in the neural activity of the resting state that, therefore, in a virtual and statistically based way, extends across different discrete points in physical time. How is such "temporal continuity" in the resting state's neural activity related to the phenomenal experience of time consciousness? Recent findings demonstrate the involvement of the midline regions in the subjective extension of time into either past or future, that is. prospection and retrospection. I now propose that such temporal extension is possible on the basis of the co-occurrence between temporal continuity and temporal change in the neural activity of the resting state. This accounts well for what William James described on the phenomenal level as the co-occurrence of "sensible continuity" and "continuous change" in the "stream of consciousness."

Key Concepts and Topics Covered

Resting-state activity, Dynamic temporal network, midline regions, temporal flow, temporal continuity, cortical midline structures, temporal extension, prospection and retrospection, stream of consciousness, continuous change, sensible continuities

NEUROEMPIRICAL BACKGROUND IA: TIME AND THE "STREAM OF CONSCIOUSNESS"

The relationship between time and consciousness is a complicated one. On one hand, we presume that consciousness takes place in an external framework of time. In this sense, consciousness is based on time. We make clear at the outset that we do not intend to explore or account for this point in detail—we presume only a standard intuitive (Newtonian) conception of physical time; anything beyond that is likewise beyond our scope.

Rather, we will here concentrate our efforts on the reciprocal relationship held in the other hand, one that we do not take for granted. Namely: how, in terms of the brain and its neural activity, is time "based on" consciousness? Or to be more precise, how is our experience of time in consciousness constituted such that the (presumed) external characteristics of time are (presumably) accurately reflected?[1]

The role of time in phenomenal experience took center stage in a metaphor introduced by William James that has become ingrained in our culture. In James's "stream of consciousness," he likens the contents of consciousness—both one's environment and its events and one's inner world of thoughts, emotions, etc.—to the contents of a continuously flowing stream (time).

The popularity of this metaphor is no doubt due to its immediate intuitive clout. It seems to capture our experience of time so well and yet so simply. Taken in this sense, consciousness may be compared to a boat in the river: The contents of consciousness may correspond to the boat in a river.

At the same time, the water in the river flows continuously forward in one direction, which allows the boat to move and be part of the "stream of the river." Analogously, consciousness is based on the continuous forward movement of time, which allows its contents, the various objects and events we experience, to be part of the "stream of consciousness." The comparison of consciousness with the stream or flow of a river implies some temporal continuity. Very much as the flow of the water in the river provides some continuity, time in consciousness provides the continuity that underlies the flow of its contents. How is such continuity generated? This is the focus in this chapter.

NEUROEMPIRICAL BACKGROUND IB: CONSTITUTION OF THE TEMPORAL CONTINUITY OF CONSCIOUSNESS AND ITS NEURONAL MECHANISMS

In order to better understand how the "stream of consciousness" and its temporal continuity are generated, we may want to go back briefly to the experience of time in consciousness. Rather than experiencing each single discrete point in time in isolation from the respective others (as in what we call "physical time" in our observation), we experience a continuous flow of time across the single discrete points in physical time (see

later for details). There is thus what I describe as "temporal continuity" rather than "temporal discontinuity" in consciousness. Accordingly, the phenomenal level of consciousness can be characterized by temporal continuity, which therefore has also been described as "phenomenal time" as distinguished from physical time.

How is such temporal continuity possible? This is possible only if the single discrete points in physical time are linked and integrated so that their temporal discontinuity is transformed into temporal continuity and, ultimately, phenomenal time. Hence, there must be some mechanisms that predispose and make possible the transformation of the temporal discontinuity of physical time into the temporal continuity of the phenomenal time of consciousness.

These mechanisms are the target of this and the two subsequent chapters: I here propose that the way the neural activity in the brain's resting state is structured and organized may be of central importance in allowing for such transformation of temporal discontinuity into temporal continuity. To put it differently, I focus on the neuronal mechanisms how time in consciousness—that is, phenomenal time—is generated. I here aim for a neurophenomenal account of time; namely, how the brain's neuronal mechanisms in its resting-state activity predispose phenomenal time in general and temporal continuity in consciousness particular. Such a neurophenomenal account concerns the constitution of time in consciousness: how phenomenal time is constituted out of physical time by our brain and its resting state activity.

More specifically, I focus on the neuronal mechanisms that allow the brain's resting state to link and integrate its neural activity at single discrete points in time into a "temporal continuity" that bridges their temporal differences. What are the neuronal mechanisms underlying the constitution of such temporal continuity in the resting state's neural activity? I will provide a first general and tentative neurophenomenal overview in this chapter while leaving open many of the specific neuronal mechanisms that will be discussed in detail in Chapters 14 and 15.

Before plunging into empirical details, let me make a brief remark. My focus in this and the subsequent chapters is on how time in consciousness, or "phenomenal time," is constituted and predisposed by particular neuronal mechanisms the brain applies to structure and organize its own neural activity in the resting state. Accordingly, I focus on the neuronal mechanisms of the constitution of time: How is time in consciousness constituted, and what are the neuronal mechanisms underlying such a constitution of time?

Such a constitution of time must be distinguished from the neuronal mechanisms underlying the perception and cognition of time as they are investigated most often in neuroscience these days (see Appendix 2 of this volume for details). The central question in these accounts is, "How can we perceive and cognize time and what are the neuronal mechanisms underlying the perception and cognition of time?"

Both perception and cognition of time take time in general and phenomenal time in particular as ready-made and thus for granted and as given. They tacitly seem to consider time and its temporal continuity to be "lying dormant" in consciousness in such a way that it only needs to be "picked up" by the mechanisms underlying cognition and perception. This, however, is not the case. Time, and more specifically, phenomenal time, must be constituted, and the neuronal mechanisms underlying such constitution need to be revealed. These neuronal mechanisms are different from those underlying the subsequent perception and cognition of time. And where there are neuronal mechanisms for the constitution of time, there is the possibility of their disruption; I suggest this to be the case in psychiatric disorders like schizophrenia and depression (see Chapter 17), where abnormalities in the brain's intrinsic activity lead also to abnormal experience of time in consciousness.

Accordingly, before venturing into the perception and cognition of time, we need to understand the neuronal mechanisms underlying the constitution of time in consciousness and thus of what has also been described as "temporality" (see, e.g., Lloyd 2011). This means that a neurophenomenal investigation of time must precede neuroperceptual and neurocognitive accounts of time as in current neuroscience. My focus in this and the subsequent chapters is therefore on the neurophenomenal investigation of time and thus the constitution of time in consciousness.

In contrast, my focus is not so much on the neuroperceptual and neurocognitive accounts of time, which therefore I will discuss briefly in Appendix 2 of this volume, and especially how they stand in relation to the here-suggested neurophenomenal mechanisms. In other words, I focus here on the prephenomenal and phenomenal mechanisms that make possible the constitution of time in consciousness, but I will not discuss the postphenomenal mechanisms that allow for the perception and cognition of time (see Appendix 2 and especially Fig. A2-3 therein for the distinction between prephenomenal, phenomenal, and postphenomenal accounts of time).

On the whole, my neurophenomenal approach to time can be situated right in between the extremes of physical approaches to time on the one hand and neuroperceptual and cognitive approaches on the other. Physical approaches investigate how time in the world is constituted by itself independent of our experience and consciousness. The neurophenomenal approach, in contrast, is not concerned with the constitution of physical time. Instead, the neurophenomenal approach is more interested in the neuronal mechanisms that allow for transforming the merely physical time of the world into the phenomenal time of consciousness.

Such neurophenomenal approach has to be also distinguished from the extreme on the other end, the neuroperceptual and -cognitive approaches. Rather than on the constitution of phenomenal time with the subsequent experience of time, neurocognitive approaches focus on the perception and cognition of time and the underlying neuronal mechanisms. Most importantly, the neuronal mechanisms underlying the perception and cognition of time should not be confused with the ones related to the constitution of time. This would be to perceive and cognize time before it is constituted by itself. That though remains impossible for which reason we here focus on the neuronal mechanisms underlying the constitution of time.

NEURONAL FINDINGS IA: HOW TO INVESTIGATE TIME IN THE BRAIN AND ITS NEURAL ACTIVITY

How can we experimentally investigate the constitution of temporality? There is more than one obvious methodological obstacle to experimental access. Temporality is a constant in consciousness in the sense that it cannot simply be turned on and off in a control condition in order to compare behavioral or neural dependent variables in its present versus absence. The typical approach of a neuroimaging contrast— something like *Time* versus *No-Time*—is just not an option. Moreover, our access to temporality typically occurs in concert with, or indirectly through, perception and cognition. Temporality is implicit; it cannot easily be made explicit. So, the difficulty of disentangling the foundation of temporality in consciousness from higher time-based cognition is not trivial, since most attempts at the former would be implemented through the latter—for example, through experimental paradigms based on time-based cognitive tasks. That said, neither of these barriers is absolute. In fact, we will shortly bring into consideration studies using higher cognitive tasks such as prospection and retrospection. Nonetheless, the point remains that approaching temporality is not a straightforward problem, but rather one that requires an approach of many roads.

We begin with one road that is as direct as any one could hope to find. We turn to Dan Lloyd, originally a philosopher from Hartford, Connecticut, who turned to neuroscience to answer some of his questions about the mind. Lloyd does not forget his philosophical background but instead uses it as a template or roadmap to guide his experimental strategies. This leads him to very innovative experimental approaches, as we have already seen in the context of sparse coding (see Volume I, Chapter 6).

Now he extends his search for the neuronal mechanisms underlying consciousness to the question of temporality.

Lloyd (2002, and especially Lloyd 2011) sought to investigate correlates of temporality in neural activity recorded by functional magnetic resonance imaging (fMRI) in the resting state. His approach to the diffuse and difficult problem was reasoned as follows. A subject might lie aware in a static situation with no specific stimuli, not engaged in any specific task (any of which could involve active time-based cognition in some respect), and in particular not purposefully monitoring the passage of time—in short, in the resting state. Even under such circumstances, conscious experience will be in constant change in at least one sense: the subject will experience at a basic level the progressive flow of time. Lloyd focused on this experience as a reflection of temporality, not perfectly isolated from the confounds of higher cognition, to be sure, but at least with those confounds dimmed by virtue of being in the resting state.

For purposes of this investigation, Lloyd operationalized temporality as information in neural activity encoding time elapsed from the start of resting-state periods. Working with whole-brain time series of neural activity recorded in fMRI during multiple resting-state and stimulus- or task-related periods for each subject in the study, Lloyd used machine learning techniques to attempt to extract information from these time series about elapsed time from the beginning of any given resting-state period.

Specifically, he trained a machine learning algorithm with a set of time series corresponding to a sample of resting-state periods. He then tested those trained "machines" by setting them to predict elapsed time for frames taken from the remainder of their resting-state periods, of which they had no prior knowledge. The successful prediction of elapsed time in the test condition was an indication that information as to elapsed time was available, embedded, in the neural activity on which the machines had trained.

Lloyd was able to ask which patterns of voxels— that is, brain regions—contained the most information that the machines had used (see Lloyd 2011). In other words, he determined which brain regions were most responsible for encoding elapsed time in their BOLD activity insofar as removal of the activity variance in those regions from the machines' training most negatively impacted the accuracy of their predictions in testing.

He simply took all the images acquired during the course of scanning from both task-related and resting-state studies. Instead of comparing task- versus non-task periods and resting state as a whole, he compared the neuronal changes from one image/scan to the next subsequent image/scan across both task- and resting-state periods. Thereby, depending on what is called "repetition time in imaging," the images/scans were parsed 2–3 seconds apart from each other, and comparing them allowed him to account for their difference in activity levels (see Lloyd 2011).

Why did he choose such an approach? Lloyd proposed that the activity differences between subsequent images/scans signify the spontaneous activity changes and thus the temporal structure generated by the brain's intrinsic activity itself, independent of resting-state or stimulus-induced activity. He was thus interested in revealing the spontaneous temporal flow of the brain's intrinsic activity as distinguished from the temporal pattern of the extrinsic stimuli or tasks and their imposition upon the brain's intrinsic activity and its own temporal structure.

Neuronal Findings IB: Spontaneous Activity Changes in Cortical Midline Structures Shape a "Dynamic Temporal Network"

What did his data show? Lloyd's analysis (Lloyd 2011) showed that especially cortical midline regions like the ventromedial prefrontal cortex (VMPFC), the perigenual anterior cingulate cortex (PACC), the medial temporal cortex (MT), including the hippocampus, and, though weaker, also the posterior cortical midline regions (like the posterior cingulate cortex) and the subcortical midline regions (like the dorsomedial thalamus) showed the strongest signs of spontaneous activity changes; namely, temporality. In contrast, lateral cortical regions like the dorsolateral prefrontal cortex and others did not contribute to the same extent.

Lloyd characterized the implicated midline regions as the "dynamic temporality network" (DTN) (Fig. 13-1). What Lloyd calls the DTN obviously closely overlaps with the default-mode network (DMN) and cortical midline structures (CMS) (see Volume I, Chapter 4). One obvious objection that could be raised in response to these findings is that since the study analyzed resting-state data and the DMN is already well implicated in the resting state, perhaps the DMN-like pattern that emerged from Lloyd's analysis emerged simply "by default" on this basis.

Lloyd forestalled this concern by underscoring the fact that the activity time series comprised activity variance that was widespread across the whole brain. Recall that the DMN is established as more active than other regions during the resting state (see Chapter 4 in Volume I), but other regions are by no means inactive. Moreover, information that might yield to machine learning is not necessarily tied to amplitude—it could well have been less pronounced activity in disparate regions that embedded elapsed time information in its complex spatiotemporal patterns.

What exactly do these spontaneous activity changes mean? These spontaneous activity changes reflect, as Lloyd himself says, the "brain's intrinsic flow of time" or the "temporality of its own neuronal activity". By continuously changing its neuronal activity from one discrete point in time to the next subsequent one, the brain itself generates a flow of time or temporality. The terms "flow of time"/"temporal flow" or "temporality" describe the intrinsically generated changes in neuronal activity across different discrete points in physical time. Accordingly, the concept of "temporal flow" refers to the degree of change in the brain's neural activity (see below for a more detailed definition of "temporal flow").

The temporal flow or temporality of the brain's intrinsic neuronal activity seems to be the strongest in the midline regions, while the intrinsic temporal flow or temporality appears to be rather weak in lateral cortical regions. Lloyd therefore describes these midline regions as the "dynamic temporality network" (DTN) (Lloyd 2011). Thus, that Lloyd's machine-learning approach isolated the strongest neural activity changes in a pattern of regions centering on CMS

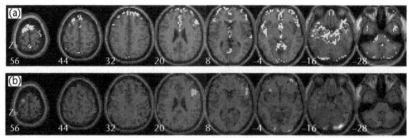

Figure 13-1 Fluctuation of neural activity in cortical midline regions. Changing regions underlying temporal information encoding, compared with aggregate default mode network in 25 subjects, 2 runs each. (*a*) Standard deviation of dynamic change in temporal components in fifty runs. For each run (two per subject), voxels above the 95th percentile in standard deviation were noted. The aggregate image here displays voxels above the 95th percentile from the first pass. Thus, voxels in the image represent the top 0.25% of standard deviation values. Voxels in light color fell in the top 0.25% standard deviation in one to fifteen runs. Voxels in darker color were in the top 0.25% in more than 15 runs. (*b*) Aggregate best-match default mode components in fifty runs, showing voxels above the 95th percentile, activated (darker) and deactivated (darkest). Reprinted with permission of Elsevier, from Lloyd D. (2011). Neural correlates of temporality: Default mode variability and temporal awareness. *Conscious Cogn, 21*(2), 695–703.

that closely resemble the default-mode network (DMN) does suggest that it is the midline structures in particular that are implicated in temporality, at least as operationalized in this study.

Implication of default-mode intrinsic activity, omnipresent and predisposing a wide range of (or all) higher cognition (see below, as well as Oestby et al. 2012), parallels nicely the omnipresent character of temporality in consciousness, as we will see in the next sections. However, before linking the spontaneous activity changes in the midline structures to the temporality in consciousness, we have to be clear about the neuronal mechanisms themselves; this is the focus in the next section.

Neuronal Hypothesis IA: Anatomical Structure Mediates a Particular Input Structure

How can we characterize the DTN and its possible ongoing neuronal processes in further detail? As stated previously, the DTN is characterized by cortical (and subcortical) midline regions that are part of what I, anatomically, subsumed under the inner and middle ring (see Chapter 4 in Volume I).

In a nutshell, the inner ring contains the cortical and subcortical regions that are directly adjacent to the ventricles; the inner ring includes mainly the anterior and posterior cingulate on the cortical level. The middle ring is located directly adjacent to

the inner ring, including cortically, for instance, the VMPFC, dorsomedial prefrontal cortex (DMPFC), and precuneus. As such, the regions of the inner and middle rings must be distinguished from the regions of the outer ring that are at the outer surface of the brain, like the sensory regions and the lateral prefrontal and parietal cortices.

How, now, is it possible that the regions of the inner and middle ring especially show strong activity changes across the different discrete points in time? Besides their anatomical location, one main difference between the different rings is the different inputs they receive: the inner ring receives predominantly interoceptive input from the body, while the outer ring is characterized by exteroceptive input (see Chapter 4 in Volume I). The middle ring, in contrast, does not receive any direct input from outside the brain, while the inner ring is characterized by strong interoceptive input from the body.

Neuronal Hypothesis IB: Extrinsic Inputs Perturb the Temporal Flow of the Brain's Intrinsic Activity

How, then, is this input structure related to the observation of strong activity changes across time? Unlike the inner and outer rings' regions, the midline regions of the middle ring do not receive any direct input from extrinsic stimuli originating in either the body or the environment, so the regions' intrinsic activity remains unperturbed by those extrinsic stimuli. The middle ring's intrinsic activity may thus most closely reflect the brain's intrinsic activity by itself, independent of extrinsic stimuli from either the body or the environment.

In other words, the middle ring's spontaneous changes in neural activity across the different discrete points in physical time are the least perturbed and disrupted by the single discrete points (in physical time) associated with the occurrence of the extrinsic stimuli. There should therefore be a high degree of temporal flow in the intrinsic activity in the middle ring's regions as sustained by strong neural activity changes across different discrete points in physical time. That is exactly what Lloyd observed when he subsumed the midline regions under the concept of the "dynamic temporal network."

In contrast, the encounter of the various exteroceptive inputs at different discrete points in physical time in especially the outer ring may strongly disrupt these regions' spontaneous temporal flow of their intrinsic neural activity. The outer rings' lateral cortical regions should consequently not show such strong degree of spontaneous activity changes across different discrete points in physical time as the middle rings' midline regions. This is indeed in accordance with the data.

This leads me to postulate the following hypothesis about the relationship between spontaneous neural activity changes and intero- and exteroceptive input: the less extrinsic intero- or exteroceptive inputs at their single discrete points in physical time perturb the spontaneous intrinsic neural activity changes across different discrete points in physical time, the better and thus higher degrees of temporal flow of neural activity can be generated in the respective regions/networks.

NEURONAL HYPOTHESIS IC: DEGREE OF DIFFERENCES BETWEEN EXTRINSIC INPUTS AND INTRINSIC ACTIVITY CONSTITUTE THE TEMPORAL FLOW OF NEURAL ACTIVITY

Why are there activity changes across time in regions like the PACC and the posterior cingulate cortex (PCC) that are part of the inner ring? As the regions of the inner ring, these regions also receive strong input: interoceptive input

from the body. This interoceptive input should disrupt the spontaneous activity changes across time in the inner ring like the exteroceptive input does in the outer ring. This, however, does not seem to be the case, since the inner ring's regions, like PACC and PCC, are apparently part of the DTN.

How is that possible? I tentatively propose that the interface between the body's interoceptive input and the brain's intrinsic activity is much stronger than the one between exteroceptive input and neuronal input. The interoceptive input from the body is much more continuous and rhythmic than the exteroceptive input from the environment.

That makes it possible for the brain and its intrinsic activity to better link and integrate the extrinsic stimuli into its own ongoing spontaneous activity changes. This is indeed empirically supported by recent results that showed co-variation between heart rate variability and changes in functional connectivity in particularly the inner (and middle) ring's subcortical and cortical regions (see Chang et al. 2012, as well as Chapter 4 [Volume I] and Chapter 32 [this volume] for more details on the integration of the brain's activity and the body's interoceptive input; as well as Chapter 20 in this volume for the alignment of brain's intrinsic activity to the onset of extrinsic stimuli from body and environment).

If my hypothesis of strong integration between the inner and middle rings' neural activities holds, one would expect the degree of neural activity changes in the inner ring—that is, PACC and PCC—to closely resemble the ones in the middle ring; that is, the VMPFC, DMPFC, and so on.

In contrast, due to the different structure of their exteroceptive input, the outer ring's lateral regions should differ in their degree of spontaneous activity changes from both inner and outer rings' regions. And that is exactly what the data by Lloyd indicate. This implies the following hypothesis: the more closely the temporal distribution of the respective extrinsic input (that is its statistically frequency distribution or its temporal statistics; see volume I) is related and thus corresponds to the continuously ongoing intrinsic neural activity changes, the better the intrinsic activity changes can align and link themselves to the extrinsic input, and the higher the degree of temporal flow in the brain's intrinsic activity.

Accordingly, small differences in the temporal frequency distribution (that is the temporal statistics) between extrinsic input and intrinsic activity changes will perturb the ongoing spontaneous activity changes in the brain's intrinsic activity to a lesser degree when compared to large discrepancies. Such a lower degree of perturbation by extrinsic stimuli will in turn lead to higher degrees of temporal flow in the intrinsic neural activity (see Figure 13-2a).

NEURONAL HYPOTHESIS IIA: PREDOMINANCE OF LOW FREQUENCY FLUCTUATIONS IN CORTICAL MIDLINE REGIONS

The brain's neural activity can be characterized by fluctuations in its degree of neural activity; that is, frequency fluctuations. Frequency fluctuations reflect fluctuations of neural activity in different frequency ranges (see Chapter 5 in Volume I for details) and may thus specify in a physiological sense what Lloyd describes (more statistically) as neural activity changes across different discrete points in physical time. We also showed that extrinsic stimuli and their single discrete points in physical time perturb the long phase durations of the low-frequency fluctuations by partitioning them into higher frequency fluctuations with shorter phase durations (see Chapter 5).

How, then, is all that related to the midline regions? In addition to their high resting-state activity (see Chapter 4 in Volume I) and their high degree of activity changes across time (see earlier), the midline regions also show particularly strong power in their low-frequency fluctuations (<0.001 – 0.1 Hz) (see Chapter 5 in Volume I). Why do the midline regions show such strong low-frequency fluctuations?

One possible reason could be that the original low-frequency fluctuations may be related to the intrinsic activity changes independently of any extrinsic input. If so, the midline regions' low-frequency fluctuations should be less perturbed by extrinsic input compared to

the other rings' regions. Due to the absence of direct input, such temporal partitioning may occur to a lesser degree in the midline regions, compared to other regions that receive direct extrinsic inputs. This entails a predominance of lower frequency fluctuations in the midline regions, while their higher frequency fluctuations should be weaker. That is exactly what can be observed, as was discussed in more detail in Chapter 5 in Volume I.

How, exactly, does the extrinsic input interfere with the low-frequency fluctuations? By imposing their single discrete time points onto the broader temporal windows of the lower frequency fluctuations, the stimuli partitions the low-frequency fluctuations' long phase durations into shorter time windows and thus higher frequency fluctuations with shorter phase durations. This may shift the balance of the power from lower to higher frequency fluctuations, especially in the regions that receive strong extrinsic input, like the lateral cortical regions, as can indeed be observed (see Chapter 5, as well as Chapters 18 and 19 in this volume, for more details).

NEURONAL HYPOTHESIS IIB: LOW-FREQUENCY FLUCTUATIONS CONSTITUTE TEMPORAL CONTINUITY OF NEURAL ACTIVITY

What does the predominance of low-frequency fluctuations in the midline regions imply for the temporal flow of their neural activity? Lower frequency fluctuations imply longer time windows, meaning that the phase durations of their activity fluctuation are longer. Conversely, this means that their ongoing neural activity is less interrupted or perturbed by changes as induced either spontaneously or by intero- or exteroceptive stimuli.

Decreased degrees of interruption or perturbation imply that the level or degree of neural activity does not change and remains continuously the same. There is thus what can be referred to as a "temporal continuity" of neural activity. The concept of "temporal continuity" means that the degree and level of neural activity does not change; this distinguishes temporal continuity from its sibling, "temporal flow," which refers

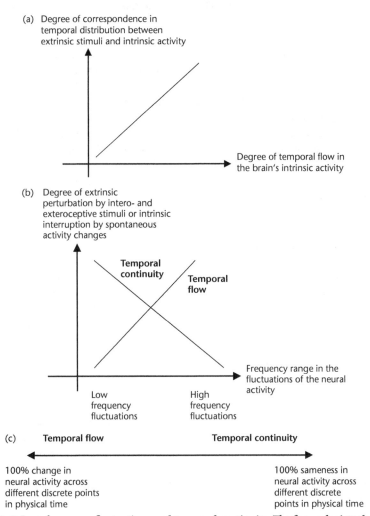

Figure 13-2a-c Low-frequency fluctuations and temporal continuity. The figure depicts the relationship between perturbation by stimuli, temporal flow of intrinsic activity (*a*); and the range of frequency fluctuation, its relationship to temporal continuity and discontinuity of the intrinsic activity (*b*); and the latter's relationship to the neuronal continuum of intrinsic activity changes (*c*). (*a*) The figure shows the relationship between the degree of temporal flow of the intrinsic activity and its correspondence to the temporal distribution of extrinsic stimuli (intero- and exteroceptive): the more extrinsic stimuli and intrinsic activity correspond in their temporal distribution, the higher the degree of temporal flow in the brain's intrinsic activity. (*b*) The figure shows the relationship between the degree of perturbation by extrinsic stimuli (intero- and exteroceptive) and the frequency ranges of the fluctuations in neural activity (during both resting-state and stimulus-induced activity): The greater the perturbation by extrinsic stimuli, the more the low-frequency fluctuations become temporally partitioned and the higher the degree of the frequency range in the activity fluctuations. Temporal continuity of neural activity is thus preserved by low degrees of extrinsic perturbation, while temporal flow of neural activity predominates in high degrees of extrinsic perturbation. Note the opposite curves between temporal continuity and discontinuity of neural activity, with both ranging on a neuronal continuum. (*c*) The figure shows the neuronal continuum of neural activity changes (including both resting-state and stimulus-induced activity) ranging from 0% to 100%. Here 100% indicates continuous activity change from each discrete time point to the next discrete time point of neural activity, while 0% describes the lack of any change in intrinsic (and extrinsic) activity from each discrete time point to the next discrete time point. The upper arrows describe the opposite directions of temporal continuity and temporal flow of neural activity toward 0% and 100% of changes in changes in intrinsic (and extrinsic) activity. That indicates a reciprocal balance between temporal continuity and the flow of neural activity with, for instance, increases in one accompanying decreases in the other (and vise versa).

to the degree of change in neural activity rather than its degree of sameness (see the next section for a more refined conceptual discussion of both terms).

Based on these considerations, I propose the following. I hypothesize that the degree of temporal continuity in neural activity depends on the range of frequency fluctuations: lower frequency ranges are proposed to go along with higher degrees of temporal continuity, while higher frequency ranges may reduce the degree of temporal continuity in neural activity. Strong power in low-frequency fluctuations as in midline regions may thus be indicative of a high degree of temporal continuity in neural activity, whereas strong power in high-frequency fluctuations may rather go along with a high degree of temporal flow (see Fig. 13-2b).

NEURONAL HYPOTHESIS IIC: RECIPROCAL BALANCE BETWEEN "TEMPORAL CONTINUITY" AND "TEMPORAL FLOW" IN THE BRAIN'S INTRINSIC ACTIVITY

We should note that the term "temporal continuity" is taken in a purely neuronal sense: the concept of temporal continuity means that the neuronal activity remains the same and does not change across those different discrete points in physical time, as they are, for instance, included within phase durations of the low- and high-frequency fluctuations in neural activity. In short, the term "temporal continuity" refers to the degree of sameness of neural activity.

The term "temporal continuity" describes the counterpart to "temporal flow," as used earlier. Like the concept of temporal continuity, the term "temporal flow" is used in a purely neuronal context, too: it describes the changes (rather than the non-change as in continuity) of neural activity across different discrete points in physical time, as discussed earlier. Accordingly, the term "temporal flow" describes the degree of change in neural activity rather than its degree of sameness.

Rather than the number of time points *during which* neural activity remains the same, as in temporal continuity, the concept of the temporal flow refers to the number of time points *after which* neural activity changes. Accordingly, the concepts of temporal flow and temporal continuity describe, metaphorically, the two sides of the same coin and can thus be compared to *yin* and *yang* in the Chinese tradition. This leads me to the following purely neuronal hypothesis about the relationship between temporal continuity and temporal flow: lower frequency fluctuations and their longer phase durations (including a higher number of discrete time points) should go along with a higher degree of temporal continuity and a lower degree of temporal flow.

In contrast, higher frequency fluctuations (and their short phase durations with their lower number of discrete time points) should be characterized by the converse pattern, with a high degree of temporal flow and a low degree of temporal continuity. In short, I propose that both temporal flow and temporal continuity depend on higher and lower frequency fluctuations, though in a converse way, as we can well see in the preceding figure (Fig. 13-2b). As pointed out earlier, high-frequency fluctuations may be generated by partitioning the low-frequency fluctuations. The high-frequency fluctuations and their shorter phase durations are thus generated on the expense of the lower frequency fluctuations and their longer phase durations. This implies that temporal flow and temporal continuity are intimately linked and, more specifically, reciprocally dependent on each other: an increase in one entails a decrease in the other, and vice versa.

Temporal continuity and temporal flow reciprocally balance each other: they must be regarded as the opposite ends of a neuronal continuum, signifying the reciprocal relationship between the degrees of sameness and change in neural activity across different discrete points in physical time. Depending on the degree of extrinsic stimulus input, this reciprocal balance between temporal continuity and temporal flow in the brain's neural activity is continuously changing. The degrees of both temporal continuity ("wow", this is boring, time has stopped) and temporal flow ("wow", time went by so fast) are thus dynamic and transitory, rather than static and fixed (see Fig. 13-2c).

NEURONAL FINDINGS IIA: FROM "TEMPORAL CONTINUITY AND FLOW" OF THE BRAIN'S NEURAL ACTIVITY TO "TEMPORAL EXTENSION" IN CONSCIOUSNESS

How can we relate the purely neuronally defined concepts of temporal flow and temporal continuity to the experience of time in consciousness and thus the phenomenal level? Lloyd's empirical data of continuous change, especially in the midline structures, the "dynamic temporality network" as he calls it, provide direct empirical evidence for particular a neuronal mechanism. This concerned the degree of change and sameness of neural activity and thus the latter's temporal flow and continuity across different discrete points in physical time, as I described it.

However, in contrast to the neuronal mechanisms, Lloyd's data leave open how the temporal flow and continuity are related to the experience of time in consciousness. His results may thus be only neuronally but not phenomenally relevant. Lloyd himself (2011) remarks that he infers the phenomenal relevance of the DTN for consciousness from its reported involvement in the consciousness of internal (like dreaming, mind-wandering, etc.; see Chapter 26) and external contents (see Chapters 28–30).

How can we now bridge the gap from the neuronal level of the brain, including the temporal flow and continuity of its neural activity, to the phenomenal level of consciousness? For that, I turn to Antoine d'Argembeau. Antoine d'Argembeau is a Belgian psychologist who conducted imaging studies on autobiographical memory, which let him investigate the relationship between self and time—that is, past and future—in a series of human imaging studies (see below for empirical support from others' studies). These studies (d'Argembeau et al. 2008a and b, 2010a and b) tested the subjects' ability to imagine themselves in either the future (i.e., prospection) or past (i.e., retrospection) and thus to "extend time" in either direction. The ability to anticipate the future or imagine the past is called "mental time travel" in the current neuroscientific literature (see below for further references). Subjects have to extend themselves mentally from their present point in time to either the future or the past; they thus have to mentally stretch (or extend) their current discrete point in physical time to the future or the past. This presupposes what I later describe as "temporal extension."

NEURONAL FINDINGS IIB: NEURAL ACTIVITY IN CORTICAL MIDLINE REGIONS MEDIATE "MENTAL TIME TRAVEL"

In a study on the interaction between prospection into the future and self (see d'Argembeau et al. 2010a), d'Argembeau included three conditions: imagination of future events that are relevant to one's personal goals, imagination of future events unrelated to one's own person, and imagination of routine activities. All three types of mental operations were cued and selected on the basis of a prescan interview.

What did d'Argembeau observe in his results? When comparing the two conditions related to the anticipation of the future (personally and non-personally relevant) with those of daily routine activities, he observed strong activity changes in anterior and posterior cortical midline structures (VMPFC, PACC, PCC). The same was the case when comparing both "future conditions" (personally and non-personally relevant) separately from that of routine activities. Accordingly, the anticipation of the future requiring extension or prospection of time was related to strong activity changes in the midline regions.

In addition to the temporal effects related to the future, the midline regions' neural activity was also modulated by the degree of personal relevance. Personally relevant items led to stronger activity changes in the midline regions than non-personally relevant ones (see Chapters 23 and 24 for details on the neural mechanisms underlying personal relevance and thus self-relatedness).

These effects were not as strong, however, as the ones related to the anticipation of events in the future (see Fig. 13-3). This means that the anticipation of events in the future was the "driving factor" of neural activity changes in the midline regions, whereas their degree of personal relevance was more a "modulatory factor" (see

Personal future events > routine activities

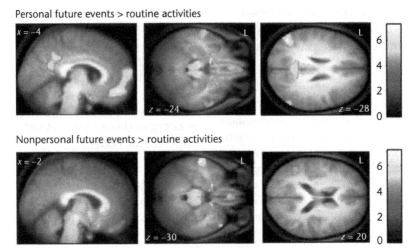

Nonpersonal future events > routine activities

Figure 13-3 Neural activity during prospection into the future. The imagination of nonpersonal future events versus routine activities was associated with activation in a smaller portion of MPFC. Foci of activation were also detected in lateral temporal lobe and temporoparietal junction. Displayed at $p < 0.001$ (uncorrected) on the mean structural MRI of all participants. Reprinted with permission of MIT Press, from D'Argembeau A, Stawarczyk D, Majerus S, Collette F, Van der Linden M, Feyers D, Maquet P, Salmon E.: The neural basis of personal goal processing when envisioning future events. *J Cogn Neurosci.* 2010 Aug;22(8):1701–13.

also Chapter 10 in Volume I for an analogous distinction between "driving and modulatory factors" in the context of cross-modal interaction).

Does the degree of temporal extension into the near and far future make a neural difference? Interestingly, events pertaining to the far future induced more neural activity in the VMPFC when compared to those in the near future (see also Wittmann et al. 2010, who, conducting a study on subjective time dilation, also observed the involvement of cortical midline regions in subjective time extension or dilation). In contrast, a subcortical region, the caudate, was more active during events in the near future when compared to those in the far future. This suggests that cortical regions may be able to extend time (on a phenomenal level) to a wider degree than subcortical regions.

How about the extension of time into the past? Another study by d'Argembeau tested the comparison between present and past events being either personally related or not (d'Argembeau et al. 2008a, see also d'Àrgembeau et al. 2010b). Subjects had to view adjectives and judge whether these described their present or past self, or past or present traits of an intimate

other. All four conditions recruited neuronal activity in the anterior and posterior midline structures. However, the degree of midline neural activity differed between the four conditions. The present self induced the strongest activity changes in the VMPFC, the DMPFC, and the PCC when compared to past self, and present and past other.

These findings are further confirmed by fMRI studies from other authors. Addis et al. (2007; see also Schacter et al. 2007; Szpunar et al. 2007; Buckner and Carrol 2007; Abraham et al. 2008) investigated the ability of subjects to project or anticipate events into the future and to recall events from the past. Interestingly, they observed a strong overlap between prospection and retrospection, especially in the anterior and posterior cortical midline structures (i.e., PACC, VMPFC, DMPFC, SACC, PCC, precuneus).

Taken together, these results demonstrate the central involvement of cortical midline structures in the subjective extension of time into either future (i.e., prospection) or past (i.e., retrospection). Neural activity in the cortical midline structures seems to be essential in extending the time point of our present moment into both temporal directions, the past and the future. In short, neural activity in the midline regions seems to account for temporal extension (see below for an exact definition of the latter term).

Metaphorically put, the midline structures' neural activity seems to continuously stretch and extend the single discrete points in physical time in very much the same way that we like to stretch and extend our chewing gum into one long band. The only difference consists of the difference between mouth and brain: we use the tongue in our mouth to extend the chewing gum, while we require our brain in the case of temporal extension in consciousness.

NEURONAL FINDINGS
IIC: RESTING-STATE ACTIVITY MEDIATES "TEMPORAL EXTENSION"

The findings by d'Argembeau and others show predominant involvement of cortical midline regions during the subjective extension of time into either the past or the future. Interestingly, these studies testing for the extrinsic stimulus–triggered prospection or retrospection of time showed exactly the same regions as the studies by Lloyd (see earlier), who focused more on the intrinsic neural activity changes across time.

Both sets of studies may thus be complementary in two aspects. First, they address distinct states. D'Argembeau focuses on the neuronal states underlying particular mental states, or mental time travel, implicated in temporal extension, while Lloyd targets only neuronal states independent of mental states. Second, Lloyd focuses on intrinsic neuronal activity changes in the resting-state of the brain, whereas d'Argembeau investigates extrinsically triggered mental states and their underlying stimulus-induced (or task-related) activity.

One may therefore be inclined to propose the following: the intrinsic neuronal activity changes in the midline regions, as described by Lloyd, may be related to the degree of "temporal extension" on the phenomenal level of consciousness. In short, I postulate that temporal extension to already occur in the resting-state and thus during the intrinsic activity in the midline regions especially.

This is indeed supported by a study by Oestby et al. (2012). They demonstrated neural overlap between resting-state activity in the default-mode network and the neural activity changes during prospection (of the future) and retrospection (of the past) especially in the midline regions: the degree of resting-state functional connectivity in the midline regions predicted the degree of neural activity changes in the same regions during both remembering the past and imagining the future.

This strongly suggests that the extension of time and thus what is called "mental time travel" (in the psychological context) is indeed closely related to the resting-state activity in the midline regions as suggested above. The neural activity in the resting-state may already by itself constitute (or at least predispose) what on the phenomenal level is described as "temporal extension" and psychologically as "mental time travel." Accordingly, I hypothesize that temporal extension and mental time travel are already present in the resting-state activity of the brain itself. We will see later that this hypothesis is indeed supported by, for instance, the occurrence of abnormal "inner time consciousness" in dreams (see Chapter 25 for details).

NEUROPHENOMENAL HYPOTHESIS IA: LOW AND HIGH-FREQUENCY FLUCTUATIONS MEDIATE DIFFERENT DEGREES OF "TEMPORAL EXTENSION" IN CONSCIOUSNESS

What exactly is meant by the concept of "temporal extension"? And how does the temporal extension in consciousness relates to the "temporal flow and continuity" of the brain's neural activity? Let us start with the first question.

The concept of "temporal extension" describes the ability to "stretch" the current actual single discrete point in physical time into either the future or the past and thus to connect and link yourself (or others) with other single discrete points in physical time. As such, the concept of temporal extension must be considered a phenomenal concept that describes our ability to link different discrete points in physical time in our consciousness and thus to stretch and extend ourselves and our actual point in time into both past and future. Such stretching or extension is, however, possible only if present and past or future discrete points in physical time can be linked and integrated.

Let us compare the situation to a bridge spanning across a river. If I want to extend my reach to the other side of the river, I need to build a bridge and then cross it. The two sides of the river now correspond to the different single discrete points in physical time in the present and the future or past. In contrast, the river itself corresponds to the temporal gap between the single discrete points in the present and the future or past. If we now want to extend our actual discrete point in physical time and thus travel mentally to another one in the future, we need to link and integrate both discrete points in order to bridge their temporal gap.

How can we link and integrate and thus bridge the temporal gap between the different discrete points in the present and the future or past? In the case of the river this is easy. One takes a boat and cross the river from the one side to the other. In the case of consciousness, this is the question for the mechanisms that underlie the temporal extension of the present single discrete point in physical time to the ones in the future and past. As the results show, changes in the neural activity in the midline regions during both resting-state and stimulus-induced activity seem to play an essential role here. What, however, must happen in the neural activity changes of the midline ranges to allow for such temporal extension?

This is the moment where the earlier-described concepts of temporal continuity and temporal flow come in. As we will recall, temporal continuity was determined by the number of discrete points across time *during which* no change in neural activity occurred. Temporal flow, in contrast, was characterized by the number of discrete points across time *after which* neural activity changes occurred. In short, temporal flow concerns the change in neural activity, while temporal continuity refers to its degree of sameness.

What does that imply for the temporal extension? Temporal continuity allows us to link different discrete points in time into one neural activity by remaining the same across different discrete points in physical time. We recall from earlier that the long phase durations of the low-frequency fluctuations allow the neural activity to remain the same, entailing a high degree of temporal continuity. Since the neural activity remains the same during the low-frequency fluctuations' phase duration, the single discrete point in physical time can be extended to the discrete points in physical time that are still included in the period of the phase durations of the low-frequency fluctuations. Hence, sameness of neural activity can go along with temporal extension of the single discrete point in physical time to others.

How about high-frequency fluctuations? Here, the phase durations are much shorter. This means that the number or degree of other single discrete points included in the phase durations is much lower than in the case of the longer phase durations of the low-frequency fluctuations. Since the neural activity changes much quicker here, the degree of possible temporal extension of the single discrete point in physical time to others is much lower in high-frequency fluctuations when compared to the low ones.

This leads me to the following hypothesis. I suggest that the possible degree of temporal extension in consciousness is directly proportional to the degree of the phase duration in the fluctuations of the brain's neural activity. High-frequency fluctuations show shorter phase duration, which decreases the possible degree of temporal extension, whereas the longer phase durations of low-frequency fluctuations allow a larger degree of temporal extension in consciousness.

We have to be aware that this is hypothesis is tentative at this point in time. While several studies investigated mental time travel as described earlier, they focused only on the stimulus-induced activity in different regions; not investigating the relationship of mental time travel to the degree of low and high-frequency fluctuations. Moreover, studies on the subjective experience of time during the resting-state activity itself, where low-frequency fluctuations dominate, are still missing. These studies would be needed to provide experimental support for our neurophenomenal hypothesis, which therefore remains tentative.

NEUROPHENOMENAL HYPOTHESIS
IB: RECIPROCAL BALANCE BETWEEN
TEMPORAL CONTINUITY AND FLOW OF
NEURAL ACTIVITY IS NECESSARY FOR THE
CONSTITUTION OF TEMPORAL EXTENSION IN
CONSCIOUSNESS

We should be careful, however. Temporal extension cannot be identified exclusively with either temporal flow or temporal continuity. Instead, it is the balance between them that accounts for temporal extension. Without temporal continuity and the sameness of neural activity, there would be no "stretching" of the neural activity to different discrete points in physical time in either past or future. This is neuronally well reflected in the long phase durations especially of low-frequency fluctuations.

Conversely, without temporal flow and the change in neural activity, there would be no dynamic in neural activity that is necessary to connect and bridge the temporal gaps between the different discrete points in physical time as provided by temporal continuity (see below for further explanation of this point). This is neuronally manifested especially in the partitioning of the low-frequency fluctuations' long phase durations by the short ones of the high-frequency fluctuations (see Chapter 5 in Volume I, as well as Chapters 14 and 15 in this volume for more details and experimental support on such partitioning of low frequency fluctuations) (see Fig. 13-4a).

Why does temporal continuity (the sameness of neural activity) require temporal flow (the change in neural activity) to yield temporal extension? If there is only temporal continuity, with the neural activity remaining the same, different discrete points in physical time can be included. This is indeed the case in the resting-state activity where the long phase durations of the low-frequency fluctuations dominate the high-frequency fluctuations.

Due to the sameness of the neural activity underlying the different included discrete points in physical time, they are all experienced in the same way, without any differentiation anymore between present, past, and future ones. This, for instance, seems to be the case in depression, where abnormally high resting-state activity

with strong low-frequency fluctuations goes along with alterations in "inner time consciousness": these patients temporally experience everything in the same way, indicating that their stream of consciousness "no longer flows but stands still" (see Chapter 17 for details).

This psychiatric observation suggests that temporal continuity alone is not sufficient to constitute temporal extension. For that, one also needs temporal flow and thus changes in neural activity. However, temporal flow alone is not sufficient either. In the case of abnormally high degrees of temporal flow with strong changes in neural activity and strong high-frequency fluctuations, as for instance in mania or schizophrenia, temporal extension becomes impossible too, with the "inner time consciousness" and especially the "stream of consciousness" being continuously disrupted (see Chapter 17 for details) (see Fig. 13-4b).

I proposed temporal continuity and temporal flow to be central in constituting temporal extension. The question now is how such temporal extension is manifested in our experience and thus in the phenomenal features of consciousness. For the answer, we briefly turn to the phenomenal features of consciousness, and more specifically to the experience of time. As already mentioned earlier, William James spoke of the "stream of consciousness." How can we characterize the stream of consciousness? James (1890) distinguished between the "substantive and transitive parts" in the stream of consciousness. "Substantive parts" concern the contents of consciousness, while the "transitive parts" provide the linkage and thus the transition between the different contents. Together, substantive and transitive parts form a homogenous stream, the "stream of consciousness." Let us focus on the transitive parts for now (the contents of consciousness and thus substantive parts will be discussed in Chapters 18, 19, and 25). How can we describe the "transitive parts" in further phenomenal detail? James (1890, I, 225) points out several

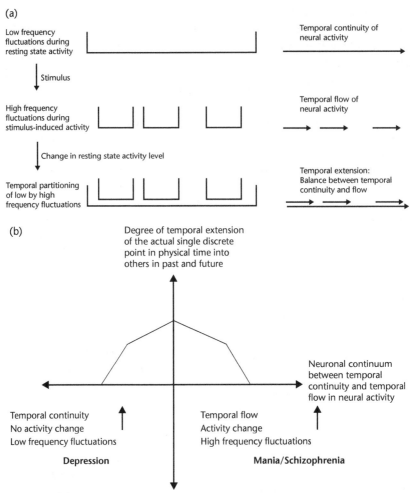

Figure 13-4a and b Frequency fluctuations and temporal extension. The figure depicts the relationship between changes in neural activity and temporal extension and how they are modulated by high- and low-frequency fluctuations (*a*) and the continuum of changes in neural activity (*b*). (*a*) The figure shows how the resting-state's low-frequency fluctuations (upper left) provide temporal continuity of neural activity (upper right) on the basis of their long phase durations, as symbolized by the length of the interval. The low-frequency fluctuations are then complemented by the stimulus-related high-frequency fluctuations (middle left) that show much shorter phase durations and allow for temporal flow of neural activity (middle right). Taken together, this implies the temporal partitioning of the resting-state's long phase durations (lower left), which leads to temporal extension of the stimulus' present discrete time point into past and future ones (lower right). (*b*) The figure depicts the relationship between the degree of temporal extension into past and future (y-axis) and the neuronal balance or continuum between temporal flow and continuity of neural activity of neural activity (x-axis). Temporal extension is based on a balance between temporal flow and continuity of neural activity, as reflected in the inverted U-shaped curve. Extremes in either direction—that is, toward predominant temporal continuity or temporal flow of neural activity—lead to psychiatric disturbances like depression and schizophrenia.

features, of which two, "sensible continuity" and "continuous changes," are particularly relevant to our discussion. "Sensible continuity" means that no phenomenal state vanishes or perishes instantaneously. Instead, there are continuous transitions between different phenomenal states that glide or slide into each other: there is a transition from moment to moment with the transitive parts especially allowing such smooth transition.

I suggest that there is a close relationship between temporal continuity on the neuronal level and sensible continuity on the phenomenal level of consciousness, with the latter being dependent upon the former. I propose that what is described as "sensible continuity" on the phenomenal level of consciousness can be traced to the temporal continuity on the level of the brain's neural activity. More specifically, I hypothesize that the temporal continuity of neural activity is a necessary (rather than sufficient) condition and thus a neural predisposition of possible (rather than actual) sensible continuity in consciousness. Most importantly, my hypothesis of temporal continuity being a neural predisposition of sensible continuity implies direct linkage between neuronal and phenomenal levels as distinguished from mere correspondence (see below for more extensive discussion of this point) as for instance suggested in the neural correlates (see Introduction I).

Neurophenomenal Hypothesis IIB: Co-occurrence between "Physical Absence" and "Neuronal Presence" of Stimuli Predisposes "Sensible Continuity" in Consciousness

How can we explain the relationship between temporal continuity and sensible continuity in further detail? During the phase duration of the activity fluctuations, the neural activity remains the same across different discrete points in physical time. As described earlier, the sameness of neural activity makes it possible to link and integrate the stimuli and their different discrete points in physical time within the respective phase durations of the frequency fluctuation. This makes it possible to constitute what I described as the temporal continuity of neural activity.

I propose that such linkage and integration of different stimuli on the neuronal level resurfaces on the phenomenal level of consciousness in "sensible continuity." The neural activity associated with the single stimulus is continued and thus extended beyond the stimulus' single discrete point in physical time.

Such an extension and continuation of the single stimulus' neural activity makes it impossible for the single stimulus and its associated content to disappear right away in the precise instant of its physical disappearance. Accordingly, even though the stimulus has already disappeared physically, it is still present neuronally in the temporal extension of its neural activity, the temporal continuity. Most important, the extension of the stimulus' neural activity may still be ongoing when the next stimulus arrives at a later single discrete point in physical time. The physically absent previous stimulus is thus still somehow present neuronally during the physical presence of the next stimulus, which again induces changes in neural activity. This means that the extended neural activity of the previous stimulus (that is already absent) is modulated by the neural activity of the present stimulus (that is present now).

Such modulation of the former stimulus' neural activity by that of the later stimulus allows the continuous transition from one stimulus to the next one. The neural activities of both stimuli are thus combined, which accounts for exactly what William James himself (1890, I, 248, 82) described as a "summation of stimuli in the same nerve tract." Accordingly, the temporal continuity of neural activity related to single stimulus predisposes or makes possible the "sensible continuity" (between different contents) on the phenomenal level of consciousness.

Neurophenomenal Hypothesis IIC: Spontaneous Changes in the Brain's Neural Activity Predispose Continuous Change in Consciousness

How about the second feature James attributes to the transitive part, "continuous change"? There is constant change in consciousness and, more specifically, in the contents of our consciousness, as pointed out by James and his concept of "continuous changes" (see earlier). We never experience our consciousness in exactly the same way twice; instead, there is "continuous change." Hence, consciousness can be characterized by what philosopher Robert van Gulick (2004) calls "dynamic flow," where continuity, that is, "sensible continuity," goes along with "continuous change."

We already postulated that the "sensible continuity" is predisposed by the temporal continuity of the brain's neural activity. How can we relate what James described as "continuous change" on the phenomenal level to the neuronal mechanisms discussed earlier? We recall from earlier that Dan Lloyd's empirical data showed particularly strong spontaneous neural activity changes, especially in the midline structures, the "dynamic temporality network," as he called it. This provides direct empirical evidence for continuous change in neural activity, which I have described as the "temporal flow" of neural activity. Unlike the temporal continuity that describes the degree of sameness of neural activity, temporal flow refers to the degree of change of neural activity.

I now postulate that the temporal flow of neural activity predisposes and thus makes possible the occurrence of "continuous change" on the phenomenal level of consciousness. As in the case of temporal continuity (see earlier), my neurophenomenal hypothesis goes beyond mere correspondence between neuronal and phenomenal levels. Rather than mere neurophenomenal correspondence, I claim that the temporal flow of neural activity makes necessary and unavoidable, and thus predisposes by default, the occurrence of "continuous change" in consciousness.

NEUROPHENOMENAL HYPOTHESIS IID: MODULATION OF STIMULUS-INDUCED ACTIVITY BY SPONTANEOUS CHANGES IN THE BRAIN'S INTRINSIC ACTIVITY PREDISPOSES "CONTINUOUS CHANGE" IN CONSCIOUSNESS

How can we explicate the role of the spontaneous activity changes in further detail? We associated the temporal flow of neural activity with the relationship between low and high-frequency fluctuations in neural activity. The shorter phase durations of high-frequency fluctuations partition the longer phase durations of low-frequency fluctuations. This may occur either during spontaneous activity in the resting-state itself, or during the encounter of extrinsic stimuli, which can both introduce change and thus a temporal flow in neural activity.

The resting-state activity itself and especially the one in the midline regions is characterized by continuous changes in its neural activity, as demonstrated by Lloyd and his data. Since the changes in neural activity are spontaneous, they cannot be avoided. Any extrinsic stimulus and its associated neural activity, or stimulus-induced activity, is therefore also subject to this spontaneous change and cannot avoid being modulated by it. This means that the resulting stimulus-induced activity is determined not only by the stimulus itself and its physical presence, but also by the degree of spontaneous change in the ongoing intrinsic activity of the brain.

What does this imply for the stimulus-induced activity? The necessary and thus unavoidable modulation of stimulus-induced activity by the neural activity changes of the ongoing intrinsic activity predisposes change in the stimulus-induced activity: even if the extrinsic stimulus is still physically present, the changes in the brain's intrinsic activity will modulate its associated stimulus-induced activity and thus change how the stimulus is processed.

Even worse, the continuous activity changes may bias or predispose the intrinsic activity for the processing of a different stimulus that either already disappeared (as past stimuli) or is not yet physically present; for example, to predict or anticipate the next stimulus (as postulated in predictive coding; see Chapters 7–9, Volume I). This means that the stimulus-induced activity associated with the physically still-present stimulus cannot avoid interfering with the neural processing of both past and future stimuli: the resulting stimulus-induced activity though elicited by the currently present stimulus consequently provides the transition to other stimuli in either past or future that are physically absent in the present moment.

How is such continuous change in neural activity and its transition between different stimuli that are either physically present or absent manifested on the phenomenal level of consciousness? The continuous change on the neural level will be accompanied by continuous change on the phenomenal level in that the stimuli and their associated contents cannot avoid continuously changing (and thus "flowing") in consciousness. In other words, the occurrence of temporal flow of neural activity predisposes the "continuous change" on the phenomenal level of consciousness. As we will see later, the necessary or unavoidable association of the temporal flow of the neural activity holds, not only during stimulus-induced activity, but also during resting-state activity, as it is phenomenally manifested in (for instance) the experience of time in dreams (see Chapter 25).

NEUROPHENOMENAL HYPOTHESIS IIIA: RECIPROCAL BALANCE BETWEEN TEMPORAL FLOW AND CONTINUITY OF NEURAL ACTIVITY PREDISPOSES RECIPROCAL BALANCE BETWEEN "SENSIBLE CONTINUITY" AND "CONTINUOUS CHANGE" IN CONSCIOUSNESS

We recall from our earlier discussion that the degree of temporal extension of a single discrete point in physical time into others in the past and future depends on the reciprocal balance between temporal flow and continuity of neural activity. What does this imply for the relationship between "sensible continuity" and "continuous changes" on the phenomenal level of consciousness?

We postulated that "sensible continuity" is predisposed by the temporal continuity of neural activity, while "continuous changes" were traceable to temporal flow. One could consequently suggest that the reciprocal balance between temporal flow and continuity of neural activity is manifested on the phenomenal level in a reciprocal balance between "sensible continuity" and "continuous change."

How can we detail that further? We recall that the impact of "temporal continuity" on "sensible continuity" is supposed to be predisposed by the low-frequency fluctuations' long phase durations, while the "temporal flow" makes possible "continuous change" via spontaneous activity changes (see Fig. 13-5).

Put together, this means that the spontaneous activity changes limit the low-frequency fluctuations' phase durations by partitioning them into the shorter ones of high-frequency fluctuations. The spontaneous activity changes consequently shorten not only the phase duration, but also the degree of sameness of neural activity as it is associated with the stimulus-induced activity and its relation to physically absent stimuli.

There is thus direct interaction between "sensible continuity" and "continuous change" with the latter determining the range of the former: the higher the degree of "continuous change", the shorter the temporal extension of the "sensible continuity". Accordingly, very much like temporal flow and continuity on the neural level, I propose "sensible continuity" and "continuous change" to be reciprocally dependent upon each other.

NEUROPHENOMENAL HYPOTHESIS IIIB: RECIPROCAL BALANCE BETWEEN "SENSIBLE CONTINUITY" AND "CONTINUOUS CHANGE" PREDISPOSES THE "STREAM OF CONSCIOUSNESS"

How is this reciprocal balance between "sensible continuity" and "continuous change" manifested on the phenomenal level of consciousness? I propose that the reciprocal balance between them is manifested in the degree of temporal extension—the degree to which the actual discrete point in physical time can be extended and stretched into others in the past and future. And most importantly, I suggest the degree of temporal extension to be manifested in what phenomenally has been described as a "stream of consciousness" or "dynamic flow" (see earlier).

How can we specify these relationships? The more the reciprocal balance tilts toward temporal continuity at the expense of temporal flow in neural activity, the larger the possible degree of temporal extension, and the slower the "stream of consciousness" and its "dynamic flow" on the phenomenal level. Psychologically, this may be

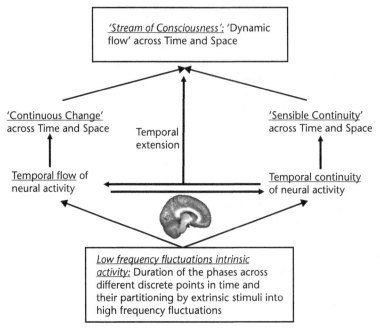

Figure 13-5 Low-frequency fluctuations and the "stream of consciousness." The figure illustrates how the two main components of the "stream of consciousness"—"sensible continuity" and "continuous change" (upper part)—supposedly depend on the duration of the phases of the low-frequency fluctuations in the brain's neural activity during both resting-state and stimulus-induced activity (lower part). I propose that what is described as "continuous change" on the phenomenal level of consciousness is predisposed by the constitution of the temporal flow of neural activity across different discrete points in physical time (middle left). I also suggest what is phenomenally described as "sensible continuity" is predisposed by the temporal continuity of neural activity (middle right). I thus propose that the temporal continuity and temporal flow of neural activity that are already present in the brain's intrinsic activity predispose, and thus make necessary or unavoidable, what phenomenally is described by "sensible continuity" and "continuous change" and hence ultimately as the "stream of consciousness" by William James.

manifested in a reduced capacity to perform mental time travel, especially toward the future. As we have discussed earlier, the extreme case here may be depression, wherein the "stream of consciousness" comes to almost a "standstill," with no flow of time being experienced by these patients.

Conversely, the more the reciprocal balance tilts toward temporal flow at the expense of temporal continuity in neural activity, the lower the possible degree of temporal extension, and the faster the "stream of consciousness" and its "dynamic flow." Psychologically, this may lead to an increased ability to perform mental time travel into both past and future; this is indeed abnormally increased in patients with mania

and schizophrenia, who can imagine themselves in temporally rather distant events in past or future.

NEUROPHENOMENAL HYPOTHESIS IIIC: RECIPROCAL BALANCE BETWEEN "SENSIBLE CONTINUITY" AND "CONTINUOUS CHANGE" OPERATES ACROSS THE DISTINCTION BETWEEN RESTING-STATE AND STIMULUS-INDUCED ACTIVITY

Finally, it should be pointed out that reciprocal balance between "sensible continuity" and "continuous change" holds during both resting-state activity and stimulus-induced activity. Like the reciprocal balance between temporal flow and continuity, I propose the one between "sensible continuity" and "continuous change" to also hold across the boundaries between resting-state and stimulus-induced activity.

If so, one would expect that both resting-state and stimulus-induced activity should be characterized by more or less the same experiences of time in consciousness, albeit in different degrees. This can indeed be supported, since, for instance, dreams show essentially the same kind of time experience during resting-state activity as we experience in the awake state during stimulus-induced activity (see Chapters 25 and 26).

Intrinsic activity, or resting-state activity, and extrinsic neural activity, or stimulus-induced activity, may then be considered just two sides of the same coin on both neural and phenomenal levels. This is well expressed by Dan Lloyd himself, though in slightly different terms:

> The temporal analysis here does not contradict the other research on the cognitive functions of the default-mode. Rather, temporality reconciles the tension between inner mentation and environmental monitoring. In this experiment, elapsed time is not signalled by the environment, entailing that it must arise endogenously. But it is a property of (our perception and cognition) environmental objects—an endogenous construct applied to the outside world. (Lloyd 2011, 8)

NEUROPHENOMENAL HYPOTHESIS IIID: NEUROPHENOMENAL VERSUS NEUROCOGNITIVE ACCOUNTS OF MENTAL TIME TRAVEL

I here suggest a neurophenomenal account of mental time travel. That can be characterized by the assumption that the constitution of time precedes the anticipation of events and their respective contents in our cognition. The anticipated contents are supposed to be linked and integrated within the ongoing constitution of time as it is predisposed by the brain's resting state activity.

This leads me to the claim that mental "time travel" and its respective cognitive functions like prospection/anticipation and retrospection are possible only on the basis of their here-described neuronal mechanisms that allow for the constitution of time. In other words, the cognitive function of prospection/anticipation and retrospection must be based on and be preceded by the constitution of time and its phenomenal features by the brain's resting state activity. On a more general level this means that neurophenomenal function must precede neurocognitive function which entails a neurophenomenal approach to mental time travel.

Such neurophenomenal approach contrasts with a neurocognitive approach to mental time travel. The neurocognitive approach claims that the constitution of time is based on the imagination of particular contents. Cognition of contents in time precedes the constitution of time in the neurocognitive approach: by imagining particular contents, they are temporally signified, which allows their extension into either past or future.

That reverses the stance of the neurophenomenal approach, where the time and its extension of the single discrete points in time into both past and future ones continues independently of any stimuli, whether real or imagined, and their subsequent cognitive processing as contents. Put in a nutshell, the neurocognitive approach claims contents to be processed first before time can be assigned to them whereas the neurophenomenal approach suggests the constitution of time to be basic and fundamental for any subsequent processing of contents.

Which approach holds, the neurophenomenal or the neurocognitive one? Does content follow time, as postulated by the neurophenomenal account? Or does time follow content, as suggested in the neurocognitive approach? In order to address these questions, we need to go into further detail about the neuronal mechanisms underlying "inner time consciousness." This will be done in the next two chapters, after which we will be able to decide whether the neurophenomenal or the neurocognitive approach holds in the case of mental time travel. We will therefore come back to the interpretation of mental time travel as either neurophenomenal or neurocognitive at the end of Chapter 15.

Open Questions

> The first open question raises the role of the midline regions and the rest of the brain in

constituting temporal continuity of neural activity, and how that, in turn, impacts the perception and cognition of time.

One issue in this context is the search for the maximal and minimal biophysical-computational limits beneath and above which temporal differences can no longer be integrated and linked. The closer the resting-state activity level operates to its minimal and maximal biophysical-computational limits, the lower the possible degree of temporal extension and the less development of the "stream of consciousness" and its "dynamic flow" during both resting-state and stimulus-induced activity (see Chapters 28 and 29 for details).

Hence, the resting-state activity itself may be able to impact, or predispose, the possible degrees of temporal continuity. Thereby the resting-state activity seems to provide a "window of spatiotemporal opportunity" for the degree of the "stream of consciousness" (see Chapters 28 and 29 for more details, as well as Volume I, Chapters 11 and 12). We will see later that the resting-state's "window of spatiotemporal opportunity" is almost completely closed in patients with disorders of consciousness like the vegetative state (see Chapters 28 and 29).

Another question arises from the phenomenal side. There is a double relationship between time and consciousness. On one hand, consciousness is based on the constitution of time, with the latter providing a matrix or grid for the former. In short, consciousness is based on time rather, than time being based on consciousness. This is well reflected in the concept of the "stream of consciousness," as discussed in this chapter.

At the same time, we experience time in consciousness, resulting in what is called an "inner time consciousness" (see Chapter 14). In short, time is based here on consciousness, rather than consciousness being based on time. This will be discussed in the Chapters 14 and 15, which are devoted to distinct phenomenal features of "inner time consciousness." And we also need to distinguish such inner time consciousness from the perception and cognition of time. This is related to our perceptual and cognitive functions. That will be discussed in full detail in Appendix 2.

Finally another open question pertains to the exact neuronal mechanisms of how the high resting-state activity in the midline regions constitutes temporal continuity of neural activity. While these regions show predominantly low-frequency fluctuations, it remains unclear how these are related to the kind of temporal synthesis we experience in what is phenomenally described as "inner time consciousness." The more detailed processes and mechanisms of the constitution of such temporal continuity in our consciousness will be the subject of the next two chapters.

NOTE

1. That said, it's not obvious that the two "hands" can be easily disentangled. At least the standard Newtonian physical model of time as a one-dimensional continuum is strongly, if not entirely, developed based on our subjective experience. This approach is based on the assumption that subjective experience accurately reflects physical reality to at least a reasonable extent.

CHAPTER 14
Slow Cortical Potentials and "Width of Present"

Summary

Chapter 13 focused on how the brain's intrinsic activity undergoes continuous changes in its neural activity, thereby making possible what I described as the "temporal flow" and "temporal continuity." of its neural activity These, in turn, were considered to predispose the constitution of what phenomenally is described as the flow of time, or the "stream of consciousness," including its "sensible continuity" and "continuous change." A special role is proposed for temporal continuity of neural activity in predisposing the stream of consciousness. Therefore, the present chapter focuses on the way the brain's neural activity needs to be encoded in order to make possible the "stream of consciousness." This leads us again to the low-frequency fluctuations of the brain's neural activity and more specifically to slow cortical potentials (SCPs). Due to their long phase duration as low-frequency fluctuations, SCPs can integrate different stimuli and their associated neural activity from different regions in one converging region. Such integration may be central for consciousness to occur, as it recently postulated by He and Raichle. They leave open, however, the question of the exact neuronal mechanisms, like the encoding strategy, that make possible the association of the otherwise purely neuronal SCP with consciousness and its phenomenal features. I hypothesize that SCPs allow for linking and connecting different discrete points in physical time by encoding their statistically based temporal differences rather than the single discrete time points by themselves. This presupposes difference-based coding rather than stimulus-based coding. The encoding of such statistically based temporal differences makes it possible to "go beyond" the merely physical features of the stimuli; that is, their single discrete

time points and their conduction delays (as related to their neural processing in the brain). This, in turn, makes possible the constitution of "local temporal continuity" of neural activity in one particular region. The concept of "local temporal continuity" signifies the linkage and integration of different discrete time points into one neural activity in a particular region. How does such local temporal continuity predispose the experience of time in consciousness? For that, I turn to phenomenological philosopher Edmund Husserl and his description of what he calls "inner time consciousness."(Husserl 1990). One hallmark of humans' "inner time consciousness" is that we experience events and objects in succession and duration in our consciousness; according to Husserl, this amounts to what he calls the "width of [the] present." The concept of the width of present describes the extension of the present beyond the single discrete time point, such as, for instance, when we perceive different tones as a melody. I now hypothesize the degree of the width of present to be directly dependent upon and thus predisposed by the degree of the temporal differences between two (or more) discrete time points as they are encoded into neural activity. I therefore conclude that the SCPs and their encoding of neural activity in terms of temporal differences must be regarded a neural predisposition of consciousness (NPC) as distinguished from a neural correlate of consciousness (NCC).

Key Concepts and Topics Covered

Slow cortical potentials, low-frequency fluctuations, resting state, slow wave activity, NREM sleep, difference-based coding, "going beyond," statistically based coding, temporal continuity, width of present, neural correlates of consciousness, neural predisposition of consciousness

Neuroempirical Background: Encoding of Neural Activity Predisposes Temporal Integration

In Chapter 13, I pointed out the central role of the brain's intrinsic activity and its continuous changes in constituting the temporal flow and temporal continuity of neural activity. The "temporal flow" is the intrinsic changes of neural activity across different discrete points in physical time. "Temporal continuity," in contrast, was associated with the duration of the phases, especially in the low-frequency fluctuations of the intrinsic activity. In short, temporal flow refers to the degree of change in neural activity, while temporal continuity describes its degree of sameness.

Most important, the neuronal mechanisms underlying temporal flow and temporal continuity were suggested to predispose the constitution of what William James described as "sensible continuity" and "continuous change" as phenomenal hallmarks of the "stream of consciousness." "Sensible continuity" referred to the transitions between different contents in consciousness, which I proposed to be related to the degree of temporal continuity and thus the degree of sameness of neural activity. In contrast, "continuous change" described the disappearance or fleeting character of the contents in consciousness; that was traced back to the temporal flow and thus the degree of change in neural activity. Central to the constitution of the "stream of consciousness" was the linkage and integration between different discrete points in physical time in the resulting neural activity that, as I suggested, results in temporal continuity.

How, though, is such an integration between different discrete points in physical time possible in neural activity? I hypothesized in the last chapter that low-frequency fluctuations, and more specifically the long phase duration and their large number of different discrete time points, may be central here. This explains the inclusion of different discrete time points, but it leaves open the question of how the different discrete time points within one phase duration are linked and integrated into each other.

There must be a special neuronal mechanism and, more specifically, a particular coding strategy at work in how the brain encodes its neural activity during the long phase durations of the low-frequency fluctuations. This is the focus in the present chapter. I will postulate that the temporal integration between different discrete points in physical time, such as within one phase duration, is made possible only by encoding temporal differences into neural activity. This presupposes difference-based coding as distinguished from stimulus-based coding (see Volume I for details).

Most important, I will suggest that such difference-based coding predisposes not only the temporal continuity of neural activity, but also temporal integration on the phenomenal level of consciousness. In order to illustrate this in neuroscientific (and later in neurophenomenal) detail, I now turn to neuroscientist B. J. He. She, together with M. E. Raichle, developed a special hypothesis about the relevance of the resting-state activity for consciousness in a recent paper (see He and Raichle 2009).

Neuronal Findings IA: Intrinsic Activity and Slow Cortical Potentials

Interestingly, in the footnote to that article, B. J. He thanks the U.S. immigration office for preventing her from returning to the United States. She explains that this provided her with the geographical and mental distance she needed to think outside the constraints of her university and to develop the resting-state hypothesis of consciousness. This documents well that sometimes unexpected circumstances not anticipated as contents in our consciousness are apparently needed to produce excellent hypotheses about consciousness itself.

Let us now turn from the travels of Be He to her neuroscientific results and hypotheses. He et al. (2008) investigated neurosurgical patients electrophysiologically with electroencephalography (EEG) in three different states of consciousness sequentially: wakefulness, slow wave sleep (SWS), and rapid eye movement sleep (REM). The data were low-pass filtered at <0.5 Hz to yield low-frequency fluctuations and, more specifically, spontaneous slow cortical potentials (SCPs). The correlation of SCPs across all electrodes was calculated by computing Pearson correlation coefficients between the SCPs in a seed electrode and all other electrodes.

What are SCPs? They are specific electrophysiological potentials in the low-frequency range (<0.5 Hz) and can thus be regarded as a form of low-frequency fluctuation (see Chapter 5 in Volume I for details as well van Someren et al. 2011; Riedner et al. 2011; and Mascettiet al. 2011 for excellent overviews). By correlating the SCP across different electrodes, she obtained correlation maps of SCP, signifying the occurrence of the SCP in the whole brain.

In addition, the patients also underwent resting-state functional magnetic resonance imaging (fMRI) to measure spontaneous resting-state activity and its low-frequency fluctuations. All voxels observed in fMRI that centered on a specific electrode (as the seed electrodes) were then correlated with those associated with the respective other electrodes. This yielded relationships between the SCPs' correlation maps as generated in EEG and the spontaneous BOLD correlation maps from the fMRI.

How were now the fMRI-BOLD signals related to the SCPs during the three different states of consciousness? SCP-fMRI correlation was observed in all three states: wakefulness, SWS, and REM. This distinguished the SCPs from higher frequency oscillations as the gamma oscillations (20–40 Hz). Unlike the SCP, the gamma oscillations only correlated with the BOLD signal in the awake state and during REM sleep, but not during SWS, that is, NREM sleep, where consciousness is lost.

This let the author propose that the SCPs may be a very fundamental feature of neural activity. The SCPs as low-frequency fluctuations of neural activity may reflect the intrinsic organization of the brain's neural activity independently of its kind of neural activity, that is, resting-state or stimulus-induced activity (Fig. 14-1a–c; see also He et al. 2010; van Someren et al. 2011; Riedner et al. 2011; Mascetti et al. 2011).

NEURONAL FINDINGS IB: SLOW CORTICAL POTENTIALS AND INFORMATION INTEGRATION

How can we determine the SCPs in further physiological detail? Negative shifts in the SCPs are supposed to index increases in cortical excitability. Such changes in cortical excitability have been shown to originate predominantly from synaptic activities at apical dendrites in superficial layers of the cortex where they reflect long-lasting excitatory postsynaptic potentials (EPSPs). In short, SCPs are closely related to the EPSPs in the superficial layers (layers 1 and 2) in the cortex.

Where do the superficial layers and thus the EPSPs get their input from? They get a major input from the lower layers of the cortex, layers 4, 5, and 6, that receive plenty of inputs from the thalamus (and other subcortical regions) leading subsequently to the excitation of the pyramidal cells, especially in layer 4. In addition to the lower layers' input, the superficial layers 1 and 2 also receive strong inputs from other cortical regions whose afferences terminate directly in layers 1 and 2. These cortico-cortical afferences and their respective neural excitation are then integrated and processed further in the superficial layers' abundant GABAergic inhibitory interneurons (see Chapters 2, 6, and 12 for the role of GABA in mediating neural activity).

Let us sketch the pathway of neuronal processing by taking the example of thalamic input. The input from thalamic regions is first processed in deeper cortical layers, layers 4 and 5 and 6, which leads subsequently to the excitation of the here located pyramidal cells. While also producing EPSPs, these deeper cortical signals have less impact on the activity changes in the superficial layers as measured in the SCPs. Besides the pyramidal cells, there are also many interneurons, GABAergic and inhibitory neurons in especially the superficial cortical layers. Due to their rather low amplitude of membrane flow changes, these interneurons do seem to have a minor impact, if at all, on the SCPs in particular and the local field potentials in general.

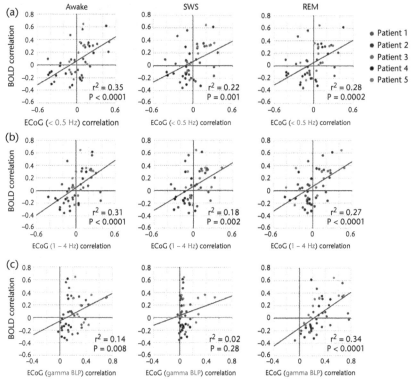

Figure 14-1 Integration of information by slow cortical potentials. BOLD vs. ECoG cross-correlation function peak values. Peak correlations of filtered (< 0.5 Hz and 1–4 Hz) ECoG activity were evaluated for lags in the range < 500 ms. Peak correlations of BOLD and γ-BLP (both sampled at 2-s intervals) were evaluated at zero-lag. Each ROI pair is represented by one symbol. All sensorimotor-sensorimotor and sensorimotor-control ROI pairs from all patients are shown. In Patient 2, the ECoG derivation was modified Laplacian; in all other patients, it was average reference. (*a*) < 0.5 Hz ECoG. (*b*) 1–4 Hz EcoG. (*c*) γ-BLP EcoG. *P* values represent the significance of the measured correlation between BOLD and ECoG peak correlations. Reprinted with permission of *Proceedings of the National Academy of Sciences*, from He BJ, Snyder AZ, Zempel JM, Smyth MD, Raichle ME. Electrophysiological correlates of the brain's intrinsic large-scale functional architecture. *Proc Natl Acad Sci USA.* 2008 Oct 14;105(41):16039–44.

Taken together, this lets one propose that the SCPs as low-frequency fluctuations are related predominantly to long-lasting depolarization of apical dendrites in superficial cortical layers. Besides the thalamic input, which enters via deeper layers like layers 4 and 5, other long-range intracortical and cortico-cortical connections preferentially terminate in these superficial layers, layers 1 and 2. This means that the SCPs cannot be associated with the information from a single stimulus. Instead, they reflect rather the summation of many stimuli as conveyed by the different connections, intracortically and

cortico-cortically, all terminating in the superficial layers.

Based on the connectivity pattern of the superficial layers and the long-lasting depolarization, the EPSPs, the resulting SCPs must reflect the integration of information from different stimuli processed in different cortical regions. This is quite compatible with the earlier reported correlation between the cortico-cortical (e.g., electrode-electrode) correlation maps of both SCP and fMRI signals. The aforementioned results are possible only if signals from different regions as measured in fMRI are integrated into the locally measured SCPs. The BOLD signals of the fMRI result from the integration of neural activity of different regions so that the correlating SCPs, as locally measured, must be related to integration of neural activities from different regions.

NEURONAL FINDINGS IC: SLOW CORTICAL POTENTIALS AND CONSCIOUSNESS

What do the SCPs as low-frequency fluctuations in the brain's resting state entail for the phenomenal features of consciousness? He and Raichle (2009) hypothesize that the SCPs are the neural correlate of consciousness and are therefore a minimally sufficient neural condition of the contents in consciousness (see the second Introduction for the exact definition of the term "correlate"). More specifically, SCPs carry information from different cortical regions. The slow time scale, the slow frequency character (< 0.5 Hz), and the integration of long-range intra- and cortico-cortical connections may allow the SCPs to temporally integrate and synchronize stimuli and thus information processed in different regions (despite the respective conduction delays) and sources.

Following He and Raichle, such integration may well account for the experience of a "unitary and undivided whole" in consciousness. This is supported, according to them, by recent findings from perception, attention, volition, and unconscious states (anesthesia, vegetative state) that all go along with changes in the SCPs and the level of consciousness (see He and Raichle 2009; see also Riedner et al. 2011 and Mascetti et al. 2011 for further empirical support as well as Chapters 15, 28, and 29 for more details on the vegetative state and anesthesia).

The exact neuronal mechanisms underlying such integration and synchronization of information in SCPs remain unclear, however. More specifically, He and Raichle leave open the question of the way that the neural activity related to the SCP must be encoded and thus generated in order to allow for the alleged integration and synchronization of the stimuli and their different discrete points in physical time. This will be the focus of my first neuronal hypothesis.

NEURONAL HYPOTHESIS IA: SLOW CORTICAL POTENTIALS MEDIATE "DOUBLE TEMPORAL INTEGRATION"

How does such local integration of transregional activity come about? He and Raichle claim that, due to their broad time window, the SCPs as low-frequency fluctuations are ideal candidates to integrate information from different regions. But how such purely neuronal integration leads to consciousness and its phenomenal features remains unclear. For that, as I claim, we need to go into further detail about the exact neuronal mechanisms of such temporal integration and, more specifically, the way neural activity during the SCP is encoded and thus generated.

What do I mean by "temporal integration"? I will distinguish between two different kinds of temporal information that need to be integrated—the temporal information related to the stimuli themselves, and the temporal information related to the brain's neural processing of the stimuli. This shall be explicated in the following discussion.

First, the temporal information related to stimuli and their different temporal properties must be integrated within the SCPs. More specifically, the stimuli and their respective information conveyed in the cortico-cortical connections are scaled on different discrete points in physical time. For instance, stimulus a may occur at time point x while stimulus b may occur at time point y. There are thus different discrete points in physical time associated with the occurrence of the different stimuli that need to be integrated in the superficial layers of the cortex where the SCPs are generated.

Second, different stimuli may be processed in varying degrees in different regions; this may occur closer or further away from the region where they are temporally integrated into an SCP. The differences in distance and regions may imply different biophysical-computational conduction delays (see also Chapters 1, 6, and 12 in Volume I) between the region processing the stimulus and the one where it is temporally integrated with other stimuli.

For instance, stimulus *a* may be first processed in region *m*, which is closer to the integrating region *i* than the region *n* where stimulus *b* is processed. This means that the different biophysical-computational conduction delays associated with different stimuli and their respective regions must also be integrated in the superficial layers where the SCPs are generated. There is consequently a need for what I describe in the following discussion as "double temporal integration": the different discrete points of the different stimuli's occurrence in physical time need to be integrated in the same way the biophysical-computational conduction delays related to the stimuli's neural processing in the brain require integration.

Accordingly, the different discrete points in physical time related to both stimuli and the brain's conduction delays need to be integrated in neural activity. One may consecutively want to speak of "double temporal integration": the concept of "double temporal integration" describes the need to integrate both the stimuli's different discrete points in their occurrence in physical time and the biophysical-computational conduction delays during their neural processing in the brain.

Neuronal Hypothesis IB: Difference-Based Coding Mediates "Double Temporal Integration"

How is such "double temporal integration" possible? I propose that the encoding of neural activity in terms of temporal differences between different discrete points in physical time as related to both the stimuli and the biophysical-computational conduction delays may be central here. In short, I suggest difference-based coding to be a necessary condition and thus a neural predisposition of "double temporal integration" in the brain's neural activity. If, in contrast, there were stimulus- rather than difference-based coding, such "double temporal integration" in neural activity would remain impossible.

How can we describe difference-based coding in the here presupposed temporal context in more detail? I hypothesize that difference-based coding (as distinguished from stimulus-based coding) allows for encoding the temporal differences between different stimuli's occurrence at different discrete time points (as it is symbolically rather than mathematically expressed by letters and numbers in the following).

Let us start with the encoding of the temporal information related to the stimulus itself. What is encoded into neural activity is not the time point x of the stimulus a and the time point $(x + 1)$ of the stimulus b but rather the temporal difference between the time points x and $(x + 1)$. Hence, the subsequently resulting neural activity neither reflects the time point x nor $(x + 1)$ but rather their temporal difference or integral, for example, $x - (x + 1)$.

This means that the neural activity does not correspond to (nor represent, as the philosophers may want to say) the discrete time point of the single stimulus by itself in an isolated and independent way. Instead, the neural activity may rather mirror the temporal difference between two (or more) discrete time points associated with different (or the same) stimuli across different discrete points in physical time. The single stimulus is thus no longer encoded into neural activity as isolated and independent from other stimuli as in stimulus-based coding. Instead, it is encoded into neural activity in relative temporal difference to other stimuli and thus in a relational and interdependent way.

How about the temporal information from the brain's biophysical-computational conduction delays? The same is supposed to apply for the temporal differences resulting from the brain's transregional processing, that is, the conduction delays, during the neural processing of stimuli a and b in regions m and n to region i: what is encoded and integrated in the region yielding the SCPs may be not so much the conduction delay from region m to region i and the one from region n to region i (as one would suggest in the case of stimulus-based coding).

Instead, what is encoded into the neural activity of region i, the one that yields the SCPs, may be the difference in conduction delays (that is, $[(i - m) - (i - n)]$), rather than the conduction delays themselves (that is, from m to i and from n to i). Accordingly, I propose difference-based coding to apply also to the neural processing of the biophysical-computational conduction delays related to the brain's neural processing of stimuli.

Taken together, both the different stimuli's different discrete points in physical time and their different biophysical-computational conduction delays in their associated neural processing are proposed to be encoded into neural activity in terms of temporal differences. Such encoding in terms of temporal differences makes it possible to integrate the different discrete points in time related to both the different stimuli and the different conduction delays. I thus hypothesize difference-based coding rather than stimulus-based coding to predispose or make possible the temporal integration of both the different stimuli's time points and the different conduction delays in the brain's neural activity.

Neuronal Hypothesis IC: "Double Temporal Integration" and Difference-Based Coding as Intrinsic Features of the Brain's Neural Activity

We have focused so far on the temporal integration of the different discrete time points related to both stimuli and conduction delays. This, though, has left open the question of how stimuli and conduction delays as different kinds of information with different origins can be temporally linked and integrated with each other.

How are stimuli and conduction delays temporally integrated in the neural activity of region i? The encoding of both stimuli and conduction delays in terms of temporal differences into neural activity provides a common format for both, a temporal difference. This allows them to be integrated despite their occurrence at different discrete points in physical time.

The neural activity of region i, the integrating region that yields the SCPs, may consecutively be characterized by "double temporal integration" as signified by ($[x − (x + 1)] − [(m − i) − (n − i)]$). Accordingly, the encoding of neural activity in terms of temporal differences allows the brain's neural activity to integrate the different kinds of information related to stimuli and conduction delays into one common format, temporal differences; this in turn makes possible their

integration into one neural activity, the neural activity of the region that yields the SCP.

One may now be inclined to object that this may well hold for stimulus-induced activity as, for instance, the contingent negative variation (CNV; see Chapter 5 in Volume I) that can be characterized as stimulus-related SCPs while it may not apply to spontaneous SCPs generated intrinsically in the resting state itself. Why? Because the resting state can not be simply characterized by stimuli but rather the absence of stimuli. One would thus wonder why there are SCPs at all in the resting state characterizing the brain's intrinsic activity.

This however, as detailed in Volume I, Chapter 4, does not hold. Even the resting state itself receives plenty of input from stimuli generated intrinsically in the brain itself, the neuronal stimuli as I described them. In addition, the resting state receives continuous interoceptive stimuli from the body and the unspecific exteroceptive sensory stimuli from the environment (see Chapter 4, Volume I for details). And very much like specific exteroceptive stimuli in the case of the CNV, these different stimuli—that is, their distinct time points and processing times—need to undergo "double temporal integration."

I consequently hypothesize that the spontaneous SCPs, as, for instance, observed by He at al. (2008) (and others like van Someren et al. 2011; Riedner et al. 2011; and Mascetti et al. 2011), can be traced back to the "double temporal integration" during the encoding of the various stimuli in terms of temporal differences into neural activity during the resting state. This means that difference-based coding and "double temporal integration" operate continuously during both resting-state and stimulus-induced activity.

Both resting state and stimulus-induced activity must therefore be regarded as intrinsic features of the brain's operation, meaning that the brain cannot avoid encoding any kind of its neural activity in terms of difference-based coding and subsequent "double temporal integration." Accordingly, I postulate that difference-based coding and "double temporal integration" are necessary and therefore unavoidable features of the brain's neural activity in general including both resting state and stimulus-induced activity.

NEURONAL HYPOTHESIS IIA: ENCODING OF THE STIMULI'S NATURAL STATISTICS PREDISPOSES NEURAL ACTIVITY TO "GOING BEYOND" THE SINGLE STIMULUS

How is the alleged encoding of temporal differences into the brain's neural activity, that is, difference-based coding, manifest in the phenomenal features of consciousness? Let us consider what happens in difference-based coding. By encoding differences between different discrete points in physical time (and conduction delays) rather than the actual discrete time points themselves, the purely physical characterization of the single stimuli, for example, their discrete points in physical time and their respective conduction delays, is resolved into a difference, that is, a temporal difference. Hence, the encoding of the stimuli (and conduction delays) in terms of temporal differences allows for "going beyond" the single stimuli's physical features, that is, their different discrete points in physical time and their conduction delay.

What exactly do I mean by "going beyond"? By encoding the single stimuli's discrete points in physical time in relation to those of other stimuli, the resulting neural activity no longer reflects (*represents* as the philosophers may want to say) exclusively the single stimulus itself. Instead, the resulting neural activity contains some information about the same stimulus at other discrete points in physical time and/or other stimuli and their specific time points. The resulting neural activity thus "goes beyond" the single stimulus itself and its particular discrete point in time.

This means that the stimuli's distribution across the different discrete points in physical time and thus their "temporal statistics" is encoded into the brain's neural activity. Rather than reflecting the single stimulus itself, neural activity encodes the stimuli "statistical frequency distribution that is the stimuli's natural statistics" or more specifically their "temporal statistics" (see Chapter 1 in Volume I). Accordingly, due to its encoding of the stimuli's "natural statistics," the neural activity "goes beyond" the single stimulus itself (see later for more details on the "going beyond").

NEURONAL HYPOTHESIS IIB: DIFFERENT DEGREES OF DIFFERENCE-BASED CODING DURING THE ENCODING OF NEURAL ACTIVITY

How can we further specify the encoding of the stimuli's "natural statistics" with regard to the here-discussed "double temporal integration"? Since it concerns the encoding of the stimuli's and their respective conduction delays' different discrete points in physical time, one may want to speak of "temporal statistics." The concept of temporal statistics describes the distribution and thus the frequency of different discrete points of time across physical time and their subsequent encoding into the brain's neural activity.

By encoding the stimuli's and their conduction delays' temporal statistics, the single stimulus and its respective conduction delays are encoded relative to the occurrence of itself and other stimuli at the same or different discrete points in physical time. This means that the single stimulus' physical features are no longer encoded as such, that is in an isolated and independent way: the single stimulus' physical features concern its specific discrete point in time and its specific conduction delay.

If these physical features are now no longer encoded in an isolated and independent way, the resulting neural activity cannot be based exclusively on the stimulus' physical features themselves. Instead of the stimuli's physical features themselves, their temporal relations, that is, temporal differences, and thus their temporal statistics are encoded into neural activity. What is encoded into neural activity is thus no longer stimulus and physically based but rather difference and statistically based (see Fig. 14-2a, b).

One should notice, however, that the distinction between physically and statistically based encoding strategies does not obey the law of all or nothing: either physically based encoding to 100% or statistically based encoding to 100% (See Chapter 1 in Volume I for details). Instead, there is rather a more-or-less distinction with a reciprocal balance between the possible degrees

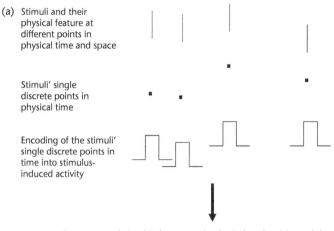

(a) Stimuli and their physical feature at different points in physical time and space

Stimuli' single discrete points in physical time

Encoding of the stimuli' single discrete points in time into stimulus-induced activity

One-to-one relationship between stimulus-induced activity and the stimuli' physical features (via their single discrete points in physical time)

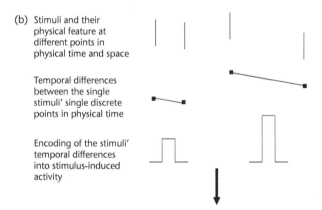

(b) Stimuli and their physical feature at different points in physical time and space

Temporal differences between the single stimuli' single discrete points in physical time

Encoding of the stimuli' temporal differences into stimulus-induced activity

Many-to-one relationship between the stimuli' physical features (via their single discrete points in time) and the stimulus-induced activity": "Going beyond" the single stimulus and its physical features by encoding its temporal difference to other single stimuli' physical features at different discrete points in physical time

Figure 14-2a-d Different encoding strategies. The figure depicts different strategies of encoding stimuli and their different discrete points in physical time (and space) into neural activity. (*a*) This figure shows the strategy of physically based encoding. Here the stimuli, including their physical features, are encoded into neural activity in orientation on their different single discrete points in physical time (and space). There is thus one-to-one correspondence between the stimuli's discrete points in physical time and the number of stimulus-induced activities. The stimulus-induced activity thus corresponds in a one-to-one way to the stimulus, its physical features, and its single discrete point in physical time. Therefore, the physically based encoding strategy can be described as stimulus-based coding. (*b*) This is different in statistically based encoding. Here, the temporal differences between the stimuli's different discrete points in physical time are encoded into neural activity. Depending on the degree of temporal difference, the resulting stimulus-induced activity will vary in its degree. The encoding of neural activity depends here no longer on the single stimulus itself and its discrete point in physical time but rather on the occurrence of stimuli across different discrete time points and thus on the stimuli's statistical frequency distribution; hence the name "statistically based." This means that the encoding of temporal differences into neural activity, or difference-based coding, is a statistically based coding strategy that makes possible the encoding of the stimuli's statistical frequency distribution—their "natural statistics." The figure depicts different strategies of encoding stimuli and their different discrete points in physical time (and space) into neural activity. (*c*) The figure depicts the relationship between physically based

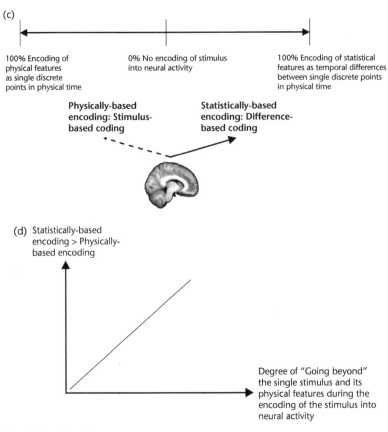

Figure 14-2a-d (Continued)

and statistically based encoding strategies. There is a balance between both with increases in the degree of the one going along with decreases in the respective other. The dotted line and the weaker characters on the side of stimulus-based coding, compared to the other side of difference-based coding, indicates that usually the balance is tilted toward difference-based coding at the expense of stimulus-based coding. (*d*) The figure shows the relationship between the different encoding strategies and the degree of "going beyond" the single stimulus and its physical features. The higher the degree of statistically based encoding when compared to physically based encoding (y-axis), the higher the degree to which the resulting stimulus-induced activity goes beyond the single stimulus and its physical features (x-axis). Hence, I propose that what metaphorically is described by "going beyond" has its origin in the balance between physically and statistically based coding strategies.

of physically and statistically based encoding and thus between stimulus- and difference-based coding: The more the stimuli's different discrete points in physical time are encoded in terms of temporal differences, the more this balance will be shifted toward the statistically based pole; that is, difference-based coding.

How will the balance be shifted in the converse case of increased encoding of the stimuli's discrete points in physical time? Most likely, the balance will be tilted toward the physically based pole; that is, stimulus-based coding. One may consequently propose a continuum of different possible degrees of statistically based encoding, or difference-based coding, that may be reciprocally related to the possible degrees of physically based encoding and thus stimulus-based coding (see Fig. 14-2c).

NEURONAL HYPOTHESIS IIC: DIFFERENCE-BASED CODING PREDISPOSES NEURAL ACTIVITY TO "GOING BEYOND" THE SINGLE STIMULUS

Such statistically based encoding of the stimulus in relation to itself and others across different discrete points in physical time implies that the resulting neural activity "goes beyond" the single stimulus' physical features. The physical features of the single stimulus are somehow preserved in the encoded neural activity, not as isolated and independent features but rather as relative to the ones of the same or other stimuli across different discrete points in physical time.

To put the same idea in a different way: The single stimulus' physical features are not lost in the encoded neural activity but rather put in the wider context of the same and other stimuli's physical features occurring at the same and other discrete points in time. Accordingly, the encoded neural activity can be characterized by what I call "going beyond" in the following.

What does "going beyond" mean? Going beyond means that the encoded neural activity includes the physical features of the stimuli themselves, though in a wider way in relative difference from other stimuli by applying a statistically based rather than physically based encoding strategy. The neural activity induced by a single stimulus thus contains more information than the one related to that particular stimulus itself; the encoded neural activity thus "goes beyond" the single stimulus and its temporal (and spatial) information.

Such going beyond the encoded neural activity is well reflected in the following quote by Buzsaki (2006, 275): "Because of the additive contribution of the brain, the behavior of a neuron or local network does not faithfully reflect the physical features of the input." What Buzsaki describes as the "additive contribution of the brain" may be closely related to the brain's application of a particular encoding strategy—difference-based and statistically based encoding, as distinguished from stimulus-based and physically based encoding.

How does such an encoding strategy lead to what Buszaki describes as "additive contribution of the brain"? Rather than encoding the stimuli's discrete points in time, the brain prefers to encode their temporal differences across different discrete points in physical time into its neural activity. This adds something to the single stimulus itself; namely, that the resulting neural activity "goes beyond" the single stimulus itself by encoding the single stimulus' temporal relation to itself and others across time.

Taken all together, this leads me to suggest the following hypothesis. I propose the degree of the going beyond to be directly dependent upon the balance between statistically and physically based encoding strategies: the more the balance tilts toward statistically based encoding, the more likely the resulting neural activity will go beyond the single stimulus. But the converse case of the balance shifting toward physically based encoding will go along with a reduced degree of going beyond the single stimulus in the resulting neural activity (see Fig. 14-2d).

NEURONAL HYPOTHESIS IIIA: LOW-FREQUENCY FLUCTUATIONS ENCODE TEMPORAL DIFFERENCES

One may now want to object that some stimuli may temporally be so different, due to both different occurrence in time and different conduction delays, that their encoding into neural activity in terms of a temporal difference and thus their temporal integration remains impossible. This may be so because the time span that needs to be integrated may exceed the degree of temporal differences that can possibly be linked and integrated.

This means that the degree of temporal differences that are to be integrated may exceed the length of the phase (or cycle) durations of even the low-frequency fluctuations like the SCP. The temporal difference between the to-be-integrated different discrete points in physical time may simply exceed the one that is available within one phase duration of the SCP. Integration of the different discrete time points and thus the encoding of the stimuli's temporal statistics remain impossible in this case.

What is the ultimate limit, the time window, beyond which different discrete points in time can no longer be encoded in terms of their temporal differences via difference-based coding?

I propose that the frequency range of the SCP sets biophysical-computational limits to the degree of temporal differences that can possibly be linked, integrated, and encoded into neural activity. The lower the frequency range of the SCPs, the more temporally extended are their time windows, and the longer are their phase durations.

And the longer the phase durations, the larger the temporal differences between different discrete points in time that can still be encoded in terms of temporal differences into the same neural activity change. Accordingly, longer phase duration predisposes the brain's neural activity to integrate temporally more distant stimuli under the umbrella of the same neural activity change.

Conversely, higher frequency ranges above the SCPs go along with shorter phase durations (for example, time windows) and can therefore encode only smaller temporal differences (see Fig. 14-3a). This means that temporally more distant stimuli can no longer be linked and integrated into the same neural activity and do instead induce rather two (or more) different neural activity changes.

I propose the following hypothesis: the lower the frequency range in the fluctuations of the neural activity, the larger the temporal differences that can possibly be encoded into neural activity. And the larger temporal differences can be encoded into neural activity, the higher the possible degrees of statistically based encoding (while at the same time decreasing the possible degrees of physically based encoding).

NEURONAL HYPOTHESIS IIIB: FROM THE ENCODING OF TEMPORAL DIFFERENCES TO LOCAL AND GLOBAL TEMPORAL CONTINUITY OF NEURAL ACTIVITY

Based on these considerations, I propose stronger (and lower) low-frequency fluctuations to go along with higher possible degrees of going beyond, while the possible degree of going beyond may decrease when the higher frequency fluctuations are stronger (see Fig. 14-3b).

By allowing for the encoding of larger temporal differences in the low-frequency fluctuations' longer phase durations, the different discrete points in physical time become linked and connected to each other and thus integrated. The physically based temporal discontinuity of the stimuli themselves becomes consequently superseded by their processing in terms of the statistically based temporal continuity in the brain's neural activity.

Stronger degrees, that is, power and range, of low-frequency fluctuations should then go along with higher degrees of statistically based encoding and going beyond, which ultimately leads to higher degrees of temporal continuity. Accordingly, I propose the possible degree of temporal continuity of neural activity to be directly dependent upon the range and power of low-frequency fluctuations and the degree of difference-based and statistically based encoding (see Fig. 14-3c, d).

In sum, I propose that "temporal continuity of neural activity" refers to the difference-based and statistically based temporal integration between the different stimuli's different discrete points in physical time during their encoding into the brain's neural activity. Hence, I regard the concept of temporal continuity to be a purely neuronal concept. As such, it is based on the specific encoding strategy the brain applies to encode and generate its own neural activity during both resting state and stimulus-induced activity when processing the different stimuli (or its own intrinsic activity changes) and their different discrete points in physical time.

Finally, one may also need to further distinguish between "local" and "global" temporal continuity of neural activity. "Local" temporal continuity concerns the statistically based integration between different particular stimuli in a specific region; that is, like the region *i*, and its superficial layers with the consecutive generation of a regionally specific SCP. "Global" temporal continuity, in contrast, refers to the integration of all stimuli the brain encounters across time and its different regions' neural activities as, for instance, manifest in its low-frequency fluctuations. I focused so far only on the neuronal mechanisms of local temporal continuity, which in the further course of this chapter shall be complemented in phenomenal regard. But I did not discuss those yielding global temporal continuity, which will be the focus of the next chapter.

Phenomenological Excursion IA: "Width of Present"

How is the local temporal continuity, as a purely neuronal feature of the brain's intrinsic activity, manifest in experience and thus consciousness?

This is the question for the phenomenal manifestation of the neuronal mechanisms underlying the constitution of local temporal continuity. For that, I turn to phenomenological philosophy, which provides excellent descriptions of the experience of time in consciousness.

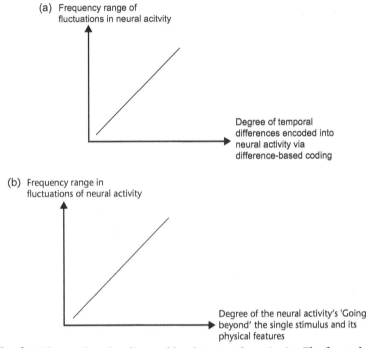

Figure 14-3a-d Difference-based coding and local temporal continuity. The figure depicts the relationship between difference-based coding and the constitution of local temporal continuity of neural activity. (*a*) The figure shows the relationship between the frequency range of fluctuations in the neural activity (i.e., the differences in the time span of the phase durations between the highest and the lowest frequency fluctuations) and the degree of temporal differences that can possibly be encoded into neural activity. The larger the degree of frequency ranges in the fluctuations of the neural activity, the larger the degree of temporal differences across different discrete points in physical time that can possibly be encoded into neural activity. (*b*) The figure shows the relationship between the frequency range of fluctuations in the neural activity (i.e., the differences in the time span of the phase durations between the highest and the lowest frequency fluctuation) and the degree to which the resulting stimulus-induced activity can go beyond the single stimulus and its physical features. The larger the degree of frequency ranges in the fluctuations of the neural activity, the larger the degree of going beyond the single stimulus and its physical features in the resulting stimulus-induced activity. (*c*) The figure shows the relationship between the frequency range of fluctuations in the neural activity (i.e., the differences in the time span of the phase durations between the highest and the lowest frequency fluctuation) and the degree of temporal continuity of neural activity. The larger the degree—that is, power and range—of frequency fluctuations in the neural activity, the larger the degree of temporal continuity of neural activity across different discrete points in physical time. (*d*) The figure shows the relationship between the degree of difference-based coding and the degree of temporal continuity of neural activity. The larger the degree of difference-based coding (when compared to stimulus-based coding), the larger the degree of temporal continuity of neural activity across different discrete points in physical time.

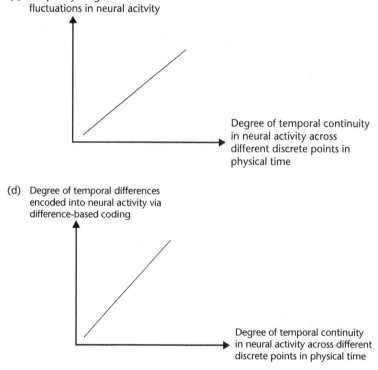

Figure 14-3a-d (Continued)

The chief founder of phenomenological philosophy was E. Husserl, who found successors, among others, in M. Merleau-Ponty, Jean-Paul Sartre, and Martin Heidegger as well as more current ones like Dan Zahavi, Alva Noe, and Evan Thompson (and see also Dainton 2008). Among other phenomenal features of consciousness like intentionality, they aim to reveal the specific structure of time in experience and thus in consciousness, that is, phenomenal time, what Husserl (1990) described as "inner time consciousness."

What is "inner time consciousness"?[1] We perceive and experience objects in the world in succession; that is, we perceive a flow of changing objects independent of whether they are stable or changing—there is continuous temporal flux entailing change and thus succession. On the other hand, we perceive and experience fixed and stable objects, objects persisting over time, implying temporal extension and duration. Succession and duration can be considered crucial features of our subjective experience of objects in time and thus of our inner time consciousness. This was already discussed in Chapter 13 when we referred to William James and his description of a "stream of consciousness."

Consider Husserl's (1990) example of a melody. We experience tones in continuous succession and change with one tone leading to the next tone. At the time, however, we retain the melody with the tones becoming temporally extended, overlapping and superseding each other. This first and foremost makes possible the experience of a melody while hearing the tones. Succession and duration of the melody imply that our consciousness must encompass more than that which is given right now. This means that the present moment cannot be considered an isolated and punctual moment detached from both the previous and the next moment.

Instead of being isolated and punctual, the present moment may be characterized by what

Husserl called the "width of present."[2] The concept of the width of present describes our ability to experience objects and events in our consciousness for a certain duration while succeeding the previous ones. "Succession" and "duration" do consecutively characterize the width of present in our experience of objects and events in consciousness.

PHENOMENOLOGICAL EXCURSION IB: "WIDTH OF PRESENT" VERSUS "KNIFE-EDGE PRESENT"

Both succession and duration would remain impossible if the present lacked any "width of present"; the present of objects and events in consciousness would then be characterized as "knife-edge present," which includes only one single discrete point in time, rather than as the "width of present" and its inclusion of several integrated single discrete points in time.

Let us detail this aspect further. Both succession and duration would be impossible if consciousness provided us only with access to the pure now-points of the objects. The same would hold if our experience were a mere series of unconnected now-points of experiences. This would resemble the loss of pearls when the chain is taken away. In this case we would be confronted with a series of isolated, punctual states without any interconnections. This would make both change, for example, succession, and duration and thus width impossible. Experience and thus consciousness would altogether be impossible in this case.

Let us apply this to our example of the melody. If our consciousness provided us with merely isolated and punctual states, that is, single discrete points in time, experience of a melody would become impossible. The experience of change and succession, which are essential to reveal a melody across the series of different tones, would no longer be given. The experience of a melody would then be replaced by hearing merely isolated and unconnected tones. There would no longer be any succession. In short: no succession, no melody.

At the same time, no tone would be temporally extended anymore in our experience. That would make any overlap and superseding of the tone right now with previous and next tones impossible. Hence, there would be no duration either. Due to the absence of both duration and succession, there would only be a series of right-now tones, which we would no longer be able to link and connect to a melody. In short, we would hear only tones but no melody. There would be no longer any width of present but only knife-edge present.

NEUROPHENOMENAL HYPOTHESIS IA: ENCODING OF TEMPORAL DIFFERENCES INTO NEURAL ACTIVITY PREDISPOSES "SUCCESSION" IN CONSCIOUSNESS

How now does the phenomenal concept of the "width of present" stand in relation to the neuronal concept of local temporal continuity? Let us recall: Local temporal continuity described the integration (linkage and connection) of different discrete points in physical time into statistically based temporal differences. The phenomenal concept of the width of present in contrast can be characterized by two phenomenal features, succession and duration.

How are neuronal and phenomenal descriptions related to each other? I hypothesize that the encoding of statistically based temporal differences in neural activity predisposes and thus makes possible not only the constitution of temporal continuity of neural activity, but also of both succession and duration, and thus ultimately of the width of present on the phenomenal level of consciousness.

Let me be more specific. By linking and connecting two different discrete points in physical time and their respectively associated tones, the two tones can no longer be segregated from each other in the resulting neural activity. This is so because the tones are encoded into neural activity in terms of their temporal difference from other that is past and future, tones, so that the neural activity "goes beyond" the single tone itself.

This implies that the tone occurring at a later discrete point in physical time is no longer arbitrarily and purely contingently tied to the previous tone and its particular discrete point in physical time. Instead, the later discrete point in time seems to be specifically tied to the preceding one, as defined by their specific temporal difference as distinguished from others. How is such non-arbitrary and non-contingent linkage between the two different tones possible? By encoding their specific temporal difference, the later tone is put into a relationship to its preceding tone. Most important, this relationship and thus their temporal difference are specific for the relationship between these two tones and may not hold for the same tone's relationship to another tone. This decreases the degree of contingency, or arbitrariness, in their relationship. Therefore, the later tone and its particular discrete point in time cannot avoid anymore to stand in a relationship of succession to the previous tone and its particular discrete point in physical time.

Accordingly, by encoding the different tones in terms of their temporal differences, the resulting neural activity "glues" (links and integrates) different tones together and generates a neural relationship between them that supersedes their physical features. Such a neural relationship in turn predisposes and thus makes possible a non-arbitrary and non-contingent relationship between the different tones in our experience; that is, in our consciousness.

How is that related to the degree of the encoding of statistically based temporal differences into neural activity? I propose the following: the more distinct and specific the degree of the encoded temporal difference between earlier and later tones is when compared to other temporal differences (between the same and other tones), the lower the degree of contingency and the higher the degree of succession that can possibly be associated with that particular tone sequence. How is that manifested in phenomenal consciousness? Very simple: we will hear the tones as connected and thus as a melody.

If, conversely, many other tone sequences also encode the same temporal difference into neural activity, their degree of succession will be rather low, while their degree of contingency

will be high. In that case, the tones may not be connected to a melody in our consciousness any more. I propose the degree of succession to be directly dependent on the degree of specificity of the temporal difference encoded between two (and more) different discrete time points and their associated stimuli.

For instance, hearing the same or closely related constellation of tones over and over again will become boring so that one no longer hears any melody anymore. This is obviously different if the same constellation or sequence of tones is played only once and preceded and followed by different, more or less unrelated, tones and sequences. In that case, the particular sequence of tones stands out and may therefore be more probably experienced as melody.

NEUROPHENOMENAL HYPOTHESIS IB: ENCODING OF TEMPORAL DIFFERENCES INTO NEURAL ACTIVITY PREDISPOSES "DURATION" IN CONSCIOUSNESS

How about the second phenomenal feature of the "width of present," duration? For that, we now take the perspective of the preceding tone and its particular discrete point in physical time. By being linked to the discrete point in time of the later tone, the single discrete point in physical time associated with the previous tone becomes extended and "stretched" toward the single discrete time point of the later tone.

Thereby, the degree of extension or stretching of the earlier discrete time point may depend on the degree of temporal difference between the two discrete time points: the larger their temporal difference that is encoded into neural activity, the more the previous tone can be extended in its associated neural activity, and the longer its subsequent duration in experience. If, in contrast, the temporal difference from the next tone's discrete time point is rather small, the degree of temporal extension of the preceding tone and its duration will decrease. I thus propose the degree of duration to be directly dependent on the degrees of temporal differences encoded between two (or more) different discrete time points and their associated stimuli.

Taking all this into consideration, I postulate that the width of present is directly related to the possible degree of local temporal continuity of neural activity and, more specifically, to the degree of statistically based temporal differences during the encoding of neural activity. The encoding of larger and more specific statistically based encoded temporal differences into neural activity is supposed to predispose higher degrees of "duration" on a phenomenal level and consequently a more extended width of present in consciousness (see Fig. 14-4a).

Conversely, the encoding of smaller and less specific statistically based temporal differences into neural activity leads to lower degrees of succession and duration on the phenomenal level of consciousness. This implies a lower degree of the width of present with reduced temporal extension and thus a higher degree of knife-edge present. The less the encoded neural activity "goes beyond" the stimulus' single discrete point in physical time, the more likely the present moment will shrink to a knife-edge present in consciousness. (see Fig. 14-4b–d).

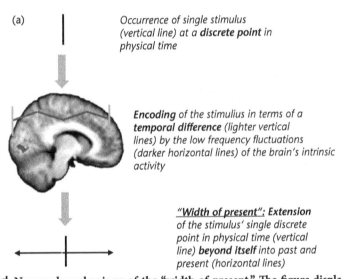

(a) Occurrence of single stimulus (vertical line) at a **discrete point** in physical time

Encoding of the stimulius in terms of a **temporal difference** (lighter vertical lines) by the low frequency fluctuations (darker horizontal lines) of the brain's intrinsic activity

"Width of present": Extension of the stimulus' single discrete point in physical time (vertical line) **beyond itself** into past and present (horizontal lines)

Figure 14-4a-d Neuronal mechanisms of the "width of present." The figure displays the neuronal mechanisms (*a*); that is, difference-based coding (*b*), low-frequency fluctuations (*c*), and local temporal continuities of neural activities (*d*) of the constitution of the width of present in inner time consciousness. (*a*) The figure shows the different stages from the extrinsic stimulus' occurrence (upper level) via its encoding into the brain's intrinsic activity in terms of a temporal difference (middle level) and the "width of present" (lower level). The most important step is here the encoding of the stimulus' discrete point in physical time in terms of a temporal difference by the brain's intrinsic activity. That makes it possible to extend or stretch the single discrete point in time beyond itself, as indicated in the "width of present," which corresponds to the regional activity in the brain. Note that the degree of the temporal differences by means of the single stimulus is encoded (as indicated by the lighter lines in the middle level) corresponds to the degree of time to which the single stimulus' discrete point in time can be extended beyond itself in both direction (past and future) as indicated by the line in the lower level. (*b*) The figure shows the relationship between the degree of temporal differences encoded into neural activity via difference-based coding and the degree of temporal extension ("succession" and "duration") of the width of present in inner time consciousness; that is, the latter's extension beyond the single discrete time point in the present moment. The higher the degree of temporal differences encoded into neural activity, the more the single discrete time point can be extended beyond its present moment. I propose a low degree of temporal differences being encoded in neural activity in vegetative state, anesthesia, and NREM sleep, which thus leads to a low degree of temporal extension in the width of present (and consequently to reduced inner time consciousness). (*c*) The figure shows the relationship between the

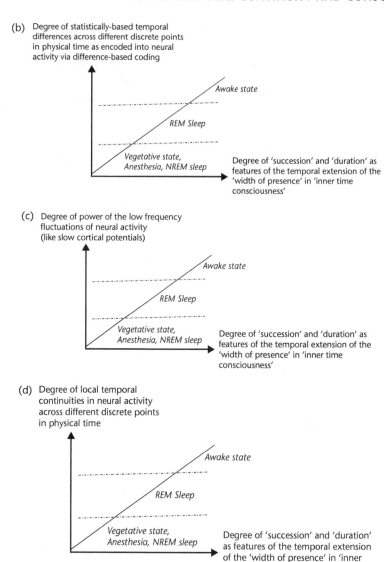

Figure 14-4a-d (Continued)
power of low-frequency fluctuations and the degree of temporal extension of the width of present in inner time consciousness; that is, the latter's extension beyond the single discrete time point in the present moment. The higher the power of low-frequency fluctuations, the more the single discrete time point can be extended beyond the present moment. I propose a low degree of difference-based coding in neural activity in vegetative state, anesthesia, and NREM sleep, which thus leads to a low degree of temporal extension in the width of present (and consecutively reduced inner time consciousness). (*d*) The figure shows the relationship between the degree of local temporal continuity of neural activity and the degree of temporal extension of the width of present in inner time consciousness; that is, the latter's extension beyond the single discrete time point in the present moment. The higher the degree of local temporal continuity of regional neural activity across different discrete points in physical time, the more the single discrete time point can be extended beyond the present moment. I propose a low degree of local temporal continuity of regional neural activity in vegetative state, anesthesia, and NREM sleep, which thus leads to a low degree of temporal extension in the width of present (and consequently to reduced inner time consciousness).

NEUROPHENOMENAL HYPOTHESIS IC: ENCODING OF TEMPORAL DIFFERENCES INTO NEURAL ACTIVITY DETERMINES THE LEVEL OR STATE OF CONSCIOUSNESS

I have so far focused only on the temporal characterization of the contents in consciousness, while I neglected its second dimension—the level or state of consciousness (see Introduction, this volume). The "level or state" means the degree of consciousness by itself and thus in terms of what psychologically is described as "arousal" independent of any contents (see Introduction, and Northoff 201).

How is my neurophenomenal hypothesis related to the level or state of consciousness? Following the phenomenological philosophers, higher degrees of the width of present should go along with higher degrees of (possible) consciousness. Conversely, this means that lower degrees of the width of present and consecutively higher degrees of the knife-edge present should lead to a decrease in, and ultimately loss of, consciousness.

I consequently claim that disorders of consciousness like the vegetative state and being under anesthesia should show lower degrees of succession and duration with subsequently low degrees of width of present and high degrees of knife-edge present. If so, they should show low degrees of difference-based and statistically based encoding of stimuli, while at the same time exhibiting a high degree of stimulus-based and physically based encoding of the stimuli's single discrete points in time. They should consequently show low degrees of temporal continuity in their neural activity.

This is exactly what can indeed be observed neuronally in these patients, as will be reported in full detail in Chapters 28 and 29. And that, by definition, goes along with extreme reduction in the level or state of consciousness. Accordingly, the example of disorders of consciousness provides empirical support (albeit indirectly) to my neurophenomenal hypothesis of the relationship between difference-based coding, temporal continuity, and state/level of consciousness.

NEUROCONCEPTUAL REMARK IA: DO SLOW CORTICAL POTENTIALS PROCESS THE CONTENTS OF CONSCIOUSNESS?

I started from the SCPs and He and Raichle's assumption of SCPs being central for consciousness. Thereby I shed a more detailed light on the kind of neuronal mechanisms that must occur to predispose and thus make possible the SCP's role in consciousness. This let me propose that SCPs and low-frequency fluctuations may indeed have a central role in consciousness, more specifically in constituting the width of present as the phenomenal hallmark of inner time consciousness.

Christoph Koch (2009) critically remarks that the hypothesis of SCP as the neural correlate of consciousness cannot account for the specificity of contents in consciousness. The contents surfacing in consciousness are highly specific, and (following his argument) this content specificity must be reflected in the underlying neuronal mechanisms. Each specific phenomenal content should correspond to a specific neuronal mechanism, as is presupposed in the hypothesis of the NCC. The NCC is thus a content-based hypothesis about the neuronal mechanisms of consciousness (see, though, Haynes 2009; de Graaf et al. 2012; Aru et al. 2012; Neisser 2011a and b; Northoff 2013; Hohwy 2011, for recent discussion about the concept of NCC with criticism resembling in part the one voiced here in the Introduction).

Koch argues that the hypothesis of the SCP violates the assumption of content specificity. The content specificity on the phenomenal level does not correspond to a neuronal specificity, since the SCPs are too unspecific. Why? The SCPs integrate information from various sources; therefore, they cannot mediate any specific content and consequently remain unable to account for content specificity on the phenomenal level. The hypothesis of the SCP thus implies a mismatch between specific contents on the phenomenal level and unspecific neuronal mechanisms in the gestalt of the SCP.

Koch's argument targets the SCP hypothesis with regard to the contents of consciousness that are supposed to correspond to certain neuronal states. The contents of consciousness, including their corresponding neuronal activities, are the result of a process that generates and yields them. This process may by itself be mediated by neuronal mechanisms that precede and must therefore be distinguished from those neuronal mechanisms that are directly related to the contents (of consciousness) themselves.

One may consequently need to distinguish between the encoding of neural activity as it is generated for the subsequent processing of any kind of content from the neuronal activities related to the actual processing of a specific content: I suppose the former, the encoding strategy during the generation of neural activity, to predispose consciousness itself independent of any particular contents. In contrast, the latter, the neuronal activities related to the actual processing of specific contents, are the neural correlates of the contents of consciousness rather than of consciousness itself. This shall be more explicated in further detail in the last section.

Neuroconceptual Remark IB: Slow Cortical Potentials are Neural Predisposition of Consciousness!

What does this imply for the hypothesis of the SCP as the neural correlate of consciousness? Koch's critic targets the assumption that the SCPs are the neuronal activities that correspond to specific contents in consciousness. However, his rejection of the SCP as the neural correlate of the contents of consciousness does not rule out that they have another yet-to-be-defined role in constituting consciousness itself independent of its contents.

Accordingly, Koch may be right in that the SCPs may not be involved in the neuronal activities underlying the contents of consciousness, while he may be wrong in that they have no role in consciousness at all. I hypothesize that the SCP may be a necessary neural condition that predisposes and makes possible the subsequent association of stimuli and their related contents with consciousness.

How can the SCP a necessary condition of the possible association of stimuli with consciousness? This is possible, as I propose, by the role of the SCP in constituting local temporal continuity as neural predisposition of the width of present on the phenomenal level of consciousness. In short, the SCP and their essential role in "double temporal integration" (see earlier) are a neural predisposition of consciousness.

Accordingly, instead of accounting for the contents themselves, SCPs seem to provide the very formal temporal structure and organization within which the contents (associated with the stimuli and their different discrete time points) are integrated such that they can be associated with consciousness. This means that the SCPs and their "double temporal integration" are necessary in temporally structuring and organizing the brain's neural activity in such a way that the latter can predispose and thus make possible consciousness.

Such temporal structure in the brain's neural activity—its temporal continuity, as described earlier—provides the temporal grid or template within which the different stimuli and their different discrete time points can be linked and integrated. The linkage and integration between different discrete points in physical time predisposes and thus makes possible the temporal extension of the contents in consciousness, the "width of present." Accordingly, to deny the SCP a role in consciousness is not only to confuse neural correlates and the neural predisposition of consciousness, but also to false positively identify contents in consciousness with consciousness itself and its particular temporal structure.

Open Questions

The first question pertains to the exact limits of possible temporal integration of neural activity. How large can the temporal differences between distinct discrete time points be that our brain can still integrate and link in one neural activity change? This is not only a question about the neuronal mechanisms but also one about the minimal and maximal biophysical-computational limits of our brain's neural processing and thus of difference-based coding. While phenomenal investigation may give us some hint here, detailed experimental procedures and possibly neural network simulation will be necessary to determine the exact biophysical-computational limits of the possible degree of temporal differences that can be encoded into neural activity on which the degree of width of present and its balance with the knife-edge present depends.

The second question concerns the concept of the width of present. While I described it in some detail, the exact characterization of its phenomenal features—succession and duration—remains unclear. Besides their conceptual-phenomenological description, one would like to also see an operationalization that allows them to be quantified and consecutively to be measured and investigated experimentally. This would be necessary to lend direct empirical support to the here suggested neurophenomenal hypotheses.

A region in the brain that has recently been closely associated with time experience and especially "present" is the insula in conjunction with the cortical midline regions (Wittmann 2009; Wittmann et al. 2010; Meissner and Wittmann 2011; Craig 2009, 2010a-c, 2011; van Wassenhove et al. 2011; Seth et al. 2011). Experimentally this has been realized by so-called subjective time dilation where the same stimulus (like a visual disc) is presented in different contexts so that it appears to be looming or receding.

This reveals strong activation activity changes in the insula and the cortical midline regions (see Wittmann et al. 2010; van Wassenhove et al. 2011; see Appendix 2 for further discussion). What is described as "subjective time dilation" in the experimental context may well correspond to what I here referred to as "width of present" within the phenomenal context (see also Appendix 2 for discussing Craig's cinemascopic theory of time and consciousness for which the insula is proposed to be central).

Finally, we here focused only on local temporal continuity, suggesting it to be central for what

phenomenally is described as width of present. The question is now how the constitution of several local temporal continuities in the different regions of the brain is connected and linked and integrated into the neural activity of neural networks and ultimately the whole brain, which can be described as "global temporal continuity." Global temporal continuity is constituted across all stimuli and regions and networks linking and integrating their respective different discrete points in physical time. This will be the focus of the next chapter.

Notes

1. It is clear that a full and detailed account of all aspects of this subject would be beyond the scope of this book. The focus on particular aspects of Husserl's account may confuse some philosophical experts, who may think that such isolation from the context impedes the exact characterization of the aspects in question, too. Right they are, but, as I said, a full account would be beyond the scope of this book. Hence, I leave it to future philosophers to put the here-proposed neurophenomenal hypotheses into the wider context of Husserl's and other authors' accounts of inner time consciousness.

2. The concept of the "width of present" may also very much resemble what William James (1890) described as "the specious present," which he described as the short duration of which we are immediately and instantaneously sensible (see also Dainton 2010 for a nice overview of time and consciousness, as well as Lloyd 2011, footnotes 1 and 2 especially, about James and Husserl on the concept of the "precious present").

CHAPTER 15
Temporal Nestedness and "Duration Bloc"

Summary

I discussed the neuronal mechanisms of the "width of present" in Chapter 14. The width of present was associated with the constitution of "local" temporal continuities of the neural activity in different regions. This raises the question how the different regions' local temporal continuities are linked and connected to each other and ultimately integrated into a more "global" temporal continuity. I here discuss findings that show each region to display a specific and idiosyncratic temporal pattern of neural activity. This will be complemented by showing that loss of consciousness is associated with decreased linkage and integration between high- and low-frequency fluctuations; that is, temporal nestedness. This leads me to hypothesize that consciousness is directly related to the degree of temporal nestedness between high- and low-frequency fluctuations. How is temporal nestedness constituted? I propose that the temporal nestedness may directly depend on difference-based coding. The larger the temporal differences encoded into neural activity via difference-based coding, the higher the possible degrees of both temporal nestedness and global temporal continuity of neural activity. And that in turn leads to increased degrees of consciousness. How is the global temporal continuity manifested in experience and thus in consciousness on the phenomenal level? I propose that the global temporal continuity of neural activity predisposes on the phenomenal level what phenomenological philosopher E. Husserl called "duration bloc." The concept of the duration bloc describes the integration of past, present, and future into one homogenous (though threefold) experience of time in consciousness. I hypothesize that the "global" temporal continuity of neural activity predisposes and makes possible such extension of the present into past and future on the phenomenal level of consciousness. By temporally structuring and organizing neural activity in a particular way, the global temporal continuity of the brain's neural activity makes necessary and unavoidable the constitution of the threefold temporal structure with past, present, and future, the duration bloc, on the phenomenal level of consciousness.

Key Concepts and Topics Covered

Temporal pattern of neural activity, low-frequency fluctuations, NREM sleep, resting state, slow wave activity, slow cortical potentials, temporal nestedness, difference-based coding, duration bloc, global temporal continuity

NEUROEMPIRICAL BACKGROUND IA: REGION-SPECIFIC TEMPORAL PATTERNS AND "LOCAL TEMPORAL CONTINUITIES"

Chapter 14 discussed slow cortical potentials and how they are related to the constitution of local temporal continuity of neural activity. Thereby, the concept of local temporal continuity referred to the integration of the different discrete time points of different stimuli in the neural activity of one particular region; that is, especially in its superficial layers 1 and 2 as manifested in slow cortical potentials (SCP) (see Chapter 14).

One may now propose the same process of temporal integration to occur in the various regions of the brain. Do the different regions' neural activities show the same local temporal continuities in their neural activities or different ones? This will be the focus of the present section. And one wants to know how that is related to the experience of time and thus to consciousness;

that is, "inner time consciousness." This will be discussed in the subsequent sections.

Let us start with the empirical data. Different regions receive different inputs and stimuli that differ in their respective statistical frequency distribution across different discrete points in physical time. As shown in Chapter 14, the constitution of local temporal continuity of neural activity is supposed to be based on the encoding of the stimuli's "temporal statistics"; that is, their statistical frequency distribution across different discrete points in physical time. Due to their different inputs and stimuli, one may consequently propose that the different regions show, not only different degrees of neural activity, but also different degrees of "local" temporal continuities. Different regions may thus show a different temporal pattern in their neural activities. This seems to be indeed the case, as is proposed by Bartels and Zeki (2004, 2005).

Bartels and Zeki (2004) investigated the visual cortex during conventional and natural stimulation in fMRI. Applying a model-free data-driven, that is, independent component analysis to their fMRI data, they observed that distinct subregions in the visual cortex show distinct time courses. For instance, the primary visual cortex (V1 and V2) showed negative signal changes during the stimulus period while returning afterward back to a high resting-state activity level. In contrast, signal changes and thus the waveform in V5 were very different from the one in V1/V2. Unlike V1/2, V5 exhibited lower resting-state activity and higher stimulus-induced activity.

Most important, the waveforms and thus the activity time curves (ATCs) were specific for each area/region, thereby distinguishing them in temporal regard. Furthermore, the time activity curves for each area were consistent across subjects. This is evidenced by the fact that the different subjects' ATCs in the same; that is, corresponding areas/regions highly correlated with each other. In contrast, the correlation of the ATCs between different areas/regions within the same subject was much lower than the correlation between the same regions across subjects. Finally, no correlation at all could be observed between different regions' ATCs from different subjects.

Taken together, this suggests area- or region-specific time curves that hold specifically for one particular region across different subjects. Moreover, since the correlation between the different regions within the same subjects was rather low when compared to the one of the same region across different subjects, Bartels and Zeki (2004) propose functional independence between the different regions in at least temporal regard.

NEUROEMPIRICAL BACKGROUND IB: FROM "LOCAL" TO "GLOBAL" TEMPORAL CONTINUITIES

The different regions of the brain do thus seem to have their specific temporal pattern of neuronal activity, which may distinguish them from each other. When conducted for the whole brain, this may ultimately generate what Bartels and Zeki (2004) call "chronoarchtitectonic maps." A chronoarchitectonic map is a time-based map of the brain's neural activity that illustrates the different temporal patterns in the different regions' neuronal activities.

What does the assumption of such region-specific different temporal patterns of neural activity imply for the constitution of local temporal continuity? Following the assumption of difference-based coding, different temporal patterns of neural activity are supposed to reflect the encoding of different degrees of temporal differences into the neural activities in the different regions. The temporal differences and consequently the respective stimuli's temporal statistics as the input to the different regions should therefore differ in the different regions. This implies that the resulting "local temporal continuities" for each region's neural activity should also differ from region to region.

More specifically, the degree of temporal extension of neural activity should be different between the different regions. Regions that encode larger temporal differences between their predominant stimulus' inputs may show a more extended "local" temporal continuity.

In contrast, local temporal continuity of neural activity may be less extended in those regions where the temporal differences between the predominant stimulus' inputs are shorter.

How are the different local temporal continuities from the different regions linked and connected to each other and how that is related to consciousness? For that, I now turn to sleep, specifically NREM sleep, and its slow wave activity.

NEURONAL FINDINGS IA: SLOW WAVE ACTIVITY IN NON–RAPID EYE MOVEMENT SLEEP

Sleep has been much investigated and is often considered a paradigmatic example of unconsciousness. One has to differentiate between different phases of sleep, however. There are early and late sleep stages where one cannot find rapid eye movements (REM), which led to the characterization of these phases as non-REM (NREM). The NREM sleep has to be distinguished from stages (in the middle of the night) with strong rapid eye movements (REM). Both NREM and REM have also been distinguished on phenomenal and electrophysiological grounds. (I here follow the traditional and broadly known classification with the distinction between REM and NREM sleep rather than adhering the most recent re-classification of the different sleep stages, which is known more to insiders at this point in time.)

The REM sleep has traditionally been associated with dreams (see Chapters 25 and 26 for details on dreams), while the NREM sleep is usually characterized by the absence of dreams, but this theory has been questioned more recently (see Nir and Tononi 2010). I here focus on NREM sleep and how it is distinguished from REM sleep; dreams will be investigated separately in Chapter 26.

How can we characterize NREM sleep? Electrophysiologically, NREM sleep can be distinguished by two particular features from REM sleep: NREM sleep shows slow wave activity (SWA) that is characterized by slow oscillations (<1 Hz) that usually last for around a second (see also Riedner et al. 2011 for an overview). These slow oscillations are supposed to be related to synchronization of the majority of cortical neurons, which oscillate between a depolarized upstate and a hyperpolarized downstate. In addition to the slow oscillations, one can also observe spindles that peak at 13–14 Hz and can be considered the second electrophysiological hallmark feature of NREM sleep.

NEURONAL FINDINGS IB: SLOW WAVE ACTIVITY (SWA) VERSUS SLOW CORTICAL POTENTIALS (SCP)

How are these SWA in NREM sleep related to the slow cortical potentials (SCPs) discussed in Chapter 14? SWA are spontaneous rhythmic oscillations of the membrane potential between a hyperpolarized downstate and a hypopolarized upstate. In addition to NREM sleep, SWA can also occur during anesthesia, where they are supposed to reflect the absence of specific attentional and other cognitive functions.

Are the SWA identical to the SCPs? He et al. (2008 supplementary material, note 3; see also He and Raichle 2009) deny that and distinguish between SWA and SCP for various reasons. First, their frequency ranges differ: SCPs show a large frequency spectrum ranging from 0.3 Hz to 4 Hz, while the one of SWA is rather narrow, centering around 0.8 Hz. Second, SWA are observed only during NREM sleep but neither in REM sleep nor in the awake state. This distinguishes them from SCPs, which, as described in Chapter 14, occur during all three, REM and NREM sleep and in the awake state (see also He et al. 2008; van Someren et al. 2011; Riedner et al. 2011; and Mascetti et al. 2011).

Third, the distribution of the SWA seems to be more or less independent of the underlying functional anatomy in that they seem to occur throughout the whole brain. In contrast, the SCPs are closely related to especially the midline regions of the default-mode network as discussed in Chapter 14 (see He and Raichle 2009). Fourth, SCPs may modulate the SWA so that the latter may be considered to be dependent upon the former.

Finally, in the preceding chapters we spoke of "fluctuations," whereas now we use the term "oscillation." What is the difference between fluctuations and oscillations? He and Raichle (2009) make a principal distinction between fluctuations and oscillations: oscillations describe rhythmic activity in EEG that centers on a specific frequency. This is the case in SWA that describe oscillatory activity centering on 0.8 Hz.

SCPs, in contrast, do not describe such oscillatory activity. Instead, they reflect fluctuations of neuronal activity that are not yet rhythmic but still arrhythmic. Hence, to equate SWA with SCPs would be to confuse rhythmic and arrhythmic neural activity and thus oscillations and fluctuations. Following this distinction, I here focus on SWA as oscillations, while the preceding chapter targeted fluctuations when discussing SCPs. (However, I will follow this distinction only rather loosely in this and the following chapters where I speak predominantly of fluctuations.)

NEURONAL FINDINGS IC: SLOW WAVE ACTIVITY AND MIDLINE REGIONS

Let us go back to the NREM sleep and its electrophysiological patterns. G. Tononi is a researcher from Italy. After having studied with Gerald Edelman and his theory of re-entrant connections (see Introduction I in Volume II), Tononi widened and extended that approach to information integration as a neural correlate of consciousness (see Appendix 1 for a detailed discussion of his information integration theory). In that context he is also very much interested in sleep and its loss of consciousness, especially during NREM sleep.

Tononi and his group applied 256-channel high-density electroencephalography (EEG). This use of such special EEG allows for high spatial resolution with the determination of the spatial and thus anatomical location of the signal, thereby complementing the high temporal resolution of the EEG. Concerning sleep, this makes it possible to localize the origin of SWA

and to investigate their spread and distribution across the rest of the brain; that is, their traveling waves (see Tononi 2009; Massimini et al. 2009, 2012, Nir et al. 2011; Riedner et al. 2011; Mascetti et al. 2011).

The data from the group around Tononi (see also Nir et al. 2011; Riedner et al. 2011; Mascetti et al. 2011) show the predominantly local origin of SWA: large currents of SWA (around 0.8 Hz, range between 0.3 and 6 Hz) appeared predominantly in the midline structures, including the anterior cingulate cortex, the posterior cingulate cortex, and the precuneus. From there the SWA seem to propagate preferentially to medial temporal regions, including the hippocampus (see Nir et al. 2011 for details). Hence, the midline regions seem to have a special role in constituting and processing SWA, in particular, and the low-frequency fluctuations in general (see Fig. 15-1).

What do these findings tell us? They show the regions that are implicated in generating the SWA. In contrast, the findings do not reveal themselves the kind of neuronal processes involved. How are SWA generated? They are generated locally and seem to reflect predominantly synaptic strength and thus local synaptic changes as shown in a combination of electrophysiological and simulation experiments (see Tononi 2009; Nir et al. 2011; Riedner et al. 2011). Let me specify this in the following.

Taken all these findings together as obtained in simulation models, rat's electrophysiological recordings, and human EEG let the authors suggest what they call "synaptic homeostasis hypothesis" (see Tononi 2009 as well as Tononi and Cirelli, 2003). The "synaptic homeostasis hypothesis" proposes that the SWA in NREM sleep may reflect the local synaptic strength and its decrease in sleep. Such synaptic decrease may serve the more general functional purpose of recalibrating neuronal circuits during sleep by desaturating them. This may prepare the neural circuits well for novel saturation in the subsequent awake state (see also Chapter 16 for more extensive discussion of physiological mechanisms).

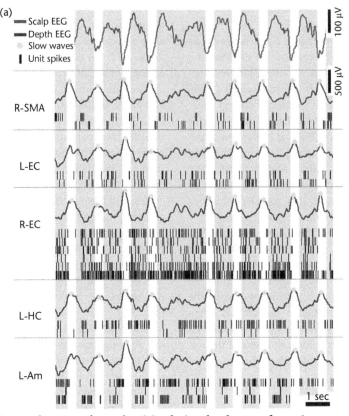

Figure 15-1 Temporal pattern of neural activity during the absence of consciousness. (*a*) Example of EEG and single-unit activity during global sleep slow waves. Example of EEG and unit activities in multiple brain regions during 11.5 s of deep NREM sleep in one individual. Rows (top to bottom) depict activity in scalp EEG (Cz), right supplementary motor area (R-SMA), left entorhinal cortex (L-EC), right entorhinal cortex (R-EC), left hippocampus (L-HC), and left amygdala (L-Am). Horizontal line in dark gray, scalp EEG; horizontal line in black, depth EEG; Vertical lines, unit spikes. Rounds dots in gray show individual slow waves detected automatically in each channel separately. Gray and white vertical bars through out the whole figure mark ON and OFF periods occurring in unison across multiple brain regions. (*b*) Sleep slow waves propagate across typical paths. (A) *Left*: Average-depth EEG slow waves in different brain structures of one individual illustrate propagation from frontal cortex to MTL. All slow waves are triggered by scalp EEG negativity. Black, scalp mean waveform. *Right*: Distributions of time lags for individual waves in supplementary motor area (SM) and hippocampus (HC) relative to scalp. (B) Mean position in sequences of propagating waves in all 129 electrodes across 13 individuals. Each circle denotes one depth electrode according to its precise anatomical location.. (C) Quantitative analysis: mean position in propagation sequences as a function of brain region. *Abbreviations*: SM, supplementary motor area; PC, posterior cingulate; OF, orbitofrontal cortex; AC, anterior cingulate; ST, superior temporal gyrus; EC, entorhinal cortex; Am, amygdala; HC, hippocampus; PH, parahippocampal gyrus. (D) An example of individual slow waves propagating from frontal cortex to MTL. Rows (top to bottom) depict activity in scalp EEG (Cz), supplementary motor area (SM), entorhinal cortex (EC), hippocampus (HC), and amygdala (Am).The dots mark center of OFF periods in each brain region based on the middle of silent intervals as defined by last and first spikes across the local population. Diagonal lines are fitted to OFF period times via linear regression and illustrate propagation trend. (E) Left: The average unit activity in frontal cortex (top, n = 76) and MTL (bottom, n = 155), triggered by the same scalp slow waves reveals a robust time delay (illustrated by vertical arrow). Right: Distribution of time delays in individual frontal (top) and MTL (bottom) units reveals a time delay of 187 ms. Red vertical arrows denote mean time offset relative to scalp EEG. Reprinted with permission of Cell Press, from Nir Y, Staba RJ, Andrillon T, Vyazovskiy VV, Cirelli C, Fried I, Tononi G. Regional slow waves and spindles in human sleep. *Neuron*. 2011 Apr 14;70(1):153–69.

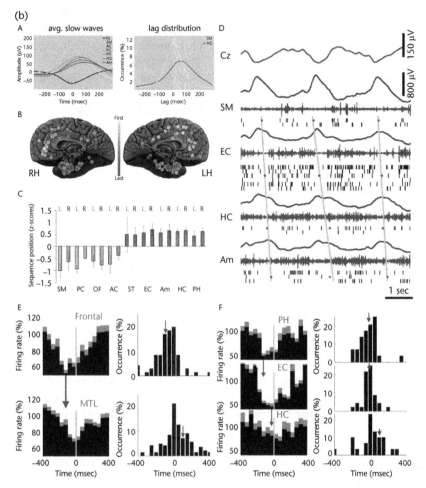

Figure 15-1 (Continued)

NEURONAL HYPOTHESIS

IA: "TEMPORAL NESTEDNESS" MEDIATES THE LEVEL/STATE OF CONSCIOUSNESS

What do these findings entail for the present and absence of consciousness? First and foremost, the SWA is by itself not sufficient to induce consciousness. Otherwise, there would be no loss of consciousness in NREM sleep that is characterized by predominance of SWA. This is further supported by the occurrence of SWA in another nonconscious state; namely, anesthesia, which, like NREM sleep, is also characterized by loss of consciousness.

How is it possible that we lose consciousness in NREM sleep (and anesthesia) despite the present of SWA? Let us recount. SWA describe oscillations in the lower frequency range centered around 0.8 Hz, which predominate during NREM sleep. In contrast, other higher frequency oscillations are rather rare in NREM sleep, with the exception of the aforementioned sleep spindles (12–13 Hz) and some slow waves with multiple negative peaks in the upper delta frequency range (2–4 Hz); that is, delta waves.

How do these waves, the spindles and the multiple negative peaks, occur? They seem to be closely related to the occurrence of SWA and may be quasi-nested in them. More specifically, Tononi (2009) proposes that the delta waves are generated on the basis of asynchronous SWA with different regional origins and/or different transregional propagation (see also Nir et al. 2011; Riedner et al. 2011; van Someren et al. 2011; Mascetti et al. 2011). If so, the delta waves simply represent an overlay or nesting of different SWAs and thus of multiple slow oscillations with distinct spatial and temporal features. In short, the delta waves may result from the temporal nesting of higher in lower frequency oscillations.

Interestingly, an almost analogous temporal nesting of different frequency waves was already described in the previous section on slow cortical potentials (SCP). Here too, based on He et al. (2010), higher frequency oscillations were proposed to be nested within lower frequency oscillations and ultimately within slow wave fluctuations like the SCP.

What then is the main difference between NREM sleep and the awake state and thus between absence and presence of consciousness? I hypothesize that the difference may consist in the degree of temporal nestedness between different frequency ranges. Higher degrees of temporal nestedness between high- and low-frequency fluctuations may go along with a higher degree in the level or state of consciousness as in the awake state. Conversely, lower degrees of temporal nestedness should lead to lower degrees in the level or state of consciousness as in NREM sleep.

NEURONAL HYPOTHESIS
IB: CONSCIOUSNESS IS LIKE THE RUSSIAN DOLLS

What exactly do I mean by "temporal nestedness"? The concept of temporal nestedness describes the relationship between high- and low-frequency fluctuations in the neural activity of the brain. It is important to note that temporal nestedness goes beyond mere co-occurrence of high- and low-frequency fluctuations.

In addition to the presence of both high- and low-frequency fluctuations, they also need to be directly connected and linked, that is, integrated. The smaller time windows of the high-frequency fluctuations should be integrated and situated; that is, nested, within the longer phase durations of the low-frequency fluctuations. Such temporal nesting is supposed to be mediated, in part, by the temporal alignment of low frequency fluctuations' phase onsets to the high frequency

fluctuations, including their phase onsets and power: their cross-frequency phase-phase and phase-power coupling (see Chapter 5 as well as Chapters 19 and 20 for details).

How can we better illustrate such temporal nestedness? Let us compare the difference between temporal nestedness and temporal co-occurrence to the well-known Russian dolls. Usually, there is one large Russian doll, which, if we open its head, contains another slightly smaller Russian doll, and so forth. The Russian dolls are thus nested within each other. If one puts different Russian dolls of different sizes on the table, they can be said to merely co-occur, while they are not nested into each other.

The same is the case in the low- and high-frequency fluctuations. If the high-frequency fluctuations are integrated in the longer phases of the lower frequency fluctuations, one can speak of temporal nestedness. This corresponds to the sorting the Russian dolls according to their size and ultimately putting them all together into one big doll. If, in contrast, there is no such integration, high- and low-frequency fluctuations stand only side by side, just like the different Russian dolls of different sizes lying beside each other on the table.

Based on these considerations, I suggest the following. I hypothesize that the difference in the degree of temporal nestedness between different frequency ranges predisposes the absence or presence of consciousness: the higher the degree of temporal nestedness between different—lower and higher—frequency ranges, the more likely consciousness is to occur and thus to be present. This parallels the case when we find 20 Russian dolls within one big one (see Fig. 15-2a).

Conversely, the lower the degree of temporal nestedness between different—lower and higher frequency—ranges, the more likely consciousness will remain absent. This parallels the situation when there are only two Russian dolls within one big one, or all three lying side by side on the table. That may, for instance, be the case in NREM sleep, anesthesia, and vegetative state, where consciousness remains absent.

Metaphorically speaking, it is the number of dolls and how they are linked that ultimately

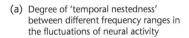
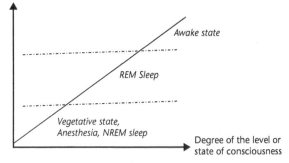

(a) Degree of 'temporal nestedness' between different frequency ranges in the fluctuations of neural activity

Awake state

REM Sleep

Vegetative state, Anesthesia, NREM sleep

Degree of the level or state of consciousness

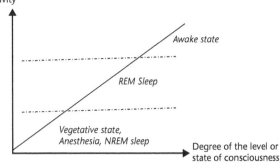

(b) Degree of temporal differences between the different frequency ranges in the fluctuations as they are encoded into neural activity

Awake state

REM Sleep

Vegetative state, Anesthesia, NREM sleep

Degree of the level or state of consciousness

Figure 15-2a and b Temporal nestedness and consciousness. The figure displays the relationship between the fluctuations of neural activity and the degree of consciousness. (*a*) The figure shows the dependence of the degree of the state or level of consciousness on the degree of temporal nestedness between different frequency ranges in the fluctuations of the neural activity. The better the high and thus shorter frequency fluctuations are linked and connected and thus nested into the longer phases of the low-frequency fluctuations, the higher the degree of the level or state of consciousness that can possibly be constituted. Hence, a lower degree of such temporal nestedness will then go along with low degrees in the level or state of consciousness, as in vegetative state, anesthesia, and NREM sleep. (*b*) The figure shows the dependence of the degree of the state or level of consciousness on the degree of temporal differences as they are encoded between the different frequency ranges in the fluctuations of the neural activity. The higher the degree or range of the temporal differences between the different frequency ranges in the neural activity fluctuations that can possibly be encoded into neural activity, the higher the possible degree of the level or state of consciousness that can be constituted. Hence, lower degrees or ranges of encoded temporal differences should go along with lower degrees of the level or state of consciousness as in vegetative state, anesthesia, and NREM sleep.

predisposes whether consciousness will be present or remain absent. Accordingly, the Russian dolls are not just traditional symbols of Russian culture, but also a wonderful (metaphorical) symbol of consciousness itself and its particular temporal (and spatial) structure.

NEURONAL HYPOTHESIS IC: DIFFERENCE- VERSUS STIMULUS-BASED CODING

Now let us go back to NREM sleep and consciousness. As described earlier, NREM sleep can be characterized by the predominance of local and asynchronous out-of-phase SWA and the concurrent absence of higher frequency waves in its resting-state activity; that is, in the absence of specific extrinsic stimuli (see also Nir at al. 2011). In contrast, higher frequency waves are well present and very abundant in the awake state during its resting-state activity. Accordingly, the resting-state activity's degree of temporal nestedness between different frequency ranges may be much higher in the awake state when compared to NREM sleep.

Due to its different resting-state activity pattern, neural activity during NREM sleep may no longer be able to properly process extrinsic stimuli. A 2011 fMRI-EEG investigation by Dang-Vu et al. (2011) demonstrated less consistent neuronal responses in auditory cortex and thalamus during auditory stimulation in NREM sleep. The neural processing of the auditory stimulus was severely hampered by the slow wave oscillations and the spindles typically occurring in the NREM sleep.

Accordingly, the ongoing rather slow resting-state activity in NREM seems to prevent the auditory stimulus from being properly processed in the brain. This may make it impossible for the stimulus to become linked and integrated into the brain's ongoing intrinsic activity; that in turn, could be crucial for the association of the resulting stimulus-induced activity with consciousness (see Chapters 11 and 29 for the detailed neuronal and neurophenomenal mechanisms of such rest–stimulus interaction).

What does this mean exactly? The auditory stimulus may not be properly processed in the brain anymore because it cannot be linked and connected to the brain's intrinsic activity. Why? The brain and its intrinsic activity are busy with other things; the SWA, and, metaphorically speaking, "have no time to take care of the extrinsic stimulus." More specifically, the auditory stimulus cannot be encoded into neural activity relative to the resting-state activity level. The degree of difference-based coding of the auditory stimulus will consequently be rather low which, as we have seen in Volume I (see Chapter 1), goes along with a high degree of stimulus-based coding. Even if the auditory stimulus induces some activity changes in the brain, these may only be related to the stimulus itself while remaining independent of the brain's intrinsic activity.

Why does the resulting stimulus-induced activity remain more or less independent of the brain's intrinsic activity? The stimulus is no longer encoded into neural activity in relative difference to the intrinsic activity but is rather independent of it in a more stimulus-based way. Accordingly, the neural processing of the stimulus may then be characterized by a low degree of difference-based coding and a rather high degree of stimulus-based coding.

NEURONAL HYPOTHESIS ID: DIFFERENCE-BASED CODING MEDIATES THE LEVEL/STATE OF CONSCIOUSNESS

This leads me to the following hypothesis. I propose the hypothesized relationship between temporal nestedness and consciousness to be mediated by difference-based coding. The encoding of temporal differences between high- and low-frequency fluctuations allows for integration of the different frequency ranges and thus for their temporal nesting. Higher degrees of difference-based coding should thus go along with higher degrees of temporal nestedness between high- and low-frequency fluctuations and consequently with higher degrees in the level or state of consciousness.

In contrast, lower degrees of temporal nestedness (and consequently higher degrees of mere temporal co-occurrence) may signify a high degree of stimulus-based coding. The balance between difference- and stimulus-based coding is here shifted toward the latter, which in turn decreases the likelihood that the resulting neural activity is associated with a high level or state of consciousness. That may, for instance, be the case in NREM sleep, anesthesia, and vegetative state, with all three supposedly showing a high degree of stimulus-based coding (when compared to the degree of difference-based coding) and rather low, if not absent, level or state of consciousness (see Chapters 28 and 29 for details).

This amounts to the following relationship between difference-based coding and the state or level of consciousness: the higher the degree of difference-based coding (and the lower the degree of stimulus-based coding) in the neural coding between high- and low-frequency fluctuations, the higher the degree of the level or state of consciousness. Accordingly, I propose the degree of consciousness to be directly related to the degree of the encoding of temporal differences into neural activity; that is, difference-based coding.

Conversely, low degrees of difference-based coding and consequently high degrees of stimulus-based coding should decrease the likelihood of high degrees in the level or state of consciousness. In the extreme case of abnormally high degrees of stimulus-based coding, one would expect loss of consciousness, which is exactly what one observes in NREM sleep, anesthesia, and vegetative state (see Fig. 15-2b; and see Chapters 28 and 29 for details).

Neuronal Hypothesis
IIA: DIFFERENCE-BASED CODING AND TEMPORAL NESTEDNESS

Why do I propose that the degree of temporal nestedness between the different frequency ranges predisposes consciousness? Let me first detail what temporal nestedness implies in neuronal terms. During the resting-state activity, temporal nestedness between different frequency ranges may be traced back to the neural overlay of extrinsic stimulus-triggered high-frequency fluctuations onto the intrinsic low-frequency fluctuations (see Chapter 5 in Volume I for details as well as Part VI in Volume II).

This means that the resulting higher frequency wave must really be considered the product of a temporal difference: the temporal difference between the phase onset and duration of the low-frequency fluctuations on the one hand and the discrete point in physical time associated with the stimulus on the other. The encoding of the temporal difference between the intrinsic activity's phase onset and the extrinsic stimulus' discrete time point is possible, however, only on the basis of difference-based coding, whereas it remains impossible in the case of stimulus-based coding.

I consequently hypothesize that the temporal nestedness of different frequency waves may directly depend on the degree of temporal differences encoded into neural activity via difference-based coding: The more fine-grained the temporal differences are encoded into neural activity via difference-based coding, the higher degrees of temporal nestedness between different ranges of frequency fluctuations can be constituted in the resulting neural activity.

Consider again the analogous example of the Russian dolls. The smaller the differences in size between the different dolls, the more dolls that can be fitted within the largest one, resulting in a higher degree of nestedness. The same now applies to the degree of temporal differences between the different ranges of frequency fluctuations as they are encoded into neural activity. As in the case of the Russian dolls, the encoding of more fine-grained and thus smaller temporal differences results in higher degrees of temporal nestedness.

Neuronal Hypothesis IIB: Encoding of Temporal Differences by the Intrinsic Activity's Low-Frequency Fluctuations

In addition to the different degrees of temporal differences between different ranges of frequency fluctuations, the brain is also confronted with different degrees of temporal differences as encoded in the different regions' intrinsic activities. We recall the findings from Bartels and Zeki, who showed that each region has its specific temporal pattern of neural activity.

This indicates that the degree of temporal differences encoded into the regions' neural activities must differ between the different regions. Some regions may predominantly encode larger temporal difference, while other regions, based on the temporal statistics of their predominant stimulus input, may encode smaller and more fine-grained temporal differences (see earlier for details).

How are the different regions' different temporal activity patterns and thus their different local temporal continuities linked and connected to each other? For that, the fluctuations in neural activity may be central. The fluctuations in neural activity, especially the low-frequency fluctuations, operate across different regions and their respective local temporal continuities.

If now the fluctuations show a broad frequency range with many intermediate frequency ranges, they will be well able to link and connect a higher multitude of local regional temporal differences and thus different local temporal continuities. I consequently propose a broad frequency range and a high variability in the frequency range to be central for the integration of neural activities in different regions (see also Garrett et al. 2011; as well as McDonnell and Ward 2011, for the relevance of variability).

This leads me to the following hypothesis. I propose that the degree to which the different regions' temporal differences can be linked and connected to each other depends very much on the degree of the range in the fluctuations' frequencies. A higher range of the fluctuations' frequencies implies a large difference between the highest and lowest frequencies with many intermediate frequency ranges.

That makes it more likely that the different regions' temporal differences can be matched and thus be connected to each other. The diverse "local" temporal continuities can consequently be integrated and nested into one "global" temporal continuity. The concept of global temporal continuity describes the linkage, integration, and ultimately synchronization between the local temporal activities of the different regions.

Neuronal Hypothesis IIc: "Global" Temporal Continuity of Neural Activity Mediates the Level/State of Consciousness

"Global" temporal continuity in this sense comes close to what is described as the "global neuronal workspace" in the current neuroscience literature on consciousness (see Baars 2005; Dehaene and Changeux 2011), though specified in temporal regard (see Chapters 18 and 19 and also Appendix 1 for a detailed discussion of the concept of the global neuronal workspace in relation to my neurophenomenal account).

Why is the global temporal continuity important? The global temporal continuity may predispose the association of the resulting neural activity with consciousness, as is the case in the awake state and, to some degree, also during dreams in REM sleep. The converse case is the one when the range of the fluctuations' frequencies is rather low. This means that the difference between the highest and lowest frequencies is rather small and/or that not many intermediate frequency ranges are present. Such a lower frequency range is less likely to be able to link the different regions' different temporal differences to each other. (see Fig. 15-3a).

The different regions' local temporal continuities may therefore no longer be well integrated and thus nested into each other so that the degree of the resulting global temporal continuity is rather low. That in turn decreases the likelihood of associating the respective neural activity with a high level or state of consciousness, as can indeed be observed in NREM sleep, anesthesia, and vegetative state (see also Chapter 16 as well as Chapters 28 and 29 for more detail). This is well in accordance with the observation of decreased spatial and temporal spread and propagation of externally induced neural activity changes these three states, as will be described in further detail in Chapter 16 (for NREM sleep and anesthesia) and Chapters 28 and 29 (for vegetative state) (see Fig. 15-3b).

In sum, I propose the number and the degree of temporal differences that are encoded into neural activity via difference-based coding to predict the degree to which the different regions' "local" temporal continuities are extended into a more "global" temporal continuity. That, in turn, may predispose the possible degree of the state or level of consciousness: higher degrees of global continuity of neural activity make more likely the association of a higher degree of the level or state of consciousness. Accordingly, larger degrees of temporal differences during the encoding of neural activity predispose a higher degree of global temporal continuity and consequently a higher level or state of consciousness.

Phenomenological Excursion Ia: "Inner Time Consciousness" and "Duration Bloc"

The question now is how such "global" temporal continuity of the brain's neural activity is manifested in our experience and thus in consciousness. Recall from the previous chapter that the

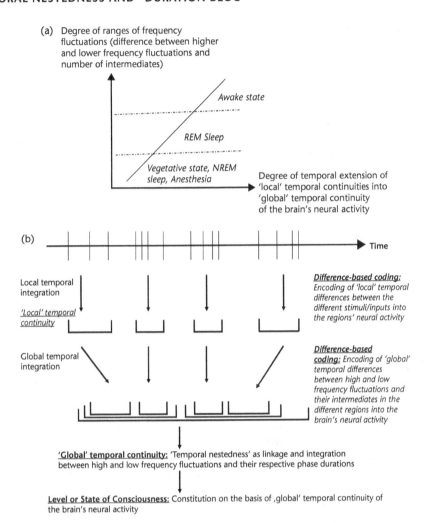

(a) Degree of ranges of frequency
    fluctuations (difference between higher
    and lower frequency fluctuations and
    number of intermediates)

Awake state

REM Sleep

Vegetative state, NREM
sleep, Anesthesia

Degree of temporal extension of
'local' temporal continuities into
'global' temporal continuity
of the brain's neural activity

(b)   Time

Local temporal
integration

'Local' temporal
continuity

Difference-based coding:
Encoding of 'local' temporal
differences between the
different stimuli/inputs into
the regions' neural activity

Global temporal
integration

Difference-based
coding: Encoding of 'global'
temporal differences
between high and low
frequency fluctuations and
their intermediates in the
different regions into the
brain's neural activity

'Global' temporal continuity: 'Temporal nestedness' as linkage and integration
between high and low frequency fluctuations and their respective phase durations

Level or State of Consciousness: Constitution on the basis of 'global' temporal continuity of
the brain's neural activity

Figure 15-3a and b Temporal nestedness and "global" temporal continuity. The figure depicts the relationship between temporal nestedness of different frequency ranges and the degree of "global" temporal continuity of the brain's neural activity. (*a*) The figure shows the dependence of the degree of temporal extension of local temporal continuities into a more "global" temporal continuity on the degree of frequency ranges in the fluctuations of the brain's neural activity. The higher the degree of frequency ranges (i.e., differences between highest and lowest) and the number of intermediate frequency ranges, the more the "local" temporal continuities (from the different regions/networks of the brain) can possibly be integrated and extended into a more "global" temporal continuity that spans across the whole brain and all its regions' neural activities. I propose the range of frequency fluctuations to be rather low in vegetative state, anesthesia, and NREM sleep (see Chapters 28 and 29 for empirical support), which consequently go along with lower degrees of temporal extension from "local" temporal continuities to a more "global" temporal continuity in the brain's neural activity. The extension from "local" to "global" temporal continuity of neural activity is supposed to be mediated by difference-based coding; for example, by encoding the temporal differences between the regions' different inputs (bars in uppermost line on the time arrow and second-highest line as well as right upper part). (*b*) The figure demonstrates how various "local" temporal continuities in particular regions (upper and middle upper part) are integrated by connecting high- and low-frequency fluctuations to each other, resulting in temporal nestedness with "global" temporal continuity of neural activity and, ultimately, consciousness (middle and lower part). This is supposed to be mediated by difference-based coding; for example, by encoding the temporal differences between different stimuli (right upper part) and the different frequency ranges into the resulting neural activity (right lower part).

local temporal continuity was associated phenomenally with what phenomenological philosopher E. Husserl described as the "width of the present" (see Chapter 14). The question now is how what I described as the "global" temporal continuity is manifested in "inner time consciousness." For the answer, I again turn to Husserl.

Husserl argues that the width of the present can be stretched and extended deeply into both past and future (we remember, for instance, the imaging findings on "prospection" and retrospection as described in Chapter 13). Such extension and stretching of the width of the present into the future and past may result in what Husserl described as "duration bloc." The duration bloc comprises and interconnects previous, present, and next moments, reflecting the three temporal modes of past, present, and future (Husserl 1991, 23, 113–114). Husserl calls these three temporal modes of the duration bloc "primal presentation," "protention," and "retention" which shall be described briefly in the following explanation.

Let us start with the "primal presentation." The duration bloc includes the right-now moment, the moment the object appears or when the tone is actually played—this may be called "primal presentation" (Zahavi 2005, 56). The here and now of the primal presentation is, however, not abstracted and isolated from the previous and next here-and-now moments, which are built into and thus enclosed in the current right-now moment.

How is such integration possible? In addition to primal presentation, there is a second element in the duration bloc: namely, retention. Retention is the component that provides us with conscious access to the just-elapsed phase of the preceding object, the previous moment that occurred just before the current right-now moment. The preceding object is retained and can therefore be carried over to the current object and thus be enclosed in the experience of the current right-now moment object. This comes close to what we, relying on William James, described as "sensible continuity" in Chapter 13.

Due to retention (and "sensible continuity"), we hear the current tone in relation to the previous one, with this temporal connection between past and present tones enabling us to decipher both previous and current tones as part of a melody. The previous tone is carried over to the current one. Without such retention both tones could not be connected in consciousness, which in turn would make experience of the tones as a melody impossible.[1]

In addition to retention of previous tones, we also anticipate the next tone, which enables us to complement the melody, even if not all tones are actually played. This leads to the third element of the duration bloc: *protention* (Husserl 1991). Listening to a melody, we often anticipate; we expect a particular tone and will be surprised if the anticipated tone does not match with the actually occurring next tone. Similar to retention, "protention" is connected to the current object while at the same time extending it to the beyond the actually occurring right-now moment to the next not-yet occurred moment.

Phenomenological Excursion
1B: THREEFOLD TEMPORAL STRUCTURE AND MUTUAL MODULATION

Let me now shed a more detailed light on how the three elements, primal presentation, retention, and protention, are related to each other. We listen to the actually occurring tone within the context of the potentially occurring (anticipated) next tone. This enables us to decipher the present tone as part of a continuous melody extending from the past, over the present, to the future. If, for example, we anticipate the tone E after C, we listen to C in relation to the (potential) tone E.

If we anticipate another C rather than E, we would listen to the present C in a completely different way than when we were anticipating E or F. The primal presentation is thus strongly impacted, modulated, and changed by protention. The anticipated tone seems to have some feedback effect (as one may call it) upon the present tone in our perception. And the same holds for retention. There is thus not only connection but mutual modulation between primal presentation, retention, and protention. The concept of mutual modulation describes that all three, presentation, retention, and protention are interdependent on each other with the constitution of the one being intrinsically related to the respective others and vice versa.

Let us describe such mutual modulation in more detail. Go one step further and imagine you anticipated E and now finally the real tone kicks in. If it is indeed the tone E, you are happy and continue singing the melody.

If, in contrast, it is not the tone E but another one, there are two options. Either the next tone is not E but F, which may continue the melody, but in an unexpected way. You are then surprised and are probably unable to sing the melody completely, but your attention is nevertheless caught by the unexpected turn of the melody. Alternatively, the next tone may be C, which does not continue the melody at all, but rather disrupts and terminates it completely. You may be disappointed and turn your attention away from the tones and stop listening altogether.

Taken together, this results in what Husserl described as the threefold structure of our experience of objects in time, including primal presentation, retention, and protention:

> In this way, it becomes evident that concrete perception as original consciousness (original givenness) of a temporally extended object is structured internally as itself a streaming system of momentary perceptions (so-called primal impressions). But each such momentary perception is the nuclear phase of a continuity, a continuity of momentary graded retentions on the one side, and a horizon of what is coming on the other side: a horizon of "protention," which is disclosed to be characterized as a constantly graded coming. (Husserl 1977, 202)

NEUROPHENOMENAL HYPOTHESIS IA: "GLOBAL" TEMPORAL CONTINUITY OF NEURAL ACTIVITY MEDIATES THE "DURATION BLOC" IN CONSCIOUSNESS

How, then, is what Husserl describes as "duration bloc" on the phenomenal level of consciousness related to the neuronal processes in the brain? First, I propose that the duration bloc corresponds well to what I described earlier as "global" temporal continuity of neural activity. The duration bloc describes the continuity

between past, present, and future on the phenomenal level of consciousness.

How does that relate to the global temporal continuity of neural activity? The concept of the global temporal continuity concerns the integration of different local temporal continuities into one more general and thus "global" temporal continuity. As such, the "global" temporal continuity is supposed to span the different regions' local temporal continuities in their neural activities, including their respective different temporal differences.

By integrating different "local" temporal continuities, the "global" temporal continuity links and connects different temporal differences. The more diverse temporal differences are linked and connected, the more the resulting "global" temporal continuity can extend across different discrete points in physical time from the present into both past and future discrete points in physical time. In short, higher degrees of "global" temporal continuity lead to higher degrees of temporal extension of neural activity.

How is that related to the "threefold temporal structure" and thus the "duration bloc" on the phenomenal level of consciousness? The higher the degree of temporal extension of the "global" neural activity from present into past and future, the more and better the threefold structure of time, with present, past, and future, can be constituted and therefore comes close to what Husserl described as a "duration bloc" (see Fig. 15-4a).

Based on these considerations, I propose that the degree of "global" temporal continuity of neural activity predisposes the degree of the "duration bloc" on the phenomenal level of consciousness: the higher degree of "global" temporal continuity in the brain's neural activity, the higher the possible degree of the "duration bloc" on the phenomenal level of consciousness. If, in contrast, the degree of "global" temporal continuity is rather low, the degree of temporal extension of the "duration bloc" will abnormally shrink, with a more limited time range between past and future (see Fig. 15-4b).

We have seen earlier that the "global" temporal continuity of the brain's neural activity ultimately depends on the degree of the

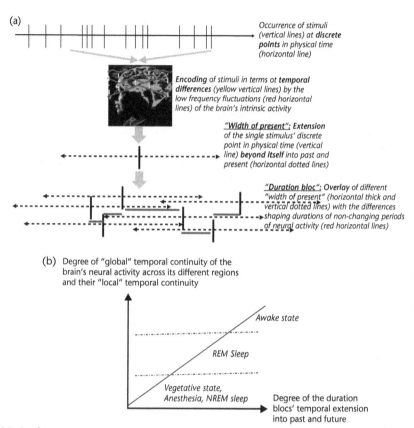

Figure 15-4a-d Neural predispositions of the "duration bloc." The figure displays how different neuronal mechanisms (*a, b, c, d*) predispose the degree of the temporal extension of the duration bloc from the present into the past and future. (*a*) The figure shows the different stages from the extrinsic stimuli's occurrence (upper level) via their encoding into the brain's intrinsic activity in terms of temporal differences (second from upper level) and the "width of present" (second from lower level) to the constitution of the "duration bloc" (lower level). The most important step is here the encoding of the different stimuli's discrete points in physical time in terms of temporal differences by the brain's intrinsic activity and its low-frequency fluctuations. That makes it possible to extend or "stretch" the single discrete point in time beyond itself, as indicated in the "width of present," which corresponds to the regional activity in the brain. The overlay of the different regional activities and their respectively associated "width of present" leads to the "duration bloc"; the concept of "duration" describes temporally homogenous stretches of neural activity where it does not change, which corresponds to phase durations that are not interrupted either by other frequencies or stimuli (see horizontal lines in the lower part). (*b*) The figure shows the dependence of the degree of the temporal extension of the duration bloc from the present into the past and future on the degree of the "global" temporal continuity of the brain's neural activity. The higher the degree and the larger the extension of the "global" temporal continuity of the brain's neural activity, the higher the number of past and future discrete time points covered by the neural activity, and the larger the possible extension of the duration bloc in "inner time consciousness." (*c*) The figure shows the dependence of the degree of the temporal extension of the duration bloc into past and future on the degree of the temporal differences between the different frequency ranges in the fluctuations as they are encoded into neural activity. The higher the degree (and number) of temporal differences encoded into neural activity, the more the actual discrete time points in the present can be extended into future and past ones, which predisposes a larger extension of the duration bloc in inner time consciousness. (*d*) The figure shows the dependence of the degree of the temporal extension of the duration bloc into past and future on the degree of temporal nestedness between the different frequency ranges in the fluctuations

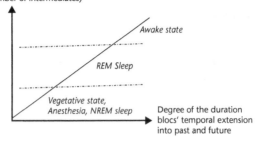

(c) Degree of temporal differences between the different frequency ranges in the fluctuations of neural activity (differences between highest and lowest and number of intermediates)

Awake state

REM Sleep

Vegetative state, Anesthesia, NREM sleep

Degree of the duration blocs' temporal extension into past and future

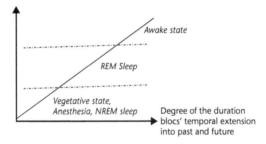

(d) Degree of temporal nestedness between the different frequency ranges in the fluctuations of neural activity (i.e., phase-locking)

Awake state

REM Sleep

Vegetative state, Anesthesia, NREM sleep

Degree of the duration blocs' temporal extension into past and future

Figure 15-4a-d (Continued)
of neural activity; that is, phase-phase or phase-power coupling. The higher the degree of temporal nestedness, the more the actual discrete time points in the present can be extended into future and past ones, which predisposes a larger extension of the duration bloc in inner time consciousness.

temporal differences encoded into neural activity and the range of the different frequency fluctuations. This implies that the degree of the "duration bloc" on the phenomenal level of consciousness is ultimately predisposed by the degree of temporal differences encoded into neural activity via difference-based coding and the range of different frequency fluctuations and their degree of temporal nestedness (see Fig. 15-4 c, d).

NEUROPHENOMENAL HYPOTHESIS
IB: PREDICTIVE CODING VERSUS "GLOBAL" TEMPORAL CONTINUITY

One may now be surprised to see the parallels of (especially) the protention in the threefold temporal structure to the assumption of a predicted input as in predictive coding. We recall from Chapters 7 through 9 in Volume I where we discussed predictive coding. Predictive coding means that the brain generates a predicted input, an anticipation of the forthcoming or expected stimulus, that is then compared and matched with the actual input. The result is described as the "prediction error," which is supposed to determine the degree of stimulus-induced activity.

How is such predictive coding, and especially the predicted input, related to the protention in the threefold temporal structure of the "duration bloc"? First and foremost, the concept of predictive coding is a functional concept that is applied to the brain and its neural activity. This distinguishes the concept of predictive coding from those of "duration bloc" and "protention," which are phenomenal rather than functional concepts. As such, both need to be distinguished from my concept of "global" temporal continuity, which is a purely neuronal concept.

How does my concept of "global" temporal continuity stand in relation to predictive coding? As detailed in Chapters 7 through 9 in Volume I, predictive coding presupposes the processing of contents and thus stimulus-induced activity, while largely neglecting the relevance of the brain's intrinsic activity independent of any stimulus processing (whether real or anticipated). This is different in my concept of "global" temporal continuity, which is supposed to operate across the boundaries of resting-state and stimulus-induced activity. Even stronger, "global" temporal continuity is supposed to be already at work in the resting-state activity of the brain itself and therefore characterizes the temporal structure of the brain's intrinsic activity.

That has important implications. The extrinsic stimulus does by itself not generate the "global" temporal continuity (or a global neuronal workspace), as seems to be often presupposed in predictive coding and also by the proponents of the global workspace theory of consciousness. Instead, the extrinsic stimulus encounters an already existing "global" temporal continuity when it interacts with the brain's intrinsic activity. This means that the stimulus must be linked and integrated into the already existing "virtual" temporal structure of the brain's intrinsic activity.

Such linkage and integration is accounted neuronally for by what I described as "rest–stimulus interaction" in Volume 1 (see Chapter 11). I now propose that such rest–stimulus interaction is central for associating the newly resulting stimulus-induced activity with consciousness and thus the "duration bloc".

How is such association of the purely neuronal stimulus-induced activity with a phenomenal state that is consciousness possible? The degree of integration between extrinsic stimulus and intrinsic activity predisposes the degree to which the intrinsic activity's temporal structure is transferred to the extrinsic stimulus and its stimulus-induced activity. The degree of the "duration bloc" in consciousness may thus ultimately depend on the degree of rest–stimulus interaction and more specifically its degree

of GABA-ergic mediated nonlinearity (see Chapter 29 for neurophenomenal details).

How now is my neurophenomenal account related to predictive coding? I assume that the here-suggested neurophenomenal mechanisms precede and are thus more basic than the cognitive processing of contents as focused upon in predictive coding and its generation of the prediction error (see Chapter 9 for an extensive discussion).

NEUROPHENOMENAL HYPOTHESIS IIA: NEUROCOGNITIVE VERSUS NEUROPHENOMENAL APPROACHES TO MENTAL "TIME TRAVEL"

How does my neurophenomenal (rather than neurocognitive account) of the "duration bloc" stand in relation to the results of mental time travel as discussed in Chapter 13? Let us recall the imaging experiments by the Belgian scientist d'Argembeau from Chapter 13, where subjects had to actively "prospect" future events or "retrospect" past events. He showed that the neural activity in the midline regions was central in the temporal extension to past and future during mental imagery.

What exactly happens during such mental time travel? The proponents of predictive coding and the global workspace theory would probably suggest that the strong neural activity changes in the midline regions are due to the mental imagination of particular stimuli and their respective contents; that is, the events or objects the subjects imagined. The temporal signature of the mentally imagined events or objects and thus the respective stimuli themselves, including their discrete points in physical time, are then supposed to cause the neural activity in the midline regions. The contents themselves and their processing are thus supposed to cause the neural activity changes in the midline regions which in turn makes possible the mental time travel with prospection and retrospection. Contents are thus processed first while their temporal signaturing comes second.

Moreover, the observed neural activity may probably be assumed to reflect a predicted input as described in predictive coding (see

Chapters 7–9 for details). Psychologically, this may correspond to the anticipation or expectation of a particular event in response to a particular cue. The anticipation of the event and its particular content is supposed to cause the extension into the future time. Hence the temporal extension and associated "inner time consciousness" follow the imagination and prospection of the contents. Accordingly, time follows the processing of contents in predictive coding and any other neurocognitive account of mental time travel.

How does such neurocognitive account stand in relation to my neurophenomenal approach? I do not deny that subjects imagine the event and that there is anticipation of particular contents. But, and this is important, the event and the anticipation of the respective contents do not cause by themselves the temporal extension as suggested in the neurocognitive account. Instead, the events and thus the contents follow the degree of neurotemporal extension that is predisposed in the midline network, the "dynamic temporal network" as Lloyd called it (see Chapter 13).

Accordingly, the neurophenomenal account claims that the processing of contents follows the prior and more basic constitution of time. This is clearly different from the neurocognitive approach where the contents are supposed to be processed first while their temporal signaturing occurs only after that in a second step. The neurophenomenal approach thus reverses the neurocognitive account: instead of temporal extension following the anticipation of content, the anticipation of the content follows the temporal extension of the midline regions' intrinsic activity and their degree of global temporal continuity. To put it more strongly still, the neurophenomenal approach considers the temporal extension provided by the intrinsic activity's degree of global temporal continuity to be a necessary condition of the possible anticipation of contents.

If there were no such underlying global temporal continuity in the brain's intrinsic activity, the subjects could probably still imagine the event. But, and this is important, they would no longer be able to anticipate the event and thus to shift its mental occurrence into the future. Why? There would be no longer a temporal matrix that allows the subjects to link their present discrete point in physical time with the ones in the future as presupposed in the anticipation of the event. Due to the lack of such a linkage, anticipation of the event would remain impossible. This is what the neurophenomenal account postulates.

Neurophenomenal Hypothesis IIB: Empirical Plausibility of the Neurophenomenal Approach to Mental Time Travel

How can we decide between neurocognitive and neurophenomenal approaches to mental time travel? The data themselves shall decide. The neurophenomenal approach claims that temporal extension is related to the brain's intrinsic activity and provides the very basis for the subsequent anticipation of future events in mental time travel. One would consequently expect neural overlap between mental time travel and intrinsic activity, especially in the midline regions.

If, in contrast, one favors the neurocognitive approach, one would expect the temporal extension to be based on the stimulus-induced or task-related activity associated with the anticipated event itself, rather than the brain's intrinsic activity. There should thus be no neural overlap between intrinsic activity and mental time travel which may then be considered as two distinct dissociable neural processes. These are clear hypotheses that can be tested and have indeed been addressed in the study by Oestby et al. (2012; see also Chapter 13).

We recall from Chapter 13 that Oestby et al. (2012) observed strong neural overlap between the midline activity during mental time travel and the same regions' high activity during the resting state (see Chapter 13 for details). This means that the resting-state activity itself must already contain some information about the temporal extension into past and future as it is applied to specific contents during mental time travel. Otherwise there would be no such neural overlap between mental time travel and intrinsic activity.

How is such a neural overlap between mental time travel and intrinsic activity possible? I suggest that this can be explained only in the neurophenomenal rather than the neurocognitive model. More specifically, we need to postulate a particular temporal structure in the neural activity of the resting-state activity itself. This temporal structure, as detailed earlier, is supposed to be manifested in the "local" and "global" temporal continuity of the neural activity in the resting state.

The subject's instruction to perform mental time travel by imagining certain extrinsic events or objects therefore only modulates the preexisting temporal structure of the brain's intrinsic activity (rather than causing it as presupposed in the neurocognitive model). By modulating the resting state's temporal structure, the event and thus the content becomes integrated into the already existing temporal structure of the brain's resting state; this in turn makes possible to extend the imagined event in time and to shift it from the present to the future.

Most importantly, the shift of the content from the present into the future allow us to anticipate or prospect the respective content. The neurocognitive function of anticipation is thus directly dependent upon the more basic neurophenomenal function of the constitution of time. Put conversely, the constitution of time—namely, the extension of the present time point into future ones— provides the basis here for the subsequent cognitive function, the anticipation or prospection.

NEUROPHENOMENAL HYPOTHESIS
IIC: "COGNITION FOLLOWS PHENOMENOLOGY" RATHER THAN "PHENOMENOLOGY FOLLOWS COGNITION"

Let us summarize. Constitution of time precedes anticipation of events in time. Since the constitution of time is associated with "inner time consciousness," neurophenomenal functions precede neurocognitive functions like anticipation or prospection. Cognition follows phenomenology, rather than the reverse, phenomenology following cognition (as it is tacitly presupposed in the neurocognitive approach).

I postulate that it is necessary and unavoidable that cognition follows phenomenology. Why? Our brain and its intrinsic activity operate in such a way that it is necessary and unavoidable. Due to the way the brain encodes its neural activity, including its own intrinsic activity, the constitution of global temporal continuity and consequently of "threefold temporal structure" and the "duration bloc" occur by default.

Since any stimulus or event, even imagined ones, cannot avoid interacting with the brain's intrinsic activity and its temporal structure, the cognition of the event, as in anticipation or prospection, has to follow the phenomenology: the consciousness of that same event. There is thus priority of time and phenomenology rather than priority of contents and cognition. This implies what I will describe as the "priority hypothesis" in Chapter 17 when discussing the relationship between cognition and the loss of consciousness in anesthesia.

Put in a nutshell, the "priority hypothesis" basically postulates that we need to switch our allegiances and follow the brain itself (and its intrinsic activity) rather than our cognition (of contents and their events and their related extrinsic or stimulus-induced activity in the brain). I provided empirical evidence for the priority of time and phenomenology over the cognition of contents in time. How about phenomenal evidence? If the brain's intrinsic activity does indeed provide temporal extension by means of its global temporal continuity, one would expect that, even in the resting state, we should be prone to continuously shifting and extending our present point in physical time to future ones.

This is indeed the case, as is well described by Blaise Pascal in the following quote where he distinguishes between "physical present" and "subjective present," with the latter obviously coming close to what I described as the "threefold temporal structure" of "inner time consciousness": "We never keep to the present. We anticipate the future as we find it too slow in coming and we are trying to hurry it up, or we recall the past as if to stay its too rapid flight" (Pascal 1966, 47).

Open Questions

We here propose temporal nestedness between high- and low-frequency fluctuations to be central in constituting "global" temporal continuity of neural activity and ultimately the "duration bloc" on the phenomenal level of consciousness.

However, we were not able to provide direct empirical evidence to support our neurophenomenal hypothesis.

One of the problems here is that the respective neuronal and phenomenal variables have not yet been operationalized. We need to develop a measure, an index of the degree of temporal nestedness between different frequency waves.

One would also need to relate the index of temporal nestedness to the degree of the duration bloc. One possible measure of the duration bloc could be the degree of temporal extension into both future and past during the experience of, for instance, mental time travel. Once these variables are operationalized and quantified, they may be tested in different states of consciousness, in awake state and in REM and NREM sleep, as well as in disorders of consciousness like vegetative state.

Another interesting question is the one for the degrees of "global" temporal continuity and the duration bloc in species other than humans. Other species may, for instance, show a lower degree of temporal extension into past and future of their "global" temporal continuity. If so, one would expect a lower degree of temporal nestedness, a lower number and less fine-grained temporal differences that can possibly be encoded in neural activity, and a lower number in the ranges of the fluctuations' frequencies in the brain's neural activity of these species. These are testable hypotheses and may be related to the degree of how deeply and extended animals can reach in their behavior into past and future (see also Chapter 31 for the discussion of consciousness in animals).

Finally, one may want to know how my neurophenomenal hypothesis stands in relation to other hypotheses about time and neural processing postulated by other neuroscientists. F. J. Varela, for instance, developed a neurophenomenological hypothesis of the neural mechanisms underlying Husserl's concept of the duration bloc. S. Gallagher also oriented himself strongly on the phenomenological model of time, as have others like J. Fuster and, in part, also E. Poeppel, M. Wittmann, and A. C. Craig. For the discussion of their hypotheses and how they compare to the one put forward here, I devote a separate appendix to them (see Appendix 2).

Note

1. Dainton (2008) contrasted Husserl's retentional concept of temporality with an extensional one. The extensional model claims that there needs to be only an overlap of both past and future with the present in order to establish temporal continuity, while the retentional model argues for complete integration of past and future into the retentional (and "protential") temporal structure. I here follow the Husserlian model of retention since it seems to be more in accordance with the complete integration of low- and high-frequency waves yielding temporal nestedness and "global" temporal continuity. This, however, does not necessarily exclude the model by Dainton of only partial overlap. Neuronally, both complete and partial integration can coexist in terms of different degrees of the same neuronal mechanisms (like temporal nestedness), even if on a conceptual level they seem to be contradictory.

CHAPTER 16
Functional Connectivity and "Inner Space Consciousness"

Summary

In the preceding chapters I focused on time and proposed specific neuronal mechanisms to underlie the constitution of temporal continuity and "inner time consciousness." I almost completely neglected the dimension of space, however, which is the focus of the present chapter. I propose that the constitution of what can be described as "spatial continuity" of neural activity and "inner space consciousness" on the phenomenal level are predisposed by functional and effective connectivity between different regions' neural activities. This is supported by the observation that decreased functional (i.e., mere correlation) and effective (i.e., causal impact) connectivity between the different regions' neural activities is accompanied by extreme reduction or even complete loss of consciousness as in anesthesia, vegetative state, and NREM sleep. What are the underlying neuronal mechanisms? Decrease in functional connectivity may lead to a decrease in the degree of spatial continuity of neural activity during the resting state. This, in turn, may make the constitution of what I describe as "local" and "global" spatial continuity of neural activity during subsequent rest–stimulus interaction impossible. Analogous to temporal continuity, I here propose "local" and "global" spatial continuity of neural activity to be constituted already by the resting-state activity itself and to predispose the possible degree of the level or state of consciousness and more specifically its degree of "inner space consciousness." "Local" and "global" spatial continuities of neural activity do not constitute "inner space consciousness" by themselves and can therefore not be considered neural correlates of consciousness. Instead, they only predispose and thus make unavoidable the possible constitution of "inner space consciousness" and the level or state of consciousness by constituting a spatial grid or template. Accordingly, rather than being a neural correlate, spatial continuity of neural activity as established by resting-state functional connectivity may better be considered a neural predisposition of consciousness.

Key Concepts and Topics Covered

Functional and effective connectivity, local and global spatial continuity, NREM sleep, REM sleep, anesthesia, vegetative state, amplification and condensation hypothesis, difference-based coding, information integration theory, coding hypothesis of consciousness

NEUROEMPIRICAL BACKGROUND
IA: CONSTITUTION OF SPACE VERSUS PERCEPTION AND COGNITION OF SPACE

So far, I have considered only temporal continuity of neural activity (Chapters 13–15) and how it predisposes "inner time consciousness." There is, however, also spatial continuity of neural activity that spans across different discrete points in physical space and may thereby predispose our experience of space in consciousness, or "inner space consciousness."

What do I mean by "inner space consciousness"? Rather than experiencing the different discrete points in physical space as single, discrete and separate points by themselves, our consciousness provides us with a link and connection between the different discrete points in physical space: we experience the different discrete points in physical space as discrete pearls of a continuous string that spans the different discrete pearls and their discrete points in physical space. Analogous to the temporal dimension and its "inner time consciousness," we may therefore propose an "inner space consciousness."

We are thus confronted with the question about the constitution of space by our brain's neural activity as the very basis, the predisposition, of the phenomenal features of consciousness and its "inner space consciousness." As in the case of time (see Chapters 13–15 and Appendix 2), we need to distinguish such "constitution of space" from the "perception and cognition of space" (see, e.g., Lloyd 2009). The constitution of space focuses on the neuronal mechanisms of how the brain's neural activity transforms the merely physical space of the world into the phenomenal space of consciousness. Metaphorically put, the constitution of space targets the string itself on which the different pearls hang.

In contrast, the perception and cognition of space targets the neuronal mechanisms that underlie our perception and cognition of the different "pearls" themselves and how they and their discrete positions in physical space are perceived and cognized as integrated into a continuous string. My focus in this chapter is on the first, the neuronal mechanisms underlying the constitution of space; while I set aside the neuronal mechanisms related to the perception and cognition of space.

NEUROEMPIRICAL BACKGROUND IB: SPATIAL (AND TEMPORAL) CONTINUITY OF NEURAL ACTIVITY AND THE LEVEL OR STATE OF CONSCIOUSNESS

Why do I focus on the constitution rather than the perception and cognition of space? I suggest that the constitution of space (and time) provides the very basis for the possibility of any subsequent consciousness.

Let me explicate that hypothesis. Like the constitution of time leads to the constitution of a temporal grid or template, the constitution of space also provides a spatial template or grid. Such spatial grid or template is purely neuronal by itself and is, I propose, closely related to the spatial continuity of neural activity (like the temporal grid or template is related to the temporal continuity of neural activity; see Chapters 13–15). Such spatial (and temporal) continuity of neural activity is already established in the resting state itself and must therefore be regarded a neuronal feature of the brain's intrinsic activity.

How is the purely neuronal spatial continuity of the brain's intrinsic activity and its spatial grid related to consciousness? Any subsequent change in neural activity as induced either by extrinsic stimuli or by the intrinsic activity itself (and its continuous spontaneous activity changes; see Chapters 4, 5, and 13) must be linked and integrated into the already existing and ongoing spatial (and temporal) continuity of the brain's intrinsic activity. In other words, any activity change must be encoded in relation to the ongoing spatial (and temporal) continuity of the intrinsic activity's spatial (and temporal) grid.

I now propose that a proper encoding of any kind of neural activity change (related to either extrinsic stimuli or the intrinsic activity itself) makes possible the association of the newly resulting neural activity level with consciousness. Proper encoding means that the activity change must be linked to and integrated with the intrinsic activity and its spatial and temporal continuity. Without such proper linkage and integration and, even more important, without the constitution of proper spatial continuity of the neural activity in the resting state, such an association with consciousness would remain impossible.

We will here focus on the spatial continuity itself and how it is constituted in the following sections whereas the exact neuronal mechanisms of such linkage and integration that is rest-stimulus interaction will be discussed later (see Chapters 28 and 29). First, though, we have to briefly consider what we introduced as the "level" or "state" of consciousness. We recall from the Introduction that "the level or state of consciousness" refers to arousal, while "the contents of consciousness" describes the objects, persons, or events we experience in consciousness. I now propose that the spatial continuity of neural activity predisposes the level or state of consciousness in very much the same way that the temporal continuity of neural activity is closely related to the level or state of consciousness, as we have seen in (especially) Chapter 15.

Decreases in the degree of the intrinsic activity's spatial continuity should then accompany decreases in the degree of the level or state of consciousness. This can indeed be observed in the case of the decreased temporal continuity of neural activity, as in the vegetative state (VS), under anesthesia, or NREM sleep (see Chapter 15). As in Chapter 15, my empirical account will therefore strongly rely on the findings of functional connectivity in these states.

NEUROEMPIRICAL BACKGROUND IC: "CONSTITUTION OF CONSCIOUSNESS IN (PHYSICAL) SPACE (AND TIME)" VERSUS "CONSTITUTION OF (PHENOMENAL) SPACE (AND TIME) IN CONSCIOUSNESS"

I proposed that the level or state of consciousness is predisposed by the degree of spatial (and temporal) continuity of neural activity. This means that (the level or state of) consciousness can ultimately be traced back to the constitution of the intrinsic activity's spatial (and temporal) continuity.

How is such spatial (and temporal) continuity of the brain's neural activity related to the physical space of the world? The constitution of the intrinsic activity's spatial (and temporal) continuity by the brain takes place within the physical space (and time) of the world the brain is part of. This means that, ultimately, consciousness and the intrinsic activity's spatial (and temporal) continuity are constituted within the physical space (and time) of the brain and the world. In short, there is constitution of an "inner space consciousness" in (physical) space (and time).

Such constitution of consciousness in (physical) space (and time) must be distinguished from the experience of space (and time) in consciousness. The experience of space (and time) in consciousness is expressed by the term "inner space consciousness" (and "inner time

consciousness"). Here, unlike in the constitution of consciousness in (physical) space (and time), we no longer refer to space (and time) as physical but rather as phenomenal. One may thus say that (phenomenal) space (and time) are constituted in consciousness. Accordingly, we have to distinguish between the "constitution of (phenomenal) space (and time) in consciousness" and the "constitution of consciousness in (physical) space (and time)."

Both are closely linked, however: since the "constitution of (phenomenal) space (and time) in consciousness" presupposes consciousness itself, it can be considered the output or result of the "constitution of consciousness in (physical) space (and time)." The focus in this (as in the preceding discussions with regard to time) is therefore on how the "constitution of consciousness in (physical) space" leads to the "constitution of (phenomenal) space in consciousness," that is, "inner space consciousness."

One may even further specify their relationship. The constitution of phenomenal space and time lays the very basis of the subsequent constitution of consciousness in general. Phenomenal space and time provide the spatial and temporal grid into which any content must be integrated and linked in order to become associated with consciousness. Metaphorically speaking, phenomenal time and space can be considered the skeleton of consciousness without which consciousness itself would remain impossible altogether.

This means that the constitution of phenomenal time and space provide the bridge between the physical space and time of the physical world on one hand and the phenomenal features of consciousness on the other. To put it slightly differently, the transformation of the different discrete points in the physical time and space of the physical world into the spatial and temporal continuity of the brain's intrinsic activity predisposes the subsequent constitution of consciousness and its various phenomenal features. Therefore, I speak of a neurophenomenal account of space and time, which I believe mediates the transition from the physical world of nonconsciousness to the phenomenal world of consciousness.

NEURONAL FINDINGS IA: SLOW WAVE ACTIVITY AND NREM SLEEP

Sleep, especially NREM sleep, can be characterized by slow wave activity (SWA) (see Chapter 15 herein for more details). Why is SWA important in the present context of consciousness? As described in Chapter 15, SWA occurs in the early (and late) sleep stages, the NREM sleep, where one is not conscious at all. This distinguishes NREM sleep from REM sleep, where one regains consciousness. NREM sleep, and its electrophysiological hallmark SWA, may therefore be considered a paradigm of unconsciousness and its distinction from consciousness; for example, REM sleep. This is why the group around Tononi have studied NREM sleep extensively, as described in Chapter 15.

What are the SWA's specific neuronal mechanisms that prevent us from becoming conscious? This amounts to the question of why we lose consciousness in the early stages of sleep where SWAs predominate. Several hypotheses have been suggested.

First, a general metabolic decrease has been suggested to underlie the slip into unconsciousness during NREM sleep. However, NREM sleep can be characterized by cross-regional redistribution of neural activity rather than by global reduction of neuronal activity and metabolism (as can be observed in VS; see Chapter 28). Such cross-regional redistribution of neural activity is mediated by the degree of functional connectivity between the different regions. Rather than the global reduction of neuronal and metabolic activity, the changes in the functional connectivity itself may be central for the loss of consciousness in NREM sleep.

Second, a blockade of sensory input (olfactory, auditory, gustatory, tactile), for example, exteroceptive stimuli, has often been proposed to be central. However, there are still exteroceptive stimuli processed in sleep since the sensory processing (tactile, gustatory, auditory, olfactory) is not completely shut off even if the visual processing is reduced due to the eyes being closed. There may thus still be subconscious sensory processing going on even in NREM sleep.

Finally, decrease in gamma activity and neuronal synchronization has often been proposed to be central for the loss of consciousness in NREM sleep. However, gamma is particularly low during REM sleep and dreams where consciousness is regained; this means that gamma decrease cannot account for the loss of consciousness in NREM sleep, since one would then expect increased rather than decreased gamma in consciousness during REM sleep.

NEURONAL FINDINGS IB: FUNCTIONAL CONNECTIVITY IN NON–RAPID EYE MOVEMENT SLEEP (NREM)

What causes the slip into nonconsciousness in NREM sleep? Tononi and his group conducted several experiments in NREM and REM sleep (see Massimini et al. 2009, 2012; and Riedner et al. 2011, for an overview). They applied high-frequency (25–30 Hz) transcranial magnetic stimulation (TMS) in the rostral premotor cortex, and electroencephalography (EEG) in the awake state as well as during NREM and REM sleep (with subjects being unaware of the TMS impulse due to noise-masking and other procedures).

When applied in the awake state and in REM sleep, premotor 25–30 Hz TMS stimulation (with an intensity corresponding to the motor threshold) triggered a series of low-amplitude and high-frequency (25–30 Hz) waves of activity. These waves spread and propagated along long-range ipsilateral and transcallosal connections over 250 ms subsequent to stimulation (see Fig. 16-1). Thereby the site of maximum activation (as measured with simultaneous EEG) differed anatomically regionally from the site of stimulation at almost all time points beyond 50 ms (i.e., 100 ms, 150 ms, 250 ms; see Esser et al. 2009; Massimini et al. 2010; Mascetti et al. 2011; Riedner et al. 2011).

The same procedure (TMS stimulation in premotor cortex) was applied in the same subjects 15 minutes later during NREM sleep (stages 3 and 4). This resulted in a different spatiotemporal activation pattern. Instead of predominantly high-frequency (25–30 Hz) waves of neural activity, TMS now triggered stronger low-frequency waves that, unlike in the awake state, did not spread and propagate to other regions at all.

More specifically, the waves remained more or less stationary at the site of stimulation and dissipated rapidly, within 250 ms. Due to the absence of such regional spread and extension of neural activity, the site of maximum activation was therefore more or less identical to the site of stimulation. The premotor cortex was still reactive in the NREM sleep by showing local activity change, which, however, was no longer connected to other regions. This indicates a loss of functional connectivity between the neural activity in the premotor cortex and the other regions (see Chapter 5 for a detailed discussion of functional connectivity), which prevented

the transregional propagation of TMS-triggered activity waves into other regions.

NEURONAL FINDINGS IC: BREAKDOWN OF FUNCTIONAL CONNECTIVITY IN NON–RAPID EYE MOVEMENT SLEEP (NREM)

How is such a breakdown of functional connectivity in NREM sleep possible? Regions like the premotor cortex receive major afferent input from the thalamus and also send efferent output back to the thalamus. This has been described as the "thalamo-cortical circuit." If the activity induced in premotor cortex no longer propagates to other regions, its functional connectivity to the thalamus and hence the

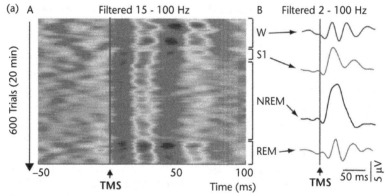

Figure 16-1a-c Spatial propagation of neural activity during the absence of consciousness. (*a*) (A) Single trial TMS-evoked responses are recorded from one channel located under the stimulator (FC2) while a subject transitions from wakefulness (W), through sleep stage 1 (S1) and NREM sleep (NREM) to REM sleep. The line with the letter TMS beneath marks the onset time of TMS. Single-trial EEG data are band-pass filtered (15 to 100 Hz). (B) The averaged responses (filtered from 2 to 100 Hz) calculated in the four vigilance states are depicted. The onset of REM sleep is associated with a resumption of TMS-evoked fast oscillations. (*b*) The averaged responses obtained in all subjects during wakefulness (W), NREM sleep (NREM) and REM sleep (REM traces) are compared. The vertical line marks the onset time of TMS. TMS-evoked potentials undergo systematic changes across states of vigilances. (*c*) (A) The TMS-evoked potentials recorded from one subject, in whom a long stretch of REM sleep could be recorded, are displayed (W: wakefulness, NREM sleep, REM sleep). The traces were recorded from the channels indicated by the dots in the upper left panel, where the site of stimulation on the subject's MRI is also indicated by (arrow). (B) Spatiotemporal cortical maps of TMS-evoked cortical activation during wakefulness, NREM, and REM sleep. For each significant time sample, maximum current sources were plotted and color-coded according to their latency of activation (0 milliseconds; 300 milliseconds). The cross marks the TMS target on the cortical surface. During REM sleep, the resumption of TMS-evoked fast oscillations was associated with a partial recovery of cortical effective connectivity. Reprinted with permission, from Massimini M, Ferrarelli F, Murphy M, Huber R, Riedner B, Casarotto S, Tononi G. Cortical reactivity and effective connectivity during REM sleep in humans. *Cogn Neurosci.* 2010 Sep;1(3):176–83.

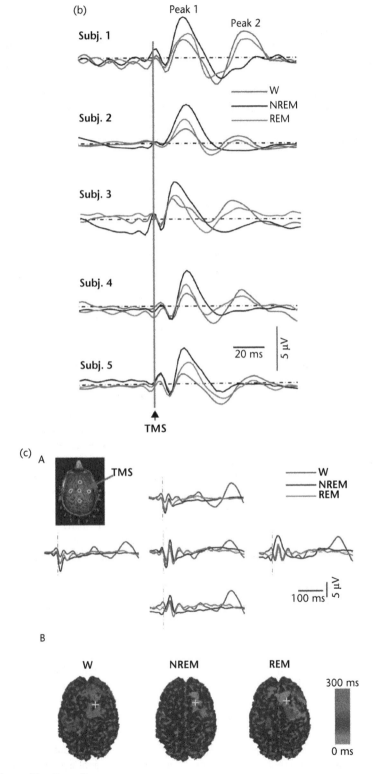

Figure 16-1a-c (Continued)

thalamo-cortical circuits may be disrupted in NREM sleep. The triggered activity in premotor cortex has then "no chance other than to stay local without having the opportunity anymore of being spread and extended to other cortical regions." One may thus say that the premotor cortex behaves like an isolated region that is disconnected from its neuronal environment, the thalamo-cortical circuits, and the other regions in the rest of the brain.

Such a breakdown of functional connectivity is not limited to the premotor cortex. In addition to the premotor cortex, the group around Tononi also stimulated the sensory cortex—the mesial parietal cortex—during both REM and NREM sleep. As in the premotor cortex, a complex pattern of low- and high-frequency activity waves with a sophisticated and time- and region-varying propagation could be induced in REM sleep over the medial parietal cortex. Hence, as in premotor cortex, there was a clear difference and thus dissociation between maximum activation and stimulation site in REM sleep.

The case was different during NREM sleep. Here, only stereotypical slow waves could be induced in mesial parietal cortex. These waves did not really propagate to other regions anymore, as indicated by the lack of regional difference between site of maximum activation and site of stimulation (which were more or less identical). What could be observed, however, was a very unspecific oil-spot-like spread of cortical currents to most of the rest of the cortex, remaining there more or less consistently over the 250 milliseconds following the stimulation. This indicates an undifferentiated and unspecific global response pattern that must be due to the disruption of functional connectivity in general and of thalamo-cortical circuits in particular.

Taken together, these experiments show that the spatiotemporal response pattern during NREM sleep is not as complex and sophisticated as during REM sleep. Instead of a time- and region-varying propagation of activity waves, as in REM sleep, neural activity in NREM sleep stayed either local without any propagation at all, or it was propagated in a very unspecific and stereotypical way to all other cortical sites.

These fiindings suggest a bistable monotonous activation pattern during NREM sleep as distinct from the multistable and complex activation pattern in REM sleep and the awake state. Since analogous results were obtained in midazolam-induced loss of consciousness mirroring anesthesia (see Ferrarelli et al. 2010) and vegetative state (see Rosanova et al. 2012 as described in detail in Chapter 29), the existence of a multistable and complex activation pattern seems to make possible the presence of consciousness while its loss leads to the absence of consciousness.

NEURONAL HYPOTHESIS IA: "EFFECTIVE CONNECTIVITY" VERSUS "INEFFECTIVE CONNECTIVITY"

Taken together, the findings show neural activity during NREM sleep (see earlier), anesthesia (see Ferrarelli et al. 2010), and vegetative state (see Rosanova et al. 2012; and see Chapter 29 herein for details) to remain local and nonpropagated, while it is more globally spread, that is, distributed and propagated, during REM sleep when consciousness is recovered (Massimini et al. 2010). This suggests that the degree of global distribution of neural activity in a time- and region-varying way is needed to induce a high level or state of consciousness.

The global distribution of neural activity is supposed to be mediated by effective and functional connectivity. What is "effective connectivity"? The concept of effective connectivity describes the causal impact of one region's neural activity on that of another region. Such a causal impact must be distinguished from mere correlation, as indicated by the term "*functional connectivity*" (see also Chapter 4 and especially Chapter 5 in Volume I).

What neuronal purpose does effective connectivity serve? Tononi and many others show and argue that it serves the neuronal communication between different regions' neural activities by allowing for time- and region-varying propagation of neuronal activity waves in a complex and sophisticated way. This is well supported by the impressive TMS stimulation results in NREM and REM sleep as well as the ones in anesthesia as described in Chapter 15.

What remains unclear, however, is how such effective connectivity between different regions can lead to better neuronal communication between them. In other words, we have to raise the question of why such connectivity is effective (i.e., having a causal impact from one region to another).

What is the mechanisms that turn merely functional into effective connectivity? This targets the neuronal mechanisms and processes by means of which the merely functional (and thus correlational) connectivity can become effective (and thus causal) for the neuronal communication between different regions' neural activities. Accordingly, we must distinguish the effective connectivity itself as the output or results of a prior neuronal process that turns mere functional connectivity that is ineffective into effective connectivity.

NEURONAL HYPOTHESIS IB: "SPATIAL AMPLIFICATION" MEDIATES THE "EFFECTIVENESS" OF "EFFECTIVE CONNECTIVITY"

What are the neural processes that transform "ineffective" into "effective connectivity"? Functional connectivity allows the neuronal communication between different regions' neural activities. How does that neuronal communication take place? As detailed in Chapters 4 and 5 in Volume I, I hypothesize that the neuronal communication between different regions is encoded into neural activity in terms of spatial and temporal differences.

The spatial differences in neural activity levels between, for instance, two different regions may be integrated into one difference-based value. This spatial difference between the two regions' neural activities is then further processed across other regions' neural activities, which are encoded relative to the preceding spatial differences, which leads to the constitution of novel spatial differences in neural activity and so forth. There is thus what I described as the encoding of spatial differences into neural activity, which presupposes difference-based coding in spatial

terms on a regional level of neural activity (see Chapter 3, Volume I, for details).

Difference-based coding enables the amplification of spatial differences during the processing of neural activity across the different regions' neural activities. This is what I subsume under what I call the "amplification hypothesis" (see also Chapter 3 in Volume I). The "amplification hypothesis" describes the continuous encoding and constitution of novel spatial (and temporal) differences into neural activity during the spread and propagation of neural activity across the various regions' neural activities.

Since the spread of neural activity across the different discrete spatial positions of the various regions' neural activities is central, one may further specify the "amplification hypothesis" by what I describe as "spatial amplification." The concept of "spatial amplification" describes the constitution of novel spatial differences between different the different discrete spatial positions of the different regions' neural activities.

Based on the spatial amplification via the constitution of novel spatial differences, I propose what I call the "spatial amplification hypothesis" of difference-based coding (see also Chapter 3 for a related amplification hypothesis in the context of sparse coding). The spatial amplification hypothesis proposes a direct relationship between the degree of amplification of spatial differences across the different regions' neural activities and the degree of effectiveness of connectivity: the higher the degree of amplification of spatial differences across the different regions' neural activities, the higher the degree of effectiveness of their effective connectivity.

This means that lower degrees in the amplification of spatial differences across the different regions' neural activities may be accompanied by lower degrees in the effectiveness of effective connectivity. As the data suggest, this is apparently the case in VS, anesthesia, and NREM sleep. In contrast, higher degrees in the amplification of neural differences are supposedly accompanied by higher degrees in the effectiveness of effective connectivity, as can be observed during REM sleep and in the awake state (see Fig. 16-2a).

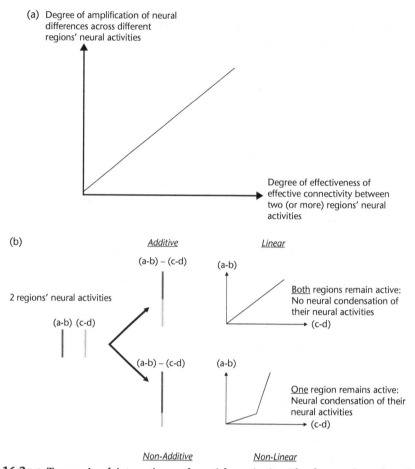

Figure 16-2a-c Transregional interaction and spatial continuity. The figures show the relationship between the neuronal mechanisms underlying interaction between different regions' neural activities and the constitution of spatial continuity of neural activity. (*a*) This figure depicts the relationship between the degree of spatial amplification of the encoded spatial differences across different regions' neural activities and the degree of functional connectivity. The more the encoded spatial differences are amplified across the different regions' neural activities, the higher their degree of functional connectivity. (*b*) This figure shows two regions' neural activities with each based on the encoding of a spatial difference (a – b, c – d) by itself (bars on the left). Two different ways of interaction are possible. One possibility is that the two regions' neural activities interact linearly and additively (upper middle and right part). In this case the neural activities of the two regions are merely added and superimposed upon each other, resulting in a linear relationship between their activities (bars in the upper middle part). This means that both regions remain active when they interact with each other, showing a linear relationship (graph in right upper part). There is no condensation of the two regions' neural activities. The situation is different in case of nonlinear and nonadditive interaction (lower middle and right part). In this case the original neural activities of both regions are changed during their interaction as indicated by the bars (lower middle part). That means that only one region may remain active during their interaction, entailing condensation of the two regions' neural activities into one region's neural activity (graph in lower right part). (*c*) This figure shows the relationship between the degree of "spatial amplification" of the encoded spatial differences across different regions' neural activities and the degree of their subsequent condensation in a lower number of regions' neural activities. The higher the degree of amplification of the encoded spatial differences across different regions' neural activities, the higher the degree to which the neural differences can possibly be condensed in a lower number of regions' neural activities. That, in turn, makes possible the constitution of spatial continuity across the different regions' neural activities; spatial continuity is manifest in the linkage and continuous transitions of neural activities across different discrete points in physical space as associated with the different regions.

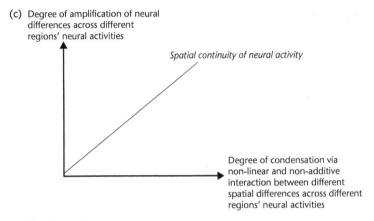

Figure 16-2a-c (Continued)

NEURONAL HYPOTHESIS IIA: ENCODING OF SPATIAL DIFFERENCES AND PARALLEL-SEGREGATED PROCESSING

The hypothesis of the spatial amplification of neural activity proposes a direct relationship between the degree of difference-based coding and the degree of effective connectivity. The encoding of spatial differences into the different regions' neural activities signifies difference-based coding (as distinguished from stimulus-based coding), which is thus linked directly to functional and, most importantly, effective connectivity (see also Chapter 5).

How can this relationship between difference-based coding and effective connectivity impact consciousness that is the presence or absence of consciousness? For the answer, we need to go into the details of what exactly happens during the encoding of spatial differences into neural activity and how these are spread and propagated across the different regions.

What exactly happens during the encoding of spatial differences into the regions' neural activities? A certain activity level and local activity propagation within a particular region x may be related to a particular spatial difference $(a - b)$ as encoded into its neural activity by difference-based coding. And, of course, the same holds true for another region that encodes a different spatial difference $(c - d)$ into its neural activity.

When the first region's particular activity level $x(1)$ is linked to the one of another region y with a different activity level 2, that is, $y(2)$, it means that the first region's encoded difference $(a - b)$ will encounter the second region's encoded difference $(c - d)$. Due to the modulation and adjustment between $x(1)$ and $y(2)$, the encoded difference $(a - b)$ becomes linked to the encoded difference $(c - d)$, resulting in the encoding of a novel difference $[(a - b) - (c - d)]$ into neural activity (the formula is here meant in a symbolic rather than strictly mathematical sense).

How can we describe $[(a - b) - (c - d)]$, in further detail? Different models are possible. The formula $[(a - b) - (c - d)]$ could reflect that the old encoded differences $(a - b)$ and $(c - d)$ are now just standing (or processed) side by side. Instead of being processed in two different regions' neural activities that are spatially apart from each other, they are now processed side by side within the same region's neural activity, while (and this is important) remaining unchanged by themselves. They are thus processed in a parallel and segregated way.

Due to the absence of any interaction, one would then need to write $[(a - b) (c - d)]$ rather than $[(a - b) - (c - d)]$ to make it more correct. Though possible, such a scenario is rather unlikely because effective connectivity especially is defined by one region's neural activity causally impacting and modulating the other region's activity level. This means that such parallel and segregated processing of the different encoded spatial differences within one region's neural activity (or between different regions) is empirically rather implausible (at least when there is effective connectivity).

NEURONAL HYPOTHESIS IIB: NONLINEAR INTERACTION MEDIATES "SPATIAL CONDENSATION" OF NEURAL ACTIVITY ACROSS DIFFERENT REGIONS

One may instead propose a direct interaction between $(a - b)$ and $(c - d)$. This interaction may now be either additive and linear, or rather nonadditive and nonlinear. In the case of an additive and linear interaction, one would propose that $(a - b)$ is merely added to $(c - d)$ so that the $[(a - b) - (c - d)]$ would better be signified as $[(a - b) + (c - d)]$.

In this case, neither $(a - b)$ nor $(c - d)$ becomes really changed by itself but is more or less preserved. Unlike in the first case, they are put together into an additive whole. Since they interact, the regions' neural activities no longer operate in parallel; they are not integrated, however, and thus remain recognizable and segregated in an isolated and independent way. However, as pointed out by the data on effective connectivity data described earlier and elsewhere (see Volume I, Chapters 10 and 11), the interaction between different regions' neural activities seems to be rather nonadditive and nonlinear. This means that $(a - b)$ from region $x(1)$ is changed and modulated by the encounter with $(c - d)$ from $y(2)$ with the latter also changing (i.e., $c - d$). This implies that neither $(a - b)$ nor $(c - d)$ can be recognized anymore nor segregated from each other since both are fused and merged into a novel difference $[(a - b) - (c - d)]$. Hence, the result of such interaction is $\{[x(1) - y(2)] [(a - b) - (c - d)]\}$ rather than $\{[x(1)(a - b)] [y(2)(c - d)]\}$ or $\{[x(1)(a - b)] + [y(2) (c - d)]\}$.

Such fusion as the merging and integration between two (or more) encoded spatial differences into one novel spatial difference is proposed to be possible only on the basis of nonlinear and nonadditive interaction.

I consecutively propose that such a nonadditive and nonlinear interaction between the different regions' neural activities and their respective encoded spatial differences, $(a - b)$ and $(c - d)$, corresponds to what I described as the "condensation hypothesis" in the purely neuronal context of Volume I (see Chapter 3). In a nutshell, the "condensation hypothesis" holds that the amplified neural activity is condensed in both spatial and temporal terms by focusing changes in neural activity on particular regions and time points (see Chapter 3 for a related condensation hypothesis in the purely neuronal context of sparse coding).

I now elaborate this hypothesis with particular regard to the spatial dimension. There is an integration and thus condensation of spatial differences from different regions' neural activities into a novel spatial difference that spans across a smaller number of regions' neural activities. Since the number of regions and their associated different discrete points in physical space are reduced or condensed, I speak of a spatial condensation hypothesis in the following discussion (see Fig. 16-2b).

The spatial condensation hypothesis is that the amplification of encoded spatial differences across different regions' neural activities accompanies the condensation of neural activity in a smaller number of regions (see Chapter 3 in Volume I). Since it allows neural activity to condense, that is, to integrate two (or more) different spatial differences and their respective regions' neural activities into the neural activity of one region, I propose that nonlinear and nonadditive interaction is necessary for the spatial condensation of neural activity across different regions' neural activities (Fig. 16-2c; see also Chapters 10 and 11 in Volume I, as well as Chapter 29 in this volume for more details on nonlinear interaction).

NEURONAL FINDINGS IIA: FUNCTIONAL CONNECTIVITY IN ANESTHESIA

Let us go beyond the NREM sleep to findings of functional connectivity in anesthesia and vegetative state. Anesthesia may serve as an indirect model of consciousness since the anesthetized patient is unconscious, which is essential to perform surgical procedures. One may therefore want to look into the results of how particular regions' neural activities and, even more important, their functional connectivity patterns change during anesthesia (see Alkire et al. 2008a and b; Nallasamy and Tsao 2011; and Bonhomme et al. 2011, for a recent review).

While the imaging results in the anesthetized state are not fully consistent, posterior midline regions like the posterior cingulate cortex (PCC), the medial parietal cortex (MPC), and the precuneus seem to be deactivated, showing lower neural activity levels. How about the functional connectivity between these regions? One of the main observations concerns the default-mode network (DMN). Even during the anesthetized state, the functional connectivity within the DMN (i.e., between PCC, medial prefrontal cortex, precuneus, and bilateral inferior parietal cortex) seems to be more or less preserved, as could be observed in both monkeys (Vincent et al. 2007) and humans (Greicius et al. 2008). However, some differences could be observed, as shall be described in the following.

Using midazolam in lower doses causing only light rather than full anesthetic sedation, Greicius et al. (2008) observed a local decrease in functional connectivity in the PCC in sedated subjects compared to the non-sedated ones. Furthermore, they observed an increase in local functional connectivity within a sensorimotor network (somatosensory and motor cortex and midcingulate cortex) in the sedated subjects.

A recent functional magnetic resonance imaging (fMRI) investigation in propofol-induced loss of consciousness demonstrated significant reduction in total integration (i.e., an index of overall functional connectivity) within as well as between different regions and networks (see Schrouff et al. 2011). Thereby, functional connectivity broke down, especially between frontal and parietal networks, the latter including the PCC (see also Stamatakis et al. 2011).

However, results concerning activity level and functional connectivity are not fully consistent among the various imaging studies during anesthesia. Some studies show no changes or reduction in activity levels, while other studies report increases or decreases in functional connectivity, sometimes even side by side, as in the study reported above (see Martuzzi et al. 2010).

In contrast, common to all results is that the basic global functional connectivity pattern, especially in the DMN, is preserved during anesthesia. This, however, seems to go along with changes in local functional connectivity as confined to particular networks like the sensorimotor network (see earlier) or the cognitive networks as the lateral cortical regions (see, for instance, Martuzzi et al. 2010).

NEURONAL FINDINGS IIB: FUNCTIONAL CONNECTIVITY IN VEGETATIVE STATE

In addition to NREM sleep and anesthesia, the neurological condition of vegetative state may serve as yet another example of a loss of consciousness. Recent investigations in vegetative, coma, and minimally conscious patients do indeed show significantly decreased functional connectivity especially within the cortical midline regions of the DMN (Vanhaudenhuyse et al. 2010; see also Cauda et al. 2009 and Boly et al. 2009) (see Chapters 28 and 29 for more details about the vegetative state).

Most important, the degree of functional connectivity between the PCC, the precuneus, and the medial prefrontal cortex correlated with the level of consciousness. The lower the degree of functional connectivity, the higher the degree of nonconsciousness, and the more likely the patient was in coma rather than in either a vegetative or minimally conscious state.

In contrast, a patient with locked-in syndrome showing preserved consciousness did not reveal any decrease in functional connectivity (see Vanhaudenhuyse et al. 2010). One should note, however, that the basic functional connectivity pattern of the DMN is still preserved even in the vegetative state, while it remained absent in a brain-dead patient (see Boly et al. 2009; see Chapters 29 and 30 for details about the vegetative state).

In addition to the functional connectivity within the DMN, one may also need to consider the functional connectivity between cortical and subcortical regions, including the brainstem. The brainstem that includes the ascending reticular activating system (ARAS) shows altered (mostly reduced) activity and metabolism in the vegetative state (see also Parvizi and Damasio 2003; as well as Chapter 31 for details about sub-cortical regions in VS). This, in turn, may lead to abnormal functional connectivity with cortical regions of the DMN like the PCC and the pre-cuneus (see Brown et al. 2010; Silva et al. 2010). Hence, we may need to consider the functional connectivity of the whole brain rather than one particular network (like the DMN or the senso-rimotor cortex) in vegetative state.

In addition to the thalamo-cortical con-nectivity, one may also need to consider the functional connectivity from the other subcor-tical regions to the thalamus. This is suggested by a recent fMRI study that used propofol to induce loss of consciousness. Applied dur-ing a verbal task, propofol induced loss of functional connectivity from putamen and pallidum to the thalamus and other regions, while thalamo-cortical functional connec-tivity remained more or less preserved (see Mhuircheartaigh et al. 2010).

These data point out the need to consider the whole brain, including the subcortical regions beneath the thalamus; I will therefore devote a whole Chapter specifically to subcortical regions and their relevance for consciousness in Chapter 31.

NEURONAL HYPOTHESIS IIIA: "SPATIAL AMPLIFICATION" MEDIATES "LOCAL" SPATIAL CONTINUITY OF NEURAL ACTIVITY

What do these findings imply for consciousness? All three states—NREM sleep, anesthesia, and vegetative state—show changes in the overall and thus global pattern of functional connec-tivity (global functional connectivity) in their resting-state activity. At the same time, the sub-jects show a highly decreased or even absent level or state of consciousness. Putting both observa-tions together, I hypothesize that the degree or level of global functional connectivity during the resting state predisposes the degree of the level or state of consciousness.

How does the global functional connectiv-ity impact neural processing in such a way that it can affect the level or state of consciousness? For that answer, we will first need to go back

to the resting state's neuronal activity itself and understand how it constitutes what I describe as "local" and "global" spatial continuity of neu-ral activity.

Let us start with the "local" spatial conti-nuity. Recall that the spatial amplification and condensation hypotheses proposed that neu-ronal differences between different regions' neural activities are amplified, that is, spread and propagated, across the whole brain. Such amplification of neural differences is then followed by the condensation of their neu-ral activity via nonlinear and nonadditive interaction.

What do "spatial amplification and conden-sation" imply for the constitution of the resting state's neural activity? "Spatial amplification" constitutes novel spatial differences between two (or more) regions' neural activities. This means that the two (or more) regions' neural activi-ties are somehow linked and connected to each other. Such linkage and connection constitutes a continuity between their respective neural activities and thus continuity of neural activity across different discrete points in physical space. Analogous to "local" temporal continuity of neu-ral activity (see Chapter 14), one may therefore want to speak of "local spatial continuity of neu-ral activity."

Local spatial continuity is a purely neuronal concept that describes the connection and ulti-mately the coordination and integration of neu-ral activities at different discrete points in the physical space of the brain. Such a link and con-nection may, for instance, be realized by func-tional and effective connectivity. The higher the degree of functional (or effective) connectivity between two (or more) regions' neural activi-ties, the higher their degree of "local" spatial continuity.

Let us elaborate upon this idea. As described earlier, functional connectivity is supposed to be dependent on the amplification of neural differ-ences across different regions' neural activities (see above). If so, the possible degree of "local" spatial continuity should be related to the degree of "spatial amplification." The higher the degree of "spatial amplification" of neural activ-ity, the higher the possible degree of functional connectivity, and consequently the higher the degree of "local" temporal continuity of neural activity between particular regions.

Note that I here do no equate "spatial amplification" and functional connectivity. Spatial amplification is considered the neural process that makes possible functional connectivity as its outcome or result.

NEURONAL HYPOTHESIS IIIB: "SPATIAL CONDENSATION" MEDIATES "GLOBAL" SPATIAL CONTINUITY OF NEURAL ACTIVITY

How about "spatial condensation" of neural activity? As proposed above, "spatial amplification" of neural activity is followed by, and goes hand in hand with, its subsequent "spatial condensation." "Spatial condensation" describes the fusion and merger of different spatial differences across different discrete points in physical space into a lower number of neural activities across a smaller number of different discrete points in physical space; that is, regions. In short, "spatial condensation" allows for the concentration of neural activity changes in a few regions.

"Spatial condensation" of neural activity in this sense implies that the different "local" spatial continuities are connected and thus fused into one larger, "global" spatial continuity. Such a "global" spatial continuity of neural activity spans a wider range of different discrete points in the space of the whole brain.

This distinguishes the "global" spatial continuity of neural activity from more "local" temporal continuities of neural activity that are restricted to continuous neural activity between particular regions, rather than involving all regions and thus the whole brain. As such, "global" spatial continuity may correspond to what I described earlier as the pattern of functional connectivity in the whole brain; that is, global functional connectivity.

I now propose the degree of "global" temporal continuity of neural activity to be directly dependent on its degree of "spatial condensation." The higher the neural activity's degree of "spatial condensation.," the higher its degree of global temporal continuity that can possibly be constituted. Since "spatial condensation"

is closely related to "global" functional connectivity, one may propose the latter to predict the degree of "global" spatial continuity of neural activity. Higher degrees of global functional connectivity should then go along with higher degrees of "global" spatial continuity (Fig. 16-3a).

NEUROPHENOMENAL HYPOTHESIS IA: "INNER TIME CONSCIOUSNESS" AND "INNER SPACE CONSCIOUSNESS"

How does such a "global" spatial continuity of neural activity predispose consciousness and particularly its spatial phenomenal features? For the answer, we need to first understand how space is constituted on the phenomenal level of consciousness; we are thus searching for what I described earlier as "the constitution of (phenomenal) space in consciousness."

The concept of "phenomenal space" refers to the subjective experience of space in consciousness, which, by analogy to time and "inner time consciousness" (see Chapters 14 and 15), one may want to describe by the term "inner space consciousness." The concept of "inner space consciousness" refers to the experience of space in consciousness and how it spatially structures and organizes our experience of the various contents; that is, objects, persons, and events, in consciousness.

We need further detail, however, and a more specific concept of "inner space consciousness." Unlike in the case of "inner time consciousness," there is not much phenomenological literature on the subjective experience of space in consciousness, or "inner space consciousness." Therefore, I here sketch a brief (and incomplete) picture of "inner space consciousness" in orientation on and analogy to "inner time consciousness."

We recall that inner time consciousness was characterized by the extension of the present, that is, the "width of present" (see Chapter 14), and a threefold temporal structure connecting past, present, and future, that is, the "duration bloc" (see Chapter 15). How does that apply to the spatial dimension? Let us start with the spatial analogy to the "width of point."

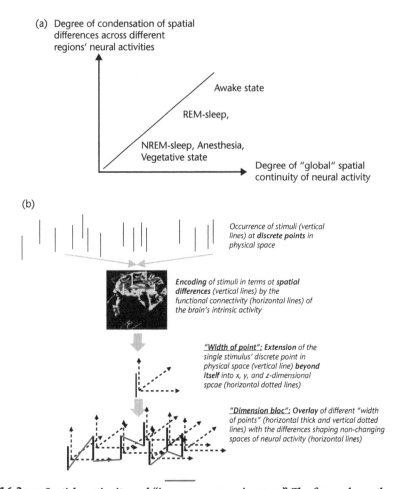

(a) Degree of condensation of spatial differences across different regions' neural activities

Awake state

REM-sleep,

NREM-sleep, Anesthesia, Vegetative state

Degree of "global" spatial continuity of neural activity

(b)

*Occurrence of stimuli (vertical lines) at **discrete points** in physical space*

***Encoding** of stimuli in terms ot **spatial differences** (vertical lines) by the functional connectivity (horizontal lines) of the brain's intrinsic activity*

***"Width of point":** Extension of the single stimulus' discrete point in physical space (vertical line) **beyond itself** into x, y, and z-dimensional spcae (horizontal dotted lines)*

***"Dimension bloc":** Overlay of different "width of points" (horizontal thick and vertical dotted lines) with the differences shaping non-changing spaces of neural activity (horizontal lines)*

Figure 16-3a-c Spatial continuity and "inner space consciousness." The figure shows the relationship between the degree of spatial continuity of neural activity (*a*) and inner space consciousness. (*b, c*). (*a*) This figure depicts the relationship between the degree of condensation between the different regions' neural activities and the degree of global spatial continuity of neural activities across the different regions of the brain. The higher the degree of condensation, the higher the degree to which the "global" spatial continuity of neural activities can extend across the different regions. The degree of condensation and consecutively the degree of "global" spatial continuity is supposed to be rather low during the loss of consciousness as in vegetative state, anesthesia, and NREM sleep, while it is intermediate in REM sleep. (*b*) The figure shows the different stages from the extrinsic stimuli's occurrence (upper level) via their encoding into the brain's intrinsic activity in terms of spatial differences (second from upper level) and the "width of point" (second from lower level) to the constitution of the "dimension bloc" (lower level). The most important step is here the encoding of the different stimuli's discrete points in physical space in terms of spatial differences by the brain's intrinsic activity and its functional connectivity. That makes it possible to extend or stretch the single discrete point in space beyond itself into three-dimensional space, as indicated in the "width of point" that corresponds to the functional connectivity between two regional activities in the brain. The overlay of the different functional connectivities and their respectively associated "widths of point" leads to the "dimension bloc"; the concept of "dimension" indicates spatially homogenous stretches of neural activity where it does not change, which corresponds to functional connectivities that are not interrupted by either other stimuli's or other regions' activities (see horizontal lines in the lower part). (*c*) This figure shows the relationship between the degree of "global" spatial continuity of neural activity across different regions and the degree of three-dimensional extension in the "dimension bloc" of inner space consciousness. The degree of "global" spatial continuity and its degree of extension in three-dimensional space is supposed to be rather low during the loss of consciousness as in vegetative state, anesthesia, and NREM sleep, while it is intermediate in REM sleep.

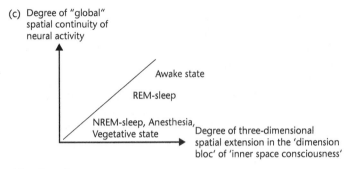

Figure 16-3a-c (Continued)

NEUROPHENOMENAL HYPOTHESIS IB: "SPATIAL AMPLIFICATION" OF NEURAL ACTIVITY AND "WIDTH OF POINT" IN "INNER SPACE CONSCIOUSNESS"

Analogous to the single discrete point in physical time in the width of present (see Chapter 14), one may propose the extension of the single discrete point in physical space beyond itself toward another single discrete point in physical space. Analogous to the width of present, one may then be inclined to speak of a "width of point. As its sibling "width of present" (Chapter 14), the "width of point" is a purely phenomenal concept that describes the experience of space and, more specifically, of a particular discrete point in physical space in our consciousness.

How is such a "width of point" predisposed by particular neuronal mechanisms? I propose that such an extension of the single discrete point beyond itself to the next one may be predisposed by the amplification of the spatial differences as encoded into the neural activity of one particular region to other regions in the brain and their respective neural activities: by amplifying the encoded spatial differences from the neural activity in one particular region and its discrete point in physical space to another region and its particular discrete point in physical space, the former regions' neural activity cannot avoid becoming spatially extended toward the neural activity in the latter region.

Therefore, the amplification of neural activity across different regions cannot avoid its own extension beyond the single discrete points in its particular region. This is manifested in what is described as *functional* connectivity, the co-variation or correlation of two (or more) regions' neural activities across time. And such functional connectivity accompanies the constitution of "local" temporal continuity of neural activity between different particular regions.

Based on these considerations, I postulate the following. I hypothesize that the degree of spatial amplification of neural activity predisposes not only the degree of "local" spatial continuity" on a neuronal level, but also the degree of the "width of point" on the phenomenal level of consciousness. The higher the degree of spatial amplification, the more likely it is that the neural activity of one particular region and its specific discrete point in physical space will be extended to other regions and their discrete point in physical space. This makes possible the constitution of "local" temporal continuity of neural activity, which I suppose to predispose the "width of point" on the phenomenal level of "inner space consciousness."

NEUROPHENOMENAL HYPOTHESIS IC: "SPATIAL CONDENSATION" OF NEURAL ACTIVITY AND "DIMENSION BLOC" IN "INNER SPACE CONSCIOUSNESS"

How about the spatial analogy to what is described as "duration bloc" in the temporal dimension of consciousness? The duration bloc can be characterized by a threefold temporal structure that spans from the past over the present to the future. Applied to the spatial dimension, this suggests a threefold spatial structure that includes all three dimensions of space by linking and connecting them. The various widths of point in space are thus extended into the three dimensions (x, y, and z) of space and can be experienced in consciousness in the gestalt of what I describe as dimension bloc.

The concept of the dimension bloc is a purely phenomenal concept that describes the experience of the extension and linkage of different discrete points in physical space into a three-dimensional space (x, y, and z-dimensions) in consciousness. The single discrete point in space is then extended (or better, projected) onto the three dimensions in space and thus "located" in the three-dimensional grid of space (Fig. 16-3b).

How about the neuronal mechanisms underlying the dimension bloc? I propose that the "global" spatial continuity of neural activity and its underlying neuronal mechanisms, "spatial condensation" and global functional connectivity (see earlier), predispose what we experience as a dimension bloc on the phenomenal level of consciousness. The higher the degree of "spatial condensation" of neural activity, the higher the degree to which the "width of point" can be extended and thus projected into the three dimensions of space, x, y, and z, of the whole brain's neural activity, and the higher the possible degree of the "dimension bloc" and its three-dimensional extension (see Fig. 16-3c).

NEUROPHENOMENAL HYPOTHESIS IIA: CROSS-MODAL INTERACTION AND THE SPATIAL CONTINUITY OF NEURAL ACTIVITY

One question that remains open in the neural regard is that of the kind of stimuli that provide the input to the constitution of the here-suggested spatial continuity of neural activity. We recall from Chapter 4 in Volume I, where I described the constitution of a virtual statistically-based spatial structure in the brain's intrinsic neural activity. I suggested that the spatial structure of the brain's intrinsic activity is based on inputs from interoceptive stimuli from the body, exteroceptive stimuli from the environment, and neural stimuli from the brain itself. This means that the constitution of the spatial continuity of neural activity presupposes the interaction among all three types of stimuli.

Let us be more specific about these interactions. There must be interactions between the different exteroceptive stimuli from the different sensory modalities: cross-modal interaction, as we described it in Chapter 11 (Volume I). Such cross-modal interaction must interact with the interoceptive stimuli, amounting to intero–extero interaction. And such intero–extero interaction must in turn be linked to the brain's intrinsic activity via stimulus–rest (and rest–stimulus) interaction. All three interactions will thus constitute the spatial continuity of the brain's intrinsic activity as sketched in this chapter.

How can we test this in experimental terms? One could hypothesize that the degree of cross-modal interaction, the linkage between different exteroceptive stimuli, may directly depend on the degree of the spatial continuity of the brain's intrinsic activity and thus its resting-state functional connectivity. For instance, the possible degrees of auditory–tactile interaction (see Chapter 11 for details) may then be predicted by the degree of the resting-state functional connectivity between the auditory and somatosensory cortices. This leads me to postulate that more generally cross-modal interaction and its interactions with interoceptive and neural stimuli are essential in constituting the spatial continuity of the brain's intrinsic activity (see also Chapter 4 in Volume I).

NEUROPHENOMENAL HYPOTHESIS IIB: CROSS-MODAL INTERACTION AND "WIDTH OF POINT" AND THE "DIMENSION BLOC" OF CONSCIOUSNESS

The foregoing was a discussion of the neuronal side. How about the phenomenal side? One could predict that the degree to which (for instance) the tactile stimulus' single discrete point in physical space is extended into a "width of point" will depend on the degree of local auditory-somatosensory cortical resting-state functional connectivity.

The higher the degree of functional connectivity between auditory and tactile cortices in the resting state, the more the tactile stimulus' single discrete point in space can be extended toward the single discrete point in space associated with the auditory stimulus, and thus the more extended the tactile stimulus' "width of point" is in consciousness. And of course the reverse also holds for the auditory stimulus and its relationship to the auditory stimulus.

Finally, the integration of auditory-somatosensory cortical resting-state functional connectivity into the more global resting-state functional connectivity of the whole brain will be relevant for the general spatial experience, the "dimension bloc." The higher the degree to which the auditory-somatosensory functional connectivity is integrated into the resting-state functional connectivity of the rest of the brain, the more likely it is that the auditory-tactile "width of point" will be integrated into a three-dimensional space of consciousness, the "dimension bloc"; and the more likely it is that the initial cross-modal auditory–tactile interaction will be associated with consciousness.

What does all this tell us about the relationship between the brain's intrinsic activity and sensory functions as implicated in cross-modal interaction? It tells us that the possible degree of cross-modal interaction and its association with consciousness depends on the local and global spatial continuity of the resting state's neural activity. More generally, one may want to say that resting-state activity exists prior to and precedes sensory functions and their cross-modal interaction. In short, sensory function follows resting-state activity.

This has important implications for the relationship between sensory functions and consciousness; that is, phenomenal functions. Since the brain's resting-state activity and its degree of spatial continuity are essential for (or better, predispose) the degree of possible consciousness that can be associated with (for instance) the tactile or auditory stimulus, the phenomenal function precedes the sensory function. Conversely, the sensory function follows the phenomenal function, rather than the latter following the former. We will see in later chapters that this holds true not only for sensory functions, but even more so for cognitive functions and their relationship to phenomenal functions.

NEUROPHENOMENAL HYPOTHESIS IIC: DISSOCIATION BETWEEN "WIDTH OF POINT" AND "DIMENSION BLOC" IN DISORDERS OF CONSCIOUSNESS

We discussed the various neuronal mechanisms underlying phenomenal features like "width of point" and "dimension bloc." What if the underlying neuronal mechanisms fail? Based on my considerations, I hypothesize that all three cases—vegetative state, NREM sleep, and anesthesia—can be characterized by a significant decrease in the degree of spatial extension of both the "global" spatial continuity of their brain's neural activity and the dimension bloc in their consciousness. Let us start with what may be preserved in these cases, which then sheds a better light what no longer works.

These patients' brains may still be able to constitute "local" temporal continuities in their different regions' neural activity. This may, for instance, be reflected in the presence of stimulus-induced activity and task-related neural activity changes in vegetative patients (see Chapter 29 for details). Phenomenally, their "width of point" may therefore still be preserved to a certain degree, which may be manifested in their ability to carry out certain sensorimotor or cognitive tasks (see Chapter 29 for details).

In contrast, these patients may no longer be able to constitute "global" temporal continuity in their brain's resting-state neural activity. This is well reflected in the earlier-described findings of decreased or nonspecific spread of neural activity across different regions as observed in VS, anesthesia, and NREM sleep by the group around Tononi.

The "width of point" can thus no longer be extended and projected into the three-dimensional space of the whole brain, which makes the constitution of the "dimension bloc" impossible. That, however, makes it altogether impossible to associate consciousness in general and its three-dimensional spatial structure in particular with the otherwise purely neuronal resting-state or stimulus-induced activity. The level or state of consciousness is consequently extremely reduced, if not completely absent, as can indeed be observed in VS, NREM sleep, and anesthesia (see Chapters 28 and 29 for details).

Neurophenomenal Hypothesis IIIA: Integration of Space and Time into "Global" Spatiotemporal Continuity of Neural Activity

One question concerns how "global" temporal and spatial continuities of neural activity are integrated into one homogenous spatiotemporal structure that characterizes consciousness. We associated "global" temporal continuity of neural activity with predominantly low-frequency fluctuations (see Chapter 15), while "global" spatial continuity was characterized by functional connectivity (see earlier). The question is now how both functional connectivity and low-frequency fluctuations are related to each other in order to understand how both spatial and temporal dimensions can be integrated on the phenomenal level of consciousness.

Low-frequency fluctuations are not purely temporal. The lower the frequency range, the more extended and spread is their operation across different regions. Hence, lower frequency ranges go along with a higher degree of spatial spread (Buzsaki 2006; Singer 1999; 2009; Buzsaki and Draguhn 2004) while the spatial spread of higher frequency fluctuations is more restricted to a single region. This means that frequency fluctuations cannot only be characterized by a temporal dimension but also by a spatial one.

The same, though in a converse way, holds for functional connectivity. Functional connectivity is defined by the degree of the temporal relationship between different regions' neural activities (see Chapters 4 and 5 in Volume I); the more their neural activities are linked and connected across their different discrete points in time, the higher the degree of their respective functional connectivity. This means that functional connectivity is inherently both spatial and temporal (see Fig. 16-4).

The intrinsic integration of spatial and temporal neuronal measures is also well reflected in the fact that there are no separate spatial and temporal codes for the encoding of neural activity (see Chapter 10 in Volume I). Both spatial and temporal dimensions are encoded into the same neural activity, as is manifested in functional connectivity and frequency fluctuations.

Accordingly, the brain itself and, more specifically, its encoding of neural activity do not make a principal difference between spatial and temporal dimensions. The distinction between spatial and temporal dimension may thus be rather related to us as outside observers of the brain's neural activity than to the brain itself and its encoding and generation of neural activity (see Appendix 3 in Volume I for more details on the distinction between *brain* and *observer*).

Neurophenomenal Hypothesis IIIB: "Global" Spatiotemporal Continuity of Neural Activity and "Inner Time-Space Consciousness"

If both low-frequency fluctuations and functional connectivity are inherently spatial and temporal, the constitution of "global" temporal continuity of neural activity "cannot avoid" going along with its "global" spatial continuity and vice versa. I therefore propose that the degree of "global" temporal continuity of neural activity is directly and positively related to its degree of "global" spatial continuity: the higher degrees of "global" temporal continuity that are constituted in neural activity, the higher its degree of "global" spatial continuity (and vice versa).

Both "global" spatial and temporal continuity of neural activity are suggested to respectively predispose the "dimension bloc" and the "duration bloc" on the phenomenal level of consciousness. One could therefore postulate an analogous direct and positive relationship between "dimension bloc" and "duration bloc" and thus between "inner time and space consciousness." The higher the degree of temporal extension of the "duration bloc" in consciousness, the higher the degree to which the "dimension bloc" can extend spatially.

Accordingly, I propose that spatial and temporal dimensions are directly and positively related to each other in consciousness. We cannot avoid experiencing spatial and temporal dimensions intimately linked in our consciousness. This implies that we remain

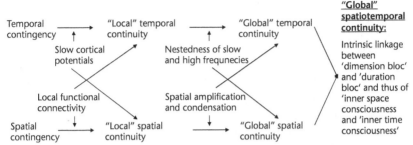

Figure 16-4 Neuronal mechanisms of spatiotemporal continuity of neural activity. The figure summarizes the neuronal mechanisms that are supposed to underlie the constitution of "local" and "global" spatial and temporal continuity of neural activity and how both are intrinsically linked and converge in "global" spatiotemporal continuity of neural activity. *Upper part*: Slow cortical potentials and temporal nestedness between high- and low-frequency fluctuations are central in yielding "local" and "global" temporal continuity of neural activity. Besides their temporal dimension, they also carry a spatial dimension and thus contribute to the constitution of "local" and "global" spatial continuity of neural activity (as indicated by the downward crossed arrows from the upper to the lower part). *Lower part*: Local functional connectivity and amplification and condensation of neural differences across different regions' neural activities are central in constituting "local" and "global" spatial continuity of neural activity. They also carry a temporal dimension and thus contribute to the constitution of "local" and "global" temporal continuity (as indicated by the upward crossed arrows from lower to upper part). *Right part*: Taken together, this results in the constitution of "global" spatiotemporal continuity of neural activity across different discrete points in both physical time and space. There is thus intrinsic and thus necessary or unavoidable linkage between spatial and temporal dimensions in the brain's neural activity. That, in turn, results in intrinsically linking "inner space consciousness," that is, the "dimension bloc," to "inner time consciousness," that is, the "duration bloc."

in principle unable to segregate and thus dissociate "inner time and space consciousness" from each other in our experience. There is thus what I describe as "inner time-space consciousness."

I suggest that such integration between time and space in our "inner time-space consciousness" is predisposed; that is, made necessary and unavoidable, by our brain and its constitution of a "global" spatiotemporal continuity of its own neural activity. Such "global" spatiotemporal continuity is based on the intrinsic linkage between spatial and temporal dimensions in the brain's neuronal measures like functional connectivity and frequency fluctuations.

Neurometaphorical Excursion
IA: DIFFERENT "EGG MODELS"

How can we further illustrate the processes underlying the constitution of "global"

spatiotemporal continuity and their relationship to consciousness? For that, I would like to invoke a figurative comparison of cooking an omelette out of two different eggs, egg A and egg B. Let us imagine different models of relationship.

The first model may be described as the "side-by-side model." This corresponds to the situation when I take egg A from the basket in the corner and put it on the table side by side with egg B from the refrigerator. That may be described as $(x(1)(a - b) (y(2)(c - d))$ or as the "table model of egg A and egg B," where both remain parallel and segregated.

The second model is the one of additive and linear interaction; this corresponds to the situation where I put egg A and egg B into the pan; they now lie on top of each other, with egg A lying on top of egg B, which I also cracked open and released into the pan before lighting the burner. Though they are now on top of each other, egg A and egg B are still essentially the same as originally. This reflects $[(x(1)(a - b) + y(2) (c - d)]$ or what can be called the "pan model of egg A and egg B," which presupposes interactive but merely additive and linear processing.

Finally, the third model corresponds to the process of cooking wherein both egg A and egg B fuse and integrate with each other, resulting in an omelette where neither the original egg AQ nor the original egg B can be recognized as such anymore. This amounts to $[(x(1) - y(2))(a{-}b) - (c{-}d)]$ or the "omelette model of egg A and egg B," which presupposes interactive and integrative processing.

NEUROMETAPHORICAL EXCURSION IB: FROM "EGG MODELS" TO "OMELETTE SPACE"

What does this metaphor imply for consciousness? Let us look at the omelette now. The omelette is spatially continuous because the originally heterogenous and discontinuous spaces occupied by egg A and egg B either on the table or in the pan (before cooking) are fused and integrated into one continuous "space," the space of the omelette. Even if egg B may somehow still be recognizable within the omelette, its space is now continuous with that of egg A, and it is this spatial continuity that identifies and characterizes the omelette *qua* omelette. The omelette can therefore be characterized by "spatial continuity" as distinguished from the "spatial discontinuity" of egg A and egg B on the table and in the pan (before cooking). One may consequently want to compare consciousness and its spatial continuity to the final omelette and its spatial continuity between egg A and egg B.

Is consciousness thus nothing but an omelette? The spatial continuity of the omelette can only be constituted on the basis of nonlinear and nonadditive interaction between egg A and egg B. Only such nonlinear and nonadditive interaction allows egg A and egg B to merge their respective spatial continuities into one unifying spatial continuity, that of the omelette, which signifies what I call "omelette space."

The same applies obviously to the brain. I proposed a nonadditive and nonlinear model of interaction, $[(x(1) - y(2))(a - b) - (c - d)]$, to hold for the amplification and subsequent condensation of neural activity across different regions of the brain. In the same way, egg A and egg B merge into one continuous space, the "omelette space."

Therefore, I suggest that the different spatial differences as encoded in the different regions' neural activities merge into a novel spatial difference, $[(x(1) - y(2))(a - b) - (c - d)]$, which then is characterized by continuity of space between $(a - b)$ and $(c - d)$. Accordingly, I propose "global" spatial continuity of neural activity between $(a - b)$ and $(c - d)$ to be manifested in the novel spatial difference of $[(x(1) - y(2))(a - b) - (c - d)]$.

NEUROMETAPHORICAL EXCURSION IC: "OMELETTE SPACE" AS "INNER SPACE CONSCIOUSNESS"

How can we further illustrate "spatial amplification and condensation" of neural activity in our omelette example? There is the space of the pan. That space is amplified by dividing it into two different spatial continuities once one puts egg A and egg B into it, the "local" spatial continuity of egg A and that of egg B. This corresponds to the "spatial amplification" of neural activity across different regions of the brain.

However, the process of cooking and heating lets both egg A and egg B, including their respective spatial continuities, merge into the omelette and its one unifying "global" spatial continuity. One can thus say that the two "local" spatial continuities of egg A and egg B are here condensed into a more "global" spatial continuity, that of the omelette and its "omelette space."

How does that relate to consciousness and especially the disorders of consciousness? NREM sleep and possibly also the vegetative state may be proposed to correspond to the situation when egg A and egg B are lying side by side. Despite strong heat from cooking, egg A and egg B do not fuse into an omelette since the former's "local" spatial continuities remain unable to merge into the more "global" spatial continuity of the latter.

Why can egg A and egg B no longer merge their "local" spatial continuities into one "global" spatial continuity, the "omelette space"? Egg A and egg B must have lost some feature that usually predisposes them to fuse into one "global" spatial continuity during heating and cooking. The analogous scenario seems to occur in the disorders of consciousness. We can now apply as much "heat," that is, extrinsic stimuli or tasks, to the subjects in NREM sleep or those who are in a vegetative state. They will not become conscious.

Why will these subjects not become conscious? The "local" spatial continuities of their brain's neural activities seem to have lost their yet-unknown neuronal feature that predisposes them to merge into a more "global" spatial continuity of neural activity. This means that their regional functional and effective connectivity that constitutes local spatial connectivity, for some yet-unknown reason, can no longer be transformed into a more global functional connectivity of neural activity.

If, however, they cannot constitute "global" spatial continuity in their brain's neural activity anymore, these patients lose their neural predisposition to consciousness in general and "inner space consciousness" in particular. Their level or state of consciousness should consequently decrease to an abnormally strong degree, which is exactly what one observes clinically.

NEUROMETAPHORICAL EXCURSION ID: DISSOCIATION BETWEEN "EGG SPACE" AND "OMELETTE SPACE" IN VEGETATIVE STATE

Finally, it should be noted that the "local" spatial continuities (of egg A and egg B) seem to be preserved in at least the vegetative state, while the "global" spatial continuity, the omelette, is disrupted in this condition. This may be manifested in the preserved stimulus- or task-related activity, as has indeed been observed in these patients (see Chapter 29 for details).

Why is this so? Let us go back to our omelette example. Due to the loss of the feature that predisposes egg A and egg B to fuse into one omelette, egg A and egg B cannot fuse into an omelette even if strong heat is applied.

Analogously, subjects in NREM sleep or vegetative state remain unable to advance from their mere neural processing of stimuli to consciousness. Due to the apparent lack of the yet-unknown neuronal feature that predisposes nonlinear interaction, the stimuli and

their associated stimulus-induced activities and "local" spatial continuities cannot be merged anymore into a more "global" spatial continuity of neural activity.

As the step from eggs and onions to the omelette is disrupted, so is the one from the regions' neural activities to consciousness. Hence, vegetative subjects still have different "eggs" like egg A and egg B; that is, different regional neural activities, while their brains remain unable to constitute "global" spatial continuity and thus to cook themselves an omelette.

Let us summarize. There is still the space of the eggs in VS, the "egg space," which accounts for their stimulus-induced or task-related activity. In contrast, the "omelette space" is lost, which makes it impossible for the patients to associate their purely neuronal stimulus-induced activity with consciousness and its phenomenal features. Accordingly, there is a dissociation between "egg space" and "omelette space" in VS. This makes it clear that without omelette, there is no consciousness either.

Open Questions

One open question concerns the phenomenal specification of our experience of space in consciousness; that is, "inner space consciousness." Unlike in time, where I ventured into the phenomenological, that is, subjective-experiential detail (see Chapters 13–15), I refrained from that in the case of space. I here restricted myself to mainly the constitution of "local" and "global" spatial continuity of neural activity, whose relationship to specific phenomenal features of spatial experience I left open for future exploration. Analogous to the case of time, it should be mentioned that my emphasis on the constitution of spatial continuity and ultimately phenomenal space must be distinguished from the perception and cognition of space as, for instance, social or interpersonal space (see Lloyd 2009). What I have here called "global" spatial continuity, which describes the constitution of neural activity, may correspond on the perceptual and especially the cognitive level to what is conceptualized as the "global workspace" or "global neuronal workspace" (Baars 2003; Deheaene and Changeux 2011). I will discuss in Chapter 24 and Appendix 1 how the latter two as perceptually and cognitively based models of consciousness stand in relation to my more neurophenomenal approach to consciousness.

Besides the link to cognitive neuroscience, there is also some implication for neurophilosophy. A 2010 investigation in animals linked especially the grid cells in the entorhinal cortex with the cognition of space (see Langston et al. 2010; Wills et al. 2010).

The commentary on the latter two papers (Palmer and Lynch 2010; see also Dehaene and Brannon 2010) points out that the neuronal mechanisms of representing space may be innate and thus independent of experience.

This is, as the authors propose, compatible with the view of the philosopher Immanuel Kant on the a priori nature of space and time. How does that fare to my approach here? What I describe as neural predisposition does, in fact, reflect the structural and functional structure and organization that is intrinsic to the brain and thus defines the brain *qua* brain (see Introduction).

Let me briefly elaborate and indicate the following. "Global" functional connectivity, difference-based coding as the encoding of spatial and temporal differences into neural activity, and the consequent "spatial amplification and condensation" of the encoded spatial and temporal differences may indeed be considered intrinsic features of the brain.

Since I consider these intrinsic features of the brain as necessary, that is, predisposing conditions of possible consciousness (see the Introduction), they may indeed be also characterized as *a priori* with regard to consciousness

(and our cognition), in very much the same way the philosopher Immanuel Kant suggested with regard to mental features of the mind like his famous categories; that is, as a necessary and unavoidable condition (in a logical and epistemic sense, as the philosophers may want to specify).

Future neurophilosophical investigation is necessary, however, to further detail and exploit the analogies between the here-suggested neurophenomenal hypotheses of space and time on one hand, and Kant's view of space and time as *a priori* intuitions on the other (see also Appendix 3 in this volume on unity, Kant, and neuroscience; as well as Northoff 2012 for a first step in this direction).

Finally, one may want to know the exact physiological and biochemical mechanisms underlying the constitution of both "global" spatial and temporal continuity of neural activity. This would well complement the rather statistically based neuronal measures like functional connectivity and frequency fluctuations on which we focused so far.

To get a better grip on their underlying physiological and biochemical mechanisms, we therefore now discuss the role of GABA and glutamate in these neuronal measures and how they predispose "inner space and time consciousness." While we discussed in Volume I the neurobiochemical mechanisms of GABA and glutamate in relation to both resting-state and stimulus-induced activity (see Chapters 3, 6, and 12 in Volume I), the next chapter extends and links them to consciousness and its phenomenal features.

CHAPTER 17
Glutamate, GABA, and "Inner Time and Space Consciousness"

Summary

The previous chapters focused on the neuronal mechanisms of spatial and temporal continuity of neural activity and their manifestation in "inner time and space consciousness." I thereby left open the biochemical mechanisms underlying difference-based coding and its constitution of spatial and temporal continuity of neural activity. Glutamate is the major excitatory transmitter that modulates functional connectivity between different regions. Since functional connectivity is hypothesized to be central for constituting spatial continuity of neural activity, I propose glutamate and neuronal excitation as crucial biochemical mechanisms in yielding spatial continuity of neural activity. GABA is the major inhibitory transmitter in the cortex that modulates the degree of neuronal inhibition within the region itself. Recent data show that GABA is central in the neuronal synchronization of neuronal activity within and across regions. This role in synchronizing neuronal activity lets me propose that GABA may be central in yielding local (regional), and ultimately global, (transregional) temporal continuity of neural activity. However, direct neurophenomenal support for the distinct roles of GABA and glutamate in temporal and spatial continuity of neural activity is rather sparse at this point. There is, however, some indirect support from neuropsychiatric disorders like depression and schizophrenia as it is discussed in the concluding sections of the chapter. Schizophrenic patients do show disruption in their "inner time consciousness" with extremely short "duration blocs" as well as decreased local and global temporal continuity of their neural activity as seemingly modulated by abnormal GABA. In contrast, patients with depression can be characterized by abnormal "inner time and space consciousness" temporal "dysbalance" between past, present, and future, as well as spatial "dysbalance" between body and environment; this may be closely related to the observed abnormal changes in glutamate in these patients.

Key Concepts and Topics Covered

Glutamate; neuronal excitation; inner time consciousness, inner space consciousness, GABA, space, neuronal inhibition, vegetative state, anesthesia, difference-based coding, sparse coding, depression, schizophrenia

Neuroempirical Background IA: From GABA and Glutamate to "Inner Time and Space Consciousness"

I have so far discussed the neuronal mechanisms that predispose—that is, make possible and thus necessary and unavoidable—the constitution of "inner time and space consciousness." The various predisposing neuronal mechanisms included temporal nestedness between low- and high-frequency fluctuations (Chapter 15), functional connectivity (Chapter 16), slow cortical potentials as low-frequency fluctuation (Chapter 14), and dynamic activity changes in the resting-state activity itself (Chapter 13). Most important, I postulated that these various neuronal mechanisms are based on the encoding of neural activity in terms of spatial and temporal differences, thus presupposing difference-based coding rather than stimulus-based coding.

Since the various neuronal mechanisms themselves are based on difference-based coding while at the same time predisposing "inner time and space consciousness," consciousness itself must be directly dependent on difference-based coding. I therefore hypothesized that the degree of temporal and spatial differences that can be encoded into the brain's neural activity predisposes the possible degree of the level or state of consciousness (see especially Chapters 14–16). The larger the temporal and spatial differences that can be encoded into neural activity during either resting state or stimulus-induced activity, the larger the possible degree of the level or state of consciousness, including the possible degree of "inner time and space consciousness."

Accordingly, I suggest that difference-based coding predisposes and makes ultimately necessary or unavoidable "inner time and space consciousness." In order to understand the neural basis of consciousness including "inner time and space consciousness," we therefore need to reveal the exact neuronal mechanisms of difference-based coding.

Difference-based coding was determined as the brain's encoding strategy, as its neural code, in Volume I. More specifically, difference-based coding described the particular encoding strategy of the brain by means of which it encodes and thus generates its own neural activity during both resting-state and stimulus-induced activity. The alternative consists in encoding the single discrete points in physical time and space by themselves into neural activity. This would be the case if there were stimulus- rather than difference-based coding. That, however, is empirically implausible given the abundance of evidence discussed in Volume I.

How are the temporal and spatial differences constituted that are encoded into neural activity? For that answer, we showed the underlying biochemical mechanisms; namely GABA and glutamate, to be central (in Chapters 2, 6, and 12 in Volume I). How though are these biochemical mechanisms that underlie the encoding of differences into neural activity related to consciousness and its phenomenal features?

I now extend the purely neuronal and biochemical claim of GABA and glutamate making possible difference-based coding to the phenomenal realm of consciousness. In a nutshell, I hypothesize that GABA and glutamate predispose "inner time and space consciousness" via their impact on difference-based coding. My neuronal and biochemical hypotheses from Volume I are thus extended to consciousness and therefore complemented by a neurophenomenal hypothesis here in Volume II.

NEUROEMPIRICAL BACKGROUND IB: GABA AND GLUTAMATE PREDISPOSE "INNER TIME AND SPACE CONSCIOUSNESS"

GABA is the main inhibitory transmitter, while glutamate is excitatory. I showed that both constitute the excitation–inhibition balance (EIB), which itself is a difference-based signal (see Chapter 2, Volume I). Despite their co-occurrence, GABA and glutamate seem to make differential contributions to the encoding of spatial and temporal differences within the EIB:

Glutamate injects early neural excitation, which then is disrupted by incoming GABA-ergic neural inhibition. Due to the higher number of interneurons, the initial glutamatergic excitation is accompanied by a disproportional increase in neural inhibition. Following Buszaki, this introduces nonlinearity into the neural system (see Chapter 2). Such nonlinearity was shown to apply to both resting-state activity (see Chapter 6, Volume I) and stimulus-induced activity (Chapter 12, Volume I).

More specifically, results on the regional level of neural activity showed that glutamate mediates neural activity and especially functional connectivity between different regions already in the resting state (see Chapters 6 and 12). At the same time, the impact of glutamatergic action seems to extend to stimulus-induced activity too, in that it apparently modulates the transition from resting state to stimulus-induced activity (see Chapter 12). How about GABA? Rather than exerting strong impact during the resting-state activity itself, GABA may predominantly modulate the stronger changes in neural activity during the transition from resting-state to stimulus-induced activity that is rest–stimulus interaction (see Chapter 12).

Though both act in conjunction when constituting the EIB, GABA and glutamate nevertheless seem to exert differential impacts on the neural activity on a regional level during both resting-state and stimulus-induced activity (see Chapters 6 and 12). While their exact differential roles remain to be determined at this point, the recent imaging data suggest different contributions of GABA and glutamate on the encoding of spatial and temporal differences into neural activity.

How now are GABA and glutamate related to "inner time and space consciousness"? Since we postulated difference-based coding to predispose "inner time and space consciousness," one may now suggest the latter to be based on both GABA and glutamate. Moreover, due to their differential neuronal effects, one may also propose that GABA and glutamate predispose distinct phenomenal features of "inner time and space consciousness."

I consequently propose different neurophenomenal roles for GABA and glutamate in "inner time and space consciousness." There is indeed some empirical support, albeit sparse and tentative, for such differential neurophenomenal roles of GABA and glutamate. This is further supported indirectly, however, by the neurophenomenal abnormalities in psychiatric disorders like schizophrenia and depression. The differential roles of GABA and glutamate in predisposing "inner time and space consciousness" will be the focus in this chapter.

NEURONAL FINDINGS IA: GLUTAMATE AND "INNER *TIME* CONSCIOUSNESS"

Let us start with glutamate. Glutamatergic-mediated transmission operates via various receptors, among which the NMDA receptor is probably the most important and influential one. Substances like ketamine antagonize the NMDA receptor and thus block glutamatergic-mediated transmission. Using ketamine in higher doses leads to anesthesia, while application of sub-anesthetic doses induces a variety of rather interesting changes in the experience of time and space; that is "inner time and space consciousness." These shall be discussed in the following section.

Pomarol-Clotet et al. (2006) investigated healthy subjects during the application of ketamine in a sub-anesthetic dose. These subjects showed a variety of interesting psychological changes when exposed to ketamine for approximately two hours. As measured with the PSE scale (present state examination), many subjects showed tiredness, poor concentration, inefficient thinking, heightened perception, and changed contents in perception.

How about phenomenal changes in "inner time and space consciousness"? The subjects' perception of time was clearly altered. Changed perception of time was, for instance, expressed in the following way by one of the subjects of that study: "It's stopped; it feels like I've been here for hours." However, the converse may also take place. Rather than slowing down of time in subjective experience, some subjects experienced an increase in the speed of subjective time during ketamine.

In addition to these temporal alterations, some subjects also showed subjective spatial alterations. This was manifest in their sense of the body; they experienced a sensation of being outside themselves and detached from the own body. This was, for instance, measured by the Clinician Administered Dissociation Symptom Scale (CADSS), where many items concerning the subject's own body are included that were affected by the application of ketamine. These items included "feeling disconnected from one's own body," "sense of body changed," and "as if looking on things from outside the body."

NEURONAL FINDINGS IB: GLUTAMATE AND "INNER *SPACE* CONSCIOUSNESS"

A subsequent study from the same group (Morgan et al. 2011) investigated the impact of ketamine in sub-anesthetic doses specifically on body ownership. While applying ketamine, they tested what is described as the "rubber hand illusion" that is a marker of body owner-ship. During the rubber hand illusion, a person feels and experiences a rubber hand lying visibly on the table (while his own hand is lying hidden and invisible beneath the table) as if it is his own hand, while both hands (i.e., his own and the rubber hand) are touched by a brush. This rub-ber hand illusion is even more pronounced when both rubber hand and the subject's own hand are stroked synchronously by the brush. Subjective measures concerned the extent and degree of the rubber hand illusion (i.e., sensation, felt rubber hand, reality of rubber hand, touch, real hand turning rubbery, etc.).

How did ketamine now affect the rubber hand illusion? Interestingly, ketamine induced a significantly stronger increase in the various subjective measures of the rubber hand illusion itself and the subsequent mislocalization of the subject's own hand in the rubber hand. Hence, the blockade of NMDA receptors by ketamine led to a significant increase in the illusion with the subsequent confusion between the subject's own hand and the rubber hand. The illusion and confusion were also observed when the strokes to the rubber hand and the real hand were set asynchronously rather than synchro-nously. That is remarkable, since, without ket-amine, both illusion and confusion significantly decrease during asynchronous strokes to real and rubber hands.

Ketamine thus seems to affect the experi-ence of time in that it abnormally constricts or extends temporal duration. Moreover, it seems to affect the experience of space in that it changes the perception of one's own body in relation to the environment, as is documented in the rubber hand illusion. This suggests a central role for glutamatergic transmission in constituting the temporal and spatial structure of consciousness; that is, "inner time and space consciousness."

Neuronal findings IIA: Glutamate and Neuroenergetic coupling

These studies used sub-anesthetic doses of ket-amine. How about anesthetic doses? Going from the lower sub-anesthetic to the much higher anesthetic doses, ketamine can induce full-blown anesthesia (see Alkire 2008; Alkire et al. 2008a and b; and Långsjö et al. 2012, for recent papers). This is in accordance with other anesthetic drugs like barbiturates, propofol, or etomidate (and the whole flurane group) that also antago-nize the NMDA receptor (thereby inhibiting glutamatergic-mediated transmission). Other receptors like muscarine, glycine, nicotine, AMPA, and serotonin are also modulated by anesthetic drugs, the main targets of anesthetic drugs are indeed NMDA and GABA-A receptors (see van Dort et al. 2008 for an overview).

How is it possible for NMDA-ergic drugs to induce anesthesia and thus loss of conscious-ness? One of the main factors may be the cou-pling of glutamate and its associated neural activity to the energy metabolism of the brain. Evidence for that comes from the group around R. G. Shulman (Shulman et al. 2003, 2006, 2009; Hyder et al. 2006, 2013).

They investigated the level of glucose and acetate and could thereby measure the cerebral energy production rates of neurons by the rate of glucose oxidation and the coupled rates of GABA and glutamate. In addition to the neu-rons' firing rates, glucose oxidation as well as GABA and glutamate were measured during different behavioral activities as well as during different degrees of anesthesia. Such combined investigation of glucose oxidation with GABA and glutamate allowed the investigators to reveal the coupling of glutamatergic-mediated neural activity to the degree of energy metabolism as signified by glucose oxidation.

How are energy and neural activity coupled? There was a clear relationship between the degree of glucose oxidation indicating energy demand and the change in the concentration of glutamate as coupled to the rate of neuronal fir-ing. Higher firing rates of the neurons increased the concentration of glutamate, which accom-panied higher degrees of glucose oxidation. This suggests close coupling between energy consumption and neural activity, with gluta-mate and glutamine seemingly mediating their relationship.

Most important, such neuroenergetic cou-pling takes place in the resting state itself. About

80%–85% of the glucose as the main energy provider was used to maintain and sustain high neuronal activity in the resting state; for example, in the absence of specific stimulation. This suggests that the high energy demand of the brain is used to maintain a continuously high level of resting-state activity so that glutamate linking energy and neural activity already has a central role in constituting the brain's resting-state activity.

NEURONAL FINDINGS IIB: GLUTAMATE AND THE LEVEL OR STATE OF CONSCIOUSNESS

How, then, does anesthesia affect the neuroenergetic coupling? Shulman remarks that the injection of anesthetic drugs led to a considerable decrease in energy consumption, which was accompanied by a decrease in the level of resting-state activity; that is, the neurons' firing rates. Since anesthesia leads to loss of consciousness, energy consumption and the energetic supply seem to be central for maintaining a high level or state of consciousness. On the basis of these findings, Shulman claims that the level or state of consciousness depends on the level of the brain's resting-state activity and its energetic metabolic supply (see Shulman et al. 2003, 2004,; Hyder et al. 2006, 2013, van Eijsden et al. 2009).

One would therefore expect extremely reduced metabolic-energetic consumption and supply to also be present in other disorders of consciousness like vegetative state (VS). This is indeed the case, as VS patients often show a 30%–50% decrease in their global metabolism (see Chapters 28 and 29 for details on the neuroenergetic coupling in VS in particular and consciousness in general).

Taken together, results from anesthesia and other disorders of consciousness indicate that glutamatergic transmission is closely related not only to energy metabolism and resting-state activity level, but also, via its modulation of the neuroenergetic coupling, to consciousness. Glutamate, and especially its precursor glutamine, are coupled to the oxidative glucose utilization that provides energy, while at the same time mediating neural activity; that is, neural excitation.

Accordingly, glutamate and glutamine modulate the brain's neuroenergetic coupling, which, as the results by Shulman and others demonstrate, predisposes the degree of the level or state of consciousness. Glutamate and its precursor glutamine have a central role in neuroenergetic coupling that provides the energy necessary for any subsequent neural activity like the encoding of spatial and temporal differences into neural activity.

In the following discussion, we will not explicitly discuss the role of neuroenergetic coupling by itself, but rather start from the encoding of spatial and temporal differences into neural activity; that is, difference-based coding. This, however, will change in Chapters 28 and 29 where we, on the basis of the findings in VS, will explicitly discuss the direct impact of glutamatergic-mediated neuroenergetic coupling on the degrees of both difference-based coding and the level or state of consciousness.

NEUROPHENOMENAL HYPOTHESIS IA: GLUTAMATE MODULATES "TEMPORAL NESTEDNESS" BETWEEN LOW- AND HIGH-FREQUENCY FLUCTUATIONS

The results of ketamine challenge demonstrated clear impact of ketamine and hence of glutamate on inner time consciousness, with the time being either extended or shrunk. This means that ketamine and thus the NMDA receptors seem to modulate the possible degree of temporal extension in "inner time consciousness" by either extending or shrinking it.

How are these effects of ketamine on "inner time consciousness" neuronally mediated? For the answer, we need to go back briefly to the neurophenomenal hypotheses postulated in the previous chapters. I proposed in Chapter 15 that the degree of the "duration bloc" as a phenomenal hallmark of "inner time consciousness" is predisposed by the degree of "global" temporal continuity of neuronal activity. The "global" temporal continuity of the brain's neural activity in turn was supposed to be related to the degree of integration, the temporal nestedness, between low- and high-frequency fluctuations and their respective phase durations.

"Temporal nestedness" describes the linkage and integration between fluctuations of different frequency ranges, such as between low and high ones. The phase onsets of the low-frequency fluctuations may be coupled to either the phases or the power/amplitude of the higher ones, resulting in what is called phase–phase and phase–power coupling (see Chapters 5 and 15). Based on its neurophenomenal effects with either extending or shrinking the "duration bloc" (see above), I now suggest that ketamine modulates the degree of temporal nestedness between high- and low-frequency fluctuations.

Ketamine should consequently change the relationship between low- and high-frequency fluctuations and more specifically their degree of phase–phase and phase–power coupling. This is indeed supported by a recent study from Hong et al. (2010), who investigated healthy subjects with sub-anesthetic doses of ketamine during an auditory task (simple tone) inducing auditory evoked potentials in electroencephalography (see also Molaee-Ardekani et al. 2007). They observed that ketamine significantly increased the power (they used the power spectrum density as main measure) of gamma fluctuations (40–80 Hz) while reducing those in the delta range (1–5 Hz) and in part also those in the theta-alpha range (5–12 Hz).

Even more interesting, both delta and gamma fluctuations and especially their ratio, that is, the ratio between gamma increase and delta decrease, correlated significantly with the severity of social withdrawal into an inner subjective world (as measured by a subjective scale) under ketamine: the higher the power in gamma and the lower the power in delta, the more subjective social withdrawal symptoms were experienced and observed.

On a whole, these results support the neuronal hypothesis that glutamate and especially the NMDA-receptors modulate the relationship between low- and high-frequency fluctuations and thus their degree of temporal nestedness. Though tentative, these results indicate changes in the degree of phase–phase and phase–power coupling between low- and high-frequency fluctuations. Unfortunately though, the study did not include more specific and direct measures of either consciousness in general or "inner time consciousness" in particular.

NEUROPHENOMENAL HYPOTHESIS IB: GLUTAMATE AND "TEMPORAL DYSBALANCE" WITHIN THE "DURATION BLOC" OF "INNER *TIME* CONSCIOUSNESS"

I have so far discussed the purely neuronal mechanisms of ketamine while leaving aside its neurophenomenal effects. I suggested in Chapter 15 that the length of the time window between the overlapping phase durations of low- and high-frequency fluctuations predisposes the degree of extension of the "duration bloc" in "inner time consciousness." Let us now discuss the neurophenomenal relevance of the time window in further detail.

Why are the overlapping phase durations of low- and high-frequency fluctuations so important for constituting the "duration bloc" of "inner time consciousness"? By coupling their phase durations with each other, low- and high-frequency fluctuations constitute a time window where their respective phase durations overlap. Within this overlapping time window, the degree of neural activity does not change. This implies that different stimuli whose discrete points fall within this time window are encoded into the same neural activity.

Such encoding results in what I described earlier as the "temporal continuity" of neural activity, the degree of sameness of neural activity during the time window of the overlapping phase durations of low- and high-frequency fluctuations (see Chapters 14 and 15). Most important, the length of this time window and thus the degree of temporal continuity was suggested to predispose the degrees of "width of the present" and "duration bloc" as phenomenal hallmarks of "inner time consciousness" (see Chapters 14 and 15).

How is that related to the neurophenomenal effects of ketamine? We recall that ketamine either extended or shrank the duration of subjectively experienced time and thus the degree of temporal extension of both "width of present" and "duration bloc." Since both "width of present" and "duration bloc" depend on the degree of temporal continuity of the neural activity, one would expect ketamine to exert its neurophenomenal effects by modulating the degree of temporal nestedness and thus the phase–phase coupling between low- and high-frequency fluctuations.

Let us detail this neurophenomenal hypothesis. The higher the degree of temporal nestedness, the longer the overlapping time window between low- and high-frequency fluctuations, the higher the degree of temporal continuity of neural activity, and the higher the degree of temporal extension of the "duration bloc." By modulating the degree of temporal nestedness, ketamine either shortens or stretches the duration of the overlapping time window and its degree of temporal continuity of neural activity; this either extends or shrinks the degree of temporal extension of the "duration bloc" in "inner time consciousness."

Accordingly, by changing the relationship between low- and high-frequency fluctuations, ketamine modulates the degree of "global" temporal continuity of neural activity across the whole brain, which then shrinks or extends the degree of the "duration bloc," as reported in the earlier-described studies. There is thus what can be described as "temporal dysbalance" within the "duration bloc" that may be shifted in an abnormal way toward either temporal dimension, past, present, or future.

NEUROPHENOMENAL HYPOTHESIS IIA: GLUTAMATE MODULATES THE EXPERIENCE OF THE BODY IN "INNER *SPACE* CONSCIOUSNESS"

What do the findings about glutamate and ketamine imply for our assumption about spatial continuity? Let us recall. When given in sub-anesthetic doses (see Pomarol-Clotet et al. 2004; Morgan et al. 2011), ketamine induced a variety of different changes that included the alteration and distortion in the degree of spatial and temporal extension of "inner time and space consciousness." I have so far focused only on "inner time consciousness" while neglecting the glutamatergic modulation of "inner space consciousness." This is the focus in the present section.

The effects of ketamine on "inner space consciousness" are well reflected in its modulation of the subjective experience of the subject's own body. One's own body as subjectively experienced is a "content" in our consciousness and is therefore linked and integrated within the spatial structure of consciousness. I characterized the spatial structure of consciousness in the preceding chapter by the "width of point" as indicating the extension beyond the single discrete point in physical space, and the "dimension bloc" that describes the extension of the former into three-dimensional space.

One's own body is subjectively experienced within this spatial structure and therefore becomes part of "inner space consciousness." As described above, ketamine lets subjects experience their body in a different way, as is manifested in illusory body ownership, a feeling of disconnection from one's own body, change in one's sense of body, and so on (see earlier). This strongly indicates that the phenomenal features of "inner space consciousness"—the "width of point" and the "dimension bloc"—must have been modulated by themselves.

This means that any modulation of the space itself, including the "width of point" and the "dimension bloc," should affect the experience of the "contents in space" like one's own body. Accordingly, in order to understand the changes in subjective perception of subjects' own bodies under ketamine, we need to go back how ketamine modulates the spatial structure of consciousness and thus "inner space consciousness." For the answer to that question, we will turn first to the neuronal effects of ketamine.

NEUROPHENOMENAL HYPOTHESIS IIB: FROM GLUTAMATE OVER FUNCTIONAL CONNECTIVITY TO SPATIAL CONTINUITY OF NEURAL ACTIVITY

We recall from Chapter 16 that "inner space consciousness" was suggested to be predisposed by the "global" spatial continuity of neural activity throughout the brain. The "global" spatial continuity of neural activity describes the distribution of neural activity across the whole brain and how it is linked and integrated, which is manifested mainly in "global" functional connectivity. How are such "global" functional connectivity and ultimately the "global" spatial continuity of neural activity related to glutamate?

Let us briefly recall our discussion from Chapter 16 (as well as from Chapters 6 and 12 in Volume I). NMDA receptors mediate neuronal excitation, especially in the cortical output layers (layer 4). Since these cortical output layers send long-range cortico-cortical and cortico-subcortical efferences to other regions (and networks), glutamatergic-mediated neuronal excitation may be central in constituting functional connectivity, thus implying an intrinsically spatial dimension in the action of glutamate. This is indeed supported by the various findings of glutamate modulating the degree of functional connectivity during both resting-state (see Chapter 6) and stimulus-induced activity (see Chapter 12).

How is functional connectivity generated? I postulated that functional connectivity results from the encoding of spatial (and temporal) differences between different regions' neural activities (see Chapter 5, Volume I). Moreover, I suggested that these spatial differences are amplified across the different regions' neural activities, leading to "spatial amplification" as I described it in Chapter 16.

If glutamate is now supposed to mediate functional connectivity, one would expect it to modulate the degree of the spatial (and temporal) differences that can be encoded into neural activity. This in turn will affect the degree of "spatial amplification" of neural activity across the different regions' neural activities, and it should be manifested in changes in their degree of functional connectivity.

This leads me to the following purely neuronal hypothesis. I hypothesize glutamatergic transmission and particularly NMDA receptors to be central in allowing the "spatial amplification" of the encoded spatial differences across the different regions' neural activities. One would therefore expect glutamate to constitute functional connectivity between different regions in both resting-state and stimulus-induced activity, which is indeed supported by the data (see Chapters 6 and 12).

What does this imply for the effects of ketamine? One would expect ketamine to modulate the degree of the encoded spatial differences and especially their degree of "spatial amplification" across the different regions' neural activities. Ketamine should impact the degree of functional connectivity during the resting-state activity (and also during stimulus-induced activity), as has indeed been reported in recent studies (see Scheidegger et al. 2012; Driesen et al. 2013; Niesters et al. 2012; Dawson et al. 2011). Such modulation, especially of resting-state functional connectivity, may be central for understanding the neurophenomenal effects of ketamine as they will be discussed in the next section.

NEUROPHENOMENAL HYPOTHESIS IIC: GLUTAMATE MODULATES THE RELATIONSHIP BETWEEN THE DIFFERENT DIRECTIONS WITHIN THE "DIMENSION BLOC" OF "INNER SPACE CONSCIOUSNESS"

How, then, is all that related to the constitution of "inner space consciousness"? Let us recall from the previous chapter that I proposed the "spatial amplification" of the encoded spatial differences across the different regions' neural activities to be essential in constituting functional connectivity and ultimately "global" spatial continuity of neural activity throughout the whole brain.

Most important, I suggested the degree of "global" spatial continuity of neural activity to predispose the degree of spatial extension of "inner space consciousness." The higher the degree of functional (and effective) connectivity between different regions in the brain, the higher the degrees of "global" spatial continuity of neural activity that can be constituted, and the higher the possible degree of spatial extension in "inner space consciousness"; namely, in the "dimension bloc."

Based on these considerations and the observed ketamine effects, I now postulate that glutamate modulates the degree of "global" spatial continuity of neural activity and thereby the degree of the possible spatial extension of "inner space consciousness" and its "dimension bloc." The "dimension bloc" concerns the extension of the single, discrete unidimensional point in space into a three-dimensional space including x, y, and z dimensions. I suggest that glutamate modulates the "dimension bloc" and its extension into three-dimensional space, which, if so, should be affected by ketamine (see Fig. 17-1a).

This is exactly the case in the earlier-described abnormal subjective experience of subjects' own bodies under ketamine. I propose that under ketamine, the extension of the three-dimensional space is by itself abnormal, which lets us experience any content like our own body in an abnormal way. Ketamine presumably changes the constellation between the x, y, and z coordinates and thus the relationship among the three different dimensions of space, the "dimension bloc" of "inner space consciousness."

The "dimension bloc" in "inner space consciousness" may thus be abnormally tilted toward any of the three directions (x, y, z) under ketamine. This entails that the relationship between one's own person/self, one's own body, and the external world as distinct "contents" within the altered three-dimensional space changes within consciousness and is consequently experienced in an abnormal way. Such an experience of an abnormal relationship between self, body, and world is well reflected in the following quote from a subject who received ketamine in sub-anesthetic dosage: "Either I am the spatial centre of the world and hence ultimately the world or the world is the centre and I no longer exist" (see Pomarol-Clotet et al. 2006, 178; Morgan et al. 2011).

How can we explain such an experience by our assumption of abnormally "tilted" x, y, and z coordinates within the "dimension bloc"? The x, y, and z coordinates, and thus the three dimensions of space, are no longer properly segregated from each other, which makes it impossible for the subject to experience herself and her own body as segregated and different from the world. The x, y, and z coordinates must have been abnormally linked and integrated due to the glutamatergic modulation by ketamine and its apparent abnormal modulation of the encoding of spatial differences and their "spatial amplification" across the different regions' neural activities (see Fig. 17-1b).

NEUROMETAPHORICAL EXCURSION: STRING AND PEARLS

Let me compare the situation to a string and pearls. You have pearls and a string lying side by side on a table. All your pearls are lying in front of you, at different discrete spatial positions on your table. Now you put them all on the string, and suddenly there is a spatial continuum between them. Most important, that changes the relationship between the pearls: they are now no longer segregated and defined by their different discrete positions in the physical space of the table. Instead, they are now defined by their relationship, that is, spatial difference, with each other on the common underlying string.

In the same way as the different pearls are now strung, the different events and objects in the world and the body (and even those occurring in the brain itself) are linked on the string of the brain itself and the spatial structure that its intrinsic activity provides. Hence, the brain's "string" consists of its intrinsic activity's spatiotemporal structure as manifested in functional connectivity and low- and high-frequency fluctuations leading to "global" spatial continuity of neural activity.

Let us go back to the pearls. If now the string itself is no longer held horizontally but tilted vertically toward one of its sides, it will affect the pearls and their spatial (and temporal) relationships, too. This is exactly what ketamine does to the brain when its shifts and "tilts" the intrinsic activity's "string," the functional connectivity and its "global" spatial continuity of neural activity, toward extreme values that are either abnormally high or abnormally low. This means that ketamine abnormally shrinks or extends the functional connectivity between the different regions' neural activities.

That, in turn, strongly affects how the different "pearls," that is, the events and objects in the body and world, can be integrated into each other. Their spatial relations to each other consequently change, too, such that suddenly the world and its various events stand in abnormally close relationship to the self, which then, off course, experiences itself as the center of the world or even as the world itself; as is vividly indicated in the earlier quote.

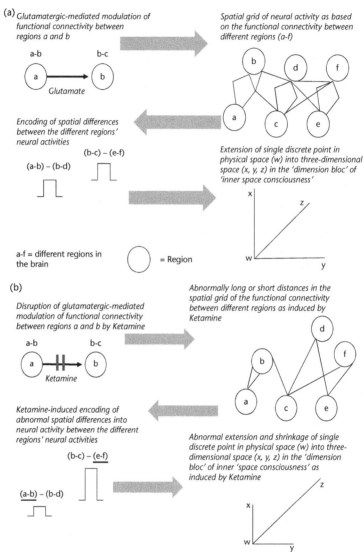

Figure 17-1a and b Glutamate and "inner space consciousness." The figures show the functional connectivity between different regions may impact our experience of space in consciousness, that is, "inner space consciousness." (*a*) This figure shows the modulation by glutamate, while (*b*) demonstrates the changes induced by blockade of glutamate as, for instance, by the NMDA receptor antagonist ketamine. (*Upper left*) The upper left part shows two regions' neural activities (*a, b*) and their functional connectivity as mediated by glutamate (*a*) as it is disrupted (bars) by ketamine (*b*). (*Lower left*) The lower left part shows the encoded spatial differences between the neural activities of the two regions in relation to each other and other regions on the basis of difference-based coding resulting in what is described as functional connectivity. (*Upper right*) Taken together with yet other regions, this leads to the constitution of a spatial grid of neural activities across the different regions of the brain as indicated on the upper right. This leads to "global" spatial continuity of neural activity across the different regions' neural activities. (*Lower right*) Such spatial grid and its "global" spatial continuity across the different regions' neural activities is manifest phenomenally in the experience of an "dimension bloc" as the extension of a single point in space (w) into a three-dimensional space (x, y, z) that constitutes inner space consciousness. Since the functional connectivity is mediated by glutamate, I propose the constitution of the dimension bloc in "inner space consciousness" to be dependent upon glutamate (*a*). Blockade of glutamate leads to an abnormally shrunk or extended extension of the single discrete point in physical space (w) into three-dimensional space in the dimension bloc of inner space consciousness during the application of ketamine (*b*).

Accordingly, in the same way the pearls' relationship to each other changes once one tilts the string, tilting the brain's string, its spatial (and temporal) structure of its intrinsic activity, by (for instance) ketamine, strongly alters and affects the relationship among the brain's pearls: the various events and objects related to self, body, and world.

NEUROPHENOMENAL HYPOTHESIS IIIA: GLUTAMATE AND HEBBIAN SYNAPSES

NMDA receptors have been shown to be central in constituting the so-called Hebbian synapse. Hebbian synapses are excitatory and activity dependent, which is based on that they increase their strength (in a nonlinear and nonadditive way) when pre- and postsynaptic activities coincide temporally. By detecting such temporal coincidence of different neurons via the increase of its own activity, the synapse is able to link and synchronize the different neurons' activities.

Such activity dependence is possible even if their respective cell bodies are spatially remote from each other thereby constituting transient and short-lived cell assemblies. This means that the Hebbian synapses are central in constituting large-scale neuronal networks and assemblies.

Based on this role of NMDA receptors in constituting transient large-scale neuronal assemblies that range across spatially distant regions and networks, German neuroscientist Hans Flohr (1995, 1998, 2006) develops his NMDA hypothesis of anesthesia. Many anesthetic drugs act directly on the NMDA receptor itself or modulate it indirectly as, for instance, GABA-A receptor antagonists. He argues that the blockade of NMDA receptors by, for instance, ketamine as NMDA receptor antagonist disrupts the constitution of activity dependence on the synaptic level and the formation of Hebbian synapses. This blocks the formation of transient large-scale neuronal assemblies (via functional connectivity).

Following Flohr, such blockade makes it impossible for the brain to generate networks that represent its own internal states as meta- or higher order (or self-referential) representation.

If, however, the own states can no longer be represented as such, constitution of consciousness remains impossible, as in anesthesia.

NEUROPHENOMENAL HYPOTHESIS IIIB: HEBBIAN SYNAPSES AND DIFFERENCE-BASED CODING

How is Flohr's hypothesis about NMDA receptors related to my neurophenomenal hypothesis of the central role of glutamate in constituting "global" spatial continuity of neural activity and the "dimension bloc" of "inner space consciousness"? By mediating activity dependence and thus the formation of Hebbian synapses via pre- and postsynaptic activity integration, the NMDA synapses encode spatial differences into their neural activity. This presupposes difference-based coding rather than stimulus-based coding. If there were stimulus-based coding, the temporal convergence of the different neurons' activities would make no difference; this, however, would make the formation of Hebbian synapses as such impossible, including their promotional role in synchronizing the neural activities from spatially distinct neurons and regions (and networks).

One may therefore propose difference-based coding on the synaptic level. This means that the Hebbian synapses' activities encode the temporal differences between pre- and postsynaptic activities rather than encoding them as separate and distinct stimuli. Such NMDA-mediated, temporally based, difference-based coding may lead to the subsequent formation of transient and short-lived neuronal assemblies; this, in turn, may allow for the constitution of both local and global temporal and spatial continuity of neural activity.

Accordingly, the Hebbian synapses presuppose a particular encoding strategy; namely, difference-based coding rather than stimulus-based coding. Since difference-based coding entails "local" and "global" spatial and temporal continuity of neural activity, my account is well compatible if not complementary to the one by Hebb and the Hebbian synapses.

What now happens in anesthesia, when the NMDA receptors are blocked? If the NMDA-mediated synapses can no longer increase their activity when pre- and postsynaptic activities coincide temporally, the encoding of temporal differences into the synapses' neural activity and thus difference-based coding are impaired.

This means that what is encoded into the synapses' neural activity reflects no longer really the difference between pre- and postsynaptic activities. Instead, the mere (linear) addition (or superposition) of the pre- and postsynaptic activities is encoded into the Hebbian synapses' activities. If this is so, one could propose a high degree of stimulus-based coding and a rather low degree of difference-based coding to operate at the synaptic level during NMDA blockade in (for instance) anesthesia.

NEUROPHENOMENAL HYPOTHESIS IIIC: NEUROPHENOMENAL VERSUS NEUROCOGNITIVE ACCOUNT OF ANESTHESIA AND CONSCIOUSNESS

Why does the NMDA-based shift from difference-based coding to stimulus-based coding lead to the loss of consciousness? Flohr proposes that this is because of the NMDA synapses' role in forming neuronal cell assemblies that mediate higher-order representation of the brain's own internal state. Lack of higher-order representation is then proposed to lead to the loss of consciousness. This is the point where I depart from Flohr. Let me detail that departure in the following explanation.

Concerning neuronal matters, I concurred with Flohr's view and complemented his suggested neuronal mechanisms, the Hebbian synapses, by difference-based coding and "global" spatial and temporal continuity of neural activity. However, when it comes to neurophenomenal matters, I depart from him.

Why do I depart from Flohr at this point? Flohr claims that the loss of cognitive mechanisms like higher-order (or self-referential) representation is the cause of the loss of consciousness. Such a neurocognitive account contrasts with my neurophenomenal approach. In my neurophenomenal account, I suggests the disruption of higher-order representation to be the consequence (rather than the cause) of

a more basic non-cognitive neurophenomenal mechanism that by itself predisposes the loss of consciousness, which in turn causes the cognitive deficits. Accordingly, my neurophenomenal approach suggests that the cognitive deficits follow the loss of consciousness whereas Flohr's neurocognitive model claims the reverse namely that the loss of consciousness follows the cognitive deficits.

Let me be more specific. I propose the disruption of those higher-order representations to be a consequence rather than the underlying cause of the loss of consciousness. NMDA synapses may no longer properly mediate difference-based coding in anesthesia; this makes the constitution of proper "local" and "global" spatial and temporal continuity of neural activity impossible. If, however, the "local" and especially the "global" spatial continuity of neural activity is no longer properly constituted, the brain's intrinsic activity can no longer constitute a proper spatial and temporal structure (see Chapters 4 and 5 for details on the spatial and temporal structure of the brain's intrinsic activity).

This makes impossible the linkage and integration of events and objects from both body and environment into the brain's intrinsic activity and its spatial and temporal structure (see Chapters 4–6 for details). If, however, the events and objects from body and environment cannot be integrated and linked anymore to the brain's intrinsic activity and its spatial and temporal structure, their related stimulus-induced activities can no longer be associated with "inner space and time consciousness." In short, "inner time and space consciousness" are supposed to be lost in anesthesia.

How is such loss of "inner space and time consciousness" related to the complete loss of consciousness in anesthesia and its "zero level" or state of consciousness? We recall from earlier in this chapter that "inner space and time consciousness" provide the very basis, the spatial and temporal grid, that makes consciousness as such—namely, its level or state—first and foremost possible. If so, the loss of "inner space and time consciousness" during NMDA-induced anesthesia should be accompanied by the complete loss of consciousness, meaning that the level or state of consciousness should tend toward zero, which is exactly what one observes in anesthesia.

NEUROPHENOMENAL HYPOTHESIS IIID: HIGHER-ORDER COGNITIVE REPRESENTATION AS CAUSE OR CONSEQUENCE OF CONSCIOUSNESS

How does my neurophenomenal approach relate to Flohr's hypothesis of the loss of higher-order (self-referential) representations as the cause of consciousness? What causes, or better, predisposes (i.e., makes necessary or unavoidable) the loss of consciousness in my neurophenomenal account is the loss of "global" temporal and spatial continuity in the brain's intrinsic activity and more specifically the loss of its spatial and temporal structure.

The loss of the intrinsic activity's spatial and temporal structure makes the association of consciousness and its phenomenal features with the otherwise purely neuronal resting-state and stimulus-induced activity impossible. The level or state of consciousness consequently remains zero, so that no experience is possible.

The loss of experience altogether, and particularly the loss of experience of one's own self in consciousness (which remains absent) may then reverberate upon the cognitive functions and their processing: if I no longer experience my self or specific environmental events in consciousness, there is no need anymore for me to recruit cognitive functions and to represent and meta-represent my self or the environmental events in higher-order representations. There is thus a loss of higher-order cognitive (and self-referential) representation that is a necessary or unavoidable consequence of the loss of consciousness, almost by default.

Accordingly, I agree with Flohr on the loss of higher-order cognitive representation in anesthesia. In contrast to him, however, I consider such cognitive loss as a consequence rather than as a cause of the loss of consciousness. Hence, I suggest the neurocognitive changes to result as an inevitable consequence and thus by default from the preceding neurophenomenal alterations, rather than the former causing the latter.

In short, I suggest that the loss of cognition follows the loss of consciousness.

NEUROPHENOMENAL HYPOTHESIS IVA: "PRIORITY HYPOTHESIS OF NEUROPHENOMENAL FUNCTION"—NEURONAL REASONS

Taking a more general perspective, I consider neurocognitive function to be necessarily dependent upon neurophenomenal functions. This reverses the traditional view. Usually, neurocognitive functions like attention, working memory, higher-order representation, etc., are considered the cause or at least a necessary condition of consciousness (see Introduction, Volume I, and Appendix 1).

I, in contrast, consider neuronal functions other than the neurocognitive functions to be necessary for consciousness; this led me from neurocognitive functions to the brain's neurophenomenal functions, which I searched for in the brain's intrinsic activity and its interaction with extrinsic stimuli. I therefore postulated different neurophenomenal functions as they were explicated with regard to "inner time and space consciousness" in this Part. Further neurophenomenal functions related to unity, self, intentionality, and qualia will be discussed in the subsequent parts of this book.

However, even more radically, I suggest those neurophenomenal functions to be more basic than, and thus to precede and operate prior to, neurocognitive functions and also all other functions like neurosensory, neuromotor, neuroaffective, and neurosocial functions (see Appendix 1 in Volume II). The neurophenomenal functions are supposed to have priority and precedence over other functions. This implies what I describe as the "priority hypothesis of neurophenomenal function" (however, see also Chapter 24 for the discussion of the relationship between neurophenomenal and other functions in a slightly different context) (see below for more explication of this hypothesis).

Why do I suggest such a radical thesis as the "priority hypothesis of neurophenomenal function"? There are both neuronal and phenomenal reasons. Let us start with the neuronal reason.

The neuronal reason consists in the simple fact that the brain's intrinsic activity occurs prior to, and is thus more basic than, any neural activity related to the sensory, motor, affective, cognitive, or social functions of the brain.

This presupposes that the brain's intrinsic activity strongly impacts the neural activity during those functions, their stimulus-induced or task-related activities, for which I provided abundant empirical evidence in Chapter 11 in Volume I. Put in a converse way, stimulus-induced or task-related neural activity is always already necessarily and unavoidably embedded into and dependent on the brain's intrinsic activity, which therefore must be given priority. Since that very same intrinsic activity predisposes consciousness and its various phenomenal features, the "priority hypothesis of neurophenomenal functions" becomes unavoidable.

NEUROPHENOMENAL HYPOTHESIS IVB: "PRIORITY HYPOTHESIS OF NEUROPHENOMENAL FUNCTION"— PHENOMENAL REASONS

How about the phenomenal reason? Very simple again. Any content related to any kind of function can in principle be associated with consciousness that is subjectively experienced. We are able to associate consciousness with the processing of sensory stimuli resulting in perception. The same holds for movements, which we also experience in consciousness as described in (for instance) agency and ownership. Emotions and affects can also be experienced as in emotional feelings (see Chapter 31 for details). The same holds for cognitive and social functions, which are often subsumed under concepts like *awareness* and *reflection*.

This means that any function and its related content are always necessarily and unavoidably embedded in experience that is consciousness. There is thus priority of consciousness (that is, "principal consciousness" as I explicated in the second Introduction) compared to the various functions on a phenomenal level. This means that the phenomenal level has priority over the sensory, motor, cognitive, affective, and social levels.

In summation, I here suggest what I describe as the "priority hypothesis of neurophenomenal function" that regards the brain's neurophenomenal functions as more basic and prior to the brain's neurosensory, neuromotor, neuroaffective, neurocognitive, and neurosocial functions. Rather than being a cause, the brain's neurosensory, neuromotor, neuroaffective, neurocognitive, and neurosocial functions must be considered the consequences of the brain's neurophenomenal functions and their intimate linkage to its intrinsic activity.

The brain's neurophenomenal functions are thus postulated to have priority over its various other functions; that is, sensory, motor, affective, cognitive, and social functions. This entails a tighter and closer link of the brain and especially its intrinsic activity with the phenomenal functions compared to its other functions (sensory, motor, affective, cognitive, social).

Finally, rather than focusing on particular neurosensory, neuromotor, neuroaffective, neurocognitive, and neurosocial functions, I will concentrate on the various neurophenomenal functions themselves in the following chapters and parts. This, admittedly, leaves open how the neurophenomenal functions impact subsequent neurosensory, neuromotor, neuroaffective, neurocognitive, and neurosocial functions; since that would be beyond the scope of this book, I leave it to others to provide such an account in the future.

NEURONAL FINDINGS IIIA: GABA AND TEMPORAL CONTINUITY OF NEURAL ACTIVITY

We focused so far on glutamate. However, glutamate operates in conjunction with GABA, both forming together what is described as the excitation–inhibition balance (EIB; see Chapters 2, 6, and 12 in Volume I). However, I delineated different roles of GABA and glutamate in constituting the spatiotemporal structure of the resting state (see Chapter 6). Since I consider the resting state's spatiotemporal structure and the temporal and spatial continuity of its neural activity to predispose consciousness, GABA should exert a differential role on the constitution of "inner space and time consciousness" when compared to glutamate.

Let us start with the modulation of the temporal processing of neural activity by GABA. As discussed in detail in Chapter 12, cortical synchronization via high-frequency fluctuations like beta and gamma bands has been shown to be related to GABA-ergic neurotransmission (see also Uhlhaas and Singer 2010 for a review). More specifically, GABA-ergic interneurons act apparently as pacemaker by producing rhythmic fast inhibitory postsynaptic potentials in pyramidal neurons in the cortical layers. This may be sufficient to synchronize the firing of a large population of pyramidal cells that determine the dominant frequency in a larger network.

These observations suggest a central role of GABA in synchronizing the time windows and thus the phases, that is, phase-locking, of especially high-frequency fluctuations (and how they are related to low-frequency fluctuations; see Chapter 12 for more details on GABA and synchronization of especially gamma fluctuations). By exerting inhibitory and synchronizing impact, GABA was supposed to be central in encoding spatial and temporal differences into neural activity, that is, the EIB.

This means that GABA has a strong impact on the degree of temporal differences that are encoded into neural activity (see Chapters 2 and 12 in Volume I). That suggests that GABA has a strong impact on constituting "local" and "global" temporal continuity of neural activity and consequently on "inner time consciousness," as we will discuss in the next section.

NEURONAL FINDINGS IIIB: GABA AND SPATIAL CONTINUITY OF NEURAL ACTIVITY

How about the spatial effects of GABA? For that, I turn to the effects of GABA-ergic drugs on consciousness. Drugs targeting GABA-A receptors can induce loss of consciousness and subsequent anesthesia (see also Shulman et al. 2003, 2006; Alkire et al. 2008; Brown et al. 2010).

Midazolam, a short-acting GABA-ergic drug, leads indeed to disruption of functional connectivity and consciousness (see Ferrarelli et al. 2010; see Chapters 15 and 16 for more details).

When given midazolam, TMS impulses no longer induces propagation and spread of neural activity across different regions; instead neural activity remains basically local and shorter (see Chapter 16 for details). Since the very same subjects also lost their consciousness during the application of midazolam, these data support a central role of GABA in constituting consciousness.

How about GABA and the vegetative state? One early study (see Rudolf et al. 2000; see also Clauss 2010) investigated the density of GABA-A receptors in nine drug-free vegetative patients using 11-C-Flumazenil. Compared to healthy subjects, the vegetative patients showed an overall global reduction of GABA-A receptor density in all cortical regions (while only sparing the cerebellum).

In contrast to the global effects, no specific focal or regional deficits in GABA-A receptor density could be observed in vegetative patients (Fig. 17-2; see Rudolf et al. 2000). Moreover, the global reduction in GABA-A receptor density accompanied a global reduction in overall glucose metabolism (see Rudolf et al. 2002). The correspondence between GABA-A receptors and glucose metabolism means that the metabolism reduction seems to be directly related to neuronal function; for example, to inhibitory function as mediated by GABA and GABA-A receptors (see Figure 17-2).

Further support for altered GABA in vegetative states comes from the therapeutic effectiveness of GABA-ergic drugs in these patients (see Taira 2009; see also Brown et al. 2010; and see Chapter 29 for more details).

Taken together, the findings suggest a central role for GABA in constituting the temporal and spatial structure of neural activity. This suggests that GABA is critically involved in constituting "local" and "global" temporal and spatial continuity of neural activity and thereby predisposes "inner time and space consciousness."

NEUROPHENOMENAL HYPOTHESIS VA: GABA AND "TEMPORAL DISRUPTION" IN "INNER *TIME* CONSCIOUSNESS"

Based on these considerations, GABA may be central for consciousness, as has been suggested

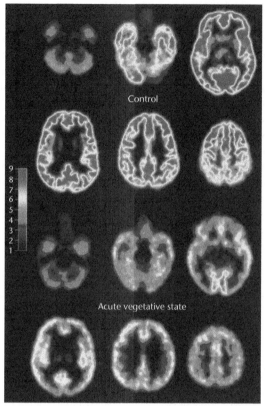

Figure 17-2 Metabolism and GABA-A receptors in vegetative state. Cortical flumazenil binding in a healthy control and a patient in an acute vegetative state Black to white scaling; values relative to average white-matter activity. Reprinted with permission of Elsevier, from Rudolf J, Sobesky J, Grond M, Heiss WD. Identification by positron emission tomography of neuronal loss in acute vegetative state. *Lancet.* 2000 Jan 8;355(9198):115–6.

by a recent review (Changeux and Lou 2011, who propose a central role for GABA in gamma synchronization and consciousness; see Chapter 19 for gamma as well as Chapter 29 for GABA and consciousness) and a study on visual awareness and GABA in visual cortex (van Loon et al. 2012; see also Qin et al. 2012, for GABA and visual cortex). However, to my knowledge, there are no findings reported on the role of GABA specifically in "inner time and space consciousness."

How is GABA now involved in constituting "inner time consciousness"? Changes in GABA, such as a deficit on the basis of GABA-A receptor blockade, may disrupt neuronal synchronization and ultimately the encoding of temporal differences into neural activity and difference-based coding. Due to altered GABA-ergic neural inhibition, the phase-locking between high- and

low-frequency fluctuation may be disrupted, entailing that the cycles of high- and low-frequency fluctuations may no longer share a common phase and thus an overlapping time window between their phase durations (see Fig. 17-3a).

This means that, ultimately, neural activity at a discrete point in physical time has a lower likelihood of being linked to a particular phase duration and a longer overlapping time window; the probability of becoming extended beyond itself to other discrete points in physical time (that is, those within the respective phase duration and its overlapping time window) is thus considerably decreased. If, however, linkage of single neural activities to a particular phase of the activity's fluctuations remains impossible, the constitution of "local" and "global" temporal continuity of neural activity is disrupted. This

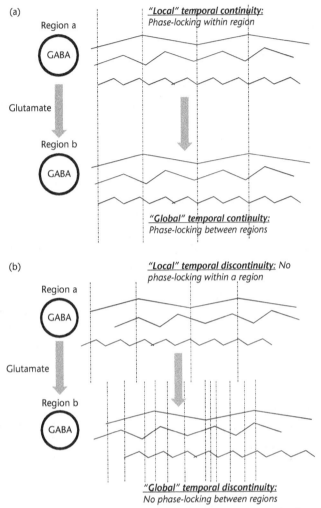

Figure 17-3a and b GABA and temporal continuity of neural activity. The figure demonstrates the relationship between GABA and temporal continuity of neural activity (*a*) and the effects of dysfunction of GABA on the constitution of time, resulting in "temporal discontinuity" of neural activity (*b*). The figures show the impact of local regional GABA on the neural activity in other regions (*left part*). The impact of these neurons/regions' activities on the fluctuations of neuronal activities is demonstrated on the right as indicated by the horizontal lines/curves in different frequency ranges (*right part*). The overlap in the phases between the different frequency ranges is indicated by the vertical dotted lines. These temporal overlaps provide overlapping time windows for the possible integration of stimuli and their different discrete points in physical time; this is manifested in "global" temporal continuity of neural activity. If GABA functions well, there are temporal overlaps and thus overlapping time windows between the different regions' GABA-ergic-modulated phase durations. This is indicated by the vertical dotted line that spans across the different neurons/regions. That allows the extension of the "local" temporal continuity to other regions and thus the "global" temporal continuity of neural activity, which in turn predisposes the degree of temporal extension of the present into past and future within the "duration bloc" of "inner time consciousness." If, in contrast, GABA does not function well, there are no temporal overlaps and thus overlapping time windows between the different regions and their GABA-ergic-modulated phase durations. This is indicated by the vertical dotted line that no longer spans across the different neurons/regions' neural activities. This leads to disruption of temporal continuity of neural activity with consequent temporal discontinuity of neural activity; that entails disruption of the linkage between past, present, and future within the duration bloc of inner time consciousness.

leads to "temporal discontinuity" rather than "temporal continuity" of neural activity. There is consequently no longer any linkage and integration between the different discrete time points of previous, present, and future neural activities, which ultimately results in a "global" temporal discontinuity of neural activity.

Such "global" temporal discontinuity of neural activity makes impossible the extension of the different single discrete time points in the present to those in the past and the future. This means that there is no longer any neural activity that can predispose the integration of past, present, and future into the "duration bloc." The "inner time consciousness" is consequently disrupted; metaphorically speaking, the "duration bloc" is scattered into different bits and pieces of time. I therefore hypothesize that disruption of GABA leads to the disruption of the duration bloc and thus of inner time consciousness. In short, I suggest changes in GABA to predispose "temporal disruption" in the "duration bloc" of "inner time consciousness" (see Fig. 17-3b).

Neurophenomenal Hypothesis VB: "Temporal Disruption" versus "Temporal Dysbalance" in Inner *Time* Consciousness

Such GABA-ergic-mediated "temporal disruption" on the phenomenal level of "inner time consciousness" must be distinguished from glutamatergic-mediated "temporal dysbalance" in "inner time consciousness"; that is, temporal extension and temporal shrinkage (see earlier). In the case of an experience of "temporal disruption" on the phenomenal level of consciousness, different discrete temporal (and spatial) positions are no longer linked to each other during the encoding of neural activity. The degree of difference-based coding when compared to stimulus-based coding may consequently be rather low. Difference-based coding is thus by itself abnormally altered: that is, disrupted.

This contrasts with "temporal dysbalance" on the phenomenal level of "inner time consciousness." In the case of temporal dysbalance, difference-based coding is still preserved but

operates by encoding either abnormally large or small spatial and temporal differences into neural activity (see above). I thus hypothesize that "temporal disruption" is related to abnormalities in GABA-ergic-mediated transmission, while "temporal dysbalance" may be associated with changes in glutamatergic-mediated transmission.

Let us invoke our earlier neurometaphorical example with the string and the pearls. We recall that glutamate tilts the string in an abnormal way in either direction. The pearls remain on the string but are abnormally close to or distant from each other. There is thus an imbalance that corresponds to the "temporal dysbalance" induced by, for instance, an NMDA antagonist like ketamine. Such a "temporal dysbalance" can indeed be experienced, as is observed in the neurophenomenal abnormalities in the neuropsychiatric disorder of depression (see below).

This is different in the case of GABA. Here, the string is not merely tilted but rather disrupted and thus "cut" by itself. The string is, figuratively, cut and sliced into bits and pieces. There is thus "temporal discontinuity" rather than mere "temporal dysbalance." And, even worse, the pearls no longer stay on the chain in their original sequence (though too close or too distant from each other) but get off and wander around, resulting in chaos and disorder.

In very much the same way as the different pearls would then lie scattered on the floor, different bits and pieces of time (and space) are "flying around" in a rather confusing and chaotic way. We will see later that this is indeed the case, as can be supported by the neuropsychiatric disorder of schizophrenia.

Neurophenomenal Hypothesis VIA: GABA and the "Dimension Bloc" of "Inner *Space* Consciousness"

How about the effects of GABA on "inner space consciousness"? For that, let us revisit the discussion in Chapter 16. Besides "spatial amplification" of the encoded spatial differences across the neural activities of different regions, I hypothesized "spatial condensation" to be essential. If two regions' neural differences are propagated, they may interact with each other via nonlinear and nonadditive interaction. This may condense the two regions' neural activities into the same neural activity of one region. If, in contrast, there is mere linear and additive interaction, such spatial condensation of neural activity remains impossible, since each region's neural activity is then carried out by itself in separate ways.

How is such nonlinear and nonadditive interaction between different regions' neural activities modulated? GABA seems to be central here, as we discussed in full neuronal detail in Chapters 2, 6, and 12 in Volume I. In a nutshell, Buszaki argues that GABA introduces nonlinearity into the glutamatergic-mediated excitatory system. Due to the higher number of GABA-ergic inhibitory interneurons when compared to the number of glutamatergic-mediated excitatory pyramidal cells, the degree of neural inhibition, as induced by the excitatory glutamate, is much higher; that is, nonlinearly higher than the initial degree of neural excitation (see especially Chapter 2 for details).

What does this imply for the neural activity that is spatially amplified across different regions' neural activities? Such GABA-ergic mediated nonlinear interaction entails that the once-amplified neural activity may be abnormally condensed into a few or even into the same neural activity, thus entailing what I described as "spatial condensation" of neural activity into a few or one region (see Chapter 16).

I hypothesized in Chapter 16 the degree of spatial condensation as mediated by nonlinear and nonadditive interaction to be directly related to the degree of global spatial continuity. The more the initially amplified neural activities from different regions can be nonlinearly condensed, the higher the degree of "global" spatial continuity between the different regions' neural activities.

If GABA is now supposed to be central in mediating nonlinear interaction and thus spatial condensation, one would expect it to have a major impact on the degree of "spatial condensation" and ultimately the "global" spatial continuity of neural activity. I therefore hypothesize that the degree of "spatial condensation" and ultimately the "global" spatial continuity of neural activity are directly dependent upon the degree of

nonlinear and nonadditive interaction as mediated by GABA-ergic mediated neural inhibition.

Abnormal alteration of GABA consequently leads to abnormal spatial condensation, which ultimately disrupts the constitution of the "global" spatial continuity of neural activity. This may severely affect the possible degree of spatial extension into three-dimensional space and thus what I described as the "dimension bloc" of "inner space consciousness" (see Chapter 16). Accordingly, as in the case of "temporal disruption" of the "duration bloc" in "inner time consciousness," abnormal GABA and its abnormal nonlinearity disrupt the three-dimensional spatial extension and thus the "dimension bloc" of "inner space consciousness."

NEUROPHENOMENAL HYPOTHESIS VIB: GABA AND NEURAL INHIBITION IN VEGETATIVE STATE

Based on these findings, I would propose that the loss of GABA in vegetative state patients disrupts their ability to constitute "global" spatial and temporal continuity of neural activity. Due to the lack of GABA and neural inhibition, neither spatial nor temporal differences can be properly encoded into neural activity anymore. This is, I propose, related to the lack of usually GABA-ergic mediated neural inhibition (see also Chapter 29 for more details).

Due to the lack of GABA-ergic mediated neural inhibition, the single stimulus and its particular discrete point in physical space and time are no longer encoded into neural activity in terms of spatial and temporal differences to other stimuli. The lack of GABA-ergic mediated neural inhibition increases thus the degree of stimulus-based coding, while abnormally decreasing the degree of difference-based coding (see Fig. 17-4a).

The increased degree of stimulus-based coding makes the constitution of "local" and ultimately "global" spatial continuity of neural activity less likely and ultimately impossible. That, however, makes impossible the spatial extension of the single discrete point in space into a three-dimensional space and thus the "dimension bloc" as the phenomenal hallmark of inner space consciousness.(see Fig. 17-4b-c).

If the level or state of consciousness is by itself preserved, the originally three-dimensional space is experienced, to speak metaphorically, in "bits and pieces of space" in a rather chaotic and disordered way. This means that the respective contents in consciousness, like objects and events in one's own body, oneself, or the environment can no longer be properly experienced in a spatially continuous and three-dimensional way. We will see that this is

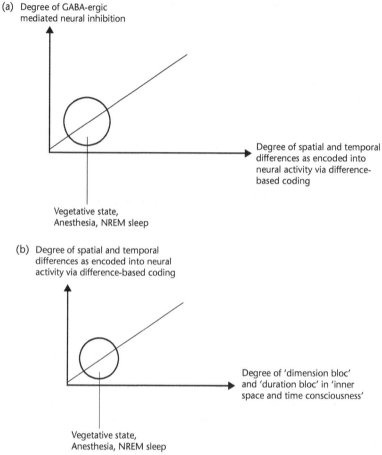

Figure 17-4a-c GABA and consciousness. The figures show the relationship between GABA-ergic-mediated neural inhibition and consciousness as mediated via difference-based coding. More specifically, I suppose GABA-ergic-mediated neural inhibition to modulate the degree of spatial and temporal differences that can be encoded into neural activity via difference-based coding. If the degree of neural inhibition is low, the degree of encoded spatial and temporal differences is rather low, as I proposed it to be the case in vegetative state, anesthesia, and NREM sleep. The degree of spatial and temporal differences encoded into neural activity does, in turn, predispose the possible degree of temporal and spatial extension in the "duration bloc" and the "dimension bloc" as phenomenal hallmarks of "inner time and space consciousness." If the degree of encoded spatial and temporal differences is rather low, the degree of the spatial and temporal extension of the "duration bloc" and the "dimension bloc," which, in the most extreme case, leads to the loss of consciousness as in vegetative state, anesthesia, and NREM sleep. Taking (a) and (b) and (c) together, one must assume that the degree of temporal and spatial extension in the duration bloc and the dimension bloc as measures of inner time and space consciousness is dependent upon the degree of GABA-ergic-mediated neural inhibition. I thus propose the loss of inner time and space consciousness in NREM sleep, vegetative state, and anesthesia to be related to the loss of GABA-ergic-mediated neural inhibition in these disorders of consciousness.

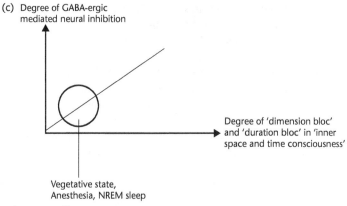

Figure 17-4a-c (Continued)

indeed the case, as one can observe in patients with schizophrenia.

NEUROPSYCHIATRIC SUPPORT
IA: NEUROPHENOMENAL EVIDENCE FROM PSYCHIATRIC DISORDERS

How can we support my neurophenomenal hypotheses about GABA and glutamate? There is no direct evidence besides the evidence I have discussed. However, there is some indirect empirical and phenomenal evidence from neuropsychiatric disorders like depression and schizophrenia.

Both depression and schizophrenia show abnormal spatiotemporal continuity in neural activity. And most important, unlike in anesthesia, NREM sleep, or vegetative state, the level or state of consciousness is still preserved by itself. This means that neuropsychiatric disorders can provide not only neuronal support as the disorders of consciousness, but also neurophenomenal evidence, since the patients are still able to subjectively experience and report how the contents in their consciousness are spatially and temporally structured.

If my hypothesis holds, one would propose primary changes in GABA to accompany "temporal and spatial disruption" in the "dimension bloc" and the "duration bloc" of "inner time and space consciousness." I propose this to be the case in schizophrenia (see also Chapters 22 and 27 for more details on the neurophenomenology of schizophrenia). In contrast, predominant changes in glutamate should lead to "spatial and temporal dysbalance," which I propose to be the case in depression (see also Chapter 27 for more neurophenomenal detail on depression).

NEUROPSYCHIATRIC SUPPORT IB: "TEMPORAL DISRUPTION" IN "INNER TIME CONSCIOUSNESS" IN SCHIZOPHRENIA

Let us start with schizophrenia and the phenomenological side. Schizophrenic patients show that they suffer a disruption of time and space that they subjectively experience in a very fragmented way. The duration bloc as phenomenally manifested in retention, presence, and protention (see Chapter 15, this volume) is disturbed in schizophrenia: the patients no longer experience the temporal extension from one discrete point in physical time to others, so the present is no longer extended into past and future anymore in their subjective experience. Instead, the different discrete time points are disconnected from each other in subjective experience, amounting to "temporal disruption" (see Northoff 2011, Chapter 11, for a much more detailed phenomenological description of schizophrenia).

Let me describe such "temporal disruption" in further detail. Thomas Fuchs, who is a German psychiatrist and philosopher from the phenomenological tradition, aims to understand the experience and consciousness of schizophrenic and depressed patients. Fuchs (2007) proposes fragmentation of "inner time consciousness" and hence disruption of the temporal continuum between retention, the present, and protention in schizophrenic patients' subjective experience.

This is reflected in the following description by a schizophrenic patient as recounted in Fuchs (2007): "When I move quickly, it is a strain on me. Things go too quickly for my mind. They get blurred and it is like being blind. It's as if you were seeing a picture one moment and another picture the next." Fuchs claims that these changes in the subjective experience of time, the abnormal inner time consciousness, are at the very root of many of the often rather bizarre schizophrenic symptoms like ego disorders, thought disorders, hallucinations, and delusions.

This fits well with my earlier described "priority hypothesis of neurophenomenal function," which claims neurophenomenal functions are more basic and take precedence over neurocognitive (and neuroaffective, neurosensory, neuromotor, and neurosocial) functions. The various schizophrenic symptoms indicate changes in neurosensory, neuroaffective, neurocognitive, and neurosocial functions whose changes may result as necessary or unavoidable consequences (rather than as causes) of the preceding and therefore more basic underlying neurophenomenal abnormalities.

NEUROPSYCHIATRIC SUPPORT IC: GABA AND "TEMPORAL DISRUPTION" IN SCHIZOPHRENIA

If my hypothesis of GABA mediating the constitution of the degree of temporal extension in the "duration bloc" is correct, one would expect changes in GABA in schizophrenia. Although there are plenty of studies (to report them would be beyond the scope of this chapter), I here focus on the ones by the group around Harvard psychiatrist Francis Benes. She conducted several postmortem studies in which they observed altered GABA-ergic interneurons in typical DMN regions like the anterior cingulate cortex and the hippocampus (see Benes 2009, 2010, for reviews).

Such alteration of GABA-ergic interneurons also holds true for other regions like the sensory cortex and the dorsolateral prefrontal cortex (see Benes 2009, 2010; Gonzales-Burgos and Lewis 2008, 2012; Lewis et al. 2012; Sullivan and O'Donnell 2012; Gonzalez-Burgos et al. 2011). More specifically, a specific subset of GABA-ergic interneurons has been found to be altered in psychosis, particularly those that contain and express mitochondrial RNA (mRNA) for NMDA receptors (Gonzalez-Burgos et al. 2012, for review). Besides these predominantly postmortem findings, alterations of GABA have also been observed in other domains. A pharmacological challenge study by Ahn et al. (2011) lends further support to the assumption of a GABA-ergic deficit in schizophrenia. They gave healthy subjects and (chronic) schizophrenic patients a dose (3.7 µg/kg) of iomazenil, a GABA-ergic substance, and compared its effects with placebo. Iomazenil induced increases in psychotic symptoms (as measured with the Brief Psychiatric Rating Scale, BPRS) only in schizophrenic patients but not in healthy subjects. This suggests abnormal GABA-A receptors in schizophrenia (see also Gonzalez-Burgos et al. 2011; Lewis et al. 2012; and Sullivan and O'Donnell 2012).

Alterations in GABA have also been related to deficits in neuronal synchronization in schizophrenia (see Gonzales-Burgos et al. 2011). More specifically, deficits in GABA-ergic interneurons in prefrontal cortex and/or the thalamus (reticular nucleus) may accompany deficits in especially gamma frequency fluctuations (30–80 Hz; see Gonzales-Burgos et al. 2011; Lewis et al. 2012; Ferrarelli and Tononi 2011; Ferrarelli et al. 2012; Guller et al. 2012). If so, one would expect altered ratio between low- and high-frequency fluctuations with the lower predominating, which is indeed supported by the current results.[1]

Taken together, though tentative at this point, schizophrenia can be characterized phenomenally by "temporal disruption" (rather than mere "temporal dysbalance"; see earlier and later) in inner time consciousness. Neuronally and biochemically, changes in both GABA and low- and high-frequency fluctuations can indeed be observed (as well as changes in glutamate).

How are these neuronal and biochemical changes related to the phenomenal abnormalities, the "temporal disruption" in the "duration bloc" of "inner time consciousness"? We currently do not know. However, despite the absence of evidence for the direct neurophenomenal link between altered GABA and "temporal disruption," schizophrenia may be regarded as a paradigmatic model to at least indirectly support my neurophenomenal hypothesis about GABA and "inner time consciousness" in further detail in the future.

NEUROPSYCHIATRIC SUPPORT IIA: "TEMPORAL DYSBALANCE" IN "INNER TIME CONSCIOUSNESS" IN DEPRESSION

Let us now consider the second case: depression. If my hypothesis holds, primary abnormalities in glutamate should be accompanied by "temporal dysbalance" with either temporal extension or temporal shrinkage of the "duration bloc" toward either the past or the future (see earlier). Such "temporal dysbalance" is to be distinguished from the "temporal disruption" of the "duration bloc," as can be observed in schizophrenia.

The "temporal dysbalance" in depression can be characterized by an abnormal focus on the past at the expense of the future. These patients are locked in their past; they constantly ruminate and think about past events, while at the same time having no subjective-experiential access to the future anymore. They remain unable to feel or experience the future or that events could possibly happen in the future. More specifically, the depressed patients' subjective time and thus their "inner time consciousness" is shifted unilaterally toward the past, with retention predominating and protention vanishing (see Fuchs 2011, as well as Northoff 2011; see Chapter 10, Volume I, for a more detailed phenomenological description of depression).

One can thus speak of "temporal dysbalance" between past and future in the "duration bloc" of "inner time consciousness" in these patients. There is a strong focus on the past, while the future diminishes more and more and ultimately becomes blocked, which may lead to affective-emotional symptoms like hopelessness (see Northoff et al. 2011a and b; Hasler and Northoff 2011). Rather

than the time and its passive synthesis shifting back and forth between past and future in subjective experience as in healthy subjects, inner time consciousness in depressed patients becomes static and quasi-frozen or locked into the past.

The opposite is the case in mania. Here, subjective experience is abnormally extended toward the future at the expense of the past. The patient's "inner time consciousness" is almost exclusively focused on the future, while the present, and even more the past, are no longer experienced as such. Hence, mania can be considered as the opposite extreme of the same underlying neurophenomenal process, that is abnormal "temporal dysbalance" "between past, present, and future within the "duration bloc" of "inner time consciousness."

NEUROPSYCHIATRIC SUPPORT IIB: GLUTAMATE AND "TEMPORAL DYSBALANCE" IN DEPRESSION

How about glutamate in depression? Giving a short and incomplete overview, human depression shows reduced levels of glutamate/glutamine as measured with magnetic resonance spectroscopy (MRS). This was observed in regions like the dorsomedial prefrontal cortex, the hippocampus, the perigenual anterior cingulate cortex (PACC), and the occipital cortex (Alcaro et al. 2010; Hasler et al. 2007; Price and Drevets 2010; Sanacora et al. 2004, 2012; Sanacora 2010; Walter et al. 2009; Hasler and Northoff 2011). Animal models of depression have also exhibited abnormal concentrations of glutamate in these regions (and other subcortical regions like the raphe nuclei) and, quite consistently, abnormal upregulation of the NMDA receptor in various cortical paralimbic and subcortical core-paracore regions (see Fig. 17-5a; Alcaro et al. 2010).

The crucial role of NMDA receptors is further supported by recent studies showing that the NMDA receptor antagonist ketamine can reverse pretreatment hyperfunction of the PACC during either emotional or cognitive tasks (Salvadore et al. 2009, 2010, 2012). Unfortunately, though, imaging of NMDA receptors in human depression remains to be reported. Other components of glutamatergic transmission like the glutamate

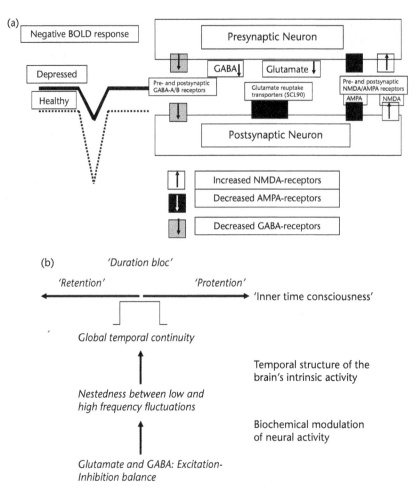

Figure 17-5a-c GABA, glutamate, and "inner time consciousness" in depression. The figures show the abnormal biochemical and temporal mechanisms of neural activity (*a*) and inner time consciousness (*b*, *c*) in depression. (*a*) On the right, the figure shows the abnormal changes in GABA, including GABA-A and -B receptors and the different glutamatergic receptors (AMPA, NMDA) in depression as based on animal and human findings (see Alcaro et al. 2010, and Hasler and Northoff 2011 for details). On the left one sees the decreased BOLD response in fMRI in anterior midline regions, indicating increased resting-state activity in the perigenual anterior cingulate cortex in depression.(*b*) The figure shows how GABA and glutamate and their resulting excitation-inhibition balance modulate "global" temporal continuity of neural activity (via temporal nestedness of high- and low-frequency fluctuations) and ultimately the balance between protention and retention in the duration bloc of inner time consciousness. (*c*) There is a dysbalance between GABA and glutamate and thus an excitation-inhibition dysbalance, which leads to a dysbalance between high- and low-frequency fluctuations and ultimately between protention and retention within the duration bloc of the inner time consciousness. There is an abnormal increase in retention with patients abnormally strongly experiencing the past at the expense of their subjective outreach to the future, so that they remain unable to project themselves into the future.

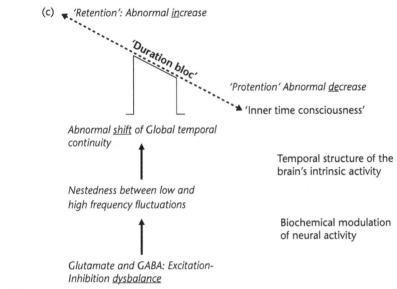

(c) 'Retention': Abnormal *increase*

'Duration bloc'

'Protention' Abnormal *decrease*

'Inner time consciousness'

Abnormal *shift* of Global temporal continuity

Temporal structure of the brain's intrinsic activity

Nestedness between low and high frequency fluctuations

Biochemical modulation of neural activity

Glutamate and GABA: Excitation-Inhibition *dysbalance*

Figure 17-5a-c (Continued)

transporter and glutamate synthetase have also been observed to be abnormal in depression (Banasr et al. 2010; Walter et al. 2009). Taken together, these results suggest abnormal glutamate-mediated neural excitation in subcortical-cortical regions, including limbic and cortical midline regions.[2]

How are the abnormalities in glutamate (and GABA[3]) related to the "temporal dysbalance" in "inner time consciousness"? As said earlier, subjective time experience in depression is abnormally shifted toward the past at the expense of the future. There is thus "temporal dysbalance." We remember from Chapter 13 that the experience of time and especially the projection into the future is apparently related to neural activity in the midline regions, specifically in the anterior midline regions like the PACC and the ventromedial prefrontal cortex (VMPFC; see Chapter 13).

These regions show abnormal hyperactivity in the resting state in depression, and that seems to be related abnormally to glutamate rather than GABA (see Walter et al. 2009; Northoff et al. 2011a and b; Hasler and Northoff 2011; Grimm et al. 2009, 2011). There seems to be abnormally strong glutamatergic-mediated

neural excitation, while the degree of GABA-ergic-mediated neural inhibition may be rather low in anterior cortical midline regions (see Walter et al. 2009, Northoff et al. 2011).

Most important, the degree of resting-state hyperactivity in PACC and VMPFC predicted the degree of hopelessness, the ability to extend oneself into the future (Grimm et al. 2009, 2011; Lemogne et al. 2012; Kuhn and Gallinat 2011): the higher the degree of resting-state activity in these regions, the higher the degree of hopelessness and thus the inability to project oneself into the future.

This suggests that the glutamatergic-mediated modulation of the abnormally high resting-state activity in these regions may be related to the "temporal dysbalance" between past and future in the "duration bloc" of "inner time consciousness." Accordingly, the case of depression lends some indirect and tentative support to the assumption that glutamate may indeed be central in balancing future, present, and past within the "duration bloc" of "inner time consciousness" (see Fig. 17-5b,c).

Open Questions

The first main question concerns the relationship between GABA and glutamate. Both act together and cannot really be separated from each other. Despite their conjunction in the EIB, I nevertheless treated them separately here for methodological and experimental purposes. Future studies may want to measure both and calculate their ratios and relate those to behavioral and phenomenal measures.

Furthermore, we may need to study the interaction between GABA and glutamate, which has rarely been done, especially in humans (see Heinzel et al. 2008 for an exception). That study needs to be combined with subjective measures of inner time and space consciousness, as the latter has especially been neglected in most current studies. Finally, one would expect this interaction between GABA and glutamate to be special in the anterior cortical midline regions that have been shown to be central in constituting spatial and temporal continuity of neural activity and inner time and space consciousness (see Chapter 13).

The second issue pertains to the question of sparse coding. I pointed out that the temporal and spatial sparsening, that is, sparse coding, of neural activity results from the modulation by GABA and glutamate (see Chapters 2, 6, and 12 in Volume I). Since I associate the action of GABA and glutamate with both sparse coding and "inner time and space consciousness," one would propose the degree of sparse coding to predict the degree of inner time and space consciousness.

More specifically, one may suggest that the degree of temporal and spatial sparsening of neural activity may be directly related to the degree to which the single discrete points of neural activities (in physical time and space) can be extended beyond themselves with the ultimate constitution of the "duration bloc" and the "dimension bloc." In other words, I propose the degree of sparse coding to predict the degree of temporal and spatial extension of "inner time and space consciousness." If so, the degree of sparse coding on a regional level of neural activity should be abnormally reduced in disorders of consciousness like vegetative state and anesthesia (see Chapters 28 and 29 for details).

Notes

1. In addition to GABA, deficits in glutamate have also been observed in schizophrenia with glutamate being apparently decreased in especially medial prefrontal cortex (see Marsman

et al. 2011 for a meta-analysis). Since glutamate affects the functional connectivity, a so-called dysconnectivity hypothesis has been postulated in psychosis (see Stephan et al. 2009 for a recent review, and Ellison-Wright and Bullmore 2009 for a meta-analysis). In a nutshell, the "dysconnectivity hypothesis" postulates abnormal functional interaction and integration between different regions in the brain. Such abnormal functional integration and interaction between different regions is supposed to mediated by glutamate, which is thus proposed to be abnormal.

How could such abnormal functional connectivity be related to the deficits in GABA? GABAergic interneurons in upper cortical layers (like layers 2, 3, and 4 as observed by Benes) modulate and control long-range glutamatergic cortico-cortical connections in lower layers (i.e., layers 3–5). The deficits in GABA may thus affect cortico-cortical connectivity via glutamatergic mediation and NMDA receptors, which have also been observed to be hypofunctional in psychosis (see Lisman et al. 2008; Corlett et al. 2009a and b). The combined involvement of GABA and glutamate may also distinguish the ketamine-induced psychosis from the psychosis in schizophrenia, since both show differences in psychotic symptoms.

2. The question of the relationship of GABA/glutamate to serotonin deserves attention, especially since serotonin is the most studied player in the genesis of depression. There is abundant evidence for serotonergic abnormalities in major depressive disorder, including synaptic levels of serotonin and specific serotonergic receptors (5HT-1a, 5HT-1b, etc.) in subcortical and cortical midline regions (see Savitz and Drevets 2009b for a review of the genetic side), and how that is related to GABA and glutamate transmission. GABA-ergic and glutamatergic neuron systems are ubiquitous throughout the cortex and in most subcortical regions. This distinguishes them from more specific neuromodulatory systems like serotonergic and adrenergic-noradrenergic systems, whose neurons are situated in subcortical regions (raphe nuclei, locus coeruleus) and are connected via long axons to forebrain-limbic regions as well as paralimbic and midline regions, especially in anterior parts of the cortex like the VMPFC and the PACC (Morgane et al., 2005). However, serotonergic neurons are connected to GABA-ergic interneurons on both subcortical and cortical levels, which may suggest that

alterations in one, for example, the serotonergic systems, entails changes in the other, for example GABA-ergic and glutamatergic systems.

3. How about GABA? Although studies of brain GABA in living human brains are sparse, there is some evidence for both reduced and normal intra- and extracellular concentrations in paralimbic and midline regions like the PACC and the dorsomedial prefrontal cortex as well as in lateral regions like the occipital cortex (Sanacora etal. 2004, 2012; Alcaro et al. 2010; Hasler et al. 2007; Hasler and Northoff 2011). The crucial role of GABA and GABA-ergic inhibition in depression is further corroborated by results from transcranial magnetic stimulation (TMS). TMS allows measurement of resting-state activity in terms of neural inhibition in techniques like "silent period" and "paired pulse" techniques. Severely depressed MDD patients show deficits in both measures in motor cortex, which is indicative of a deficit of cortical inhibition as mediated by both GABA-A and GABA-B receptors (see Sanacora 2010). Post-mortem findings report deficits in the GAD—glutamate decarboxylase-67—the enzyme that converts glutamate into GABA (see Sanacora 2010). There is further evidence from two post-mortem studies for GABA-ergic abnormalities; they show that the mRNA expression of specific subunits of the GABA-A receptor (e.g., alpha 1, 3, 4, and delta) are reduced in cortical and subcortical regions in depressed suicide victims. Finally, animal studies demonstrate decreased GABA concentration and reduced GABA-A/B receptor sensitivity and expression in many paralimbic and midline cortical regions as well as in subcortical regions (Alcaro et al. 2010; Northoff et al. 2011; Hasler and Northoff 2011).

PART VI
Spatiotemporal Unity and Consciousness

Part V focused on the constitution of spatiotemporal continuity and how that predisposes and affects consciousness. I described how various neuronal mechanisms like low-frequency fluctuations, temporal nestedness, and functional connectivity constitute spatial and temporal continuity of neural activity across different discrete points in physical time and space. Thereby I distinguished between "local" and "global" spatiotemporal continuity of neural activity. "Local" spatiotemporal continuity concerned the integration of different stimuli into the neural activity of a single region, while "global" spatiotemporal continuity allowed for the integration of the different regions' neural activities across their different discrete points in physical time and space.

"Local" and "global" spatiotemporal continuities describe the result of purely neuronal mechanisms. The question is how such neuronal continuity in spatial and temporal regard is manifested in consciousness and thus on a phenomenal level. I hypothesized in Part V that spatiotemporal continuity of neural activity across different points in physical space and time corresponds on the phenomenal level of experience to what has been described as "inner time and space consciousness."

Inner time and space consciousness describes the temporal and spatial structure of consciousness. More specifically, it refers to the spatial and temporal grid within which the objects and events in our consciousness are always already integrated. This leaves open, however, how the objects and events themselves are constituted in such way that it is possible for them to be associated with consciousness. How must objects and events be constituted in order for them to become conscious? This is the question for the constitution of the contents of consciousness, the *phenomenal contents*, which is the first main focus in this part.

Besides the phenomenal contents, there is also the form of consciousness that describes the structure and organization of the contents in spatial and temporal terms. This leads me to the second question: how must consciousness itself be structured and organized in order to allow for its contents, that is, the events and objects, to become associated with consciousness? This concerns the form or structure of consciousness as the third dimension besides contents and level/state of consciousness (see Introduction, Volume II, as well as Northoff 2013).

One of the central features of the form or structure of consciousness is unity. What is unity? We experience objects and events in consciousness. These events and objects are composites of different stimuli and their various features. For instance, a book consists of different sensory stimuli that show different features like color, motion, luminance, etc., that are integrated and unified when we experience the book as a book. The different stimuli and their various features are thus unified into one object, the book. This can be described as the "unity of phenomenal contents" of consciousness.

How is such a "unity of phenomenal contents" of consciousness constituted? This has been much debated in recent neuroscience under the umbrella of the so-called binding problem.

The problem of unity is also discussed in philosophy. Past and present philosophers, like Immanuel Kant and John Searle, also attribute unity to consciousness. However, unlike in neuroscience, their concept of unity does not concern the unity of different stimuli and their features and thus the "unity of phenomenal contents." Instead, their concept of unity addresses a unity that is prior to and occurs independently of the contents. This more basic unity of is often subsumed under the concept of "phenomenal unity," which describes the form or structure rather than the contents of consciousness; one can therefore also speak of a "unity of the phenomenal state" of consciousness.

The question now is how the "unity of the phenomenal state" of consciousness itself is related to the "unity of the phenomenal contents": for instance, the latter can be subsumed under the former, or vice versa; or both forms of unity can also be independent of each other. The focus in this part is on the investigation of both the "unity of phenomenal contents" and the "unity of the phenomenal state" of consciousness and how they must be related and linked to each other to make consciousness possible.

GENERAL OVERVIEW

Chapter 18 focuses on the neuronal mechanisms that must precede the constitution of both phenomenal contents and phenomenal state in consciousness in order for them to be possible. This leads me to recent data showing how the preceding resting state's low-frequency fluctuations modulate and entrain subsequent stimulus-induced activity and its higher-frequency fluctuations. This will reveal that the stimulus-induced activity and its associated degree of consciousness are dependent upon the phases of the preceding resting state's low-frequency fluctuations.

The phenomenal unity associated with the stimulus and its stimulus-induced activity must consequently be predisposed by the presence of some kind of neuronal unity in the preceding resting state. Since this neuronal unity cannot be experienced directly as such, i.e., by itself, while at the same time predisposing unity on the phenomenal level, I characterize such unity in the resting state as "prephenomenal unity." This leads me to propose what I describe as "resting-state–based hypothesis of prephenomenal unity."

Chapter 19 shifts from the resting-state activity to stimulus-induced activity. That leads me to discuss the neuronal mechanisms underlying the constitution of objects and events and thus of the unity of phenomenal contents in consciousness. Therefore, I focus on neuronal mechanisms like the synchronization of neural activity across different regions and time points (in physical space and time) that allow the binding of different stimuli and their respective features into objects and contents. The question for the mechanisms underlying the binding of different stimuli is described as "binding problem" and "binding by synchronization."

Both "binding problem" and "binding by synchronization" were already discussed in the neuronal context of the brain's neural code in Volume I. Now both neuronal mechanisms resurface and are put into the phenomenal context of consciousness where they are supposed to predispose the constitution of the "unity of phenomenal contents."

Why and how, though, is the "unity of phenomenal contents" associated with consciousness? For that answer, I propose that the unity of phenomenal contents must be linked and integrated with the pre-phenomenal unity of the resting state and the temporal and spatial continuity of its neural activity. This leads me to propose what I call "continuity-based hypothesis of phenomenal unity" that describes the continuity between resting-state and stimulus-induced activity with regard to unity.

Chapter 20 turns from stimulus-induced activity back to the resting-state activity and raises the issue of how its prephenomenal unity can be constituted. What are the neuronal mechanisms that allow the constitution of the resting state's low-frequency fluctuations and its associated prephenomenal unity?

This leads me back to sparse coding (see Part I in Volume I). Sparse coding describes the encoding of the stimuli from the environment in orientation to their statistical frequency distribution, that is, natural statistics, into the brain's neural activity. If so, the resting state's neural activity and especially the phases of its low-frequency fluctuations must correspond (more or less) to the stimuli's statistical frequency distribution in the environment.

This implies that there must be some kind of statistically and spatiotemporally based unity between brain and environment, the "environment–brain unity" as I call it. The concept of environment–brain unity refers to a statistically and spatiotemporally based unity between brain and environment in the gestalt of a virtual spatial and temporal grid between brain and environment. The focus in Chapter 20 is on the description of the neuronal mechanisms underlying such environment–brain unity. The capacity of the resting-state activity's low-frequency fluctuations to shift the onset of their phases in orientation on the onset of social and thus environmental stimuli may be especially central here. This is called "phase shifting," which will be detailed in Chapter 20.

How can we describe such environment–brain unity in more conceptual detail? That is the focus in Chapter 21. Chapter 21 discusses the conceptual ground in that the concept of the environment–brain unity is here linked to

the concept of subjectivity. Subjectivity is here understood in a very basic sense, as a point of view an organism takes within the world as distinguished from other possible points of view other species take. What is described here on the conceptual side as *subjectivity* and *point of view* is proposed to correspond on the empirical side to the environment–brain unity and its underlying neuronal mechanisms, like phase shifting.

Subjectivity in this sense is regarded as a core feature of unity and thus of consciousness. If there were no subjectivity, unity and consciousness would remain impossible. Unity and subjectivity do consequently seem to be closely and intrinsically linked in consciousness. However, they cannot be identified with each other, either, since subjectivity as a point of view can well occur without and thus dissociate from consciousness. This is the focus of Chapter 21.

Chapter 22 provides some indirect empirical support to my assumption of the relationship between environment–brain unity, subjectivity, and consciousness. The neuropsychiatric disorder of schizophrenia shows abnormal phenomenal contents in consciousness as well as an abnormal subjectivity. By discussing its underlying neuronal mechanisms and their respective phenomenal manifestation, the example of schizophrenia lends empirical support, albeit indirect, to the close and apparently intrinsic linkage between environment–brain unity and subjectivity in consciousness.

CHAPTER 18
Resting-State Activity and Prephenomenal Unity

Summary

Part V focused on the neuronal mechanisms underlying the constitution of spatial and temporal continuity of neuronal activity in the resting state and how that shapes our "inner time (and space) consciousness." However, we experience "contents" like objects and events within our stream of consciousness, rather than mere time and space in consciousness. This raises the questions of how the spatial and temporal continuity of the resting state's neural activity is related to the consciousness of these contents. We experience the diverse contents as parts or aspects of one unity in our consciousness: phenomenal unity. How, then, does the resting state itself and its spatial and temporal continuity impact the constitution of contents in such a way that the latter can be associated with consciousness? This is the focus of the present chapter. Investigations of multistable perception show that the kind of perceptual content—that is, the respective phenomenal content—is predicted by the level of the pre-stimulus resting-state activity in the sensory regions like auditory and visual cortex. The level of resting-state activity in the sensory cortex preceding the stimulus may thus have a say in selecting the phenomenal content. Furthermore, the data show that even the resting state of higher-order regions like the prefrontal cortex that are not directly involved in sensory processing predicts the subsequent content during multistable perception. Taken together, this suggests that the resting-state activity in both lower-order sensory and higher-order cognitive regions has an impact on the selection of the subsequent phenomenal contents in consciousness.

What are the exact neuronal mechanisms underlying such selection? Recent data show that the phases of the preceding resting state's low-frequency fluctuations are aligned to the power and the phases of higher-frequency oscillations during subsequent stimulus-induced activity. The data suggest that such alignment and phase synchronization across the divide of resting-state and stimulus-induced activity are relevant for the subsequent behavioral and phenomenal state and thus for consciousness.

How is it possible that the preceding resting-state activity, which is purely neuronal in itself, predisposes the phenomenal state and thus consciousness during subsequent stimulus-induced activity? I suppose that the duration of the resting state's low-frequency fluctuations provide a time window to constitute a temporal unity. This allows the resolution and integration of stimuli at different (physical) time points into one neural activity (which is then [temporal] difference- rather than stimulus-based). That, in turn, is dependent upon the degree of the preceding resting state's temporal continuity and unity of its neural activity, which is proposed to be carried over and transferred to the subsequent stimulus-induced activity. Depending on the temporal extension of the resting state's temporal unity and its alignment of subsequent stimulus-induced activity, the temporal unity will be manifested on the phenomenal level of consciousness. More specifically, I propose the duration of the resting state's temporal unity to predispose the possible degree of phenomenal features like the "nonstructural homogeneity" and "wholeness" that signify the phenomenal unity in consciousness. The same holds for the resting state's spatial unity, which can be associated with its functional connectivity pattern. Based on these considerations, I propose what I describe as a "resting-state–based hypothesis of prephenomenal unity." This hypothesis proposes that the brain's resting-state activity is characterized by a prephenomenal unity. Such prephenomenal unity consists of spatial and temporal unity of the resting state's neuronal activity as based on its coupling of fluctuations from different frequency ranges and functional connectivity spanning across different regions.

Key Concepts and Topics Covered

Entrainment of high frequencies by low frequencies, prephenomenal unity, phenomenal unity, resting state, stimulus-induced activity, spatial unity, temporal unity, functional connectivity, phase synchronization, wholeness, nonstructural homogeneity, resting state–based hypothesis of prephenomenal unity.

NEUROEMPIRICAL BACKGROUND
IA: MULTISTABLE PERCEPTION AND
PHENOMENAL DIVERSITY

So far, I have focused on the neuronal mechanisms underlying the constitution of time and space as the very basis or ground of consciousness (see Part V). Global spatial and temporal continuity of neuronal activity in the resting state was supposed to be central in constituting a temporal and spatial grid or net as the very basis of consciousness accounting for what William James described as "stream of consciousness."

How does the constitution of such temporal and spatial grid impact and predispose the experience of the contents in consciousness? We thus shift our focus from the constitution of the spatial and temporal dimension of consciousness to the experience of contents in consciousness.

For the answer, we first need to explore how the brain makes the transition from its resting-state activity to the stimulus-induced activity, as it is supposed to underlie the contents of consciousness. This will be the focus in this chapter, in which I take the phenomenon of multistable perception as a paradigmatic example.

What is *multistable perception*? Everyone knows that sometimes our perception is rather ambiguous when there are, for instance, two mutually exclusive interpretations. This is the case in the famous example of the drawing of the Rubin vase, where the viewer's perception switches back and forth between seeing either a face or a vase. Another such example is the Neckar cube, where it remains unclear and ambiguous which plane is perceived as being in front. Most important, such switching back and forth between different perceptions occurs while the purely physical stimulus remains exactly the same. This is called "multistable perception."

We are here thus confronted with an instance of physical stimulus identity and phenomenal, that is, perceptual, difference. Multistable perception raises interesting questions about the relationship between physical stimulus features and phenomenal percepts. How is it possible that we can have two distinct percepts while the physical stimulus remains exactly the same?

Moreover, it should be noted that we have only one percept at a time while the respective other one is excluded at that particular point in time. This is particularly of interest with regard to the unity of phenomenal contents in consciousness. Multistable perception seems to suggest that there is phenomenal unity of content, meaning that there can only be one rather than two "contents" in our perception and thus consciousness at one specific point in time. We perceive either the face or the vase in the case of the Rubin vase.

In contrast, having two simultaneously occurring perceptions seem to be impossible; we do not perceive face and vase at the same time, so phenomenal diversity seems to remain impossible. Accordingly, there seems to be a predisposition toward phenomenal unity rather than phenomenal diversity, with the latter remaining apparently impossible. However, even if phenomenal diversity at one point in time remains impossible, it nevertheless can well occur across different discrete points in physical time. We experience the vase in one moment, while in the next, we perceive the face. Multistable perception thus indicates phenomenal diversity across time.

NEUROEMPIRICAL BACKGROUND IB: LOWER- VERSUS HIGHER-ORDER THEORIES OF MULTISTABLE PERCEPTION

How can we neuroscientifically explain such multi- or bistable perception signifying phenomenal diversity across time? There has been much discussion about whether multistable perception is a lower- or higher-order phenomenon in neuronal terms. "Lower-order" means that it may be related to sensory cortical processing, such as, for instance, in the gestalt of mutually inhibitory suppression between the two perceptions in early visual cortex (layers V1–V5).

In contrast, higher-order mechanisms may be related to top-down modulation by, for instance, the prefrontal or parietal cortex that may modulate and thus reorganize neural activity in sensory cortex, that is, visual or auditory cortex (see Sterzer et al. 2009 for a recent review, as well as Lamme and Roelfsma 2000; Lamme 2006; see also Appendix 3 for the discussion of the position by S. Zeki and its relationship to that of philosopher Immanuel Kant).

Recent results shed a new light on the lower versus higher-order debate in multistable perception. They show that apparently both mechanisms may be involved and complemented by the involvement of the prior resting-state activity. This is the moment where Andreas Kleinschmidt comes into the picture.

Andreas Kleinschmidt is a neuroscientist who works in both France and Germany. He and his group conducted some excellent studies about multistable perception and how it relates to the resting-state activity preceding the onset of the stimulus. I here focus on the human results from his group (while neglecting others as, for instance, the earlier monkey-based studies on multistable perception by, for instance, Leopold and Logothetis, which are well in line with the data described in the following; see Leopold and Logothetis 1999 for a summary) since they show the impact of the resting state on subsequent perception in a paradigmatic way (see Chapter 11, as well as Northoff et al. 2010 for a recent review).

NEURONAL FINDINGS IA: LOCAL PRE-STIMULUS RESTING-STATE ACTIVITY IN MULTISTABLE PERCEPTION

The group around Andreas Kleinschmidt (Hesselmann et al. 2008a) investigated human subjects in functional magnetic resonance imaging (fMRI during the Rubin face-stimulus illusion where subjects perceive either a vase or a face. They first analyzed stimulus-related activity and thus those epochs where the stimulus was presented; these epochs were distinguished according to whether subjects perceived a face or a vase. Since the fusiform face area (FFA) is well known to be related to the processing of specifically faces, the focus was here on the FFA during both face and vase percepts.

What results did they obtain? The FFA showed greater stimulus-induced signal changes in those trials where subjects perceived a face when compared to the ones where they perceived a vase. The authors then went further ahead and sampled the signal changes in the FFA immediately prior to the onset of the stimulus defining a pre-stimulus baseline (or resting state) phase. Interestingly, this yielded significantly higher pre-stimulus signal changes in the right FFA during those trials where subjects perceived a face.

In contrast, such pre-stimulus signal changes were not observed in the right FFA when subjects perceived a vase rather than a face. In addition to such perceptual specificity, there was also regional specificity. The pre-stimulus resting-state signal change increases were only observed in the right FFA, while they did not occur in either other visual regions or other regions like the prefrontal cortex.

In addition to perceptual and regional spatial specificity, Hesselmann et al. (2008a) also investigated temporal specificity. They conducted an ANOVA (analysis of variance) for the interaction between time point (early and late resting-state signal changes in the FFA) and percept (vase, face). This revealed a statistically significant interaction between time point and percept. The late resting-state signal changes were more predictive of the subsequent percept; that is, face or vase, than the early ones. The resting state's neural activity at the time point immediately preceding the stimulus thus seems to contain the most information about the subsequent percept as related to stimulus-induced activity; this entails what can be described as "temporal specificity."

What does such temporal specificity imply? The authors themselves remark (Hesselmann et al. 2008a) that the immediate pre-stimulus FFA resting-state signal changes contain as much information about the percept as the stimulus-induced activity in FFA itself and the subject's verbal report. Hence the observed regional, temporal, and perceptual specificity of the pre-stimulus resting-state activity in the FFA may be of central importance for the kind of content associated with consciousness; that is, the phenomenal content.

NEURONAL FINDINGS IB: PRE-STIMULUS RESTING-STATE ACTIVITY IN LOWER-ORDER SENSORY REGIONS DURING MULTISTABLE PERCEPTION

One may now want to argue that the observed FFA differences during stimulus-induced activity between the two percepts may stem from the preceding pre-stimulus resting-state differences rather than from the stimulus itself. The pre-stimulus resting-state differences may thus simply be carried forth into the stimulus period and the stimulus-induced activity. If so, one would expect mere addition and thus linear interaction between the prior resting state and the neural activity induced by the stimulus itself. The assumption of such merely additive and linear interaction between resting state and stimulus is not in accordance, however, with the data, as will become clear in the following.

The data show that qualitatively (e.g., the pure inspection of the signal), the pre-stimulus resting-state differences disappeared more or less completely in the signals; that is, the BOLD curves, once the stimulus sets in. This argues against a simple carryover effect, in which case one would expect the differences in the preceding resting-state activity to persist during the onset of the subsequent stimulus. Interestingly, though, the signal associated with the pre-stimulus

resting-state activity seems to reappear later, during the peak amplitude of the BOLD curves during the stimulus-induced activity.

The same was observed quantitatively (i.e., by statistical calculation) when investigating statistically the interaction between time (peri-stimulus time segments and their respective signal changes before and during the onset of the stimulus-induced BOLD curve) and perception (e.g., face versus vase). As described earlier, this revealed a statistically significant interaction between time and percept. Taken together, these observations argue against a simple carry-over effect of the preceding resting-state differences into subsequent stimulus-induced activity. Instead, the results suggest an interaction between pre-stimulus resting state and stimulus along the lines of a nonlinear and thus supraadditive (rather than linear, i.e., additive) interaction (see Volume I, Chapter 11, as well as Chapter 29 for more details on nonlinearity in rest–stimulus interaction).

Analogous findings, increased pre-stimulus resting-state signal changes in stimulus-specific regions and nonlinear rest–stimulus interaction, could also be observed in other multistable perception tasks in both visual and auditory sensory modalities (see Sadaghiani et al. 2010 for a direct comparison). This included an ambiguous auditory perception task where increased pre-stimulus resting-state changes could be observed in auditory cortex. Increases in auditory cortical pre-stimulus resting-state activity predicted the hits (as distinguished from the misses) in an auditory detection task near the auditory threshold (Sadaghiani et al. 2009, 2010; Sterzer et al. 2009).

Analogously, the coherent percept in a motion decision task could also be predicted by increased pre-stimulus resting-state activity in a motion-sensitive area (hMT+) in occipito-temporal cortex (see Hesselmann et al. 2008b). In addition to the predictive effects of increased pre-stimulus resting-state activity in hMT+, nonlinear and thus nonadditive interaction between pre-stimulus and stimulus-induced activity could be observed along the lines described earlier. These findings argue against simple propagation or carryover of preceding resting-state differences into subsequent stimulus-induced activity. Instead, they let the

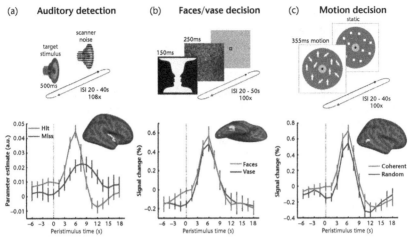

Figure 18-1 Prediction of perceptual consciousness by the preceding resting-state activity. Local spontaneous variations in ongoing activity of specialized sensory regions impact perception. The upper part illustrates the paradigm: (*a*) auditory detection experiment: in a free-response setting, subjects detected an auditory target stimulus presented at perceptual threshold. (*b*) Perceptual decision on an ambiguous figure: subjects reported either faces or vase perception in response to flashes of the faces-vase ambiguous figure. (*c*) Motion decision experiment: random dot motion was presented at motion coherence threshold, and subjects decided trial by trial whether motion was coherent or random. In all experiments, trials followed at long and unpredictable intervals. In each experiment, the pre-stimulus BOLD signal (dotted vertical line marking stimulus onset) was examined as a function of perceptual outcome and sampled from accordingly specialized sensory areas. The corresponding regions of interest (early auditory cortex, FFA and hMT+, respectively) are presented on a canonical inflated cortical surface of the right hemisphere. In all experiments, higher pre-stimulus time course in the respective sensory regions biased towards perceiving stimulus properties for which these regions are particularly sensitive. Error bars represent standard error across subjects. Reprinted from Sadaghiani S, Hesselmann G, Friston KJ, Kleinschmidt A. The relation of ongoing brain activity, evoked neural responses, and cognition. *Front Syst Neurosci.* 2010 Jun 23;4:20.

authors propose complex, that is, nonlinear, interaction between resting-state and stimulus-induced activity as distinct though interdependent components of neural activity (see Fig. 18-1).

NEURONAL FINDINGS IC: PRE-STIMULUS RESTING-STATE ACTIVITY IN HIGHER-ORDER COGNITIVE REGIONS DURING MULTISTABLE PERCEPTION

Can multistable perception thus be sufficiently explained by pre-stimulus resting-state changes and nonlinear rest–stimulus interaction in early sensory regions? No, because in addition to these lower-level sensory regions, higher-level cognitive regions like the prefrontal cortex also show differences in prior resting-state activity that also predict the subsequent percept.

This has been, for instance, demonstrated by Sterzer et al. (2007, 2009). They applied an ambiguous motion stimulus and show increased resting-state signal changes in the right inferior prefrontal cortex prior to stimulus onset. Most important, chronometric analysis (e.g., at different time points) of fMRI data revealed that such increased right inferior prefrontal cortical resting-state activity occurred prior to the onset of neural activity differences in motion-sensitive extrastriate visual cortex.

An analogous finding was made in an electroencephalography (EEG) study during visual presentation of the Necker cube (Britz et al. 2009). Here, the right inferior parietal cortex showed increased pre-stimulus resting-state activity 50 ms prior to the reversal of the perceptual content that predicted the subsequent percept.

Taken together, this suggests that pre-stimulus resting-state activity even in higher regions like the prefrontal or parietal cortex may be crucial in predicting the subsequent perception and thus the phenomenal content of consciousness. This may be possible by higher regions modulating the resting-state activity in lower sensory regions (see also Sterzer et al. 2009 for such interpretation as well as the papers by Lamme 2006; van Gaal and Lamme 2011; Lamme and Roelfsma 2000).

Accordingly, in addition to the local sensory regions, the pre-stimulus resting activity seems to operate also on a more transregional and thus global level; that is, higher- and lower-order regions lie across different regions. Such trans-regional action may be relevant in determining the perception and thus the phenomenal content during multistable perception.

NEURONAL HYPOTHESIS IA: "IDEAL" AND "WORST" PHASES IN THE PRE-STIMULUS RESTING-STATE ACTIVITY

The findings clearly demonstrate that the pre-stimulus resting-state activity predicts the subsequent perception, e.g., the phenomenal content. More specifically, the resting-state activity predicts the content of the subsequent perception like whether one perceives a face or vase. I hence focus on the contents of consciousness, the phenomenal contents, in the following discussion.

Let us go into more neuronal detail. The pre-stimulus resting-state activity indicates regional specificity, meaning that only the FFA but no other region showed increased signal changes. These increases were observed only during the subsequent perception of a face while they did not occur when subjects perceived a vase. And there was also temporal specificity with the late phases of the preceding resting state predicting the subsequent percept much better than early resting-state phases.

How can we relate these findings to the constitution of contents in perception and thus to the phenomenal content in consciousness as implicated during perception? Resting-state activity seems to bias and thus predispose the subsequent perception toward a specific phenomenal content, a face rather than a vase.

More specifically, the fluctuations in the FFA's resting-state activity level seem to be the central variable here. If the stimulus arrives at a time point of high resting-state activity in the FFA, one may perceive it as face. If, in contrast, the resting-state activity in the FFA is rather low at that point in time, one may perceive the same stimulus as vase.

There may thus be "ideal" and "worst" phases in the resting-state activity level of the FFA for the stimulus to be perceived as face (or vase). "Ideal" phases bias the phenomenal content of the subsequent perception toward the face, while "worst" phases bias the phenomenal content toward the vase. One may consequently propose the level of the resting state to be a necessary predisposing condition for determining the specific kind of phenomenal content.

This bias or predisposition of the resting state may conceptually also be described by the term "window of opportunity" that, in our specific case, may be either open or closed for either faces or vases. The resting state's neural activity may thus provide what one can describe as the "spatiotemporal window of opportunity" (see Fig. 18-2).

NEURONAL HYPOTHESIS IB: PRE-STIMULUS RESTING-STATE ACTIVITY PROVIDES A "SPATIOTEMPORAL WINDOW OF OPPORTUNITY" FOR EXTRINSIC STIMULI

However, the temporal course of the resting-state activity level and its "ideal" and "worst" phases do not determine the phenomenal content alone. In addition, the timing of the stimulus relative to the resting state's temporal course is also central and cannot be neglected, either. If the stimulus arrives at an "ideal phase" of the resting-state activity, it has a higher likelihood of becoming the content of consciousness (see later for details) when compared to its timing at the "worst phase." This means that neither the resting state alone, nor the stimulus and its specific point in time and space, can be regarded as sufficient conditions of consciousness by themselves. Only the conjunction of resting state and stimulus and, more specifically, their particular constellation may be sufficient to select and generate specific phenomenal contents.

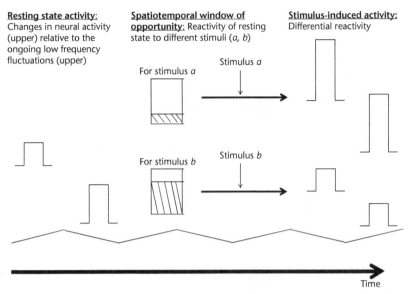

Figure 18-2 Resting-state activity and its "spatiotemporal window of opportunity." The figure demonstrates how neural activity changes in the resting state (*left*) provide a "spatiotemporal window of opportunity" (*middle*) in terms of neural reactivity for particular stimuli (*right*). (*Left*): The two bars indicate changes in neural activity, while the lower line symbolizes the ongoing low-frequency fluctuations of the resting-state activity. The two neural activity changes occur at different discrete points in physical time and space. (*Middle*): That provides a "spatiotemporal window of opportunity" of the intrinsic activity for different extrinsic stimuli to elicit strong or weak neural activity changes in the resting-state activity. The boxes shall indicate such a window while their shaded lines illustrate the degree to which the "spatiotemporal window of opportunity" is open or closed for the stimulus; it is wide open for stimulus *a* and not very open for stimulus *b*. Hence, the resting state provides what Buszaki (2006) calls "input selection." (*Right*): Following the resting state's "spatiotemporal window of opportunity," stimulus *a* elicits major changes in neural activity (large bars), while stimulus *b* does not trigger many changes in the ongoing resting-state activity (low bars). Such "input selection" by the resting state's "spatiotemporal window of opportunity" strongly impacts which stimuli and ultimately contents are selected for consciousness. Hence, the resting state is proposed to have a role in the selection of the phenomenal contents of consciousness (see text for details).

Taken together, the resting-state activity by itself is consequently only a necessary condition and thus a neural predisposition of consciousness (and its phenomenal contents). This means that the resting-state activity offers what I described in Chapter 11 in Volume I as "spatiotemporal window of opportunity" for the subsequent processing of extrinsic stimuli and their possible association with consciousness.

Such a "spatiotemporal window of opportunity" may be either less or more "open" and can thereby impact the degree to which the extrinsic stimuli are processed in the brain. This implies that neither the intrinsic resting-state activity by itself nor the extrinsic stimulus alone

(independent of the resting state) can then be regarded as a sufficient condition and thus neural correlate of (the phenomenal contents of) consciousness. Therefore, rather than being a neural correlate, the resting-state activity must then be considered a neural predisposition of the phenomenal contents of consciousness.

NEURONAL HYPOTHESIS IC: "SPATIOTEMPORAL WINDOW OF OPPORTUNITY" PROVIDES "INPUT SELECTION" AS "CONTENT SELECTION"

Let me illustrate the resting-state activity's neural predisposition in further neuronal detail by going briefly to the cellular level of neural activity. Schroeder et al. (2008) discuss four rules of neuronal oscillations, of which the first one concerns the resting state's neuronal oscillations. The (stimulus-related) firing rate of neurons, that is, their action potentials, are often related to a specific phase, that is, ascending and descending phases, of the ongoing (resting state's) oscillation as measured by local field potentials.

For instance, in macaque, negative deflections and current sinks in theta oscillations in auditory cortex go along with increased firing rates and action potentials, whereas the opposite, that is, decreased single-unit firing rates and action potentials, was observed in positive deflections and current sources of the theta oscillations (Lakatos et al. 2005a and b, 2007).

Similar observations have been made in the visual cortex with regard to gamma oscillations (30–50Hz) and single-unit firing rates (see, for instance, Fries 2005 as well as Chapter 12 in Volume I) as well as for very low frequencies (<1 Hz) by Steriade et al. (1993). Obviously, the duration of the time intervals for "ideal" and "worst" phases does differ between the different frequency bands with the temporal windows being shorter for high than for low frequencies (see also Buzsaki and Draguhn 2004 and Buzsaki 2006 for the details of such "input selection" as they call it): the lower the frequency fluctuation, the longer the time windows for ideal and worst phases for the processing of stimuli. One may consequently say that the resting state provides a "temporal (and spatial) window of opportunity" for subsequent neuronal activity changes.

How now do these observations on the cellular level stand to the aforementioned findings on the regional level? On the cellular level the resting state's frequency fluctuations provide "ideal" and "worst" phases for subsequent stimulus-induced activity; for example, its firing rates and action potentials. Analogously, the resting-state activity level on a regional level seems to provide "ideal" and "worst" phases for the association of the stimulus with particular phenomenal contents as distinguished from others.

The resting-state activity preceding the stimulus may thus provide a "temporal (and spatial) window of opportunity" for the association of the stimulus with particular contents

in consciousness; e.g., phenomenal contents. In other words, the resting state predisposes the selection of phenomenal contents. There is thus what Buzsaki (2006) (see also Buzsaki and Draguhn 2004) describes as "input selection," which may be specified in the present context as "content selection. The concept of "content selection" refers to the mechanisms and criteria on the basis of which contents in consciousness are chosen and thus selected.

I therefore propose the resting-state activity to be an essential, that is, necessary, predisposing neural condition, in selecting the contents that can possibly be associated with the extrinsic stimulus and ultimately with consciousness itself. By providing "ideal" and "worst" phases for particular phenomenal contents, the resting-state activity exerts a predisposing impact on which phenomenal content can possibly be selected and associated with the stimulus, implying "input or content selection."

NEURONAL FINDINGS IIA: FLUCTUATIONS IN THE RESTING STATE ACTIVITY

In addition to the selection of the phenomenal content, the pre-stimulus resting-state activity may also contribute to the instantiation of the phenomenal state during rest–stimulus interaction. This raises the question about the neuronal features of the resting state itself: what kind of neuronal features must the resting state show in order to predispose the instantiation of a phenomenal state and ultimately phenomenal unity during the subsequent encounter with a stimulus?

We recall that resting-state activity is characterized by predominantly low-frequency fluctuations, while stimulus-induced activity shows rather high-frequency fluctuations (see Parts I and II in Volume I). One may consequently investigate how both high- and low-frequency fluctuations are related to each other and how that relationship is involved in constituting consciousness, including both its contents and state.

To reveal the exact neuronal mechanisms of the coupling between high- and low-frequency fluctuations, I first turn to the cellular and population level of neural activity in this section.

Humans and consciousness will be discussed in the next section. While neglecting other studies (see Canolty and Knight 2010; Sauseng and Klimesch 2008; Klimesch et al. 2010, for excellent reviews), I here focus on a monkey-based study by Lakatos et al. (2008) that shows the relationship between higher- and lower-frequency ranges in a paradigmatic way. Together P. Lakatos and C. Schroeder made major contributions in clarifying the relationship between high- and low-frequency fluctuations and how they relate to perception and attention (see also Schroeder and Lakatos 2009a and b; as well as Chapter 20 herein).

Lakatos et al. (2008) investigated the primary visual cortex (V1) in two macaque monkeys (see Besle et al. 2011 for more or less corresponding experiments in human subjects undergoing intracranial recording in various sites). The monkeys were trained to perform an intermodal selection task in which auditory (beeps) and visual (flashes) target stimuli were presented with random stimulus-onset synchronies (between 500ms and 800 ms with a mean of 6.50 ms corresponding to 1.5 Hz delta frequency).

These target stimuli, beeps and flashes, were embedded in a rhythmic stream of auditory and visual stimuli. Monkeys had to either attend to the visual (AV: attention to visual stimulus) or the auditory (AA: attention to auditory stimulus) target stimulus. Multi-unit activity (MUA) measuring local field potentials and current source density (CSD) recording oscillatory activity were obtained. They focused on MUA and CSD activity during the onset of the stimulus in particular in order to reveal the contributions of the ongoing preceding resting-state activity to the subsequent stimulus-induced activity.

NEURONAL FINDINGS IIB: ENTRAINMENT OF HIGHER- BY LOWER-FREQUENCY FLUCTUATIONS

What are the results of the study by Lakatos et al. (2008)? As expected, MUA was larger, and CSD response amplitude in V1, the primary visual cortex, was stronger in the AV condition when compared to the AA condition. How does such stimulus-induced activity relate to the preceding resting-state activity, the baseline, and its

predominant lower-frequency oscillations like delta? For that, they focused on the neuronal changes during stimulus onset since that reveals the contributions of the preceding resting-state activity.

Visual cortical CSD activity (which measures oscillatory activity and its different phases) showed opposite signs (in supra- and infragranular layers but not in granular layers) during the onset of the stimulus in AA and AV. This indicates different phases during the ongoing delta oscillation in the preceding resting state and thus what is described as *phase difference* or *phase shift* during AA and AV.

Let me be more specific. The phases were 180 degree out of phase, that is, shifted, during the onset of the stimulus in AA and AV. The phase at visual stimulus onset was close to the negative peak in the AV condition, while the opposite was the case in the AA condition, where it was in the phase close to the positive peak.

One may now want to argue that the phase shift is related to the different sensory modalities, that is, the visual and auditory stimulus. This, however, was not the case. Rather than being dependent upon the sensory modality of the stimulus, the phase shift was related to whether the stimulus was attended. Hence, the phase shift may signal the degree of attention one devotes to the stimulus whatever its sensory modality, auditory or visual.

Where does the phase shift, the phase difference between AV and AA at stimulus onset, come from? The results demonstrate that the gamma and MUA differences between AA and AV (as described above) were related to their differential entrainment by the preceding resting state's delta oscillation phase.

Higher and lower amplitudes of MUA and CSD were related to a specific phase in the pre-stimulus delta oscillation. The largest MUA and CSD amplitudes occurred close to the negative peak of the preceding delta oscillation, indicating a high excitability phase, while the lowest MUA and CSD amplitudes were rather related to a positive peak in the delta oscillation being indicative of rather low excitability. This means that the stimulus-induced amplitude in MUA and CSD was very much dependent upon the pre-stimulus phase of the delta oscillation in the preceding resting state (Fig. 18-3).

Finally, the phase of the preceding resting-state delta oscillation did not just predict and thus entrain the higher frequencies and the MUA during stimulus-induced activity. Additionally, the resting state's delta phases determined the subsequent behavior, the reaction time by means of which the monkeys responded to the respective stimuli. The fastest reaction times occurred during the negative peak of pre-stimulus delta oscillation, while the reaction times were longer when a positive peak of the delta oscillation preceded in the resting state. This means that the phase of the delta oscillation does not only predict and entrain higher frequencies and MUA but also the behavior; for example, the reaction time.

Taken together, these findings show the relevance of low-frequency oscillations in the resting state preceding the onset of the stimulus and its stimulus-induced activity. More specifically, the resting state's phase of delta-band oscillation predicted higher-frequency oscillation (CSD), MUA, and even behavioral measures (like reaction time) during subsequent stimulus-induced activity.

The amplitude and phase of higher frequencies like gamma during stimulus-induced activity consequently seem to follow the phase of the ongoing underlying low-frequency oscillation, that is, delta, in the preceding resting state. Accordingly, to put it conversely, the resting state's slow-frequency oscillation phase entrains and thus "enslaves" the power and phases of the higher-frequency oscillations and their associated behavior during subsequent stimulus-induced activity.

NEURONAL FINDINGS IIC: ENTRAINMENT AND CONSCIOUSNESS

The data demonstrate that the phases of the resting state's low-frequency oscillations, such as delta, entrain the higher-frequency oscillations, such as theta and gamma, during subsequent stimulus-induced activity. This raises two questions. First, the resting state in humans shows even lower-frequency ranges as in the infraslow range (<0.1 Hz). Do these infraslow frequencies also (like the delta oscillations) entrain higher-frequency oscillations related to stimuli?

Secondly, while Lakatos et al. showed the behavioral relevance of such low-high-frequency entrainment in monkeys, its phenomenal relevance for human consciousness remains unclear. To address both questions, I turn to a study by Monto et al. (2008) (while there do not seem to be many other studies addressing low-high-frequency entrainment and consciousness in the healthy awake subject).

Monto et al. (2008) investigated high and infraslow frequencies using EEG in human subjects. Subjects were delivered a somatosensory stimulus at random intervals (1.5. to 4.5 s) with a current directed towards and targeting their right index finger. The current was adjusted so that the subjects were able to detect only 50% of the applied stimuli; that is, hits and misses. Hits indicated conscious detection of the current, while misses reflected unconsciousness, with subjects remaining unaware that a current was applied. Besides 1–40 Hz oscillations, the EEG also recorded infraslow-frequency (ISF) oscillations between 0.01 and 0.1 Hz.

What are the results? As expected (see also Buzsaki and Draguhn 2004), general power during the task was increased in low-frequency oscillation, while it was decreased in high-frequency oscillation. Most important, a clear coupling and thus correlation of the phase of the ISF to the hits and misses in the detection of the stimulus could be observed. The probability of a hit was highest during the rising phases of the ISF, while it was lowest during the falling ISF phases at the central (Cz) and fronto-central (Fpz) anterior midline electrodes. In contrast to the hits and misses, rising and falling phases were not associated with different reaction times (see later for discussion).

Unlike the phase of the ISF, neither its amplitude nor its absolute measures, the "real part," e.g., the actual time point and course, of the ISF predicted either the behavioral choice (hit probability) or the reaction time. Hence, only the timing of the phase of the resting state's slow/infraslow oscillation in relation to the timing of the stimulus predicted subsequent stimulus-related behavioral performance; that is, hits and misses. This suggests a special

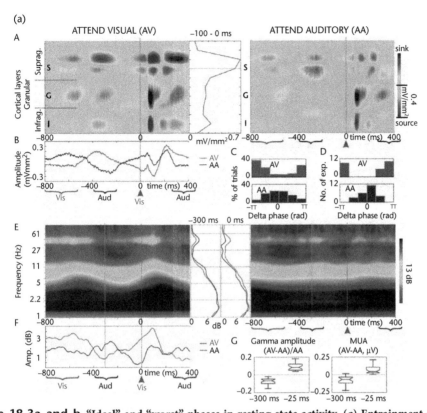

Figure 18-3a and b "Ideal" and "worst" phases in resting-state activity. (*a*) Entrainment and the oscillatory hierarchy. (A) Color maps show CSD profiles related to standard visual stimuli in the AV and AA conditions for the −800 to +400 ms time frame from a representative experiment. Traces between the CSD maps show the laminar profile of prestimulus oscillation amplitude based on the Hilbert transform of the CSD (−100 to 0 ms). The arrowhead indicates the visual event used as trigger (0 ms). The brackets indicate the time frames in which adjoining auditory and visual events occur, respectively. (B) CSD from supragranular electrode "S" in the AV and AA conditions. (C) Distribution of single-trial supragranular prestimulus (0 ms) delta oscillatory phases in the same experiment. (D) Pooled prestimulus mean (across trials) delta phase for all experiments (*n* = 24). (E) Time-frequency plots display the average oscillatory amplitude of the wavelet-transformed single trials in the selected supragranular site in (A). Traces in the middle show prestimulus amplitude spectra in the AV and AA conditions at −300 and 0 ms. (F) Time courses of the averaged (37 to 57 Hz) gamma amplitudes. (G) Pooled (*n* = 24) normalized gamma-amplitude and MUA differences between AV and AA conditions [(AV-AA)/AA)] for the −325 to −275 and −50 to 0 ms time frames. Notches in the boxes indicate a 95% confidence interval about the median of each distribution. Whiskers extend to the most extreme values. (*b*) Prestimulus delta phase and its effect on the visual event-related response. (A) Laminar CSD (top) and MUA (bottom) profiles elicited by standard visual stimuli in a representative experiment. The bars between the maps represent response amplitudes for the 50 to 135 ms time interval in the AV and AA conditions, respectively ("real" average). (B) Response amplitudes sorted into six bins on the basis of prestimulus delta phase. The bars at right represent response amplitudes averaged across the bins using the mean of each bin ("simulated" average). Error bars indicate SE. (C) Pooled (*n* = 24) normalized CSD and MUA response amplitude differences between AV and AA conditions [(AV-AA)/AA)] for real and simulated averages [see (A) and (B)]. Notches in the boxes indicate a 95% confidence interval about the median. Whiskers extend to the most extreme values. (D) Distribution of single-trial supragranular prestimulus (0 ms) delta phases in the same experiment. Reprinted with permission of *Science,* from Lakatos P, Karmos G, Mehta AD, Ulbert I, Schroeder CE. Entrainment of neuronal oscillations as a mechanism of attentional selection. *Science.* 2008 Apr 4;320(5872):110–3.

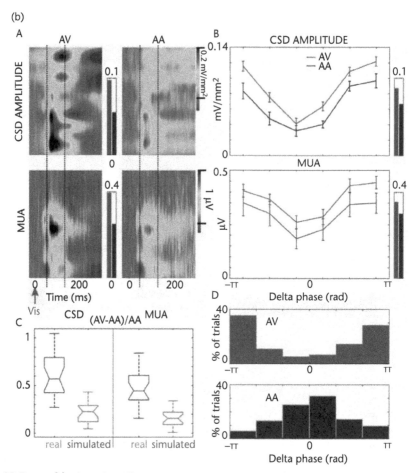

Figure 18-3a and b (Continued)

significance of the resting state's low-frequency fluctuations' phases for consciousness.

What about the relationship between high and low frequencies? In addition to its entrainment of behavioral performance, that is, hits and misses, ISF phases also entrained high-frequency oscillations in the range between 1 to 40 Hz at Fpz and Cz. Amplitudes in the 1–40 Hz oscillations were highest in the rising phases of the ISF, while they were rather low in the falling ISF phases. This suggests that the stimulus-related higher frequencies are entrained by or nested in the phases of the lower ones in the ongoing resting state.

Taken together, these findings clearly indicate the central role of the resting state's infraslow-frequency oscillations. The rising phases of the ISF

were associated with hits and higher amplitudes in the higher frequencies, while the falling phases of the ISF were rather related to misses and low amplitudes in higher frequencies. Accordingly, the phase of the ongoing ISF seems to provide a time window that is relevant for both the amplitude of high-frequency oscillations and behavioral performance, that is, conscious detection.

NEUROPHENOMENAL HYPOTHESIS IA: NEURONAL, BEHAVIORAL, AND PHENOMENAL RELEVANCE OF THE LOW-FREQUENCY FLUCTUATIONS IN THE RESTING-STATE ACTIVITY

Both animal and human data show that the amplitude of high-frequency oscillations seems to be related to and thus entrained by the phase of low-frequency oscillations including both delta (as in Lakatos et al. 2008) and infraslow frequencies (as in Monto et al. 2008). Such entrainment seems to operate across the boundaries between resting-state and stimulus-induced activity.

This must be proposed because the stimulus-induced high-frequency oscillations follow in their phase and amplitude the ongoing low-frequency oscillations in the resting state. Taken together, these data clearly indicate the neuronal relevance of the phases in the resting state's low frequencies for the stimulus-related higher frequencies.

Let me be more specific about the neuronal relevance of the resting state's low frequencies. The phasing and cycling of the low-frequency oscillations in the resting state provide a time window for the stimulus that may either be "ideal" or "worst" for the stimulus to induce neuronal activity (see earlier for "ideal" and "worst" phases). This was clearly demonstrated in the findings by Lakatos et al. (2008). The amplitude of both high-frequency oscillations (CSD) and MUA were predisposed or biased by the phase of the underlying ongoing delta oscillation in the resting state.

The study by Monto et al. (2008) complements these observations by showing that even infraslow-frequency oscillations (0.01–0.1 Hz) entrain higher ones and that this is mediated specifically by their phase rather than their amplitudes. Taken together, these data clearly demonstrate the preceding resting-state activity to bias or predispose subsequent stimulus-induced activity. Hence, the resting state's low-frequency oscillation and, more specifically, its phases are neuronally relevant for the higher-frequency oscillation's phases and amplitudes during subsequent stimulus-induced activity.

What exactly do I mean by "neuronal relevance"? The concept of neuronal relevance describes the importance of one neuronal measure for another neuronal measure. In our case I demonstrated that the resting state's low-frequency oscillations are neuronally relevant for the high-frequency fluctuations as elicited by the stimulus.

In addition to their neuronal relevance, one may also raise the question for the behavioral relevance of the resting state's low frequencies. The concept of behavioral relevance means that a specific neuronal measure impacts and modulates behavioral performance like detection of hits and misses or reaction time. Interestingly, both studies showed dependence of behavioral measures on the phases of the resting state's low-frequency oscillations. Lakatos et al. (2008) demonstrated that the reaction times in response to the stimuli were predicted by the phase of the ongoing delta oscillation in the resting state.

Such prediction of reaction times by the phase of the resting state's low-frequency oscillation was not observed, however, by Monto et al. (2008). Instead, Monto et al. (2008) observed that the detection of the stimulus, the hits and misses, was predicted by specifically the phases (and not the amplitude) of the infraslow-frequency oscillations. Rising phases were associated with hits, while falling phases made misses more likely. This clearly indicates behavioral relevance. Hence, the resting state's low-frequency oscillations are behaviorally relevant with regard to hits/misses, while they remain irrelevant for the reaction times.

However, the relevance of the resting-state activity's low-frequency fluctuations goes even beyond the merely behavioral domain. The hits reflect the detection of the stimulus when it was applied in a suprathreshold way, while misses occurred during subthreshold stimulus application. Subjects must have been conscious of the stimulus in order to detect and thus hit it (given also the adjustment to the individual subjects' threshold; see earlier). Hence, the behavioral relevance extends here to phenomenal relevance. This will be discussed in the next sections.

NEUROPHENOMENAL HYPOTHESIS IB: RESTING-STATE ACTIVITY PREDISPOSES THE PREPHENOMENAL UNITY

How can we define the concept of "phenomenal relevance"? The concept of phenomenal relevance describes that a particular neuronal mechanism may be relevant for and thus contribute to the constitution of consciousness and its phenomenal features. The neuronal mechanism can, for instance, concern the phases of the resting state's low-frequency oscillations, while the phenomenal feature may, for instance, be the phenomenal unity, including its phenomenal contents and phenomenal state.

The above described findings imply that the phase of the resting state's low-frequency oscillations at the stimulus-onset biases and predisposes the occurrence of subsequent consciousness and its phenomenal hallmark of phenomenal unity. The phase of the low-frequency oscillations reflects their ongoing phasing and cycling in the preceding resting-state period. Therefore, one must propose that the resting state itself biases and predisposes the constitution of consciousness and thus phenomenal unity during the subsequent stimulus-induced activity.

What does such bias or predisposition toward phenomenal unity mean? The low-frequency oscillation phase in the preceding resting-state period may bias and predispose a subsequent stimulus to be associated or not associated with phenomenal unity (which in turn paves the way for consciousness).

How is such association of a mere stimulus with phenomenal unity possible? I propose that the "right" phases of the resting-state activity's low-frequency fluctuations biase and predispose the carryover and transfer of the resting state's temporal and spatial continuity of its neural activity to the subsequent stimulus-induced activity. Thereby, the encounter with the extrinsic stimulus transforms the intrinsic activity's spatial and temporal continuity into spatial and temporal unity, as is manifested in the phenomenal unity of consciousness.

Based on these considerations, I propose that the actual phenomenal unity as associated with a particular extrinsic stimulus and its stimulus-induced activity is predisposed by the brain's intrinsic activity and the spatial and temporal continuity of its neural activity. More specifically, in order to transform the intrinsic activity's spatial and temporal continuity into the phenomenal unity as associated with an extrinsic stimulus, the extrinsic stimulus must occur in relation to the "right" phase of the intrinsic resting-state activity's low-frequency fluctuations.

NEUROMETAPHORICAL EXCURSION: HOW EXTRINSIC KEYS LEAD TO THE CARRYOVER AND TRANSFER OF THE BRAIN'S INTRINSIC ACTIVITY TO THE "LIVING ROOM OF CONSCIOUSNESS"

How can we illustrate the situation better? For that, I turn to a metaphorical comparison of intrinsic and extrinsic neural activity with the keyhole and key of a door. The intrinsic activity and thus the resting-state activity's temporal and spatial continuity are "the door" that is closed. In order to open the door, the "right" key is needed, a key that fits into the keyhole of the door.

What is the key, and what is the keyhole? The keyhole is an intrinsic part of the door, e.g., the intrinsic activity, and may therefore correspond to the phases of the resting-state activity's low-frequency fluctuations. The key, in contrast, is not part of the door and is therefore extrinsic to it. The key corresponds to the extrinsic stimulus, which must be timed in the "right" way to fit the phases of the resting-state activity's low-frequency fluctuations and their phase onsets.

Once the extrinsic stimulus and the intrinsic low-frequency fluctuations' phase onsets match and thus fit with each other, the door opens and provides access to the room. The opened door is moved into and thus carried over and transferred from the hallway to the now-accessible "living room of consciousness." Analogously, the temporal and spatial continuity of the intrinsic activity is carried over and transferred to the extrinsic stimulus-induced activity where, in the ideal case, it resurfaces as a phenomenal unity, as the living room of consciousness (see Chapter 30 for a more detailed discussion of such carryover and transfer).

NEUROPHENOMENAL HYPOTHESIS IC: "RESTING-STATE–BASED HYPOTHESIS OF PREPHENOMENAL UNITY"

What does this scenario imply for the conceptual characterization of the resting-state activity itself? Such a carryover and transfer imply that the resting-state activity itself—more specifically, the phases of its low-frequency oscillations—must already show some kind of unity.

However, unlike the phenomenal unity of consciousness, this unity of the resting state is not yet experienced as such and is therefore not phenomenal by itself.

At the same time, however, it already biases and predisposes the subsequent stimulus-induced activity toward temporal and spatial unity and thus phenomenal unity. This makes it impossible to render it as merely nonphenomenal. I therefore speak of a "prephenomenal unity."

How can we determine the concept of "prephenomenal unity" in further detail? The concept of "unity" in "prephenomenal unity" refers to a spatial and temporal unity that is based upon the resting state's spatial and temporal continuity as discussed in the previous part. The concept of "prephenomenal" describes two aspects: the prefix "pre" indicates that the unity cannot be experienced as such, thus remaining nonphenomenal. However, at the same time, the alleged temporal and spatial unity of the resting state is already related to the phenomenal unity in consciousness, albeit indirectly, which makes its characterization as completely non-phenomenal impossible, too.

This double characterization of the resting-state activity's spatial and temporal unity as "non-experienced" by itself but as biasing and predisposing subsequent experience can conceptually best be described by the term "prephenomenal unity," as distinguished from both phenomenal unity and nonphenomenal unity. Accordingly, the concept of the "resting state's prephenomenal unity" describes how the resting states' neuronal activity biases and predisposes the association of subsequent stimulus-induced activity with phenomenal unity and thus consciousness.

This leads me to the following neurophenomenal hypothesis. I propose that the phases of the resting state's low-frequency oscillations are phenomenally relevant in that they contribute to the constitution of the phenomenal unity of consciousness. I therefore speak of what I describe as "resting state–based hypothesis of prephenomenal unity."

More specifically, I hypothesize the phases of the resting state's low-frequency fluctuations to predispose the degree of the phenomenal unity of consciousness that can possibly be elicited during subsequent stimulus-induced activity (see Fig. 18-4a). As such, the resting state's low-frequency fluctuations and their phases are a neural predisposition of consciousness (NPC), the *necessary* neural conditions of possible consciousness, rather than its neural correlate of consciousness (NCC), the *sufficient* neural condition of actual consciousness.

We have now cleared the empirical and conceptual ground of the resting state–based hypothesis of prephenomenal unity. However, we left open the exact phenomenal features in consciousness that are predisposed and biased by the resting state's prephenomenal unity. For that, we need to briefly venture into phenomenological territory to be clearer about the exact phenomenal features indicating phenomenal unity in consciousness. This will allow us to investigate how these phenomenal features are biased and predisposed by the resting-state activity's neuronal mechanisms and its prephenomenal unity.

PHENOMENOLOGICAL EXCURSION: "LACK OF INTERNAL STRUCTURE" AND "LACK OF PROCESSUALITY"

To better understand the prephenomenal unity and what exactly it biases and predisposes, we need to provide further phenomenological detail about the phenomenal unity itself. More specifically, we need to detail what exactly is meant by the term "unity" in phenomenological regard; that is, how we experience unity and what kind of phenomenal features we attribute to it.

What is unity? Following the philosopher J. R. Searle, unity describes that we cannot experience separate aspects of objects with only one becoming conscious and the other not. Instead, we experience all aspects at the same time in a unified manner without any distinction between different sensory modalities and domains: "We do not perceive just the colour or shape, or the sound, of an object, we perceive all these simultaneously in a unified, conscious experience" (Searle 1998, p. 2075).

Unity in this sense entails what is often described as "wholeness." The concept of wholeness refers to the observation that conscious experience cannot be separated and reduced to distinct structures, parts, or elements. This

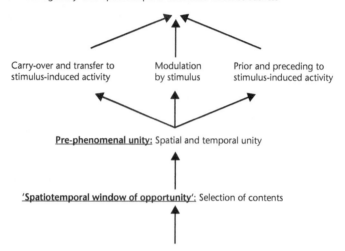

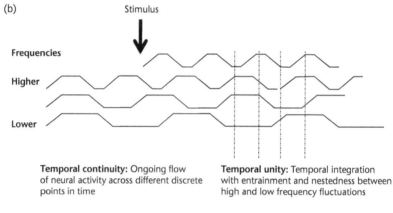

Figure 18-4a-e "Resting-state–based hypothesis of prephenomenal unity." The figure demonstrates distinct aspects of the resting state–based hypothesis of prephenomenal unity. (*a*) The figure illustrates how the phenomenal unity and its phenomenal features in experience (*upper part*) are based on the resting-state activity (*lower part*) as suggested by the "resting state–based hypothesis of prephenomenal unity." The resting state shows spatiotemporal continuity of its neural activity, which provides a spatiotemporal window for neural activity changes during the constitution of spatial and temporal unity (*middle*). That makes possible the selection of contents that can possibly be associated with the subsequent extrinsic stimulus implying "input or content selection." This spatial and temporal unity predisposes the constitution of phenomenal unity during subsequent stimulus-induced activity; the resting-state activity's spatial and temporal unity can therefore be characterized as prephenomenal unity. The intrinsic resting state's prephenomenal unity is carried over and transferred to the subsequent extrinsic stimulus-induced activity (*middle-upper left*) and, at the same time, is modulated and thus changed by itself by the extrinsic stimulus (*middle-upper middle*). This results in the constitution of phenomenal unity and its phenomenal features like "lack of internal temporal and spatial structure and processuality," that is, "nonstructural homogeneity" and "spatiotemporal wholeness" in experience and

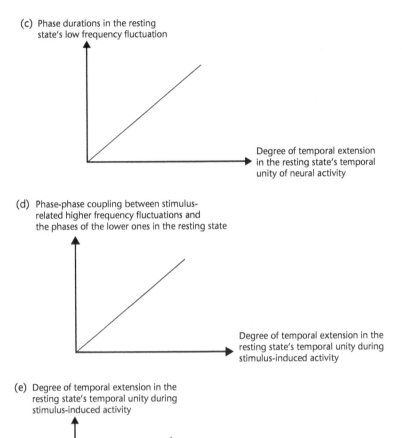

(c) Phase durations in the resting state's low frequency fluctuation

Degree of temporal extension in the resting state's temporal unity of neural activity

(d) Phase-phase coupling between stimulus-related higher frequency fluctuations and the phases of the lower ones in the resting state

Degree of temporal extension in the resting state's temporal unity during stimulus-induced activity

(e) Degree of temporal extension in the resting state's temporal unity during stimulus-induced activity

Degree of 'lack of internal temporal structure and processuality', i.e., temporal wholeness' and 'non-structural temporal homogeneity' in experience associated with stimulus-induced activity

Figure 18-4a-e (Continued)

thus in consciousness. (*b*) The figure demonstrates how the stimulus entrains and aligns the phase onsets between high- and low-frequency fluctuations. Thereby transitory temporal unities are constituted across the different discrete points in physical time associated with high- and low-frequency fluctuations. (*c–e*) The relationship of the resting state's low-frequency fluctuations and their phase durations (*c*) to phenomenal features of phenomenal unity, "lack of internal temporal structure and processuality," that is, "nonstructural temporal homogeneity" and "temporal wholeness," (*e*) via the degree of temporal extension and smoothing during resting state and stimulus-induced activity (*d*) are shown. The longer the phase durations of the resting-state activity's low-frequency fluctuations, the more temporal extension and smoothing are possible during both resting-state (*c*) and stimulus-induced activity (*d*), and the higher the possible degrees of "lack of internal temporal structure and processuality," that is, "nonstructural temporal homogeneity" and "temporal wholeness" (*e*) during the experience associated with stimulus-induced activity.

wholeness and inseparability has also been called "nonstructural homogeneity" (Metzinger 2003; Northoff and Heinzel 2003; Northoff 2004a and b). "Nonstructural homogeneity" means that experience shows no internal structure or heterogeneity, being rather smooth (Metzinger 2003, 190) or, as Sellars (1963, 26) said, "ultimately homogenous." Such smoothness and homogeneity of experience shall be described as a "lack of internal structure" in the following explanation.

In addition to the lack of internal structure, nonstructural homogeneity can be characterized by the absence of change and process. We do not experience the processing of the stimuli themselves; we only experience the outcome or results of these processes, that is, the objects and events. In contrast, we remain unable to experience the respectively underlying and preceding neuronal processes themselves (because of, as I propose, difference-based coding rather than stimulus-based coding; see Volume I as well as below; and Northoff 2011, chapter 2).

Due to our lack of experience of the underlying processes themselves, one may characterize the experience of the phenomenal unity in consciousness as result based rather than process based. There is thus what Metzinger (2003, 192) describes as "lack of processuality." We experience the ready and finished results, while the processes that lead to that result remain hidden and inaccessible to us in our experience and thus to our consciousness.

I therefore characterize the phenomenal unity of consciousness by the phenomenal features of wholeness and nonstructural homogeneity. This implies that we neither experience an internal structure nor any processes. The phenomenal unity of consciousness must consequently be characterized by lack of internal structure and lack of processuality.

Neuronal Hypothesis IIA: Low-Frequency Fluctuations Allow "Temporal Smoothing" of Neural Activity

We now have gathered all the neuronal and phenomenal tools needed to characterize the resting state's prephenomenal unity in further detail. How exactly can the resting state's

neuronal mechanisms predispose the phenomenal features that characterize the phenomenal unity? In other words, we now need to develop specific neurophenomenal hypotheses about the relationship between the resting state's low-frequency oscillations and the phenomenal features of lack of internal structure and lack of processuality. Metaphorically speaking, we need to put more phenomenal meat to the resting state–based hypothesis of prephenomenal unity.

Let us start again with the neuronal side of things and develop the necessary neuronal hypotheses, as shall be done in this and the following sections, which will then enable us to develop specific neurophenomenal hypotheses.

Based on their data, Schroeder et al. (2008) calculate the time window within which different frequency oscillations can integrate stimuli with different temporal onsets. Thereby, stimuli within the time window of half a cycle of a frequency oscillation can be integrated across time. Why only half the cycle and not the full cycle? Because their data (see earlier) clearly show that rising and falling slopes, or positive and negative deflections, of the phase of an oscillation are associated with different states of excitability, that is, ideal and worst, for possible stimulus-induced activity.

We need to detail the mechanisms with regard to the temporal integration of stimuli. The ideal or worst time windows for integrating stimuli across time depends on the frequency range of the oscillation, with high and low frequencies implying different time windows. Higher-frequency oscillations accompany shorter time windows, while low-frequency oscillations entail longer time windows. For instance, delta (1–4 Hz) and theta (4–8 Hz) oscillations would then entail time windows of 125–250ms (delta) and 70–100 ms (theta). In contrast, gamma oscillations show much shorter time windows, with 12.5ms (because 12.5ms is just half the period or cycle of a 40Hz oscillation).

What do these oscillation-based time windows, or phase durations, imply for the timing of the stimulus? They imply that stimuli occurring at different discrete positions in (physical) time can be integrated within a certain time window, i.e., the one provided by the phases of the resting state's fluctuations.

This means that, within this time window, all the stimuli are processed neuronally in the same way, regardless and independently of their respectively different discrete points in (physical) time. That obviously holds true only for the respective time window as provided by the different frequency fluctuations' phases in the resting state. In other words, there is some kind of temporal "smoothing" of the extrinsic stimuli's discrete time points by the time windows; that is, the phase durations of the low-frequency fluctuations in the resting-state activity.

NEURONAL HYPOTHESIS IIB: "TEMPORAL SMOOTHING" PREDISPOSES "TEMPORAL UNITY" OF NEURAL ACTIVITY

We need to be more specific, however. The different discrete time points of the stimuli are integrated within one particular time window; this is made possible by processing the different stimuli (within that time window) in terms of temporal differences presupposing difference-based coding (see Part V here as well as Volume I for more details about difference-based coding). The differences between the different stimuli's time points are consequently resolved, embedded, and unified into one temporal difference (see Fig. 18-4b-c).

Such integration and resolution, i.e., the temporal smoothing, make possible the integration of the different stimuli's discrete time points into one temporal unity (as distinguished from temporal diversity; see also Chapter 19 for details). The longer the time window (that is, phase durations) provided by the resting-state activity's frequency fluctuations, the stronger the stimuli's discrete time points can be extended and smoothed into each other. I consequently propose the degree of possible temporal extension of the temporal unity to be dependent on (and thus predisposed by) the degree of the phase durations of the resting-state activity's low-frequency oscillations (see later for details).

How is such temporal unity related to the phases of the resting-state activity's low-frequency oscillations? As I said earlier, the phases last for a certain duration. The lower the frequency range of the oscillations, the longer the duration of their phases. And the longer the

duration of the phases, the longer the time window within which stimuli from different discrete time points can be integrated and thus temporally smoothed into one temporal unity.

I consequently hypothesize the degree of temporal extension of the temporal unity to be directly dependent on the phase durations of the low-frequency oscillations. This means that lower-frequency oscillations make possible longer temporal unities. The lower the frequency range of the intrinsic resting-state activity's oscillation, the longer the duration of its phases, and the longer the possible temporal unity within which extrinsic stimuli and their discrete time points can be integrated, extended, and smoothed.

NEURONAL HYPOTHESIS IIC: "PHASE ALIGNMENT" AND "TEMPORAL UNITY" OF NEURAL ACTIVITY

So far, we have remained on a purely neuronal ground when discussing the relationship between low-frequency oscillations' phases in the resting-state activity and temporal unity during stimulus-induced activity. What exactly happens neuronally, however, during the encounter between intrinsic resting-state activity and extrinsic stimulus? For the answer, we turn to what we described in Chapter 11 as rest–stimulus interaction, which now shall be specified in temporal terms.

We recall that both studies described earlier (and many others) observed that the phases of the resting state's low-frequency oscillations were aligned to the phases and power of the higher-frequency oscillations during subsequent stimulus-induced activity. What does this mean for the temporal unity described earlier?

The temporal unity's degree of temporal extension was proposed to correspond to the phase duration of the low-frequency oscillations. If now the stimulus-induced high-frequency oscillations are well aligned to the phases of the low-frequency fluctuations, the time windows of the latter are more or less preserved. The degree of temporal extension of the temporal unity is not so much affected by the stimulus and its associated high-frequency oscillations. The lower-frequency oscillations thus remain more or less the same.

This changes, however, once the higher frequencies are no longer so well aligned to the phases of the lower ones. In that case, the time window provided by the low-frequency oscillations' phase durations will be sliced into bits and pieces, resulting in much shorter phase durations. This, in turn, will considerably reduce the degree of temporal extension of the resting-state activity's temporal unity.

Based on these considerations, I suggest the following neuronal hypothesis: the more aligned and thus phase-synchronized stimulus-induced higher frequencies are to the phases of the low-frequency oscillations in the resting-state activity, the longer and more extended the temporal unity for the subsequent integration of stimuli across different discrete time points (see Fig. 18-4d).

Conversely, the less aligned and synchronized the stimulus-induced higher frequencies are to the phases of the low-frequency oscillations in the resting-state activity, the smaller the possible temporal unity for the subsequent integration of stimuli occurring at different discrete time points. I therefore propose the degree of temporal smoothing and extension of the temporal unity during stimulus-induced activity to be directly dependent on the degree of alignment (or entrainment) between high- and low-frequency oscillations in the preceding resting-state activity.

NEUROPHENOMENAL HYPOTHESIS IIA: DIFFERENCE-BASED CODING PREDISPOSES PHASE ALIGNMENT

How, then, are these neuronal mechanisms related to the phenomenal features of the phenomenal unity described earlier? We recall that phenomenal unity could be characterized by "wholeness" and "nonstructural homogeneity" as well as by "lack of internal structure" and "lack of processuality." In the following discussion, I focus on the temporal domain while leaving the spatial domain for the subsequent section.

How are these phenomenal features related to the earlier-postulated temporal unity as the neuronal result of high-low-frequency entrainment? Within the duration of the resting state's temporal unity, all stimuli are processed together in terms of one temporal difference, regardless and

independently of their different discrete time points (see earlier). The stimuli's different time points are thus subsumed, or better, "smoothed," into one whole within the temporal unity, resulting in "temporal wholeness" and a "lack of internal temporal structure."

Moreover, the different stimuli's time points are not processed anymore by themselves in distinct and separate forms of neuronal activity. Instead, they are coded and processed from the very beginning in terms of one unifying temporal difference, e.g., in relation to and thus difference from the resting-state activity and the phase onsets and durations of its frequency fluctuations. If two stimuli and their different discrete time points fall within one and the same phase duration, they are encoded into neural activity in terms of the same temporal difference. That, though, means that both stimuli are integrated and smoothed into one and the same stimulus-induced activity.

Such difference-based coding must be distinguished from stimulus-based coding. In that case, each stimulus and its respective discrete time point would be encoded separately and independently of whether the different stimuli fall into the same phase duration or not. This means that, in any case, the two stimuli would lead to two different stimulus-induced activities.

The main distinguishing criterion for the encoding of neural activity is here the stimulus' discrete time point. This reflects stimulus-based coding. That is to be distinguished from difference-based coding, where the main distinguishing criterion is the phase duration of the intrinsic resting-state activity and its temporal relationship to the extrinsic stimuli's discrete time points. Hence, the alleged temporal unity between intrinsic activity and extrinsic stimuli is possible only in the case of difference-based coding, whereas it remains impossible in stimulus-based coding.

NEUROPHENOMENAL HYPOTHESIS IIB: PHASE ALIGNMENT PREDISPOSES "LACK OF INTERNAL TEMPORAL STRUCTURE AND PROCESSUALITY"

What does such difference-based coding and the subsequent constitution of temporal unity in neural activity imply in phenomenal terms?

This means that the stimuli's single discrete time points themselves, as well as the processes of their integrated encoding into a temporal differences value, are lost in the resulting neuronal activity and its temporal unity. The neuronal activity of the temporal unity reflects consequently the result, but not the process, of encoding by itself; it is therefore result-based rather than process-based.

This entails "nonstructural temporal homogeneity" and "lack of temporal processuality." The phenomenal features of "nonstructural temporal homogeneity" and "lack of temporal processuality" are thus proposed to be predisposed by the loss of separate neural processing of the single stimuli's different discrete time points by the intrinsic activity and its frequency fluctuations. In other words, I suggest difference-based coding to predispose "nonstructural temporal homogeneity" and "lack of temporal processuality," which would both remain impossible if there were stimulus-based coding. Taken together with the above-suggested neuronal hypothesis, this leads me to the following neurophenomenal hypothesis: the higher the degree of alignment and phase synchronization between the phases of the resting state's low-frequency oscillations and the stimulus-related high-frequency oscillations, the more the temporal unity can be extended and smoothed (across different discrete time points) in subsequent consciousness. And higher degrees of temporal unity, as I suppose, go along phenomenally with higher possible degrees of temporal wholeness and nonstructural temporal homogeneity and thus lack of internal temporal structure and processuality in the phenomenal unity of consciousness.

Conversely, this means that lower degrees of alignment and phase synchronization will lead to lower degrees of extension and smoothing of the temporal unity. This, in turn, implies phenomenally lower degrees of temporal wholeness and nonstructural temporal homogeneity, that is, lack of internal temporal structure and processuality in the phenomenal unity of consciousness. I therefore propose the degree of phenomenal unity and its phenomenal features to be directly

dependent on the degree of alignment of the stimulus-induced activity to the resting state's low-frequency oscillations (see Fig. 18-4e).

Considering the central role of the resting state's low-frequency oscillations, our hypothesis may now be extended in the following way: the lower the frequency ranges of the resting state's oscillations, the longer their phases; the longer the subsequent temporal unity can possibly be extended and smoothed (across different discrete time points); and the higher the possible degrees of temporal wholeness and nonstructural temporal homogeneity. I consequently propose the possible degrees of the features of the phenomenal unity to be predisposed by the resting state's phase duration and its respective frequency ranges.

This specifies well what I described earlier as the resting state–based hypothesis of prephenomenal unity in temporal and phenomenal terms. More specifically, the resting state–based hypothesis of prephenomenal unity proposes the resting state's phases and its frequency ranges to provide a neural predisposition for the phenomenal unity and its phenomenal features like nonstructural homogeneity. The resting state itself can therefore be characterized by a prephenomenal temporal (and spatial) unity in the earlier described sense (see Fig. 18-4a).

Neurophenomenal Hypothesis IIIA: Functional Connectivity Predisposes "Spatial Unity" of Neural Activity during Rest–Stimulus Interaction

So far, I have focused only on the temporal dimension of the resting state's prephenomenal unity, while I neglected its spatial dimension almost completely (see though Chapter 16 for details, as well as Chapter 4 in Volume I). This, and especially the integration between spatial and temporal dimensions, shall be the focus of this section.

We postulated "global" spatial continuity of neural activity across different regions of the brain (see Chapter 16), which was proposed to be based on functional connectivity. Functional connectivity describes the temporal synchronization of the neural activities between different regions (see Chapter 4 in Volume I as well as Chapter 16 for details). The more temporally synchronized different regions' neural activities, the higher degrees of functional connectivity can be observed between them. This means that functional connectivity and consequently the global spatial continuity of neural activity contain an inherent temporal dimension (see also Chapters 5 and 16).

What does such global spatial continuity of neural activity mean exactly? It means that the regions whose neural activities are functionally connected act together and thus form a spatial unity. As we already discussed in Part V, the resting state itself shows a very high degree of functional connectivity and thus a high degree of global spatial continuity. This means that the resting state itself can be characterized by spatial unity, a linkage and integration between spatially separate points (or better, regions) of neural activity.

How, then, do the extrinsic stimuli interfere with the intrinsic resting state's functional connectivity and spatial unity? As in the case of the temporal unity, the stimulus, depending on its features, may fit/match better or worse with the resting state's functional connectivity pattern and its spatial unity. The better the different stimuli fit and match with the resting state's functional connectivity pattern, the more they will be connected and linked to each other during subsequent neural processing of their associated stimulus-induced activity (see Chapter 11 for more detailed results on rest–stimulus interaction and functional connectivity).

NEUROPHENOMENAL HYPOTHESIS IIIB: FUNCTIONAL CONNECTIVITY PREDISPOSES "LACK OF INTERNAL SPATIAL STRUCTURE AND PROCESSUALITY"

What does such a spatial connection and linkage between different stimuli imply for the phenomenal level? The stimuli will consequently be integrated to a high degree into the resting state's spatial unity. I propose that this results phenomenally in increased degrees of spatial wholeness and nonstructural spatial homogeneity. as well as lack of internal spatial structure and lack of spatial processuality.

If, in contrast, the stimuli strongly disrupt the resting state's functional connectivity pattern, they can no longer be well integrated into the resting state's spatial unity. That, in turn, will go along, as I propose, with decreased degrees of spatial wholeness and nonstructural spatial homogeneity as well as lack of internal spatial structure and lack of spatial processuality. I consequently propose the degree of the phenomenal features, that is, spatial wholeness and nonstructural spatial homogeneity, to be directly dependent on the degree to which the stimuli disrupt the resting state's functional connectivity pattern and thus its spatial unity.

This neurophenomenal hypothesis implies that the resting-state activity itself and more specifically its functional connectivity pattern and spatial unity have a strong say in constituting the degree of the phenomenal features. Higher degrees of the resting state's functional connectivity and its spatial unity entail higher possible degrees in the phenomenal features associated with subsequent stimulus-induced activity. The resting state and more specifically its functional connectivity pattern and its spatial unity provide a neural predisposition for the phenomenal unity and its phenomenal features.

The resting state can therefore be characterized by a prephenomenal spatial unity that I propose to consist in the resting state's spatial unity as based on its functional connectivity pattern. This specifies what I earlier described as the resting state–based hypothesis of prephenomenal unity in spatial and phenomenal terms.

Open Questions

One of the main problems I am facing here is the lack of quantitative measurements of phenomenal unity. We would need detailed measures of, for instance, nonstructural homogeneity and "wholeness". I supposed that the degree of such measures may be predicted by the phases of the resting state's low-frequency fluctuations and the resting state's functional connectivity pattern. If so, this would lend empirical support albeit indirectly to my assumption of the resting state constituting what I here described as prephenomenal unity.

We also left open the neuronal mechanisms underlying the constitution of the resting state's low-frequency oscillations and its functional connectivity pattern. I discussed in Volume I how their constitution is based on a particular coding strategy, difference-based coding rather than stimulus-based coding. We now want to question where, for instance, the phase durations and thus the frequency ranges of the resting-state activity come from by themselves. And, most important, whether that is relevant and thus important for constituting the resting state's prephenomenal unity and ultimately the phenomenal unity of consciousness. This will be the focus of Chapter 20 in this part.

Finally, the exact neuronal mechanisms that allow for transforming the purely neuronal spatial and temporal unities of the resting state into a phenomenal unity in consciousness remain unclear. I could associate the phenomenal features of wholeness and nonstructural homogeneity with specific neuronal mechanisms. In contrast, it remains unclear why the supposed rest–stimulus interaction goes along with a transformation of the underlying neuronal state into a phenomenal state.

One may propose the resting-state activity's prephenomenal unity, including its prephenomenal spatial and temporal unity, to be central here. They may be carried over and transferred to the subsequent stimulus-induced activity. Why such carryover and transfer go along with a transformation of a neuronal into a phenomenal state remains unclear, however. For that, we need to go into more detail about what happens once the stimulus encounters the resting state. This will be the focus of the next chapter.

CHAPTER 19
Gamma and Phenomenal Unity

Summary

One of the central hallmarks of consciousness is the subjective experience of unity, i.e., phenomenal unity. The concept of "unity" refers to the integration and convergence of different objects and events into one unified experience by one particular subject. What are the neuronal mechanisms of such phenomenal unity? Recent findings demonstrate that visible and thus conscious objects are associated with early (40–140 ms after stimulus onset) increases in neuronal synchronization between the phases of especially gamma (40 Hz) oscillations when compared to invisible; that is, unconscious, objects. I propose these early changes to be related to what is described conceptually as "objectual unity." The concept of objectual unity refers to the binding of different stimuli and their respective features into one object or event that then surfaces as content, e.g., phenomenal content in consciousness. In addition to such early neuronal changes and their associated objectual unity, later changes (240–300 ms after stimulus onset) in neural activity are also observed in the visible, that is, conscious, stimuli. I propose that these later changes correspond to what conceptually has been described as "cognitive unity," the conjunction and integration of various cognitive functions like attention, working memory, and so on. By providing cognitive unity, the associated cognitive functions may allow us to access the contents, the phenomenal contents, we experience in consciousness; the cognitive unity may thus be related to what is described conceptually as "access unity," the unity of access consciousness. How are these neuronal mechanisms related to the phenomenal unity as manifest in phenomenal consciousness? I propose what I describe as the "continuity-based hypothesis of phenomenal unity." The continuity-based hypothesis of phenomenal unity proposes that the phenomenal unity is based on and supersedes the already constituted spatial and temporal continuity in the ongoing resting-state activity. More specifically, the stimulus may be linked to the resting state's ongoing spatial and temporal continuity. Such linkage in turn makes possible the constitution of temporal and spatial unity on the grounds of what we described as "duration bloc" and "dimension bloc" in the previous Part on "inner time and space consciousness" By superimposing its particular discrete point in (physical) time and space onto the spatial and temporal continuity of the resting state's neural activity, the stimulus elicits or triggers the constitution of spatial and temporal unity. That, in turn, is supposed to make possible the association of the stimulus and its otherwise purely neuronal stimulus-induced activity with phenomenal unity in particular, and consciousness in general, e.g., phenomenal consciousness.

Key Concepts and Topics Covered

Neuronal oscillation, synchronization, gamma oscillation, phenomenal unity, objectual unity, access unity, rest–stimulus interaction, phenomenal state, phenomenal content, phenomenal consciousness, access consciousness

NEUROEMPIRICAL BACKGROUND IA: STIMULUS-INDUCED ACTIVITY AND CONSCIOUSNESS

Chapter 18 highlighted the relevance of the resting-state activity and its low-frequency fluctuations for consciousness. This let me suggest what I described as the "resting state–based hypothesis of prephenomenal unity." The resting-state-based hypothesis of prephenomenal unity proposes that the resting-state activity by itself, its spatial and temporal measures of neuronal activity, exerts a predisposing and biasing impact on the selection of contents, e.g., phenomenal contents, that will be associated with consciousness during subsequent stimulus-induced activity. In other words, I proposed the resting state's prephenomenal unity to predispose the selection of contents with which the stimuli and their stimulus-induced activity will be associated in consciousness.

How is the resting state's prephenomenal unity manifest in stimulus-induced activity and the associated consciousness? For that, I now turn to stimulus-induced activity and how it is related to consciousness. Currently, this is probably the most extensive area of neuroscientific research on consciousness. Several experimental paradigms have been developed and conducted to reveal the neuronal mechanisms underlying the difference between unconscious and conscious processing of contents during stimulus-induced (or task-related) activity.

The focus on stimulus-induced activity (which is taken as synonymous with task-related activity throughout this volume unless indicated otherwise) is the hallmark of most theories under the umbrella of the NCC, the neural correlates of consciousness (see also the Introduction to Volume II). The traditional comparison here is the comparison between unconscious and conscious presentation of the same stimulus and how the underlying neuronal effects differ from each other. This raises the question of the kind of experimental paradigms to use, as shall be dealt with briefly in the next section.

NEUROEMPIRICAL BACKGROUND
IB: EXPERIMENTAL PARADIGMS IN THE INVESTIGATION OF CONSCIOUSNESS

Dehaene and Changeux (2011) broadly categorize the different experimental paradigms into subliminal and inattentional tasks (see also Kouider and Dehaene 2009). Subliminal paradigms are those where the stimulus is presented

as weak and short as possible (usually by using masking) such as that it is still processed in the brain's neural activity while not yet being associated with consciousness. Following Kouider and Dehaene (2007; see also Kouider et al. 2010), the effects are rather weak and more difficult to obtain for phonological and semantic processing, while they are more easily acquired for motor, lexical (i.e., single letters), and orthographic (i.e., words) stimuli.

This is different in the other type of paradigm, the inattentional paradigm. Here the stimulus is presented longer and stronger while being accompanied by a simultaneous attention-demanding task. This pulls attention away from the stimulus so that it is processed but does not enter consciousness. Due to the longer and stronger stimulus presentation, results are more apparent and easy to obtain for both phonological and semantic levels of processing.

This rather short and obviously incomplete overview of the main experimental paradigms makes it already clear that the focus is here on the stimulus itself and the neural activity it elicits in the brain. In short, the focus is here on stimulus-induced activity. What must the stimulus-induced activity be like in order to associate the respective stimulus with consciousness?

As indicated earlier, there is an abundance of different studies using different experimental paradigms (like inattentional vs. subliminal) and testing for different levels of neural processing (like motor, lexical, orthographic, semantic, and phonological). To give a complete review of all the studies and their intricate details is beyond the scope of this chapter for which reason I refer to the excellent most recent review paper by Dehaene and Changeux (2011).

Instead of giving a complete overview, I here focus on the least controversial findings holding across the various studies. For that, I will present one particular study as a paradigm. This serves as a starting point to discuss its implications for the unity of consciousness. As we will see, this raises further neuroscientific questions venturing into more debated and controversial empirical territory.

NEURONAL FINDINGS IA: INVISIBLE VERSUS VISIBLE PRESENTATION OF STIMULI

As stated above, there have been several studies on stimulus-induced activity and how it is related to whether the stimulus is associated with consciousness. Since the detailed description of all these studies is beyond this chapter (see Dehaene and Changeux 2011 for an excellent review), I here discuss one representative example that shows paradigmatic findings, the study by Melloni et al. (2007).

Melloni et al. (2007) investigated human subjects with electroencephalography (EEG) during the presentation of words. The words were presented for 33 ms ("sample word") and were preceded and followed by masking stimuli (67 ms) that, due to luminance, rendered the sample word either visible or invisible. This allowed them to test the same stimulus in either a conscious (i.e., visible) or unconscious (i.e., invisible) mode.

The same or a different word was also presented 533 ms later in each trial ("test word"). The subjects had to decide whether the test word was the same as the sample word. That allowed to test for behavioral measures of conscious perception (see below). Control conditions for both visible and invisible words consisted of presenting the sample word after a masking screen as well as directly before the test word presentation; this yielded perceptual similarity to the experimental condition (as described above), while differing in the degree of consciousness.

How do conscious and unconscious presentation, e.g., visible and invisible stimuli, differ in their associated behavioral and neuronal measures? Let us start with the behavioral data. Behavioral data based on the judgement of the test word showed that responses in the invisible condition were at chance level (50% correct and 50% incorrect). This indicates unconscious perception. In contrast, the visible condition yielded 94% correct responses, which is indicative of conscious perception. Hence, the difference between visible and invisible stimuli and thus between consciousness and unconsciousness is well reflected in the responses of the subjects.

The question is now whether subjects were processing the invisible stimulus at all. The chance level of their responses could be simply due to the fact that the invisible stimulus was not processed at all by the brain's neural activity. Alternatively, the stimulus may be processed neuronally though not strongly enough to enter consciousness; as in the case of non-processing, such a scenario would also go along with a chance level in the subjects' responses.

To rule out the first possibility—no neuronal processing of the stimulus—the authors conducted yet another behavioral experiment. They added a priming task using the same stimuli, that is, the sample word, to test whether the unconscious word was still processed. In the priming task, the invisible sample word was associated with another word in order to test whether the former exerts some effects on the latter; if so, one would propose that the invisible stimulus must have been processed neuronally. The additional priming tasks' results clearly revealed strong priming effects of the unconscious words, especially in trials with high semantic congruency between the invisible sample word and the visible target word: Subjects showed faster reaction times in those conditions where the invisible sample word and the visible target word were semantically congruent (i.e., same semantic categories) when compared to semantically incongruent trials (i.e., different semantic categories). This suggests that the invisible and thus unconscious sample word was still processed neuronally, while not yet reaching consciousness.

NEURONAL FINDINGS IB: LATE CHANGES DURING STIMULUS-INDUCED ACTIVITY AND CONSCIOUSNESS

How about the EEG results? In addition to early changes (80–130 ms) in phase synchrony (see later), later changes were also observed that were clearly distinguished from the earlier ones. The mean amplitude of the P300 at around 240–300 ms after sample word presentation was significantly larger for the visible than the invisible condition. Besides the P300 amplitude, the amplitude of theta oscillations (5–6 Hz) also increased over especially frontal electrodes in the same time interval during the visible condition (see Fig. 19-1a).

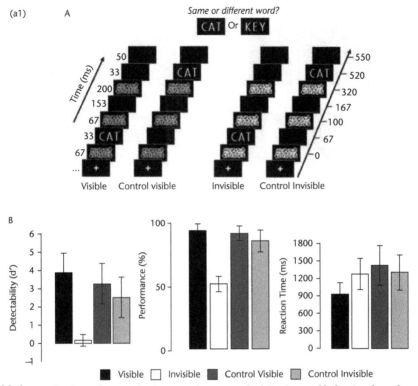

Figure 19-1a Early phase changes during consciousness. (*a1*) Design and behavioral results of experiment. *A*, Stimulus sequence. The task was to compare a briefly presented word (sample word) with a subsequent word (test word). The sample word visibility was controlled by changing the luminance of the masks. Control conditions were created to assess the brain response to the mask stream. The left timeline shows the duration of each stimulus. The right timeline shows the cumulative time. *B*, Behavioral performance. The left plot shows stimulus detectability for all conditions, expressed as detectability index (*d*), and the middle plot is the success rate. The right plot shows the reaction time for all conditions. Plots indicate mean performance ±1 SD. (*a2*) Spectral power and phase synchrony to visible and invisible words. The visible condition (visible – control_visible) and invisible condition (invisible – control_invisible) are shown. The time-frequency plot shows the grand average of all electrodes. The phase-synchrony plot shows the grand average for all of the electrode pairs. The scale indicates amplitude in SD, calculated over a 500 ms baseline. Zero corresponds to first mask onset. Vertical lines indicate sample- and test-word presentation. *A*, Time – frequency plot. Two increments of gamma-power emission are visible. The first is only present in the visible condition, and the second is present in both conditions. *B*, Phase synchrony. There are three statistically significant bursts of synchronous activity. The first and second peaks occur only in the visible condition. No significant differences were found for the last peak. (*a3*) ERPs elicited by visible and invisible words. *A*, Time course of responses to visible and invisible words at different electrodes. The *x*-axis shows time, and the *y*-axis shows electrodes; the color scale is expressed in microvolts. Zero represents the first mask onset. Vertical lines indicate sample-word and test-word presentation. Small lines at the top of the graph code for the two time windows corresponding to the voltage scalp maps in *B*. *B*, Voltage scalp map for two windows indicated for visible and invisible conditions. The first difference started at 130 ms after sample-word presentation, as a P300a-like component. Then, a P1-like component was observed ~200 ms after test-word presentation, for both conditions. *C*, Time course of the signal recorded from left frontal electrode F3. (*a4*) Scalp topography of induced gamma power and phase synchrony for the visible and invisible condition. Top row: Visible condition. Bottom row: Invisible condition. The background color indicates induced gamma power averaged in a 50–57 Hz frequency range. Each head represents the average of a 150 ms

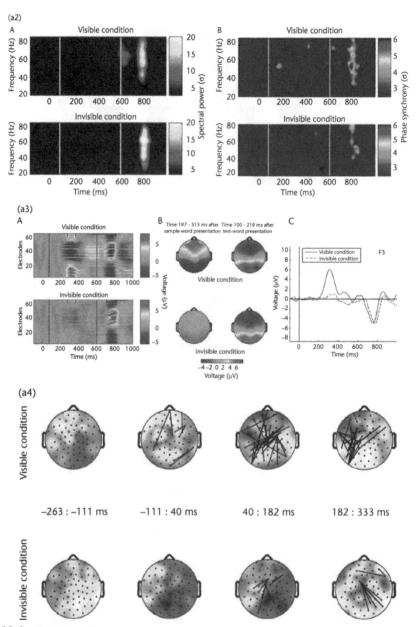

Figure 19-1a (Continued)

time window. Time 0 indicates the onset of the sample word. Lines connect pairs of electrodes display-ing significant synchronization ($p < 0.000001$). Gamma activity does not statistically differ between visible and invisible conditions. In contrast, phase synchrony is stronger in the visible condition dur-ing the 40–180 ms time window involving occipito, parieto, and frontal electrodes, with intrahemi-spheric and interhemispheric connections. In the window between 180 and 330 ms, the pattern of phase synchrony lateralizes over the left hemisphere and restricts to occipitoparietal electrodes. Reprinted with permission, from Melloni L, Molina C, Pena M, Torres D, Singer W, Rodriguez E. Synchronization of neural activity across cortical areas correlates with conscious perception. *J Neurosci.* 2007 Mar 14;27(11):2858–65.

What do these neuronal changes, the P300 and the theta oscillations, signify in functional terms? As discussed by the authors themselves, both changes, P300 and theta oscillations, may be related to cognitive processes like attention (i.e., P300) and working memory (i.e., theta oscillations) that have previously been associated with these measures (see Buzsaki and Draguhn 2004; Buzsaki 2006). Hence, cognitive functions may be involved in facilitating the distinction between conscious and unconscious sample words. Finally, even more delayed differences were observed 10–40 ms after the test word presentation, where both power and synchrony of gamma oscillations (67–80 Hz) were significantly increased for the visible words compared to the invisible ones.

What exactly do these late neuronal changes that have been observed in this and many other studies imply for consciousness? These late neuronal changes around 300ms after stimulus onset have been most consistently observed in different studies and must therefore be considered a robust finding. This distinguishes them from the earlier changes at around 80–130ms that are more controversial and less consistently observed in different studies. In the following discussion, I will focus on the late changes, while the earlier changes will be discussed in later sections.

Later changes at around 300ms have been observed most consistently in the different studies on unconscious and conscious processing. Following Dehaene and Changeux (2011), this seems to hold true across different paradigms (i.e., inattentional, subliminal), different stimuli (i.e., visual, auditory, tactile), and different levels of processing (motor, lexical, orthographic, semantic, phonological). Such late changes are usually associated with long-distance neuronal synchronization at beta and gamma frequencies, and the recruitment of a fronto-parietal network beyond the respective sensory and posterior cortical regions.

The later changes in neuronal activity are, following Deheaene and Changeux (2011), most often observed in studies testing for conscious versus unconscious access to contents (see below for the concept of the "conscious access"). They may therefore be associated with what conceptually has been described as "access consciousness"

(see later). Before though plunging into more detailed conceptual discussion, more empirical findings need to be described.

NEURONAL FINDINGS IIA: PREFRONTO-PARIETAL NETWORK AND GLOBAL NEURONAL WORKSPACE (GNW)

Based on the findings of late neuronal changes (at around 300ms after stimulus onset), Dehaene (together with Changeux) developed what he calls the global neuronal workspace (GNW) theory (Dehaene and Changeux 2005, 2011). The GNW proposes that cortical pyramidal cells with long-range excitatory axons in especially layer II and III are most abundant in prefrontal and parietal cortex. There they form what he calls "a neuronal workspace" that links and integrates the different modules or processors, that is, the other regions and networks (evaluation/value, motor, sensory, attention), together.

By interconnecting the multiple highly specialized "automatic nonconscious processors" and the underlying regions or networks, their respectively processed stimuli and contents can access consciousness. Since the GNW includes the neurons and regions associated with verbal-linguistic skills like the frontal and the parietal cortex (see later), the conscious contents can also be reported verbally. Hence, Dehaenes's characterization of consciousness by reporting about the subjectively experienced contents (see later).

How can we further characterize the GNW? The GNW is based on the global workspace theory as initially developed by B. Baars (see Appendix 1 for detailed discussion). By shifting from the purely cognitive level of Baars's global workspace theory to the neuronal level, the GNW can be regarded as the neuronal extension of the former. Thereby it specifies the regions and the neuronal mechanisms that are supposedly sufficient to associate a stimulus and its contents (see later for the discussion of the transition from stimulus to content) with consciousness.

To elaborate: the GNW attributes a central role to prefrontal and parietal cortical activity, since they bind together the neuronal activities of the different regions and networks. Since they link regions and networks from all over the brain, the term *global neuronal workspace* is used to describe their neural activity. The global neuronal workspace as provided by prefrontal and parietal cortical activity is often considered sufficient to associate the stimuli and their respective contents with consciousness.

NEURONAL FINDINGS IIB: SUBLIMINAL VERSUS PRECONSCIOUS NEURAL PROCESSING

How exactly does the prefrontal-parietal network function as the global neuronal workspace of the brain? Dehaene and Changeux (2011) distinguish consciousness from the preconscious and the subliminal (see also Kouider and Dehaene 2009). The "subliminal" is characterized by a weak stimulus input, which by itself is not strong enough to elicit sufficient bottom-up modulation from the respective sensory cortex to the fronto-parietal cortex.

Accordingly, the stimulus by itself "has no chance of entering" the global neuronal workspace, e.g., the prefronto-parietal network, and thus to become associated with consciousness. Therefore the stimulus remains subliminal rather than being associated with consciousness.

This is different in the case of the "preconscious." Here, the stimulus itself and its bottom-up modulation from sensory to prefronto-parietal cortex are strong enough to elicit changes in prefronto-parietal cortical activity. However, the prefronto-parietal cortex is not ready at that moment to be "ignited" by the stimulus. Why? The prefronto-parietal cortical activity is not "free"; it is busy with "other things" like the processing of another stimulus or strong spontaneous activity changes.

In this case, the neuronal resources of the prefronto-parietal network itself and its top-down modulation (as is psychologically manifested in the degree of attention) are too limited to allow the stimulus to access it. This, however, makes conscious processing of the stimulus impossible. The stimulus is thus no longer subliminal, but it is not conscious, either; it is therefore "preconscious" (see also Kouider and Dehaene 2009).

If, in contrast, both conditions—that is, strong enough stimulus and "free" prefronto-parietal network—are met, the stimulus can access the prefronto-parietal network and thus conscious processing. This, Dehaene and Changeux propose, is the case when we are able to report the presence of the stimulus in our experience (see Fig. 19-1b).

NEURONAL FINDINGS IIC: GLOBAL NEURONAL WORKSPACE (GNW) AND THE PHENOMENAL FEATURES OF CONSCIOUSNESS

How does the GNW stand in relation to consciousness and its phenomenal features? The GNW details the regions and the neuronal mechanisms that are supposedly implicated in the contents that are associated with consciousness. The GNW is thus a purely neuronal hypothesis about consciousness and its contents. The GNW is considered to be a theory about the "conscious access" to information. It is about whether and how information and thus content can gain access to conscious processing, which Dehaene and Changeux (2005, 2011) define as "reportable subjective experience." Everything we can report and thus put into verbal terms is considered a subjective experience, e.g., consciousness.

This implies, as they themselves say explicitly (Dehaene and Changeux 2011, 200), a focus on the contents of consciousness. Accordingly, the GNW aims to describe those neuronal mechanisms by means of which we are able to access the contents in consciousness, e.g., phenomenal contents; such conscious access must be distinguished from lack of access, in which case the contents remain unconscious. In short, the GNW is about the access to contents in consciousness.

In contrast to the contents, the GNW does not address the state or level of consciousness, as is altered in the disorders of consciousness. This means that the GNW does not explain how the phenomenal state itself with which the contents are associated is generated. The neuronal mechanisms underlying the phenomenal state itself and its various phenomenal features irrespective of their association with contents consequently remain unclear.

Rather than explaining how the phenomenal features themselves, like the phenomenal unity, are generated, the GNW seems to presuppose them as ready-made, thus taking them as given. That,

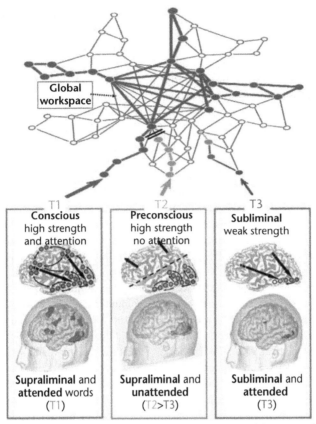

Figure 19-1b Frontal cortical involvement during consciousness. Taxonomy between conscious, preconscious, and subliminal processing, based on the theoretical proposal by Dehaene et al. (2006). This distinction stipulates the existence of three types of brain states associated with conscious report, non-conscious perception due to inattention (preconscious state), and nonconscious perception due to masking (subliminal perception; Dehaene et al. 2001, 2006). Reprinted with permission of Royal Society Publishing, from Kouider S, Dehaene S. Levels of processing during nonconscious perception: A critical review of visual masking. *Philos Trans R Soc Lond B Biol Sci.* 2007 May 29;362(1481):857–75.

though, leaves open the question of which neuronal mechanisms first and foremost make possible and thus predispose the constitution of the phenomenal unity in a necessary and unavoidable way. This is important to determine in order to understand the neuronal mechanisms that allow for the association of consciousness with the contents and our access to them, as investigated in the GNW.

NEURONAL FINDINGS IID: NEUROCOGNITIVE VERSUS NEUROPHENOMENAL APPROACHES TO CONSCIOUSNESS

Put differently, the GNW is a neurocognitive theory about contents and how we can access

them so that we can report them. It focuses on the neurocognitive mechanisms that allow us to access the contents in our consciousness and to report them. For that, the GNW compares accessible (reportable) and non-accessible (non-reportable) contents in its experimental paradigms. Neuronally, the prefrontal-parietal cortical activity as global neuronal workspace is supposed to be central in allowing such access and reporting.

This, however, presupposes consciousness, and especially "phenomenal consciousness" (see below for a definition of this concept and its distinction from "access consciousness"), rather than identifying them and their neuronal mechanisms. Before accessing and reporting the contents, we first need to experience and thus associate them with phenomenal consciousness. Therefore, the difference between accessibility/reporting and non-accessibility/non-reporting cannot be equated or identified with the distinction between experience/consciousness and non-experience/nonconscious.

Instead, non-experience/nonconscious presupposes experience/consciousness: this means that the phenomenal functions — experience and thus consciousness—precede the cognitive functions like access and reporting. Accordingly, we cannot identify the neuronal mechanisms underlying the phenomenal state of consciousness by searching for those related to access to and reporting of contents. We therefore need to complement the neurocognitive account of the GNW (and many other theories of consciousness) by a neurophenomenal approach, which is the focus in this volume (see also the first Introduction in Volume II and Appendix 1 in Volume II).

How can we pursue such a neurophenomenal approach that will allow us to reveal the neuronal mechanisms underlying the constitution of the phenomenal state itself, including its phenomenal unity while remaining independent of the contents themselves? In order to gain insight into the neuronal mechanisms underlying the generation of the phenomenal unity of consciousness, we will now make a brief neuroconceptual excursion into philosophy of mind and discuss two different forms of consciousness and their respective unities.

NEUROCONCEPTUAL EXCURSION:
PHENOMENAL UNITY AND ACCESS UNITY

Australian philosophers Tim Bayne and David Chalmers (2003) distinguish between phenomenal and access unity that is based on the work of American philosopher Ned Block and his conceptual distinction between *phenomenal consciousness* and *access consciousness* (Block 1995, 2005). Let us start with briefly defining the latter, access consciousness. Based on Block, access consciousness can be defined by the access to the contents of consciousness if one is for instance is able to report what one experiences which

presupposes the access to the phenomenal contents in consciousness."

The access to the phenomenal contents of consciousness must be distinguished from the experience of the very same phenomenal contents. The phenomenal contents are experienced, with this experience being characterized by a phenomenal state. Such a phenomenal state is hallmarked by the phenomenal feature of "what it is like" going along with a particular point of view (Nagel 1974; see Chapter 21 as well as Chapter 30 for more details).

Let us give an example. I am aware of sitting in front of the computer while typing these lines. I thus access the phenomenal contents of my consciousness, which is made possible by access consciousness. That needs to be distinguished, however, from my experience of the very same computer and my writing, which is described by the "what it is like" and ultimately *qualia* (as qualitative-phenomenal feature) of experience and thus of phenomenal states (see Chapter 30 for details on *qualia*). This is what Block calls "phenomenal consciousness." My "access consciousness" of my computer as phenomenal content must thus be distinguished from my experience of that phenomenal content in terms of "what it is like," my "phenomenal consciousness."

How, then, is the distinction between phenomenal and access consciousness related to the concept of unity? Relying on Block's distinction, Bayne and Chalmers speak of access and phenomenal unity. There is access unity if the subject has access to the contents of two (or more) states, such as, for instance, when I am aware that the book is both red (rather than blue) and rectangular (rather than round). And there is phenomenal unity when one has an experience and thus a phenomenal state characterized by "what it is like," signifying, for instance, the redness of the book in my experience.

NEURONAL HYPOTHESIS
IA: PREFRONTO-PARIETAL CORTEX
CONSTITUTES "COGNITIVE UNITY"

How can we now link the different concepts of unity to the empirical findings reported above? The paradigmatic empirical data by Melloni et al. (2007) (see Chapters 16 and 19, as well as Dehaene and Changeux 2011, for more empirical evidence) showed late differences at around 240–300 ms after stimulus onset between visible and invisible words. The question is how these late changes may be related to the different concepts of unity as described above. Thereby, I here focus on the late changes that are the most robust findings and the least controversial (see above) while coming to the early differences in the next section.

The later differences between visible and invisible words occurred at around 240–300 ms after stimulus onset. They concerned the amplitude of the P300 and the power of theta oscillations, which both were significantly higher in visible than invisible words. Moreover, even later changes were observed concerning higher gamma power in visible words 10–40 ms after the test word presentation.

How are these late neuronal differences related to the concept of unity? These neuronal measures like the P300 and the theta oscillations are proposed to be related to cognitive processes like attention and working memory. The different cognitive functions seem to act in conjunction during consciousness showing simultaneous occurrence in time at around 240–300 ms (after which their neuronal indices disappear). There is thus a clear time frame with minimal and maximal temporal borders. This time frame on the neuronal level may correspond to what conceptually is described as cognitive unity.

How can we define the concept of "cognitive unity"? The concept of cognitive unity (see also Tye 2003; Brook and Raymont 2010) describes the linkage and integration between different cognitive functions like working memory, attention, and executive function. Their integration and linkage makes it possible for them to act in conjunction during their processing of their respective stimuli and the associated particular objects or events (and states).

Accordingly, the cognitive unity seems to consist of the integration and linkage and thus the conjunction between attention and working memory within that specific time interval of neuronal processing in prefrontal and parietal cortical activity. That is also compatible with the well-known association of these (and other) cognitive functions with the prefrontal and parietal cortex, which further supports these regions' central role in consciousness as suggested by the GNW (see earlier and later discussion for details).

How does the cognitive unity stand in relation to the global workspace model of consciousness? The concept of cognitive unity is often associated with the central role of the global workspace in consciousness. By distributing information of the stimuli globally, that information becomes available for processing by the various cognitive functions.

Such distribution and availability of the stimuli to different cognitive function is suggested to allow the stimuli to be associated with consciousness (see Appendix 1 for a more extensive discussion of the global workspace model; see also Dehaene and Changeux 2011, for an excellent review). Accordingly, I propose that the concept of cognitive unity may correspond on the conceptual side to what empirically has been described by the neuronal processes in prefrontal-parietal cortical activity and their function as global neuronal workspace.

Neuronal Hypothesis IB: Cognitive Unity Constitutes "Access Unity"

How does the assumption of the cognitive unity stand in relation to the concepts of phenomenal and access unity as discussed earlier? Cognitive functions like working memory and attention are definitely needed for making a judgement about the respective stimuli and thus the content, regardless of whether it was perceived. The cognitive functions may thus allow for accessing the phenomenal content and meta-representing it by means of which the content becomes available for detection, judgement, and evaluation.

As pointed out earlier, a judgement was indeed required in the earlier described experiment by Melloni. One may consecutively associate the late changes he and others observed with the access to the phenomenal content and thus with what Chalmers and Bayne describe conceptually as "access unity." The assumption of such detection, judgement, and evaluation is also compatible with the GNW that focuses on the "conscious access" as "reporting of subjective experience" (see above). Since such conscious access, and especially the "reporting," requires exactly cognitive functions like attention and working memory, one may propose the GNW and its fronto-parietal network to also be compatible with the concept of access unity.

Based on these considerations, I suggest the following neuronal, or better, neurocognitive, hypothesis. I propose that there is a close relationship between fronto-parietal cortex, cognitive unity, and access unity. The neural activity in fronto-parietal cortex makes possible cognitive unity, which in turn may be regarded as at least a necessary, if not sufficient, condition of access

unity. That means that, without fronto-parietal cortical activity, cognitive unity and consequently access unity, remain impossible. Following the GNW, what is conceptually described as access unity is supposed to be based empirically on a global neuronal workspace for which the fronto-parietal cortex is central (see Fig. 19-2).

Let us now characterize the access unity in further detail. The access unity must be described in spatiotemporal terms. Spatially, it may involve a more global (rather than regional) distribution of neural activity as postulated by the global workspace model and the GNW. Temporally, the access unity may occur rather late, some 240–300 ms after stimulus onset. Moreover, the access

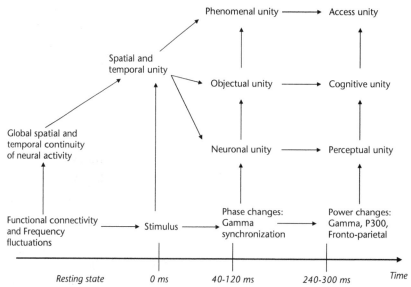

Figure 19-2 Timing of neural activity and different forms of unity. The figure shows the relationship between the timing of neural activity during the transition from resting-state activity to stimulus-induced activity. The time axis is shown below (horizontal axis). The most significant time points (0 = stimulus onset, 40–120 ms = early gamma synchronization, and 240–300 ms = late power changes) and P300 changes are marked. The early and late neuronal mechanisms lead to different forms of unity (vertical arrows), which, by building on each other, lead ultimately to the phenomenal unity and the access unity of consciousness (*upper part*). The constitution of stimulus-related unities (*right part*) is based on the preceding intrinsic resting-state activity and the constitution of global temporal and spatial continuity of its neural activity (*left part*). That, in turn, makes possible the constitution of objectual and neuronal unity as triggered by the extrinsic stimulus and ultimately the constitution of phenomenal unity. This is indicated by the arrows leading from the global spatial and temporal continuity to all three, neuronal, objectual, and phenomenal unity (*middle*). These, in turn, provide the basis for the constitution of subsequent later unities related to perceptual and cognitive processing, resulting in perceptual unity, cognitive unity, and access unity (*far right*).

unity is temporally transitory in that it seems to last only for about 100 to 300 milliseconds.

The access unity may be characterized empirically as transitory, late, and spatiotemporal. Finally, in neuronal terms, the concept of the access unity seems to correspond well to the GNW and its emphasis on the fronto-parietal cortex and the late synchronization in beta and gamma ranges (see earlier).

How is such empirically defined access unity related to other philosophical theories of consciousness that emphasize the central role of higher-order thoughts and meta-representation for consciousness? The here-suggested neuro-cognitive characterization of the access unity may provide some kind of bridge to these philosophical theories. However, further empirical and conceptual details would need to be discussed in order to make this assumption more plausible; this, though, is beyond the scope of this book and must therefore remain open at this point.

Instead of venturing into such higher-order cognitive territory, we prefer to go into the opposite direction, towards the lower-order mechanisms. More specifically, we shift our focus now from the late neuronal changes during stimulus-induced activity to the earlier ones that occur immediately after stimulus onset, in order to get a grip on phenomenal unity (as distinguished from access unity).

NEURONAL FINDINGS IIIA: EARLY CHANGES DURING STIMULUS-INDUCED ACTIVITY MEDIATE CONSCIOUSNESS

Let us return to the above-described study by Melloni et al. (2007). In addition to the later changes at around 240–300 ms (see earlier), the EEG data showed an early difference between visible and invisible sample words at around 80 to 130 milliseconds. During this early period, the phase synchrony of 50–57 Hz (i.e., gamma oscillations and their synchronization across different regions or electrodes) over all electrodes was significantly higher for the visible than the invisible words.

Phase synchronization in this early time period, that is, between 40 ms and 180ms after sample word presentation, was observed only between few electrode pairs in the invisible

condition. This contrasted with numerous electrode pairs between frontal, occipital, and parietal pairs showing phase-locking and thus phase synchronization in the visible condition.

These results suggest that increased global, that is, transcortical, synchronization occurs in the visible and thus the conscious condition. Such global synchronization must be distinguished from the more local synchronization in the invisible, that is, unconscious mode (see also Hipp et al. 2011 for further empirical support in this direction).

Moreover, such increased global synchronization via phase synchrony can neither be related to changes in power, that is, amplitude, of gamma oscillations nor to differences in the mean event-related potentials (ERPs). Why? Because both measures, that is, power and ERP, did not show any differences between visible and invisible conditions. This further underlines the specific role and importance of early phase synchrony (as distinguished from mere power) in yielding consciousness.

We have to be careful, however. In contrast to the late changes that are well established in the neuroscientific research on consciousness (see earlier), the early changes at around 100 ms as reported by Melloni et al. are highly debated. They are usually very small. And, even more important, we can currently not exclude the possibility that the early changes may result from differences in the preceding spontaneous activity; there they may reflect predictions of the expected stimulus and thus what is described as "pre-stimulus priors" (see Melloni et al. 2011; del Cul et al.2007; see especially Chapters 7–9 for extensive discussion of predictive coding and "empirical priors").

Accordingly, the early changes at around 50–140ms may be related to either the stimulus itself, to its association with consciousness, or to the preceding resting-state activity. Which of these possible origins of the early changes is central for consciousness remains unclear at this point, however.

NEURONAL FINDINGS IIIB: EARLY NEURONAL SYNCHRONIZATION MEDIATES CONSCIOUSNESS

Despite the not fully resolved situation about the early changes at around 100 ms, they cannot be neglected. This is even more the case given that, as reported in Chapter 18, prestimulus resting-state activity may already impact subsequent consciousness. While this makes it unclear whether the early changes are activity changes in their own right, that is, independent of the preceding resting state, the prestimulus resting-state activity changes highlight the early changes' importance for consciousness.

Even if the early changes reflect mere neural overlaps or carryovers from the preceding resting-state activity, its spontaneous fluctuations (see Dehaene and Changeux 2005; as well as Chapter 18) or predictive inputs and thus the prior expectations (see Melloni et al. 2011 as well as Part III on predictive coding in Volume I), they may nevertheless be relevant for consciousness. Therefore, I will devote this section to them.

What do the early changes tell us about neuronal synchronization and consciousness? The occurrence of early phase synchrony independent of any power changes, that is, amplitude, underlines the crucial role of the oscillations' phases (as distinct from their power) and their synchronization (phase synchronization).

We thereby must distinguish between local and global synchronization. "Local neuronal synchronization" refers to the time-locking of the neural activities and thus the phases of the oscillations related to different stimuli (at different discrete points in physical time) in one particular region, while "global neuronal synchronization" describes the time-locking of the neural activities, the phases, from different regions and networks across the brain.

The study by Melloni et al. (2007) shows the early global synchronization (at around 80–140 ms) across wide-ranging electrode pairs to be central for the visible conditions and thus for consciousness (see many other studies for empirical support as described in Chapter 15; as well as Dehaene and Changeux 2011, for their excellent review). In contrast, local synchronization was also observed in the invisible condition, which, however, unlike the visible conditions, lacked the global synchronization.

How can we further characterize the global neuronal synchronization during consciousness? As suggested by the data, the global neuronal synchronization is temporally transient. Phase synchrony occurred early and lasted only for about 100 ms before it disappeared. One may consecutively speak of transient global neuronal synchronization. The transient nature of long-range synchronization, as Melloni et al. (2007) themselves remark, distinguishes them from the global workspace model of consciousness (see Appendix 1 for discussion of the global workspace model) that would predict a longer and thus temporally more sustained occurrence of global phase synchrony.

In addition to its temporally transient nature, the early global phase synchronization seems to trigger a cascade of later electrophysiological events like increased P300 and theta amplitudes. These later changes are most likely related to cognitive processes like working memory and attention, as pointed out at the very end of the preceding section.

Electrophysiologically, the later changes seem to be instantiated only when phase synchronization occurs earlier. The early global synchronization may consecutively be regarded a necessary neural condition or predisposition for the later electrophysiological events and their associated cognitive functions to occur. We need to be careful, however, because the exact causal relationship between early and late processes remains to be demonstrated.

NEURONAL FINDINGS IIIC: EARLY NEURONAL SYNCHRONIZATION AND STATE VERSUS CONTENT OF CONSCIOUSNESS

Another question concerns whether the early and transient global synchronization is related to the constitution of either the phenomenal contents in consciousness, that is, the visible words, or, alternatively, the phenomenal state of consciousness. This difficulty in distinguishing between phenomenal content and phenomenal state is paradigmatically reflected in another study by Sehatpour et al. (2008). They conducted intracranial recordings in three human subjects from lateral occipital, medial temporal, and prefrontal cortex.

What did the authors observe in their results? First and foremost, subjects perceived scrambled or unscrambled line drawings with only the latter, the unscrambled ones, allowing some (conscious) object recognition. Electrophysiologically, significant differences between unscrambled and scrambled conditions were observed for all three subjects in most electrodes at around 140–400 ms after stimulus onset in especially the beta-frequency band (14–26 Hz) (see also Engel and Fries 2010 for a recent review about the beta band).

The data indicate global neuronal synchronization across the different electrode sites. This further underlines the relevance and importance of long-distance and thus global synchronization for conscious perception (see also Uhlhass et al. 2009a and b for a recent review).

Is such early global neuronal synchronization related to the phenomenal content or rather to the phenomenal state itself? It remains unclear, however, whether the early neuronal synchronization is related to the constitution of the unscrambled line drawings as visible object and thus as phenomenal content in consciousness (see the next section for the exact definition of the concept of "phenomenal content"). In that case, one would need to raise the question of what mechanisms allow the transformation of single stimuli into the objects or events we experience as contents in consciousness.

Or one may propose that the global neuronal synchronization is associated with the instantiation of the state of consciousness, the phenomenal state, rather than with the constitution of its objects, the phenomenal contents. In this case one would need to determine the concept of the phenomenal state and its features like the phenomenal unity in more detail, which will be the focus in the subsequent sections.

NEURONAL HYPOTHESIS IIA: EARLY "NEURONAL UNITY" IS A SPATIOTEMPORAL UNITY OF NEURONAL ACTIVITY

The access unity seems to presuppose prior processes. Melloni et al. (2007) suggest the later processes around 240–300ms to be possibly dependent upon the earlier ones (>40ms after stimulus onset), for example, the early phase synchrony. While neuronally this claim needs to be supported by more evidence in the future, it raises some important questions in conceptual terms, such as: Which kind of unity can be associated with these earlier processes?

One could now argue that the earlier processes already reflect the access unity. That, however, is empirically implausible, given that early and late neuronal changes are characterized by different neuronal mechanisms (see later) and that the earlier changes are not as robust as the later ones. Hence, we must search for the kind of unity that may possibly be associated with the earlier processes, the phase synchrony. This will be the subject in this and the following sections.

How is the described early global neuronal synchronization, the phase-locking in the gamma frequencies, related to the concept of unity? First, the early global neuronal synchronization corresponds well on the empirical, that is, the neuronal side, to what conceptually can be described as "neuronal unity."

What does the concept of "neuronal unity" refer to? The concept of neuronal unity describes the integration and convergence between different neural activities, such as, for instance, from the different regions or networks of the brain (and their respective electrodes as measured in EEG; see Bayne and Chalmers 2003; Bayne 2010, for the definition of the concept of "neuronal unity"). Neuronal unity in this sense is clearly constituted by the early global neuronal synchronization that synchronizes and thereby unifies the neuronal activities of different regions.

Considered purely conceptually (and logically), the concept of neuronal unity implies temporally (and spatially) defined borders and limits, since otherwise there would be no unity. If there were no boundaries, unity would be impossible. How are the temporal and spatial boundaries of such neuronal unity manifested empirically? The temporal borders and limits are empirically well manifested in the findings of specific time windows.

For instance, the early global neuronal synchronization occurred within a certain time window, between 40 and 140 ms. Since the early global neuronal synchronization in the gamma range is signified by a particular time window, one may characterize it conceptually as neuronal unity (see Fig. 19-2). The alleged neuronal unity is thus manifested as temporal unity.

Analogously, the phase synchronization extends to particular regions and networks while excluding others; there is thus spatial unity, which specifies the neuronal unity in spatial terms.

NEURONAL HYPOTHESIS IIB: CONTINUOUS CHANGES AND THE DYNAMIC NATURE OF THE "NEURONAL UNITY"

How can we describe the spatial and temporal unity of the neuronal unity in further detail? The neuronal unity is characterized by a particular degree of spatial and temporal extension within which neural activities at different discrete points in (physical) time and space are linked and integrated.. The neuronal unity is thus intrinsically spatiotemporal with spatial unity and temporal unity, which implies that there are clearly demarcated spatial and temporal boundaries.

In addition to spatial and temporal unity, one may also characterize the neuronal unity by continuous change. The earlier-described data show that the neuronal unity occurs both spatially and temporally in a limited frame; both spatial and temporal unity are thus dynamic and transient rather than static and enduring.

This dynamic nature, as Melloni et al. (2007) themselves remark (see earlier), distinguishes the concept of proposed neuronal unity from the global workspace model of consciousness, which seems to be more static. Rather than corresponding to the global workspace model, the here-proposed concept of neuronal unity may better be compared with what empirically has been described as *microstates* or *neuronal transients* (see Britz et al. 2010; van den Ville et al. 2010; Lehmann et al. 1998, 2010; Lehmann and Michel 2010; Friston 1995, 1997; see also Volume I for details).

The empirical concepts of "microstates" and "neuronal transients" refer to specific constellations of neuronal activity that occur within a limited spatial and temporal frame and are subject to continuous change (across both time and space). In short, both microstates and neuronal transients are dynamic and transient. Therefore, these concepts may resemble on the empirical side what I described conceptually by the term "neuronal unity."

NEURONAL HYPOTHESIS IIIA: GAMMA AND "BINDING" OF THE CONTENTS OF CONSCIOUSNESS

How is such neuronal unity now related to consciousness? The findings show clear differences in the degree of global neuronal synchronization between visible and invisible words. One may consecutively propose gamma oscillations in general and their phase-locking in particular to be central for consciousness. This has been, for instance, suggested by Francis Crick and Christoph Koch.

Let me briefly provide some biographical details of Francis Crick and Christoph Koch. Francis Crick discovered, together with James Watson, the genetic code, the DNA. After he revealed the genes of life, he strived to decode the neural germs of consciousness. Before many others in neuroscience, he ventured into the field of consciousness and developed neuronal hypotheses about it (Crick 1994). Thereby, he collaborated together with a German scientist working in California, Christoph Koch. Together (Crick and Koch 2003), they proposed the 40 Hz gamma oscillations to be central for consciousness, more specifically as a sufficient condition and thus as neural correlate of consciousness (NCC).

How now does their hypothesis stand in relation to the data? For that, we need to distinguish between different concepts and processes. There is, for instance, binding-by-synchronization as discussed in the previous sections and in Volume I (and see Chapter 28 herein). Binding-by-synchronization allows the binding and linking of the neural activities of different cells/populations and/or regions in the brain. Binding-by-synchronization is thus a purely neuronal (rather than phenomenal or neurophenomenal) concept that may therefore be associated with what I earlier described as neuronal unity.

Such binding-by-synchronization must be distinguished from what is simply called "binding." Binding describes the linkage and connections between different features and stimuli into one object or event. Rather than being a purely neuronal concept like binding-by-synchronization, the concept of binding refers to the linkage and integration of different stimuli into one object or event as the content of consciousness.

Since it refers to the contents of consciousness, the concept of binding can no longer be regarded as a purely neuronal concept. As such, binding may be proposed to correspond on the empirical side to what conceptually has been described by the term "objectual unity," the unity of the object or content of consciousness. That assumption needs to be detailed further, though, both empirically and conceptually, which will be discussed in the next section.

NEURONAL HYPOTHESIS IIIB: "BINDING" AS NEUROPHENOMENAL CONCEPT

We have so far remained within the purely neuronal realm when describing the neuronal unity and its underlying neuronal mechanisms, the binding-by-synchronization. This left open empirical data that lend support to the assumption of linking and integrating, e.g., binding, different stimuli into one object or content of consciousness. We mentioned earlier the study on scrambled and unscrambled items. Here, 40 Hz oscillations and global synchronization were only associated with the items, the unscrambled ones, that could be put together into an object.

In contrast, 40 Hz oscillations and global synchronization remained absent in scrambled items that could not be put together into an object. Hence, the constitution of an object and thus of objectual unity was possible only when 40 Hz oscillations and global synchronization occurred. This makes it likely that the purely neuronal binding-by-synchronization is central for the constitution of an object and its objectual unity, thus implying what is described by the concept of binding.

What exactly does the concept of "objectual unity" refer to? The philosophers T. Bayne and D. Chalmers (2003) propose the concept of "objectual unity" to describe the unification of different features into one object. For instance, when seeing a red book, one has to link the color red to the rectangular shape and the paper pages. All three—red, rectangularity, and paper pages—are then integrated and linked when the reader experiences the book in consciousness. The book is thus experienced as an object of consciousness, presupposing what is described as objectual unity.

The concept of objectual unity resurfaces in the "binding problem" as was discussed in Volume I as "binding-by-synchronization" (see also Chapter 10, Volume I). Binding-by-synchronization describes how the neuronal activity of different neurons and cell assemblies can be linked and connected. The concept of binding-by-synchronization is thus a purely neuronal concept as stated above.

However, binding-by-synchronization goes beyond the purely neuronal domain. By synchronizing neuronal activity in space and time, binding-by-synchronization allows for the binding and linking together and thus connecting of the different stimuli and their respective features associated with the different neuronal activities. The "binding problem" thus refers to the binding between different stimuli into one object or event, thereby resulting in what is described conceptually as "objectual unity." Since such objectual unity is proposed to be central for consciousness, the concept of binding can no longer regarded a purely neuronal concept, like binding-by-synchronization, but rather a neurophenomenal (or better, neurocognitive; see below) concept.

How does binding in this sense stand in relation to the hypothesis by Crick and Koch? Crick and Koch propose the 40Hz oscillations to be central in binding and for objectual unity. Since they regard the binding problem and thus objectual unity as being at the very core of consciousness, they propose the 40Hz oscillation to be a sufficient condition or neural correlate of consciousness. Crick and Koch would thus determine the concept of binding indeed as a neurophenomenal (rather than purely neuronal) concept that as such is relevant for consciousness.

NEURONAL HYPOTHESIS IIIC: "BINDING" AS NEUROCOGNITIVE CONCEPT

Are 40 Hz oscillations and thus binding and objectual unity indeed sufficient for consciousness to occur? Recent studies by Revonsuo (2006) and Zmigrod and Hommel (2011) demonstrate that binding of different features and stimuli into one object is indeed associated with 40 Hz oscillations. However, such binding is possible also in the absence of consciousness, thus remaining unconscious.

Different stimuli or features can well be linked and thus bound together into one object and thus constitute objectual unity, even if they are not associated with consciousness. The constitution of objectual unity therefore does not seem to be related to the association of consciousness to the respective object. In other words, an object and its objectual unity can dissociate from consciousness and its phenomenal unity.

That, though, sheds some doubt on whether binding is indeed a sufficient neural condition of consciousness and thus a truly neurophenomenal concept. Instead, the concept of binding seems to refer rather to the cognitive processes that link and integrate different stimuli into one object and its unity, the objectual unity independent of their subsequent association with consciousness. This means that binding must be characterized as a neurocognitive rather than neurophenomenal concept (see Fig. 19-2).

What does this imply for our concepts of neuronal and objectual unity? The 40 Hz oscillations and binding may account for neuronal unity, the unity of neuronal processes, and objectual unity, the unity of the object in consciousness, while 40 Hz and thus gamma oscillations may not account for the association of neuronal unity and objectual unity with consciousness and its phenomenal unity. In other words, 40 Hz oscillations and their neuronal unity are not a sufficient condition of the phenomenal unity of consciousness.

Nor is the objectual unity by itself a sufficient condition of phenomenal unity and thus of consciousness in general. Both concepts, neuronal and objectual unity, may therefore be regarded to be purely neuronal (or at best neurocognitive) concepts rather than being neurophenomenal. And the same holds for their respectively underlying neuronal mechanisms, binding-by-synchronization and binding, which then must be determined as purely neuronal (or neurocognitive) rather than neurophenomenal concepts.

We have so far determined that the concepts of binding and binding-by-synchronization are purely neuronal (or neurocognitive) concepts and associated them with neuronal and objectual unity. This, however, leaves open the question of which neuronal mechanisms are central in constituting the phenomenal state of consciousness and, more specifically, its phenomenal unity.

In other words, we need to develop a truly neurophenomenal hypothesis, rather than remain within the bounds of neuronal and neurocognitive hypotheses. For that, we have to turn back to the brain's intrinsic activity by itself and the spatial and temporal unity of its neural activity.

NEUROPHENOMENAL HYPOTHESIS IA: SPATIOTEMPORAL CHARACTERIZATION OF THE "PHENOMENAL UNITY" OF CONSCIOUSNESS

So far, I have discussed different forms of unity, cognitive and access unity as well as neuronal unity and objectual unity, which I associated with specific neuronal mechanisms. While the different mechanisms and their respective associated unities are neuronally relevant, they turned out to be insufficient to induce the phenomenal unity of consciousness, thus being neurophenomenally irrelevant. In other words, I left open the question of the neuronal mechanisms underlying what I described earlier as phenomenal unity.

What exactly is meant by the concept of "phenomenal unity"? Recalling from earlier, the concept of phenomenal unity describes the unity associated with the subjective experience of consciousness itself independent of any subsequent reporting and cognitive recruitment. What are the neuronal mechanisms underlying such phenomenal unity? For that, I turn briefly to part V and the discussion of temporal and spatial continuity of neural activity in the resting state.

We recall that phenomenally, the "stream of consciousness" can be characterized in temporal terms by the "duration bloc" (see Chapter 15) and spatially by the "dimension bloc" (see Chapter 16). The phenomenal concept of the duration bloc describes the extension of inner time consciousness beyond specific single discrete points in (physical) time.

I proposed that the phenomenal duration bloc can be traced back to the neuronal constitution of global temporal continuity of neural activity by the nestedness between high- and low-frequency fluctuations in the resting-state activity (see Chapter 15). The phenomenal concept of the "dimension bloc" refers to the extension of "inner space consciousness" beyond single discrete points in (physical) space. As such, the dimension bloc was proposed to be related to the neuronal constitution of global spatial continuity via functional connectivity between different regions' neural activities in the resting state (see Chapter 16).

Neurophenomenal Hypothesis IB: From the "Spatial and Temporal Continuity" of Resting-State Activity to the Neuronal Unity During Stimulus-Induced Activity

How, then, is such spatial and temporal continuity related to the neuronal unity described earlier? I thus raise the question of how the neuronal constitution of spatial and temporal continuity in the resting state is related to the constitution of spatial and temporal unity in neuronal unity during stimulus-induced activity. Let us start with the spatial unity.

Spatial unity may be constituted by demarcating spatial boundaries; every region included within the range of the functional connectivity is part of a spatial unity of neuronal activity. In contrast, the regions outside that range are not part of the spatial unity of neuronal activity. Spatial unity can thus be defined by spatial demarcation and boundaries. How is such spatial unity related to the spatial continuity of neuronal activity? Even if there is spatial continuity of neuronal activity, there may nevertheless not yet be some kind of spatial demarcation or boundary. That may be the case if there are lower degrees of functional connectivity between particular regions, which may prevent the respective regions from being included within a specific spatial unity of neuronal activity.

What does this imply for the relationship between spatial continuity and spatial unity? By demarcating spatial boundaries of functional connectivity via (for instance) the comparison of different connectivities' strengths, the underlying spatial continuity is structured and organized into different spatial unities. Conceptually, one may therefore say that the spatial unity supersedes and imposes itself upon the underlying spatial continuity.

Empirically, the resting state's spatial continuity of its neural activity may provide the very basis or grid (or template) upon which the extrinsic stimulus can demarcate the resting state's spatial continuity into a spatial unity by setting spatial boundaries (see below for details). The extrinsic stimulus and its particular discrete point in (physical) space may spatially demarcate the ongoing spatial continuity in the resting state's neural activity and thereby transform the latter into spatial unity (during stimulus-induced activity). This transformation needs to be detailed further, though, which will be the focus in the next section.

Neurophenomenal Hypothesis IC: From the Spatial Continuity of the Brain's Intrinsic Activity to the Spatial Unity of Phenomenal Consciousness

How can we describe the concept of spatial unity in more detail? We recall that the concept of "objectual unity" refers to the linkage between different stimuli and their respective features into one object. This is possible, however, only if the different features are set into one common space, which presupposes what Tim Bayne and David Chalmers (2003; see also Bayne 2010) call "spatial unity."

The concept of spatial unity means that different features, stimuli, objects, and/or events seem to occur in the same space in our experience in consciousness. The spatial unity can thus be compared to a spatial grid or template into which the different features, stimuli, or objects are woven (see Fig. 19-2).

How can we describe the relationship between the spatial grid or template and the extrinsic stimuli in further detail? Let us consider the following example. My experience of my car and my experience of a tree concern different objects and thus different objectual unities. Despite referring to different objects, they are nevertheless experienced in the same commonly underlying space. This is possible only when there is some degree of commonly underlying spatial continuity (which predisposes the constitution of spatial unity).

The same holds for auditory and visual objects. Despite being different and concerning different objects—that is, auditory and visual—they are nevertheless experienced as integrated and linked as distinct aspects of a commonly underlying space. Auditory and visual object senses must thus presuppose one and the same space, a common space with spatial continuity, which, for instance, makes cross-modal interaction first and foremost possible (see Chapter 10, Volume I, for details on cross-modal interaction).

How does all that relate to the concept of spatial unity as advanced by Bayne and Chalmers? They describe the concept of spatial unity as a phenomenal concept, one that characterizes and describes our subjective experience. Following them experience is possible only if we experience a unified space: spatial unity.

How, though, is such spatial unity in a phenomenal sense constituted? That is where the resting state and the spatial continuity of its neuronal activity come in. I propose the intrinsic resting state's spatial continuity of its neuronal activity to provide the spatial "grid" or "template" within which the extrinsic stimuli are integrated and woven.

Most important, by means of the extrinsic stimulus' linkage and integration into the intrinsic activity's spatial continuity, the latter is transformed into a spatial unity by the extrinsic stimulus and its spatial demarcation and boundaries in the spatial continuity of the intrinsic activity (see earlier). This implies that the resting state's neural activity and its spatial continuity are prephenomenal rather than being merely nonphenomenal; otherwise they could not predispose the constitution of spatial unity on the phenomenal level of consciousness.

NEUROPHENOMENAL HYPOTHESIS ID: FROM THE TEMPORAL CONTINUITY OF THE BRAIN'S INTRINSIC ACTIVITY TO THE TEMPORAL UNITY OF PHENOMENAL CONSCIOUSNESS

How about the temporal dimension? Analogous to the spatial dimension, I would hypothesize

that the same mechanisms, e.g., demarcating and setting boundaries, also operate in the case of temporal continuity and temporal unity. High-frequency fluctuations as introduced by extrinsic stimuli may divide the underlying low-frequency fluctuations of the resting state and its temporal continuity into different temporal unities.

By demarcating the long phase durations of low-frequency oscillation into the shorter phase durations of high-frequency fluctuations, the latter supersede and impose themselves upon the former (see Chapter 15). This implies the constitution of different temporal unities on top of the ongoing temporal continuity of the brain's intrinsic activity with the former superseding and imposing itself upon the latter (see Fig. 19-3a).

How is the constitution of such temporal and spatial unities on the basis of the spatial and temporal continuity of the brain's intrinsic activity possible? We recall from Part V that the neuronal constitution of spatial and temporal continuity was related to the continuously ongoing neuronal activity of the resting state, that is, rest–rest interaction, and its functional connectivity and low-frequency fluctuations. Stronger changes in functional connectivity and low-frequency fluctuations at more discrete points in (physical) time and space as related to single extrinsic stimuli may then lead to the partitioning of the spatial and temporal continuity into temporal and spatial unities.

How can such changes in the resting state be induced? They are usually elicited by extrinsic stimuli from body and environment. However, the same kind of stronger changes may also be induced by changes in the resting state itself, such as during exceptional circumstances like dreams (see Chapter 26).

Hence, we have to look at what happens to the resting state and its spatial and temporal continuity during the changes of its neuronal activity, as they can occur either spontaneously or during the encounter of extrinsic stimuli. This is especially necessary in order to understand how the alleged spatial and temporal unities are central in constituting the phenomenal state of consciousness including its phenomenal unity.

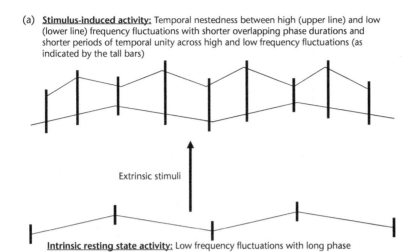

(a) **Stimulus-induced activity:** Temporal nestedness between high (upper line) and low (lower line) frequency fluctuations with shorter overlapping phase durations and shorter periods of temporal unity across high and low frequency fluctuations (as indicated by the tall bars)

Extrinsic stimuli

Intrinsic resting state activity: Low frequency fluctuations with long phase durations and periods of temporal continuity (as indicated by the small bars)

Figure 19-3a-c "Continuity-based hypothesis of phenomenal unity." The figure shows distinct aspects of the continuity-based hypothesis of phenomenal unity. The relationship between temporal continuity and unity (*a*), the basis of phenomenal unity in the intrinsic resting state's global spatiotemporal continuity of its neural activity (*b*), and the relationship between temporal nestedness and neuronal and phenomenal unity (*c*). (*a*) The figure shows how the temporal continuity of the intrinsic resting-state activity (*lower part*) is converted into temporal unity during extrinsic stimulus-induced activity (*upper part*). The intrinsic resting-state activity is mediated by the long-phase durations of the low-frequency fluctuations (*lower part*), which are supplemented by the high-frequency fluctuations (*upper part*) during extrinsic stimulus-induced activity. Due to the temporal overlap between high- and low-frequency fluctuations, short temporal periods of temporal unity are constituted. (*b*) The figure shows the relationship between the temporal nestedness of high- and low-frequency fluctuations in the resting-state activity and the degree of neuronal and phenomenal unity during subsequent changes in neural activity during either rest–rest or rest–stimulus interaction. The higher the degree of temporal nestedness mirroring temporal continuity in the resting-state activity, the more likely the activity change will be able to elicit neuronal and ultimately phenomenal unity. (*c*) The figure shows how the constitution of phenomenal unity (*upper part*) is based on the intrinsic resting-state activity and the global spatiotemporal continuity of its neural activity (*lower part*). The stimulus triggers binding by synchronization during rest–stimulus interaction (*lower right*). This leads to the subsequent constitution of neuronal unity and objectual unity (*middle right*) that provide the content to the phenomenal unity of consciousness (*upper right*). At the same time, the intrinsic resting state's spatiotemporal continuity is carried over and transferred to the extrinsic stimulus-induced activity (*lower left*), where it results in spatial and temporal unity. If this step does not take place, the stimulus' processing remains "subliminal" and thus unconscious. The constitution of the resting-state activity's spatial and temporal unity makes possible the constitution of neuronal and objectual unity during stimulus-induced activity as indicated by the weak horizontal arrows from left to right. The spatial and temporal unity also makes possible the organization of the resting-state activity in self-specific and preintentional regards (see upper left; also see Chapters 23–27 for details), which merges with the objectual unity into a phenomenal unity. Hence, both arms (right and left) and thus form and content of consciousness converge and merge in the phenomenal unity. I propose that this merger makes consciousness possible and thus necessary or unavoidable during the "right" kind of rest–stimulus interaction. If, in contrast, such a merger does not take place due to too weak (and thus too linear) rest–stimulus interaction (see Chapter 29 for details), no phenomenal unity will be constituted, resulting in the "preconscious."

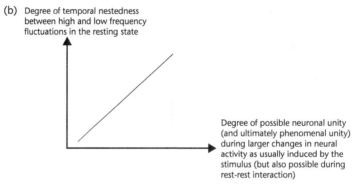

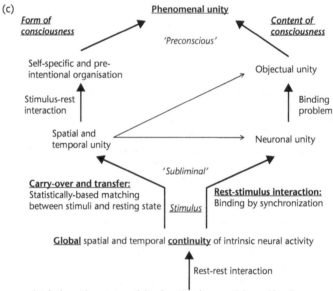

Figure 19-3a-c (Continued)

Neurophenomenal Hypothesis IIA: "Temporal and Spatial Smoothing" of Extrinsic Stimuli by the Brain's Intrinsic Activity

Where does this leave us with regard to consciousness and its phenomenal unity? So far, I have proposed the partitioning of the resting state's temporal and spatial continuity by (usually) stimuli to result in the constitution of spatial and temporal unity.

In contrast, I neglected what such spatial and temporal partitioning of the intrinsic resting state's spatial and temporal continuity implies for the extrinsic stimulus itself. Though the extrinsic stimulus triggers the demarcation of spatial and temporal boundaries in the resting state's neural activity, the extrinsic stimulus itself nevertheless becomes integrated and linked to the intrinsic spatial and temporal continuity, which in turn transform the latter into temporal and spatial unity.

More specifically, the stimulus' discrete point in (physical) time and space is thereby resolved and embedded (or nested) within the temporal and spatial continuity and the superseding temporal and spatial unity of the brain's intrinsic activity (as now modulated by the stimulus and its stimulus-induced activity).Let us put this in a slightly different way. Earlier I said that the extrinsic stimulus imposes its discrete point in (physical) time and space upon the ongoing spatial and temporal continuity in the intrinsic resting-state activity. This leads to the demarcation of spatial and temporal boundaries with the subsequent constitution of spatial and temporal unities that thus supersede and impose themselves upon the spatial and temporal continuity.

However, superseding and imposition are bilateral. As the extrinsic stimulus impinges itself upon the intrinsic resting state, the intrinsic resting state imposes itself upon the extrinsic stimulus and its stimulus-induced activity. More specifically, the resting state's spatial and temporal continuity imposes itself on the stimulus and its discrete point in (physical) time and space by means of which the latter becomes resolved into the former. In other words, the stimulus' discrete point in (physical) space and time becomes linked to and integrated in the resting state's temporal and spatial continuity and is subsequently embedded within resulting spatial and temporal unity.

The embedding and resolution of the stimulus's discrete point in (physical) time and space into the spatial and temporal continuity and its consequent embedding within the resulting temporal and spatial unity implies that the stimulus itself and its spatial and temporal features are no longer accessible as such, e.g., by themselves as discrete point in (physical) time and space. Instead, the stimulus and its distinct discrete point in (physical) time and space become smoothed, merged, and unified with other discrete points in (physical) time and space.

Metaphorically speaking, the extrinsic stimulus' discrete point in (physical) time and space becomes smoothed and extended in space and time in the same way that we extend and stretch chewing gum in our mouth. The mouth and its tongue correspond then to the brain's resting-state activity and its spatial and temporal continuity, while the chewing gum takes on the role of the extrinsic stimulus in our metaphorical comparison. In the same way as our mouth and tongue manipulate the spatial and temporal configuration of the chewing gum, the brain's intrinsic activity extends and thus changes the spatial and temporal features of the

extrinsic stimuli; namely, their discrete points in physical time and space, by integrating and linking them to itself.

NEUROPHENOMENAL HYPOTHESIS IIB: REST–STIMULUS INTERACTION AS SUFFICIENT NEURAL CONDITION OF PHENOMENAL UNITY

What, now, exactly happens during the encounter of the stimulus with the resting-state activity such that the phenomenal state of consciousness is generated? The resting state's temporal and spatial continuity are transformed into spatial and temporal unity, as we discussed earlier. This may be possibly manifest in the early and late changes during stimulus-induced activity (see above). Thereby the different stimuli become integrated and unified into one particular content, the phenomenal content of consciousness (see Chapter 25 for more discussion of the constitution of contents). This is reflected in the neuronal synchronization that makes possible the "binding" and objectual unity (see Fig. 19-2).

At the same time, the resting-state activity's spatial and temporal continuity is carried over and transferred so that it interacts with the stimulus, resulting in what we observe as stimulus-induced activity (see Chapters 28 and 29 for details). The degree and the manner in which both resting state and stimulus interact with each other determine the degree to which the stimulus is associated with phenomenal unity and thus the degree or level of consciousness.

This is reflected empirically in the degree to which the stimulus interacts with the intrinsic resting-state activity and its spatial and temporal continuity. Most importantly, the degree of stimulus-induced activity is dependent upon both the state or level of the resting-state activity and the strength of the extrinsic stimulus by itself. The constitution of phenomenal unity must thus be related to all three: the resting-state activity, the stimulus, and their interaction.

This implies that any one of the three, resting-state activity, stimulus, and stimulus-induced activity, can by itself be regarded only as a necessary (but not a sufficient) neural condition of phenomenal unity. In contrast, the specific kind and degree of their interaction (see Chapters 11 and 29 for different kinds of rest–stimulus interaction), namely rest–stimulus interaction, must be regarded a sufficient neural condition of actual phenomenal unity.

NEUROPHENOMENAL HYPOTHESIS IIIA: THE CONTINUITY-BASED HYPOTHESIS OF PHENOMENAL UNITY

Based on the earlier-discussed considerations, I suggest what I describe as the continuity-based hypothesis of phenomenal unity. The continuity-based hypothesis of phenomenal unity proposes the constitution of spatial and temporal unity and ultimately the phenomenal unity of consciousness to be based upon and predisposed by the resting state's spatial and temporal continuity and its respective neuronal processes, that is, functional connectivity and low-frequency fluctuations.

How can we further specify the continuity-based hypothesis of phenomenal unity in both empirical and conceptual regard? Let's start with the empirical side of things (see Fig. 19-3b).

Empirically, the continuity-based hypothesis of phenomenal unity implies the following: the higher, for instance, the resting state's degree of temporal continuity, that is, the temporal nestedness between high- and low-frequency fluctuations, the more likely the extrinsic stimulus will be able to trigger the constitution of a higher degree of neuronal unity, that is, global neuronal synchronization in the gamma range during stimulus-induced activity. And the higher the degree of neuronal unity elicited by the stimulus, the more likely the resulting temporal and spatial unity can be smoothed and extended beyond the stimulus' discrete point in (physical) time and space.

How does my continuity-based hypothesis of phenomenal unity stand in relation to the earlier described data? I propose that the early phase synchrony as demonstrated by Melloni is very much dependent on the resting-state activity preceding the stimulus onset. At the same time, the early phase synchrony is supposed to also depend on the specific timing of the stimulus' occurrence relative to the phases of the resting state's ongoing low-frequency fluctuations.

This can be tested in the future. As we saw in Chapter 18, there is indeed empirical support for the prestimulus resting state impacting subsequent neuronal activity and consciousness. The continuity-based hypothesis of phenomenal unity can thus be regarded as the extension of the resting state–based hypothesis of prephenomenal unity (see Chapter 13) onto the level of stimulus-induced activity.

NEUROPHENOMENAL HYPOTHESIS IIIB: CONTINUITY-BASED HYPOTHESIS OF PHENOMENAL UNITY VERSUS "GLOBAL NEURONAL WORKSPACE" (GNW)

What about the GNW theory (see earlier) in the context of the continuity-based hypothesis of phenomenal unity? We recall that the GNW distinguishes between the "subliminal," the "preconscious," and the full-blown consciousness. Our investigation revealed the full-blown consciousness in the GNW to correspond to cognitive and access unity and thus to access consciousness. This, however, left open the quest for phenomenal unity and phenomenal consciousness.

That is where the continuity-based hypothesis of phenomenal unity fits in. Rather than subsuming phenomenal unity and consciousness under the preconscious as in the GNW (see Box 4 in Dehaene et al. 2006), I consider phenomenal unity and consciousness to be distinct from both preconscious and access consciousness. They must be distinguished not only conceptually but also phenomenally, and, most importantly, empirically that is neuronally. Let me detail this distinction in the following.

Both *preconscious* and *access consciousness* refer mainly to stimulus-induced activity, as I pointed out earlier. This distinguishes them from the phenomenal unity that, as suggested here, results from a specific (yet to be determined) form of rest–stimulus interaction (see Chapter 29). Accordingly, the continuity-based hypothesis of phenomenal unity fills in a gap, the gap of the phenomenal unity, that the GNW leaves open and unexplained (due to its predominant focus on contents and its neurocognitive rather than neurophenomenal approach; see earlier).

Let me be more specific. The GNW addresses mere "conscious access" as defined by "subjective reporting," which implies access consciousness (see earlier). This is different in the continuity-based hypothesis of phenomenal unity, which instead targets phenomenal unity and thus phenomenal consciousness as defined by experience rather than access.

Such phenomenal unity and consciousness is supposed to be based by itself on the preconscious while serving as the basis for subsequent access unity and consciousness. Hence, the continuity-based hypothesis of phenomenal unity claims to close the phenomenal gap between the preconscious and the access consciousness as was left open in the GNW. Such a closure of the phenomenal gap is made possible, I propose, by closing the empirical, e.g., neuronal gap between intrinsic resting-state activity and extrinsic stimulus-induced activity.

The continuity-based hypothesis of phenomenal unity proposes that the phenomenal unity and thus phenomenal consciousness are dependent upon the "right" kind of interaction between extrinsic stimulus and intrinsic resting-state activity; that is, rest–stimulus interaction. The stimulus is central in that it triggers a particular neuronal organization, spatial and temporal unity, on the very basis of the resting state's neural predisposition, the spatial and temporal continuity of its neural activity.

This means that the resting state's spatial and temporal continuity is a necessary and unavoidable neural condition and thus neural predisposition of (possible) phenomenal unity. In contrast, the extrinsic stimulus and its particular kind of rest–stimulus interaction, including the associated stimulus-related changes, are sufficient neural conditions and thus neural correlates of (actual) phenomenal unity.

NEUROPHENOMENAL HYPOTHESIS IIIC: "SUBLIMINAL" AND "PRECONSCIOUS" IN THE "CONTINUITY-BASED HYPOTHESIS OF PHENOMENAL UNITY"

How does the continuity-based hypothesis of phenomenal unity account for the preconscious and the subliminal? We recall that the GNW

associated the subliminal with a too weak stimulus while the preconscious was related to a closed fronto-parietal network (see earlier). I here propose the "subliminal" to be related to the inability of the extrinsic stimulus to transform the intrinsic resting state's spatial and temporal continuity into spatial and temporal unity.

More specifically, the stimulus may interact with the resting state, but this rest–stimulus interaction may be too weak to demarcate clear spatial and temporal boundaries in the spatial and temporal continuity of the resting state's neural activity. This may be due to either the stimulus itself being too weak (as the GNW proposes; see earlier). Or it may be related to the resting state itself that may no longer be reactive to the stimulus, irrespective of its being either weak or strong (as may be the case in vegetative state; see Chapters 28 and 29; see Fig. 19-3c).

How about the preconscious? Here the stimulus may be able to trigger the transformation of the resting state's spatial and temporal continuity into spatial and temporal unity of neural activity. The resting state's spatial and temporal continuity may, however, not be transformed yet into full-blown phenomenal unity and thus consciousness. Hence, metaphorically put, the resting state may be ready by providing spatial and temporal unity. And the stimulus itself may also be ready by being associated with objectual unity. However, the merger of spatial and temporal unity and objectual unity into full-blown phenomenal unity may not take place.

Let us describe this situation in more detail. Everything is ready, but the "final push" is missing. The GNW associates the final push with the fronto-parietal network's availability. The continuity-based hypothesis of phenomenal unity, in contrast, proposes this final push to be associated with the specific form of rest–stimulus interaction, namely GABA-ergic mediated degree of nonlinearity during rest–stimulus interaction. Unlike in the case of the GNW and its focus on the prefrontal and parietal cortex, such nonlinear rest–stimulus interaction is not confined to a particular region or network in the brain. Why? I propose that the non-linear rest-stimulus interaction can occur in any region or network of the brain, including sensory cortical regions, subcortical regions, and the fronto-parietal network (and all others; see Chapter 29 for details).

NEUROPHENOMENAL HYPOTHESIS IIID: GAMMA AND THE "CONTINUITY-BASED HYPOTHESIS OF PHENOMENAL UNITY"

We may also want to briefly mention how the continuity-based hypothesis of phenomenal unity stands in relation to Crick and Koch's suggestions of gamma as a neural correlate of consciousness (see earlier). Does my continuity-based hypothesis of phenomenal unity commit the same conceptual confusion as Crick and Koch? On the basis of their false-positive identification between objectual unity and phenomenal unity, they proposed the 40 Hz oscillations to be a sufficient condition and thus a neural correlate of consciousness (see earlier).

My continuity-based hypothesis of phenomenal unity differs in several regards from the one by Crick and Koch. First, unlike them, I do not associate stimulus-induced activity with consciousness and its phenomenal unity. Instead, I rather propose the phenomenal unity of consciousness to be related to a specific form of rest–stimulus interaction, thus considering both resting-state activity and stimulus-induced activity. Secondly, unlike Crick and Koch, I do not target the sufficient conditions and thus neural correlates of (actual) consciousness but only the necessary conditions and thus the neural predispositions of (possible) consciousness.

Finally, unlike Crick and Koch, I do not identify the objectual unity with the phenomenal unity of consciousness. However, I do propose the spatial and temporal unity in the earlier mentioned sense to be a central feature of the phenomenal unity of consciousness. However, spatial and temporal unity can neither be identified with objectual unity (see earlier) nor with the phenomenal unity of consciousness (see also Appendix 3).

This raises the question for the additional neuronal ingredients that are necessary to constitute the phenomenal unity of consciousness as

distinguished from both neuronal and objectual unity (see also Appendix 3 for the discussion of the position by S. Zeki and its relation to the philosopher Immanuel Kant). For that, as I propose, we need to better understand what exactly happens in the resting state itself and how it aligns itself to the environment. This will be the subject in Chapter 20.

Open Questions

One question pertains to how the stimulus interacts with the resting-state activity's temporal and spatial continuity so that it triggers the constitution of temporal and spatial unity. Schroeder and Lakatos (2007) describe different rules of oscillations during rest–stimulus interaction. One rule concerns phase resetting: an extrinsic stimulus can shift the phase of the ongoing intrinsic synchronized fluctuations toward either a more hyperpolarized or a more depolarized state. Thereby, it makes subsequent stimulus-induced activity either more or less likely. This is, for instance, the case in cross-modal interaction between auditory and visual cortex. Visual stimuli do not elicit action potentials in auditory cortex or changes in the power of ongoing oscillations (Lakatos et al. 2005a and b, 2007, 2008, 2009). However, they affect the phase of the ongoing synchronized fluctuations by shifting it towards more depolarized states.

This, in turn, makes it easier, that is, more likely, for an accompanying auditory stimulus to induce an action potential and thus stimulus-induced activity (see Volume I, Chapter 10 for details). Analogous phase resetting was observed also in the visual cortex itself where stimuli modulate the ongoing phase of the gamma oscillations, leading to what in Volume I was described as "gamma shift" (see Volume I, Chapters 10 and 12 for details).

While described well on a neuronal level, the implications of this rule of neuronal oscillation for constituting the phenomenal unity of consciousness remain unclear. Such phase resetting suggests that the stimulus has a strong impact on the resting state in that it resets the temporal and spatial measures of the resting state's global spatial and temporal continuity.

By resetting the phases of the resting state's low-frequency fluctuations, the stimulus may trigger the demarcation of temporal boundaries and consequently the constitution of temporal boundaries with subsequent temporal unity. One may thus propose that phase resetting may be a central mechanism in how the extrinsic stimulus triggers the constitution of temporal unity on the basis of the intrinsic resting state's ongoing temporal continuity. That, however, is a tentative hypothesis at this point.

This leads me to the second question. As described in the previous and this chapter, the resting-state activity seems to have a central role in selecting the phenomenal content and instantiating a phenomenal state. How is it possible that the resting-state activity has a say in selecting phenomenal contents while being devoid of any phenomenal or nonphenomenal contents itself? Therefore, we must investigate how the resting-state and the spatial and temporal continuity of its neuronal activity are related to contents; this will be the main focus in Chapter 20.

Moreover, we must investigate how the resting-state activity makes it possible for, that is, predisposes, the stimulus and the respective contents to become associated with a phenomenal unity and ultimately with a phenomenal state and thus consciousness during rest–stimulus interaction. This will be another focus in Chapter 20.

CHAPTER 20
"Neurosocial Activity" and "Environment–Brain Unity"

Summary

So far, I have discussed the neuronal mechanisms that allow the constitution of phenomenal unity (Chapter 19) and prephenomenal unity (Chapter 18). However, I claim that we need to go one step even further by tracing back the prephenomenal unity to a preceding more basic virtual unity, the spatial and temporal unity between environment and brain, which I describe as "environment–brain unity." The concept of "environment–brain unity" refers to a virtual statistically based linkage between the brain's intrinsic activity and the environment's occurrence of extrinsic stimuli across different discrete points in (physical) time and space. An analogous linkage may be proposed to hold true for the relationship between the bodily stimuli and the brain's intrinsic activity, so that one may speak of a body–brain unity. Since empirical data are sparse in this case, however, we will here focus mainly on the environment–brain unity. The assumption of such a virtual statistically-based environment–brain unity is based on empirical findings that the brain's resting-state encodes into its neural activity the statistical frequency distribution of the stimuli in the environment. That means that the resting-state activity and, more specifically, the phases of its low-frequency oscillations encode the statistically-based temporal and spatial differences of the stimuli's occurrences in the environment across different discrete points in (physical) time and space. Such difference-based encoding of the environment's statistical structure, that is, the natural and social statistics, by the brain's intrinsic activity is indeed empirically supported. This has, as I hypothesize, far-reaching neuronal, phenomenal, and conceptual implications. More specifically, the statistically based encoding of the extrinsic stimuli's statistical structure and thus their natural and social statistics into the brain's intrinsic resting-state activity makes possible the constitution of a virtual statistically based spatio-temporal unity between brain and environment, the environment–brain unity. Such an environment–brain unity may serve as a base, ground, or predisposition for the subsequent constitution of the prephenomenal unity by the resting-state activity. This leads me to propose what I describe as the "environment-based hypothesis of prephenomenal unity." The "environment-based hypothesis of prephenomenal unity" suggests that both phenomenal and prephenomenal unity are ultimately based on and predisposed by the virtual statistically based unity between the environmental stimuli's natural and social statistics and the brain's intrinsic activity, the environment-brain unity: The more the resting state's low-frequency oscillations shift towards and align themselves to the environmental (and bodily) stimuli's statistical occurrences across the different discrete points in (physical) time and space, the stronger the degree of the environment–brain unity, and the higher the possible degree of both prephenomenal and ultimately phenomenal unity including consciousness. Accordingly, a strong or high degree of environment–brain unity predisposes an increased probability of possible phenomenal unity and thus of consciousness. In contrast, a low or weak environment–brain unity decreases the probability of possible consciousness.

Key Concepts and Topics Covered

Natural statistics, rhythmic and continuous mode, environment–brain unity, low-frequency oscillations, phases, difference-based coding, temporal differences, prephenomenal unity, resting state, phenomenal unity, environment-based hypothesis of prephenomenal unity

NEUROEMPIRICAL BACKGROUND IA: FROM THE NEURAL TO THE NEUROSOCIAL CHARACTERIZATION OF THE BRAIN'S INTRINSIC ACTIVITY

I discussed the neuronal mechanisms underlying the constitution of the phenomenal unity of consciousness (see Chapter 19) and the prephenomenal unity of the resting-state activity (see Chapter 18). This led me to characterize the resting state in neuronal and prephenomenal terms.

Neuronally, the resting state can be characterized by spatial and temporal continuity of its neuronal activity. This differs from its prephenomenal description. Here, the resting-state activity may be described by prephenomenal unity as predisposition for a virtual unity that spans across the different discrete points in (physical) time and space. Most important, I demonstrated that the resting-state activity's prephenomenal unity and its underlying neuronal mechanisms are central in making possible and thus predisposing consciousness and its phenomenal unity (see Chapters 18 and 19).

That, however, left open the question of how the prephenomenal unity itself is constituted by the intrinsic activity in the brain's resting state. In other words, I am now searching for the necessary and thus predisposing conditions that make possible the resting-state activity's constitution of a prephenomenal unity. This is the focus in the present chapter.

Where can we find the necessary conditions that predispose the constitution of the prephenomenal unity by the brain's intrinsic activity? Rather than searching in the brain and its neural activity itself, we may need to broaden our perspective and consider the brain's intrinsic activity in its environmental context. How must the brain and its intrinsic activity be related to its environmental (and bodily) context in order to make possible the constitution of the prephenomenal unity?

This shifts the focus from the brain itself to how the brain's resting-state activity and its low-frequency oscillations are aligned and relate to the environment (and the body). We therefore have to consider the brain's intrinsic activity no longer in isolation, but rather in relation to the environment. Instead of investigating the brain and its intrinsic activity in a purely neuronal way, we are now taking a broader perspective and considering the brain in the social context of the environment. In other words, we turn from the purely neural description to the neurosocial characterization of the brain's intrinsic activity.

NEUROEMPIRICAL BACKGROUND IB: NEUROSOCIAL CHARACTERIZATION OF THE BRAIN'S NEURAL ACTIVITY

How can we characterize the brain's intrinsic activity in neurosocial rather than in purely neural terms? The first intuition coming to mind is to revert to social neuroscience. Social neuroscience investigates how different social processes, like empathy, "mind reading," buying and selling, moral judgment, and many others as well as cultural differences are mediated neuronally (see also Han and Northoff 2008 ; and Han et al. 2013, for the extension of social neuroscience into the cultural domain).

How does social neuroscience characterize stimulus-induced activity? Wihin the context of social neuroscience, stimulus-induced and task-related activity are associated with specific social functions as distinguished from, for instance, cognitive and affective functions. The focus is here on distinguishing the kinds of stimulus-induced and task-related activities that are related to specific social functions..

Are we targeting in this chapter the social functions of the brain and their related stimulus-induced and task-related activities? No, the aim we are pursuing here is much deeper and more profound. We do not target specific social functions of the brain and their associated extrinsic stimulus-induced or task-related activity. Instead, we want to show that the brain's generation of its own neural activity in general, including both intrinsic and extrinsic activity, is necessary and unavoidably tied to its social context, the environment.

I therefore postulate that any neural activity, independently of whether it is intrinsic or extrinsic, must be characterized as neurosocial rather than purely neural. We now seek to discover the neuronal mechanisms that make it necessary and unavoidable for the brain's intrinsic and extrinsic activities to be neurosocial rather than merely neural.

NEUROEMPIRICAL BACKGROUND IC: FROM THE ENCODING OF THE SPATIAL AND TEMPORAL CONTEXT TO THE NEUROSOCIAL CHARACTERIZATION OF THE BRAIN'S ACTIVITY

What are the neuronal mechanisms that make possible the neurosocial character of the brain's neural activity? One possible neural candidate is the low-frequency fluctuations. We demonstrated that the brain's intrinsic activity is characterized by activity fluctuations in the low-frequency range (< 4 Hz or even < 0.1 Hz; see Chapter 5). How do these low-frequency fluctuations stand in relation to the social processes in the environment? This will be the first major focus in the present chapter.

Another neural candidate is the strategy by means of which the brain encodes its neural activity. We discussed in length in Volume I the fact that the brain encodes the statistical frequency distribution of the different stimuli rather than the stimuli themselves. This included the encoding of the stimuli's natural statistics, social statistics, vegetative statistics, and neuronal statistics (see Chapters 1–2 and 8–9).

The concept of "natural statistics" describes the statistical frequency distribution of the exteroceptive target stimuli, while "social statistics" refers to the relationship of the target stimulus to its respective social context and thus other stimuli. The terms "vegetative statistics" and "neuronal statistics" concern the statistical frequency distributions of interoceptive stimuli from the body and neuronal stimuli from the brain's intrinsic activity.

What does such a statistically based encoding strategy imply for the characterization of the brain's neural activity? The encoding of statistical frequency distributions implies that any neural activity including both intrinsic and extrinsic activity is generated in dependence on its respective spatial and temporal context and consequently its social context. The resulting neural activity is consequently intrinsically neurosocial rather than purely neural.

Let us explicate what exactly is meant by the term "neurosocial." There is no way to generate neural activity other than in dependence on its spatial and temporal context. This means, however, that even the encoding and thus the generation of the brain's intrinsic activity must be dependent on its respective spatial and temporal contexts. What, then, is the spatial and temporal context for the brain's intrinsic activity? The spatial and temporal context for the brain's intrinsic activity consists of the body, the vegetative context, and the environment, or the social context.

I will here focus on the latter—the environment and the social context it provides for the brain's intrinsic activity—while I will neglect the body and its vegetative context (see, though, Chapter 32 for extensive discussion of the body and its relation to consciousness). We will demonstrate that the brain's intrinsic activity can by default not avoid aligning itself with the ongoing stimuli in its social environmental context. The here-suggested neurosocial character of the brain's neural activity can then be traced back to its particular encoding strategy; namely, that the brain encodes its neural activity in direct dependence on its respective social contexts.

NEUROEMPIRICAL BACKGROUND ID: THE "NEUROSOCIAL CHARACTER" OF THE BRAIN'S NEURAL ACTIVITY PREDISPOSES CONSCIOUSNESS

How is the brain's intrinsic activity dependent upon the social context in the environment? This can be explored in two steps. The first step is to show some of the neuronal mechanisms that can align the brain's intrinsic activity with the social environment. For that purpose we will discuss a recent study by Stefanics et al. (2010) in a more detailed way that shows the alignment of the intrinsic resting-state activity's delta phase oscillations to the statistical frequency distribution of the extrinsic stimuli in the environment.

The focus on neuronal mechanisms will be complemented in a second step by recent results from social neuroscience that show the neural activity in one subject to be directly related to the neural activity in another subject. This extends into the domain of social (and cultural) neuroscience and how brains from different subjects synchronize their neural activity with each other (see Saenger et al. 2011; Hasson et al. 2012; Han, Northoff, et al. 2013; Han and Northoff 2008). These data lend empirical support to the here suggested neurosocial character of the brain's intrinsic activity. In the subsequent neuronal—or better, neurosocial—hypotheses, I will argue that these results can only be explained by assuming the "neurosocial character" of the brain's neural activity, including intrinsic resting-state activity and extrinsic-stimulus-induced activity.

What do I mean by the concept of "neurosocial character" of the brain's neural activity? The concept of the "neurosocial character" of the brain's neural activity describes a necessary or unavoidable linkage and alignment between the brain's "neural activity" and the environment's "social activity."

More specifically, the environment's "social activity" is directly involved in generating and thus shaping the brain's neural activity. The resulting neural activity is therefore not purely neural nor completely social in its origin but rather "neurosocial". Most important, I postulate that the neurosocial character of the brain's neural activity first and foremost makes possible and thus predisposes consciousness, especially its prephenomenal and phenomenal unity. This will be explained in full detail in the last sections of this chapter.

Neuronal Findings IA: Delta Oscillations Lock Their Phase Onsets to Extrinsic Stimuli

In order to better understand the neuronal mechanism of the relationship between the brain's intrinsic activity and its alignment to extrinsic stimuli, let us discuss one interesting study in this context, the study by Stefanics et al. (2010; and while there do not seem to be many other studies in this regard, especially ones focusing on the relationship between rhythmic stimulus presentation and consciousness; see Tecchio et al. 2000, for an earlier study).

Stefanics et al. (2010) conducted an electroencephalographic (EEG) study in healthy human subjects. Subjects were presented with target tones to which they had to react by pressing a button, thus yielding a reaction time. Preceding the target tone, the investigators presented different cue stimuli (also tones, though with a different frequency than the target tone) that indicated the probability of the subsequent target tone's occurrence.

In the first experiment, four different cue tones were presented, one indicating 10%; the second, 37%; the third, 64%; and the fourth, 91% probability of the target tone's occurrence. Depending on the degree of probability indicated by the cue tone, it was followed either by a target tone or by another cue tone (see Fig. 20-1a).

Following the hypothesis of Schroeder and Lakatos (2009a and b; and see above and Chapter 19), the authors focused on especially low-frequency oscillations in the delta range and their entrainment by higher-frequency oscillations (like gamma). Why? Because they suspected the high-low-frequency entrainment and thus the shifting of the low frequency's phase onsets to be related to the statistical probability of the stimulus' occurrence across time.

What behavioral results did they obtain? As expected, they demonstrated that the reaction time (i.e., time needed for the response to target tones) was significantly faster in those trials (i.e., target tones) where the preceding cue tones indicated higher probability. The higher the probability indicated by the cue tone, the faster subjects were able to react, resulting in shorter reaction time to the target tone. This pattern was observed in both experiments.

How about the EEG data and more specifically the delta phase and its entrainment to the stimuli's different degrees of probability? The phase of delta oscillation was significantly entrained to the onset of the target tone as manifest in a significant phase preference. The target tone's onset was especially locked to the negative phase; that is, the negative deflection, the "right" phase value, in the ongoing cycle of the fluctuations in the delta range.

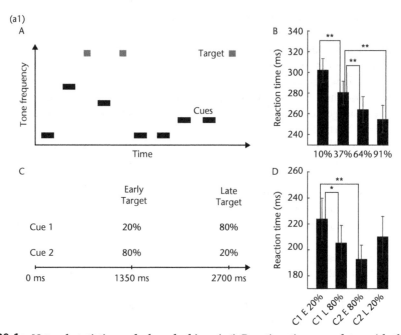

Figure 20-1a Natural statistics and phase locking. (*a1*) Reaction time correlates with the level of expectancy. (*A*) Auditory target detection paradigm of experiment 1. Four different cue tones (black) predicted the target tone (gray) to be the next stimulus with increasing probability paralleling the increase of cue-tone frequencies (p = 0.1, p = 0.37, p = 0.64, and p = 0.91). Participants were to press a response key to the target tone. (*B*) Reaction times (RT) significantly decreased with increasing predictability of the target (n = 13; ANOVA, $p < 10^{-9}$, with Tukey's *post hoc* tests, $p < 0.01$). Error bars indicate SEM. (*C*) In experiment 2, two different cue tones predicted the timing of the target tone with different probabilities. An early target (1350 ms after the cue) was delivered with p = 0.2 after cue 1 and with p = 0.8 after cue 2. On trials with no early target, a late target (2700 ms after the cue) was delivered (p = 0.8 after cue 1 and p = 0.2 after cue 2). (*D*) The early-target RT was significantly shorter after cue 2 (p = 0.8 probability, third bar) than after cue 1 (p = 0.2 probability, first bar) (p = 0.01, Tukey's *post hoc* test). In the absence of an early target, delivery of the late target could be predicted with 100% certainty, resulting in faster RTs compared with the early target with p = 0.2 (following cue 1, $p < 0.05$ and cue 2, p = 0.08). C1, cue 1; C2, cue 2; E, early target; L, late target. *$p < 0.05$; **$p < 0.01$. (*a2*) Phase entrainment of the cortical delta oscillation. (*A–D*) Distributions of delta phase values (measured at Cz) at target onset are presented on rose diagrams with the radial extent of the circle segments representing the probability of the given phase range. Trials with 10% (*A*), 37% (*B*), 64% (*C*), and 91% (*D*) target probabilities were separately pooled from all (n = 13) participants. (*E–H*) Individual (gray) and average (black) phase histograms for the four different target probabilities (two cycles; idealized delta waves in the upper gray line in *E*; negativity is upward). Unimodal phase preference of the distributions is clearly visible, with the mean phases near the negative peak of the delta waves (from 10% to 91%, in radians: 2.56, 2.85, 3.10, –3.03). The accuracy of phase entrainment (measured as the concentration (sharpness, κ) of phase histograms) increased with increasing levels of target predictability (κ values from 10% to 91%: 0.74, 0.82, 1.07, 1.19). The difference between the 37% and 64% as well as between the 64% and 91% conditions was significant (permutation tests with p values for the comparisons of 10% vs 37%, 37% vs 64%, and 64% vs 91%: 0.094, 0.0001, 0.036, respectively). (*I, J*) Distribution of delta-phase values (measured at Cz) at the time of the expected delivery of the early target in experiment 2. Trials from late-target trials (i.e., no early target was delivered) were pooled separately for p = 0.2 (*I*) and p = 0.8 (*J*) early-target probability from all participants (n = 11). (*K, L*) Individual (gray) and average (black) phase histograms for p = 0.2 (*K*) and p = 0.8 (*L*) target probabilities. Phase values were significantly more concentrated for high- than for low-probability targets (p = 0.024, permutation test; κ (mean phase): 0.27 (–2.84)

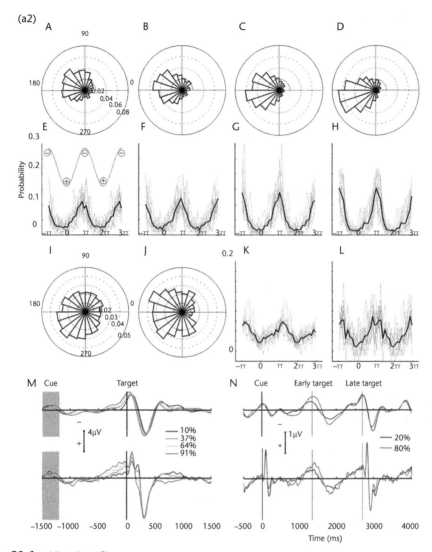

Figure 20-1a (Continued)

and 0.40 (–3.04), for the 20% and 80% target probabilities, respectively). (*M*) Average EEG traces from experiment 1 aligned at target onset (0 ms), filtered between 0.5–3 Hz (top) and 0.5–20 Hz (bottom). The traces were averaged separately for the four different levels of target predictability (10%; 37%; 64%; 91%). Note the amplitude increase at target onset with increasing levels of target predictability. (*N*) Average filtered EEG traces from experiment 2 aligned at the presentation of the cue tone, shown separately for the two different cue tones (late-target trials, only), filtered between 0.5–3 Hz (top) and 0.5–20 Hz (bottom). The average delta-wave amplitude was markedly higher at 1350 ms post-cue (the expected onset of the early target marked by the vertical dotted line) for cue 2 (early target by *p* = 0.8; vertical line) than for cue 1 trials (*p* = 0.2; vertical line). Reprinted with permission, from Stefanics G, Hangya B, Hernádi I, Winkler I, Lakatos P, Ulbert I. Phase entrainment of human delta oscillations can mediate the effects of expectation on reaction speed. *J Neurosci.* 2010 Oct 13;30(41):13578-85. Erratum in: *J Neurosci.* 2011 Jan 26;31(4):1559.

Most interestingly, such phase-locking significantly increased from the cue tone indicating 37% probability over the medium ones to the one signifying 91% target tone probability. The higher the predictability of the target tone as indicated by the cue tone in the phase preceding the target tone, the more the delta oscillations' phase onset was locked to the expected time of the target tone's onset.

How is such phase-locking possible? It is possibly only if the phases of the delta oscillations actively shift their onsets toward the predicted or expected onsets of the target tone. Higher predictability of the target tone's onset as indicated by the cue tone must have induced higher degrees of phase shifting of the delta oscillation's phase onset.

The phase onset of the delta oscillations thus followed the expected natural statistics of the target tone: different probabilities of the target tone's occurrence led consequently to different degrees of phase shifting. The results thus provide strong empirical support to the encoding of the stimuli's natural statistics by the phase shifting of especially low-frequency fluctuations like delta oscillations.

NEURONAL FINDINGS IB: ENCODING OF NATURAL STATISTICS INTO DELTA PHASE OSCILLATIONS

These results were demonstrated in the first experiment by Stefanics et al. (2010), where the prediction and thus the expected onset fell together with the onset of the presentation of the target tone. Hence, it remains impossible to disentangle the effects of the preceding resting state from the ones induced by the target tone itself. To distinguish both preceding resting-state and stimulus-induced activity, the investigators conducted a second experiment.

The second experiment presented the same target tone but now varied its temporal relationship to the cue tones by presenting the target tone either early, right after the cue tone, or rather late, with some temporal delay before the cue tone. Both early and late target presentations were preceded by two different cue tones that either indicated 20% or 80% target tone occurrence.

This allowed them to investigate especially the late-target tone trials where an early target tone was expected (with especially high probability of 80%) but not delivered. That made it possible to disentangle preceding resting-state activity and subsequent rest–stimulus interaction, including stimulus-induced activity.

How about the delta phase entrainment during those trials where a target tone was expected but not delivered? This pertains to those trials where a cue tone indicating high probability (80%) was followed by a late (rather than early) target tone. Delta oscillations were now locked in their phase to the expected onset of the target (i.e., the onset of the early target tone) even though it was not delivered (because it was a late target tone trial).

Such delta phase entrainment was observed in both conditions where cue tones (20%, 80%) were followed by late target trials (rather than early target trials). And as in experiment 1, the phase locking to the expected target tone onset was significantly higher in those trials with high-probability cue tones (80%) when compared to those with low-probability cues (20%; see Fig. 20-1b). The delta oscillations' phase onsets were thus shifted to the expected target tone onsets, even if the latter were not actually delivered.

NEURONAL FINDINGS IC: BEHAVIORAL RELEVANCE OF DELTA PHASE LOCKING

How is such delta phase locking related to behavior, that is, reaction times? Stefanics et al. (2010) conducted a correlation analysis between reaction time and delta oscillation phase. They observed that the delta phase locking at the onset of the target tone, independently of whether it was actually delivered (Experiment 1) or not, e.g., just expected (Experiment 2), significantly correlated with the reaction time in response to the respective target tones. The stronger the delta oscillation was phase-locked to the target tone onset (expected or presented), the shorter the reaction times. And as expected the correlation became stronger with increasing probability indicated by the cue tone.

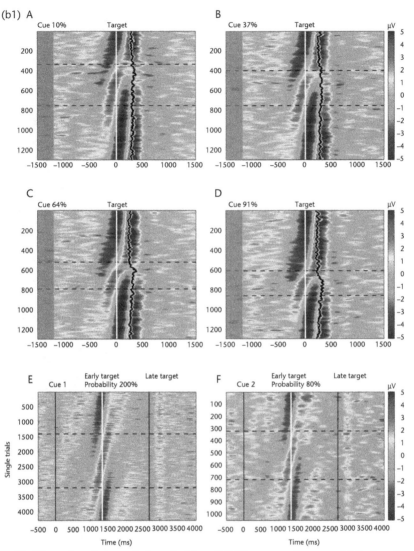

Figure 20-1b Natural statistics and phase locking. (*b1*) Phase-entrainment of delta-band EEG oscillations. (*A–D*) ERP images of single-trial responses filtered between 0.5 and 3 Hz from experiment 1, sorted by phase-values from –Π to Π at target onset time. Trials from all 13 subjects at Cz site from 10%, 37%, 64%, and 91% probability conditions are shown in plots *A–D*, respectively. *X*-axis: time in ms, *y*-axis: individual EEG traces, colors represent amplitude values. Shaded areas mark the random interval where the cues were presented between –1500 and –1200 ms preceding the target. Data were smoothed using a vertical window of 20 trials. Vertical white line at 0 ms represents the onset of the target tone, curved vertical black lines show single reaction time values, gray lines show SEM. Area between horizontal dashed lines contains trials with positive amplitude at target onset. Note the reduction of trials falling into this region with increasing target probability and the presence of oscillatory activity during the whole epochs. (*E, F*) ERP images of single-trial responses from experiment 2 from all 11 subjects, similar to plots *A–D*. Epochs from late-target trials, when no early target was delivered, are sorted by delta-phase values at the early (1350 ms) expected onset time (marked by vertical white lines); cue (0 ms) and late target (2700 ms) onset times are indicated by vertical black lines. Twenty percent and 80% expectancy conditions at Position 1 are shown in *E* and *F*, respectively. The proportionally smaller number of trials with less favorable phase values (between the horizontal dashed lines) in the

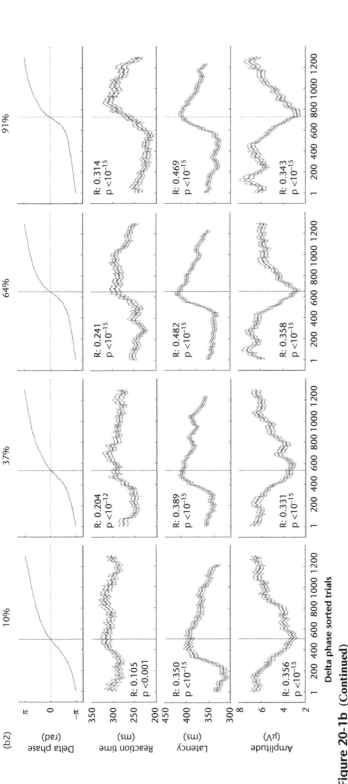

Figure 20-1b (Continued)

80% condition demonstrates that the accuracy of delta-phase entrainment increased at higher target probability. (*b2*) Task performance is correlated with delta phase modulation. First row: Central (Cz) delta-phase values measured at target onset, pooled, and sorted in ascending order from all trials of all participants in experiment 1 (1300 trials), separately for the four levels of target probability (from the left: 10%, 37%, 64%, 91%). The nonlinearity of the curves is the consequence of phase entrainment. Second row: RTs arranged in the same way. Data were smoothed for visualization using a 100-point sliding window (gray lines, SEM resulting from the smoothing). RTs significantly correlated with the delta phase at target onset (circular-linear correlation coefficients and *p* values are indicated on the plots). Fastest reactions were observed when the delta phase at the target onset fell on the rising slope of delta oscillation, near the negative peak (delta phase in radians at the minimal reaction time, from 10% to 91%: −2.76, −2.68, −2.56, −1.98, respectively). Third and forth rows: Latency and amplitude of the delta-peak component arranged similarly as in the rows above. These measures also correlated with the delta phase at the target onset, with minimal latency and maximal amplitude near the negative peak of delta oscillation (delta phase at the minimal latency, from 10% to 91%: −2.71, −2.57, −2.14, −2.13, respectively; delta phase at maximal amplitude, from 10% to 91%: −3.12, −3.11, −2.96, −2.93, respectively). Reprinted with permission, from Stefanics G, Hangya B, Hernádi I, Winkler I, Lakatos P, Ulbert I. Phase entrainment of human delta oscillations can mediate the effects of expectation on reaction speed. *J Neurosci.* 2010 Oct 13;30(41):13578−85. Erratum in: *J Neurosci.* 2011 Jan 26;31(4):1559.

The same relationship between phase locking and reaction time also holds true when subsequent event-related potentials like the P300 and their latency were included as possible covariates. This makes it unlikely that the reaction time was related to specific components of the stimulus-induced activity like the P300 and the latency. Instead, the behavioral measure, like the reaction time, must be related to the preceding resting state and the phase-locking of its delta oscillations.

Finally, the authors observed some regional specificity of these effects. The reported effects were observed in midline electrodes, Cz, Fz, and Pz. The authors also conducted the very same analyses in lateral electrodes (C3 and C4) to exclude effects related to motor readiness (and motor cortex as indicated by C3 and C4). Unlike in the midline electrodes, delta phase-locking was not observed in these more lateral electrodes. This suggests that the dependence of delta phase locking on the target tone's probability is rather unlikely to be related to motor readiness.

Taken together, the findings show that the phases of the delta oscillations in the resting state follow the statistical probability of the stimulus; e.g., its natural statistics. This means that the stimuli's statistical frequency distribution across their different discrete points in (physical) time rather than their actual discrete point in (physical) time is encoded by the phase onsets of the resting state's delta oscillations. More generally, these findings suggest the encoding of the stimuli's natural statistics, for example, their statistical frequency distribution (see Part I in Volume I for details), into the resting-state activity in general and its low-frequency fluctuations in particular.

Neuronal Hypothesis IA: Encoding of Natural Statistics into the Phase Onsets of the Delta Oscillations in the Resting State

We already discussed the encoding of neural activity at full length in Volume I and suggested difference-based coding as distinguished from stimulus-based coding to be the main encoding strategy of the brain (see Chapters 1–3). This applied to both resting-state activity (see Chapters 4–6) and stimulus-induced activity (see Chapters 10–12). Most important, such difference-based coding was supposed to enable the encoding of the stimuli's statistical frequency distribution and thus their natural statistics into the brain's neural activity.

In the following discussion, we will illustrate this by the results from the study by Stefanics et al. (2010). The findings from both studies by Stefanics et al. (2010) clearly demonstrate that delta phases entrain to the statistical frequency distribution of the stimuli. This is possible only by encoding the temporal differences between the stimuli's occurrence across their different discrete points in time. Most important, this also holds true in the absence of the stimulus, as demonstrated in the second experiment.

What is here encoded into neural activity is thus not the stimulus itself and its specific discrete point in time but rather the probability of its occurrence across different discrete points in physical time and space. How is the encoding of such probability possible? This is possible only by encoding the temporal difference between the stimulus' last occurrence and the stimulus' next expected occurrence as based on the previous temporal differences in the stimulus' occurrence.

This means that the encoding strategy is statistically based rather than physically based. Rather than encoding the physical features of the stimulus like its specific point in time, the delta phase encodes the stimulus' statistical frequency distribution across different discrete points in time and space. Only such statistically based coding strategy can account for the results in the second experiment, which otherwise should not show the alignment of the delta phases to the expected rather than the actual onset (see Part I in Volume I for details).

Let us summarize. What is encoded into the resting state's neural activity are the statistical frequency distributions of the stimuli's occurrence, that is, their probability, across different points in time and space. In contrast, the stimulus' physical features themselves are not encoded into the resting state's delta phase (see also Chapter 1, Volume I, for more details). Nor is a cognitive representation of the stimulus (and its physical features) encoded into the resting-state activity. Stefanics et al. (2010) tested for that by taking a cognitive potential, the P300, as covariate, which did not change the results. While this does not fully exclude cognitive encoding strategies, it makes them rather unlikely. This means that we have to search for neuronal mechanisms other than neurocognitive functions.

NEURONAL HYPOTHESIS IB: DIFFERENCE-BASED CODING MEDIATES THE ENCODING OF NATURAL STATISTICS INTO THE PHASE ONSETS OF THE DELTA OSCILLATIONS

What exactly is encoded in the resting state's neural activity? What is encoded in the resting state's neural activity is the temporal (and spatial) structure of the stimulus' statistical frequency distribution. We recall that there was not only delta phase locking in orientation to the onset of the target stimulus, which implies encoding of the stimuli's natural statistics. In addition, the authors also observed that the degree of this delta phase locking was very much dependent upon the degree of probability of the target stimulus' occurrence. This implies that the anticipated or expected natural statistics of the stimuli, rather than their actual natural statistics, are encoded into the resting state's neural activity.

Let me detail this assumption of the encoding of the expected or anticipated natural statistics. As the authors (Stefanics et al. 2010) themselves emphasize, their findings imply that the encoding process is not only passive and purely mechanistically based on the actual occurrence of the stimulus at its actual discrete points in (physical) time and space.

Instead, the resting state's encoding strategy is rather active in that it extracts and anticipates its probability and more specifically the expected or anticipated degree or statistical frequency distribution of the stimulus' occurrence across its different discrete points in (physical) time and space. Accordingly, what is encoded concerns the expected or anticipated natural statistics of the stimulus and thus their possible (or probable) natural statistics rather than the actual natural statistics.

Let me explain this a little further. Stefanics et al. (2010) observed clear dependence of the degree of delta phase locking on the statistical probability of the target tones' occurrence. The higher the latter's statistical probability, the higher the degree of delta phase locking.

How is such a relationship between delta phase locking and statistical probability possible? This is only possible if the delta oscillations encode the occurrence of the stimulus (independently of whether it is actually presented or is just expected) across different discrete points in (physical) time, thereby yielding a measure of its degree of statistical probability (as here operationalized in the experiment with the different cue tones).

How can the delta oscillations' phase encode the stimulus' occurrence across different discrete points in (physical) time? I hypothesize that the delta oscillations' phase encodes the temporal differences of the stimulus' occurrence across different discrete points in (physical) time, thus presupposing difference-based coding. Difference-based coding (in temporal regard) must be distinguished from stimulus-based coding, where only the discrete time point of the single stimulus itself, independently of its occurrence across time, is encoded into neural activity.

Finally, such a coding strategy, e.g., the encoding of the stimuli's natural and social statistics, can also be demonstrated in humans, such as, for instance, in auditory and visual cortex (Luo et al. 2010; Lakatos et al. 2008) and even in higher cognitive functions like speech and language (Schroeder et al. 2008; Howard and Poeppel 2010).

NEURONAL HYPOTHESIS IC: DIFFERENCE-BASED CODING VERSUS STIMULUS-BASED CODING IN THE PHASE ONSETS OF THE DELTA OSCILLATIONS

How can we further illustrate the difference between difference- and stimulus-based coding in the present context? Let us imagine the following highly simplified scenario. The larger the temporal difference between the occurrence of the same stimulus a across different discrete points in (physical) time, that is, time points $a(x)$ and $a(x + 3)$, the lower the statistical probability of its actual occurrence. Conversely, the smaller the temporal difference between the occurrence of the same stimulus a across different discrete points in (physical) time, that is, time points $a(x)$ and $a(x + 1)$, the higher the statistical probability of the occurrence.

How does that scenario relate to the observed results? The degree of delta phase locking was dependent upon the degree of the stimulus' degree of statistical probability. This is possible only when the delta oscillations' phase encodes the temporal difference between the same (and different) stimuli across different discrete points in (physical) time. Thereby the encoded temporal differences are based on the relative temporal positions of the stimuli to each other, that is, their temporal difference.

In contrast, these findings, that is, the similar results in experiments 1 and 2, are not compatible with the encoding of the stimulus' absolute temporal position by itself; that is, its single discrete point in (physical) time, independent of its occurrence later (or earlier) in time. The observed delta phase locking thus presupposes the encoding of temporal differences, that is, difference-based coding, rather than the encoding of the single discrete stimulus by itself, that is, stimulus-based coding (see Part I in Volume I for details).

In summary, the low-frequency oscillations' phase encodes and entrains very much the natural statistics and thus the temporal structure of stimuli rather than the stimulus itself and its discrete point in time. This is possible only on the basis of difference—rather than stimulus-based coding, which would make the encoding of the stimuli's natural statistics impossible (see also Volume I, Part I, for further details of the relationship between difference-based coding and natural statistics).

Neuroempirical Background II: From *Neuronal* Activity *in the Single* Brain to *Neurosocial* Activity *Between Different* Brains

I have so far discussed neuronal findings and hypotheses concerning the encoding of the stimuli's natural statistics into the brain's neural activity. This accounts for the encoding of the stimuli themselves, their natural statistics. In contrast, it leaves open whether the relationship

of the stimuli to other stimuli that constitute the respective social context is also encoded into neural activity (see Chapter 8 for details). In addition to the stimuli's natural statistics, its statistical relationship to others, their social statistics as I described it in Chapter 8, may also be encoded into neural activity. This will be the focus in the following sections.

How can the brain encode the social statistics of its environment into its neural activity? Due to the encoding of social statistics, the brain's neural activity is strongly dependent on its particular social context (in a non-instrumental way; see Chapter 8 in Volume I). For instance, the neural activity in one subject's brain may depend on what another subject is doing and its brain's activity. This is what I described in Chapter 8 as "context-dependence," which refers to the encoding of the spatial and temporal context of stimuli into the brain's neural activity.

I now want to expand the concept of such social context-dependence by showing tight if not intrinsic linkage between the brain's neural activity and the environment's social context. Several studies have been conducted that measure neural activity simultaneously in socially interacting subjects (see Lindenberger et al. 2011; and Hasson et al. 2012, for recent reviews). I here focus on two particular studies, one in fMRI during presentation of movies on different subjects, and another one using EEG in two guitar players. Let us start with the fMRI study.

Neurosocial Findings IA: Cortical Synchronization Between Different Brains' Neural Activities

Hasson et al. (2004) investigated five subjects in fMRI while they were all freely watching the same audiovisual movie for 30 minutes without any interruption. After having analyzed the regional activities in the brain of each subject by itself, they correlated each voxel in the brain of one subject, the "source subject," with the corresponding voxel in the same region in the other subject, the "target subject" (they had a total of 10 unique pairwise comparisons).

How are the neural activities of the two brains related to each other? The investigators observed highly significant correlations between source and target brains in the voxels and their time course of activity (across the 30 minutes of the movie). Twenty-nine percent +/– SD of all voxels on the cortical surface correlated between the two subjects' brains. The correlating voxels included both nonselective and selective regions. The nonselective regions spread beyond the audiovisual cortex to voxels in the ventro- and dorso-occipitotemporal cortex where intra- and intersubjective correlations could be observed. The authors suggested that these voxels reflect global activation that remains unspecific.

In contrast, the selective regions whose activities correlated between subjects were limited to specific regions; these included the superior temporal sulcus, the lateral sulcus, the retrosplenial cortex, and the secondary somatosensory cortex. In addition, the investigators also observed certain regions whose voxels did not correlate at all between the brains of both subjects. These noncorrelating regions included the supramarginal gyrus, the angular gyrus, and the prefrontal cortex.

Based on the distinction between regions that correlated between subjects and those that did not, the authors suggest a distinction between externally and internally oriented regions in the brain: the externally oriented regions follow the environmental stimuli and therefore synchronize their activity between subjects and their brains. Such synchronization can, in contrast, not be observed in those regions whose voxel did not correlate between the subjects' brains. Unlike the synchronizing and eternally-oriented regions, these regions' activities seem to be driven by the persons' internal processes rather than the external environmental stimuli.

Finally, the authors also investigated whether the time course of the regional activities predicted the contents in the movie (which they call a "reverse correlation approach," since usually the stimuli are assumed to predict the voxels' time courses rather than the voxels' time course predicting the stimuli). They looked at the time courses of the regions' activity and selected the strong peaks in their time course (while discarding the weak ones) during the 30 minutes' viewing of the movie.

This revealed strong activity peaks, especially during the emotionally charged and surprising moments in the movie. More specifically, activity peaks in the fusiform face area (FFA) occurred at exactly those time points when faces were presented in the movie. The same was observed in a building-related area, the collateral sulcus, whose activity peaked during indoor and outdoor scenes and building presentations in the movie.

Taken together, this study demonstrated cortical synchronization in the neural activity between different subjects' brains while watching an audiovisual movie. Since then, other studies have demonstrated similar synchronization in neural activity between different subjects and their brains during other tasks, such as during speaking and listening (see Stephans et al. 2010), music-making in different subjects (see Kokal et al. 2011, Lindenberger et al. 2009, Saenger et al. 2012), and various neuro-economic games (see Hasson et al. 2012, Saenger et al. 2011 for reviews). This suggests that there is indeed some kind of cortical synchronization between the brain's neural activities of different subjects. The exact neuronal mechanisms of such "neurosocial synchronization" remain unclear, however; this will be the focus in the next section.

NEUROSOCIAL FINDINGS IB: PHASE SHIFTING AS AN ACTIVE CONTRIBUTION OF THE BRAIN'S INTRINSIC ACTIVITY TO CORTICAL SYNCHRONIZATION BETWEEN DIFFERENT BRAINS

How is such cortical synchronization between the neural activities of different subjects' brains possible? One could first argue that the subjects were exposed to the same stimulus, the audiovisual movie, which elicited the same neural activity in different subjects. Cortical synchronization is therefore related completely and exclusively to the stimulus (or the task) itself, without any active contribution by of the brain itself.

However, we saw in the earlier-described study by Stefanics et al. (2010) that the brain's neural activity may indeed be able to actively interfere and shift, for instance, the phase onsets of its delta oscillations in dependence on the onset of the extrinsic stimuli in the environment. Such phase shifting may also underlie the observed cortical synchronization between the neural activities in the brains of different subjects.

Phase shifting would then be an active contribution by the brain itself that enable its alignment to its current social context. In contrast phase shifting could then no longer be regarded as the brain's merely passive processing of the extrinsic stimuli and their onsets. Is the assumption of phase shifting as an active (rather than passive) neuronal mechanism that underlies the cortical synchronization between different brains empirically plausible? This has been investigated in two studies on guitar players by Lindenberger et al. (2009) and Saenger et al. 2012). First, though, we need to briefly revisit the resting-state activity itself.

How can we support the claim that it is really the intrinsic activity that contributes to the social character of the brain's neural activity? If the intrinsic activity does indeed contribute to the social character of the brain's neural activity, one would expect neural overlap between resting-state activity and the neural activity during social-cognitive tasks.

This was investigated in a meta-analysis by Schilbach et al. (2012). They conducted a meta-analysis including imaging studies from all three kinds of studies, resting state, emotional tasks, and social-cognitive studies. In a first step, they analyzed the regions implicated in each of the three kinds of studies. This yielded significant recruitment of neural activity, especially in the midline regions like the ventro- and dorsomedial prefrontal cortex and the posterior cingulate cortex (bordering to the precuneus). In addition, neural activity in the temporo-parietal junction and the middle temporal gyrus was observed.

In a second step, they overlaid the results from the three kind of studies—emotional, social-cognitive, and resting state—in order to detect commonly underlying areas. This indeed revealed the midline regions, the dorsomedial prefrontal cortex and the posterior cingulate cortex, to be commonly shared among emotional and social-cognitive tasks and the resting-state activity. Based on this neural overlap, the authors suggested that there may be an intrinsically social dimension in our brain's neural activity in general and its intrinsic activity in particular (see also Schilbach et al. 2013; Pfeiffer et al. 2013).

The authors concluded that this neurosocial character of our brain's intrinsic activity may be central for consciousness,. They however let open the question of the exact neuronal mechanisms. This is the moment where the phase shifting described earlier may be relevant. We therefore now turn back to the phase shifting in an explicitly social context.

NEUROSOCIAL FINDINGS IC: PHASE LOCKING *WITHIN* BRAINS AND PHASE COHERENCE *BETWEEN* BRAINS

We have so far shown that the brain's intrinsic activity seems to have a social character. The exact neuronal mechanisms by means of which especially the intrinsic activity connects to the social environment remain unclear, however. For that answer, we now turn to a study investigating social interaction in EEG.

Lindenberger et al. (2009) investigated eight pairs of guitarists in EEG while playing together the same melody (in "60 trials," meaning 60 repetitions), a modern jazz fusion piece in E-minor with four quarters per measure. In each of the eight pairs of guitarists, they selected one lead guitarist, with the other one following. Before playing, they included a preparatory period where the two guitarists listened to a metronome and its beat.

Using EEG, they determined the "phase locking index" (PLI); they measured the invariance of phases across different trials from single electrodes within one subject's brain. This served to determine the degree of cortical synchronization between different electrodes within one particular brain related to one subject.

In addition, they calculated what they call "interbrain phase coherence" (IPC). The IPC measures the degree of constancy in phase differences across different trials in the same electrode from two different brains (of the two subjects in each pair) simultaneously. This served to determine the degree of cortical synchronization between the different subjects' brains in one particular electrode. They time-locked the periods around the onset of the metronome beat in the preparatory period and the play onset of the lead guitarists (three-second sequences with one second before onset and two seconds after). Based on prior considerations, they focused on lower and midrange frequencies up to 20 Hz.

What are the results? They observed increase in phase synchronization between the different electrodes within each subject thus reflecting the PLI. Such locking of the phase onsets between the different electrodes' activities within the subjects' brains was especially observed in the theta range (4–8 Hz) in fronto-central electrodes during both the onset of the metronome beats and the play onset of the lead guitarist. The task thus led to increased cortical synchronization between the different electrodes within the subjects' brains.

How about the cortical synchronization between the different subjects' brains? The increase in PLI in the brain of each subject was accompanied by an increase in IPC, the measure of the coherence of the phases between the brains of the two subjects. The fronto-central electrodes in particular showed increased phase coherence, especially in the delta range, between the brains of the two subjects while they were playing. Most interesting, such delta coherence between different subjects' brains was observed in relationship to the play onset of the lead guitarist and his starting gesture immediately prior to play onset. These data indicate increased cortical phase coherence between the neural activities in the different subjects' brains.

Taken together, the data show both increased cortical synchronization; that is, phase locking within subjects' brains (PLI), as well as increased phase coherence between different subjects' brains (IPC). How are both intra- and intersubject measures of neural activity related to each other? Interestingly, intrasubject phase locking and intersubject phase coherence were positively correlated: the higher the degree of the PLI; that is, the intrasubject phase locking, the higher the degree of the IPC; that is, the intersubject phase coherence.

Neurosocial findings id: phase coherence as an *active* contribution of the *single* brain to its relationship with *different* brains

One may now want to argue that such phase coherence between the different subjects' brains

can be traced to the similarity of stimuli (the guitarists were playing the same piece) with consequently the same perception, proprioception, and movements in both subjects. For that purpose, the same group conducted another study where they let the guitarists play different segments from the same piece: this time a classical piece, a rondo from an earlier composer (see Saenger et al. 2012). By letting the different guitarists play different segments of the same piece, they could control for the similarity or identity of the stimuli and tasks.

This allowed them to distinguish between "stimulus-related effects" and "brain-related effects" in the investigation of the neural similarities between the different subjects' neural activities. "Stimulus-related effects" concern the neural similarities between different subjects' neural activities that can be traced back to the exposure of the same stimulus to the different subjects. In contrast, the term "brain-related effects" refers to the neural similarities between different subjects' neural activities that can be traced back to the brain itself and an active contribution from its intrinsic activity, rather than to the exposure to the same stimulus material.

Let us return to the study that, as said, controlled well for stimulus-related effects in neural similarities between the different subjects' neural activities. The study investigated 32 guitarists with 16 overlapping duets and measured their neural activity in EEG while the guitarists were playing together. Unlike in the previous study, the investigators also manipulated the roles of leader and follower across the 16 pairs of guitarists. As in the previous study, PLI and IPC (and other whole-brain measures like small-network organization (which I only peripherally touch on here) were measured.

What are the results? This second study showed more or less the same results as in the first study. There was again increased phase-locking between electrodes (PLI) in the theta range in the brains of the single subjects during both the preparatory period and the playing period.

Moreover, the investigators observed a difference between leader and follower, with the leader showing strong PLI in the preparatory period, while the follower's PLI was rather strong in the playing period. Such intra-brain phase locking was, as in the previous study, accompanied by inter-brain phase coherence. There was phase coherence between the different subjects' brains (IPC) in frontocentral electrodes, especially in the delta range. As in the previous study, this suggests that intersubject phase coherence occurs mainly in lower-frequency ranges; namely, delta ranges, when compared to intrasubject phase synchronization that seems to be related rather to higher frequency ranges.

NEUROSOCIAL HYPOTHESIS IA: PHASE SHIFTING IN LOWER-FREQUENCY FLUCTUATIONS AS "BRAIN-RELATED EFFECT"

What are the neuronal mechanisms underlying the neurosocial communication between different brains? Let us start simply, with the neuronal mechanisms for which we consider both lines of studies, the one by Stefanics about phase shifting, and the ones about neurosocial communication between different brains.

The central finding in the neurosocial studies was the increased phase coherence between the different subjects' brains. This may be related either to the similarity in the stimulus material, to a stimulus-related effect, or to an active contribution by the brain itself: a brain-related effect (see earlier for this distinction).

Is the increased phase coherence between the subjects' neural activities a stimulus- or brain-related effect? Since Saenger et al. (2012) controlled well for stimulus similarity when letting the guitarists play different segments of the same melody, stimulus-related effects are rather unlikely. This means that the observed phase coherence between the different subjects' neural activities must be traced back to the brain itself thus entailing brain-related rather than stimulus-related effects.

Where does the brain-related effect come from? The single brain itself seems to provide an input that enables its phase coherence with other brains. The observed intersubject phase coherence must consequently be considered a brain- rather than stimulus-related effect. Let us specify the brain-related effect. The two neurosocial studies on the guitarists observed phase

coherence mainly in delta oscillations (as distinguished from the intrasubject phase-locking that occurred in the theta range). That meshes nicely with the earlier-described mechanisms of phase shifting in the delta frequency range as observed in the study by Stefanics et al. (2010). There the phase shifting in the delta oscillations was identified as a neuronal mechanism by means of which the brain's intrinsic activity can actively shifts its phase onsets towards the onsets of the stimuli.

Taking the results from both the Steanics' and the Saenger study leads me to the following tentative hypothesis. The lower-frequency ranges like the delta frequency seem to be specifically related to the neurosocial communication between the brains of different subjects because of their active phase shifting toward the stimuli onsets. Phase shifting in low-frequency ranges like delta thus seems to provide an active contribution of the brain itself, a brain-related effect, to the neurosocial communications between different brains. This, however, warrants future empirical investigation for support. Moreover, it remains to be investigated whether even lower-frequency fluctuations like < 0.1 Hz also provide such active phase shifting and thus brain-related effects.

NEUROSOCIAL HYPOTHESIS IB: ENCODING OF "NATURAL STATISTICS" DURING THE NEUROSOCIAL COMMUNICATION BETWEEN DIFFERENT SUBJECTS' BRAINS

What exactly does the phase shifting of the delta oscillations imply for the encoding of neural activity? As discussed earlier, phase shifting presupposes the encoding of the stimuli's statistical frequency distribution across their different discrete points in (physical) time and space. What is encoded into the brain's neural activity is not so much the single stimulus itself and its particular discrete point in (physical) time and space; instead, it is the statistical structure of the stimuli, their "natural statistics."

How does the assumption of the encoding of the stimuli's natural statistics stand in relation to the earlier-described results in the various neurosocial studies? Let us start with the fMRI study on the movie. The earlier described data show strong cortical synchronization between different subjects' brains when watching the same movie. The neural activity in a particular region in one subject predicted the same region's activity in another subject while watching the same movie.

How is that possible? I postulate that this is possible only by the encoding of the stimuli's natural statistics into the neural activity of the brains in the different subjects. While the subjects were watching the same movie, the stimuli showed the same statistical frequency distribution, which, if encoded into the neural activity of the different subjects' brains, should lead to the same kind of neural activity and thus to correlations in the regional neural activities between the different subjects.

That is exactly what the fMRI study during the watching of a movie by different subjects observed. Their data thus lend support, albeit indirectly, to the existence of encoding of the same natural statistics into the brain's neural activities of different subjects. Accordingly, by encoding the same stimuli in the same way, that is, in terms of their natural statistics, the brains of the different subjects can connect their neural activities.

NEUROSOCIAL HYPOTHESIS IC: STIMULUS-RELATED EFFECTS VERSUS BRAIN-RELATED EFFECTS

However, things are more complicated. In addition to the stimuli's natural statistics, their relationship to other stimuli is also encoded into the brain's neural activity. This, as discussed in Chapter 8, means that the stimulus' social context, like their relation and co-occurrence with other stimuli, is also encoded into the resulting neural activity. I therefore spoke of the encoding of the stimuli's "social statistics" into the brain's neural activity.

How does the encoding of the stimuli's social statistics stand in relation to the here described data on neurosocial communication? Our description has so far focused only on the encoding of natural statistics while leaving open the question of social statistics. The first study, the one on movie-watching in fMRI, cannot make any assumptions about that, because the

investigators did not control for stimulus-related effects as distinguished from brain-related effects.

We therefore cannot know whether the observed neural similarities between different brains are traceable to the stimuli themselves and the encoding of their natural statistics as stimulus-related effects; or alternatively whether the neural similarities are related to an active contribution by the brain, a brain-related effect that could (for instance) consist in encoding the social relations of the stimuli, their social statistics.

In contrast, the second study, the EEG study with the guitar players, controlled well for stimulus similarity and was therefore able to distinguish between stimulus- and brain-related effects. The increased phase coherence between the different subjects' brain must be considered an active contribution of the brain itself, a brain-related effect, rather than a stimulus-related effect. If so, one would expect that especially the social context of the stimuli, their social statistics, determines the neural similarities between the different subjects; that is, their phase coherence.

NEUROSOCIAL HYPOTHESIS ID: ENCODING OF *SOCIAL STATISTICS* DURING THE NEUROSOCIAL COMMUNICATION BETWEEN DIFFERENT SUBJECTS' BRAINS

Let us be more specific. We recall that the phases of the guitar player following the leader cohered and thus synchronized with those of the lead guitar player. The phases in the following guitar player synchronize in relation to their social context; namely, the rhythm of the tones as played by the lead guitar player.

Such phase coherence is possible only by encoding both natural and social statistics: The following guitar players hear the tones from the lead guitar player and encode their natural statistics into their own brain's neural activity. At the same time, though, the following guitar player also encodes the social context of the tones, that is with whom the tones are related, and where they come from, amounting to the tones' social statistics, into his neural activity. I consequently propose that the observed phase coherence between following and leading guitar players is only possible by encoding both natural and social statistics into neural activity.

This leads me to make the following neurosocial hypothesis. I postulate that the degrees of regional correlation and phase coherence between different subjects' neural activities is directly dependent upon the degree to which the stimuli's natural and social statistics is encoded into neural activity: the larger the degree of especially the stimuli's social statistics that is encoded into the brains' neural activity, the larger the degree of regional correlations and phase synchronizations between the neural activities in the different subjects' brains (see Fig. 20-2a).

We have to be again careful, however. The data (as described here, and some others; see Saenger et al. 2011, for an excellent review) show phase coherence between the different subjects' brains. While we may infer from the results a particular encoding strategy, namely, the encoding of both natural and social statistics, we still lack direct empirical support for the encoding of the stimuli's social statistics. Future experimenters may therefore want to test whether the observed inter-subject phase coherence corresponds to the statistical frequency distribution of the social context as related to the target stimuli and their natural statistics.

Finally, we also have to consider that neither of the neurosocial studies really distinguished between resting-state and stimulus-induced activity. If the encoding of social statistics is indeed an active contribution of the brain itself and thus a brain-related effect, one would expect it to be related to some neuronal feature in the intrinsic activity itself. This neuronal feature must characterize the intrinsic activity which in turn makes possible the active phase shifting and consequently the encoding of both natural and social statistics.

NEUROSOCIAL HYPOTHESIS IIA: THE BRAIN'S NEURAL ACTIVITY IS NECESSARILY NEUROSOCIAL BY DEFAULT

The encoding of both natural and social statistics has major reverberations for the characterization of the brain's neural activity in general and its intrinsic activity in particular. Since the encoding

of the stimuli's social statistics apparently cannot be avoided and occurs by default, the generated activity must be characterized as neurosocial rather than as merely neural. I consequently speak of 'neurosocial activity' in the following.

What exactly do I mean by the concept of "neurosocial activity"? The concept of "neurosocial activity" describes that the brain's neural activity is necessarily dependent upon its social context, thus reflecting what I describe as "social context-dependence" (see also Chapter 8). This means that the brain's neural activity is necessarily and unavoidably encoded and thus generated in relation to the brain's social context, its environment. The brain's activity can thus neither be characterized as exclusively neural nor as exclusively social but rather as neurosocial where both neural and social aspects are intrinsically tied together (see below for details).

Where does the neurosocial nature of the brain's activity come from? I postulate that the neurosocial nature of the brain's neural activity is predisposed by its particular coding strategy; namely, the encoding of the stimuli's social statistics. What is encoded into neural activity is not the single stimulus itself, but rather its spatial and temporal relationships to other stimuli. These spatial and temporal relationships to other stimuli signify the social context and marks the subsequently resulting activity as neurosocial rather than merely neural.

However, there may be different balances between natural and social statistics and their encoding into neural activity. The social statistics may be rather strong, in which case the natural statistics may be not as strongly encoded into the brain's activity. The converse case, with stronger natural statistics and weaker social statistics, may also be true (see Fig. 20-2b).

Put that into the context of different subjects and their respective brains, and it may lead to different constellations where different balances between natural and social statistics are encoded into the brain's activity. The encoded neural activity can thus be considered an amalgam of both neural and social components in different balances and constellations. This is what I mean when I characterize the brain's neural activity as "neurosocial."

(a)

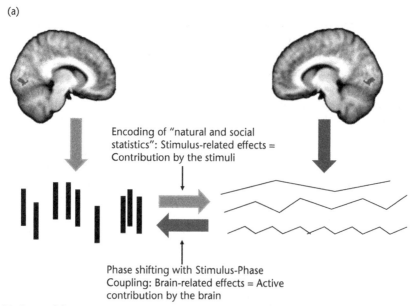

Encoding of "natural and social statistics": Stimulus-related effects = Contribution by the stimuli

Phase shifting with Stimulus-Phase Coupling: Brain-related effects = Active contribution by the brain

Figure 20-2a and b Interaction between different subjects' brains and the generation of "neuroso-cial activity." The figure illustrates the interaction between two different subjects' brains (*a*) and how that can lead to different modes of their brains' operation on a continuum between rhythmic and continuous modes (*b*). (*a*) The figure illustrates two different brains and how they interact. The left subject's' brain sends out some stimuli (lower left with vertical blue arrow) with a particular statistical-frequency distribution across different discrete points in physical time and space. Such "natural and social statistics" is encoded into the neural activity of the right subject's brain as indicated by the horizontal light gray arrow. The stimuli induce stimulus-related effects reflecting the effects of the stimuli in the other person's brain. The right subject's brain shows its own intrinsic activity as for instance its low and high-frequency fluctuations as indicated on the lower right with the vertical dark gray arrow. In order to adapt to the other subject and its brain, the right subject's brain shifts the onset of its phases of especially its low-frequency fluctuations in orientation on the statistical-frequency distribution of the stimuli send out by the left subject's brain; this is indicated by the horizontal dark gray arrow. This reflects the active contribution of the brain itself and thus brain-related effects rather than stimulus-related effects. Such phase shifting with stimulus-phase coupling happens off course also in the left subject's brain in orientation on the statistical-frequency distribution of the stimuli send out by the right subject's brain. That however, for the sake of simplicity, is not indicated here. The result of which is that the neural activity as generated in both subject's brain is intrinsically neurosocial rather than being merely neuronal. (*b*) The figure illustrates different modes of neural operation (rhythmic, continuous) in the subjects' different brains during their interaction. The degree of interaction for each subject is indicated by the arrows between them mirroring their degree of brain-to-brain coupling. Their respectively resulting neural activity may include both components neuronal (NN) and neurosocial (NS) components with both varying in different degrees in dependence on the mode of neural operation. Three different scenarios are sketched here. One subject may couple strongly while the other may not couple much entailing a rhythmic mode in the latter (with a high degree of the neurosocial component in their neural activity) and a continuous in the former (with a high degree of the neuronal component in their neural activity) (first scenario). Both subjects may not couple at all entailing a continuous mode in both subjects' brains (with a high degree of the neuronal component in their neural activity) (second scenario). And finally both subjects' brain may couple strongly with both brains being in a rhythmic mode (with a high degree of the neurosocial component in their neural activity) (third scenario).

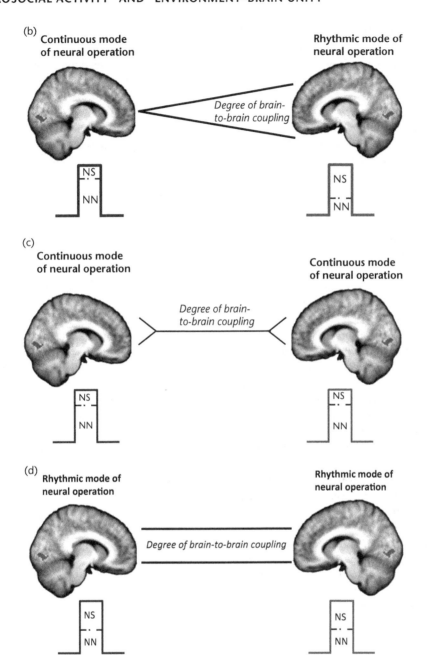

Figure 20-2a and b (Continued)

NEUROSOCIAL HYPOTHESIS
IIB: "NEUROSOCIAL ACTIVITY" VERSUS "NEUROSOCIAL FUNCTION"

Why do I postulate such a strong hypothesis that claims that any kind of neural activity is necessarily neurosocial? One could probably more easily swallow a weaker version of the same hypothesis; namely, that particular types or kinds of neural activity are related to specific social functions of the brain. The neurosocial character of the brain's activity would then be limited to the brain's neurosocial function, while it would not apply to the neural activities that are not related to the brain's neurosocial functions. This would amount to a narrow version of my neurosocial hypothesis as distinguished from a broader one.

Why do I prefer the broader to the narrow version? This shall be explicated in the following. My broader hypothesis is about how the brain generates neural activity, and by what kind of encoding strategy. I determined the brain's encoding strategy by difference-based coding that allows for the encoding of the stimuli's natural and social statistics. Since the encoding concerns all neural activity, my assumption of its necessary neurosocial character applies to any neural activity, including both intrinsic and extrinsic activity as well as any function ranging from sensory over affective, to cognitive and social functions of the brain.

This means that any neural activity that is encoded in terms of difference-based coding must be necessarily neurosocial. Since, however, difference-based coding comes in degrees and in reciprocal balance with stimulus-based coding (see Volume I), the neurosocial character of the brain's neural activity also comes in degrees, as described earlier. There is no purely neural or completely social activity that is encoded and generated. Instead, there are different degrees to which the generated neural activity is neurosocial.

On a whole, the difference between the broader and narrow versions of the neurosocial characterization of the brain's neural activity can be traced back to the distinction between "generation of activity" and "generation of function." (see also Introduction in Volume I for this distinction). The broader version is about the "generation of neural activity" and therefore concerns any neural activity including both intrinsic and extrinsic activity. This is different from the narrow version, which is rather about the "generation of function" and describes therefore only the neural activities that are specifically related to the brain's neurosocial functions that concern only stimulus-induced activity that is, extrinsic activity.

How are both broader and narrow versions related to each other? The "generation of function" presupposes the generation of neural activity, the "generation of activity", which therefore must be considered more basic and fundamental. Without generating neural activity, no function at all (including social functions) could get off the ground. Reflecting the generation of any kind of activity, the neurosocial character of the brain's activity must thus be assumed to provides the basis or blueprint for the subsequent generation of any kind of function, including social (and cognitive) functions as investigated in social and cognitive neuroscience.

NEUROSOCIAL FINDINGS IIA: "RHYTHMIC MODE" OF BRAIN FUNCTION

Both the neuronal findings by Stefanics and the various neurosocial results suggest that the neural processes in the brain of one subject are actively related to those in other subjects' brains. One may thus want to suggest that there is a "multi-brain frame of reference" rather than a "single-brain reference" (see Hasson et al. 2012).

This means that the neural processes in one brain are linked to the processes in another brain. There is therefore what can be described as "brain-to-brain coupling," which, as I will point out in the following explanation, has major implications for how we characterize the brain itself and its neural activity. This in turn is essential to understanding how the brain and its neural activity can predispose consciousness and its phenomenal unity.

What do these findings imply with regard to the characterization of the brain itself and its mode of neural operation? Based on their own findings, Schroeder and Lakatos (Schroeder et al. 2008; Schroeder and Lakatos 2009a and b, 2012; Lakatos et al. 2005, 2008, 2009; Schroeder et al. 2010) distinguish between a rhythmic and a continuous mode of neural operation by the brain, which nicely complements the here-described neurosocial findings. Let us start with the rhythmic mode.

In the case of a rhythmic mode, the brain's low-frequency fluctuations can align their phases with the statistical frequency distribution of the stimuli; e.g., their occurrence across different discrete points in (physical) time and space. The brain's intrinsic activity can *quasi* follow what occurs in the environment. In such a "rhythmic mode" of neural operation, the high-frequency oscillations during stimulus-induced activity are more or less aligned to the low-frequency fluctuations and their phase alignment to the statistical structure of the stimuli in the environment (see also Canolty and Knight 2010; Canolty et al. 2012; Sauseng and Klimesch 2008; Klimesch et al. 2010, for excellent and critical reviews of such stimulus-phase coupling).

There are two distinct processes in play in the rhythmic mode of brain function. First, there is the cross-frequency coupling that allows for coupling and linking—that is, entraining—high-frequency oscillations and even behavior to the phase of the ongoing low-frequency oscillation in the resting state. And secondly, there is the coupling or alignment of the resting state's low-frequency oscillations and especially their phases to the onset of the rhythmic or statistical structure of the stimuli's occurrence in the environment (see earlier and later for details).

NEUROSOCIAL FINDINGS IIB: "CONTINUOUS MODE" OF BRAIN FUNCTION

However, there are not always rhythmic stimuli in the environment that the brain and its intrinsic activity can align to. The rhythmic mode must therefore be distinguished from a more "continuous mode" of neural operation (Schroeder and Lakatos 2009a and b).

Unlike in the rhythmic mode, there seems to be no particular rhythm or statistical structure in the stimulus presentation to which the resting-state activity's low-frequency oscillations (and subsequently the higher frequencies and behavior) can entrain and align their phase onsets. In other words, the brain is now "left to itself" and must therefore by itself actively structure and organize its own intrinsic activity.

How can the brain structure and organize its own intrinsic activity? The brain can no longer rely on the rhythmic presentation of the stimuli and process them passively but must become active itself; that is, continuously active. Instead of adapting the high-frequency oscillations to the lower ones, as in the rhythmic mode, the stimulus-induced high-frequency oscillations are now "on their own" in the continuous mode.

This means that the stimulus-induced high-frequency oscillations must account for the stimulus independently of the resting-state activity's low-frequency oscillations and their phase onsets because the latter are no longer aligned to the statistical structure of the stimuli. Rather than being helpful by aligning themselves to the extrinsic stimuli as in the rhythmic mode, the resting-state activity's low-frequency oscillations may now stand in the way of the stimulus-induced high-frequency oscillations.

Increased higher frequencies like gamma may thus be accompanied by their decreased cross-frequency coupling to lower frequencies and their phase onsets. This is exactly what has been observed in paradigms without rhythmic presentation of stimuli to which the delta (and subsequently gamma) oscillations of the resting state can entrain (see, for instance, Fries et al. 2001; see also the next sections for more details).

The low-frequency fluctuations are consequently suppressed, while the high-frequency fluctuations are strengthened in order to process the stimuli. The temporal pattern in the "continuous mode" is thus the reverse of the one in the "rhythmic mode," where the low-frequency fluctuations are strong and the high-frequency fluctuations are rather weak.

NEUROMETAPHORICAL EXCURSION IA: TOKYO IN A "RHYTHMIC MODE"

How can we further illustrate the rhythmic and continuous modes of brain function? Besides the earlier described findings of phase coherence between different subjects' brains, let us imagine that you are in the middle of Tokyo with a good friend who knows the city well. Will you study maps and search the Internet for travel tips? No, you will simply follow your friend who knows the city well.

Nor will you think much? about the way he leads you. Hence, you will not spend much mental effort to figure out the exact way to your destination as long as you can follow your friend. Your friend will set the pace and you will adapt, rather than setting your own pace. Why waste your precious cognitive and mental resources if you do not need to do so?

This is exactly what the brain seems to "think," too. Why shall it waste its neuronal resources when it can simply follow the rhythmic presentation of the stimuli and thus the statistical structure of their occurrence in the environment? Instead of actively structuring its low-frequency oscillations by itself and its own resources, the resting-state activity simply follows passively the statistical structure of the stimuli's occurrence in the environment.

Accordingly, in the same way that you follow your friend's pace and rhythm of steps in Tokyo, the phases of the resting-state activity's low-frequency oscillations follow the pace and intervals, or rhythms, of the stimuli's occurrence in the environment. The same may also hold true in the case of the body's predominantly interoceptive stimuli: the brain's resting-state activity may simply follow their rhythm, like the rhythm of the heart, for which there is indeed some recent empirical support (see Chang et al. 2012).

What does this tell us about the brain and its intrinsic activity? Both exteroceptive stimuli in the environment and interoceptive stimuli in the body may serve as "pacemakers" for the brain's intrinsic activity in the same way your friend in Tokyo serves as a "pacemaker" for your own intrinsic physical and mental activity (as well as for your brain's neuronal activity). Why should the brain be different from us as persons, after all?

Neurometaphorical Excursion
IB: Paris in a "Continuous Mode"

How does the continuous mode of brain function compare to our metaphorical example? You are now in Paris, and you do not know anyone there. You are on your own and must find your way by yourself. You also forgot your iPhone so that you cannot "google." Nor do you speak French or English; hence, there is no way for you to communicate with other people. And there is no Internet café around, either.

What now? You are lost in the mass of similar-looking streets. How to get back to your hotel? You have no idea. You recruit all your cognitive and mental efforts to figure out the way. You become continuously active by yourself to find your way back to the hotel. You are thus no longer passively in a "following mode" as corresponding to the brain's "rhythmic mode," but rather active in a "continuous mode."

The same is true again in the case of the brain. If there are no rhythmic stimuli in the environment, the brain's intrinsic activity can no longer follow and align itself to them. The only option for the brain's intrinsic activity is thus to become "active by itself," meaning continuously active. The brain must thus revert from a "rhythmic mode" to a "continuous mode" in its neural operation.

Let us carry your brain back to Paris. You are still in Paris and haven't found your way yet back to the hotel. You become exhausted. Spontaneously, you have the urge to follow somebody. This would make your life easier and would relieve you of all your cognitive and mental efforts to find the way by yourself. But that is dangerous, since you do not know where the person is heading.

And asking the person is no option either, because you speak neither English nor French. Hence, you try to suppress that urge. Your attention will be refocused from following other people to detecting some signposts that may guide you on the "right" way toward your hotel.

This is exactly what the brain is doing in the case of a non-rhythmic structure of stimuli. In the same way as you suppressed your urge to follow another person, the brain suppresses its own low-frequency oscillations, including the alignment of their phase onsets; they are then no longer in the way of the stimulus-induced high-frequency oscillations that may make possible the detection of signposts for the "right" way. This means that high-frequency oscillations like gamma become more independent and consequently stronger in their power with decreased synchronization of their phases and power to the phases of the lower-frequency oscillations.

Neurophenomenal Hypothesis IA: Phase Locking and Consciousness

Where are we now? We showed that the brain's intrinsic activity, its delta oscillations, align their phase onsets to the onsets of the extrinsic stimuli in the environment. These findings by Stefanics were complemented by results from neurosocial communication that showed direct cortical synchronization and phase coherence between different subjects' brains. This was suggested to lead to different modes of brain function, *rhythmic* and *continuous*. Taken together, this suggests that the brain's neural activity is intrinsically neurosocial as it is related to the encoding of the respective spatial and temporal contexts.

How, then, are the intrinsically neurosocial character of the brain's neural activity and its different modes of operation related to consciousness and its phenomenal unity? Unfortunately, neither of the earlier-described studies included any measures of consciousness, so the exact relationship between neurosocial activity and consciousness remains unclear at this point. In order to develop specific neurophenomenal hypotheses, we here rewind briefly to the phenomenal unity and the prephenomenal unity as discussed in the previous chapters.

The concept of phenomenal unity describes the unity that we experience when a particular object or event consisting of a multitude of stimuli becomes conscious. Thereby the phenomenal unity was characterized by both phenomenal content and phenomenal state. Both phenomenal state and phenomenal content were shown to be predisposed by the resting state preceding the stimulus onset (see Chapters 18 and 19).

This let me consider the resting-state activity itself in further detail (see Chapter 19). The phases of the resting-state activity's low-frequency fluctuations entrain the stimulus-induced high-frequency oscillations. This makes possible the constitution of the carryover and transfer of the resting-state activity's spatial and temporal continuity to the stimulus and the subsequent integration of its discrete point in physical time and space into the statistically based spatial and temporal unity of neuronal activity (during stimulus-induced activity).

What does our characterization of the brain's intrinsic activity as neurosocial imply for the carry-over and transfer? The low frequency fluctuations of the resting state do not only entrain the higher frequency fluctuations of the specific stimulus but are by themselves entrained by the frequency distribution of the ongoing stimuli in the environment. This relation of the resting state's low frequency fluctuations to the environment is consequently carried-over and transferred to the resting state itself from where it is carried-over and transferred to the stimulus-induced activity.

The resulting neuronal unity of the stimulus-induced activity is thus build not only on the pre-phenomenal unity of the resting state itself but also on the resting state's alignment with the environment and its natural and social statistics, an "environment-brain unity" as I will call it in the following. I now postulate that the "environment-brain unity" that is, the resting state's degree of phase locking to the onset of the environmental stimuli, is directly relevant for consciousness: the better the phases of the resting state's low frequency fluctuations are locked to the onset of the environmental stimuli, the higher the possible degree of consciousness that can be associated with specific stimuli. In short, I hypothesize that the environment-brain unity predisposes consciousness. In order to better understand this rather daring hypothesis, we must characterize the concept of the environment-brain unity in more empirical detail.

NEUROPHENOMENAL HYPOTHESIS IB: ENCODING OF NATURAL AND SOCIAL STATISTICS AND THE "ENVIRONMENT–BRAIN UNITY"

How can we describe the postulated "environment-brain unity" in further detail? The resting-state activity's temporal and spatial unity is supposed to predispose the degree of phenomenal unity associated with the subsequent stimulus-induced activity.

The stronger the carryover and transfer of the resting-state activity's temporal and spatial unity, the more the unity associated with the stimulus-induced activity will be extended in space and time, and the more likely a phenomenal state and thus consciousness will be associated with the respective stimulus and its stimulus-induced activity. The resting-state activity's spatial and temporal unity can therefore be characterized as a prephenomenal unity that as such predisposes the degree to which a phenomenal unity can possibly be associated with the stimulus and its stimulus-induced activity.

How is the resting state's prephenomenal unity related to the resting state's statistically based encoding strategy, the difference-based coding as the encoding of the stimuli's natural and social statistics? The statistically based encoding strategy implies that the duration of the resting state's low-frequency oscillations may correspond to the temporal (and spatial) differences between the stimuli's statistically based occurrence in the environment; that is, their natural and social statistics. If the stimuli occur rhythmically though slowly, with larger temporal differences between them, the resting-state activity's phase onsets will align and thus entrain to them by recruiting and shifting the phase onsets of its lowest-frequency oscillations (like the frequencies lower than delta in the range of 0.001–0.01 Hz).

If, in contrast, the stimuli occur rhythmically but in a fast pace with small temporal differences, the resting-state activity will recruit, shift, and align the phases of its higher-frequency oscillations (like delta and higher) because of the shorter duration of their phases. The recruitment, shifting, and alignment of the low-frequency fluctuations' phase onsets and durations in the resting-state activity may thus depend upon the statistically based temporal (and spatial) differences of the stimuli's occurrence across different discrete point in (physical) time (and space) in the environment.

What does the statistically-based encoding of the environment's natural and social statistics imply for the brain's relationship to the environment? The brain's resting-state activity is always already connected to the environment in a statistically based and thus virtual way. There is thus a certain statistically based virtual unity between environment and brain, which I describe by the concept of "environment–brain unity."

This statistically-based virtual unity between environment and brain is natural and social at the same time. It is based on the encoding of the natural statistics of the stimuli themselves which makes the environment-brain unity natural. At the same time, the relation of the natural stimuli to the other stimuli and thus their social statistics is also encoded into the resting state's neural activity. This makes the environment-brain unity not only natural but also social. Metaphorically speaking, the environment–brain unity can therefore be considered an amalgam of intrinsically interwoven and inseparable natural and social features.

NEUROPHENOMENAL HYPOTHESIS IC: THE "ENVIRONMENT–BRAIN UNITY" IS STATISTICALLY AND SPATIOTEMPORALLY BASED

How now can we characterize the environment-brain unity in further detail?

The concept of the environment–brain unity[1] describes a virtual statistically based spatiotemporal linkage and integration (and thus unification) between the environmental stimuli and the brain's resting-state activity. More specifically, the temporal (and spatial) differences in the environmental stimuli's occurrences across different discrete points in (physical) time and space are proposed to correspond to the temporal duration (and the spatial extension) of the resting-state activity's low-frequency phase durations (and distances between regions in functional connectivity).

This signifies the environment–brain unity as spatiotemporal. The spatiotemporal character of the environment-brain unity refers to the fact that the environment-brain unity is based on spatial and temporal differences rather than on single discrete points in time and space. The environment-brain unity is thus difference-based rather than stimulus-based. If the environment-brain unity were indeed stimulus-based, it would be atemporal and aspatial rather than temporal and spatial.

There is however more to consider. Since the brain's encodes the natural and social statistics of the stimuli in the environment, the environment–brain unity is not only spatiotemporally based but also statistically based[2]. The statistically-based nature of the environment-brain unity must be distinguished from a merely physically-based nature where it would be based on the physical features of the stimuli themselves rather than their statistical frequency distribution. This however is not the case. Instead, the statistical frequency distribution is encoded into the environment-brain unity. Since the stimuli and their statistical frequency distribution in the environment continuously change, the encoded neural activity and consequently the environment-brain unity too continuously change. This makes the environment-brain unity and its related activity like its degree of phase locking flexible and dynamic rather than being merely static and fixed. (see Fig. 20-3).

Neurophenomenal Hypothesis
IIA: Modes of Brain Functions and the "Environment–Brain Unity"

I so far characterized only the environment-brain unity while leaving open its relationship to consciousness. This shall be the focus in the remaining sections.

How does the statistically- and spatiotemporally-based environment-brain unity stand in relation to the different modes of brain function as described by Schroeder and Lakatos? I suggest that both rhythmic and continuous modes can be regarded extremes on a continuum of different possible relationships between brain and environment. They thus signify the dynamic and flexible nature of the environment–brain unity.

More specifically, rhythmic and continuous modes of the brain's operation reflect different relationships between natural and social statistics during the encoding of neural activity. The rhythmic mode can be characterized by a strong encoding of social statistics, whereas the degree of the encoded social statistics is rather low in the continuous mode. The different modes do consequently reflect different constellations in

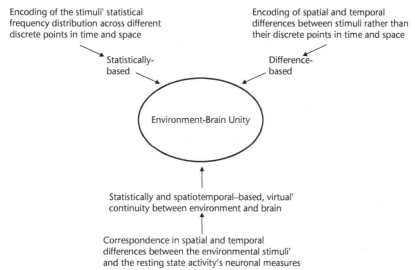

Figure 20-3 Characterization of the environment-brain unity. The figure shows central features of the environment–brain unity. It is based on the encoding of the stimuli's statistical-frequency distribution across their discrete points in time and space, their natural and social statistics (*upper left*). This implies a statistically rather than physically based encoding strategy, one that is based on the statistical rather than physical features of the stimuli. That is possible by encoding temporal and spatial differences between different stimuli across their different discrete points in physical time and space (*upper right*). That implies difference-based coding as distinguished from stimulus-based coding. The resting state aligns its spatial and temporal measures to the onset of the stimuli in the environment (*lower part*). This results in statistically and spatiotemporal correspondence and continuity between the environment's and the resting state's spatial and temporal measures. The resulting environment–brain unity can thus be characterized as statistically and spatiotemporally based and thus as "virtual."

the degrees of natural and social statistics during the encoding of neural activity (see earlier).

This leads me to the following hypothesis. The two different modes of neural operation, rhythmic and continuous, entail different degrees of the environment–brain unity: the more rhythmic the environmental stimuli, the better the resting state's low frequency fluctuations can lock their phase onsets to the stimuli and encode their natural and social statistics, the higher the degree of a rhythmic mode, and the higher the subsequent degree of the environment–brain unity.

In contrast, a less rhythmic stimulus occurrence in the environment makes both phase-locking and encoding of natural and social statistics more difficult for the resting state's low frequency fluctuations. This increases the degree of the resting state's continuous mode which in turn lowers the degree of the environment–brain unity. Accordingly, I propose both the degree of the environment–brain unity to be dependent upon the environmental stimuli's degree of rhythmicity and the subsequent degrees of phase-locking and encoding of natural and social statistics by the resting state activity (see Fig. 20-4a).

NEUROPHENOMENAL HYPOTHESIS IIB: THE "ENVIRONMENT-BASED HYPOTHESIS OF PREPHENOMENAL UNITY"

How do the different degrees of the environment–brain unity stand in relation to the prephenomenal unity of the resting-state activity? As shown earlier, the environment–brain unity can be characterized as virtual statistically based spatiotemporal unity; this is supposedly manifested in the shifting of the phase durations of the resting-state activity's low-frequency oscillations (and the spatial extension of its functional connectivity) in orientation on the stimuli's natural and social statistics.

As such, the resting-state activity's temporal (and spatial) unity with the environment (as constituted by the low-frequency oscillations and the functional connectivity) sets the temporal (and spatial) frame within which the prephenomenal unity can be constituted. This means that the degree of statistically based temporal

(and spatial) extension of the environment–brain unity predisposes the possible degrees of the prephenomenal unity and its spatiotemporal extension that can be constituted by the brain's resting-state activity. Let us exemplify this by the temporal dimension. The statistically based temporal unity of the environment–brain unity is determined by the shifting of the phase duration of the resting-state activity's low-frequency oscillations as manifested in how well their phase onsets align to the natural and social statistics of the stimuli in the environment.

The shifting of the phase onsets and subsequently of the low-frequency oscillations' phase durations provides, in turn, the time window within which high--frequency oscillations and their shorter phase durations can be aligned and thus entrained during the resting-state activity (see Chapters 18 and 19 for details). Since the resting-state activity's prephenomenal unity can be defined by the degree of alignment between high- and low-frequency oscillations, the temporal unity of the environment–brain unity must predispose the possible degree of the temporal extension of the prephenomenal unity.

Based on these considerations, I claim that the statistically based virtual environment–brain unity predisposes the possible degree of temporal and spatial extension of the prephenomenal unity. Accordingly, I propose the environment–brain unity to be a necessary condition and thus a neural predisposition of the possible constitution of the prephenomenal unity by the resting-state activity.

And since the prephenomenal unity is by itself a neural predisposition for the phenomenal unity of consciousness (see Chapters 18 and 19), the environment–brain unity must be suggested to predispose the phenomenal unity of consciousness (albeit indirectly via the prephenomenal unity). I consequently speak of what I describe as the "environment-based hypothesis of prephenomenal (and phenomenal) unity."

What do I mean by the "environment-based hypothesis of prephenomenal unity"? The environment-based hypothesis of prephenomenal unity proposes the statistically based spatiotemporal relationship of the brain's intrinsic activity to the environment to first and foremost

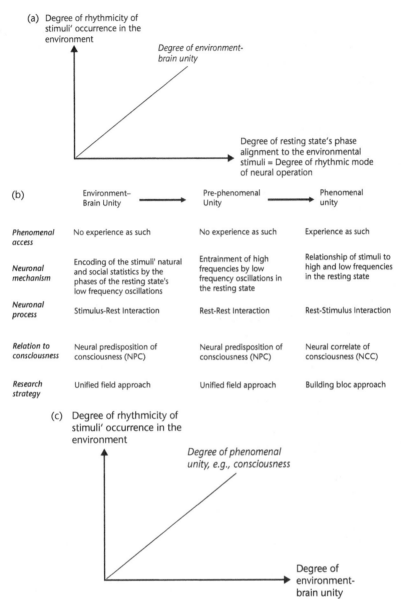

Figure 20-4a-c "Environment–brain-based hypothesis of prephenomenal unity." (*a*) The figure shows distinct aspects of the environment-based hypothesis of prephenomenal unity. The degree to which the resting-state activity can align its phase onsets to the stimuli in the environment very much depends on the degree to which the latter occur in a rhythmic way. The more rhythmic the environmental stimuli occur, the more likely the resting-state activity can align its low-frequency fluctuations' phase onsets to them, and the higher the degree of the statistically and spatiotemporally based virtual environment–brain unity. (*b*) The figure demonstrates how the phenomenal unity and its underlying neuronal mechanisms (*right part*) are based on the resting-state activity's prephenomenal unity (*middle part*), which in turn is based on the environment–brain unity (*left part*). The figure can be read from left to right; this will provide a forward movement from neuronal mechanisms to the phenomenal unity of consciousness. (*c*) The figure shows the dependence of the degree of phenomenal unity on both the degree of the environment–brain unity and the degree of rhythmicity of the stimuli's occurrence in the environment. The more rhythmic the stimuli occur in the environment, the higher the degree of the environment–brain unity, and the higher the possible degree of the phenomenal unity and thus consciousness.

make possible and thus to predispose the possible constitution of the phenomenal unity of consciousness. Accordingly, the environment-based hypothesis of prephenomenal unity describes a neural predisposition rather than a neural correlate of consciousness.

NEUROPHENOMENAL HYPOTHESIS IIC: ENVIRONMENT-BRAIN UNITY AND THE PHENOMENAL UNITY OF CONSCIOUSNESS

How does my "environment-based hypothesis of prephenomenal unity" stand compared to my other neurophenomenal hypotheses? The environment-based hypothesis of prephenomenal unity complements my "continuity-based hypothesis of phenomenal unity" (see Chapter 19) and my "resting state–based hypothesis of prephenomenal unity" (see Chapter 18).

How exactly are these three hypotheses related to each other? The environment-based hypothesis of prephenomenal unity is the most basic one, since it provides the predisposing ground upon which the two other hypotheses stand: both prephenomenal unity and phenomenal unity are suggested to be possible only on the ground or basis of the environment–brain unity. Without the latter, the former would simply remain impossible. Therefore, I propose the "continuity-based hypothesis of phenomenal unity" to be nested within the "resting state-based hypothesis of prephenomenal unity", which in turn is nested within and thus based on the "environment-based hypothesis of prephenomenal unity" (see Fig. 20-4b).

How are environment–brain unity and phenomenal unity related to each other in more detail? One may want to propose the following relationship: The higher the degrees of rhythmic stimulus presentation and the associated environment–brain unity, the higher the probability that higher degrees of the phenomenal unity and thus of consciousness can possibly be associated with the respective stimuli.[3] In contrast, lower degrees of rhythmic stimulus presentation and environment–brain unity may decrease the possible degrees and thus the probability of the subsequent association with phenomenal unity in particular and consciousness in general.

This implies that the degree of the phenomenal features (of the phenomenal unity) like wholeness and non-structural homogeneity (see Chapters 18 and 19) may be dependent upon the degree of both rhythmic stimulus presentation and the associated environment–brain unity: A high degree of wholeness and nonstructural homogeneity (as phenomenal features of phenomenal unity; see Chapters 18 and 19) will more likely occur in the case of high degrees of rhythmic stimulus presentation and environment–brain unity (see Fig. 20-4c).

Taken together, this amounts to the following. A more rhythmic mode of stimulus presentation in the environment is more likely to go along with a higher probability of phenomenal unity and thus of consciousness of the respective objects or events in the environment. Accordingly, a more rhythmic mode of neural operation will be more likely associated with a high degree of consciousness of the respective environmental object or event than a continuous mode. In short, rhythmic stimulus presentation and a rhythmic mode of neural operation make phenomenal unity and thus consciousness more likely than a non-rhythmic mode.

How can we support this empirically? Very simple. We all know only too well that a rhythmic presentation of stimuli like in music (if not too repetitive though), considerably enhances our consciousness of that melody. The melody stays with us, its tunes reverberate in our mind. And, if shared with others, we all make the same movements and dance with each other as in the case of drumming. The phenomenal unity of consciousness is here accompanied by a social unity with shared consciousness among different subjects.

How is such sharing of experience possible? I suggest that such shared experiences can ultimately be traced back to the degree to which our brain's resting state activity can lock its phase onsets to the onsets of the environmental stimuli and thereby encode their natural and social statistics. The environment-brain unity is thus a shared unity that not only unifies our brain with the environment but also different subjects within that very same environment in a statistically- and spatiotemporally-based way. The environment-brain unity is consequently neurosocial and that is, as I suggest here, central for making possible and thus predisposing consciousness. Accordingly, without the neurosocial character of our brain's activity and its environment-brain unity, we would not be able to develop any consciousness at all.

Open Questions

One of the main questions is how we can experimentally investigate this environment–brain unity. I gave clear neuronal criteria like the degree of correspondence between the environmental stimuli's statistically based temporal differences and the shifting of the phase duration (via the shifting of the phase onsets) of the resting state's low-frequency oscillations. Further criteria need to be developed in the future, however.

There is a strong debate in the current literature about whether event-related potentials as measured with EEG can be traced back to phase shift with phase resetting or to the activity evoked by the stimulus itself (see Sauseng and Klimesch 2008). The debate is still open and yet unresolved. What is clear is that the phase shift or phase resetting as induced by the stimulus is a central and generally acknowledged neuronal mechanisms that has been observed especially in the context of memory in prefrontal cortex and hippocampus (Fell and Axmacher 2011; Sauseng and Klimesch 2008; Klimesch et al. 2010; Canolty and Knight 2010).

Moreover, one would like to investigate different degrees of the environment–brain unity in relation to consciousness. This could be done by, for instance, testing the impact of rhythmic and non-rhythmic stimulus presentation on the degree of the phenomenal features of phenomenal unity, that is, wholeness and nonstructural homogeneity (see Chapter 30 for details about these phenomenal features). That would allow for testing the following hypothesis: the more rhythmic the stimulus presentation, the higher the degree of the environment–brain unity, and the higher the possible degrees of wholeness and nonstructural homogeneity in consciousness.

Conceptually, we should be careful not to confuse the concept of the neurosocial activity with the philosophical concept of intersubjectivity. Traditionally, the concept of "intersubjectivity" describes the relationship between different subjects and is therefore a cognitive or phenomenal concept. In contrast, "neurosocial activity" is an empirical concept that describes the brain's neural activity. To confuse intersubjectivity and neurosocial activity is thus to confuse phenomenal/cognitive and empirical/neural concepts. However, the neurosocial activity predisposes possible intersubjectivity and can therefore be considered a neural predisposition (rather than neural correlate) of possible (rather than actual) intersubjectivity.

Another issue is of a more methodological nature, in that it concerns the principal research strategy. Searle (2004, 105–108) distinguishes between the "building block approach" and the "unified field approach" in current neuroscience. The building block approach presupposes that one particular form of consciousness, such as, for instance, visual consciousness and its neuronal mechanisms, can be investigated. From there one may infer the neuronal mechanisms underlying other forms of consciousness like auditory consciousness or even self-consciousness and ultimately consciousness as such. This research strategy thus proceeds as if there are different unities or blocks of consciousness, hence the name "building block approach."

The assumption of such different unities or blocks is denied in the unified field approach. Here, the research into the neuronal mechanisms underlying specific forms of consciousness will tell us something about that particular modality or form of consciousness but not about consciousness as such. For that, one may, following Searle, need to investigate the unity by itself that underlies any and thus all specific forms of consciousness. Hence, the strategy here is to investigate the unified field that supposedly underlies all forms of consciousness, which then serves as the very basis for understanding the neuronal mechanisms underlying the different forms of consciousness.

How do these approaches stand in relation to my distinction between different unities, environment–brain, prephenomenal, and phenomenal? The building-block approach targets the phenomenal unity and the neuronal processing of specific phenomenal contents regardless of whether they enter consciousness. The "unified field approach" seems to be compatible with the "environment-brain unity" and the "prephenomenal unity" (see also Fig. 20-3b). This, however, must be debated in the future.

One may also want to raise an even more theoretical question, the one for the conceptual characterization of the brain. In the context of the philosophy of mind, there have been approaches that characterize the concept of mind as extended; they describe the mind as closely related to the environment, thus reaching beyond itself. Considering the suggested close statistically and spatiotemporally based unity between environment and brain, one may be inclined to speak of a concept of the "extended brain." Analogously to the concept of the extended mind, the one of the brain describes the brain's intrinsic linkage to the environment. That, however, dents deeply into the conceptual determination of the brain (see also Chapters 1 and 2 in Northoff 2011), which is beyond the scope of this chapter and book.

Finally, one may want to propose that the neural principles underlying the constitution of the environment–brain unity may also operate in the case of the alignment of the brain's intrinsic activity to the input from its own body. Unlike the environmental stimuli, the stimuli from the brain's own body, like the ones from the heart, occur in a much more rhythmic way. One may thus propose the rhythmic mode to be predominant in the case of the body–brain unity, which, like the environment–brain unity, may be virtual, statistically based, and spatiotemporal.

There may thus be no principal difference between environment–brain unity and body–brain unity, with both showing the same basic features and being based on the same encoding strategy. There may, however, be a difference in degree between both unities: Due to the higher degree of rhythmic occurrence of the bodily stimuli when compared to the environmental stimuli, the body–brain unity may show a higher degree of unity than the environment–brain unity. This is why we experience our own body as much closer to us and ourselves than the environment.

NOTES

1. The conceptually minded philosopher might want to remark on the particular sequence of the terms "environment" and "brain" in my concept of "environment–brain unity." Why not "brain-environment unity" rather than "environment–brain unity"? This is based on the empirical considerations because, as the data show, it is the brain's low-frequency oscillation phase that seems to adapt to the statistical structure of the stimuli in the environment rather than vice versa. Due to the fact that the adaptation process proceeds from the environment to the brain rather than from the latter to the former, I here prefer to call this unity "environment-brain unity" rather than "brain-environment unity." This, however, should not suggest that the brain is enslaved by the environment; this is neither empirically plausible, as shown by rest–stimulus interaction, nor conceptually plausible, as we will see later.

2. Such statistical basis of the environment–brain unity must be distinguished from other possible bases for unities like physically, cognitively, or representationally based unities, which cannot be explained in further detail here.

3. This may be also the case in the relationship between brain and body. Analogous to the relationship between environment and brain, I also propose a statistically based unity between body and brain, a "body-brain unity." Since the bodily stimuli occur often in a highly rhythmic way, one may propose a high degree of alignment of the resting state's oscillations to them and consecutively a high degree of consciousness of the body.

CHAPTER 21
Unity and Subjectivity

Summary

I suggested the constitution of different unities, phenomenal unity, prephenomenal unity, and environment–brain unities, in the previous chapters and associated them with different neuronal mechanisms. What do these different unities imply for the characterization of consciousness? The answer pertains to more conceptual and theoretical and thus philosophical issues that shall be the focus in this chapter. First, I discuss the different concepts of unities—phenomenal unity, prephenomenal unity, and environment–brain unities—in the context of the current discussion of the philosophy of mind. That allows me to compare the philosophical concept to the here-suggested three different unities, thus putting my empirically based concepts into a more conceptual and thus philosophical context. This raises the question of the exact determination of subjectivity as another hallmark of consciousness. Based on the assumption of the environment–brain unity, I distinguish between different concepts of subjectivity. The concept of "biophysically based subjectivity" refers to the specific biophysical properties of the brain, which predispose the possible range and scope of the environment–brain unity and consequently the point of view that can possibly be taken (and constituted) by any member of a particular species; whether human or nonhuman. Since they show different biophysical properties of their brains, I postulate that the biophysically based subjectivity differs in range and scope in different species. Different species can consequently be characterized by different points of view and different kinds of biophysically based subjectivity. Most important, I suggest that the more (neuro)philosophical concept of biophysically based subjectivity corresponds to the neuroscientific concept of the environment–brain unity within the empirical context of the brain. Characterized by the species-specific biophysical features of the brain and the respectively associated possible environment–brain unities, the concept of "biophysically based subjectivity" must be distinguished from the subjectivity associated with experience of a particular individual and its phenomenal states of consciousness. Therefore, I speak of "phenomenally based subjectivity," which also needs to be distinguished from "cognition-based subjectivity." In contrast to biophysically based subjectivity, which cannot be experienced as such and is thus phenomenally inaccessible, "phenomenally based subjectivity" can easily be experienced and is often considered the phenomenal hallmark of consciousness. I propose that such phenomenally based subjectivity must be associated with the phenomenal unity of consciousness rather than the environment–brain unity. Finally, I discuss the question of how these two concepts of subjectivity, biophysically based and phenomenally based subjectivity, stand in relation to the different concepts of unity as suggested in recent philosophical discussions. I conclude that both unity and subjectivity are co-constituted and co-occurrent, which makes impossible their clear-cut distinction and separate determination.

Key Concepts and Topics Covered

Unity, experiential parts view, no experiential parts view, environment–brain unity, prephenomenal unity, phenomenal unity, consciousness, subjectivity, point of view, biophysically based subjectivity, phenomenally based subjectivity, biophysical convergence zones

PHILOSOPHICAL BACKGROUND
IA: CONSCIOUSNESS AND SUBJECTIVITY

Unity is considered central for consciousness. Many philosophical authors ranging from Immanuel Kant to John Searle regard unity as *the* hallmark feature of consciousness. The here suggested introduction of different forms of unity, phenomenal unity, prephenomenal unity, and environment–brain unity, may thus have major implications and consequences for how we conceive and determine the concept of consciousness.

Though this is a more conceptual and theoretical, and thus philosophical, issue, it will have major reverberations for our empirical search for the neural predispositions and correlates of consciousness. Rather than focusing on empirical data and studies, the present chapter therefore concentrates on discussing the theoretical implications of the different concepts of unity for the characterization of consciousness and its subjective nature.

In addition to unity, subjectivity is often regarded as yet another hallmark of consciousness (see the beginning of the first Introduction in this Volume I). Both current neuroscientific and philosophical discussions seem to tacitly consider the concept of *consciousness* as placeholder for the concept of *subjectivity* when using both terms (more or less) interchangeably. Accordingly, if we want to reveal the neuronal mechanisms underlying consciousness, we cannot avoid addressing the question of whether the very same neuronal mechanisms can also account for the subjective nature of consciousness in particular and subjectivity in general. That, though, will first entail a more theoretical discussion of how the concept of consciousness is related to the concept of subjectivity. This will be the purpose in this chapter.

PHILOSOPHICAL BACKGROUND IB: RELEVANCE OF (NEURO)PHILOSOPHY FOR THE NEUROSCIENCE OF CONSCIOUSNESS

More neuroscientifically minded and data-driven readers may be inclined to skip this chapter and go straight to Chapter 22, where I resume exploring empirical findings about subjectivity.

More specifically, I will discuss abnormal alterations in subjectivity in the psychiatric disorder of schizophrenia which serves to reveal some of the neuronal mechanisms underlying the constitution of subjectivity. However, to fully understand the implications of the environment–brain unity (as in Chapter 20) for consciousness, we first need to make this more theoretical-conceptual detour into the terrain of philosophy, or better, neurophilosophy, to be more specific.

I have to give a warning. Due to space constraints, I will not be able to venture into full philosophical detail as the academic philosophers might expect. However, even such brief philosophical detour will help us nevertheless to shed a better light on our empirical findings in neuroscience. Most important, my neurophilosophical excursion will make us better understand why and how consciousness is intrinsically, i.e., unavoidably and thus necessarily, subjective and why our brain, due to its intrinsic features, makes it impossible for us to not generate subjectivity and consciousness, including their intrinsic coupling.

The theoretical-conceptual discussion is not only helpful for better understanding the neuronal mechanisms underlying the unity and subjectivity of consciousness. In addition, the exact conceptual-theoretical definition of unity has major reverberations upon the kind of experimental strategy one chooses to empirically investigate the underlying neuronal mechanisms. If, for instance, we have to redefine the concept of consciousness in terms of the different kinds of unities, we may also need to tailor our experimental approaches accordingly in order for them to target the "right" kind of unity.

Accordingly, empirical-experimental approaches and designs cannot be considered in isolation from conceptual-theoretical issues (in the same way the latter cannot be isolated from the former either; see Northoff et al. 2010a and b; chapter 3 in Northoff 2011, for details). Therefore, I focus in the present chapter on the conceptual-theoretical implications of the different kinds of unities for the concept of consciousness before I return to more empirical and thus neuronal issues in Chapter 22.

CONCEPTUAL BACKGROUND
IA: THE "EXPERIENTIAL PARTS VIEW"
AND THE UNITY OF CONSCIOUSNESS

What does the introduction of novel concepts like "prephenomenal unity" and "environment–brain unity" (see Chapters 19 and 20) imply conceptually for the characterization of our experience? There has been much discussion in current philosophy about whether experience and thus consciousness consist of parts.

This amounts to the question of whether there are parts within the phenomenal unity of our experience, i.e., consciousness. Those who postulate that there are parts within the phenomenal unity of consciousness advocate what is called an "experiential parts view." Others who deny that there are parts at all in the phenomenal unity of consciousness advocate what is called the "no experiential parts view" (see Brook and Raymont 2010 for a recent overview).

Let us start with the experiential parts view. The experiential parts view considers experience as a composite with different parts; this raises the question about the relation between the different conscious experiential parts. Bayne and Chalmers (2003), for example, advocate the experiential parts view (others include Shoemaker, Dainton, and Lockwood).

They argue that when two different experiences, A and B, are unified, they are "aspects of a single encompassing state of consciousness." Both experiences are then "subsumed by a single state of consciousness," which results in the simultaneous experience of both with the one subsumed under the other.

This comes close to co-consciousness, indicating that we can be co-conscious of A and B as, for instance, we can be of visual and auditory stimuli at the same time. Consciousness, however, cannot be identified with co-consciousness. This is so because there may be instances of consciousness without such a co-relationship, that is, consciousness without co-consciousness. This may, for instance, be the case in self-consciousness, as argued by some authors (Brook and Raymont 2006; see Fig. 21-1a); this is so because the self is homogenous and unified in itself and consists consequently only of one rather than two or more experiences.

CONCEPTUAL BACKGROUND IB: THE "NO EXPERIENTIAL PARTS VIEW" AND THE UNITY OF CONSCIOUSNESS

The alternative view, the "no experiential parts view" (Brook and Raymond 2006), postulates that experience is not a composite and has no "parts."[1] The American philosopher John Searle (2000) is one leading advocate of this view. He (Searle 2000) defines conscious experience as having "one unified conscious field": "A conscious state, in short, is by definition unified, and the unity will follow from the subjectivity and the qualitativeness because there is no way you could have subjectivity and qualitativeness except with that particular form of unity" (Searle 2000, 562).

The American philosopher Michael Tye is another current proponent of the no experiential parts view, which rejects any combination, be it subsumption or co-consciousness:

> There are not five different or separate simultaneous experiences somehow combined together to produce a new unified experience. Nor are there multiple unified experiences within each sense....But there is just one experience here, an experience that can be described less fully as my experience of a bright red shape or as my experience of fruity taste, etc. (Tye 2003, 27; see also Fig. 21-1a).

Tye indicates one important implication of the no experiential parts view. Experience and consciousness cannot be separated according to the different sensory modalities and domains. Instead, the experience of different senses is phenomenally unified:

> On this view, there really are no such entities as purely visual experience or purely auditory experiences of purely olfactory experiences in normal, everyday consciousness. When there is phenomenological unity across sense modalities, sense-specific experiences do not exist. They are the figments of the philosophers' and psychologists' imaginations. And there is no problem,

thus, of unifying these experiences. There are no experiences to be unified. Likewise within each sense: there are not many simultaneous visual experiences, for example combined together to form a complex visual experience. There is a single multimodal experience, describable in more or less rich ways. (Tye 2003, 28)

In summary, the current philosophical discussion considers the phenomenal unity of consciousness to consist of either different parts, the "experiential parts view," or to be completely unified with no parts at all, the "no experiential parts view." This shows that the concept of unity in the phenomenal unity of consciousness can be considered in different ways, at least conceptually.

The question now is which of the conceptual characterizations of the concept of unity is the most plausible one when compared to the empirical, i.e., neuronal mechanisms. In order to test for what may be described as the empirical plausibility of philosophical concepts, we now consider both views, experiential parts view and no experiential parts view, within the empirical context of the neuronal mechanisms as postulated in the preceding chapters.

We are thus testing for the empirical, neuronal plausibility of a particular concept as discussed in philosophy. I will speak of "neuroconceptual plausibility" in the following discussion (see Northoff 2011, chapter 3, for such a methodology in the context of neuropsychoanalysis).

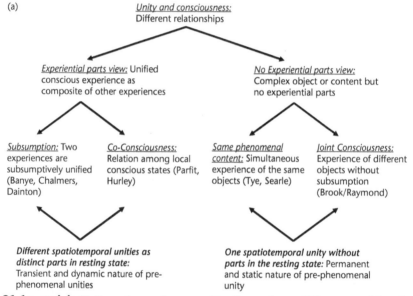

Figure 21-1a and b Unity and consciousness. The figure shows different possible relationships between unity and consciousness (a) and that the phenomenal unity of consciousness is ultimately nested in and based on the environment–brain unity (b). (a) The figure demonstrates two different ways of unity being either a composite of different parts (upper left) or consisting of no parts (upper right) as discussed in current philosophy of mind. This is related to different ways of how the content is constituted in consciousness (subsumption, same phenomenal content), implying different forms of consciousness (co-consciousness, joint consciousness) (middle left and right). I postulate that the two different tracks (parts, no parts) in the relationship between consciousness and unity may be traced back to two different ways of how spatiotemporal continuity of neural activity is constituted by the resting-state activity of the brain (lower left and right) (see later sections in this chapter). (b) The figure shows that the phenomenal unity of consciousness can ultimately be traced back to the environment–brain unity that is statistically and spatiotemporally based. The alignment of the resting state's spatial and temporal measures to the spatial and temporal distribution of environmental stimuli within the physical world is indicated by the dotted lines both horizontally (thick) and vertically (thin).

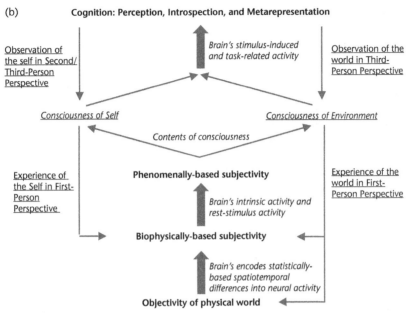

(b)   **Cognition: Perception, Introspection, and Metarepresentation**

Brain's stimulus-induced and task-related activity

Observation of the self in Second/Third-Person Perspective

Observation of the world in Third-Person Perspective

Consciousness of Self   *Consciousness of Environment*

Contents of consciousness

Experience of the Self in First-Person Perspective

Phenomenally-based subjectivity

Experience of the world in First-Person Perspective

Brain's intrinsic activity and rest-stimulus activity

Biophysically-based subjectivity

Brain's encodes statistically-based spatiotemporal differences into neural activity

Objectivity of physical world

Figure 21-1a and b (Continued)

NEUROCONCEPTUAL PLAUSIBILITY IA: PREPHENOMENAL UNITY AND THE "EXPERIENTIAL PARTS VIEW"

How do both views stand in relation to the concept of prephenomenal unity? Does my amplification of the unity into prephenomenal and phenomenal unity fit better with the experiential parts view or the no experiential parts view? I suggest that both views are right and wrong, meaning that they are both empirically, i.e., neuronally, plausible and implausible at the same time.

Let us first have a closer look at the prephenomenal unity. The concept of prephenomenal unity denotes a spatiotemporal unity that is already present in the resting state itself, where it predisposes the constitution of phenomenal unity during subsequent stimulus-induced activity. Since it cannot be phenomenally experienced by itself, I described this unity as prephenomenal.

Most importantly, the prephenomenal unity must be regarded as dynamic and flexible rather than being rigid and static. The dynamic and flexible nature of the prephenomenal unity is neuronally well reflected in the continuously changing constellations of the phase-coupling between high- and low-frequency oscillations.

This means that the spatiotemporal window for the constitution of the prephenomenal unity as spatiotemporal unity is dynamic and flexible rather than static and rigid.

What does the dynamic and flexible nature of the prephenomenal unity as spatiotemporal unity imply for the conceptual discussion? It means that there is not one spatiotemporal unity but rather several or multiple unities across different discrete points in (physical) time and space. This seems to accord rather with the experiential parts view than with the no experiential parts view. The empirically based different spatiotemporal unities may then be taken to correspond to what conceptually is described as distinct parts in the "experiential parts view."

We have to be careful, however. The experiential parts view claims that there are different parts that are linked, that is, subsumed or conjoined, together into one unity, the phenomenal unity of consciousness. There are, however, no such different spatiotemporal unities in the prephenomenal unity. Unlike in the "experiential parts view," clear-cut segregation and distinction between different spatiotemporal unities remains impossible in the case of the prephenomenal unity.

This is so because the spatiotemporal unity in the prephenomenal unity is based on the spatial and temporal continuity of the resting state's neural activity. There is thus a commonly underlying spatiotemporal continuity that binds the different spatiotemporal unities (see Chapters 18 and 19 for details).

This is well reflected in my continuity-based hypothesis of phenomenal unity (see Chapter 19). Due to the assumption of such a basic, commonly underlying spatiotemporal continuity of neural activity in the resting state, there are no real "parts" as segregated and distinguishable spatiotemporal unities within the prephenomenal unity. Therefore, the prephenomenal unity cannot be postulated to correspond to what conceptually has been described as "experiential parts view," which consequently must be considered as empirically (i.e., neuronally) rather implausible.

Neuroconceptual plausibility IB: Prephenomenal unity and the "no experiential parts view"

Is the assumption of a prephenomenal unity thus more compatible with the no experiential parts view? The fact that the prephenomenal unity is based on the spatiotemporal continuity of the resting state's neuronal activity seems to speak in favor of this assumption. There is only one unity in the prephenomenal unity of the resting state, and that is carried over and transferred onto the stimulus-induced activity where it constitutes phenomenal unity and thus consciousness.

There are no experiential parts in the resting state's prephenomenal unity, in very much the same way as Tye and Searle describe it in the above-cited quotations. The concept of prephenomenal unity and its predisposing role for the phenomenal unity seems compatible with the no experiential parts view, which therefore must be deemed to be empirically, i.e., neuronally plausible.

We again have to be careful, however. The conceptual characterization of the prephenomenal unity by the "no experiential parts view" ignores the transient nature of the spatiotemporal unity. As described earlier, the spatiotemporal unity is highly dynamic and flexible. This means that there are varieties of distinct spatiotemporal unities over the course of time and space with each spatiotemporal unity being only of transient occurrence.

The question now is whether the various transient spatiotemporal unities are variants of one and the same spatiotemporal unity. This would still be compatible with the "no experiential parts view." Or whether the transient spatiotemporal unities are different spatiotemporal unities amounting to different parts in experience, entailing the "experiential parts view." The answer to this question depends on the criteria one postulates for identity and difference between distinct spatiotemporal unities. These are rather conceptual and logical issues that remain beyond the scope of this book.

What is clear, however, is that both conceptual views, experiential parts and no experiential parts views, seem to be empirically plausible in some regards and empirically implausible in others, as indicated above. The discussion also makes it clear that we need to consider the temporal and spatial dimensions when discussing the empirical and conceptual plausibility of both views.

What does it mean to "consider the temporal and spatial dimensions" in investigating the empirical plausibility of concepts? Just like the brain and its resting-state structures its neural activity in temporal and spatial terms, we have to put our investigations of the possibly corresponding concepts into a spatial and temporal context. Otherwise, the discussion and the answers we provide may be more related to us as observers and our concepts than to the brain itself and its very neuronal mechanisms. Our concepts may then turn out to be more observer-based than brain-based (see Appendix 3 in Volume I for this distinction).

For instance, our investigation demonstrates that the conceptual distinction between the "no experiential parts view" and the "experiential parts view" may not be an all-or-nothing distinction where one has to decide between either view. Instead, the empirical data suggest a continuum rather than an all-or-nothing distinction between both views. Such a continuum between both views must be considered more empirically plausible and thus as brain-based rather than observer-based (see Appendix 3 in Volume I for this distinction).

Neuroconceptual Plausibility IIA: Nesting of "Prephenomenal Unity," and "Phenomenal Unity" within the "Environment–Brain Unity"

How about the third unity, the environment–brain unity, we suggested in Chapter 20? How does the environment–brain unity stand in relation to the two views about the unity of consciousness? At first glance, one may suggest that the three different unities, the environment–brain unity, the prephenomenal unity, and the phenomenal unity, may be conjoined into one unity. For instance, the phenomenal unity may be regarded as the subsumption or co-joining of the other two unities, the prephenomenal unity and the environment–brain unity. That would presuppose that all three unities are different unities that need to be integrated in order to become one unity.

This is not the case empirically, however. The environment–brain unity is not principally different from the prephenomenal unity and the phenomenal unity. Instead of being segregated and operating in parallel, both the environment–brain unity and the prephenomenal unity build on each other and are thus nested within each other. More specifically, the environment–brain unity provides the very ground or framework and thus the neural predisposition within which the resting-state activity can constitute its prephenomenal unity.

And that, in turn, provides the predisposition for the subsequent constitution of the phenomenal unity during stimulus-induced activity. Hence, rather than being different and segregated unities, all three unities are necessarily dependent upon each other while still being distinct. In other terms, the environment–brain unity predisposes the prephenomenal unity, which in turn predisposes the phenomenal unity.

What exactly do I mean by the concept of predisposition in this context? The term "predisposition" describes the necessary but non-sufficient conditions. By being necessary but nonsufficient, the environment–brain unity provides the very ground and basic framework, the basic spatiotemporal grid or template upon which the resting state can constitute its prephenomenal unity. The environment–brain unity thus provides, metaphorically speaking, a space

for the possible constitution of the subsequent prephenomenal unity.

Accordingly, when I speak of predisposition, I refer to the possible (rather than the actual) constitution of (for instance) the prephenomenal unity that is made possible and thus predisposed by the environment–brain unity. In order to turn the possible constitution of the prephenomenal unity into an actual one, additional conditions besides the environment–brain unity must be met (see Fig. 21-1b).

How can we better illustrate such a predisposing relationship among the three unities? The relationship among the three different unities can be compared to the famous Russian nested dolls. The largest doll provides the largest number of possibilities for the other dolls of smaller size to be integrated. The number of possibilities is smaller for the next-smaller doll, and so forth. Analogously, the environment–brain unity provides the largest number of possibilities for the subsequent prephenomenal unity. And the prephenomenal unity provides a yet-smaller number of possibilities for the constitution of the subsequent phenomenal unity.

Taken in this sense, the three different unities may be characterized by different degrees of possibility and specification. Corresponding to the largest Russian doll, the environment–brain unity carries the highest number of possibilities but the lowest degree of specification, while the prephenomenal unity contains a lower number of possibilities but a higher degree of specification. Finally, the phenomenal unity, corresponding to he smallest Russian doll, can be characterized by the highest degree of specification and the number of possibilities' tending toward zero. The three unities are thus nested in each other in very much the same way the Russian dolls are nested in each other.

Neuroconceptual Plausibility IIB: "Environment–Brain Unity" and the "Experiential Parts View" versus the "No Experiential Parts View"

What does such a nested relationship among the three unities tell us about the relationship of the environment–brain unity to the two views about the unity of experience? Assuming nestedness between the three unities excludes the possibility that the three different unities can be regarded as different parts as presupposed in the experiential parts view. Does this mean that the no experiential parts view holds?

In that case, one would postulate all three unities to be identical and/or be derivatives of one and the same unity. But this is not the case, either. Instead, all three unities can be distinguished from each other in terms of possibility and specification, as described earlier. At the same time they build on and predispose each other. Hence, the three different unities are both distinct and necessarily (though not sufficiently) dependent on each other. They are consequently fully compatible with neither the "experiential parts view" nor the "no experiential parts view."

Taken together, the assumption of three different unities, environment–brain unity, prephenomenal unity, and phenomenal unity, does not seem to be compatible with either view, the experiential parts view or the no experiential parts view. Based on the previous chapters, I postulate that the distinction and dependence between the three unities is highly empirically, i.e., neuronally, plausible.

If the conceptual distinction between these views does not properly correspond to or match with the empirical distinction between the three unities and their relationship to each other, one may consider the former, the conceptual distinction between the two views, to be empirically implausible. This means, however, that the conceptual distinction may be more related to us as observers and philosophers and consequently to the way we develop concepts. In contrast, the distinction between the two views may be less related to the brain itself and its neuronal mechanisms independent of us and our observation of them and the kind of concepts we use to describe them.

We therefore can currently not exclude that our conceptual distinction between experiential and no experiential parts views turns out to be more observer based than brain based. If so, the conceptual characterization of the relationship between experience and unity as discussed in the two views in current philosophy may need to be revised and adapted to the three unities as postulated on empirical grounds. That in turn would increase the empirical plausibility of the conceptual account of the relationship between experience and unity.

PHILOSOPHICAL EXCURSION
IA: SUBJECTIVITY AND CONSCIOUSNESS

In addition to unity, consciousness provides another tough nut to crack. Consciousness is generally considered the paradigmatic example of subjectivity, if not its (phenomenal) placeholder (whatever it means; see later for its definition), since both terms are often used interchangeably in the current neuroscientific and philosophical discussions (see the beginning of the first Introduction to Volume II).

What is meant by "the subjectivity of consciousness"? Our experience is *subjective* in that it is restricted to me and no one else. I am conscious of reading this book, and this experience cannot be shared by the person sitting beside me. That makes experience, and thus consciousness, essentially subjective. And it distinguishes the phenomenal states of consciousness from the neuronal states of the brain (and other physical states). Neuronal states can be observed by many persons at the same time in the same way and must therefore be considered objective rather than subjective.

How now are the subjectivity of consciousness and its phenomenal states constituted by the merely objective neuronal states of the brain? The assumption of different unities, phenomenal unity, prephenomenal unity, and environment–brain unity, may be central in this regard. In other words, I postulate the constitution of these different unities to go hand in hand with the constitution of subjectivity. To understand that, we first have to discuss the concept of subjectivity in more conceptual detail, which will be the focus in the following sections. This will be followed later by discussing briefly how subjectivity and unity are related to each other.

PHILOSOPHICAL EXCURSION
IB: SUBJECTIVITY AND POINT OF VIEW

The concept of subjectivity is usually associated with the first-person perspective (FPP) as distinguished from the third-person perspective (TPP), and with intra-individual rather than inter-individual access. However, the notion of "what it is like" as introduced by American philosopher T. Nagel (1974, 2012) carries a broader implication that reaches beyond the FPP.

Nagel exemplified this broader implication by the example of the bat: we as humans are not able to take the point of view of the bat and thus to experience "what life is like" for the bat. We remain unable to access, share, and ultimately experience the bat's experience. Why are we unable to take the point of view of the bat? Because the bat possesses different biophysical features than humans, which, for instance, allow the bat to perceive ultrasonic waves that we as humans are unable to access at all.

Following Nagel's account, the concept of subjectivity is here associated with a point of view rather than the FPP. This is important to note, since both FPP and TPP presuppose a point of view. This means that a point of view includes both FPP and TPP, whereas exactly that is denied when subjectivity is equated with FPP alone.

Accordingly, the characterization of subjectivity by a point of view rather than by FPP alone is more basic and far-reaching than its determination by FPP alone. A point of view is like an anchor from which we can experience the world in FPP and, at the same time, observe it in TPP. Hence, to equate point of view with FPP alone would be to neglect the very basis and thus the necessary conditions upon which FPP itself (and also TPP) stands.

What does this imply for the definition of the concept of subjectivity? The concept of subjectivity may be defined in either a broader or a narrow way. In the broader sense, the concept of subjectivity refers to the subject's point of view and includes thereby both FPP and TPP. In contrast, a narrower definition bases subjectivity on FPP alone, while distinguishing it from TPP as being objective (rather than subjective). We will see in the following remarks how these two definitions of the concept of subjectivity can be distinguished and specified in further detail.

Philosophical Excursion IIA: Concept of "Biophysically Based Subjectivity"

How can we describe the concept of point of view in further detail? If the concept of point of view is more basic and far reaching than the one of FPP alone, it should also refer to some features

other than those that can be accessed in FPP. Let us compare the "what it is like" of bats and their point of view with the one of humans.

In addition to their different experiences, bats and humans also differ in their basic biophysical equipment. The bat's auditory system, for instance, is very well tuned to ultrasonic frequencies, which we as humans are unable to detect, given our auditory system and its specific tuning. Accordingly, different species like humans and bats may be characterized by biophysical differences.

What do such biophysical differences between different species entail for the concept of subjectivity? The concept of subjectivity in Nagel's example of the bat is no longer defined by and based on FPP and intra-individual access alone. This implies the rejection of what can be described as an individually specific concept of subjectivity, a concept of subjectivity that is based on the individual and its FPP alone.

Instead, Nagel's concept of subjectivity seems to be based on the biophysical spectrum within which a particular species, like the bat or the human, can process a particular range of stimuli from the environment. The concept of subjectivity is thus species-specific rather than individually specific.

Let us reformulate the same idea in slightly different terms. I postulate that differences in biophysical equipment entail different points of view and consequently a difference subjectivity. This means that the concept of subjectivity must be defined not only by a point of view but also by the respective organism's biophysical equipment and thus in a biophysically based way. I therefore speak of the concept of "biophysically based subjectivity" in the following.

How can we define the concept of biophysically based subjectivity? The concept of biophysically based subjectivity refers to the characterization of a particular species rather than concerning one specific individual member within a particular species. There is thus species specificity rather than individual specificity. Moreover, the concept of biophysically based subjectivity refers to the biophysical equipment that defines and is specific to all the individual members of that species. It is thus biophysically based, hence its name (see Fig. 21-2a).

Such a biophysical basis for the concept of subjectivity must be distinguished from other kinds of possible basis, which shall only briefly be indicated here. The possible basis could include a phenomenal basis in consciousness, thus referring to experience, a mental basis when assuming a mind, a cognitive basis referring to cognitive functions, and a representational basis that associates subjectivity with a specific type of representation. As it is clear, I reject either of these assumptions for a possible basis of subjectivity. Why? Because they are not compatible with the empirical data as laid out in the chapters throughout this book.

I am aware though that even such rejection of the alternative assumptions would require detailed arguments. However, I will not go into the detailed discussion of these different forms of subjectivity here; I leave that to the philosophers. Moreover, I will not discuss here the relationship between subjectivity and self, which will be touched upon in Part VII. Instead, I here focus on how subjectivity is related to consciousness.

PHILOSOPHICAL EXCURSION IIB: "BIOPHYSICALLY BASED SUBJECTIVITY" PREDISPOSES CONSCIOUSNESS

What does the concept of biophysically based subjectivity imply for the organism's stance in relation to the world? The species-specific biophysical equipment makes it possible for the organism to take a certain point of view, which anchors it in the world. Such a point of view must be distinguished from the points of view other organisms (other species) are able to take on the basis of their species-specific biophysical equipment.

The presence of such point of view must be distinguished from the absence of any point of view. Such a lack of any kind of point of view is, for instance, often ascribed to God, who by definition cannot have a "point of view" in this sense because, among other reasons, he is lacking any biophysical equipment that would anchor him in the world. The presence of such a biophysically based point of view makes it possible for the organism to experience the world from its particular species-specific point of view. This is what Thomas Nagel referred to when he characterized subjectivity by a point of view.

The concept of biophysically based subjectivity predisposes the range of possible experience a species can (possibly) make. Such a predisposition of possible experience by biophysically based subjectivity must be distinguished from the conditions that allow for the actual experience in FPP, which may be associated with the individually rather than species-specific concept of subjectivity (see later for details).

In addition to predisposing possible experience in FPP, biophysically based subjectivity may also predispose the possible distinction between experience in FPP and observation in TPP. If so, the species-specific biophysically based subjectivity must be considered more basic and fundamental than both experience in FPP and observation in TPP alone that are rather individually than species-specific.

I therefore characterize the concept of biophysically based subjectivity by species specificity, a particular biophysical spectrum, and a point of view.[2] As such, the concept must be distinguished from concepts of subjectivity that postulate a phenomenal, mental, cognitive, or representational rather than biophysical basis, and consequently an individually rather than species-specific determination[3]. Most important, by providing a point of view, biophysically based subjectivity in this sense predisposes; that is, makes necessary and unavoidable, the possible constitution of consciousness.

PHILOSOPHICAL EXCURSION IIC: CONCEPT OF "PHENOMENALLY BASED SUBJECTIVITY"

The concept of biophysically based subjectivity must be distinguished from the concept of subjectivity that is implied by the experience and thus by consciousness itself. When one considers experience and thus consciousness in isolation from their very basis, e.g., biophysically based subjectivity and the point of view, one may restrict the concept of subjectivity to FPP alone as distinguished from TPP. This, however, means that subjectivity can then no longer be defined by a species-specific point of view (which includes both FPP and TPP) but rather by an individually specific FPP.

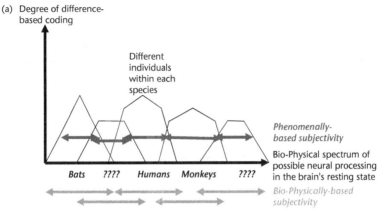

Figure 21-2a-g Brain and subjectivity. The figures show different concepts of subjectivity and their philosophical and neurophilosophical characterization. (*a*) This figure shows the relationship between the encoding of spatial and temporal differences into neural activity and the species-specific biophysical spectrum. Difference-based coding is supposed to operate in all species and thus across different biophysical spectra in the different species (x-axis). This, in turn, is supposed to be dependent on the physical features of the stimuli in the environment, including their spatial and temporal differences (see y-axis). (*b*) The figure illustrates the relationship between biophysically based subjectivity, phenomenally based subjectivity, and consciousness of self and the environment, as suggested here. Biophysically based subjectivity results from the interaction between brain and environment as characterized by how the brain encodes its neural activity (lower part). This is species-specific rather than individually specific. Additional processes by the brain's intrinsic activity and its interaction with specific extrinsic stimuli lead from biophysically based to phenomenally based subjectivity (see middle lower part). That provides the basis or correlate of consciousness of both self (left) and environment (right in upper middle part) in first-person perspective. Cognition then makes it possible to cognize and thus observe both self and the environment in third-person perspective (right and left upper part). (*c*) The figure illustrates the relationship between the brain and consciousness in cognition-based approaches. They assume that the physical objectivity of the world directly translates into the neuronal objectivity of the brain (lower part). This gives rise to the third-person perspective (middle part). The reflection upon its own neuronal states by the brain (shown by arrow), its own mental states (not shown here), and the vegetative state of its body (not shown here) is supposed to give rise to consciousness and subjectivity, with the experience of the self in first-person perspective (left part). In the meantime, the third-person perspective allows an objective observation of both brain and world (right part) that seemingly does not implicate consciousness (right part).(*d*) The figure demonstrates the different concepts of subjectivity: biophysically, phenomenally, and cognition-based. They are all based on each other and related to each other, as indicated by the dotted horizontal lines. This means that they are nested within each other, as indicated by the vertical lines. Ultimately, they are all based on the physical world and its physically based objectivity. As indicated on the left, the different concepts of subjectivity are related to different domains: metaphysical-epistemic, phenomenal, and empirical (cognitive). (*e*) The figure shows the characterization of biophysically based subjectivity by the brain's resting-state activity and its biophysical-computational features, like its ranges of high- and low-frequency fluctuations, which may differ between different species. The concept of biophysically based subjectivity describes the relationship between a particular species and the rest of the physical world, thus being species-specific. On the basis of that specificity, each individual or member within a particular species develops its own individually specific phenomenally based subjectivity that describes its degree of actual consciousness. The x-axis describes different biophysical-computational properties in the different species' brains and their respective resting-state activities. The y-axis concerns the degree of difference-based coding relative to stimulus-based coding, which I postulate to be central in constituting biophysically based subjectivity. (*f*) The figure shows the correspondence (arrows) between the different concepts of subjectivity (left) and unity (right). The biophysically based subjectivity corresponds to the environment–brain unity, the phenomenally based subjectivity to the phenomenal unity, and the cognition-based subjectivity to the cognitive unity. (*g*) This figure shows how the biophysical convergence zones (right middle) allow for the

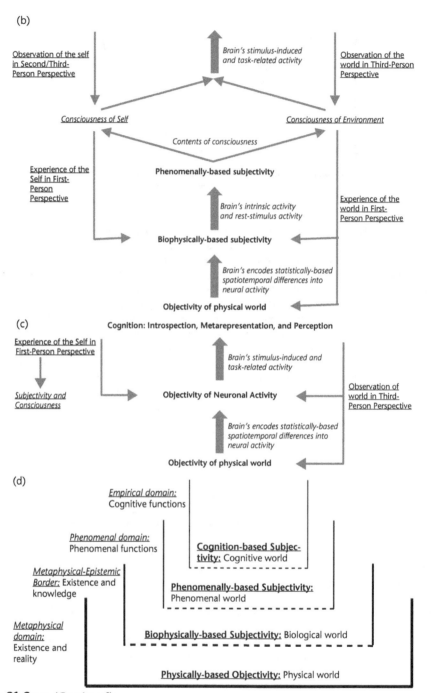

Figure 21-2a-g (Continued)
statistically and spatiotemporally based alignment between the resting state's activity and the physical world's spatial and temporal measures (thick vertical lines between the physical world [lower part] and the environment–brain unity [upper part]). This, in turn, makes possible the constitution of a statistically and spatiotemporally based virtual environment–brain unity where the respective spatial and temporal trajectories converge onto a point of view (see right upper part). A point of view provides a statistically and spatiotemporally based, virtual, species-specific stance within the physical world; that is, biophysically based subjectivity. This provides the stance from which each individual member can then experience the physical world in an individually specific way; that is, phenomenally based subjectivity.

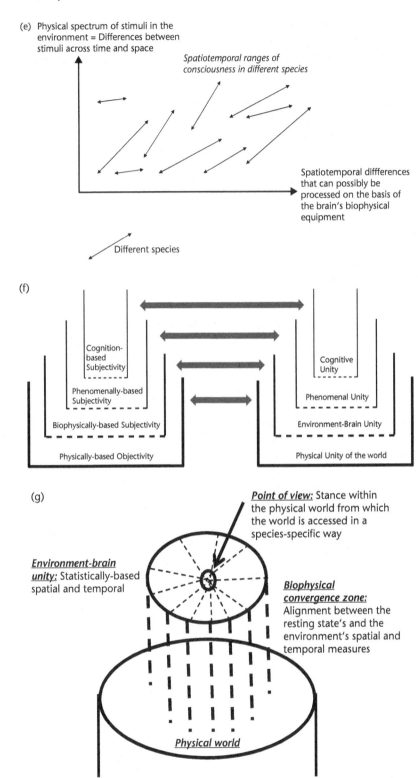

Figure 21-2a-g (Continued)

How does such individually specific determination of subjectivity by FPP stand in relation to the biophysically based subjectivity as implied by Nagel and his example of the bat? What Nagel calls "point of view" is not to be confused with the FPP: the point of view is prior to (and more basic than) the distinction between FPP and TPP because the species-specific biophysical spectrum may affect both FPP and TPP.

Moreover, the biophysically based subjectivity is not tied to one particular individual but rather to all individuals within one particular species, thus being species-specific rather than individually specific. This is different when one restricts subjectivity to FPP. Then, subjectivity concerns only one specific individual member within all the individuals and members of a particular species.

The main difference then is no longer between the different biophysical equipment in different species but rather between different phenomenal states in different individual members of the same species. There is consequently individual specificity rather than species specificity. Rather than being determined biophysically as biophysically based subjectivity, such individually specific subjectivity is determined by the respective individuals' phenomenal states. One may consequently want to speak of what I describe as "phenomenally based subjectivity" (see later for an exact definition).

The concept of phenomenally based subjectivity describes an FPP-based and individual-specific concept of subjectivity that is based on the phenomenal states of consciousness, e.g., experiences in the FPP of the respective individuals, rather on the species' biophysical equipment. Since such a concept of subjectivity is phenomenally rather than biophysically based, I introduce the term *phenomenally based subjectivity* in order to distinguish it from *biophysically based subjectivity*.

I therefore postulate what I describe as "phenomenally based subjectivity." The concept of phenomenally based subjectivity can be characterized by individual specificity rather than species specificity, phenomenal states rather than biophysical equipment, and FPP rather than a point of view (which provides the basis for both FPP and TPP).[4] It must therefore be distinguished from the concept of biophysically based subjectivity.[5]

Philosophical Excursion IID: *Phenomenal Correlate* versus *Prephenomenal Predisposition* of Self and Consciousness

How do the concepts of "biophysically based subjectivity" and "phenomenally based subjectivity" relate to the concepts of consciousness and self? Let us start with consciousness.

The concept of "phenomenally based subjectivity" implies and thus necessarily entails consciousness, as indicated by the prefix "phenomenally." Most important, this refers to any kind of consciousness, including both consciousness of the environment and consciousness of the self; that is, self-consciousness. This means that the concept of phenomenally based subjectivity is closely related to both self and consciousness. Without phenomenally based subjectivity, neither "self" nor consciousness would be possible. Therefore, phenomenally based subjectivity can be considered a sufficient phenomenal condition or correlate of both sense of self and consciousness (see Fig. 21-2b).

This is different in the case of "biophysically based subjectivity." Unlike in the case of "phenomenally based subjectivity," "biophysically based subjectivity" is associated neither with self nor with consciousness. There can be "biophysically based subjectivity" without either self or consciousness. This means that biophysically based subjectivity is not a sufficient condition and thus correlate of self and consciousness.

However, as spelled out earlier, biophysically based subjectivity *predisposes* both self and consciousness. It predisposes the self by providing a point of view, which, pending individualization, will be transformed into a self (see Chapters 23 and 24 for details of such individualization of the point of view). In addition, the biophysically based subjectivity predisposes consciousness by providing the kind of spatiotemporalization (see later) that makes possible the association of both environmental stimuli and the point of view, (including its individualized self) with the phenomenal features of consciousness (see Chapter 24 for details).

Without biophysically based subjectivity, we would have neither consciousness nor a self. If there is no point of view, no self could develop at all, because there would be nothing to individualize. Most important, without the spatiotemporal nature of the biophysically based subjectivity (see later), the association of both environmental stimuli and the point of view with consciousness would remain impossible. There would consequently neither be consciousness of the environment nor of a self.

This makes it clear that biophysically based subjectivity provides the necessary condition of the possibility of both consciousness and self. While not being phenomenal by itself, biophysically based subjectivity nevertheless provides the predisposition of consciousness and self and must therefore be characterized as prephenomenal rather than nonphenomenal.

PHILOSOPHICAL EXCURSION IIIA: CONCEPT OF "COGNITION-BASED SUBJECTIVITY"

We already indicated at several points that the concept of biophysically based subjectivity must be distinguished from cognitive concepts of subjectivity. How can we now characterize such cognitive concepts of subjectivity? Cognitive concepts of subjectivity suggest that subjectivity is limited to a certain mode of cognition; namely, in the first-person perspective. Cognition in the mode of the first-person perspective is subjective, whereas cognition in the mode of the third-person perspective is objective.

What, then, distinguishes both modes of cognition? Cognition in the third-person perspective targets contents in the world, as it is independent of ourselves, which accounts for the objective character of this mode of cognition. This is different from the cognition in the first-person perspective which targets our own contents like our own body and our brain, as we perceive and cognize them in first-person perspective.

How is such cognition of our own contents possible? The modern neurophilosophical proponents of such a view, like Thomas Metzinger (2003) and Patricia Churchland (2002) and many others, assume integration and coordination of all the information and processes in brain and body to be essential. Such integration and coordination is possible by either representation/meta-representation in higher-order cognition functions (Churchland 2002, Metzinger 2003,

and many other philosophers), or by perception of one's own inner bodily and mental states (as, for instance, suggested by Damasio 1999, 2010).

What does such integration look like? Take all the information from the body and brain, coordinate and integrate it, and then you have a cognition of your own brain and body and their respective processes in first-person perspective. In more technical terms, our own brain and body are represented in the neuronal activity of the brain. And such representation is the model of your own brain and body, so that one can speak of self-representation. Self-representation, and therefore subjectivity, is nothing but an inner model of the integrated and summarized version of your own brain and body's information processing (see Fig. 21-2c).

What we cognize in first-person perspective is thus the self-representation of our own brain and body. And it is this cognition of our own self-representation that, following these models, yields subjectivity in our first-person based cognition, as distinguished from the objectivity in our cognition in third-person perspective. The subjectivity here is thus based on cognition, and for that reason I speak of "cognition-based subjectivity." The concept of "cognition-based subjectivity" describes the definition of subjectivity by cognition and more specifically by a particular mode of cognition: cognition in the first-person perspective.

PHILOSOPHICAL EXCURSION IIIB: "COGNITION-BASED SUBJECTIVITY" PRESUPPOSES RATHER THAN PRODUCES CONSCIOUSNESS

How is the concept of "cognition-based subjectivity" related to consciousness? Let us briefly recapitulate the other concepts of subjectivity in this regard. The concept of "biophysically based subjectivity" is supposed to predispose consciousness as the necessary condition of its possible existence. Without "biophysically based subjectivity," consciousness remains impossible. However, consciousness cannot be found in "biophysically based subjectivity."

This is different from the concept of "phenomenally based subjectivity." Rather than preceding and being more basic than consciousness, like "biophysically based subjectivity," "phenomenally based subjectivity" operates within consciousness itself. "Phenomenally based subjectivity" describes the subjectivity of consciousness itself, meaning that consciousness is unavoidably and necessarily subjective.

How about "cognition-based subjectivity"? "Cognition-based subjectivity" concerns neither the basis nor the predisposition of possible consciousness like "biophysically based subjectivity." Nor does it describe the intrinsically subjective nature of consciousness as implied by the concept of "phenomenally based subjectivity." Instead, "cognition-based subjectivity" describes how we cognize our own brain and body within and thus on the basis of consciousness. In other words, "cognition-based subjectivity" operates on the basis of, and thus presupposes, consciousness.

Put in a nutshell, "biophysically based subjectivity" predisposes consciousness, "phenomenally based subjectivity" describes consciousness, and "cognition-based subjectivity" presupposes consciousness. There is thus what can be described as "nestedness" between the different concepts of subjectivity (see Fig. 21-2d).

Putting all this together, one may characterize the different concepts in the following way. "Biophysically based subjectivity" is a wide concept of subjectivity that can be "located" at the border between metaphysical and epistemological domains of existence/reality and knowledge; "phenomenally based subjectivity" is a more narrow concept of subjectivity that refers to the phenomenal domain of consciousness; and "cognition-based subjectivity" is an even more limited concept of subjectivity that implicates the empirical domain of cognition. Based on their different scopes, the different concepts of subjectivity are nested within each other.

NEUROPHILOSOPHICAL EXCURSION
IA: "ENVIRONMENT–BRAIN UNITY"
IS BIOPHYSICALLY BASED AND
STATISTICALLY BASED

Due to its most basic and fundamental character, I will now focus on the neurophilosophical investigation of the concept of biophysically based subjectivity and how it stands in relation to the environment–brain unity and its underlying neuronal mechanisms. The exact neuronal mechanisms of the phenomenally based subjectivity will be explained in Chapter 25 in full detail, when I show how subjectivity and consciousness become integrated and linked. Due to my neurophenomenal focus, I leave open the exact neuronal, or better, neurocognitive, mechanisms of the cognition-based subjectivity.

Before starting with the biophysically based subjectivity, we need to make a short remark. Methodologically, this detour leads me to directly compare a theoretical concept, biophysically based subjectivity, with the empirical mechanisms underlying the "environment–brain unity." This means that I now test whether the theoretical concept of biophysically based subjectivity is compatible and in accordance with the empirical, that is neuronal, data. I thus test for the empirical, that is neuronal, plausibility of the theoretical concept of biophysically based subjectivity.

We recall that the concept of "environment–brain unity" described the correspondence and convergence between the environmental stimuli's temporal/spatial differences and the brain's encoding and processing of temporal and spatial differences into the neural activity of its resting state (see Chapter 20). How, then, is such difference-based environment–brain unity related to the concept of biophysically based subjectivity?

To answer that question, we need to go into more detail about the environment–brain unity. The environment–brain unity consists of the encoding of the environmental stimuli's statistical frequency distribution, e.g., their natural statistics, by the resting state's low-frequency fluctuations and their phases.

Such encoding of the stimuli's natural statistics is possible only on the basis of encoding temporal and spatial differences between different stimuli across their different discrete points in (physical) time and space. This presupposes difference-based coding rather than stimulus-based coding where the stimuli's discrete points in (physical) time and space would be encoded by themselves in isolation of each other and thus independently of their differences.

If the temporal and spatial differences in the resting state's neural activity correspond to the one between the stimuli's occurrence in the environment, environment and brain are unified in a statistically based way. More specifically, together they constitute a difference- and statistically based temporal and spatial unity and thus what I described as environment–brain unity (see Chapter 20).

In sum, the environment–brain unity is based on the encoding of spatial and temporal differences between organism and environment into the brain's neural activity. Such encoding is statistically based, while the degree of spatial and temporal differences themselves is based on the biophysical equipment of the respective species' brains. In short, the environment–brain unity is biophysically and statistically based.

Neurophilosophical Excursion Ib: Spatiotemporal Structure of the Environment–Brain Unity Is Species-Specific

How does such environment–brain unity as difference- and statistically based temporal and spatial unity relate to the concept of biophysically based subjectivity? We recall that I defined the concept of biophysical subjectivity by the respective species' biophysical equipment. The biophysical equipment determines, for instance, the possible spectrum or range of frequencies that can possibly be perceived by the respective species.

Depending on the spectrum or range of its respective biophysical equipment, one species may show a rather low range of possible frequencies in the neuronal fluctuations of their brain's resting-state activity. In contrast, other species may be characterized by a larger biophysical spectrum with a higher range of possible frequencies in their brain's resting state's neuronal fluctuations.

How, then, is the range of the frequencies that can possibly be processed by the brain's resting-state activity involved in the organism's relationship to the world? The range of the frequencies that can possibly be processed by the brain's resting-state activity predisposes the particular species to align its resting state to the corresponding differences and thus the respective statistical frequency ranges

of the stimuli's occurrences in the environment. At the same time, the species-specific biophysical spectrum excludes the frequency ranges of the stimuli's occurrences in the environment that do not fall within the possible range of the spectrum of the species' biophysical equipment.

What does the dependence upon the biophysical spectrum imply for the constitution of the temporal and spatial unity by the brain's resting-state activity? The species' biophysical equipment presupposes its brain's resting state to a particular species-specific duration and extension of its temporal and spatial unity with the environment and its stimuli. The spatial and temporal range and extension of the environment–brain unity is thus very much dependent upon the spectrum of the biophysical equipment of the respective species.

I consequently postulate the exact structure of the environment–brain unity—for example, its possible degree of spatial extension and temporal duration of its spatial and temporal unity—to be specific for a particular species. Accordingly, the environment–brain unity is species-specific and therefore depends on the temporal and spatial features of the biophysical spectrum of the respective species.

Neurophilosophical Excursion Ic: Species-Specific "Biophysical Convergence Zones" Between Environment and Brain

What does the relevance of the brain's biophysical spectrum imply for the relationship between the environment and the brain? There seem to be what I call "biophysical convergence zones" between the environment's stimuli and the organism's biophysical equipment; that is, its species-specific biophysical spectrum.

The concept of "biophysical convergence zones" describes the possible ranges and degrees of correspondence between the spatiotemporal features of the environmental stimuli and the species-specific spatiotemporal spectrum in the neural processing of the brain's resting state. Such convergence is postulated to be based on the encoding of spatial and temporal differences between the environmental stimuli's (statistical) occurrences across time and space, i.e., their natural statistics, into the resting-state activity of the organism's brain. In short, I postulate the biophysical convergence zones to be difference- and statistically based as well as species-specific (see Fig. 21-2e).

How do such biophysical convergence zones impact the constitution of the environment–brain unity? Within the spatial and temporal ranges of the species-specific biophysical convergence zones, difference-based coding can take place (though probably with varying degrees in the gestalt of a U-shape; see later), while outside each species-specific biophysical convergence zone, neither difference-based coding nor any encoding of the stimuli by the brain and its resting-state activity are possible anymore.

How can we further illustrate the here-suggested concept of biophysical convergence zones? The concept of biophysical convergence zones closely resembles what American psychologist James Gibson described as "affordance," the mutual match between the organism's behavior and its ecological niche; that is, its environmental context.

What Gibson describes in a behavioral and evolutionary context is rephrased here in the neuronal context of the brain's biophysical equipment and its possible relationship to the environment. Future investigations, both empirical and theoretical, may want to further develop my concept of biophysical convergence zones in a more evolutionary and also behavioral context, for which Gibson's concept of affordance may provide a useful roadmap. One question occurring in this context is whether other species, like the bat, also operate on the basis of difference- rather than stimulus-based coding.

Let us recall from Volume I the many examples of sparse coding stemming from different animals, including mice, rats, and monkeys (see Chapter 1). Since sparse coding presupposes difference- rather than stimulus-based coding, these examples may be seen to support the assumption of difference-based coding holding in other species, too. If so, we must postulate that difference-based coding is the neural code of the brain in general—that is, cross-species—which

may operate within (and thus across) different biophysical convergence zones and their different biophysical spectra in different species.

Based on the statistically based encoding of the stimuli's natural statistics, I here postulate that different species show different biophysical convergence zones between brain and environment. Since the environment–brain unity is based on the biophysical convergence zone, it must be postulated to differ between different species, thus implying species specificity. Putting all together, our little excursion into the theoretical realms of subjectivity has revealed three further characterizations of the environment–brain unity: for example, biophysically based subjectivity, point of view, and biophysical convergence zones.

NEUROPHILOSOPHICAL EXCURSION IIA: "ENVIRONMENT–BRAIN UNITY" AND "BIOPHYSICALLY BASED SUBJECTIVITY"

The determination of the environment–brain unity as biophysically based converges with the concept of biophysically based subjectivity. The biophysical spectrum of the species determines the spatial and temporal range and extension of both the unity in the environment–brain unity and the subjectivity in the biophysically based subjectivity. If so, the concept of environment–brain unity may correspond on the empirical, i.e., neuronal side to what philosophically is described by the concept of biophysically based subjectivity (see Fig. 21-2f).

I have already suggested that the concept of biophysically based subjectivity finds its empirical sibling in the environment–brain unity. How about the other concepts of subjectivity? The phenomenally based subjectivity described the subjectivity of consciousness and must therefore be related to what I described earlier as the "phenomenal unity" (see also Chapters 18 and 19). Finally, the concept of cognition-based subjectivity concerns cognitive unity as related to cognition (see Chapters 18 and 19 as well as earlier in this chapter).

How can we specify the relationship between environment–brain unity and biophysically based subjectivity? The environment–brain unity may be suggested to constitute on empirical, i.e., statistical, grounds what Thomas Nagel described conceptually by "point of view": This means that the species-specific environment–brain unity may constitute the point of view from which the particular species can possibly experience and observe the world in a species-specific way.

Let us describe the relationship between environment–brain unity and point of view by Nagel's example of the bat: postulate Due to its different biophysical equipment, the bat may encode different stimuli with different spatial and temporal features and thus different statistical frequency distributions, i.e., natural statistics, into its resting-state activity when compared to humans. This gives the bat a different point of view and thus a different biophysically based subjectivity as it is empirically manifested in an environment–brain unity with different spatial and temporal features.

In sum, I postulate that the neuronal, that is, empirical mechanisms underlying the species-specific environment–brain unity make possible the constitution of what theoretically is described by the concept of "the point of view" of a particular species and its species-specific biophysically based subjectivity.

Neurophilosophical Excursion
IIB: Difference- versus Stimulus-based Point of View

How can we further describe the relationship between environment–brain unity and point of view? Metaphorically speaking, the environment–brain unity anchors the organism in the world by giving it a point of view from which it can experience and observe the world. That means that I postulate the absence or disruption of the environment–brain unity to go along with the absence or disruption of the point of view (and consequently with alterations in both FPP and TPP). This can indeed be supported empirically, as I will discuss in Chapter 22 in more detail with the example of schizophrenia.

However, we do not need to remain in the metaphorical realm anymore when describing the concept of point of view. If the

environment–brain unity is supposed to constitute the point of view, we can now characterize the concept of point of view in further detail. Point of view may be postulated to be based on differences, temporal and spatial differences between the stimuli's occurrences in the environment as they are encoded into the brain's resting state and its neural activity. The point of view is thus difference-based.

The difference-based nature of the point of view must be distinguished from its possible stimulus-based nature. In the case of a stimulus-based rather than difference-based nature of the resting state's neural activity, the latter would be based on the encoding of single discrete points (rather than the difference between them) in (physical) time and space.

Since this makes impossible the constitution of spatial and temporal unity between brain and environment, i.e., the environment–brain unity, any kind of point of view would remain absent in such cases of stimulus- rather than difference-based coding. Accordingly, a stimulus-based "point of view" would remain impossible (at least in our actual natural world while it may be possible a purely logical world), with any such concept being not only empirically implausible but also logically incoherent (within the framework of at least our actual natural world) (see Fig. 21-2g).

Let us further explicate this. I postulate that the point of view is statistically based (rather than being physically based; see later). This concerns the statistical frequency distribution of stimuli and the encoding of their natural statistics into the resting state's neural activity across different discrete points in (physical) time and space. That characterizes the point of view as statistically based rather than physically based, which then also applies to the biophysically based subjectivity.

If, in contrast, the encoding of stimuli into the resting state's neural activity were physically rather than statistically based, i.e., based on the encoding of the stimuli's discrete points in (physical) time and space, the constitution of an environment–brain unity, and consequently of a point of view, would remain impossible. There would thus no longer be any point of view, which would also make the constitution of bio-physically based subjectivity (and consequently, consciousness) impossible altogether.

NEUROPHILOSOPHICAL EXCURSION
IIC: POINT OF VIEW AND BIOPHYSICALLY
BASED SUBJECTIVITY ARE INTRINSICALLY
SPATIAL AND TEMPORAL

How does the point of view relate to the temporal and spatial dimensions of the environment–brain unity? I postulate that the point of view can be characterized by spatial extension and temporal duration and ultimately by the virtual statistically based temporal and spatial unity between organism and environment.

More specifically, I suggest that the degree of both spatial extension and temporal duration depends on the degree of correspondence between environmental stimuli's occurrence and the resting state's range of low frequency fluctuations and thus ultimately on the brain's biophysical range or spectrum. The larger the spatial and temporal extension of the environment–brain unity, the more extended and longer lasting the spatial and temporal unity of the point of view. What does such characterization of a point of view entail for the concept of biophysically based subjectivity? Since a point of view is a hallmark of biophysically based subjectivity, the features of the former are also supposed to be ascribed to the latter. I hence postulate the concept of biophysically based subjectivity to be difference- and statistically based and to be characterized by the virtual statistically based temporal and spatial unity between organism and environment, i.e., the environment–brain unity.

Finally, we should also note that neither biophysically based subjectivity nor the point of view should be confused with the self. Both biophysically based subjectivity and point of view describe a species-specific stance of a biophysical organism in the physical world. Such a species-specific stance must be distinguished from an individually specific self that distinguishes one individual from another one within one species, rather than a species from another species.

In order to understand the self, we must account for the mechanisms and processes that allow it to individualize the point of view and make it individually-specific, which is accompanied by the transition from biophysically to phenomenally based subjectivity. This will be the topic in Chapter 24, which focuses on self-specificity and self, and how they stand in relation to consciousness.

CONCEPTUAL BACKGROUND
IIA: DEPENDENCE OF UNITY ON
SUBJECTIVITY—"AVAILABILITY THESIS"

How is subjectivity related to unity? Subjectivity is a hallmark of consciousness, with the concept of "consciousness" often even being regarded as the (phenomenal) placeholder for the former; that is, "subjectivity." We therefore made a little theoretical excursion into the concept of subjectivity. The question now is how the two concepts of subjectivity as discussed here relate to the concept of unity as the other hallmark of consciousness. For that, I briefly tap into the current philosophical discussion about the relationship between unity and subjectivity.

Different positions on the relationship between unity and subjectivity have been put forward in the current philosophical discussion.[6] Here I provide only a rough outline of the main positions and their main advocates, while a more sophisticated account of the different positions remains beyond the scope of this book.

Some authors like British philosopher Susan Hurley (1998) argue that unity and subjectivity remain independent of each other. The unity of consciousness is not subjective and remains independent of the "what it is like"; therefore, the concept of unity must be considered in objective rather than subjective terms. This is contrasted by views where either unity is postulated to be dependent on subjectivity as put forward by Bayne and Chalmers (2003; Bayne 2007, 2010), or that subjectivity is based on unity as, for instance, suggested by Searle (2004).

Let's briefly explain the latter two positions. Bayne and Chalmers (2003; Bayne 2007, 2010) suggest what they call the "unity thesis." They discuss different possibilities for how the unity of consciousness (e.g., what I call phenomenal unity) can be generated.

One option is to generate unity by accessing different contents that may be globally available; this is, for instance, presupposed by the global workspace hypothesis (see appendix 1 for the discussion of the global workspace hypothesis). The better and the more different contents are available and the more global such access, the more likely one is able to generate a phenomenal unity and thus consciousness. Hence, unity is here based on availability and global access, which Bayne and Chalmers describe as the "availability thesis."

CONCEPTUAL BACKGROUND
IIB: DEPENDENCE OF UNITY ON SUBJECTIVITY—"CONSISTENCY THESIS"

The "availability thesis" must be distinguished from the "consistency thesis":? The "consistency thesis" postulates that unity is not based on availability and global access but rather on the consistency between different contents: The more consistent and overlapping different contents are, the more likely the phenomenal unity of consciousness may be generated.

Hence, unity is based here upon consistency rather than availability. Following Bayne and Chalmers (2003; Bayne 2007, 2010), both the availability thesis and consistency thesis are implausible, however, both empirically and conceptually (for reasons I will not discuss here).

They instead suggest an alternative thesis, the "unity thesis" that they deem to be more empirically and conceptually plausible. The unity thesis claims that the unity of consciousness is generated on the basis that different contents in experience are unified by their reference to one and the same subject who experiences them. Hence, the unity of consciousness is here based on the unity of the experiencing subject, subject unity, rather than on either the availability or consistency of the contents themselves.

This implies that the unity as presupposed in the unity thesis is based and necessarily dependent upon the unity of the subject, the "subject unity" (see Chapter 19 for the different concepts of unity). Without subjectivity and subject unity, no phenomenal unity and thus consciousness can be constituted, while conversely there could still be subjectivity and subject unity without phenomenal unity and consciousness.

CONCEPTUAL BACKGROUND
IIC: DEPENDENCE OF SUBJECTIVITY ON UNITY—SEARLE

Such unilateral dependence of phenomenal unity on subject unity and hence on subjectivity is rejected by John Searle, who argues for exactly the opposite relationship. Following him (Searle 2004), subjectivity and hence subject unity are very much based and dependent upon the phenomenal unity of consciousness, rather than the latter being based upon the former.

How can we further explain Searle's position? Searle (2004, 93–101) distinguishes between essential and nonessential features of consciousness. Essential features are those that are intrinsic and defining to consciousness since without them consciousness would cease to be consciousness. Searle considers qualitativeness, subjectivity,[7] and unity as essential and thus intrinsic features of consciousness. However, unity seems to be even more basic to consciousness than the other two essential features of consciousness.

This is well reflected in the following quote by Searle:

> I used to think that these three features, qualitativeness, subjectivity, and unity, could be described as distinct features of consciousness. It now seems to me that that is a mistake; they are all aspects of the same phenomenon. Consciousness by its very essence is qualitative, subjective, and unified. There is no way that a state could be qualitative, in the sense that I have introduced, without it also being subjective in the sense that I have explained. But there is no way that the state could be both qualitative and subjective, without having the kind of unity that I have been describing. You can see the last point if you try to imagine your present state of consciousness broken into 17 independent bits. If this occurred, you would have no conscious state with 17 parts; rather there would be 17 independent consciousness, 17 different loci of consciousness. It is absolutely essential to understand that consciousness is not divisible in the way that physical objects typically are; rather, consciousness always comes in discrete units of unified conscious fields. (Searle 2004, 95–96)

Taken together, there are three main positions in the current philosophical debate about the relationship between subjectivity and phenomenal unity. Either both unity and subjectivity are considered independently (Hurley), or they are postulated to be unilaterally dependent on each other in either direction (Searle, Bayne/Chalmers). How does that relate to the here-suggested characterization of the "environmental-brain unity"? This is the focus of the next section.

Neuroconceptual Plausibility IIIA: Biophysically Based Subjectivity and the Different Relationships Between Subjectivity and Unity

How does my distinction between biophysically and phenomenally based subjectivity stand in relation to the three possible relationships between phenomenal unity and subjectivity raised in the current philosophical discussion: What is now based on what: subjectivity on unity, or unity on subjectivity? Or do both unity and subjectivity remain unrelated and thus independent of each other?

Let me sketch three different possible scenarios. Either the environment-brain unity is based on the biophysical convergence zone which ultimately entails a necessary dependence of phenomenal unity on biophysically based subjectivity. This would come close to the unity thesis suggested by Bayne and Chalmers that claims the dependence of unity on subjectivity. Or the biophysical-based subjectivity is dependent upon the environment-brain unity. This would correspond to Searle's view of subjectivity being based upon phenomenal unity. Alternatively, both environment-brain unity and biophysical-based subjectivity may also be independent of each other. This would come close to the independence thesis between phenomenal unity and subjectivity as advocated by Hurley.

What is clear is that the species-specific environment-brain unity depends very much on the respective species and its brain's biophysical equipment and thus its biophysical convergence zone. Since the biophysical convergence zone is supposed to account for the point of view as hallmark of subjectivity, that is, biophysically based subjectivity, this scenario seems to support the unity thesis of Bayne and Chalmers who argue for the dependence of unity on subjectivity. Conceptually unity is then based on biophysically based subjectivity in the same way as empirically the environment–brain unity is based on the biophysical convergence zones.

Bayne and Chalmers' unity thesis seems to hold, however, only for the concept of biophysically based subjectivity, while it does not apply to the one of phenomenally based subjectivity. Phenomenally based subjectivity and thus the phenomenal unity of consciousness are supposed to be based on, for example, predisposed by, the prephenomenal unity and thus ultimately on the environment–brain unity. Here unity seems to come first and subjectivity second, thus supporting Searle's position rather than the one of Bayne and Chalmers. Hence, Searle's assumption of unity being more basic may be right, that is, empirically plausible, in the case of phenomenally based subjectivity, while it may not apply to biophysically based subjectivity.

This means that Searle's and Bayne/Chalmers' positions are both right and wrong, i.e., empirically plausible and implausible. Their assumption of subjectivity being more basic than unity applies to biophysically based subjectivity but not to phenomenally based subjectivity. While Searle's assumption that unity is more basic than subjectivity holds for phenomenally based subjectivity, whereas it is not plausible in the context of biophysically based subjectivity.

Neuroconceptual Plausibility IIIB: "Co-Occurrence and Co-Constitution" Between Unity and Subjectivity

Finally, one may want to raise the question whether priority in the directionality between unity and subjectivity can be postulated at all. Let us go back to the biophysical convergence zones and the environment–brain unity. Who is first and who comes second? Does the environment–brain unity come first and allow subsequently for the secondary constitution of biophysical convergence zone? Or vice versa?

Especially when considering evolution-ary mechanisms, we may remain unable to set both apart and segregate them from each other. The particular biophysical convergence zone of a specific species may have been constituted on the basis of a particular environment–brain unity that, due to the environmental and ecolog-ical circumstances, may have been favorable. At the same time the environment–brain unity may have been constituted on the basis of the avail-able biophysical spectrum of the respective spe-cies and thus its biophysical convergence zone.

Who comes first and who is second? We may ultimately remain unable to tell and thus cannot give a clear unidirectional and causal account of the relation between unity and subjectivity. Instead, all we can say and know is that there seems to be co-constitution and co-occurrence (see Northoff 2004a and b) between unity and subjectivity, that is, between environment–brain unity and the biophysically based subjectivity (as manifested in the biophysical convergence zone).

The assumption of co-occurrence co-constitution implies that any specific unilateral directionality in the relation between unity and subjectivity may not be empirically plausible. Hence, assumptions of unilateral dependence, as suggested by both Searle and Bayne/Chalmers (though in opposite directions), may be more related to their conceptual (and logical) equip-ment as philosophers, rather than to the brain itself and its resting state's neuronal mechanisms by means of which it relates to the environment.

Accordingly, the positions assuming uni-lateral dependence in either direction may be more related to the philosopher than to the brain itself as it functions independently of our observation and conceptualization. In short, I postulate these conceptual assumptions to be more observer based than brain based (see Appendix 4 in Volume I for the introduction of this distinction).

Open Questions

One issue concerns the implication of both environment–brain unity and biophysically based subjectivity for the concept of the brain. Usually the brain is defined as a physical organ, as reflected in the title of a recent book by P. M.

Churchland: *Plato's Camera: How the* Physical Brain *Captures a Landscape of Abstract Universals* (emphasis mine).

If the brain does indeed encode spatial and temporal differences between different stimuli rather than the stimuli themselves and their discrete points in physical space and time, the brain cannot be regarded as a purely physical organ but must also be a statistical organ. This, as Churchland would probably remark, does not invalidate the claim of the brain's being a physical organ, however.

Since such difference-based coding predis-poses the intrinsic relationship of the brain and its resting-state activity to the environment, the brain must also be regarded as a biological organ. Again, such a biological characterization does not falsify the description of the brain as a physical organ. It does, however, complement its meaning that a purely physical characteriza-tion of the brain remains incomplete. Therefore, I determine that the brain is a biophysical rather than merely a physical organ (see also Northoff 2011 and 2012 for further elaboration on the concept of "the brain").

The concept of such a biophysical brain implies a non-reductive account of subjectivity. Due to the inclusion of the biological component, the brain as biophysical organ is intrinsically and neces-sarily linked to the environment. This means that the "localization" of biophysically based subjectivity within the brain itself in terms of some kind of representation remains impossible. Rather than being located in and reduced to the brain itself, as is often assumed in the case of a physical brain (see, e.g., Metzinger 2003), bio-physically based subjectivity is supposed to be only based on, but not reduced to, the brain. One may therefore speak of a "brain-based" rather than a "brain-reductive" account of biophysically based subjectivity in particular, and subjectivity in general.

I shall also note that the concept of biophysically based subjectivity predisposes the concept of intersubjectivity, while it cannot be considered a sufficient condition and thus a correlate. Without biophysically based subjectivity, any intersubjec-tivity would be impossible. If there were physi-cal objectivity rather than biophysically based subjectivity, for instance, any kind of intersub-jectivity would remain impossible. However, the presence of biophysically based subjectivity alone does not entail the presence of intersubjectivity.

Another question concerns the here proposed theory of subjectivity and its related neuronal mechanisms, conceptual distinctions, and phenomenal features. I here considered the concept of subjectivity only to specify my concept of environment–brain unity as distinguished from the ones of prephenomenal and phenomenal unity. That led me to distinguish between biophysically and phenomenally based subjectivity that mirrors more or less the distinction between point of view and first-person perspective. While I am aware that many authors these days (see, for instance, Metzinger 2003) equate both point of view and first-person perspective with each other, I here refrain from such identification. This, however, already demonstrates how slippery the conceptual territory is when it comes to subjectivity and theories about it. Since I here focus mainly on empirical aspects, I leave a more detailed conceptual and theoretical elaboration of a theory of subjectivity to future investigation. This leads me to yet another problem; namely, how we can garner empirical support in favor of the distinction between biophysically and phenomenally based subjectivity. Experimentally, one would require double dissociation. One would need to manipulate phenomenally -based subjectivity while keeping biophysically based subjectivity constant. This is given in different species that show different forms of biophysically based subjectivity as related to their respective biophysical convergence zones.

The reverse scenario, keeping phenomenally based subjectivity constant while manipulating biophysically based subjectivity, remains impossible, however. Why? Because phenomenally based subjectivity is unilaterally dependent on and thus nested in biophysically based subjectivity. Hence, differences in biophysically based subjectivity entail (necessarily) differences in phenomenally based subjectivity. This is, I postulate, reflected in the differences in phenomenal consciousness between different species.

These constraints force us to consider the reverse case, manipulating phenomenally based subjectivity while keeping biophysically based subjectivity constant. There are indeed disorders that meet these criteria. Disorders of consciousness like vegetative state can be characterized by loss of phenomenally based subjectivity while their biophysically based subjectivity is still intact. Due to the fact that these patients' resting state operates close to its minimal biophysical limits,

they are no longer able to instantiate the degree of difference-based coding and thus the kind of spatial and temporal differences that are necessary to constitute the prephenomenal and ultimately the phenomenal unity. They are thus losing their phenomenally based subjectivity and ultimately consciousness altogether (see Part VIII for details).

Other examples are neuropsychiatric disorders, like schizophrenia. Unlike in disorders of consciousness, the phenomenally based subjectivity is instantiated here though in an abnormal sense. Schizophrenic patient may lose the ability to distinguish between first- and third-person perspective and may thereby develop an altered sense of phenomenally based subjectivity. This may be traced back possibly to neurodevelopmental alterations with early trauma in their childhood that leads to the constitution of an already volatile (and possibly flawed) environment–brain unity. Based on their alterations, schizophrenia may thus provide some empirical support albeit indirect to my neurophenomenal hypotheses of phenomenally based subjectivity and its dependence upon prior environment–brain unity and biophysically based subjectivity. I will therefore elaborate on this in Chapter 22.

Notes

1. Other views include the *internal links theory*, which postulates a phenomenally evident relationship among parts within a unified phenomenal space (Revensuo 2006), and the *co-ownership theory*, which is based on the assumption "that experiences had by the same subject involve their attribution to the same extra-phenomenal substrate or bearer of experiences, one that can be individuated independently of what is to be found in experience, and thus independently of the notion of a unified field of conscious contents" (Brook and Raymond 2006, 22).

2. The characterization of biophysically based subjectivity by a point of view sets it apart from the concept of subjectivity as suggested by John Searle, who associates it with the first-person perspective exclusively. He understands subjectivity in an ontological sense; that is, ontological subjectivity, meaning that consciousness is defined by first-person ontology. Following him, consciousness exists exclusively in the experience by a human or animal subject, and as such, it exists only in first-person perspective,

so it can ontologically be characterized in a twofold way by experience and first-person perspective. This feature of first-person ontology must be distinguished from the epistemic characterization of consciousness, which can be investigated and well accounted for in an epistemically objective way and thus in TPP, which makes it accessible to science. A subjective, first-person, experiential ontological feature of reality like consciousness can thus be investigated objectively by epistemic access to third-person observation in science: "The mode of existence of conscious states is indeed ontologically subjective but ontological subjectivity of the subject matter does not preclude an epistemically objective science of that very subject matter" (Searle 2004, 95).

3. One may also be reminded of Alfred Whitehead when I talk about biophysically based subjectivity. Alfred North Whitehead pursues a metaphysical approach to reality. Unlike traditional metaphysics, he rejects the concept of substances and replaces it by the concept of process. Everything is dynamic and changes continuously, and in this change, the true essence of nature, its existence and reality, can be found. There are processes overall and these processes define existence and reality, i.e., they are metaphysically relevant.

Physical reality is no longer determined by a static physical substance or physical properties as the modern derivative of the former. Instead, physical reality, as especially visible in the quantum physics of his time, is in itself dynamic and underlies continuous change. Change itself and thus the respective processes must consequently characterize the existence and reality of the physical world. Whitehead thus presupposes a process-based characterization of existence and reality.

As described so far, Whitehead's characterization of the physical remains within the bounds of the objective world as a hallmark of our current description of the physical. However, Whitehead departs from the assumption that the physical world is purely objective as we conceive of it. Instead, he argues that the physical world and its processes already contain the germ of subjectivity in its various processes. The continuous change and processes allow the continuous constitution of subjectivity out of the objective physical world, which therefore can no longer be regarded as purely objective in itself.

Whitehead thus focuses on the processes that constitute something subjective out of the objective physical world, with the latter predisposing the former. Does this mean that the objective physical world is not only subjective but also experiential and thus "conscious" in itself? Do we have to assume "panpsychism" with consciousness being present already in the lowest levels of the physical? Whitehead thus raises the question of whether there is subjectivity and thus consciousness in physical reality and existence itself. This is what many authors assume who see panpsychism as an absurd assumption that lets one suggest that stones can "experience" and thus be conscious.

However, to understand Whitehead in this way would be to misunderstand him. He argues that the physical world is indeed subjective and therefore an experiential world. This, however, does not imply that the physical world is conscious. Why? Because Whitehead assumes consciousness to be a higher-order function that comes later and builds on the more basic lower-order function of experience. In other words, there may be subjectivity and experience without consciousness, which violates one of the central presuppositions of the hard problem. Therefore, one may characterize, if one wants to do so, Whitehead's position as pansubjectivism and panexperientialism, but not as panpsychism (see also Griffin 1998).

How does Whitehead's position compare to the concept of "biophysically based subjectivity"? Both "locate" subjectivity in the world. However, the extent of that location is different. Whitehead considers the physical world to be subjective by itself. This includes any physical process independent of any biological organism. One may therefore speak of a "physically based subjectivity" that applies to any species within our physical world. "Physically based subjectivity" is thus not specific to a particular species and is therefore species-unspecific. Instead, it is specific for a particular world, the natural world as the physical world we live in, as distinguished from other natural worlds (or logically conceivable worlds). There is thus world-specificity rather than species-specificity.

The concept of biophysically based subjectivity differs. Here, the physical world is assumed to be objective, rather than subjective as in Whitehead. It is rather the transition from the physical world to the organism and their biophysical world and their brains that brings in subjectivity. I therefore speak of "biophysically based subjectivity" rather than "physically based subjectivity." This makes it clear that Whitehead's concept of "physically based subjectivity" is much more far-reaching and extensive than that of "biophysically based subjectivity." That is also why Whitehead determines his concept of "physically based subjectivity" as metaphysical or ontological. In contrast, my concept of "biophysically based subjectivity" must be "located' right at the border between metaphysical and epistemological domains in very much the same way as Kant's distinction between noumenal and phenomenal worlds can be found at exactly the same border.

4. Both concepts of subjectivity—phenomenally and biophysically based subjectivity—must be further distinguished in epistemological regard. This can be best illustrated by sketching their respective opposites. The opposite of phenomenally based subjectivity is objectivity. This sense of objectivity relies on the observation of physical states rather than the experience of phenomenal states. This sense of objectivity is thus no longer phenomenally based but physically based. And it is observer based rather than experience based. Such an observer-based and physically based concept of objectivity is associated with TPP rather than FPP.

The observer-based and physically based concept of objectivity is the epistemological opposite to the concept of phenomenally based subjectivity.

This distinguishes it from the concept of objectivity that is opposite to the biophysically based subjectivity. Objectivity in this sense can no longer be physically based nor be based on a point of view. It rather describes the absence of any point of view as well as the absence of any physical equipment, which is usually associated with God. Since this reaches beyond the limits of our possible knowledge, we remain unable to characterize this sense of objectivity in more positive detail. The only thing we seem able to know is that it must be different from the observer-based and physically based concept of objectivity.

5. There is another difference between both concepts of subjectivity not yet mentioned. The phenomenally based subjectivity is well compatible with objectivity of knowledge since the latter is delegated here to the third-person perspective. This contrasts with the biophysically based subjectivity where the subjectivity affects both first- and third-person perspective and thus all our possible knowledge. Subjectivity in the latter sense is thus epistemically relevant while in the former sense it is not (only being empirically relevant but not epistemically) when presupposing epistemological relevance in a Kantian sense. Many of the ambivalences in the interpretation of Kant's philosophy may stem from the confusion between these two notions of subjectivity. When Kant, for instance, claims for principal limits in our possible knowledge, he must presuppose what I here describe as biophysically based subjectivity that by definition is epistemically relevant. In contrast, his description of how consciousness is constituted seems to presuppose rather the concept of phenomenally based subjectivity; that, however, is only empirically but not epistemically relevant. Hence, his epistemological distinction between noumenal and phenomenal worlds can only be made on the basis of biophysically based subjectivity, while it remains impossible and nonsensical when presupposing phenomenally based subjectivity.

6. Again I leave it to the philosophers to go into detail here; I can only roughly sketch the main positions.

7. As detailed in a prior note, Searle understands subjectivity in an ontological sense, that is, ontological subjectivity, describing that consciousness is defined by first-person ontology. Consciousness exists only in experience by a human or animal subject and as such it exists only in first-person perspective so that it can ontologically be characterized in a two-fold way by experience and first-person perspective. This feature of first-person ontology must be distinguished from the epistemic characterization of consciousness that can well be investigated and accounted for in an epistemically objective way and thus in TPP that makes it accessible to science.

CHAPTER 22
Unity and Subjectivity in Schizophrenia

Summary

I discussed the neuronal mechanisms underlying what I described as the environment–brain unity (Chapter 20) and associated it with what conceptually has been described as point of view and subjectivity as hallmark feature of consciousness (Chapter 21). The question now is how we can gather empirical support in favor of this assumption that subjectivity and unity go hand in hand. For that, I turn to the neuropsychiatric disorder of schizophrenia. Patients with schizophrenia do indeed experience a disruption in their relationship to the environment, a lack of attunement, as it is described in phenomenological approaches. Neuronally, schizophrenia can be characterized by deficits in early sensory processing, as they are, for instance, manifest in a specific electrophysiological potential, the mismatch negativity (MMN), and frequency phase synchronization. Based on these findings, I hypothesize abnormal encoding of the statistical structure of bodily and environmental stimuli in schizophrenia, which I subsume under what I describe as the "encoding hypothesis" ("EC hypothesis"). Such abnormal encoding leads, in turn, to the neural coding of abnormal differences in neural activity that are either abnormally high or low. Difference-based coding is consequently abnormal amounting to what I describe as "difference-based coding hypothesis" of schizophrenia ("DC hypothesis"). How is such abnormal encoding of the statistical structure (and thus their natural statistics) of (bodily and) environmental stimuli and subsequent abnormal difference-based coding possible? Based on neurodevelopmental evidence, I postulate biopsychosocial trauma in early infancy and social isolation to be central here. Taking all this together, one may postulate abnormal statistically based spatiotemporal configuration in the environment–brain unity and consecutively in the brain's resting state in schizophrenia. This, in turn, leads to abnormal phenomenally based subjectivity in these patients as manifested in their bizarre symptoms like auditory hallucinations, paranoid delusions, thought disorders, and ego disturbances. Hence, the example of schizophrenia lends empirical and phenomenal support, albeit indirectly, to my neurophenomenal hypothesis of the close relationship between environment–brain unity and subjectivity.

Key Concepts and Topics Covered

Schizophrenia, environment-brain unity, low-frequency fluctuations, encoding hypothesis, difference-based coding hypothesis, social deafferentiation, early trauma

NEUROEMPIRICAL BACKGROUND I: WHAT SCHIZOPHRENIA CAN TELL US ABOUT THE RELATIONSHIP BETWEEN SUBJECTIVITY AND UNITY

I have discussed different forms of unity—phenomenal unity, prephenomenal unity, and environment–brain unity in the preceding chapters. Therein, environment–brain unity especially remained rather abstract, and its impact on our phenomenal consciousness was not made clear. This is the focus of the present chapter.

Herein I pursue an indirect approach, namely taking the detour through a neuropsychiatric disorder, schizophrenia.[1] Schizophrenia may tell us something about the environment–brain unity and how and why it predisposes and is thus necessary to yield the phenomenal unity and the phenomenally based subjectivity of consciousness. For that, I will go into detail

about schizophrenia both neuronally and phenomenally. This, in turn, will allow me to draw
inferences about the features and role of the
environment–brain unity for phenomenal unity
and phenomenally based subjectivity and thus
for phenomenal consciousness in general.

What is schizophrenia? Schizophrenia is a
complex neuropsychiatric disorder in which
patients experience bizarre symptoms like auditory hallucinations, paranoid delusions, thought
disorders, ego disturbances, avolition, and lack
of affect. Various neuronal functions and mechanisms have been investigated and found to be
abnormal. One major focus is the neuronal processes underlying early sensory processing.

Unlike the neuronal mechanisms underlying
early sensory processing, those related to affective and cognitive changes in schizophrenia are
beyond the scope of this chapter. Chapter 27 will
focus on the neuronal mechanisms underlying
the abnormal self in schizophrenia, while I leave
open completely the neuronal mechanisms of
the affective and cognitive symptoms in schizophrenia in this book.

Moreover, I mainly focus on imaging studies while the many postmortem and animal
studies on schizophrenia are neglected. Recall
that I indicated some of the biochemical abnormalities of schizophrenia with regard to GABA
and glutamate in Chapter 17, when discussing
abnormal experience of time and space.

NEURONAL FINDINGS IA: ABNORMAL EARLY PREATTENTIVE AUDITORY PROCESSING IN SCHIZOPHRENIA

Let us now focus on sensory processing and their
neuronal mechanisms in schizophrenia. One
early electrophysiological potential related to
sensory processing in auditory cortex is the mismatch negativity (MMN). The MMN is an electrophysiological potential that can be measured
when a deviant (i.e., oddball) auditory stimulus
occurs embedded in a stream of familiar or standard auditory stimuli. The MMN can be measured in both electroencephalography (EEG)
and magnetoencephalography (MEG) as a negative waveform that results from subtracting the

event-related response to the standard event
from the response to the deviant event.

Elicited by sudden changes in auditory stimuli, the MMN occurs about 100–250 ms after
the onset of the deviant stimulus and is strongest over frontal and temporal regions. While
the MMN is primarily an auditory potential (see
Naatanen et al. 2007 for review), it is a matter of
debate whether potentials analogue to the MMN
also occur in other sensory modalities as, for
instance, in visual and somatosensory modalities (see Chapter 7 for a detailed discussion of
the MMN, as well as Garrido et al. 2008, 2009a–c
for review).

Numerous studies showed changes and deficits
in the MMN in schizophrenia (see Garrido et al.
2009a-c and Javitt 2009a and b for reviews). More
specifically, these studies demonstrated reduction in the amplitude of the MMN in patients
with schizophrenia, which holds for when both
the frequency and the duration of the deviant
stimulus were varied. Moreover, the amplitudes
of the deviant stimulus and thus the MMN correlate with disease severity and cognitive dysfunction in these patients; this further underlines
the crucial relevance of the MMN as marker of
altered auditory processing in schizophrenia.

NEURONAL FINDINGS IB: ALTERATIONS IN EARLY SENSORY PROCESSING IN SCHIZOPHRENIA

In addition to the MMN, other markers of early
sensory processing in auditory cortex have been
observed to be altered in schizophrenia. These
include reductions in the amplitude of even earlier auditory electrophysiological potentials like
P50 and N100 that are elicited by simple repetitive stimuli; this distinguishes them from the
MMN that are induced by a deviant stimulus
after a series of repetitive stimuli.

Both electrophysiological potentials, for
example, P50 and N100, are postulated to be
generated in auditory cortex, including both primary and secondary auditory regions (see Javitt
2009a and b and Turetsky et al. 2007a–c for recent
overviews as well as Tregallas et al. 2009 for a
recent functional magnetic resonance imaging

[fMRI] study). Taken together, these findings point to deficits in the early stages of auditory sensory processing, where the stimulus starts to be processed and evaluated in schizophrenia.

These changes are not limited to the auditory cortex but are also observed in other sensory systems like the visual cortex. Amplitudes in early visual electrophysiological potentials like the steady-state visual-evoked and auditory-evoked potentials (ssVEPs, ssAEPs), the N100, and the P100 have been found to be reduced in patients with schizophrenia (Javitt 2009a and b).

At the same time, low- and high-frequency visual stimuli induced significantly lower neural activity in primary and secondary visual cortex in patients with schizophrenia when compared to healthy subjects (Martinez et al. 2008). Since the other sensory systems (olfactory, somatosensory, gustatory) also show physiological and phenomenological abnormalities (see Javitt 2009a and b), one may postulate a general alteration in early automatic processing of sensory stimuli in the sensory cortex in schizophrenia.

NEURONAL HYPOTHESIS IA: ABNORMAL IMPLICIT AND AUTOMATIC PROCESSING IN SCHIZOPHRENIA

What do these deficits in early electrophysiological potentials mean in psychological and functional regard?

Let us go back to the MMN. Psychologically, the MMN has been associated with implicit and thus automatic processing since it occurs independent of and thus prior to attention (Garrido et al. 2008, 2009a–c). For instance, the MMN is induced when the subjects do not pay attention at all to the stimuli, whether they be standard or deviant, or when subjects perform a task completely unrelated to the stimuli. Hence, preattentive cognitive processes that allow for the detection of deviant stimuli (in the midst of repetitive stimuli) have been postulated to underlie the MMN.

The independence of the MMN from attention is further underlined by its occurrence in sleep and even in comatose patients in vegetative states who by definition do not show consciousness (see Qin et al. 2008). This strongly indicates that the MMN does not only occur prior to attention but remains also independent of consciousness altogether.

In sum, psychologically the MMN seems to mirror an early stage of sensory processing that may be independent of and prior to both attention and consciousness. The observation of an abnormal MMN in schizophrenia means that these early implicit and automatic processes may be disrupted in this disorder.

NEURONAL HYPOTHESIS IB: ABNORMAL DIFFERENCE-BASED CODING IN SCHIZOPHRENIA

What processes cause the MMN? The MMN results from the mismatch between the deviant, for example, present, and the standard, for example, previous, auditory stimuli, hence the name mismatch negativity. This implies, most important, that the MMN must be considered a potential that results from a difference between different stimuli, that is, deviant and repetitive stimulus, rather than from a single stimulus alone. And it is this difference between the two stimuli that induces an electrophysiological potential, the MMN (see also Chapter 7, Volume I, for a more detailed account of the MMN).

The MMN thus presupposes difference-based coding as distinguished from mere stimulus-based coding. Hence, the fact that the amplitude of the MMN is reduced in schizophrenia tells us that these patients are apparently no longer able to generate proper neural differences between different stimuli, entailing altered difference-based coding.

Let's be more precise. How exactly is the difference between deviant and repetitive stimuli generated in the MMN? Neural coding of the difference between the deviant and repetitive stimulus presupposes first inhibition of any response to the repetitive stimulus and second detection of the deviant stimulus as deviant (see Turetsky et al. 2007a–c. While the inhibition of repetitive stimuli is mirrored by early potentials like the P50 and N100 (and the prepulse inhibition), detection of the deviant stimulus is supposed to be related to the MMN itself and even later potentials like the P300. In sum, the abnormalities in the various electrophysiological potentials described earlier lend evidence to the view that schizophrenia can be characterized by failures in both inhibition of repetitive stimuli and detection of deviant stimuli in early automatic sensory processing (see Javitt 2009a and b and Turetsky et al. 2007a–c). The deficits in both inhibition and detection may lead to reduced neuronal differentiation and thus to the encoding of smaller spatial and temporal differences in early processing into sensory cortical neural activity in schizophrenia. This inclines me to postulate that the automatic generation of early spatial and temporal differences between different stimuli in terms of difference-based coding may be reduced and thus abnormal in schizophrenia.

NEURONAL FINDINGS IIA: ABNORMAL *HIGH*-FREQUENCY FLUCTUATIONS IN SCHIZOPHRENIA

In addition to the changes in the early event-related potentials, abnormal changes in high and low-frequency oscillation amplitudes and phase synchrony have also been observed in schizophrenia. Studies by Spencer et al. (2003, 2008, 2009; see Spencer 2009 as well as Moran and Hong 2011 for reviews) observed reduced phase locking and amplitude in especially gamma oscillations in visual and auditory cortical sites in patients with schizophrenia during auditory or visual tasks.

Let us be more specific. Mulert et al. (2010) observed a significant correlation between the severity of auditory hallucinations and phase synchronization in the gamma range between the bilateral primary auditory cortices: the higher the gamma phase synchronization between right and left auditory cortex, the higher the score for auditory hallucinations.

In addition to the changes in sensory functions, abnormal power and phase synchrony in high-frequency fluctuations like gamma has also been observed in schizophrenia during a variety of cognitive paradigms (attention, working memory, executive functions, etc.) over especially frontal and temporal electrodes (see Uhlhaas and Singer 2010 for a recent review).

NEURONAL FINDINGS IIB: ABNORMAL *LOW*-FREQUENCY FLUCTUATIONS IN SCHIZOPHRENIA

I have focused thus far on higher-frequency fluctuations like gamma in schizophrenia. What about low-frequency fluctuations like < 0.01? A recent fMRI resting-state study (6 minutes eyes closed) compared 29 medicated patients with schizophrenia with healthy subjects with regard to their low-frequency fluctuations (see Hoptman et al. 2010). Thereby, the ratio of the amplitude in a low-frequency band to the amplitude in the total frequency band (fALFF = fractional, i.e., relative, amplitude of low-frequency fluctuation) and as absolute amplitude of the low-frequency fluctuation itself (ALFF) were calculated. Frequency ranges calculated here were between 0.02 to 0.07 Hz.

Patients with schizophrenia showed significantly decreased fALFF and ALFF values in the left insula, the cuneus, precuneus, the middle occipital cortex, the posterior cingulate cortex, precentral and postcentral cortex, and the caudate. As the authors themselves remark, this concerns especially those regions involved in early sensory and motor processing, which is consistent with the findings in the early event-related potentials reported earlier (though the exact relationship between low-frequency fluctuations and event-related potentials remains a matter of debate).

In contrast, significantly increased amplitudes in low-frequency fluctuations in schizophrenia were observed in the parahippocampus/hippocampus as well as in various spots in the medial prefrontal cortex, including the dorsomedial prefrontal cortex and the anterior cingulate cortex. Hippocampal dysfunction is well known in schizophrenia and the medial cortical changes suggest abnormalities in the default-mode network in schizophrenia, which will be discussed in further detail in the parts on self-perspectival organization and intentionality (see Part VII).

Another fMRI study (Rotarska-Jagiela et al. 2010) investigated the relation between low-frequency fluctuations and psychopathological symptoms scores in the resting state. They observed that the power spectral density (PSD) of low-frequency fluctuations (< 0.06 Hz) was positively related to the severity of positive symptoms like disorganization and delusions. The higher the PSD of the low-frequency fluctuations in the superior temporal gyrus and anterior cingulate cortex (and the hippocampus/amygdale), the more the patients suffered from a higher degree of severity of the respective symptoms of disorganization and/or delusion.

NEURONAL FINDINGS IIC: ABNORMAL PHASE SYNCHRONY IN SCHIZOPHRENIA

Recent EEG studies investigated patients with schizophrenia during an auditory oddball task. Here abnormalities in the phase-resetting of delta (1–4 Hz) and theta (4–8 Hz) frequencies could be observed (see Doege et al. 2010). Especially the phase resetting of the delta phase was related to symptoms of disorganization, hence corroborating the evidence that low-frequency fluctuations and especially their phases are related to positive symptoms (e.g., delusions, hallucinations, thought and ego disorders) in schizophrenia. Interestingly these abnormalities were most pronounced in the midline electrodes (Fz, Cz, Pz), further suggesting changes in the cortical midline structures in schizophrenia (see Chapter 23 for more details).

These findings indicate alterations in the infraslow-frequency fluctuations (< -0.1 Hz) as well as the slow (delta and theta) and high (gamma and beta) frequency fluctuations. They concern both power, that is, amplitude, and phase synchrony, which is indicative of abnormal regional and global neuronal coordination in both resting state and stimulus-induced activity. In addition, there seem to also be changes in gamma frequencies, which may be closely related to the changes in the lower ones (Moran and Hong 2011; Hamm et al. 2011).

Though tentative, these findings suggest abnormal increases in low-frequency fluctuations in cortical midline regions of the default-mode network while they seem to be rather decreased in sensory and motor regions. Finally, changes in the low-frequency fluctuations (< 4Hz) seem to be directly related to especially positive symptoms in schizophrenia. However, at this point in time, these findings

have to be considered preliminary, awaiting further support and experimental investigation.

NEURONAL HYPOTHESIS IIA: "CONTINUOUS" RATHER THAN "RHYTHMIC" MODE OF BRAIN FUNCTION IN SCHIZOPHRENIA

The neuronal findings in schizophrenia clearly demonstrate early abnormalities in sensory processing and low- and high-frequency fluctuations' amplitude and phase in schizophrenia. Why are both early sensory processing and especially low-frequency fluctuations abnormal in schizophrenia? First of all, difference-based coding may be abnormal, as mentioned previously.

Where does such abnormal difference-based coding stem from? The differences coded in neural activity in schizophrenia may be either abnormally low or extremely high, while the intermediate range of differences seems to be rarely utilized anymore. I postulate that the coding of abnormal differences in difference-based coding may stem from abnormalities in the encoding of the environmental stimuli's statistical frequency distribution, i.e., their natural statistics, into the resting state's neural activity (see Dias et al. 2011 for a recent study that indirectly supports the assumption of an encoding deficit in schizophrenia).

To explain this in more detail, let us recall the two modes of neural presentation, rhythmic and continuous, as described in Chapter 20. The rhythmic mode of neural operation is associated with high phase synchrony between high- and low-frequency fluctuations as well as with the matching between the rhythmic presentation of environmental stimuli (e.g., their statistical occurrence across time) and the low-frequency fluctuations' phases.

However, the encoding of the stimuli's statistical structure of their occurrence across time comes to its limits when there is no rhythmic structure as, for instance, during discontinuous and random stimulus presentation. In this case the phase synchronization of the low-frequency fluctuations and subsequently their entrainment of higher frequency fluctuations can no longer rely on the environmental stimuli and their statistical structure. The brain itself has to provide a certain structure now and this is associated with the suppression of the resting state's low-frequency fluctuations by the stimulus-induced high-frequency fluctuations. The brain is then no longer in a rhythmic mode of function but rather in a "continuous mode," where it has to be continuously active by itself.

The two modes of neural operation, rhythmic and continuous, may basically be considered opposite extremes on a continuum of different possible relationships between environmental stimuli and the resting state's low-frequency oscillations (see Chapter 20 for details). Different degrees of rhythmicity in the occurrence of environmental stimuli across time may then go along with different degrees of phase synchronization and thus different time windows in the low-frequency fluctuations' cycle. The more rhythmic the stimuli occur in the environment, the higher the likelihood that the resting state's low-frequency fluctuations can align their phase onsets to the predicted stimuli's onset (see Fig. 22-1a).

NEURONAL HYPOTHESIS IIB: "ENCODING HYPOTHESIS" OF SCHIZOPHRENIA

Based on the findings discussed earlier, I hypothesize that this matching process between the low-frequency's phase synchronization, that is, their phase alignment, and the statistical structure of the environmental stimuli is altered in schizophrenia. Unlike in healthy subjects, the phase synchronization and hence the cycle's time windows of low-frequency fluctuations, including their phase onsets, may no longer vary as a function of different degrees in the environmental stimuli's statistical structure.

Accordingly, the low-frequency fluctuations' phase onset synchronization may be decoupled from the temporal and thus the statistical structure of the environmental stimuli. In other words, the low-frequency fluctuations' phase onsets is detached from the onsets of the stimuli in the environment, i.e., their natural statistics. I therefore hypothesize that the low frequencies' phase alignment to the external stimuli is significantly reduced in schizophrenia. This means that the stimuli's natural statistics is no longer properly encoded in the resting state's neural activity,

which I describe as the "encoding hypothesis" of schizophrenia ("EC hypothesis").

The "EC hypothesis" describes the assumption that the encoding of the bodily and environmental stimuli's natural statistics, i.e., their statistical frequency distribution, is disrupted in schizophrenia. Such abnormal encoding is supposed to be manifest in abnormal difference-based coding which in turn leads to abnormal neural processing all over the brain as it shall be sketched briefly in the following.

Since the patients with schizophrenia seem to no longer encode the statistical frequency distribution of the environmental stimuli, it must be postulated that their brain and thus their resting state operate in a "continuous mode" rather than a "rhythmic mode" of neural operation. The schizophrenic patient's brain may thus remain unable to switch between the different modes of neural operation, e.g., rhythmic and continuous, and to adjust their brain's mode to the respective environmental (and bodily) demands.

NEURONAL HYPOTHESIS IIC: FALSE POSITIVE AND NEGATIVE ENCODING OF STIMULI LEADS TO THE DECOUPLING OF ENVIRONMENT AND BRAIN IN SCHIZOPHRENIA

How could we lend empirical support to the EC hypothesis of schizophrenia?

One could conduct investigations in patients with schizophrenia and animals models of schizophrenia similar to those reported earlier, especially in Chapters 19 and 20. To my knowledge, this remains to be investigated. I hypothesize decreased variation in low-frequency phase synchronization, that is, phase alignment, in response to rhythmically and nonrhythmically presented environmental stimuli. Unlike in healthy subjects, I postulate that there will be no difference in the low-frequency oscillations' phases during rhythmic and nonrhythmic stimulus presentation. In addition, I hypothesize that the actual degree of low-frequency phase synchronization will be shifted toward extreme values showing either abnormally low or extremely high values. Either the phases are abnormally synchronized with no variation between them; or they are not synchronized at all, operating

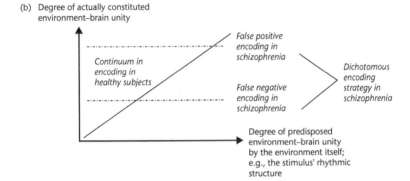

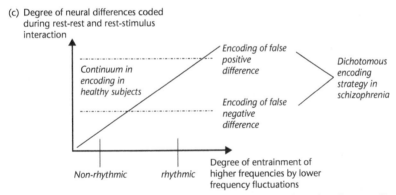

Figure 22-1a-c Encoding hypothesis in schizophrenia. The figure describes the encoding strategies of stimuli into the brain's resting-state activity in healthy and schizophrenic subjects. (*a*) The figure shows the continuous encoding of the rhythmic structure of stimuli in healthy subjects via phase alignment of their resting state's low-frequency fluctuations. Such continuous encoding is no longer possible in patients with schizophrenia who revert to a dichotomous encoding strategy with false-positives and false-negatives. (*b*) Such a change in the encoding strategy is supposed to lead to mismatches between environmental stimuli and the encoded neural activity due to encoding of false-positive and false-negative spatial and temporal differences between different stimuli into neural activity. (*c*) The implications for difference-based coding and the entrainment of higher frequency fluctuations by lower ones are already shown with the consequences of the dichotomous encoding strategy in schizophrenia.

almost completely randomly. Either extreme may make it impossible to encode the statistical structure and thus the natural statistics of environmental stimuli in a proper way.

For instance, rhythmically presented stimuli may then possibly be encoded in a false-negative way; that is, as nonrhythmic. In contrast, the opposite holds true for nonrhythmic presentations, which may then possibly be encoded in a false-positive way; that is, as rhythmic. Such false encoding means that the intrinsic activity in the schizophrenic patients' brains is no longer organized and structured in orientation to the natural and social statistics of the environmental (and bodily) stimuli. The brain's intrinsic activity is thus detached or decoupled from the environment (and the body); that is, from their natural, social, and vegetative statistics of their stimuli.

NEURONAL HYPOTHESIS IIC: MISMATCH BETWEEN "REAL" AND "ENCODED" ENVIRONMENT–BRAIN UNITY IN SCHIZOPHRENIA

What does the ED hypothesis imply for the environment–brain unity in schizophrenia? The encoding of extreme values in the low-frequency oscillations' phases implies that the environment–brain unity may be unstable, volatile, and fragile. Both brain and environment can consecutively easily be decoupled and dissociate from each other. I postulate such decoupling to be well manifested in both false-positive and false-negative encoding as described earlier.

Brain and environment become consecutively less unified, with their relationship oscillating between the extremes of false-positive and false-negative encoding strategies. Instead of spatial and temporal unity and thus environment–brain unity, there will be spatial and temporal disunity in neural activity and thus discontinuity between brain and environment (and body) in schizophrenia. The continuum in the encoding strategy of healthy subjects becomes here replaced by a dichotomous encoding strategy.

More specifically, in the case of false-positive encoding, the patient with schizophrenia may neuronally constitute a high degree of environment–brain unity when it is actually rather low in reality. In contrast, in the opposite case of false negative encoding, he fails to constitute a proper degree of environment–brain unity when in reality it is rather high. There is consecutively a mismatch between the degree of the actually encoded environment–brain unity and the degree of the "real" environment–brain unity as predisposed by the environment (and its stimuli) itself. One may thus postulate discrepancy between what is encoded in neural activity and what is predisposed by the environment itself (for subsequent encoding into the brain's intrinsic activity) (see Fig. 22-1b).

PHENOMENOLOGICAL EXCURSION: DEFICITS IN "ATTUNEMENT" AND "CRISIS OF COMMON SENSE" IN SCHIZOPHRENIA

One may be surprised by my insertion of a phenomenological account at this stage. The phenomenological account refers to how the patient perceives and experiences his symptoms, his environment, and himself in schizophrenia. As such, the phenomenological approach describes, for instance, how we (i.e., both healthy and schizophrenic subjects) experience incoming sensory stimuli as exteroceptive auditory stimuli or interoceptive stimuli from our own body in a subjective way, and thus how we can relate them to our self, the subject of experience. The linkage of sensory stimuli to the self in experience thus concerns what phenomenological accounts describe as "attunement" (see later for details; Bin Kimura 1997; Blankenburg 1969; Parnas et al. 1998; Parnas et al. 1998, 2001, 2003; Parnas 2003; Parnas and Handest 2003, Sass 2000, 2003; Sass and Parnas 2001, 2003).

Josef Parnas, who works in Copenhagen at the Centre for Subjectivity, has been one of the leading phenomenological psychiatrists in developing the phenomenology of experience in schizophrenia. He has written many papers based on patients' reports, in which he describes the phenomenology in impressive ways.

Central to Parnas's work is the concept of "attunement," which describes, most broadly, the relationship of the self to the world; for example, how the self adjusts and adapts to the various objects, events, and other persons in its various environments. Most important, phenomenologists point out that "attunement" in this sense operates already on a prereflective, implicit, or preconceptual level, which Parnas (2003) and Sass (2003) describe as "prereflective or preconceptual attunement." In the following discussion, I will use the concept of attunement to describe such prereflective, preconceptual, and implicit adaptive processes.

How is the loss of such prereflective and preconceptual attunement manifested in subjects' experience and behavior? Patients with schizophrenia seem to lose their "common sense." Such a loss of common sense may be visible when patients with schizophrenia begin to question the meaning and nature of the very objects and events of the world they experience, as well as the nature of their own self, which they can apparently no longer access in their experience.

They thus become "hyper-reflective" as Sass (1996, 2003) would say; they reflect on and ponder the reasons why the objects and events in the world are as strange as they experience and perceive them to be. Stanghellini (Stanghellini 2009; Stanghellini and Ballerini 2007, 2008) describes such a loss of "normal relation to the world" as a "crisis of common sense" or "loss of prereflective operative common sense that disrupts self-experience in the context of relatedness."

Schizophrenia may therefore be characterized phenomenologically by "disrupted attunement," which makes it impossible for the patient with schizophrenia to relate to his environment in a subjective and experiential way. This may be phenomenologically manifested in what is described as "disturbed preconceptual attunement" and "crisis of prereflective operative common sense" (see also Chapters 17 and 27; see also Northoff 2011, chapter 11, for more phenomenological details).

Neurophenomenal Hypothesis

IA: "DIFFERENCE-BASED CODING HYPOTHESIS" IN SCHIZOPHRENIA

I postulated low-frequency fluctuations to be central in schizophrenia in that they no longer allow proper encoding of the stimuli's statistical structure, i.e., their natural statistics. Such abnormal encoding, in turn, is supposed to affect the constitution of the environment–brain unity, leading to a discrepancy between actual encoding (by the brain's intrinsic activity) and real predisposition (by the environment itself).

The question now is how the abnormal encoding in the low-frequency fluctuations affects subsequent neuronal processing and the associated prephenomenal and phenomenal features as described in the preceding section. We already discussed two instances of subsequent neuronal processing: early sensory processing and high-frequency fluctuations.

Let me start with the latter, the high frequency fluctuations. As discussed especially in Chapter 19, high-frequency fluctuations are entrained by the phases of the low-frequency fluctuations. If now the low-frequency fluctuations, that is, their phases, are by themselves abnormal, their lack of proper encoding is transferred and carried forth to the high-frequency fluctuations.

What does such lack of proper encoding imply in neuronal regard? Neuronally this means that the abnormal difference-based coding as a consequence of the earlier improper encoding is amplified further in coding subsequent neural activity during the coupling of low- to high-frequency fluctuations. The assumption of such abnormal difference-based coding is well in accordance with the findings reported earlier.

I therefore postulate the improper difference-based coding during the encoding to be carried over, transferred, and thus amplified to subsequent interactions within the intrinsic activity itself, rest–rest interaction, and its low-high frequency coupling. And there is even further amplification. When the schizophrenic patient's resting state encounters a particular extrinsic stimulus, the latter and thus the stimulus-induced activity will also be affected. That is, for instance, evident in the deficits in early sensory processing described earlier that also indicate abnormal difference-based coding during rest–stimulus interaction.

Taken together, this leads me to formulate what I describe as the "difference-based coding hypothesis" of schizophrenia ("DC hypothesis"). The DC hypothesis points out that the differences coded in neural activity in schizophrenia are abnormal, being either too high or too low.

The encoding of neural activity thus follows a dichotomous rather than continuous distribution. This pertains to all three stimulus–rest, rest–rest, and rest–stimulus (and probably to stimulus–stimulus) interaction (Fig 22-1c).

NEUROPHENOMENAL HYPOTHESIS
IB: ABNORMAL "DIFFERENCE-BASED CODING HYPOTHESIS" PREDISPOSES AN ABNORMAL "PREPHENOMENAL UNITY" IN SCHIZOPHRENIA

How is such abnormal difference-based coding related to the abnormal phenomenal features in schizophrenia described earlier? The abnormal difference-based coding in the resting state leads to the constitution of an abnormal global spatiotemporal continuity with either too large or too small spatial extensions and temporal durations. The spatiotemporal continuity of the resting state constituted on the basis of rest–rest interaction (see Part V here) must therefore be postulated to be abnormal by itself in schizophrenia. This, however, affects the resting state's constitution of spatial and temporal unity of its neural activity and consecutively its prephenomenal unity (see Chapter 18 for details).

I now postulate the alterations of the resting state's prephenomenal unity, that is, the spatiotemporal continuity and unity of its neural activity, to be carried over and transferred to subsequent stimulus-induced activity and consecutively to the phenomenal unity of consciousness. The resting state's spatiotemporal continuity may, for instance, "suffer" from either too large or too small spatial and temporal differences as related to abnormal difference-based coding.

Phenomenally, this may be manifest in abnormal spatial extension and temporal duration with both being either too small or too large in inner time and space consciousness. More simply put, the spatial and temporal grid or template provided by the brain's intrinsic activity may itself be already abnormal in schizophrenia; this in turn leads to abnormal spatial and temporal continuity of its neural activity and consequently to abnormal prephenomenal unity.

How is the abnormal spatial and temporal grid or template of the brain's intrinsic activity manifested in subjective experience and thus in consciousness? The abnormal spatial grid or template may result in what phenomenologically has been described as the "lack of preconceptual attunement" and the "crisis of prereflective operative common sense.": the resting state may simply be less affected by the environmental (and bodily) stimuli, entailing reduced rest–stimulus interaction. Phenomenally this may be manifested in diminished self-affection and altered presence (see earlier), which in turn may lead to the earlier described alteration or crisis of common sense.

I therefore hypothesize that the earlier described phenomenal abnormalities in schizophrenia may be neuronally related to abnormal difference-based coding of stimulus–rest, rest–rest, and rest–stimulus interactions. These abnormal interactions may be traced back to abnormalities in spatiotemporal continuity and prephenomenal unity in the resting state that predisposes abnormal phenomenal unity during subsequent stimulus-induced activity.

Accordingly, I postulate that the phenomenal abnormalities in schizophrenia may result from the carryover and transfer of the abnormal environment–brain unity over the prephenomenal onto the phenomenal unity. Therefore, one may regard schizophrenia as a disorder of the environment–brain unity and hence as a disorder of the neural predispositions of consciousness (rather than being a disturbance of the neural correlates of consciousness themselves; see Fig. 22-2a and b).

NEURONAL FINDINGS
IIIA: NEURODEVELOPMENTAL HYPOTHESIS OF SCHIZOPHRENIA

I have so far postulated abnormal encoding of environmental (and bodily) stimuli into the brain's intrinsic activity. This, as I supposed, leads to abnormal difference-based coding with subsequent abnormalities in the prephenomenal and phenomenal unity. In contrast, I left open the reasons why there is such abnormal encoding in schizophrenia. This question shall be the focus in this and the following sections.

There is much discussion about a neurodevelopmental hypothesis in schizophrenia (see Lewis and Levitt 2002). The neurodevelopmental hypothesis argues that there may be

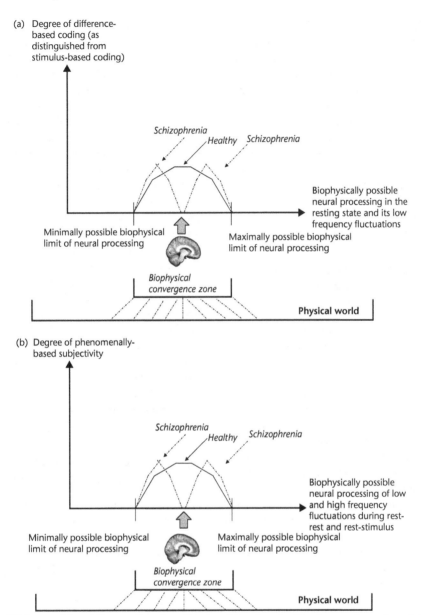

Figure 22-2a and b Difference-based coding in schizophrenia. The figures show the relationship between the biophysical convergence zones, difference-based coding, and phenomenally based subjectivity. (*a*) The figure shows the relationship between the resting state's low-frequency fluctuations within the biophysical convergence zones and the degree of difference-based coding. The higher the degree of the possible low-frequency fluctuations, the higher the degree of possible difference-based coding. While this also holds true in schizophrenia, there seems to be a dichotomous distribution rather than a continuous one as in healthy subjects. In the lower part the whole spectrum of the physical world is indicated and the brain's biophysical convergence zones align (dotted lines) to a specific segment of the whole physical spectrum in the physical world. (*b*) The same is now shown with regard to the relationship between low-high frequency entrainment and phenomenally based subjectivity. The better the higher frequencies can be entrained by the lower-frequency fluctuations, the higher the degree of phenomenally based subjectivity. This also holds true for schizophrenia, which shows a dichotomous rather than a continuous distribution.

some biological (or social) alteration in early infancy (or even prenatally) due to some genetic changes, viral infection, obstetric or gestational complications, or even more likely, some early biopyschosocial trauma. This may predispose one to develop schizophrenia later in adolescence or early adulthood.

However, schizophrenia does not become manifest before late adolescence or early adulthood, raising the question for some additional later developmental process in the human brain around that time, too. In the following discussion, I will focus on the additional development processes in late adolescence.

NEURONAL FINDINGS IIIB: ABNORMAL CORTICAL REORGANIZATION IN ADOLESCENCE IN SCHIZOPHRENIA

One empirical suggestion for such an additional later process is that the outbreak of schizophrenia in late adolescence may be related to the overpruning of synaptic contacts in late adolescence and the subsequent reorganization of the brain's wiring and its neural networks (see Lewis and Levitt 2002 for an overview). Core regions and circuits implicated in schizophrenia such as the dorsolateral prefrontal cortex, the hippocampus, the sensory cortex, and cortical midline structures have been shown to be sensitive to developmental changes in the period of late adolescence or early adulthood (see Lewis and Levitt 2002; Gonzales-Burgos and Lewis 2008, 2012, Gonzalez-Burgos et al. 2011; Lewis et al. 2012; Lipska and Weinberger 2000; Lewis 2009a–b).

While there have been a number of studies, I here focus on a 2009 study that used electroencephalography (EEG) to investigate neural synchrony in healthy subjects ranging from 6 to 21 years of age (Uhlhaas et al. 2009a–b). The authors observed that, in early adulthood, theta, beta, and gamma oscillations and their long-range synchronization increase to an enormous extent. This increase in synchronization in early adulthood is preceded by a significant reduction of beta and gamma phase synchronization during late adolescence that follows

continuous increases in phase synchronization from childhood to late adolescence.

This suggests that maturation of cortical synchronization and neural networks in early adulthood goes through a period of transient destabilization in late adolescence before being organized in the most stable and mature way in subsequent adulthood. The period of late adolescence may thus be considered a critical period for constituting stable and more precise cortico-cortical synchronization.

Some preliminary evidence suggests that the processes of transient destabilization and mature stabilization in late adolescence and early adulthood may be related to changes in cortico-cortical myelination and GABA (besides others like cannabinoids receptors). Both myelination and GABA undergo changes in exactly these time periods and may thereby significantly impact neural wiring and synchronization in early adulthood (see Uhlhaas et al. 2009a and b; Di Cristo et al. 2007). Due to its inhibitory impact, GABA may be central here in reorganizing neuronal phase synchronization (see Uhlhass et al. 2009a and b; Gonzales-Burgo and Lewis 2008; see also Chapter 17 for more details about schizophrenia and GABA).

NEURONAL FINDINGS IIIC: SOCIAL DEAFFERENTIATION IN SCHIZOPHRENIA

How does the predisposition toward neuronal desynchronization and neural destabilization and confusion relate to the biopsychosocial trauma in early infancy? For that, I turn to Ralph Hoffman. Ralph Hoffman (2007), a psychiatrist at Yale University who devotes his life and research to schizophrenia, recently postulated what he calls the "social deafferentiation hypothesis" (SAD). The SAD postulates that high levels of social withdrawal and isolation in vulnerable individuals prompt the predisposition to generate schizophrenic symptoms.

Following Hoffman, the SAD relies on several observations of the crucial nature of social isolation and withdrawal in schizophrenia. First, often the onset of auditory hallucinations, delusions, and other schizophrenic symptoms is preceded by reduced interpersonal interactions and social isolation. Thereby social isolation should not be understood in an absolute sense but rather relative to the person's standard or usual degree of social contact and hence its own prior baseline of social involvement.

Second, delusions and hallucinations produce socially and emotionally meaningful intra- or interpersonal contents that can be considered as substitutes of the real world. They may therefore be regarded as compensatory attempts to escape social isolation and withdrawal by producing some kind of relation to a world though an imaginary world as a substitute for the real world (see also McGlashan 2009, 479).

Third, sensory deafferentiation of, for instance, the visual cortex produces neuronal reorganization and complex hallucinations. Analogously, social withdrawal may also prompt neuronal reorganization with the subsequent generation of schizophrenic symptoms. Fourth, social withdrawal and isolation in critical developmental periods such as early infancy or late adolescence may significantly impact the changes in the processes of neuronal synchronization and wiring, which are already in progress during these critical time periods.

How is what Hoffman describes as "social deafferentation" related to the here-postulated alterations in the environment–brain unity? The schizophrenic patient can simply not connect his brain's resting state with the stimuli and their natural statistics as they occur in the environment. In other words, he remains unable to shift and align his resting state's low-frequency phase onsets to the onsets of the stimuli in the environment, i.e., their natural statistics.

That, however, makes it impossible for the schizophrenic patient to put his brain into a rhythmic mode (as distinguished from a continuous mode; see earlier) and to consequently constitute a stable (virtual statistically based) environment–brain unity. Yet the degree of the continuous mode of his brain's neural operation may be high, entailing discontinuity and division rather than continuity and unity in the relationship between environment (body) and brain. Accordingly, I postulate that Hoffman's hypothesis of "social deafferentiation" presupposes the kind of neuronal processes that account for the disruption of the environment–brain unity in schizophrenia.

NEUROPHENOMENAL HYPOTHESIS IIA: ABNORMAL ENVIRONMENT–BRAIN UNITY IN SCHIZOPHRENIA

I postulated the alignment of the low-frequency fluctuations' phases to the stimuli to be abnormal. As described earlier, this was supposed to provide the basis for false-positive or false-negative encoding of environmental stimuli in the resting state's low-frequency oscillations. Thereby I left open where such encoding abnormalities come from. The here described neurodevelopmental abnormalities may provide a first, albeit tentative, answer.

The early biopsychosocial trauma seems to affect the capacity of the low-frequency fluctuations' phase onsets to shift and align themselves with the onset of the stimuli. Why that is so and how it works remains unclear at this point. However, such a hypothesis is in strong agreement with the clearly observed neurodevelopmental abnormalities and the psychosocial trauma in these patients (see also Northoff 2011, chapters 11 and 12 for further details).

One may now postulate that the early trauma leads to a decrease in stimulus–rest interaction, resulting in the described encoding deficit. That, in turn, sets in motion increased rest–rest interaction and reduced rest–stimulus interaction as hypothesized earlier (see also Northoff and Qin 2011 for a more detailed account of these processes with regard to the specific symptom of auditory hallucinations).The early trauma may lead to the abnormal constitution of the environment–brain unity, which inclines the subjects to later develop schizophrenia.

How does the abnormal environment-brain unity affect the consciousness and its contents in these patients? The abnormal environment–brain unity may be carried over to the prephenomenal unity and ultimately to the phenomenal unity as described earlier. This raises the question of how schizophrenia can now lend empirical and phenomenal support to our assumption of the environment–brain unity and its characterization by subjectivity. Let me proceed in different steps.

NEUROPHENOMENAL HYPOTHESIS IIB: ABNORMAL "ENVIRONMENT–BRAIN UNITY" PREDISPOSES ABNORMAL "PHENOMENALLY BASED SUBJECTIVITY" IN SCHIZOPHRENIA

Schizophrenia is clearly a disorder of what I described as phenomenally based subjectivity in Chapter 21. The concept of phenomenally based subjectivity describes the intra-individually based experience in First-Person Perspective (FPP) as being not accessible to any other individual (of the same species). Abnormalities of such phenomenally based subjectivity are well manifest in typical schizophrenic symptoms like paranoid delusions, auditory hallucination, and ego disturbances that all reflect abnormal subjective experiences in first-person perspective.

Why is there such abnormal phenomenally based subjectivity in schizophrenia? I postulate that such altered phenomenally based subjectivity can be traced back to the abnormal encoding of the environmental stimuli by the resting state with the consecutive abnormalities in the environment–brain unity. If so, the case of schizophrenia lends empirical support albeit indirectly to the assumption that, in general, the environment–brain unity is a predisposition of phenomenally based subjectivity. Only if the environment–brain unity predisposes phenomenally based subjectivity and is thus a necessary condition of its possibility, abnormalities in the environment–brain unity can lead to the abnormal changes in the phenomenally based subjectivity as they are observed in schizophrenia (Fig. 22-3).

NEUROPHENOMENAL HYPOTHESIS IIIA: ABNORMAL OPERATION OF THE "BIOPHYSICAL CONVERGENCE ZONE" IN SCHIZOPHRENIA

I demonstrated that the alterations in the environment–brain unity in schizophrenia lead to subsequent changes in phenomenally based subjectivity and ultimately in phenomenal unity in these patients. How about the biophysically based subjectivity? We recall from Chapter 21

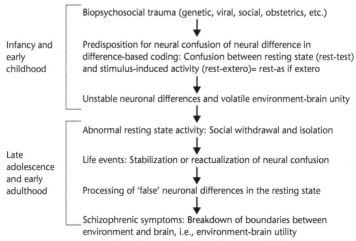

Figure 22-3 Volatile environment–brain unity and unstable neural differences in schizophrenia. The figure shows the different steps of the neurodevelopmental hypotheses, ranging from early infancy to late adolescence/early adulthood, combined with [my assumption of] the early disruption. I assume traumatic-related disruption of difference-based coding in early infancy that later then leads to the encoding of false-positive or false-negative spatial and temporal differences into neural activity. Finally, the outbreak of schizophrenic symptoms may be associated with a breakdown of the volatile environment–brain unity, which then makes impossible the distinction between inner and outer worlds, as is manifested in many schizophrenic symptoms.

that the concept of biophysically based subjectivity describes the species-specific biophysical spectrum of an organism and thus the range of physical features its brain's resting-state activity can operate on.

Since the biophysical equipment is species-specific (rather than individually specific), biophysically based subjectivity remains essentially intact in schizophrenia. Why? The biophysical spectrum is still the same in patients with schizophrenia as in healthy subjects because their basic biophysical equipment does not change when compared to healthy humans. The biophysically based subjectivity must thus be postulated to remain basically intact by itself in schizophrenia.

How however does a seemingly intact biophysically based subjectivity lead to an abnormal phenomenally based subjectivity? Patients with schizophrenia, however, seem to use the same biophysical spectrum in a different way than healthy subjects. Rather than using and operating on its different degrees in a continuous u-shape way, they seem to operate on it in a dichotomous way. This, I suppose, is well manifest in the encoding of abnormal differences, abnormally high or low, in difference-based coding. Hence, the biophysically subjectivity while remaining intact by itself is used and operated on in a different way in schizophrenia when compared to healthy subjects. How about the "biophysical convergence zone"? The concept of the "biophysical convergence zone" describes the biophysically based possible spatiotemporal correspondence between brain and environment (see Chapter 21)? The biophysical equipment and thus the biophysical convergence zone are off course the same in schizophrenic subjects as in healthy subjects. As indicated earlier, the biophysical convergence zone, or better, its biophysical spectrum, is used in a different way. Instead of using the whole continuum of the biophysical convergence as the healthy subjects do, the patients with schizophrenia seem to use only the outer extreme parts of the spectrum while leaving the intermediate range out. This is, as I said earlier, manifested in the coding of extreme differences in neural activity, with either extremely large or small differences being coded in neural activity.

Such extreme coding is, for instance, manifested in low–high-frequency coupling with high-frequency fluctuations being either abnormally strong or not all aligned to the phases of the low ones. The same holds for the use of the statistically based spectrum in the encoding of the stimuli from the environment into the brain's neural activity: the environmental stimuli and their natural statistics are encoded either in a false-positive or a false-negative way (see earlier), which is possible only on the basis of encoding either too large or too small (spatial and temporal) differences into the brain's resting-state activity.

Taking both abnormal coding and encoding together, the biophysical convergence zone of the brain's intrinsic activity to the environment and thus their commonly underlying biophysical spectrum is only exhausted in its outer, extreme ranges, whereas its middle ranges seem to be underutilized in schizophrenia (see Fig. 22-4).

NEUROPHENOMENAL HYPOTHESIS IIIB: ABNORMAL TRANSITION FROM BIOPHYSICALLY TO PHENOMENALLY BASED SUBJECTIVITY IN SCHIZOPHRENIA

How does such abnormal usage of the biophysical convergence zone and the respective biophysical spectrum affect subjectivity? The example of schizophrenia makes it clear that biophysically and phenomenally based subjectivity should not be confused with each other. As we can see in the case of schizophrenia, they can dissociate from each other. The biophysically based subjectivity remains basically intact in itself, while the phenomenally based subjectivity changes.

The possibility of their dissociation implies that we need to distinguish the neuronal mechanisms underlying the minimal and maximal biophysical limits, i.e., the biophysical spectrum, of the biophysically based subjectivity from those that allow the constitution of phenomenally based subjectivity on the basis of the former. Accordingly, we need to distinguish biophysically based subjectivity by itself from the processes that allow for the transition from biophysically to phenomenally based subjectivity.

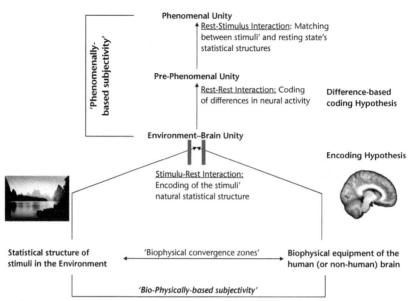

Figure 22-4 Unity and subjectivity in healthy and schizophrenic subjects. The figure shows the constitution of the environment–brain unity and how it serves as neural predisposition for the subsequent constitution of the prephenomenal unity and the phenomenal unity. Moreover, it serves as neural predisposition for the constitution of phenomenally based subjectivity as indicated on the left. The different processes (rest–rest, rest–stimulus, stimulus–rest) are marked. Moreover, the basic deficit in schizophrenia is marked by the two vertical bars (at the encoding level in the lower part of the figure); the constitution of the environment–brain unity is supposed to be disrupted. This leads me to formulate the encoding and difference-based hypotheses of schizophrenia.

What are the neuronal mechanisms that enable the transition from biophysically to phenomenally based subjectivity? I postulate that difference-based coding, and more specifically, the encoding of the environment's natural statistics, are essential for the subsequent coding of the brain's intrinsic activity in terms of differences. Such difference-based coding, in turn, enables the transformation of the purely biophysically based subjectivity into what I described as environment–brain unity, and later, into prephenomenal unity as predisposing steps toward the ultimate constitution of a phenomenal unity and thus consciousness.

NEUROPHENOMENAL HYPOTHESIS IIIC: DISTINCTION BETWEEN BIOPHYSICALLY BASED SUBJECTIVITY AND ENVIRONMENT–BRAIN UNITY

This also makes it clear that we cannot identify the concept of biophysically based subjectivity with that of environment–brain unity, as was tacitly suggested in the preceding sections. Instead, we need to differentiate between the two. Why is this so? The concept of environment–brain unity presupposes the usage of and operation on the biophysical spectrum as it signifies the biophysically based subjectivity. For instance, the concept of environment–brain unity is based on, and thus presupposes, a particular type of encoding neural activity; namely, difference-based coding rather than stimulus-based coding.

This is different in the concept of biophysically based subjectivity. The concept of biophysically based subjectivity only presupposes a particular relationship between the organism's biophysical features and the physical features of the world, as I described by the term "biophysical convergence zones." In contrast to the environment–brain unity, the biophysically based subjectivity remains independent of any particular encoding strategy by the brain of the organism. In other words, the biophysically based subjectivity must be "located" or "situated" prior to the brains' encoding of the environmental stimuli into neural activity.

The concept of biophysically based subjectivity consequently precedes and ultimately predisposes the possibility of the environment–brain unity. Accordingly, to identify the environment–brain unity with the biophysically based subjectivity would be to confuse what requires a particular predisposition, i.e., the environment–brain unity, with the predisposition itself, i.e., the biophysically based subjectivity.

Let me sketch the "location" between both concepts in a more illustrative way. The concept of biophysical subjectivity must be distinguished from the purely physical world that is objective rather than subjective. Instead, it signifies the biophysical equipment of a particular species and how that relates to the physical world. This is what I described as the biophysical convergence zone.

As soon, however, as a particular individual of that species becomes alive and encodes the world's physical features into its own brain and its resting-state activity (in accordance with its brain's biophysical spectrum), the biophysically based subjectivity is transformed into an environment–brain unity. Such environment–brain unity is manifest in the gestalt of the spatio-temporally and statistically based relationship between the brain's biophysical features and the world's physical features. Accordingly, to identify biophysically-based subjectivity with the environment–brain unity would be to conflate input and output of the transformation and to consecutively overlook what exactly happens in schizophrenia.

Open Questions

The first question pertains to the exact neuronal mechanisms in schizophrenia. Much more empirical support is needed for my encoding hypothesis as well as for the difference-based coding hypothesis. While the current data lend some indirect support, more-direct experimental testing will be necessary.

Therefore, one focus should be on low-frequency fluctuations and how their phases align with the environmental stimuli presented in different modes; that is, rhythmic or nonrhythmic. That is needed to provide experimental support to the encoding hypothesis, while a more computational approach will be needed to test the difference-based coding with the presumed bistable-dichotomous coding of either abnormally large or small differences in neural activity. While we hypothesized the resting-state activity to no longer encode the statistical frequency distribution of the environmental stimuli, or their natural statistics, direct empirical evidence remains sparse. One way to test this hypothesis would be to compare the impact of rhythmic and nonrhythmic stimulus presentation on neural activity in the resting state. One would expect schizophrenic patients to no longer show any differences in the alignment of their low-frequency oscillations' phase onsets to the stimuli's onsets in the environment during the two different kinds of stimulus presentation.

Another way is to test for sparse coding. As detailed in Volume I (see Part I), sparse coding, the coding of many stimuli into the one neural activity (many-to-one relationship between stimulus and neural activity), is closely related to the encoding of the stimuli's statistical frequency distribution across their different discrete points in (physical) time and space.

If schizophrenic patients do indeed show abnormalities in their encoding, one would expect low degrees of sparseness in both temporal, that is, lifetime sparseness, and spatial, that is, population sparseness, in their spatial and temporal neural activity pattern. And one would expect rather high degrees of local coding (one-to-one relationship between stimulus and neural activity) or even dense coding (one-to-many relationship between stimulus and neural activity).

Even more difficult will be bridging the gap from the neuronal hypotheses to the phenomenal features in schizophrenia as, for instance, described by Parnas. We can see that schizophrenia really leads us to the limits of the brain in both neuronal and phenomenal regard. Neuronally, this limit may be manifest in the predominant use of the outer ranges of the biophysical spectrum and thus the biophysical convergence zone between brain and environment. Phenomenally, the limit may be manifest in the kind of experience of the world and self beyond which any kind of experience and thus phenomenal consciousness can only but breakdown completely. The patients with schizophrenia seem to find themselves at the extremes of both their brains' possible bio-physical spectrum and their possible experience, beyond which neither any kind of neural processing, nor experience and thus consciousness as such, are possible anymore.

Note

1. The most common disorder discussed in the context of the phenomenal unity is the "split brain," in which two halves of the brain are disconnected in the corpus callosum. Some philosophers take these patients and their psychological changes as evidence for disrupting the phenomenal unity of consciousness in that they show two unities rather than one. However, the interpretation of these cases is not clear. Bayne and Chalmers (2003) and Bayne (2010) consider these cases instances of a breakdown of the access unity, while the phenomenal unity is supposed to be essentially preserved.

I follow this interpretation by pointing out that, even if the communication between the two hemispheres is disrupted in the corpus callosum, there can still be temporal synchronization among the oscillations and their phases between the two hemispheres (see Chapter 5, Volume I). And the low-frequency fluctuations in both hemispheres could still be matched with the statistical frequency distribution of the environmental stimuli, accounting for the environment–brain unity. Since the environmental stimuli are the same for both hemispheres, it is rather likely that both hemispheres encode the same temporal structure and organization in their respective low-frequency oscillations' phases. Despite being disrupted and separated, this makes it more likely that the two hemispheres constitute one environment–brain unity rather than two. To lend empirical support to such a hypothesis, one would need to investigate right- and left-hemispheric low-frequency fluctuations and their phases in dependence on the statistical distribution of the environmental stimuli (such as, for instance, during rhythmic and nonrhythmic presentations of the latter in an experimental design).

PART VII
Spatiotemporal Organization and Consciousness

Volume I discussed the neuronal mechanisms underlying the constitution of spatiotemporal continuity in the resting state. I proposed the resting-state activity's functional connectivity and low- and high-frequency fluctuations to be essential here. This purely neuronal description of the resting-state activity was then complemented in Volume II by showing its relevance to the phenomenal features of consciousness. For instance, the spatiotemporal continuity on the neuronal level of the brain's resting state was supposed to be manifested on the phenomenal level in what is described as "inner time and space consciousness" (see Part V).

This was further extended in Part VI on spatiotemporal unity and its relationship to the phenomenal unity of consciousness. I proposed the resting-state activity and, more specifically, its entrainment of higher frequencies by its own lower-frequency ranges to constitute what I described as "prephenomenal unity," which I proposed as predisposing the phenomenal unity of consciousness (see Chapter 19). However, the prephenomenal unity had to be traced back even further, to the way the brain's resting-state activity encodes the stimuli from the environment. Showing statistically based encoding of the stimuli's natural and social statistics led me to propose what I described as "environment–brain unity" (see Chapter 20).

How is the environment–brain unity related to consciousness? I propose such environment–brain unity to constitute what philosophers describe as "point of view," the stance within the world from which one experience the world (see Chapter 21). Such point of view is supposed to be based on the biophysical equipment and thus the biophysical spectrum of the brain as related to the physical properties and features of the world. The point of view provides the basis for what I described as the concept of "biophysically based subjectivity," which concerns the biophysical features of the particular species' brain and how they converge with those of the world. I propose such biophysically based subjectivity to provide the basis and thus the neural predisposition for the essentially subjective nature of consciousness.

The experience of subjectivity in consciousness was described as "phenomenally based subjectivity" since it is tied to the phenomenal state and the associated first-person perspective (FPP) of the individual person (see Chapter 21). Such phenomenally based subjectivity and its transition from biophysically based subjectivity was shown to be altered in schizophrenia; this lends further empirical support, albeit indirectly, to all three concepts: environment–brain unity as well as biophysically and phenomenally based subjectivity (see Chapter 22).

Let me summarize what I have achieved so far. We covered the spatial and temporal structure of consciousness and how it is based on and predisposed by the spatiotemporal continuity of the resting state's neuronal activity. And we demonstrated that such spatiotemporal continuity serves to constitute spatial and temporal unity between environment and brain, the environment–brain unity, as well as within the resting state itself, the prephenomenal unity.

That shed some light on the neuronal mechanisms underlying the form or structure of consciousness. However, my account has left open the question of the subject or self, the one who experiences consciousness. In short, we have not yet addressed the question of the self and how it must relate to the environment in order to experience consciousness. This is the focus of the present part.

Let us frame the same issue in slightly different terms. Despite all the ground we already covered, we still lack something essential to consciousness. What exactly is lacking? Consciousness is not only about spatiotemporal continuity and unity. There is much more to it. What is this "more"? Loosely put, somebody experiences something. This implies, as philosophers say, a subject-object structure in consciousness. There must thus be a subject, a self that experiences objects as the contents of consciousness. Where do the experiencing self and the contents it experiences come from? This is the focus of the present part.

GENERAL OVERVIEW

Chapter 23 focuses on the relationship between self and resting state. Recent data show the predominant involvement of cortical midline regions during the application of self-specific stimuli. Since the very same regions also show high resting-state activity, there seems to be a strong overlap between self and rest in midline regions. This has been confirmed and even extended to suggest that the resting-state activity level may predict the subsequent stimuli's degree of self-specificity.

On the basis of these findings, I propose the resting state to show what I refer to as "self-specific organization," the organization of the resting state's neural activity around a center

provided by the individual organism itself and its individually specific relationship to the environment. Such a self-specific organization of the resting state is, I propose, a neural predisposition of what is described as "self-perspectival organization" on the phenomenal level of consciousness, the perspectival nature of experience, i.e., consciousness, as tied to the first-person perspective of the specific individual.

Chapter 24 focuses on how the resting state's self-specific organization is carried over and transferred to subsequent stimulus-induced activity and its associated functions and tasks. This is exemplified by different psychological functions like emotions, rewards, and decision-making, which are all shown to implicate both self-specificity and the midline regions. Moreover, I will discuss recent findings on functional connectivity and low-frequency fluctuations during self-specific stimuli in order to demonstrate the spatial and temporal features of the resting state's self-specific organization. These findings suggest that the resting state's self-specific organization must be linked and integrated with the spatiotemporal continuity and unity of the resting state. That integration allows, I suggest, the conversion of the resting state's prephenomenal self-specific organization into the self-perspectival organization on the phenomenal level of consciousness.

Chapter 25 investigates recent findings on the neural balance between midline and lateral cortical networks and their association with the psychological balance between internal and external awareness. Such neural and psychological balancing occurs in both resting-state activity and stimulus-induced activity, which makes possible the assignment of an internal or external origin of the contents in consciousness. The guiding question here is: How is it possible to become conscious of external contents, as in dreams, even if external stimulus input is absent during the resting state?

I propose that the constitution of contents is based on the coding of differences between different stimuli, that is, difference based, rather than coding stimuli on the basis of their origin, that is, origin based. Such difference based constitution of contents is complemented by their designation as internal or external, which I associate with the neural balance between midline and lateral cortical networks. Finally, this neural balance is integrated with the rest of the brain and its environment–brain unity and associated point of view. Such a linkage between point of view and contents accounts for what can be described as the resting state's preintentional organization that is manifested on the phenomenal level of consciousness in the gestalt of "intentionality," the "directedness towards contents in the world."

Chapter 26 gathers further empirical evidence for the characterization of the resting state by both self-specific and preintentional organization. For that, I turn to the examples of dreams and mind wandering. Dreams are characterized by the experience of external contents, despite the absence of any external stimulus input. Recent findings do indeed show abnormal shift of neural activity toward the midline network in dreams that may account for the presence of external contents in consciousness, even though external stimulus input remains absent. There is thus still intentionality, i.e., directedness toward external contents in consciousness during dreams, despite the absence of external stimuli. This is possible only when we assume a preintentional organization in the resting state itself that predisposes the constitution of intentionality towards contents on the phenomenal level of consciousness.

How about the opposite case, of intentionality with directedness toward internal contents in the presence of external stimulus input? For that, I turn to the example of "mind wandering." Mind wandering describes the slip toward one's internal thoughts during external stimulation. Recent imaging findings implicate the midline and the lateral networks in mind wandering. This means that mind wandering is based on the recruitment of the neural balance between midline and lateral networks and taps thereby into the resting state's preintentional organization. The resting state's preintentional organization can be directed toward either internal or external contents, independently of the presence or absence of external stimuli. A shift in the neural balance between midline and lateral networks may then go along with a shift in the balance between internal and external contents. This is what I propose to happen in mind wandering, hence the focus on internal contents despite the presence of external stimuli.

Finally, Chapter 27 focuses on neuropsychiatric disorders like schizophrenia and depression to further support the assumption of the resting state's self-specific and preintentional organization. Schizophrenia shows severe alterations in the self, a basic disturbance of the self, and abnormal experience with decreased self-specificity.

I propose that these abnormalities of the self are related to abnormal resting-state activity, as observed in recent studies, and the alterations in its self-specific organization. Hence, I suggest the self-abnormalities in schizophrenia to necessarily presuppose, abnormal self-perspectival organization of the resting-state activity, which further supports such a characterization of the resting-state activity in general, albeit indirectly (via pathological changes).

How about the resting state's preintentional organization? For that I turn to the example of depression. Depression shows an abnormal shift of directedness toward internal contents like one's own self, i.e., an increased self-focus, which accompanies a shift away from the environment, i.e., a decreased environment focus. Such an abnormal shift towards internal contents may be due to an abnormal neural balance between midline and lateral networks in the resting state. Due to the abnormal neural balance, the resting state's preintentional organization may thus be abnormally shifted in depression toward internal contents (as related to the self) at the expense of external contents (as related to the environment). Hence, I suggest depression and its shifts towards internal contents to be possible only on the basis of assuming preintentional organization in the resting state, which thus lends support, albeit indirectly, to its characterization in this way in general.

CHAPTER 23
Resting-State Activity and Self-Specificity

Summary

How is it possible that our brain can constitute the experience or sense of a self as distinguished from other selves? This is not only central to the question of the neuronal mechanisms underlying the self but also for consciousness, which is often assumed to remain impossible without a self. Recent imaging studies show specifically regions in the midline of the brain to be recruited during stimuli that show high degrees of self-specificity. This concerns especially anterior midline regions like the perigenual anterior cingulate cortex and the ventromedial prefrontal cortex. Moreover, the results indicate a strong neural overlap of the neural activity elicited by especially highly self-specific stimuli with the high resting-state activity in these regions. Finally, most recent empirical data demonstrate that the resting-state activity in these regions can even predict the degree of self-specificity assigned by the subjects to the stimulus. This raises the following question: How can merely intero- and exteroceptive stimuli be transformed into self-specific stimuli? I propose what I describe as the "matching hypothesis." The matching hypothesis postulates the statistically based matching between the temporal and spatial features of the stimuli themselves and the spatial and temporal neuronal measures (like low-frequency oscillations' phases, functional connectivity) of the resting-state activity. The higher the degree of the statistically based correspondence or matching between the stimuli's spatial and temporal features and those of the resting state's neural activity, the higher the degree of self-specificity that will be assigned to that particular stimulus. This leads me to propose that the neural activity in the resting state can itself be characterized by what I refer to as "self-specific organization": the temporal and spatial structuring of the resting-state activity's neuronal measures in orientation to the stimuli that statistically match best and can thus be well aligned with the resting-state activity itself. The resting-state activity's self-specific organization makes it possible for the resting-state activity to impact and ultimately predict the subsequent stimuli's degree of self-specificity as it was observed in the data. As such, the resting-state activity's self-specific organization must be proposed to be a necessary but nonsufficient condition of what has been described as self-perspectival organization on the phenomenal level of consciousness, the organization of experience around the first-person perspective of the individual person and its self.

Key Concepts and Topics Covered

Self, self-perspectival organization, resting state, stimulus–rest interaction, rest–rest interaction, dreams, self-specificity, threefold anatomical organization, subcortical and cortical midline structures, self-specific organization, phase alignment, stimulus-phase coupling

NEUROEMPIRICAL BACKGROUND
IA: NEUROPHENOMENAL APPROACH TO THE LINKAGE BETWEEN SELF AND CONSCIOUSNESS

So far, we have covered the resting state and how the spatiotemporal continuity (see Part V) and unity (see Part VI) of its neural activity predisposes consciousness. Besides spatiotemporal continuity and unity, there is yet another important feature of consciousness, the self. There has been much discussion about what the self is and whether it exists at all, in past and present philosophy (see Kant 1998; Zahavi 2005; Metzinger 2003; Bayne 2010; Dainton 2008). This has recently been complemented by the introduction of the self into neuroscience, where it has been conceptualized and defined in different ways (see Appendix 4 for details).

The focus in the present chapter and the consecutive chapters in this part is not so much on the self itself—for example, how we can define what it is and what it is not, and which neuronal mechanisms mediate the self if it is assumed to exist (see, for instance, Metzinger 2003; Feinberg 2009; Damasio 1999a and b; Klein 2012; Klein and Gangi 2010, and obviously many others not mentioned here). Hence, I will neither discuss the full philosophical-conceptual details and definitions of the self nor the different neuronal mechanisms of the different kinds of selves as postulated by different authors.

Rather than discussing "the self," I here focus on how the self is related to consciousness. Whatever "the self" is (see later, and Chapter 24 and Appendix 4 for discussion), many philosophers such as I. Kant (1998), T. Bayne (2010), and D. Zahavi (2005), as well as neuroscientists like A. Damasio, J. Panksepp, and T. Feinberg (Damasio 1999a, 2010; Parvizi and Damasio 2001, 2003; Panksepp 1998a; Northoff and Panksepp 2008; Feinberg 2009) consider the self as necessary for consciousness. There is no consciousness without self. Accordingly, if we want to reveal the neuronal mechanisms of consciousness, we have to understand the neuronal underpinnings of the self and how they make possible its association with consciousness.

The question of the relationship between self and consciousness becomes even more contentious given recent findings in patients in vegetative state. These patients, who by definition are not conscious, still show neural activity during self-specific stimuli like hearing their own name or autobiopgraphical questions. At the same time though, the degree of neural activity when hearing their own name predicts the degree of consciousness in these patients (see Qin et al. 2010; Huang et al. 2013; as well as Chapter 29 for more details). This suggests a rather intricate relationship between self and consciousness, which seem to be both independent of and interdependent on each other.

Given these complexities in the relationship between self and consciousness, I here focus on only one particular aspect of their relationship. My aim is only to reveal the neuronal mechanisms that underlie their linkage. My focus is thus clearly empirical rather than conceptual. For that reason, I will refrain from extensive philosophical discussion about the metaphysics, the existence, and the reality of the self and its relationship to consciousness. Admittedly such a strategy still presupposes some kind of notion and concept of self, so that the issue of defining the concept of self cannot be completely avoided.

Instead of venturing into the metaphysical and epistemological territory of the philosopher, I here presuppose only a purely empirical and operationalized version of the self in terms of self-specific stimuli (see next section for definition of the concept of "self-specificity") and investigate how that is related to consciousness. Therefore, my aim is purely neurophenomenal (rather than metaphysical or epistemological): I want to show how self-specificity is mediated neuronally and how that makes it possible and thus predisposes us to experience a sense of self in our consciousness.

Such a neurophenomenal approach is to be distinguished from a neuronal approach where the self is reduced to the brain itself, independently of consciousness (as often seen in current neuroscience; Damasio 1999, 2010; Panksepp 1998a and b). My neurophenomenal approach also differs from a neurocognitive approach that associates the self with specific cognitive mechanisms like representation and meta-representation, again remaining independent of consciousness (as often seen in current neurophilosophy; e.g., Metzinger 2003, Churchland 2002). Finally, my neurophenomenal approach is also different from a neurosensory and neuromotor approach to the self as is often advocated in neurophenomenological approaches that account for the self in terms of the body (Legrand 2007a and b; Christoff et al. 2011). Finally, my neurophenomenal approach also differs from a purely phenomenological approach where the self is considered an integral part of consciousness (in the gestalt of pre-reflective self-awareness) and explored and described in purely phenomenal (rather than neurophenomenal) terms (Zahavi 2005).

The here-suggested strategy shifts the focus from the self itself and self-consciousness to its relationship to the neuronal mechanisms that link self and consciousness. Since I propose the resting-state activity to be central in consciousness, as pointed out in the previous two Parts, my first focus will be on the relationship between self and resting state. This is the subject of the present chapter, which therefore provides the prephenomenal background and thus the neural predisposition for the linkage between self and consciousness on the phenomenal level of consciousness.

We will investigate the resting-state activity in further detail this time, though in a slightly different way. The purely neuronal approach from Volume I gives way to a more neurophenomenal approach that considers the resting state activity from the perspective of consciousness and thus in phenomenal (or better pre-phenomenal) terms. Rather than discussing the spatial and temporal structure of its neural activity as in the preceding chapters 13–22, I now focus on its "organization in relation to the organism itself."

What do I mean by its "organization in relation to the organism itself"? The preceding chapters focused on time and space and how they are processed and constituted by the brain's intrinsic activity. I suggested that the brain's intrinsic activity constitutes a spatiotemporal grid or template that spans in a virtual statistically based way across the boundaries of brain, body, and environment. This left open, however, how the individual organism stands in relation to such a spatiotemporal grid or template as constituted by his brain.

How is it possible for the individual organism to relate to his brain's spatiotemporal grid or template? I suppose that we again need to go back to the brain's intrinsic activity and investigate how it processes and incorporates stimuli related to a particular individual organism. This means that we have to search for the neuronal mechanisms that underlie the processing of what can be described as "self-specific stimuli." The concept of "self-specific stimuli" refers to the stimuli that are specific for a particular organism as distinct from others. For instance, one's own name is a stimulus that is specific for a specific organism or subject. Such self-specificity and how it is generated neuronally are the topics in the present chapter, which proposes an intimate relationship between self-specificity and resting-state activity.

That will be complemented in Chapter 24 by discussing how such self-specificity can be linked to consciousness. I will then discuss how both intero- and exteroceptive stimuli from the body and environment can possibly be experienced as self-related or self-specific while we experience a "sense of self" in consciousness. This will be the focus in Chapter 24, which, by shifting to the experience of a self, a sense of self, discusses the neuronal underpinning of the relationship between self-specificity and consciousness.

NEURONAL FINDINGS IA: IS NEURAL ACTIVITY IN MIDLINE REGIONS SPECIFIC FOR SELF-SPECIFICITY?

Neuroscience in general, and functional brain imaging in particular, detected the "self" in the last decade. In the last decade years, several imaging studies on the brain's recruitment of neural activity during personally or self-specific stimuli were detected. Subjects viewed and judged words (or other stimuli like pictures or sounds) that were closely related to themselves, like, for instance, the term "piano" for a concert pianist. These self-specific words were then compared to other words unrelated and thus non-self-specific to the person (see van der Meer et al. 2010; Gillihan and Farah 2005; Legrand and Ruby 2009; Northoff et al. 2006; Qin and Northoff 2011 for reviews)

Interestingly, most of these studies observed strong activity in the anterior and posterior cortical midline regions like the perigenual anterior cingulate cortex (PACC), the supragenual anterior cingulate cortex (SACC), the ventro- and dorsomedial prefrontal cortex (VMPFC, DMPFC), the posterior cingulate cortex (PCC), the precuneus, and the retrosplenium (see Northoff and Bermpohl 2004; Northoff et al.

2006; van der Meer et al. 2011; Christoff et al. 2011; and Qin and Northoff 2011, for reviews and meta-analyses). These findings have led to the question of whether the cortical midline structures specifically process the stimuli's degree of self-specificity and can thus be considered a network specific to the self.

However, the assumption of self-specificity of these regions has been put into doubt because tasks and stimuli other than those focusing on the self also recruit these regions (Gillihan and Farah 2005; Legrand and Ruby 2009; Christoff et al. 2011). This includes various cognitive functions like mind-reading and decision making, and social functions like empathy, reward, and emotional-affective functions (see also Chapter 24).

Another observation is that self-specificity does not only recruit cortical midline structures. If self-specific stimuli are presented independently of any associated cognitive tasks (like judgment), they also elicit neural activity changes in lateral cortical regions like the ventrolateral prefrontal cortex, as well as in subcortical midline regions like the dorsomedial thalamus, the ventral striatum, the tectum, the periaqueductal gray, and the colliculi (see Northoff et al. 2009; Schneider et al. 2008; Northoff and Panksepp 2008; Panksepp and Northoff 2009).

Is there thus a subcortical-cortical midline system mediating the self? There is indeed some neuroanatomical ground justifying the assumption of such subcortical-cortical midline system (see though the critical stance of Gillihan and Farah 2005; Legrand and Ruby 2009; and Christoff et al. 2011, who consider the midline regions to be too unspecific, given their involvement in various functions, and instead suggest what they call "general evaluation function"). This is well documented in the threefold radial-concentric anatomical organization, with inner, middle, and outer rings, that spans from the subcortical to cortical regions (see Volume I, Chapter 4, for anatomical details).

We recall that the inner ring spans around the ventricles including regions like the PAG subcortically and the anterior cingulate on the cortical level. The outer ring, in contrast, concerns the regions that lie on the outer edge of both brain stem/midbrain and cortex (with the latter including sensory and lateral prefrontal cortices). Finally, the middle ring is sandwiched between inner and outer rings and includes, for instance, the medial prefrontal cortex and precuneus on the cortical level.

How are the purely anatomically and thus structurally described anatomical rings related to the functional processing of self-specific stimuli? This will be the focus in the next section.

NEURONAL FINDINGS IB: HOW DO THE DIFFERENT ANATOMICAL RINGS STAND IN RELATION TO SELF-SPECIFICITY?

How is such threefold subcortical-cortical neuroanatomical distinction related to the self? Does it map self-specificity better and more congruently than the traditional dichotomous medial-lateral distinction?

For answers to these questions, the American (or better, "New Yorkian") neurologist Todd Feinberg relies, much like traditional neurologists such as Charles Sherrington, on the careful study of neurological patients. These patients suffer from lesions in particular regions of the brain and often experience bizarre changes in their phenomenal consciousness, including their sense of self. Feinberg attempts to explain his patients' unusual experience of the self with the concept of the threefold anatomical organization (see Feinberg 2009, 2010, 2011).

How does Feinberg propose the self to be related to the three rings? Feinberg (2009, 2010) proposes that the inner ring reflects the bodily or "intero-self," while the outer ring may be rather related to the environmental self or the "extero-self." The middle ring is more related to the integration between both and thus the self proper, the "integrative self," than spans across intero- and exteroceptive stimuli and thus body and environment.

Can we gain any empirical support in favor of the different rings' association with self-specificity? Chinese postdoctoral student Pengmin Qin from my group (Northoff, Qin, et al. 2010; Qin and Northoff 2011) conducted a meta-analysis of all imaging studies on the self using self-specific, familiar, and unfamiliar stimuli. Let me briefly explain the regional effects of these three different conditions.

The self-specific condition yielded activity changes in the inner ring regions like the PACC, the insula, and the PCC as well as in the middle ring, that is, VMPFC and DMPFC. The familiarity condition, in contrast, did not yield any signal changes in the inner ring and its anterior regions; that is, insula and PACC. Instead, the familiarity condition did induce signal changes in the middle ring, VMPFC and DMPFC, as well as in the posterior regions of the inner ring, the PCC. Finally, the posterior regions of the inner

ring like the PCC were also recruited during the unfamiliar condition. Unlike familiarity, the unfamiliar condition did not recruit any other midline regions in the anterior parts but rather the temporo-parietal junction and the temporal pole (see Fig. 23-1 and Table 23-1).

Taken together, these findings suggest an inner-to-outer gradient coupled with an anterior-to-posterior gradient in the brain with regard to self-specificity. The more inner and anterior regions like the PACC and insula allow for the neural processing of high degrees of self-specificity, while the converse holds for the

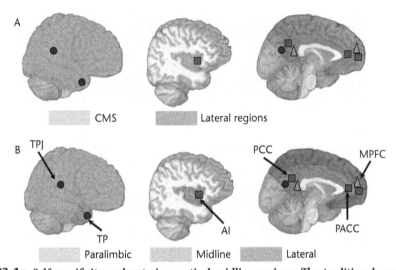

Figure 23-1a Self-specificity and anterior cortical midline regions. The traditional medial-lateral twofold anatomical dichotomy. medial with cortical midline structures (CMS); lateral regions. (B) Threefold anatomical distinction. paralimbic; midline; lateral. Squares represent the regions activated in the self condition (like own face or name) in the meta-analysis; Triangles represent the regions activated under non-self familiarity condition (like famous person) in meta-analysis; Dots represent the regions activated under other, i.e., non-self and non-familiar (like unknown person's face or voice) condition in meta-analysis. Note that the for instance the insula is classified as lateral region in the traditional medial-lateral dichotomy as visible in (a). That makes it rather difficult to explain why the insula show self-specific activity in the midst of other regions that are not self-specific. This is different once one changes the anatomical classification and reverts to a threefold anatomy with inner, middle, and outer ring. Though placed lateral (according to the medial-lateral dichotomy), the insula is now part of the inner ring and thus anatomically close (according to the threefold classification) to other paralimbic regions like the PACC that also show self-specific activity. Hence, the switch in the anatomical classification from medial-lateral to the threefold rings (inner, middle, outer) sheds a novel light and better understanding on the neural activity pattern of regions like the insula (see also Table 23-1 where the same is put into the form of a table). *Abbreviations*: TPJ = temporal-parietal junction, TP = temporal pole, AI = anterior insula, PCC = posterior cingulate cortex, MPFC = medial prefrontal cortex, PACC = pregenual anterior cingulate cortex, CMS = cortical midline structures. Reprinted with permission of Elsevier, from Northoff G, Qin P, Feinberg TE. Brain imaging of the self-conceptual, anatomical and methodological issues. *Conscious Cogn.* 2011 Mar;20(1):52–63.

Table 23-1 Comparison between the two- and three-fold anatomical characterizations with regard to meta-analytic results from self, familiarity and other.

	Self	Familiarity	Other (no-self and no familiarity)
Paralimbic regions			
Anterior	PACC, Insula	–	–
Posterior	PCC	PCC	PCC, TP
Midline regions			
Anterior	MPFC	MPFC	–
Posterior	–	–	–
Lateral	–	–	TPJ
CMS regions			
Anterior	PACC, MPFC	MPFC	–
Posterior	PCC	PCC	PCC
Lateral regions			
Anterior		–	–
Posterior	–	TPJ, TP	

The table represents the results from the metaanalyis of studies on the self when compared to non-self (familiar and non-familiar). Most important, it represents the results in a way ordered along the threefold anatomical distinction into paralimbic regions (upper), midline regions (upper middle), cortical midline structures (CMS) (lower middle), and lateral regions (lower). We can see that for instance the insula which seems to show self-specific activity is once ordered in the paralimbic regions as part of the inner ring when one presupposes the threefold anatomy with inner, middle, and outer ring. If, in contrast, one presupposes the traditional medial-lateral anatomy, the insula is listed as lateral region. This though makes it hard to understand why it shows self-specific activity since only paralimbic but not lateral regions show such activity pattern.

PACC: perigenual anterior cingulate cortex, PCC: posterior cingulate cortex, MPFC: medial prefrontal cortex, TP: temporal pole, TPJ: temporo-parietal junction.

Reprinted with permission of Elsevier from Northoff G, Qin P, Feinberg TE. Brain imaging of the self—conceptual, anatomical and methodological issues. *Conscious Cogn.* 2011 Mar;20(1):52–63.

more outer (like lateral regions) and posterior regions (like PCC and precuneus) that are more associated with low degrees of self-specificity. Simply put, one's own self is associated with inner and anterior parts in the brain, while others' selves are more related to outer and posterior parts.

NEURONAL FINDINGS

IC: SUBCORTICAL-CORTICAL MIDLINE NETWORK MEDIATES SELF-SPECIFICITY

We have to be careful, however. The aforementioned findings described concern mainly on the cortical level, while there are much less data about the subcortical regions. Hence, future investigation is needed to reveal whether, for instance, the inner-to-outer gradient also applies to the subcortical level (see Chapter 31 here for further details on subcortical regions).

One step in this direction has been taken by neuroscientist Hans Lou from Denmark. Having investigated the self in a series of excellent studies (see Lou et al. 1999, 2004, 2005, 2010a and b, 2011a and b; Luber et al. 2012, Kjaer et al. 2002), he proposes a subcortical-cortical paralimbic network to be central in mediating self and consciousness. This includes the thalamus (pulvinar), the striatum, the subgenual and pregenual anterior cingulate cortex, the medial prefrontal cortex (VMPFC, DMPFC), and the posterior cingulate cortex/precuneus (see also Northoff et al. 2009; Schneider et al. 2008; de Greck et al. 2008; for showing the processing of self-specificity in subcortical regions).

That network can be characterized as a self-reference network that may balance other networks associated with reward, emotion, and executive-cognitive functions. Lou considers the self-reference network central for consciousness (see also the later discussion of this network in further detail), though he does not give a hint about the neuronal mechanisms that link self-specificity to consciousness (see subsequent chapters in this Part).

In addition to different regions and neural networks, we also have to distinguish between the self-specificity of internal and external contents and their recruitment of midline regions. Internal contents concern one's own thoughts and one's own body, whereas external contents are related to objects and events in the environment.

The studies reported above focused mainly on the self-specificity of external contents, while leaving the neural mechanisms of self-specific internal contents open. Future studies are needed to show, I believe, that both internal and external contents with high degrees of self-specificity are processed in the subcortical-cortical midline regions (see Chapter 25 for further discussion of internal and external contents).

NEURONAL FINDINGS IIA: NEURAL OVERLAP BETWEEN RESTING-STATE ACTIVITY AND SELF-SPECIFICITY—ANTERIOR MIDLINE REGIONS

The cortical midline structures are core regions of the so-called default-mode network (DMN) that shows particularly high neural activity in the resting state (see Buckner et al. 2008; Raichle et al. 2001). Since the midline regions have been shown to be implicated in mediating self-specificity, neural activity during self-specificity may strongly overlap with the high resting-state activity in the very same regions. This is indeed the case, as recent studies demonstrated.

We remember the Belgian researcher Antoine d'Argembeau from Chapter 13 on the experience of time. He focuses on memory and its alterations in, for instance, Alzheimer's disease. Since, however, especially autobiographical memory implicates the self, he is also interested in investigating the neuronal mechanisms underlying self-specificity using functional imaging.

D'Argembeau et al. (2005) conducted an H20 positron emission tomography (PET) investigation. Subjects underwent four conditions: thinking/reflection about one's own personality traits, thinking/reflection about another person's personality traits, thinking/reflection on social issues, and a pure rest condition where subjects could relax. This design allowed to compare self- and non-self conditions as well as to investigate the relation between self-conditions and the resting state.

What about their results? The VMPFC showed significant increases in regional cerebral blood flow (rCBF) during the self condition when compared to the other and the social condition. In addition, they compared all three task-related conditions, that is, thinking/reflection about one's own personality traits, thinking/reflection about another person's personality traits, and thinking/reflection on social issues, against a rest condition. This yielded increased rCBF in the DMPFC and the temporal regions, while no differences were observed in the VMPFC. Conversely, the rest condition (when compared to the other three conditions) showed rCBF increases in a large medial fronto-parietal and posterior medial network with no differences in the VMPFC.

The separate account of self and rest allowed the authors to directly compare both conditions with each other. This yielded strong overlap in the VMPFC between both conditions, rest and self-specificity, that showed similar degrees of rCBF increases. In contrast, the other and the social condition induced rCBF decreases in the same region.

Post-scanning subjective measures demonstrated that self-referential thoughts were most abundant in the self condition while being more diminished in the other three conditions. The authors therefore correlated the post-scanning measures of self-referential thinking with the rCBF changes. This yielded a positive relationship in the VMPFC. The higher the rCBF in the VMPFC, the higher the degree of self-referentiality in the thoughts subjects reported to experience.

This strong association, that is, regional overlap, between self and rest in especially the regions of the inner ring was further confirmed by the earlier-mentioned meta-analyses by Pengmin

Qin from my group (Qin and Northoff 2011) as I will describe in the following. Pengmin Qin conducted a meta-analysis of human imaging studies on the self when compared to nonself. Most important, he also included studies on the resting state to compare their neural activity pattern to the one during self- and non-self-specific stimuli. The non-self-specific stimuli included familiar (like a famous person) and unfamiliar (an unknown non-famous person) stimuli. This allowed him to, for instance, directly compare resting state in the default-mode network (DMN) with the regions recruited during self- and non-self-specific stimuli.

What are his results? They confirm the ones observed in the study by d'Argembeau showing regional overlap between self and rest. More specifically, the regional activities during self-specific stimuli and the ones during resting state overlapped especially in the PACC extending to the VMPFC, while no such regional overlap with the resting state was observed in the non-self-specific conditions, that is, familiarity and unfamiliarity, in either the PACC or any other region (see Fig. 23-1b).

Taken together, these results suggest neural overlap between self-specificity and resting-state activity in the anterior midline regions like the PACC and the VMPFC.

Neuronal Findings IIB: Neural Overlap between Resting-State Activity and Self-Specificity—Subcortical-Cortical Midline System

The strong neural overlap between resting state and regions recruited during self-specificity was further confirmed in a recent study by Whitfield-Gabriel et al. (2011). They conducted two experiments with different subject groups. Each group underwent a self-reference task, explicit judgment of trait adjectives as self- or non-self-related, and a control task with a valence judgment of the trait adjectives as either positive or negative, and a pure resting state (of about 10 s). This allowed them to compare all three conditions/tasks (self, valence, rest) with each other and to see, in particular, how much self and rest overlap with each other.

As expected, they found in both experiments recruitment of stronger neural activity in anterior and posterior midline regions (VMPFC, DMPFC, PACC, PCC, precuneus) during the self-task when compared to the valence task. Moreover, the rest condition was associated with stronger activity than the valence task in the midline regions, whereas this was not the case for the self-task when compared to rest. The level of neural activity in the midline regions did not differ between the self-task and the resting-state condition.

The authors also conducted analyses that allowed them to directly investigate overlapping and dissociating regions between self and rest. Overlapping regions (i.e., conjunction analysis) between self and rest concerned the PACC, the VMPFC, and the PCC, while dissociating regions included the DMPFC (stronger during self) and the precuneus (stronger during rest). These findings could be confirmed in the second experiment where the relevant regions, as yielded in the first experiment, showed the same pattern of neural activity during the three conditions, self, non-self, and rest.

These findings suggest a close relationship, that is, regional overlap, between the neural activities underlying rest and self in especially the regions of the inner ring, the PACC and the PCC, while in the regions of the middle ring (precuneus, DMPFC), neural activities during self and rest seem to dissociate from each other.

The overlap between rest and self is further support by a recent magneto-encephalo-graphic (MEG) study by Lou et al. (2010a). He investigated judgment of self-related words (see Chapter 23 for details of this study) and focused on three main regions, precuneus, thalamus/pulvinar, and anterior midline regions (including VMPFC, DMPFC, and PACC). Using Granger causality analysis (which allows testing for the direction of functional connectivity), he observed that the magnetic activities in the sites (or better, sensors) related to the three regions were bi-directionally connected to each other (i.e., showing high degrees of statistical covariance in their signal changes).

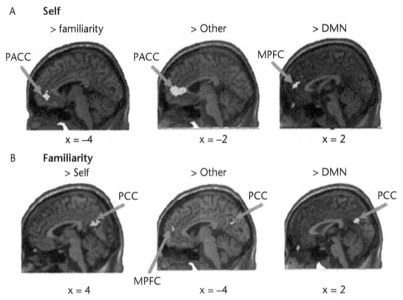

Figure 23-1b Overlap between self-specificity and high resting-state activity in anterior midline regions. The activated clusters by contrasts between each condition. A: the self condition showed stronger activation than the other three conditions (non-self familiar, non-self non-familiar = Other, resting state – default-mode network (DMN)); B: the familiarity condition showed stronger activation than the other three conditions (self, other, DMN). Note the absence of any difference in Self > DMN in the PACC (image on the upper right) when compared to the contrast Self > Familiarity (image on the upper left) in the PACC. This suggests neural overlap between self-specific activity and resting state activity (DMN) in the PACC which is further supported by the overlay of their activities (as shown in Figure 4 and 5 in that paper). *Abbreviations*: PCC = posterior cingulate cortex, MPFC = medial prefrontal cortex, PACC = pregenual anterior cingulate cortex, DMN = default-mode network. Reprinted with permission of Elsevier, from Qin P, Northoff G. How is our self related to midline regions and the default-mode network? *Neuroimage*. 2011 Aug 1;57(3):1221–33.

Most interesting, the increase in functional connectivity occurred already 900 ms before stimulus onset and thus in the resting-state period preceding the stimulus. The pre-stimulus increase in functional connectivity was then further enhanced by the onset of the stimulus and the subsequent 900 ms. Such functional connectivity was strongest in the gamma frequency range between 30 and 45 Hz before and after stimulus onset and strongest in the self-condition after stimulus onset. Hence, these results lend further support to a special relationship, i.e., a neural overlap between self-specific and resting-state activity in subcortical and anterior cortical midline regions.

These studies show strong overlap between high resting-state activity and stimulus-induced activity as elicited by high self-specific stimuli in anterior subcortical-cortical midline regions. Hence, the resting-state activity in the anterior regions of the inner ring seems to be closely related to self-specificity in as-yet-unclear ways.

NEURONAL HYPOTHESIS IA: ENCODING OF THE STIMULI'S NATURAL, SOCIAL, AND VEGETATIVE STATISTICS INTO THE BRAIN'S RESTING-STATE ACTIVITY

The findings demonstrate a clear neural overlap between high resting-state activity and self-specific activity, especially in the anterior (subcortical and) cortical midline structures like the PACC and the VMPFC. The question arising now is the following: How is such an overlap between self and rest generated? All stimuli have to be processed by the resting-state activity, which ultimately decides the degree of the resulting stimulus-induced activity. Such a neural overlap between rest and the self, however, is possible only if the resting-state activity shows a specific sensitivity and reactivity for self-specific stimuli and tasks.

How is such a special sensitivity and reactivity of the resting-state activity for self-specificity possible? For the answer, I briefly go back to the encoding of stimuli in neural activity as already discussed in Volumes I and II. I demonstrated in Chapter 1 of Volume I that stimuli are encoded in the sensory systems' neural activity in terms of their statistical frequency distribution, for example, their natural statistics. This was extended to the resting state itself that was also shown to encode the statistical frequency distribution, the natural statistics, of exteroceptive (and probably interoceptive) stimuli (see Volume I, Chapter 6).

Going beyond the purely neuronal context of the brain, the very same encoding strategy, that is, the encoding of the stimuli's natural (and social and vegetative) statistics (see chapters 8 and 20), was proposed to be relevant in the phenomenal realm of consciousness. More specifically, I proposed the encoding of the stimuli's statistical frequency distribution into the phases of the resting state's low-frequency oscillations to be central in constituting what I described as "environment–brain unity." (see Part VI)

As we will recall, the concept of the environment–brain unity describes a statistically based congruency between the spatial and temporal features of the stimuli's occurrence across the different discrete points in (physical) time and space in the environment on one hand, and the spatial and temporal features of the resting-state activity itself (i.e., functional connectivity and low-frequency fluctuations) on the other (see Chapter 20). Such virtual statistically based environment–brain unity was, in turn, proposed to predispose the prephenomenal and ultimately the phenomenal unity of consciousness (see Chapter 21).

NEURONAL HYPOTHESIS IB: PHASE ALIGNMENT OF THE BRAIN'S RESTING-STATE ACTIVITY IN THE *INNER* RING TO *INTEROCEPTIVE* STIMULI FROM THE *BODY*

What does such encoding of the stimuli's natural statistics into the resting state's neural activity imply for the assignment of self-specificity to intero- and exteroceptive stimuli? Let's start with the interoceptive stimuli from the body. The continuous interoceptive inputs from one's own body may show more or less the same statistical frequency distribution across (the different discrete points in physical) time and space. Hence, the same stimuli occur here rather regularly and frequently because after all, despite all the changes the body goes through, it is the same body the stimuli are coming and thus originating from.

What does such rhythmic occurrence of the body's interoceptive stimuli mean for the brain and its resting state? The interoceptive stimuli provide a certain rhythmic structure to which the phases of the resting state's low-frequency fluctuations can themselves easily align by shifting the onset of their phases. This leads me to the following neuronal hypothesis: I propose a high degree of phase shifting and thus stimulus-phase coupling, or phase alignment, of the resting-state activity's low-frequency fluctuations in the case of interoceptive stimuli, which consequently leads to a high degree of a rhythmic mode in the brain's neural operation (see Chapter 20; see also Chang et al. 2012 for empirical support). Since interoceptive stimuli are strongly processed in anterior midline regions, I propose such high degree of stimulus-phase coupling to be particularly strong, especially in the anterior regions of the inner ring like the PACC, the VMPC, and the insula (Fig. 23-2a; see earlier, as well as Chapter 4 in Volume I; and Chang et al. 2012).

NEURONAL HYPOTHESIS IC: PHASE ALIGNMENT OF THE BRAIN'S RESTING-STATE ACTIVITY IN THE *OUTER* RING TO *EXTEROCEPTIVE* STIMULI FROM THE *ENVIRONMENT*

How about exteroceptive stimuli? Here the statistical situation is different. Unlike the

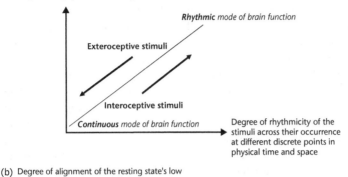

(a) Degree of alignment of the resting state's low frequency fluctuations and their phase onsets to the stimuli' onsets at their different discrete points in physical time and space

Rhythmic mode of brain function

Exteroceptive stimuli

Interoceptive stimuli

Continuous mode of brain function

Degree of rhythmicity of the stimuli across their occurrence at different discrete points in physical time and space

(b) Degree of alignment of the resting state's low frequency fluctuations and their phase onsets to the stimuli' onsets at their different discrete points in physical time and space

Degree of statistically-based matching between stimuli and phase onsets = Degree of self-specificity of stimuli or tasks

Degree of rhythmicity of the stimuli across their occurrence at different discrete points in physical time and space

Degree of statistically-based matching between stimuli and phase onsets

Degree of self-specificity of stimuli or tasks

Degree of deviation of stimulus-induced or task-related activity from the resting state activity level

Figure 23-2a and b Neuronal mechanisms of self-specificity. The figure shows the relationship between the rhythmic/statistical structure of stimuli and the degree of alignment (a) and its relationship to self-specificity and the resting-state activity level (b). (a) The more rhythmic the stimuli are presented, the more likely it is that the resting-state activity's low-frequency fluctuations (delta (1–4Hz), theta (5–8Hz), and infraslow (lower than 0.1 Hz)) can align their phases to the onsets of the stimuli. Due to the more rhythmic structure, this is more likely to occur for interoceptive stimuli, though in the right circumstances it is also possible for exteroceptive stimuli (as the interoceptive stimuli may also occur nonrhythmically); this is symbolized by the upward and downward arrows from intero- and exteroceptive stimuli. (b) The degree of alignment as related to the degree of rhythmicity in the environmental and bodily stimuli's occurrence is closely related to the degree of self-specificity assigned to the stimulus. The more aligned and rhythmic the stimulus, the higher the degree of self-specificity assigned to the stimulus (upper graph), while that goes along with an inverse relationship to the degree of deviation from the resting-state activity. The more the stimulus-induced activity deviates from the resting-state activity level, the lower the degree of self-specificity assigned to the stimulus (lower graph).

interoceptive stimuli from the body, the extero-ceptive stimuli do not come as regular and rhythmically. Why? The degree of change and inconsistency is probably much higher in the case of exteroceptive stimuli from the environ-ment when compared to the body's interocep-tive stimuli. This means that the phases of the resting state's low-frequency oscillations can no longer as easily align themselves to the extero-ceptive stimuli as to their interoceptive counter-parts. The brain reverts then to what is described as "continuous mode" of neural operation (see Chapter 20 for details).

This leads me to the following neuronal hypothesis for exteroceptive stimuli: I propose that the general degree of phase shifting and stimulus-phase coupling of the resting-state low-frequency fluctuations is lower for extero-ceptive stimuli when compared to intero-ceptive stimuli. Due to the lack of possible stimulus-phase coupling, there may thus be a higher degree of the continuous mode of neural operation in exteroceptive stimuli: The brain's resting state is thus more on its own, must become activity by itself, and remains therefore more independent of the stimuli to which it can no longer align itself as easily anymore (see Chapter 20).

Regionally, I expect the degree of stimulus-phase alignment for exteroceptive stimuli to be highest in especially the regions of the outer ring. This includes sensory cortex and higher executive regions (like the lateral prefrontal cortex) that process predominantly exterocep-tive stimuli. The regions of the outer ring may thus show lower degrees of phase shifting and stimulus-phase coupling of the resting-state activity's low frequency fluctuations when compared to those of the inner regions (see earlier).

I therefore propose that the difference in phase shifting and stimulus-phase coupling between inner and outer rings is related to the difference in the statistical structure of intero- and exteroceptive stimuli and their respective associations with the inner and the outer rings' neural activities. Accordingly, the more rhyth-mic nature of the interoceptive stimuli makes it more likely for the resting-state activity's low frequency fluctuations in the inner ring to shift their phase onset and to align them-selves to the interoceptive stimuli from one's own body.

Since they are less rhythmic, exteroceptive stimuli from the environment cannot be as well and easily aligned to by the resting-state activity in the outer ring as interoceptive stimuli in the inner ring. Such a difference in the degree of the resting-state activity's phase alignment to intero- and exteroceptive stimuli predisposes, as I claim, a difference in how closely and ultimately self-specifically we can experience our body and environment in consciousness.

NEURONAL HYPOTHESIS IIA: RESTING-STATE ACTIVITY *CONTAINS* INFORMATION ABOUT SELF-SPECIFICITY

How do such differences in phase alignment between intero- and exteroceptive stimuli trans-late into different degrees of self-specificity? Based on the observed strong overlap between resting-state activity and self-specific activity in anterior and inner regions (see earlier), one may now make the following assumption. I hypoth-esize that high phase alignment predicts high degrees of self-specificity, while low degrees of phase alignment are rather predictive of low degrees of self-specificity.

How does the phase alignment translate into self-specificity? Let us go back to the findings. We showed strong regional overlap between resting-state activity and neural activity related to self-specificity in the anterior regions of the inner ring. Going beyond such regional over-lap, we will see in the next sections that the rest-ing state seems to even predict the subsequent stimuli's degree of self-specificity (see next sections for details). This lets me propose that the resting-state activity must contain some special information about self-specificity. In other words, the neural activity in the resting state must encode in a yet-unclear way some information about self-specificity in its neural activity.

How could such information about self-specificity be encoded in the resting state's neural activity? One hallmark of the resting-state activity is its low-frequency oscillations, including delta and theta oscillations as well as infraslow oscillations (lower than 0.1 Hz; see Chapter 5, Volume I, for details). As demonstrated earlier, the resting state's low-frequency oscillations are also proposed to lock and thus entrain the higher frequency oscillations like gamma that are elicited by the stimuli. One could consequently propose that the phases (and the power) of the resting state's low-frequency oscillations may encode information related to self-specificity.

NEURONAL HYPOTHESIS IIB: PHASE ALIGNMENT *ENCODES* SELF-SPECIFICITY INTO THE BRAIN'S RESTING-STATE ACTIVITY

How can the phases of the resting-state activity's low-frequency oscillations encode self-specificity? I proposed earlier that the phases of the resting state's low-frequency oscillations align themselves to the onsets of both intero- and exteroceptive stimuli in different degrees and in different regions.

By aligning the phase onsets of its low-frequency fluctuations to the stimuli and their onsets, the resting state's low-frequency oscillations encode the temporal (and spatial) differences between the stimuli's occurrence (in environment or body) across (different discrete points in physical) time and space (see Fig. 23-2b). The temporal (and spatial) differences in the (more or less) rhythmic and regular occurrence of the stimuli and their onsets are thus encoded into the temporal duration of the low frequencies' phases (and possibly also into the spatial extension of the functional connectivity).

Such phase alignment is obviously easier to achieve when the stimuli are presented in a more rhythmic way. Rhythmic presentation means here that the stimuli display the same temporal (and spatial) differences over and over again, thus yielding a rhythmic pattern. This makes it easier for the resting-state activity's phase onsets to align themselves to the stimuli's onsets. That is the case, for instance, in interoceptive stimuli, where the degree of rhythmicity is rather high when compared to the more irregular and arrhythmic exteroceptive stimuli (see earlier). One would consequently expect strong phase shifting and stimulus-phase coupling in the case of interoceptive stimuli, as hypothesized earlier.

However, even exteroceptive stimuli can show a high degree of regularity and rhythmicity. This is, for instance, the case in one's own name. One's own name contains stimuli as, for instance, the letters and their respective context that are always set in the same way, thus displaying a specific rhythmic pattern. Statistically, this means that the stimuli and their respective context always show the same temporal (and spatial) differences (between them). Since the letters (and their respective context) as the different stimuli of one's own name always show the same temporal (and spatial) differences, the phases of the resting state can easily align themselves to the stimuli associated with one's own name.

This, in contrast, is different in another person's name. Here the temporal (and spatial) differences (for the letters and their respective context) vary in different situations, which makes it more difficult for the resting state's phases to shift and align their onsets in orientation to the stimulus' onsets. Even if the name is familiar, it may nevertheless occur in a less regular and thus rhythmic way as well as in different contexts when compared to one's own name. Hence, the spatial and temporal patterns in the stimuli of the familiar name may be less regular and rhythmic than those of one's own name. Familiar and unknown names may thus lead to lower degrees of phase shifting and stimulus-phase coupling in the resting-state activity's low-frequency fluctuations.

NEURONAL HYPOTHESIS IIC: PHASE ALIGNMENT DOES *NOT* REQUIRE THE BRAIN TO *CHANGE* ITS RESTING-STATE ACTIVITY *LEVEL*

This, however, leaves unexplained one of the major findings described above, the neural overlap in the degrees of neural activity between resting-state activity and self-specificity. Why do self-specific stimuli not induce much change in neural activity in the midline regions when compared to the resting state?

I can only speculate at this point. Once the stimulus is aligned to the resting state and its low-frequency oscillations (and functional connectivity), the resting state may no longer need to become active by itself and thus change its activity level. Due to the stimulus' alignment to the resting state, the former will then be assigned a high degree of self-specificity. I thus speculate that high self-specificity accompanies decreased deviation from the resting state.

This is different in the case of low self-specificity. Here, the resting state cannot shift and align its phase onsets to the onset of the stimuli. What, then, shall the resting state "do" with the stimulus it cannot align itself to? If the resting state cannot link to and integrate the stimulus via the phase onsets of its low-frequency fluctuations, the only way to do this is to change the level of its neural activity and thus to deviate from its resting-state activity level. The resulting neural activity level, the stimulus-induced activity, will consequently deviate significantly from the level of the preceding resting state. However, as we all know, nothing comes for free. The same holds true for the deviation from the resting-state activity: The price the stimulus has to pay for its change of the resting-state activity level may be that it will be assigned a low degree of self-specificity.

How can we further illustrate what exactly happens in the case of especially highly self-specific stimuli where the level of resting-state activity in anterior midline regions does not change and thus deviate? Metaphorically speaking, the resting state "sees no need" anymore to change its activity once it can align itself, that is, its phase onsets, to the stimuli's onsets. Isn't it more than natural to be no longer active and thus change yourself once (you think that) your job is done? Although we suggested a strong and rather tentative hypothesis, we need to gather more empirical support to back it up. In other words, we need to further tighten the link between resting-state activity and self-specificity, which will be the focus in the next sections.

NEURONAL FINDINGS IIIA: PREDICTION OF SELF-SPECIFICITY BY RESTING STATE ACTIVITY— INCREASED PRE-STIMULUS GAMMA POWER

How can we gather further empirical support for the proposed neural overlap between resting-state activity and self-specificity in the PACC? For that, we conducted an intracranial study in collaboration with the neurosurgeons in Toronto (Lipsman et al. 2013).

We first investigated nine patients with depression who underwent deep brain stimulation in the subgenual part of the anterior cingulate cortex. The cell firing rates and their frequency fluctuations during self- and non-self-specific stimuli (i.e., own versus other name presented visually) were measured as well as during the resting state (i.e., long baseline and intertribal intervals). To test for regional specificity, we undertook the same measurements in the subthalamic nucleus (STN) in patients with Parkinson's disease.

What kind of firing rates would one expect? Since a stimulus is applied when presenting names, one would expect a stimulus-related increase in the firing rates. This was indeed the case in non-self-specific stimuli. There we observed a significant increase in the firing rates. In contrast, this was not the case for self-specific stimuli, that is, one's own name. We did not observe any significant change in the cells' firing rates during self-specific stimuli, that is, one's own name, when compared to the preceding baseline. Even more interesting, this was specific for the subgenual cingulate cortex since we did not observe such firing pattern in the subthalamic nucleus where both self- and non-self-specific stimuli induced significant increases in the cells' firing rates (see Fig. 23-3a).

Since previous studies demonstrated association of increased gamma power with self-specificity (see Chapter 24 for details), we then focused our subsequent analyses on gamma power. This demonstrated increased gamma power in the subgenual cingulate cortex during self-specific stimuli and rest when compared to non-self-specific stimuli. Most interestingly, we observed increased gamma power in the resting

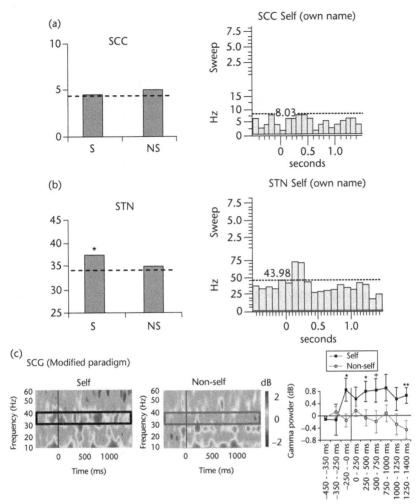

Figure 23-3a Lack of deviation of firing rates in subgenual cortex during self-specific stimuli from resting-state firing rates. There was no significant difference in firing rate in the first 500 ms of presentation of either self-relevant (S) (e.g., the own name) or non-self-relevant (NS) (e.g., another person's name) stimuli in subgenual cingulate cortex (SCG) SCG neurons, when compared to the intertrial interval (–700 ms to –300 ms; 4.88 Hz; indicated by horizontal dashed line). A sample Raster plot and peri-stimulus histogram is shown of a representative SCG neuron responding to patient's own name, with stimulus onset at time 0. The first 1.5 s of stimulus presentation is shown, as well as 0.5 s of intertrial interval (ITI), with the horizontal line representing two standard deviations above the mean firing rate in the ITI. (*b*) There was a significant difference in firing rate in subthalamic nucleus' (STN) neurons in response only to self-relevant stimuli (S), when compared to the ITI across all stimuli presentations (34.32 Hz; horizontal dashed line). Difference marked with an asterisk indicates significance at $p < .05$. Raster plots and peri-stimulus histogram for an STN neuron responding to "own" name is shown. (*c*) Time-resolved relative gamma power from baseline (–450 to –350 ms) for self-relevant stimuli versus non-self-relevant stimuli. Differences marked with an asterisk were significant at $p < .05$, + were marginal at $p < 0.1$. Error bars indicate standard error. There was significant difference between own name and other person's name in the SCC neurons when we used a modified paradigm (see text for explanation). Stimulus onset is at time 0. Line graph shows averaged gamma power in 250 ms ranges. Note the significant differentiation between self and nonself in gamma power from pre-stimulus onset (–250–0 ms) continuing into stimulus-induced activity (0–500 ms).

state preceding the onset of self-specific stimuli, while this was not the case in non-self-specific stimuli.

This raises the question of whether the increased gamma power in the preceding resting state is related to the expectation of a self-specific stimulus or is related to the ongoing spontaneous fluctuations in the resting state's gamma power independent of the presentation of subsequent stimuli. If the latter holds, one would expect high resting state gamma power to be predictive of the subsequent stimuli's degrees of self-specificity. High gamma power in the preceding resting state should then predispose the subjects to assign a high degree of self-specificity to the stimulus.

NEURONAL FINDINGS IIIB: PREDICTION OF SELF-SPECIFICITY BY RESTING-STATE ACTIVITY— INCREASED PRE-STIMULUS GAMMA POWER AND SELF-SPECIFICITY

This hypothesis was tested in three other intracranial patients from Berlin, Germany, who underwent another paradigm (Lipsman et al. 2013). Instead of the stimulus itself being self- or non-self-specific (i.e., one's own versus another's name), we let subjects themselves decide about the degree of self-specificity. For that, we presented pictures of different faces from the famous Ekman series. After an initial perception period, subjects had to judge the degree of self-specificity of the pictures whether it was high or low self-specific (while controlling for emotions and race in subsequent behavioral analysis). All that was done during the recording of the local field potentials (rather than the cells' firing rates), which allowed us to investigate the gamma power during both resting state and stimulus presentation.

What did the results show? Let us start with the changes observed during the stimulus presentation itself. The local field potentials showed significantly higher gamma power during those stimuli that were rated by the subjects as high self-specific when compared to the ones rated as low self-specific. The higher the gamma power induced by the stimulus, the higher the degree

of self-specificity assigned to the stimuli by the subject itself. This confirms the association of self-specificity with high gamma power in the PACC during stimulus-induced activity (see also Chapter 24).

Where does the high gamma power during the stimulus presentation come from? It could be induced by the stimulus itself. In that case one would expect no differences between high and low self-specific stimuli in the preceding state. Or, alternatively, it could originate in the resting state itself and thus be simply carried over and transferred to the subsequent stimulus-induced activity. In that case one would expect significant differences between high and low self-specific stimuli in the resting state period preceding the stimulus onset.

To test these alternative hypotheses, we plotted the degree of gamma power in the preceding resting state interval, the intertrial interval that precedes the onset of the stimulus. Interestingly, we could see there that up to 800 ms pre-stimulus onset, gamma power was already significantly higher in those trials where the subsequent stimulus was assigned a high degree of self-specificity, while low pre-stimulus gamma power predicted low degree of self-specificity of the subsequent stimulus. Hence, the stimulus' degree of self-specificity (rather than its emotion or race) was predicted by the degree of gamma power in the preceding resting state periods (see Fig. 23-3b).

Taken together, these findings go beyond the previous ones that showed regional overlap between resting-state activity and self-specificity in anterior regions of the inner ring, that is, PACC and insula. There is not only regional overlap but, much stronger, prediction of the stimuli's degree of self-specificity by the preceding resting-state activity level, that is, gamma power. The preceding resting state's neuronal measures like the gamma power (and possibly others) must consequently encode and thus contain some information related to self-specificity. Otherwise the here observed prediction of the stimuli's degree of self-specificity by the preceding resting-state activity would remain impossible.

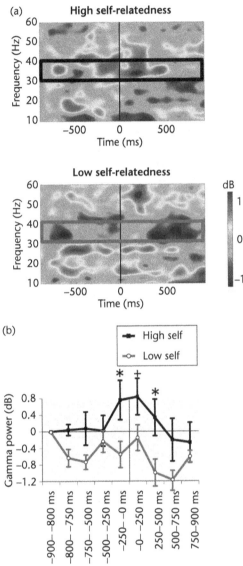

Figure 23-3b Prediction of stimuli's degree of self-specificity by the gamma power in the preceding resting state. Time-resolved relative gamma power from baseline (–900 to –800 ms). Relative powers were averaged between L03 and R03 channels for high and low self-relatedness face. Stimulus onset is at time 0. Line graph shows averaged gamma power in 250 ms ranges. Note again the significant differentiation between high- and low self-related stimuli in local field potentials and gamma power, in particular, prior to the onset of the stimuli, that is, –250–0 ms, which continues into stimulus-induced activity (0–500 ms). Hence, the degree of self-relatedness subjects assigned to the stimuli (stimuli here concerned faces which subjects had to judge for their degree of self-relatedness rather than the subject's own, or others', names as in the data presented in Fig. 23-3a). Hence, the pre-stimulus differentiation in gamma power predicts the degree of self-relatedness, that is, high or low, subjects will assign to the subsequently presented stimuli (see supplement material for exclusion of confounding factors in the stimuli).

Neuronal Findings IVA: Prediction of Resting State Activity by Self-Specificity—Stimulus–Rest Interaction During High and Low Self-Specific Stimuli

How is the information about self-specificity encoded into the resting state such that the latter can predict the subsequent stimuli's degrees of self-specificity? For that to be possible the resting-state activity must have somehow been impacted by previous stimuli and their degree of self-specificity. In other words, there must have been some kind of stimulus–rest interaction.

This hypothesis of stimulus–rest interaction was tested in a recent study of ours by Schneider et al. (2008). Schneider et al. (2008) took the neural overlap between self and rest as a starting point and investigated how the stimulus' degree of self-specificity affects the signal changes in the subsequent resting state period. They showed emotional pictures in functional magnetic resonance imaging (fMRI; pure perception without cognitive tasks) with periods of baseline/resting state (e.g., fixation cross) and afterward let subjects rate the pictures' degree of self-specificity (and affective measures like valence and intensity).

The subjective ratings were then divided into high and low self-related pictures, which allowed the comparison of the different resting state periods, or baselines, with each other. Those baselines following high self pictures, for example, "baseline high self" (as we named it), showed significantly stronger signal changes in the VMPFC, the MOFC, the DMPFC, and the PCC (as well as in parietal cortex and the left anterior insula) when compared to "baseline low self." These results were confirmed by a regression analysis with the degree of signal changes in the midline regions' resting state predicting the preceding pictures' degree of self-specificity. This means that the degree of resting-state activity following the stimuli was directly dependent upon the degree of the preceding stimuli's degree of self-specificity.

How about emotions as confounding variables? We controlled for the affective dimensions of the stimuli (valence, intensity) in our ratings. However, the resting state's activity changes were significantly more strongly related to the pictures' degree of self-specificity than to their degrees of emotional valence and intensity. This suggests that the subsequent resting state period was specifically affected by the preceding pictures' degree of self-specificity rather than their affective features (see Fig. 23-3c).

Neuronal Findings IVB: Prediction of Resting-State Activity by Self-Specificity—Distinction Between Stimulus- and Resting-State Related Effects

How could the effects of self-specificity during the subsequent resting state period be distinguished from those during the stimulus itself? We also performed direct comparison between stimulus periods and resting state periods and their respective modulation by the different degrees of self-specificity. In addition to baseline high self and baseline low self, we therefore also investigated the impact of high and low self during the stimulus period itself, "stimulus high self" and "stimulus low self."

This demonstrated that the stimuli's degree of self-specificity affected predominantly subcortical regions like the right amygdala, the tectum, and the ventral striatum (as well as the MOFC) during the stimulus presentation period itself (i.e., "stimulus high self" larger than "stimulus low self"). In contrast, signal changes in the cortical midline regions like the VMPFC, DMPFC, and PCC were specific for the effects of the preceding pictures' degree of self-specificity on the subsequent resting state period ("baseline high self" larger than "baseline low self").

Taken together, these data suggest that the anterior and posterior cortical midline regions are related specifically to self-specificity during the resting state, while subcortical midline regions seem to be more implicated during stimulus-induced periods. Hence, the neural activity in the subcortical and cortical midline regions seems to have a specific sensitivity and reactivity to be modulated by stimuli with high degrees of self-specificity. Thereby, both subcortical and cortical midline regions seem to act and

F. Schneider et al. / Neuroscience 157 (2008) 120–131

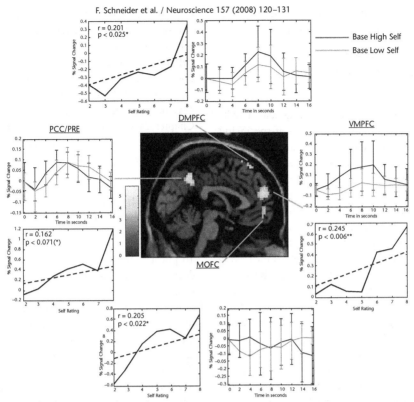

Figure 23-3c Stimulus–rest interaction for self-specificity in subcortical and cortical midline structures. Effects of self-relatedness ratings on neural activity during the subsequent baseline period. The SPM maps show the categorical comparison between the baseline periods (intertrial periods with fixation cross) following high self-related pictures and the baseline periods following low self-related pictures (Base High Self > Base Low Self). The sagittal view depicts the right hemisphere; the threshold of significance is set to $P < 0.001$ (uncorr), $k > 10$. BOLD curves (x-axis: time locked to baseline onset (t0), y-axis: % signal change) are plotted separately for baseline following high (black curve) and low (gray curve) self-related pictures. The doromedial prefrontal cortex (DMPFC) finding is reported with caution, as it is located at the periphery of the prefrontal cortex, and we cannot exclude an artifact. However, it should be noted that clusters of activation were projected on the MNI standard brain and extended into the cortex on a lower level of significance. We also plotted the correlation curves between % signal change (y-axis) and the degree of self-relatedness (based on visual analogue scale ranging from 0 to 9 with the extreme values, 0 and 9, cutoff; x-axis); the original data points as obtained by partial correlation analysis and the regression curve are shown. Correlation values are based upon Spearman correlation analysis (* $P < 0.05$, ** $P < 0.005$, (*) $P < 0.05$–0.1). Abbreviations and MNI coordinates (x, y, z, Z): Dorsomedial prefrontal cortex = DMPFC (close to premotor cortex and BA 8) (–3, 24, 66, 3.09), Medial orbital frontal cortex = MOFC (bordering to the ventromedial prefrontal cortex = VMPFC) (0, 57, –6, 2.94), VMPFC (bordering to the DMPFC) (–3, 57, 24, 3.74), Posterior cingulate cortex/ Precuneues = PCC/PRE (–3, –54, 39, 3.84). Reprinted with permission, from Schneider F, Bermpohl F, Heinzel A, Rotte M, Walter M, Tempelmann C, Wiebking C, Dobrowolny H, Heinze HJ, Northoff G. The resting brain and our self: Self-relatedness modulates resting state neural activity in cortical midline structures. *Neuroscience.* 2008 Nov 11;157(1):120–31.

operate together across the divide of resting-state activity and stimulus-induced activity.

NEURONAL HYPOTHESIS IIIA: "MATCHING HYPOTHESIS OF SELF-SPECIFICITY"

How is it possible that the resting-state activity can predict the stimuli's degrees of self-specificity? Let us recall from the earlier sections.

The previously discussed findings of the neural overlap between self and rest led me to the following neuronal hypothesis. I hypothesized that the stimuli's degree of self-specificity is directly dependent upon the degree of phase shifting and stimulus-phase coupling. The higher the degree of the coupling of the phase onsets of the resting state's low-frequency fluctuations to the stimulus' temporal features (i.e., its onset, its temporal differences in its occurrence across time, etc.), the higher the degree of self-specificity that can possibly be assigned to the stimulus. Unfortunately, no empirical data are currently available to directly support this hypothesis.

Let us explicate that hypothesis in detail. The hypothesis implies the following for high self-specific stimuli: I propose the temporal (and also spatial) differences in the high self-specific stimuli's occurrence (across discrete points in physical time and space) to correspond to a high degree with the temporal (and also spatial) differences between the phase onsets in resting-state activity's low-frequency oscillations (and functional connectivity). Accordingly, the spatial and temporal measures of both resting-state activity and stimuli seem to match and thus correspond well to each other in high self-specific stimuli. In contrast, the degree of such statistically based matching and correspondence is presumed to be rather low in the case of low self-specific stimuli.

This leads me to propose what I describe as the "matching hypothesis of self-specificity." The matching hypothesis of self-specificity proposes that the statistically based comparison, that is, matching, between the stimuli's statistical frequency distribution across space and time on one hand, and the spatial and temporal neuronal measures of the resting state, that is, its

functional connectivity and low-frequency fluctuations, on the other, determines the degree of self-specificity assigned to each stimulus: the better the statistical frequency distributions of both stimuli and resting state match with each other, the less the resulting neural activity will deviate from the preceding resting state (see Chapter 24 for details on that), and the higher the degree of self-specificity assigned to the stimulus (see Fig. 23-4a).

NEURONAL HYPOTHESIS IIIB: STATISTICALLY BASED MATCHING REQUIRES NEURAL ACTIVITY IN MIDLINE REGIONS

To put it slightly differently, I propose that the degree of such statistically based matching reflects the degree of correspondence or congruency between the environmental stimuli and the resting-state activity's neuronal measures. That degree of correspondence or congruency does in turn predict the degree of self-specificity that can possibly be assigned to the stimulus. Accordingly, the matching hypothesis proposes self-specificity to be based on a statistically based comparison process between two different statistical structures operating across different discrete points in physical time and space: one from the extrinsic stimuli, and the other from the intrinsic resting-state activity.

How is the matching hypothesis manifested in the neural activity of regions and networks in the brain? In terms of regions in the brain (and thus in spatial regard), the matching hypothesis of self-specificity proposes a central role for the subcortical-cortical midline system. This subcortical-cortical midline system concerns mainly the inner and middle rings and may therefore include what Lou describes (2010a and b, 2011a and b; see also Northoff and Panksepp 2008; Panksepp and Northoff 2009) as the "paralimbic network" (that includes PACC, the subgenual cingulate, the PCC, the precuneus, the striatum, and the thalamus; see earlier).

The above-reported findings showing neural overlap between self-specificity and resting-state activity especially in the midline regions suggest that the degree of statistically based

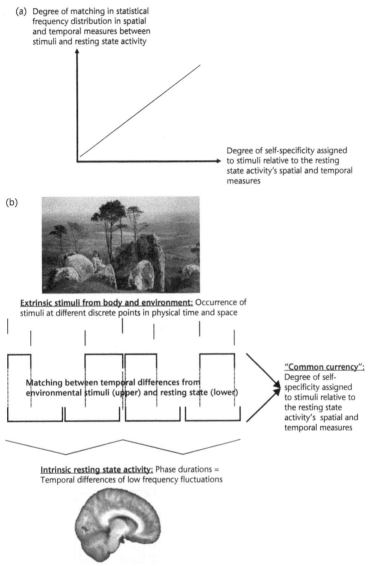

Figure 23-4a and b Matching hypothesis of self-specificity. The figure illustrates distinct aspects of the matching hypothesis of self-specificity with regard to the dependence of self-specificity on the degree of statistically based matching (*a*) and self-specificity as "common currency" between intrinsic and extrinsic activity (*b*). (*a*) The figure shows the dependence of the stimulus' degree of self-specificity on the degree of statistically and spatiotemporally based matching between the resting-state activity and stimuli's occurrence with regard to their respective spatial and temporal measures. The better both match with each other, the higher the degree of self-specificity that will be assigned to the stimulus. (*b*) The resting-state activity is characterized by predominant low-frequency fluctuations (*lowest bottom part*) that show long phase durations and thus long temporal differences between the different phases (*second to bottom*). These temporal differences from the resting-state activity are matched against the temporal differences (*second to top part*) from the stimuli's occurrence across different discrete points in physical time and space (*highest top part*). The comparison allows for a statistically and spatiotemporally based matching process between resting-state activity and stimulus-related temporal differences (*middle*). This results in the assignment of self-specificity to all stimuli relative to the resting-state activity level; the self-specificity can then be regarded as "common currency" between stimuli and resting state and thus between extrinsic stimulus-induced and intrinsic resting-state activity (see far right).

matching between extrinsic stimuli and intrinsic resting-state activity is particularly high in the subcortical-cortical midline system. The midline system may therefore be central in matching, regulating, and integrating intrinsically and extrinsically generated activities in the brain (see also Lou 2011 for a more or less analogous suggestion).

How about the temporal mechanisms of such statistically based matching? Temporally, the subcortical-cortical midline system may be characterized by a high degree of neuronal synchronization as, for instance, in the gamma range in both the resting state (see earlier) and during stimulus-induced activity (see Chapter 24 for details). This is based on the intracranial findings reported earlier and the ones by Lou et al. (2010a and b, 2011a and b; see earlier); however future investigation and support will be necessary.

What can be proposed, though, is that increased gamma synchronization may reflect the outcome of the statistically based matching process between the temporal features of extrinsic stimuli (both intero- and exteroceptive) and those of the intrinsic resting-state activity. The more the stimuli's different discrete points in (physical) time can be matched with those of the resting-state activity, the higher the degree of gamma synchronization in the subcortical-cortical midline system and the higher the stimuli's degree of self-specificity. Low degrees of gamma synchronization may thus indicate low degrees of matching and thus a high degree of temporal discrepancy between extrinsic stimuli and intrinsic activity, which consequently leads to low degrees of self-specificity.

Neuronal Hypothesis IIIC: Self-Specificity is an Extrinsic Rather than Intrinsic Feature of the Stimulus

What does the matching hypothesis imply for the determination of self-specificity? The information about self-specificity may be encoded in the temporal (and spatial) differences between the phase onsets of the resting state's low-frequency oscillations (and functional connectivity). This is, I propose, why the resting state and the phase onsets and durations of its low-frequency fluctuations predict the subsequent stimuli's degrees of self-specificity (and vice versa) as described earlier (see below in the next section for further explanation). Only if the resting state's low-frequency fluctuations, i.e., their phase onsets and phase durations, contain and encode some information about self-specificity, can the resting-state activity predict the degree of self-specificity that will be assigned to subsequent stimuli, as reported earlier.

How does that relate to the difference between intero- and exteroceptive stimuli? Due to their probably lower degrees of phase shifting and stimulus-phase coupling (see earlier), exteroceptive stimuli may be assigned a lower degree of self-specificity when compared to interoceptive stimuli. However, the reverse is also possible with exteroceptive stimuli like one's own name being highly self-specific and interoceptive stimuli becoming rather lowly self-specific (as, for instance, in certain neuropsychiatric disorders like schizophrenia in which one no longer experiences the body as self-specific, i.e., as one's own body; see subsequent chapters).

The fact that the degree of self-specificity assigned to both intero- and exteroceptive stimuli can vary suggests that self-specificity is not an intrinsic feature of the stimuli themselves (which, for instance, could be traced back to their origin in either body or environment). Instead of being intrinsic to the stimuli themselves, self-specificity must be regarded an extrinsic feature that is applied, or better, imposed, upon the stimuli by the brain and its resting-state activity.

Accordingly, self-specificity is extrinsic to the stimuli, rather than being an intrinsic feature of them in which case it would be completely and sufficiently determined by the stimulus itself. I consequently propose the matching hypothesis to apply to any kind of stimulus, whether intero- or exteroceptive, and thus to self-specificity in general, independent of the origin of the stimuli in either body or environment, that is, intero- and exteroceptive stimuli.

Neuronal Hypothesis IIID: Neuronal Versus Neurocognitive Approaches to Self-Specificity

The description of self-specificity as an extrinsic feature of the stimulus may come as a surprise. Isn't self-specificity rather an intrinsic feature of the stimuli themselves as it seems to be the case in, for instance, the own name? No, because even one's own name must be processed in certain ways in order to be associated with a high degree of self-specificity. We will see later, in Chapter 27, that these processes can be disrupted in (for instance) schizophrenia. This makes it impossible for these subjects to associate a high degree of self-specificity to even their own name, which ultimately results in their experience of being a "different person" or self.

The possible disruption of the neuronal processes underlying the generation of self-specificity is evidence enough that self-specificity does not come with the stimulus itself. Instead, self-specificity must be associated with the stimulus and is therefore an extrinsic rather than intrinsic feature. Most important, that association must be mediated by certain neuronal mechanisms, as discussed in the preceding sections.

This, however, is a presupposition that does not seem to be shared by neurocognitive approaches, among others. Neurocognitive approaches focus on the cognitive processes that are related to the subsequent neural processing of high and low self-specific stimuli. This leads them to postulate different degrees of self-reference that are associated with different cognitive processes (see Chapter 24 for the details on the distinction between *self-specificity* and *self-reference*). Briefly, the concept of self-reference describes that a stimulus is related and thereby refers to one's own self like one's own name.

The cognitive processes of self-reference and their neural correlates are supposed to "quasi-decipher" the degree of self-specificity that (as an intrinsic feature) is assumed to "lie" inherent in the stimulus itself. The neurocognitive approaches therefore seem to take the self-specificity of the stimulus as given. A person's own name has an intrinsically high degree of self-specificity (as acquired by prior learning), which only needs to be deciphered in terms of self-reference by recruiting the "right" cognitive processes.

That assumption, however, stands opposite to my neuronal hypothesis. I postulate that in each instance, independently of any prior learning processes, the degree of self-specificity of stimuli, including one's own name, must be generated anew. Certain prior learning processes may make it easier and predispose us to make the association of a high or low degree of self-specificity with the respective stimulus. However, this does "not relieve the brain" from the role of initiating the neuronal mechanisms that enable the association of self-specificity to the actual stimulus.

Even though schizophrenic patients learned that their own name carries a high degree of self-specificity, they nevertheless failed to associate it with a high degree of self-specificity in the acute psychotic state when they experienced themselves as a different self or person (see Chapter 27). This makes it clear that self-specificity cannot be taken as given as in neurocognitive approaches but must be associated to the stimuli by the brain and its neural activity. My so far purely neuronal approach to self-specificity must therefore be distinguished from neurocognitive approaches that focus more on self-reference than self-specificity.

Therefore, I am not so much interested in the subsequent cognitive processes and their neuronal correlates that underlie the subsequent processing of low and high self-specific stimuli in terms of self-reference (see Chapter 24 for the distinction between self-specificity and self-reference). Rather than investigating the subsequent neurocognitive processes with the transformation of self-specificity into self-reference, my focus is more on the preceding neuronal mechanisms that underlie the generation of self-specificity itself. How can we express this hypothesis in a more illustrative or metaphorical way? Metaphorically speaking, I target the "floor," the brain itself, and its neuronal "carpets" of self-specificity as the very ground upon which stand the various cognitive pieces of "furniture" of self-reference that the neurocognitive approach investigates .

NEURONAL HYPOTHESIS IIIE: SELF-SPECIFICITY IS THE "COMMON CURRENCY" BETWEEN INTRINSIC ACTIVITY AND EXTRINSIC STIMULI AND THUS BETWEEN BRAIN AND ENVIRONMENT

What is self-specificity, and how can we characterize it in positive terms by itself? Self-specificity seems to be a "common currency" in two distinct ways. I proposed self-specificity to result from the statistically based matching process between environmental stimuli and resting state. It may thus be a "common currency" between the extrinsic stimuli's and the intrinsic resting-state activity's spatial and temporal measures. As such, self-specificity must be assumed not only to be statistically based, but also to operate across the divide between resting-state and stimulus-induced activity.

Self-specificity must be considered a "common currency" in two slightly different ways. First, it is a "common currency" between the brain's intrinsic activity and the extrinsic stimuli themselves as originating in the environment (or the body). The "common currency" consists here of the spatiotemporal features associated with both the brain's intrinsic activity and the extrinsic stimuli. Such a "common currency" between brain and environment is supposed to be made possible by the brain's encoding of the statistical frequency distribution of the extrinsic stimuli from the environment in terms of their spatial and temporal features.

Secondly, taken in a purely neuronal sense, there is a "common currency" between the brain's intrinsic activity and its extrinsic activity, the stimulus-induced (or task-related) activity as associated with the extrinsic stimulus. This second meaning of the concept of "common currency" is purely neuronal and, unlike the first meaning, remains therefore purely within the brain itself where it describes the commonality between intrinsic and extrinsic activity.

How are both meanings of "common currency" related to each other? The second meaning, the "common currency" between intrinsic and extrinsic activity, is a direct consequence of the first meaning, the "common currency" between brain and environment. By linking both meanings of "common currency," the brain is able to directly link its intrinsic and extrinsic activity to the environment where the extrinsic stimuli originate. The glue or the bridge of this linkage is what I describe as self-specificity. Taken in this sense, self-specificity not only provides a "common currency" between the brain's intrinsic and extrinsic activity, but also, more generally, does so between brain and environment. (see Fig. 23-4b).

In addition, self-specificity can be assigned to both intero- and exteroceptive stimuli. This means that self-specificity does not operate along the divide between body and environment. Hence, by relating both intero- and exteroceptive stimuli to the brain's resting-state activity, self-specificity seems to also provide a "common currency" between body and environment. This may well imply what is conceptually described as "embodiment. In contrast, the first meaning of "common currency," the one concerning the linkage between brain and environment, may entail on the conceptual side what is referred to as "embeddedness" (see Chapter 32 as well as Appendix 1 for further discussion).

NEUROPHENOMENAL HYPOTHESIS IA: THE BRAIN'S RESTING STATE SHOWS A *"SELF-SPECIFIC ORGANIZATION"* IN ITS NEURAL ACTIVITY

How is my neuronal hypothesis about the relationship between stimulus-phase coupling and self-specificity related to the phenomenal realm of consciousness? Let's briefly review the main assumptions so far.

I proposed the stimuli's statistical frequency distribution in body and environment to be aligned to and thus carried over and transferred to the spatial and temporal features of the resting state's neuronal measures like low-frequency oscillations and functional connectivity. And, most important, I proposed the result of this carry-over and transfer, the degree of statistically based correspondence between stimuli and resting state, to be predictive of the stimulus' degree of self-specificity. The higher the degree of statistically based temporal and spatial correspondence between extrinsic stimulus and intrinsic resting-state activity, the higher the degree of self-specificity that is assigned to the stimulus.

What does such carryover and transfer of the environment's (and body's) statistical frequency distribution of their stimuli imply for the temporal and spatial organization of the resting state itself? The intrinsic resting state may then show spatial and temporal features in its neuronal measures that are (more or less) analogous to those of the extrinsic stimuli's occurrence across (the different discrete points in physical) time and space. This is what I described as "environment–brain unity" in the second part (see Chapter 20).

Since I now suggest higher degrees of such statistically based correspondence to be associated with higher degrees of self-specificity, one may propose the resting-state activity to be spatially and temporally organized in a self-specific way. What do I mean by self-specific organization? The concept of self-specific organization describes that the resting state's temporal and spatial features are structured in orientation on the statistically based correspondence between stimuli and resting state. Accordingly, I propose the resting state's self-specific organization to be statistically based and more specifically to be based on the statistical frequency and regularity of the stimuli in body and environment.

How can we explain in further detail the concept of "self-specific organization"? The concept of "organization" points to the way the spatial and temporal measures of the resting state like functional connectivity and low-frequency fluctuations are structured and organized. They are structured and organized in a certain way across the different discrete points in time and space, resulting in a particular spatiotemporal structure (see the previous parts as well as Part II in Volume I). How exactly can we characterize such a spatiotemporal structure? This shall be the focus in the next section.

Neurophenomenal hypothesis
IB: *"SELF*-SPECIFIC VERSUS *NON-SELF*-SPECIFIC ORGANIZATION" OF THE BRAIN'S RESTING STATE ACTIVITY

The concept of self-specific organization includes the concept of self. What does the concept of self stand for in this context? The concept of "self"

in "self-specific organization" does not refer to any kind of self as discussed in philosophy, be it a phenomenal self, a mental self, a representational self, a cognitive self, an affective self, or just an illusion of a self (see also Appendix 4).

Instead, the term "self" refers here to the resting state itself and more specifically to the spatial and temporal structure of its neuronal measures like functional connectivity and low-frequency fluctuations. Accordingly, the concept of "self" stands in the present context for a particular organization of the resting state's spatial and temporal neuronal measures. Metaphorically speaking, one may want to compare the self in this sense to a neuronal grid or structure into which any subsequent stimulus, function (see Chapter 24), and content (see Chapter 25) must be linked interwoven in order for it to be further processed in the brain.

What about the term "specific" in self-specific organization? The term "specific" in "self-specific organization" refers again to the resting state itself, but now, more specifically, to the particular way it structures and organizes its own neural activity. The extrinsic stimuli from the environment the intrinsic resting-state activity matches well with, that is, high self-specific stimuli, leave their strong traces in the resting state's neuronal measures. In contrast, stimuli with low degrees of statistically based matching, that is, low self-specific stimuli, do apparently not imprint themselves upon the resting state and its spatiotemporal structures (see earlier for the data). The resting state's neuronal measures become therefore organized in a way that is specific to their degree of statistically based matching with the environmental stimuli. This results in a self-specific organization.

Such self-specific organization must be distinguished from a non-self-specific organization of the resting-state activity, which we can only imagine how it may look in a thought experiment. In that case, the resting-state activity would organize and structure its own neuronal measures independently of the degree of the statistically based matching process between its own neuronal measures and the environmental stimuli. There would consequently be neither a statistically based matching process nor any self-specificity. In other words, my "matching hypothesis of self-specificity" would be obsolete and thus no longer apply in such purely imaginary scenario. This, however, is not empirically plausible, as we discussed in the preceding sections. Therefore, I leave the possibility of a non-self-specific organization behind and return to the self-specific organization.

Most important, the assumption of a self-specific organization of the resting-state activity is well in accordance with the earlier described data showing that the resting-state activity predicts the stimuli's degree of self-specificity. Due to its self-specific organization, the resting state already contains some spatial and temporal information about self-specificity. The resting-state activity's self-specific organization and thus the corresponding information can then be imposed upon the stimulus and the subsequent stimulus-induced activity and has thereby a strong say in determining the stimulus' degree of self-specificity, which in turn makes the reported prediction possible.

Neurophenomenal Hypothesis IC: Prephenomenal "Self-Specific Organization" of the Brain's Resting-State Activity and Phenomenal "Self-*Perspectival* Organization" of Consciousness

How is such self-specific organization of the resting state and its purely neuronal characterization now manifested on the phenomenal level of consciousness? I have so far proposed the resting state's neural activity to predispose various phenomenal features of consciousness, that is, inner time and space consciousness (see Part V) and phenomenal unity (see Part VI). The characterization of the resting state by self-specific organization should consequently affect, that is, predispose, specific phenomenal features of consciousness, too.

What phenomenal feature of consciousness is predisposed by the resting-state activity's self-specific organization? I propose the resting state's self-specific organization to predispose and thus be a necessary though nonsufficient condition of what is described as "self-perspectival organization" on the phenomenal level of consciousness.

What do I mean by "self-perspectival organization"? The concept of "self-perspectival organization" describes the organization of experience and thus of consciousness to be structured around and oriented on a center. This center or gravitation point provides the prephenomenal stance (rather than cognitive stance as for instance in D. Dennett) from which the contents and ultimately the world are experienced in consciousness. What I here describe as a center or gravitational point on the prephenomenal level is referred to on the phenomenal level as the "self." And what I describe by the concept of "stands from" finds its analogue in the one of "perspective" on the phenomenal level of experience, hence the name "self-perspectival organization" (see Chapter 24 for a more detailed discussion). What exactly is such "self-perspectival organization"? And how is it possible for it to be predisposed by the brain's resting-state activity and its self-specific organization? That will be the focus of Chapter 24.

Open Questions

The first main question concerns how the proposed self-perspectival organization stands in relation to the self-specificity of stimuli and even more important to the assumption of a self. The question of the self has been much debated in recent years. Some, like Thomas Metzinger (2003), propose the concept of self to be a mere illusion that has no counterpart in reality. Others, like Barry Dainton (2008), favor a phenomenally based concept of self. This is also in line (more or less) with phenomenological approaches to the self (Zahavi 2005), where the self is related to experience and thus (prereflective) self-awareness (see also Appendix 4 for the discussion of the concept of the self).

I have here distinguished the concept of "self-specificity" from that of "the self." Self-specificity concerns stimuli and how closely their statistical frequency distribution is related to that of the neuronal measures of the resting state, while the concept of "the self" may be related to the phenomenal level of consciousness, where it may signify the experience of a sense of self (see Chapter 24 for details).

One should also be careful about equating *self* and *consciousness*. Data in vegetative patients suggest that you can have neural activity related to self-specific stimuli without becoming and being phenomenally conscious of them (see chapters 28–30 for details). That argues against the identification of the self and consciousness, which leaves open the exact nature of their relationship.

I also did not focus on the relationship between self-specificity and first-person perspective as distinguished from a third-person perspective. This has been empirically investigated extensively by, for instance, Olaf Blanke (see, for instance, Blanke 2012). I propose self-specificity to be more basic and operating beneath or prior to the more cognitive distinction between first- and third-person perspectives.

I have here rather focussed on the very neuronal ground that first and foremost makes possible the constitution of phenomenal consciousness and its subsequent differentiation between first- and third-person perspectives rather than discussing how the first-person perspective itself is constituted on the ground of phenomenal consciousness.

Such differentiation is of central importance since even the constitution and acquisition of a third-person perspective is only possible on the basis of prior phenomenal consciousness: if you do not have phenomenal consciousness, you will remain unable to take not only the first-person perspective, but also the third-person perspective (see chapter 24 for more discussion of the different perspectives and their relation to consciousness).

Another question pertains to the issue that phenomenal consciousness is not only characterized by self-perspectival organization but also by directedness towards contents; that is, intentionality. Our phenomenal consciousness is also directed toward any kind of content, whether it is internal (in ourselves and our body) or external (in the environment). Such directedness toward (internal or external) contents is manifested on the phenomenal level of consciousness in what philosophers call "intentionality." What are the neuronal mechanisms underlying such directedness toward contents and thus intentionality? This will be discussed in Chapter 25 in full detail.

CHAPTER 24
Self-Specificity and Self-Perspectival Organization

Summary

I discussed the neuronal mechanisms underlying the supposedly self-specific organization of the brain's resting-state activity in Chapter 23. Now the question arises of how the resting-state activity's self-specific organization impacts subsequent stimulus-induced activity and its manifestation on the phenomenal level of consciousness. I discuss various findings from emotion, reward, and decision making to show how they are impacted by self-specificity and the midline region's activity. These findings suggest that self-specificity is indeed central in predisposing the neural activity in the various functions. Self-specificity may not be one function among others; that is, cognitive, affective, sensory, motor, and social. Instead, self-specificity may be more basic in the very same way the resting-state activity itself is basic for any stimulus-induced (or task-related) activity and the respectively associated functions, whether cognitive, affective, sensory, motor, or social. The resting-state activity's self-specific organization can thus serve as a template or measure for any subsequent stimulus-induced activity and its assignment of different degrees of self-specificity to the stimuli and their associated functions and tasks. At the same time, however, the resting-state activity's self-specific organization is integrated with the other prephenomenal structures of the resting state. The resting-state activity's self-specific organization is thus linked and integrated to the underlying spatiotemporal continuity (see Chapters 13–15). This leads me to postulate what I describe as the "continuity-based hypothesis of self-specificity." The continuity-based hypothesis of self-specificity asserts self-specificity to be based on the spatial and temporal continuity of the resting state's neural activity: the different stimulus-induced (or task-related) activities in the brain's different regions and networks are "put into the same time and space" of the resting-state activity and its temporal and spatial continuity. In short, stimulus-induced activity becomes "temporalized" and "spatialized." Such "temporalization" and "spatialization" of the neural activity related to self-specificity is supposed to predispose and thus make possible its association with consciousness. At the same time, the resting-state activity's self-specific organization must also be integrated and linked with yet another prephenomenal structure of the resting-state activity, the environment–brain unity and its point of view, as discussed in Chapters 20 and 21. Both environment–brain unity and point of view are associated with the resting-state activity's self-specific organization, which, I postulate, yields what philosophers describe as "self-perspectival organization" postulate on the phenomenal level of consciousness. Self-perspectival organization is a phenomenal concept that can be characterized in a double way by a "virtual" center, a gravitational point, and spatial and temporal trajectories leading to and from the center. I postulate that such double characterization of the self-perspectival organization by a "virtual center" and spatiotemporal trajectories can be traced back to its double origin in both the self-specific organization and the point of view as associated with the environment–brain unity. Since the environment–brain unity is central in constituting the self-perspectival organization on the phenomenal level, I am here suggesting what I refer to as an "unity based hypothesis of self-perspectival organization." The "unity based hypothesis of self-perspectival organization" means that the self-perspectival organization of consciousness, and ultimately the experience of a sense of self, can be traced back to the resting-state activity's environment–brain unity and its point of view.

Key Concepts and Topics Covered

Self-specificity, self-specific organization, resting state, rest–stimulus interaction, functional connectivity, frequency fluctuations, reward, emotions, integration hypothesis, self-perspectival organization

NEUROEMPIRICAL BACKGROUND IA: ASSIGNMENT OF SELF-SPECIFICITY TO SENSORY, AFFECTIVE, COGNITIVE, AND SOCIAL FUNCTIONS

The reader versed in the different branches of neuroscience like cognitive, affective, sensory, motor, or social neuroscience may wonder why, up to this point, I have so far not discussed the neuronal mechanisms of any of these functions and how they are related to consciousness. Instead of revealing the neural substrates of these functions and their stimulus-induced (or task-related) activities, I have focused on the resting-state activity itself and how its neural activity is structured and organized in spatial and temporal terms.

Based on my neurophenomenal approach (see Introduction 2 for definition), I postulated that the resting-state activity's spatial and temporal structure predisposes the various phenomenal features of consciousness like "inner time and space consciousness" (see Chapters 13–17), "phenomenal unity" (see Chapters 18–22), and "self-perspectival organization" (see Chapter 23). How are these neurophenomenal predispositions of the resting-state activity's spatial and temporal organization related to the various cognitive, affective, sensory, motor, and social functions of the brain that are usually associated with consciousness (see first Introduction and Appendix 1 for an overview)? This is the focus in the present chapter.

One such neurophenomenal predisposition is the resting-state activity's self-specificity or self-specific organization, as we discussed in the preceding chapter. Self-specificity describes the organization of the resting-state activity's spatial and temporal measures in orientation to its own organism and its particular needs and demands (see Chapter 23). That, as discussed in Chapter 23, makes possible the assignment of self-specificity to both intero- and exteroceptive stimuli and their respectively associated stimulus-induced activities.

How about the various functions of the brain, like cognitive, sensory, motor, affective, and social functions? Since any extrinsic stimulus and the various associated functions (or tasks—sensory, motor, cognitive, affective, social) must interact with the brain's intrinsic activity, one would postulate them to be also affected by the resting-state activity's self-specific organization. This means that even functions and tasks like reward or decision-making that do not directly target self-specificity itself should nevertheless be affected by and ultimately dependent on it.

Let me be more specific. The various cognitive, affective, social, sensory, and motor functions and their respective stimulus-induced (or task-related) activities all build and depend on the brain's resting-state activity. The respective stimulus or task must (necessarily and unavoidably) interact with the brain's resting-state activity by default in order to elicit activity changes in the brain that can then result in stimulus-induced (or task-related) activity. The associated stimuli or tasks and their related neural activities can consequently not avoid being affected by the resting-state activity's self-specific organization. This entails that the resting-state activity's self-specific organization is imposed upon the stimulus-induced or task-related activity whose associated function or task is therefore assigned some degree of self-specificity.

NEUROEMPIRICAL BACKGROUND IB: MIDLINE REGIONS MEDIATE THE ASSIGNMENT OF SELF-SPECIFICITY TO SENSORY, AFFECTIVE, COGNITIVE, AND SOCIAL FUNCTIONS

How can we support such a daring hypothesis? One may support it on both psychological and neuronal grounds. Psychologically, the various sensory, motor, affective, and cognitive functions should be susceptible to different degrees of self-specificity. For instance, different functions like emotions, reward, or decision making may be associated with different degrees of self-specificity. This is the psychological side of things.

How about the neuronal side? Since high degrees of self-specificity are associated with high degrees of neural activity in the cortical (and subcortical) midline regions (see Chapter 23), one would expect the very same regions to be also active during highly self-specific emotions, reward, or decisions. This is indeed the case, as will be discussed in full detail in the first part of this chapter. I will focus on three particular examples—emotions, decision making, and reward—in order to show how they are all affected by self-specificity and the midline regions' neural activity.

One may now want to argue that I choose, with decision making, reward, and emotions, functions that all are well known to implicate the subcortical and cortical midline regions. The real litmus test would involve the functions that do *not* implicate the midline regions. For instance, higher-order cognitive functions like working memory and attention are associated with the lateral regions in the parietal and the prefrontal cortex. And, most important, these regions, as demonstrated in Chapter 23, have not been associated with self-specificity.

Are higher-order cognitive functions thus spared from and immune to the resting-state activity's self-specific organization and consequently devoid of self-specificity? No: the lateral regions' neural activities are well balanced (reciprocally) against those of the midline regions (and vice versa), as I will discuss in Chapter 25. Due to such neural (reciprocal) balance between midline and lateral regions, even neural activity in the lateral cortex (and thus the regions of the outer ring; see Chapters 4 and 23) cannot avoid being affected by the midline regions (and thus the regions of the inner and middle ring; see Chapters 4 and 23).

How does that stand in relation to cognitive functions like working memory and attention? In addition to their recruitment of regions in lateral prefrontal and parietal cortex, they also induce activity changes in the midline regions which are described as deactivation in fMRI. Stronger degrees of cognitive load in these higher-order cognitive functions induce stronger degrees of deactivation in the midline regions. Such involvement of the midline regions means that

these higher-order cognitive functions also cannot avoid modulating the resting-state activity's self-specific organization and become affected by it themselves. Even the higher-order cognitive functions like working memory or attention are consequently assigned a certain degree of self-specificity, albeit a rather low one (due to the strong deviation from the resting-state activity).

One would thus postulate that higher-order cognitive functions like working memory, episodic memory, attention, etc., are assigned a certain degree of self-specificity, which neuronally may be related to the degree of the midline regions' involvement. To demonstrate this for the various functions is, however, beyond the scope of this chapter (and book), and I therefore leave it for future investigators.

NEUROEMPIRICAL BACKGROUND IIA: NEUROPHENOMENAL FUNCTIONS VERSUS NEUROCOGNITIVE FUNCTIONS

Why is all that relevant for our neurophenomenal account of consciousness? Every function, ranging from sensory over motor and affective to cognitive and social function, and their underlying stimulus-induced or task-related activities can be associated with consciousness. This association with consciousness is made possible, I claim, by particular neuronal mechanisms for which the resting-state activity's spatial and temporal structure is central.

How can we describe the functions of the resting-state activity in conceptual regard? Since the neuronal mechanisms concern the phenomenal features of consciousness, one may want to speak here of "neurophenomenal functions." The concept of "neurophenomenal functions" describes the neuronal mechanisms and functions related to the different phenomenal features of consciousness like "inner time and space consciousness," "phenomenal unity," "self-perspectival organization" and *qualia* (see second Introduction).

How, then, are these neurophenomenal functions related to the other functions of the brain, its neurosensory, neuromotor, neuroaffective, neurocognitive, and neurosocial functions? Most accounts of consciousness in both current neuroscience and philosophy associate consciousness with one of these functions rather than specific neuropheomenal functions. The proponents of for instance higher-order cognitive theories associate consciousness with neurocognitive functions, the social proponents with neurosocial functions, the sensorimotor advocates with neurosensory and neuromotor functions (see first Introduction and Appendix 1 for more details). This seems to entail that the phenomenal features and their underlying neurophenomenal functions are dependent upon the neurocognitive, neuroaffective, or neurosensory functions.

Are the proclaimed neurophenomenal functions thus dependent on the brain's neurocognitive, neuroaffective, or neurosensory functions? I claim for the converse in my neurophenomenal approach to consciousness. Rather than subsuming and subordinating the neurophenomenal functions under the wings of the neurosensory, neuromotor, neuroaffective, neurocognitive, or neurosocial functions of the brain, I consider the neurophenomenal functions to be the necessary condition of the other functions of the brain.

NEUROEMPIRICAL BACKGROUND IIB: NEUROPHENOMENAL FUNCTIONS ARE MORE BASIC AND FUNDAMENTAL THAN NEUROCOGNITIVE FUNCTIONS

Even more radically, I argue that the neurophenomenal functions are the most basic functions of the brain and are thus more basic and fundamental than their neurosensory, neuromotor, neuroaffective, neurocognitive, or neurosocial functions. Metaphorically put, the neurophenomenal functions are considered the "oldest sibling," which provides a blueprint or spatiotemporal template for its younger siblings, the neurosensory, neuroaffective, neurosocial and neurocognitive functions.

Why do I make such a radical claim? There are both phenomenal and neuronal reasons. The phenomenal reason concerns the fact that any function can in principle be associated with consciousness and, to put it more metaphorically, "occurs in the space of consciousness." For instance, any cognitive function presupposes

some kind of spatial and temporal continuity as constituted by "inner time and space consciousness." The same holds for affective functions, with the emotions always being already associated with some degree of spatial and temporal continuity (see Chapter 31 for details on that). This is the phenomenal reason.

How about the neuronal reason? The various functions neurosensory, neuromotor, neuroaffective, neurocognitive, or neurosocial, can be characterized by stimulus-induced or task-related activity. Stimulus-induced or task-related activity can be elicited only on the basis of the brain's resting-state activity. This means that the resting-state activity is more basic and fundamental than the stimulus-induced or task-related activity. There is no stimulus-induced or task-related activity as related to neurosensory, neuroaffective, neurosocial, and neurocognitive functions without the brain's resting state activity.

How is all that related to the neurophenomenal functions? The brain's resting-state activity is characterized by a particular spatial and temporal structure and organization (see Chapters 4–6). Most importantly, I claim that the resting-state activity's spatial and temporal structure predisposes the constitution of the various phenomenal features of consciousness and their association with the otherwise purely neuronal stimulus-induced or task-related activities (see Chapters 13–23). In other words, I associate the proclaimed neurophenomenal functions with the resting-state activity and its particular spatial and temporal structure.

Since resting-state activity is more basic than stimulus-induced or task-related activity, the neurophenomenal functions related to the former must also be more basic than the various functions associated with the latter. I suggest consequently postulate that the brain's neurophenomenal functions are more basic and fundamental than its neurosensory, neuromotor, neuroaffective, neurocognitive, and neurosocial functions.

NEUROEMPIRICAL BACKGROUND IIC: SELF AND CONSCIOUSNESS

This was the easy nut to crack—the association of stimulus-induced or task-related activity and its various functions with neurophenomenal functions and, ultimately, consciousness. Things are much more complicated, though. We thus come to the hard nut that is much more difficult to crack—the association of both consciousness and the various functions with some kind of "self."

What is "the self" and its role? We claim there is some kind of self that performs the different kinds of sensory, motor, social, affective or cognitive functions, or tasks. And even more puzzlingly, we claim such a self to have consciousness. This means that there must be some kind of self at the very bottom that first and foremost makes possible both the occurrence of consciousness and the performance of the various functions and tasks.

However, at the same time, we can access this self only in consciousness. We experience our own self, a "sense of self" (as I will say in the following), in consciousness; this amounts to what is described as *self-consciousness* in philosophy. If, in contrast, we lose our consciousness, we also lose our experience of self. Does this mean that we lose our self altogether? Some authors claim indeed that there is no such thing as the self and that our consciousness only provides us with an illusion of a self that, however, does not exist independently of our experience (see, for instance, Metzinger 2003).

This raises the question of the relationship between self and consciousness: How are *self* and *consciousness* related to each other? I demonstrated in the previous chapter that one central neurophenomenal function of the resting-state activity consists of self-specificity that, I postulated, predisposes the self-perspectival organization on the phenomenal level of consciousness. The second part of this chapter starts from there and focuses on how the resting-state activity's self-specific organization predisposes the experience of a self, a sense of self, as the subject of both consciousness and our performance of the various functions. I thus focus on how the resting state activity's self-specific organization can be associated with consciousness and how that makes possible the experience of a self, a sense of self.

NEURONAL FINDINGS IA: SELF-SPECIFICITY AND EMOTIONS

How does self-specificity permeate the different neurosensory, neuroaffective, and neurocognitive functions in both psychological and neural regard? For that I turn to three paradigmatic examples, emotions, reward, and decision making. Let us start with emotions.

Studies on the relationship between self-specificity and emotions show close linkage between both. One study by Moran et al. (2006) applied a two-by-two factorial interaction design during the judgement of stimuli (e.g., words like "lazy" or "honest" describing personality characteristics) for their emotional valence (positive or negative) and self-specificity (high and low). They showed an interaction between self-specificity and emotional valence in specifically the pregenual and subgenual anterior cingulate cortex (Moran et al. 2006).

The central involvement of these regions was further supported by a recent study of ours (Northoff et al. 2009). To exclude task-related effects like judgments (and to focus on stimulus-related effects related to perception), we let subjects merely perceive emotional pictures (e.g., International Affective Picture System) in the scanner. Afterwards outside the scanner subjects had to judge the emotional arousal (i.e., excited/aroused or not) and valence (i.e., positive or negative) as well as the degree of self-specificity of the same pictures on a visual analogue scale. The results from the subjective ratings were then parametrically correlated with the neural activity changes during the perception of the very same picture.

How are the subjective ratings of self-specificity related to the same pictures' underlying neural activity? The correlation yielded a significant relationship between the neural activity in several subcortical/cortical regions and the pictures' degree of self-specificity. Subcortical regions included tectum, colliculi, amygdala, ventral tegmental area (VTA), mediodorsal thalamus, and ventral striatum (VS), while cortical regions concerned perigenual anterior cingulate cortex (PACC), ventromedial prefrontal cortex (VMPFC), dorsomedial prefrontal cortex (DMPFC), and the posterior cingulate cortex (PCC; see Northoff et al. 2009). The higher the subjects' neural activity in these regions during perception of the emotional pictures, the higher the degree of self-specificity subjects assigned to the very same pictures. There is thus parametric dependence of the degree of self-specificity on the degree of neural activity in these subcortical-cortical midline regions (see Fig. 24-1a).

NEURONAL FINDINGS IB: CORTICAL MIDLINE ACTIVITY MEDIATES SELF-SPECIFICITY IN EMOTIONS

One may now raise the question of whether the parametric dependence of the neural activity in these midline regions is really due to the stimuli's degree of self-specificity or, rather, to their affective-emotional components, that is, emotional arousal and valence. To test for the emotional effects, we also plotted the subjective emotional ratings against the neural activity during the picture perception. This allowed us to directly compare the effects of both self-specificity and emotion dimensions (arousal, valence) on neural activity in the midline regions.

The regions whose neural activity was parametrically dependent on the degree of self-specificity also showed parametric dependence on the emotion dimensions. However, the direction of their correlation was different in cortical and subcortical regions. Cortical regions like the PACC, VMPFC, and DMPFC showed opposite directions in their dependence on self-specificity and arousal/valence. Increased degrees of self-specificity of the stimuli were associated with increased degrees of neural activity in the regions, whereas increased degrees of arousal/valence of the same stimuli led to lower degrees of neural activity in the same regions.

This contrasted with the pattern we obtained in subcortical regions. Subcortical regions like the tectum, the periaqueductal gray, and amygdala did not show such opposite directionality of self-specificity and arousal/valence. Here, both self-specificity and arousal/valence correlated with neural activity in the same direction. This means that increases in all three dimensions lead to increases in the regions' activity level (see Fig. 24-1b).

Taken together, these findings demonstrate the close relationship between emotions and self-specificity in neural activity. This concerned the subcortical and cortical midline regions, whose neural activities, while being implicated in both, are modulated in different ways by self-specificity and emotion dimensions.

NEURONAL FINDINGS IIA: SELF-SPECIFICITY AND REWARD

In addition to emotions, reward has been shown to be closely related to self-specificity, too. Moritz de Greck (de Greck et al. 2008) and Bjoern Enzi (Enzi et al. 2009) from our group conducted a study in which they directly compared rewarding and self-specific tasks using the same stimuli. They applied three different types of stimuli, alcoholic stimuli (bottles of wine, etc.), gambling stimuli (slot machines, etc.), and natural reinforces (food, etc.).

All three types of stimuli were associated with two different tasks. Subjects had to bet and thus gamble for money when they saw the stimuli—this was the reward task. And they had to judge the degree of self-specificity (high or low) of the very same stimuli. This allowed them to investigate what happens during high and low self-specific stimuli in regions recruited during reward.

What are their results? The rewarding stimuli elicited neural activity changes in the typical reward regions, VTA, VS, and VMPFC. Since he (de Greck et al. 2008) let subjects then determine the degree of self-specificity of the same stimuli, that is, the rewarding stimuli, he could see what happens in the reward regions during the processing of high and low self-specific stimuli. High self-specific stimuli elicited high degrees of neural activity in exactly those regions where reward induced strong activity changes, that is, in the VTA, the VS, and the VMPFC (see Fig. 24-1c).

Hence, there is a strong neural overlap between self-specificity and reward in the regions of the reward system that mainly consists

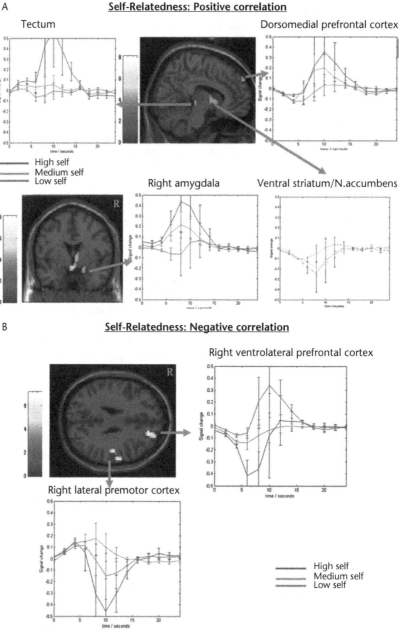

Figure 24-1a Neural activity during self-specificity of emotions. Signal intensities in positively (A) and negatively (B) correlating parametric maps of self-relatedness. The image represents all regional signal intensities that correlate either positively (A) or negatively (B) with the degree of self-relatedness (1–9 on visual analogue scale). Subject-specific partial correlation analysis of self-relatedness was done at $P < 0.001$ uncorrected with extent threshold $k = 10$ voxels. The sagittal images depict the right hemisphere. The curves (x-axis represent time and y-axis signal percent change) demonstrate the BOLD-signals for high (6–9 on visual analogue scale; upper curve), medium (4–6 on visual analogue scale, middle curve), and low (1–3 on visual analogue scale, lower curve) self-relatedness within each region. Reprinted with permission of Wiley Publishing, from Northoff G, Schneider F, Rotte M, Matthiae C, Tempelmann C, Wiebking C, Bermpohl F, Heinzel A, Danos P, Heinze HJ, Bogerts B, Walter M, Panksepp J. Differential parametric modulation of self-relatedness and emotions in different brain regions. *Hum Brain Mapp.* 2009 Feb;30(2):369–82.

X - axis = Degree of rating
Y - axis = Signal intensity
z - axis = Peristimulus time

(A) DMPFC

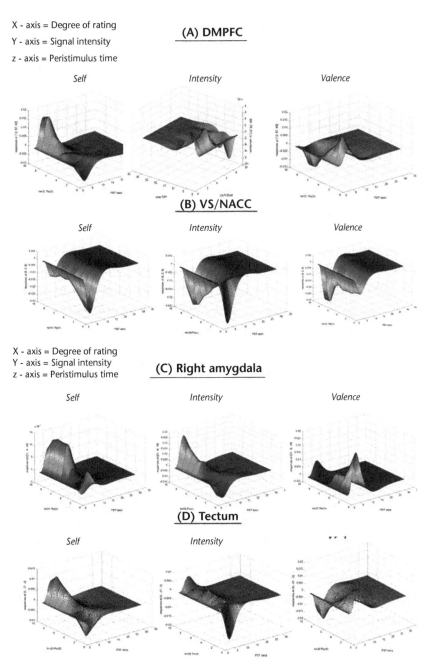

Self　　　*Intensity*　　　*Valence*

(B) VS/NACC

Self　　　*Intensity*　　　*Valence*

X - axis = Degree of rating
Y - axis = Signal intensity
z - axis = Peristimulus time

(C) Right amygdala

Self　　　*Intensity*　　　*Valence*

(D) Tectum

Self　　　*Intensity*

Figure 24-1b Interaction between self-specificity and emotion processing. Three-dimensional representation of parametric correlation of self-relatedness and emotion dimensions with regional signal changes. The figure shows the three-dimensional visualization of parametric correlation of self-relatedness, emotional valence, and emotional intensity with signal changes in different regions (A–E). The x-axis represents the subjective evaluation scores as obtained on the visual-analogue scale ranging from 1 to 9; the y-axis represents the percent signal changes; and the z-axis represents the time in seconds. *Abbreviations*: DMPFC, dorsomedial prefrontal cortex; VLPFC, ventrolateral prefrontal cortex; VS/NACC, ventral striatum/nucleus accumbens. Reprinted with permission of Wiley Publishing from Northoff G, Schneider F, Rotte M, Matthiae C, Tempelmann C, Wiebking C, Bermpohl F, Heinzel A, Danos P, Heinze HJ, Bogerts B, Walter M, Panksepp J Differential parametric modulation of self-relatedness and emotions in different brain regions. *Hum Brain Mapp.* 2009 Feb;30(2):369–82.

X - axis = Degree of rating
Y - axis = Signal intensity
z - axis = Peristimulus time

(E) Right VLPFC

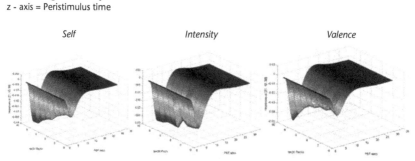

Self   *Intensity*   *Valence*

Figure 24-1b (Continued)

of subcortical-cortical midline regions. The close neural overlap between self-specificity and reward was further confirmed by another group around Ersner-Hersfield (2009). They observed interaction between temporal discounting of reward (i.e., delaying delivery of reward) and self-specificity in the PACC (see also Northoff and Hayes 2011 for a recent review).We also applied our paradigm in alcoholic and gambling patients who, in their clinical behavior, show strongly reduced loss of self-specificity in activities usually strongly related to the self. Although the reward-related activity in the reward regions was (more or less) normal in these patients, their high self-specific signals were completely depleted (see de Greck et al. 2009, 2010).

Most importantly, this suggests that reward- and self-specific-related neural activities can dissociate from each other in the reward system. This also fits well with the observation that these patients clinically lose their sense of self-specificity as manifest in their loss of interest in any formerly personally relevant activities. Taken together, these studies suggest close overlap between reward and self-specificity in the reward system in healthy subjects. Such a neural overlap suggests a close relationship between both self-specificity and reward. However, both functions can also apparently neurally dissociate from each other, as in addictions like alcoholism and gambling. Such neural dissociation between self-specificity and reward suggests that these two functions are not identical and cannot be reduced to each other.

NEURONAL FINDINGS IIB: RESTING-STATE ACTIVITY IN MIDLINE REGIONS MEDIATES SELF-SPECIFICITY IN REWARD

To further confirm the seemingly close overlap between reward and self-specificity, Niall Duncan from our group conducted a meta-analysis on functional imaging studies in humans. He took all studies on self-specificity and compared them with those probing reward (see Duncan et al. 2013). This revealed strong neural overlap between self-specificity and reward in the PACC (extending into the VMPFC) and the PCC, thus including mainly cortical midline structure in the inner ring.

Since these regions also show high resting-state activity, he then investigated the neural overlap between reward-related activity and resting-state activity. This yielded the same regions as described earlier (see Chapter 9 for details). Taken together, these results indicate strong neural overlap between rest, self-specificity, and reward in anterior and posterior midline cortical regions.

How about the neural overlap between self-specificity and resting-state activity in subcortical regions? We did not obtain any neural overlap between self-specificity, reward, and resting state in the subcortical regions. Before assuming that all three may be processed independent and parallel in subcortical regions, we may need to consider a methodological issue. The studies on self-specificity and the ones on resting-state activity usually focus almost exclusively on cortical regions. There are consequently

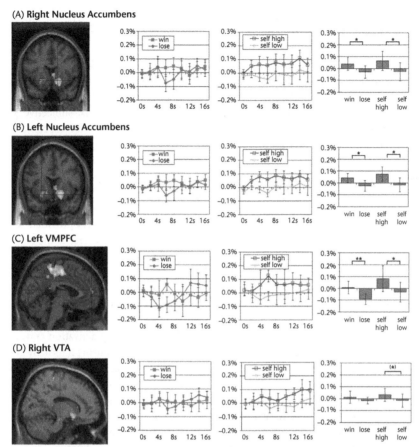

Figure 24-1c Neural activity during self-specificity in reward circuitry. Activation in reward regions during win, lose, high self, and low self events. The second-level group statistic for the contrast reward win > reward lose revealed activations in the right and left nucleus accumbens, the left ventromedial prefrontal cortex (VMPFC), and the ventral tegmental area (VTA). The left picture of each line shows the t contrast calculated with SPM2. The two diagrams in the middle of each line show the mean normalized fMRI signal changes (y-axis) for the conditions gambling win, gambling lose, high self, and low self (error bar: standard deviation) with $t = 0$ for the start of the feedback phase. The box diagram on the right pictures the mean normalized fMRI values (y-axis) for the time points 4–8 s. (A) Right nucleus accumbens (16, 14, −8). We found a higher mean fMRI signal for reward win compared with reward lose ($t(14) = 3.092$; $p = 0.008$) and a higher mean fMRI signal for high self events compared with low self events ($t(14) = 2.664$; $p = 0.019$). (B) Left nucleus accumbens (−24, 12, −12). We found greater mean fMRI signals for reward win compared with reward lose ($t(14) = 3.449$; $p = 0.004$) and for high self compared with low self events ($t(14) = 3.770$; $p = 0.002$). (C) Left VMPFC (−2, 54, 14). Reward win events compared with reward lose events caused highly significant greater fMRI signal ($t(14) = 5.320$; $p < 0.001$). The comparison of high self with low self events was significant, too ($t(14) = 2.724$; $p = 0.016$). (D) Right VTA (14, −18, −16). The contrast of reward win and reward lose failed significance ($t(14) = 1.669$; $p < 0.112$). The comparison of high self with low self events revealed a statistical trend (t(14) = 1.941; $p = 0.073$) for a higher mean fMRI signal during high self events. Abbreviations: VTA = ventral tegmental area, VMPFC = ventromedial prefrontal cortex, $^*p < 0.05$, $(^*)p < 0.1$. Reprinted with permission of Elsevier, from de Greck M, Rotte M, Paus R, Moritz D, Thiemann R, Proesch U, Bruer U, Moerth S, Tempelmann C, Bogerts B, Northoff G. Is our self based on reward? Self-relatedness recruits neural activity in the reward system. *Neuroimage.* 2008 Feb 15;39(4):2066–75.

rather sparse data if at all on subcortical regions in self-specificity and resting state. That makes a meta-analysis impossible. Moreover, it has to be said that the subcortical regions are rather difficult to scan in fMRI in a proper way, which may contribute to the lack of subcortical data on self-specificity. Hence, the absence of neural overlap between self, rest, and reward in subcortical regions may simply be due to the lack of available data.

Taken together, these findings suggest that the effect of self-specificity on reward and their associated overlap in subcortical and cortical midline regions can be mediated by the resting-state activity in the same regions. If this is so, one would expect the resting-state activity in these regions to predict the degree of reward-related activity in the same regions, which is indeed supported by recent data (see Chapter 9 for details; Duncan et al. 2013).

NEURONAL FINDINGS IIIA: SELF-SPECIFICITY AND DECISION MAKING

I demonstrated a close relationship of self-specificity with both emotions and reward. Interestingly, in both cases neural activity in the cortical midline structures was of central relevance in mediating their relationship. I now want to give a third example of how self-specificity may be implicated in other functions and modulate their underlying neural activity. For that, I turn to decision making.

When we make a decision, we usually rely on the external cues as provided by the situation and the context. We always search for those cues in our external environment to guide and help us. If, for instance, we are confronted with the alternative between right and left mouse buttons, we may look for cues that possibly indicate a higher gain in terms of, for instance, money associated with either button. But what if those external cues remain completely absent? In that case, no external cue can guide our decision making anymore. Instead, we have to rely on internal cues, the cues provided by the person itself and its internal criteria to make the decision.

This is where my former Japanese postdoctoral student Takashi Nakao, who is now Professor in Hiroshima/Japan, enters the picture. He is particularly interested in those situations when there is no external cue to guide our decisions. That is, for instance, the case in moral decision making. Moral judgments rely strongly on our internal criteria and thus what one subjectively prefers, that is, subjective preference, within a given specific cultural context.

Nakao and colleagues (2012a and b) consequently distinguish between internally and externally guided decision making. Internally guided decision making describes that we have to more strongly rely on our own internal criteria than on external criteria provided by the environment, while the reverse is the case in extrinsically guided decision making, where external criteria predominate. What does this imply for the neuronal level? Internal criteria are closely related to the person and its self and should thus show a high degree of self-specificity. If so, one would expect strong activation and recruitment of midline regions during internally guided decision making. Lateral cortical regions, in contrast, should be more strongly recruited during externally guided decision making.

To test this assumption, Nakao conducted a meta-analysis comparing studies on decision making that rely on external cues (with high or low predictability of the subsequent gain), e.g., externally guided with those where no external cues were presented (e.g., mostly studies on moral judgment), e.g., internally guided (see Nakao et al. 2012). Interestingly, externally guided decision making studies yielded significantly stronger activity changes in lateral frontal and parietal regions. In contrast, internally guided decision-making studies yielded significantly stronger activity changes in the midline regions, including PACC, VMPFC, DMPFC, PCC, and precuneus (see Fig. 24-1d).

What do these data tell us? These data strongly support the distinction between internally and externally guided decision making on a neural level. Even more important, in the present context, they lend evidence to the postulated involvement of self-specificity and midline regions in decision making. Since self-specificity overlaps strongly with the high resting-state activity in the midline regions (see Chapter 23), one may raise the question of how their involvement in internally guided decision making is affected by their resting-state activity.

NEURONAL FINDINGS

IIIB: RESTING-STATE ACTIVITY MEDIATES SELF-SPECIFICITY IN DECISION MAKING

Nakao and his colleagues (2013) tested this in an electroencephalographic (EEG) study where he compared internally versus externally guided decision-making with regard to the same stimuli, words indicating different professional occupations. The words were presented in different frequencies, and subjects had to judge which of the two presented words was presented more often. They could thus rely on external criteria for their decision making; namely, the frequency of the words.

How about the reliance on internal criteria in our experimental design? Now the same words were presented again to the subjects; however, rather than judging their frequency, subjects had to decide which profession indicated by the two words they preferred. Here, they could thus rely only on internal rather than external criteria, thus indicating internally guided decision making. During both kinds of decision making, internally and externally guided, electrophysiological activity was recorded using EEG.

More specifically, Nakao and colleagues focused on a task-related electrophysiological potential like the N200, which has been well known to be associated with decision making. In addition, they recorded electrophysiological activity during the resting state in eyes closed and eyes open (5 minutes each). This allowed them to directly relate electrophysiological task-related measures, the N200, to the strength of neural activity in the resting state as measured by the power of the various frequency bands.

How are externally and internally guided decisions related to the resting-state activity? Both internally and externally guided decision

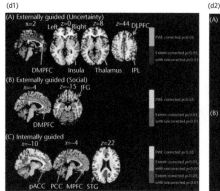
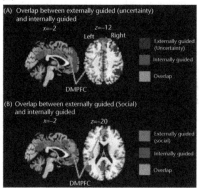

Figure 24-1d Comparison between internally and externally guided decision making. (*d*1) Multi-level kernel density analysis results for (A) externally guided decision making under uncertainty, (B) externally guided decision making in a social situation, and (C) internally guided decision making. Results from the different statistical thresholds are shown, a height threshold of familywise errorrate (FWE) corrected at $p < 0.05$;, a stringent threshold of FEW corrected for the spatial extent at $p < 0.05$ with primary thresholds of uncorrected $p < 0.001$;, a medium threshold of FEW corrected for the spatial extent at $p < 0.05$ with primary thresholds of uncorrected $p < 0.01$. No clusters were identified at the stringent threshold in externally guided decision making under uncertainty or in a social situation. *Abbreviations:* DMPFC, dorsomedial prefrontal cortex; DLPFC, dorsolateral prefrontal cortex; IPL, inferior parietal lobule; IFG, inferior frontal gyrus; pACC, perigenual anterior cingulate cortex; PCC, posterior cingulate cortex; MPFC, medial prefrontal cortex; STG, superior temporal gyrus. (*d*2) Multi-level kernel density analysis results for overlaps (A) between externally guided decision making under uncertainty and internally guided decision making and (B) between externally guided decision making in a social situation and internally guided decision making.

making induced the typical task-related potential, the N200, with no major differences between both conditions; that is, internally and externally guided decisions. How, then, is the task-related N200 potential related to the resting-state activity? This is where internally and externally guided decision making diverged. Nakao showed that the task-related potentials like the N200 during only internally, but not externally, guided decision making were related (that is they correlated) to the degree of resting-state activity as measured separately during eyes closed. The higher the power of delta, theta, and alpha frequency fluctuations in the resting state (during eyes closed), the stronger the N200 potentials that were elicited during internally guided decision making. In contrast, no such correlation was observed during externally guided decision making that was thus not predicted by the degree of power in the resting state.

This is even more interesting given that both internally and externally guided response trials concerned the same stimuli (though in different combinations) and elicited the same degree of N200. That makes it rather likely that the same output of electrophysiological and behavioral parameters, the N200 and the decision itself, was much more impacted by the resting state activity in the case of internally guided decisions, while this was apparently not the case in externally guided response trials where subjects had other resources to rely on, e.g., the stimulus itself and the external criteria it provided.

Taken together, these results do not only show the involvement of self-specificity and midline regions in decision making but also the relevance of the resting-state activity in especially internally guided decision making. Furthermore, the data suggest that the effect of self-specificity on decision making is mediated by the midline regions and their resting-state activity.

Neuroempirical Background III: Self-Specificity and Other Functions

How can we explain these data that show the effects of both self-specificity and midline activity

on emotions, reward, and decision making? In order to explain these data, we must presuppose a certain relationship between self-specificity and the different functions like reward, emotion, and decision making.

What do these results tell us about self-specificity and its relationship to the other functions? We observed considerable neural and behavioral overlap of self-specificity with other functions like emotions, reward, and decision making in especially midline regions. Although this needs to be expanded to other affective, cognitive, sensory, social, and motor functions in the future, it nevertheless raises some important questions that can be "located" at the boundary or interface between empirical and theoretical issues. These shall be discussed in the following.

How is self-specificity related to other functions? I here suggest four different possible models, the "top model," the "subsumption model," the "independence model," and the "basis model." These shall be explained in the following section with regard to self-specificity in particular as one example of a neurophenomenal function. This implies the more general question of how neurophenomenal functions (see the beginning of this chapter) stand in relation to sensory, motor, cognitive, affective, and social functions.

Neuronal Hypothesis IA: Self-Specificity as Cognitive Function—"Top Model"

Let me start with the first model, the "top model." Self-specificity is often determined as the output of all functions when they finally become related to one's own self. This presupposes self-reference and self-representation, which require higher-order cognitive functions (see Churchland 2002, Legrand and Ruby 2009). Taken in this sense, self-specificity would follow the various other functions and would therefore be, metaphorically speaking, their "highest cognitive pinnacle." Self-specificity would then stand at the top of all functions, being the highest in the hierarchy. This entails what I refer to as the "top model" (taken in both literal and figurative senses!) (see Fig 24-2a).

Let me detail the characterization of self-specificity as a cognitive function. Self-specificity is often considered a cognitive function since it allows the individual to represent stimuli as being related to one's own organism and its self. That is supposed to require representation and meta-representation of the respective stimuli as such, and such meta-representation is usually associated with higher-order cognitive functions (see, for instance, van den Meer et al. 2010 for such interpretation). Since it refers the stimuli to the self that is presupposed or taken as

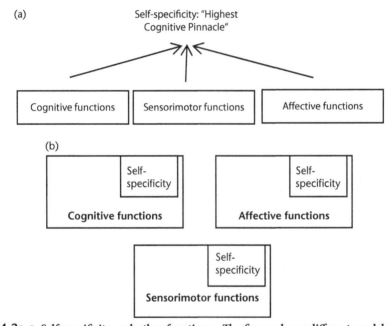

Figure 24-2a-e Self-specificity and other functions. The figure shows different models in the relationship between self-specificity and other functions (affective, sensorimotor, cognitive, and others not mentioned here). (*a*) In the "top model," self-specificity is regarded as a top function that results from the integration of cognitive, affective, and sensorimotor functions. Self-specificity is regarded as the highest and thus top form of integration between different stimuli and functions and thus as "highest cognitive pinnacle." (*b*) In the "subsumption model" self-specificity is regarded as a specific instance of either a cognitive, affective, or sensorimotor (or social) function. Self-specificity is then regarded by itself as a cognitive, affective, or sensorimotor function. (*c*) In the "independence model" self-specificity is regarded as an independent function by itself that stands side by side with affective, cognitive, and sensorimotor functions. As such, self-specificity remains essentially independent of these other functions, though of course interactions are possible (which, for sake of simplicity, are not indicated here due to the absence of arrows between the different functions). (*d*) In the "basis model," self-specificity is regarded as a basic function that as such is closely aligned to the resting-state activity. Analogous to the resting-state activity that provides the basis for any stimulus-induced activity, self-specificity is proposed to provide the very basis for any other function, whether cognitive, affective, social, or sensorimotor by interacting with the resting state activity and its self-specific organization, these functions are associated with a particular degree of self-specificity. (*e*) The figure shows how the midline regions' self-specific organization (lower part) predisposes and thus makes possible the assignment of self-specificity to the stimuli, tasks or functions (upper part). The degree of self-specificity that can possibly be assigned to the stimuli, tasks, or functions is supposed to be mediated by the degree of deviation from the midline regions' resting-state activity level. The more the midline neural activity deviates from their resting-state activity level, the more neural activity changes will be elicited by the respective stimulus, task, or function in their stimulus- or task-related regions (left graph) and the lower the degree of self-specificity that can possibly be assigned to the respective stimulus, task, or function (right graph).

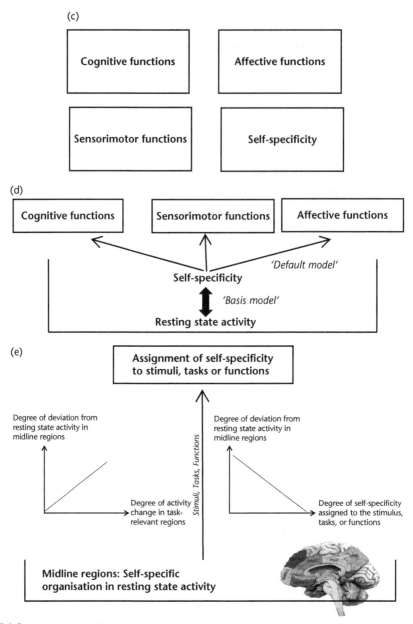

Figure 24-2a-e (Continued)

a given, one may speak here of *self-reference* or *self-referential processing* (Northoff 2007).

Such higher-order cognitive meta-representational characterization of self-reference must be distinguished from the more basic noncognitive sense of self-specificity as supposed here, where no such self or representation or meta-representation are presupposed (see Appendix 4 for a more detailed discussion of this point). Instead of being determined in a representational or meta-representational and thus cognitive way as "self-reference," I postulate self-specificity to signify the more basic and fundamental relationship of the stimuli from environment and body to the brain.

NEURONAL HYPOTHESIS IB: *SELF-SPECIFICITY* AND THE ENVIRONMENT–BRAIN RELATIONSHIP ARE MORE BASIC AND FUNDAMENTAL THAN *SELF-REFERENCE* AND REPRESENTATION

Let us explicate that in further detail. Self-specificity concerns the environment–brain relationship by itself, and is therefore neither representational nor cognitive. Self-reference, in contrast, tacitly presupposes that very same environment–brain relationship and take it for granted when claiming for representation and meta-representation of stimuli/tasks.

But what exactly is being represented or meta-represented? It is not the stimulus or task alone, independent of brain and body, that is represented or meta-represented. Instead, it is the relationship of the stimulus or task to both the body and the brain's intrinsic activity that is represented and meta-represented. What is represented and meta-represented is thus the environment–brain relationship (and body-brain relationship) the stimulus or task triggers and induces. Most importantly, that environment–brain relationship can show different degrees which are manifest in what I described as self-specificity. Accordingly, what is represented and meta-represented, the environment–brain relation, comes already by itself with a certain degree of self-specificity.

Can the stimulus or task be represented without and thus independent of the environment–brain relation? No! The stimulus or task could then not enter the brain which is only possible through the environment–brain relationship as the entrance gate. If however nothing enters the brain, there is nothing that can be represented and meta-represented. Accordingly, representation and meta-representation of stimuli or tasks necessarily presuppose the environment–brain relationship. Without such an environment–brain relationship and its associated degree of self-specificity, there would be nothing to represent or meta-represent anymore. The representation would thus remain "empty" and therefore impossible.

This has major implications for the relationship between self-specificity and self-reference. Only if stimuli are designated as self-specific can they be represented as such and yield what is described as self-reference. What though do I mean by the concept of "self-reference" and how do I distinguish it from self-specificity? Empirically, self-reference presupposes what has been described as self-referential processing in current *Cognitive Neuroscience*. Self-referential processing is usually tested for by letting subjects evaluate how much the stimuli are important, relevant or related to the own person (see Appendix 4 for details). As such, self-referential processing and thus self-reference is closely related to stimulus-induced activity and the related cognitive functions.

Self-referential processing, however, needs to be distinguished from self-specific processing. Self-specific processing is more related to the resting state, how the stimulus matches and compares to the actual resting state activity, prior to and before it induces stimulus-induced activity and the related cognitive functions. This implies that self-specific processing and consequently self-specificity are more basic and must occur prior to any subsequent self-referential processing.

Taken together, the cognitive characterization of self-specificity in terms of self-reference and representation/meta-representation must presuppose self-specificity and its associated environment–brain relationship. Without self-specificity, self-reference remains impossible, which argues against the characterization of the former in terms of the latter. To subsume self-specificity under cognitive functions and thus to opt for the top model would be to neglect the basic presupposition, the environment–brain relationship and its generation of self-specificity. Metaphorically speaking, to opt for the top model would be to reach out to the ceiling while at the same time eroding or eliminating the bottom or ground on which one stands.

NEURONAL HYPOTHESIS IC: SELF-SPECIFICITY AS AFFECTIVE OR SENSORIMOTOR FUNCTION—"SUBSUMPTION MODEL"

How about an affective rather than cognitive determination of self-specificity? Self-specificity has indeed been associated with affective functions. Emotional feelings are here postulated to be the first and most basic manifestation of self-specificity, by, for instance, Jaak Panksepp (Panksepp 1998a and b, 2011). He postulates emotions in general and emotional feelings in particular to be possible only on the basis of involving a basic version of the self, thus implying self-specificity (see Chapter 31 for more details of such "affective self"). This means that emotional feelings, the subjective experience of emotions, are assumed to always already implicate some degree of self-specificity, since otherwise the experience itself, the emotional feeling, would remain impossible.

In addition to emotions and affects, self-specificity has also been related to sensorimotor functions that postulate self-specificity to be based on perception and motor action and thus ultimately on one's own body (see Christoff et al. 2011; Legrand and Ruby 2009). Hence, the cognitive or characterization of self-specificity is here replaced by its association with sensorimotor functions that signify the body (see Appendix 4 for a more extensive discussion). What do these different characterizations of self-specificity as cognitive, affective, and sensorimotor have in common? Despite their differences, all characterizations of self-specificity, cognitive, affective, and sensorimotor function, share their association with a specific function. Self-specificity is thus subsumed under the umbrella of the respective function and considered one particular manifestation of the function in question. I therefore speak of what I describe as the subsumption model of self-specificity (see Fig. 24-2b).

How about the neuronal mechanisms of self-specificity in such a "subsumption model"? Neuronally, one would expect self-specificity to be processed in the same neural networks that mediate the respective functions. Different degrees of neural activity within the respective cognitive, affective, or sensorimotor neural networks would then be postulated to signify different degrees of self-specificity.

This raises the question of the modulation of the degree of neural activity in the neural networks related to the different functions. What modulates the degree of neural activity and its dependence on self-specificity in sensorimotor, cognitive, affective, and social networks of the brain? The earlier-described data suggest that the resting-state activity may be central here, and most likely its associated degree of self-specificity as well. That means, however, that self-specificity cannot be subsumed under the sensory, motor, affective, cognitive, or social functions in the same way that stimulus-induced activity cannot be subsumed under resting-state activity. The subsumption model thus comes to its limits here. This entails the need for a different model to describe the relationship between self-specificity and other functions.

NEURONAL HYPOTHESIS ID: SELF-SPECIFICITY AS INDEPENDENT FUNCTION—"INDEPENDENCE MODEL"

The subsumption of self-specificity under a particular function must be distinguished from another view. In this view, self-specificity is no longer subsumed under the umbrella of another function but is rather regarded a separate and independent function by itself, e.g., in its own right. Rather than being subsumed under another specific function, self-specificity is now postulated to be separate and independent, standing parallel to the other functions. I therefore speak of an "independence model" that postulates self-specificity to be a separate function in its own right as distinguished from affective, cognitive, and sensorimotor functions (see Fig. 24-2c).

How can we further specify the independence model? Self-specificity is here postulated to remain independent of affective, cognitive, and sensorimotor functions. Self-specificity is then considered an independent function, entailing its own specific psychological and neuronal mechanisms. One would therefore no longer expect the cognitive, affective, or sensorimotor networks to be implicated in self-specificity as suggested in the case of the "subsumption model." Instead, one would postulate self-specificity to be processed in a separate and distinct neural network for which the midline regions have often been regarded a viable neural candidate.

NEURONAL HYPOTHESIS IE: RESTING-STATE ACTIVITY AND SELF-SPECIFICITY ARE "EVERYWHERE AND NOWHERE" IN THE BRAIN AND ITS VARIOUS FUNCTIONS

However, as discussed in Chapter 23, the midline regions cannot be considered specific for the neural processing of self-specificity in this sense; that is, as separate and distinct function. Many other functions, like mind reading, emotion, moral judgement, etc., have been demonstrated to implicate the midline regions (see Legrand and Ruby 2009; Gillihan and Farah 2005; Amodo and Frith 2006; see Chapter 23 herein for details). This makes it clear that the midline regions cannot be regarded a network that is specifically and exclusively associated with self-specificity while not being implicated in any other function. That means, however, that self-specificity itself may not be regarded as an independent function that exists alongside other functions like sensory, motor, cognitive, affective, and social functions.

In addition, our data (see above as well as deGreck et al. 2008; Nakaso et al. 2013; Northoff et al. 2009) show that the resting-state activity in the midline regions seems to be central in mediating the impact of self-specificity on reward and decision making (and possibly also on emotions). This suggests the association of self-specificity with the resting-state activity, as we discussed it in the previous chapter in full detail (see Chapter 23). Since the resting-state activity impacts any subsequent stimulus-induced or task-related activity, self-specificity as associated with the former impacts any other functions by default and can therefore not be regarded as an independent function that stands side by side with the other functions.

In the same way that the resting-state activity does not stand side by side with the different forms of stimulus-induced activity, self-specificity as associated with the former cannot be considered to stand side by side with the other functions, either. Instead, very much like the brain's resting-state activity, self-specificity and its midline involvement seem to be "everywhere and nowhere" in both the brain and its various functions. This implies that self-specificity may be a more basic function that requires a model different from both the subsumption and the independence model.

NEURONAL HYPOTHESIS IIA: SELF-SPECIFICITY AS THE "COMMON GROUND" OF ALL FUNCTIONS—"BASIS MODEL"

What can we learn from the other models: the top model, the subsumption model, and the independence model? All three models point to a more basic role for self-specificity than for sensory, motor, cognitive, affective, and social functions. This more basic role seems to be neuronally mediated by the resting-state activity and its alleged self-specific organization, as discussed in the previous chapter. Such resting-state activity must be distinguished from the stimulus-induced or task-related functions associated with the sensory, motor, affective, cognitive, and social functions.

What does this imply for the relationship between self-specificity and the other functions? Self-specificity seems to be a more basic function compared to the other functions in the same way that the brain's resting-state activity is more basic than its stimulus-induced activity. One may consequently opt for what can be described as the "basis model," where self-specificity provides the basis or "common ground" for the various sensory, motor, affective, cognitive, and social functions (see Fig. 24-2d).

The earlier-described data on self and reward, emotion, and decision making (see above) provide the first tentative evidence for such a "basis model." They show that self-specificity permeates functions as diverse as emotions, reward, and decision making. And they demonstrate that the impact of self-specificity is mediated by the resting-state activity in especially the midline regions and its resting state activity. This in turn impacts the subsequent stimulus-induced or task-related activity in the midline and other regions and its association with the different neurosensory, neuroaffective, and neurocognitive functions.

Taken together, this strongly suggests that self-specificity and its underlying neuronal mechanisms, the resting-state activity's self-specific organization (see Chapter 23), perform a basic function of the brain compared to its other functions. This is what I mean by the "basis model," which aims to describe the relationship of self-specificity (and other phenomenal functions) to the neurosensory, neuromotor, neuroaffective, and neurocognitive functions of the brain.

NEURONAL HYPOTHESIS IIB: ASSIGNMENT OF SELF-SPECIFICITY TO STIMULI, FUNCTIONS, AND TASKS—"DEFAULT MODEL" AS THE SIBLING OF THE "BASIS MODEL"

How is self-specificity as a basic function neuronally mediated? This is the question concerning the neuronal mechanisms by means of which self-specificity as the basic function can impact all other functions. We recall from Chapters 4 and 5 in Volume I the distinction between *task-positive* and *task-negative networks*.

Task-positive networks are those wherein tasks and their associated sensory, motor, affective, cognitive, or social functions induce positive signal changes in fMRI. These include mainly the lateral prefrontal and parietal cortex as well as (in a more extended sense) the sensory cortex (and thus regions of the outer ring; see Chapters 4 and 23). In contrast, task-negative regions are regions mainly in the midline of the brain (including the inner and middle ring; see Chapters 4 and 23) wherein predominantly negative signal changes are induced by sensory, motor, affective, cognitive, or social tasks (see left graph in Fig. 24-2e).

Strong cognitive tasks (like working memory, attention, etc.) induce not only positive signal changes in the lateral prefrontal cortex, but, at the same time, negative signal changes—that is, deactivation—in the midline regions (see Shulman et al. 1997; Raichle et al. 2001; see Chapters 4 and 23 for details). At the same time, we discussed in Chapter 23 various findings that strongly suggest the degree of deviation from the resting-state activity level in the midline regions to be associated with different degrees of self-specificity. The more the stimulus-induced or task-related activity in midline regions deviates from the resting-state activity level, the lower the degree of self-specificity that is assigned to the respective stimulus or task. Conversely, lower degrees of deviation from the resting-state activity level accompany the assignment of higher degrees of self-specificity to the respective stimuli or tasks (see Fig. 24-2e, right graph).

By interacting with the midline regions' resting-state activity and its self-specific organization, the stimuli or tasks and their respectively associated functions are assigned a certain degree of self-specificity. If, for instance, the task requires a high cognitive load, there will be a high degree of deactivation in the midline regions that then will strongly deviate from their resting-state activity level. A rather low degree of self-specificity will consequently be assigned to the respective stimulus, task, or function. If, in contrast, the stimulus, task, or function induces only a low degree of deviation from the midline's resting-state activity level, they will be assigned a high degree of self-specificity (see Fig. 24-2e, upper part). This makes it clear that any stimulus, task, or function cannot avoid being assigned some degree of self-specificity, whether low or high. In the same way that any stimulus-induced or task-related activity has to "go through" and interact with the brain's resting-state activity, including the one in the midline regions, no function or task can avoid interacting with (and thus being "confounded by," if one wants to say so) the self-specificity as associated with the resting-state activity's self-specific organization.

Taken together, the "basis model" of self-specificity and its potentially underlying neuronal mechanisms postulate that the various neurosensory, neuromotor, neuroaffective, neurocognitive, and neurosocial functions cannot avoid being assigned some degree of self-specificity, whether low or high. This means that self-specificity is assigned to the various functions by default and thus in a necessary or unavoidable way. One may therefore describe this as the "default model" of self-specificity, which can be considered the sibling or the *Yang* of the "basis model" as the *Yin*.

NEUROPHENOMENAL BACKGROUND IA: ASSOCIATION OF SELF-SPECIFICITY WITH CONSCIOUSNESS AS THE *"EASY"* NUT TO CRACK

Where are we now? We have so far investigated how self-specificity permeates all other functions, including sensory, motor, affective, cognitive, and social functions, in a necessary and unavoidable way and thus by default. This was expressed in what I described as the "basis model" and the "default model." This, however, leaves two issues open. Let us start with the first issue.

The first issue pertains to the association of self-specificity with consciousness. Our account so far has shown only how self-specificity permeates and is associated with neurosensory, neuromotor, neurocognitive, neuroaffective, and neurosocial functions. Nothing in our account, however, implied anything about how and why the various more-or-less self-specific functions are associated with consciousness and its various phenomenal features.

In other words, we are looking for the neuronal mechanisms that make necessary and unavoidable the association of the various functions, whether low or high, self-specific with consciousness. How is such self-specificity as a basic function of the brain's resting-state activity associated with consciousness, and what are the neuronal mechanisms underlying such association? This is an easy nut to crack when compared to what else needs to be addressed.

I postulate that the midline regions and the self-specific organization of their neural activity must be linked to and integrated with the spatiotemporal structure of the resting-state activity of the whole brain. This will make it possible for the self-specific organization to be related to the spatial and temporal continuity and unity of the neural activity in the resting state, as discussed in the Parts V and VI.

One would consequently expect self-specificity to interact with the respectively underlying neuronal mechanisms like the low-frequency fluctuations and functional connectivity. This will be the focus of the neuronal findings in the next sections. That, however, is only the easy nut to crack. There is a much harder nut to crack, which shall be briefly described before going on.

NEUROPHENOMENAL BACKGROUND IB: ASSOCIATION OF SELF-SPECIFICITY WITH A SELF AS THE *FIRST* HALF OF THE *"HARD"* NUT TO CRACK

We have so far addressed only half of the puzzle. In addition to the association of self-specificity with consciousness, we need to investigate how self-specificity is associated with a self, and how that in turn is linked to consciousness. This raises the question of the relationship between self-specificity, self, and consciousness. That is a much more difficult question to answer, since it digs deeply into conceptual issues that have been discussed rather contentiously throughout the history of philosophy.

How are *self-specificity*, *self*, and *consciousness* related to each other? Like every nut, this rather "hard" nut consists of two halves. The first half is the question of the relationship between self-specificity and self (see later for the second half of the nut): How can self-specificity be associated with a self?

Obviously, there has been much discussion about whether a self exists at all, in both philosophy and neuroscience. If, like some philosophers (Metzinger 2003), one assumes that no such thing as a self exists, this half of the nut can be thrown into the trash can of illusory philosophical ideas. Others in current philosophy, though, claim the existence of some kind of self (see, e.g., Strawson 2009; and Dainton 2008). Further complicating things is that, especially in current neuroscience, the terms *self-specificity* and *self* are often not clearly distinguished from each other.

In neuroscience, the observation of high degrees of self-specificity is often taken to indicate the presence of some kind of self. We have to be careful, however. The concept of self-specificity (and also the one of self-reference) is an operational term that signifies stimuli, tasks, or functions in their relationship to the organism and its supposed self (see also Northoff et al. 2006, 2010;

and Northoff 2007, for further discussion of the concept of self-specificity).

Self-specificity in this sense implies something about the stimuli, tasks, or functions and how close or distant they are to the self. In contrast, it does not imply anything about the nature, existence, or experience of the self itself (see Appendix 4 for more discussion of the concept of self). Accordingly, we cannot make the direct inference from self-specificity itself to "the self." This means that we need to recruit other resources to better understand how self-specificity can be associated with a self, a sense of self, and thus a self in a phenomenal or experiential sense, as I will argue.

NEUROPHENOMENAL BACKGROUND IC: ASSOCIATION OF THE SELF WITH CONSCIOUSNESS AS THE *SECOND* HALF OF THE *"HARD"* NUT TO CRACK

This leads me to the second half of the "hard" nut to crack. The first half of the "hard" nut led us from self-specificity to self. However, such a self can be experienced in consciousness and must therefore somehow be associated with consciousness. This is the second half of the "hard" nut, which leads us into the debate about the relationship between self and consciousness.

There has been much discussion about how *self* and *consciousness* are related to each other, throughout the history of philosophy and more recently also in neuroscience. I do not aim to recount these debates and enter into the conceptual complexities of the relationship between self and consciousness. This deserves a book of its own. Instead, I will here only highlight some basics that I consider necessary to understanding the neuronal mechanisms that I will postulate to underlie the relationship between self and consciousness.

There has been a long discussion in philosophy about the relationship between self and consciousness. Past philosophers such as Rene Descartes and Immanuel Kant (though in different ways) argued for the need of a self in order to have consciousness. Following them, consciousness remains impossible without a self

that, according to their accounts, provides the basic subjectivity as the hallmark of consciousness. More present-day philosophers, such as Dan Zahavi (2005), Barry Dainton (2008), and Galen Strawson (2009), also point out the need to postulate some kind of self as the core of consciousness.

From the neuroscientific side, authors like Antonio Damasio and Jaak Panksepp have argued for the need to consider the self in consciousness (Damasio 1999a and b, 2010; Parvizi and Damasio 2001; Panksepp 1998a and b; Northoff and Panksepp 2008; Panksepp and Northoff 2009). They suggest a subcortically based "proto-self" (see below for further characterization of such a "proto-self," as well as Chapter 31) that enables the homeostatic regulation of the organism within its various environmental contexts. As can already been seen by the reference to homeostatic regulation, such a "proto-self" is closely associated with the body and is therefore often considered the "body self."

While not yet being fully conscious by itself, such a "proto-self" is nevertheless considered necessary to generate and yield consciousness, "core consciousness," as Damasio (1999a and b, 2010) says. By seemingly "driving" consciousness, the self becomes an integral part of our consciousness. That, however, leaves open the question of what exact neural mechanisms allow us and our brain to link and integrate self and consciousness. I postulate that those neuronal mechanisms can be found again in the resting-state activity itself and, more specifically, in the interaction between its different spatial and temporal structures.

NEUROPHENOMENAL BACKGROUND ID: FROM THE *"HARD"* NUT TO CRACK OVER THE BODY BACK TO THE BRAIN AND ITS INTRINSIC ACTIVITY

There is much recent literature in neuroscience about the consciousness of one's own body as "body self-consciousness" which is supposed to be also manifested in agency and ownership of the body (see, e.g., Blanke 2012 for a recent review, as well de Vignemont 2011; and Longo et al. 2010). While discussing the role of the body and especially of interoceptive awareness later (in Chapter 32), we here do not follow this literature. Instead, we argue that we aim to tap into neuronal mechanisms that are prior to and thus precede the constitution of one's own body as "content" in consciousness.

While admittedly the body is central in physiologically and metabolically constituting the self and ultimately consciousness, from the "perspective of the brain" (metaphorically speaking), the body is ultimately just one aspect of the brain's environment. In the same way that the brain's resting state matches its own neural activity with the spatial and temporal differences of the exteroceptive stimuli from the environment, I postulate that it does essentially the same with regard to the interoceptive stimuli from the body.

This means that both intero- and exteroceptive stimuli are assigned self-specificity, albeit in different degrees, as discussed in Chapter 23. I consequently postulate that there is no principal difference between intero- and exteroceptive stimuli and thus between body and environment from "the perspective of the brain" and its resting-state activity as signified by a particular spatiotemporal organization in the sense of a self-specific organization.

I postulate that both intero- and exteroceptive stimuli encounter the brain's intrinsic activity and its various processes and interactions. In order to understand how the intero- and exteroceptive stimuli and ultimately the perception and cognition of body and environment can be associated with both self and consciousness, we therefore need to investigate what exactly happens in the resting-state activity itself.

Accordingly, both halves of the "hard" nut to crack, the association of self-specificity with self and the association of the self with consciousness, lead us back to the brain itself and its intrinsic activity. More specifically, we need to investigate how the brain's intrinsic activity and its functional connectivity and low-frequency fluctuations encode self-specificity. This is important to consider, since it may reveal how the brain's intrinsic activity and its self-specific organization can predispose the self-perspectival organization and a sense of self on the phenomenal level of consciousness.

NEURONAL FINDINGS IVA: SELF-SPECIFICITY AND THE NEURONAL MEASURES OF RESTING-STATE ACTIVITY

How is self-specificity associated with consciousness? We recall from the previous parts that the brain's resting state can be characterized by the spatial and temporal continuity and unity of its neural activity. The spatial and temporal continuity and unity of the resting state neural activity was supposed to be mediated especially by low-frequency fluctuations and functional connectivity. Most important, these neuronal measures of the resting-state activity's spatial and temporal continuity and unity were suggested to predispose the association of neural activity changes (during either stimulus-induced activity or the resting state itself) with consciousness (see Chapters 13–22).

What does that imply for self-specificity? If self-specificity and its underlying neuronal mechanisms interact with these neuronal measures and thus the resting-state activity's spatial and temporal continuity and unity, one would assume it to be associated with consciousness. One would consequently expect self-specificity to modulate the functional connectivity and the low-frequency fluctuations in the neural activity of the brain and its resting state. This is indeed supported by recent findings, as they shall be described below.

We characterized the resting-state activity in the midline regions by anterior-posterior functional connectivity and strong low-frequency fluctuations (see Chapter 23 and Chapter 4 in Volume I). How are these neuronal measures of the midline regions' resting-state activity impacted by stimuli? This is the focus in the next two sections. For that, I turn to empirical findings how self-specificity is related to functional connectivity and low-frequency fluctuations in general and the midline regions in particular.

NEURONAL FINDINGS IVB: FUNCTIONAL CONNECTIVITY AND SELF-SPECIFICITY

Let us start with the findings on functional connectivity. Schmitz and Johnson (2006) conducted a functional magnetic resonance imaging (fMRI) study during judgement of words' degree of self-specificity. They observed increased functional connectivity between different midline regions like the VMPFC, the DMPFC, and the PCC during high self-specific stimuli when compared to low self-specific words. More or less similar findings were also observed by other authors like van Buuren et al. (2010), Moran et al. (2010), and Buckner et al. (2008). This means that the functional connectivity between anterior and posterior midline regions may be essential in mediating high self-specific stimuli.

Thereby the PACC/VMPFC is central in linking the midline regions to posterior regions like the PCC, while the DMPFC seems to be more closely connected to lateral regions like the dorsolateral prefrontal cortex (see Schmitz and Johnson 2006; Whitfield-Gabrieli et al. 2010). These investigations concerned functional connectivity during stimulus-induced activity, while leaving open its relationship to the resting state. We recall from the preceding chapter that neural activity in anterior midline regions elicited by self-specific stimuli overlaps with and is predicted by the resting-state activity in the same regions.

How now does the functional connectivity during stimulus-induced activity overlap with the one during resting-state activity? Whitfield-Gabrieli et al. (2010) investigated the functional connectivity during the resting state in regions that were either recruited stronger during a self-task or during rest (see Chapter 23 for details). They demonstrated that the functional connectivity between VMPFC and PCC was strong during both resting-state activity and self-task.

In contrast, the DMPFC showed stronger functional connectivity with the right and left ventrolateral prefrontal cortex during the resting state when compared to the self-task. The same holds true for the precuneus that showed higher functional connectivity with the bilateral parietal cortex and the bilateral dorsolateral prefrontal cortex during the resting state when compared to the self-task. The self-specific task thus decreased the functional connectivity between these regions compared to that in the resting state. This distinguished both DMPFC and precuneus from the VMPFC and the PCC whose functional connectivity strength did not differ between the resting state and the self-specific stimuli.

Taken together, the results show the functional connectivity between anterior and posterior midline regions to be central in mediating self-specificity. Thereby especially the functional connectivity of the very anterior regions like the PACC and the VMPFC to the PCC seems to overlap considerably between the resting state and self-specificity. This suggests that the self-specific stimuli do not seem to change much the functional connectivity of the PACC and the VMPFC, compared to that in the resting-state activity. In contrast, the resting state functional connectivity in other midline regions like the DMPFC and the precuneus is decreased by the self-task.

NEURONAL FINDINGS IVC: LOW-FREQUENCY FLUCTUATIONS AND SELF-SPECIFICITY

We have so far discussed the impact of self-specific stimuli and self-related tasks on the resting state's functional connectivity. In addition to functional connectivity, the resting state can also be characterized by low- and high-frequency fluctuations.

How do self-specific stimuli impact the low- and high-frequency fluctuations in the resting state's activity? Some indirect information about frequency fluctuations is already contained in the results on functional connectivity. Functional connectivity describes the correlation between the changes in neural activity in different regions across (different points in) time and space (see Volume I, Chapters 5 and 6). This implies a temporal dimension, but it does not specify the exact timing and thus the frequency range. We therefore need to revert to studies that directly test for frequency ranges and fluctuations during self-specificity.

Mu and Han (2010) conducted an EEG study during the presentation of self- and non-self-specific trait adjectives. Frontal theta oscillations (5–7 Hz) were associated particularly with the self-specific condition as distinguished from the non-self-specific ones. Moreover, higher frequency oscillations like alpha or beta were related to the more cognitive aspects of the self-specific stimuli like their self-awareness, evaluation, or memory retrieval (as associated with the judgement of these stimuli in the experimental paradigm) rather than to their degree of self-specificity per se (as more related to their pure perception in the experimental design). This study thus lends support to the assumption that the degree of self-specificity during stimulus-induced activity is associated rather with lower frequency ranges (i.e., theta).

Other studies reported specific effects of self-specific stimuli in the alpha band (12–14 Hz) (Hoeller et al. 2011a and b; Qin et al. 2013). For instance, Pengmin Qin (Qin et al. 2008, 2013) from our group established a "MisMatch Negativity" (MMN) paradigm for self-specificity by using self-specific and unknown names as either deviant or repetitive stimuli. He observed that when controlling for physical differences, the subject's own name elicited a specific MMN at around 140–280 ms.

Interestingly, this accompanied changes in power and synchronization (as indexed by inter-tribal coherence) in specifically the alpha frequency band (12–14 Hz). The alpha frequency band is of particular interest, since resting-state studies have shown that power in the alpha band decreases when opening the eyes (e.g., during eyes open when compared to eyes closed). Since eyes open denotes a basic form of activation (see also Chapters 4 and 5), changes in the alpha band seem to signify most basic changes in the resting-state activity itself.

Does self-specific neural activity resemble the resting state activity not only in anatomical terms (see Chapter 23) but also in electrophysiological regard? The specific involvement of alpha band changes in self-specificity suggests that self-specific stimuli can apparently elicit more or less the same kind of neuronal changes

in the resting-state activity as mere opening the eyes does. Taken in a more general way, this further underlines the close and specific relationship between resting-state activity and self-specificity as demonstrated in the preceding chapter.

NEURONAL FINDINGS IVD: HIGH-FREQUENCY FLUCTUATIONS AND SELF-SPECIFICITY

How about higher frequencies like gamma? Lou et al. (2010a) conducted a magneto-encephalo-graphic (MEG) study during the presentation of self-specific, familiar, and unfamiliar trait adjectives. They focused on those sites (or better, sensors) related to the PACC/VMPFC, the PCC/medial parietal, and the thalamus whose degree of synchronization they targeted.

What did they obtain in their results? The degree of phase synchronization in the gamma frequency range (they investigated all frequency ranges between 2 to 100 Hz) between the three sites (or better, sensors) was significantly higher during self-specific stimuli when compared to the familiar and unfamiliar stimuli. Hence, self-specific stimuli may induce increased gamma synchronization between subcortical, that is, thalamus, and cortical, that is, PACC/VMPFC and PCC/medial parietal, regions.

Presented in another paper, the same data were apparently also analyzed with regard to functional connectivity between the three main regions (see Lou et al. 2011). This yielded bi-directional functional connectivity between all three regions, which was particularly strong in the gamma range (30–45 Hz). Interestingly, increased bi-directional functional connectivity was already observed in the resting-state period prior to the onset of the stimulus (900 ms before) and continued for another 900 ms during the stimulus. Hence, the self-specific stimulus may merely accentuate the ongoing increased gamma power in the resting state in a minor way, rather than causing major changes.

Another recent study also applied self-specific, familiar, and unfamiliar trait adjectives. This was done in subjects undergoing intracranial recording in the posterior midline regions around the

PCC and the precuneus (Dastjerdi et al. 2011). The results showed increased gamma power in the self-specific condition when compared to the familiar and unfamiliar one. This is well in accordance with the earlier described findings by Lou et al. (2010a). Moreover, it blends in nicely with the observation of increased gamma power in the subgenual anterior cingulate during high self-specificity as reported in Chapter 23 (Lipsman et al. 2013).

In addition to the investigation of frequency bands in self-specific stimuli, other EEG studies focused on event-related potentials (ERP) occurring earlier like the N100 (at 100 ms) and the mismatch negativity (occurring at around 125 ms) or later ERPs like the P300 (at 300 ms). These studies demonstrated that self-specific stimuli (like one's own name) induced early changes at around 100 ms when compared to non-self-specific stimuli like famous and unknown names (Zhao et al. 2011; Qin et al. 2008).

In addition, later changes at 300 ms in, for instance, the P300 were also observed (Holeckova et al. 2008; Perrin et al. 2005). The early changes seem to be associated with the self-specific content itself, which seems to reflect the latter's pre-reflective and pre-attentive processing (see Qin et al. 2008, 2013; Tateuchi et al. 2012). In contrast, the later changes are related to cognitive—that is, reflective and attentive—processing of the self-specific content (see, e.g., Esslen et al. 2008; Mu and Han 2010; Tateuchi et al. 2012).

Taken together, the findings point out the central relevance of lower frequencies like theta and alpha as well as of synchronization in higher frequencies like gamma; that is, their power and phases, in the midline regions during self-specific stimuli. How, then, are both self-specificity and midline regions related to consciousness? This will be the focus in the next sections.

Neuronal Hypothesis IIIA: Temporal Continuity of Neural Activity in Midline Regions Predisposes "Inner Time Consciousness"

We distinguished between two different nuts that need to be cracked, an "easy nut" and a

"hard nut." The "easy nut" concerned the association of self-specificity with consciousness, while the "hard nut" was about how self-specificity is associated with a self (first half of the hard nut) and how the self is associated with consciousness (second half of the hard nut). In the following I will focus on the first nut, the "easy nut."

How can the stimulus-related self-specificity and its midline activity interact with the resting-state activity in such way that consciousness can be associated with self-specificity? For the answer, let us briefly return to the resting state itself and the temporal continuity of its neural activity. We encountered the midline regions (see Chapter 13) in what Lloyd described as the "dynamic temporal network" (DTN). The DTN, consisting mainly of midline regions, was shown to mediate the spontaneous changes in neural activity across different discrete points in (physical) time (and space). That, in turn, was postulated to be central for constituting what has been described as the "dynamic flow" of time on the phenomenal level of consciousness (see Chapter 13).

More specifically, I suggested the length in the phase durations of the resting-state activity's low-frequency oscillations and their degree of nestedness with higher frequency oscillation to constitute global temporal continuity of neural activity in the resting state (see Chapters 14 and 15). Most important, such global temporal continuity of the resting state's neural activity was postulated to be manifested on the phenomenal level in "inner time consciousness."

The resting-state activity's global temporal continuity can thus be considered to provide the temporal grid, template, or matrix into which the stimuli and their respectively associated contents (see Chapter 25 for more detail on how contents are constituted out of stimuli) must be linked and integrated in order for them to be associated with consciousness. I consequently postulated the global temporal continuity in especially the midline regions' neural activity to be a neural predisposition of consciousness in general, and of "inner time consciousness" in particular.

NEURONAL HYPOTHESIS IIIB: LINKAGE BETWEEN SELF-SPECIFICITY AND TIME IN MIDLINE REGIONS—"CONTINUITY-BASED HYPOTHESIS OF SELF-SPECIFICITY"

Why is the global temporal continuity of the resting state's neural activity in the midline regions relevant for self-specificity? The midline regions' activity is apparently involved in the constitution of both temporal continuity and self-specific organization. This is supported by the fact that the same neuronal measures, phase durations of low- and high-frequency fluctuations, are centrally involved in constituting both temporal continuity of resting-state activity (see earlier and Chapter 15) and self-specific organization of neural activity (see Chapter 23 and earlier in this chapter).

Why is such a neural overlap between temporal continuity and self-specificity in the midline regions' resting-state activity relevant for consciousness? Due to the midline's participation in both global temporal continuity and self-specificity, their self-specific organization cannot avoid becoming linked and aligned to the global temporal continuity of their neural activity and thereby predisposing consciousness. Self-specificity and temporal continuity may consequently be closely linked to each other in the neural activity of the midline regions during the resting-state activity. This may apply especially for high self-specific stimuli that, as described in the preceding chapter, do not induce much deviation from the resting-state activity. Based on these considerations, I suggest what I describe as a "continuity-based hypothesis of self-specificity."

The "continuity-based hypothesis of self-specificity" postulates that the degree of self-specificity (of stimuli, tasks, or functions) and its underlying stimulus-induced activity in the midline regions depends on the degree of temporal continuity in the resting-state activity of the midline regions: the higher the degrees of spatial and temporal continuity in the midline's neural activity of the resting state, the higher degrees of self-specificity can possibly be assigned to a stimulus (function or task).

This is the neuronal part of the "continuity-based hypothesis of self-specificity." We will see later that it has major implications for consciousness, thus concerning its phenomenal (or better, neurophenomenal) part. Before turning to the neurophenomenal implications, however, we need to describe the neuronal mechanisms in more detail.

NEURONAL HYPOTHESIS IIIC: SELF-SPECIFICITY DEPENDS ON THE LONG PHASE DURATIONS OF THE LOW-FREQUENCY FLUCTUATIONS IN THE RESTING-STATE ACTIVITY

Let us detail the neuronal mechanisms of the "continuity-based hypothesis of self-specificity." As described in Chapters 13 through 15, the global temporal continuity of neuronal activity is closely related to the phase durations of the resting-state activity's low-frequency fluctuations that may be especially strong in the midline regions. The stronger the low-frequency fluctuations' phase durations, the more their long phase durations predominate over the shorter ones of the higher frequency fluctuations, and consequently the more extended and thus the higher the degree of temporal continuity of neural activity in the midline's resting state.

How does that relate to self-specificity that is also processed in the midline regions? I demonstrated that higher degrees of self-specificity go along with lower degrees of deviation in neural activity from the resting state. This means that the neural activity in the midline regions during self-specific stimuli deviates less from, and is thus closer to, the resting-state activity, including its strong and predominant long phase durations. More specifically, lower deviation from the midline regions' low-frequency fluctuations and their long phase durations should accompany the assignment of higher degrees of self-specificity to stimuli, tasks, or functions.

I consequently postulate that the degree of self-specificity during stimulus- and task-related activity depends on the phase durations of the ongoing resting-state activity's low-frequency fluctuations and their degree of temporal continuity. The better the resting-state activity's low-frequency fluctuations and their long phase durations and thus their global temporal continuity are preserved, the higher the possible degrees of self-specificity that can be assigned to the respective stimuli, functions, or tasks.

NEURONAL HYPOTHESIS IIID: GAMMA SYNCHRONIZATION MEDIATES DECREASED DEVIATION FROM RESTING-STATE ACTIVITY AND INCREASED SELF-SPECIFICITY

How is that observation related to the above-described findings of increased gamma synchronization during self-specific stimuli and tasks? Increased gamma synchronization signifies increased temporal homogeneity and thus increased alignment between the gamma phase durations across the different regions. The increased gamma synchronization makes it easier for and thus more likely that the gamma phase durations will be aligned to and thus be entrained by the ongoing low-frequency fluctuations and their longer phase durations.

One may consequently postulate increased cross-frequency phase-phase (and phase-power) coupling between (the stimulus-induced) gamma and the (resting state's ongoing) lower frequency fluctuations' longer phase durations during high self-specific stimuli (compared to low self-specific stimuli). Let me explicate that. Increased phase-phase (and phase-power) coupling between (the stimulus-induced) gamma and the (resting state's ongoing) lower-frequency fluctuations implies that the latter and especially their long phase durations are better preserved. This means that the long low frequencies' phase durations deviate less from their original temporal configuration in the resting state prior to the onset of the stimulus. And such decreased deviation from the resting state's ongoing low-frequency fluctuations, in turn, makes possible, I argue, the assignment of high degrees of self-specificity to the stimulus (functions or tasks).

If the increased gamma synchronization does indeed reflect increased cross-frequency phase-phase (and phase-power) coupling, it signifies the decreased deviation from the resting state's low-frequency fluctuations and consequently decreased stimulus-induced activity. This sounds paradoxical, though, since one would associate increased gamma synchronization with increased rather than decreased deviation from the resting-state activity and thus to mirror increased (rather than decreased) stimulus-induced activity.

That, however, stands opposite to the results described earlier that show high degrees of self-specificity to go along with decreased rather than increased stimulus-induced activity. Accordingly, the data seem to favor the first interpretation of increased gamma synchronization's signifying decreased deviation from resting-state activity and decreased stimulus-induced activity during high self-specific stimuli (functions or tasks).

NEURO-PHENOMENAL HYPOTHESIS IA: "TEMPORALIZATION OF SELF-SPECIFICITY"

We so far postulated the "continuity-based hypothesis of self-specificity" as a purely neuronal hypothesis. In addition to specific neuronal mechanisms, this hypothesis also postulates the association of the latter with particular phenomenal features. This shall be the focus in the following discussion, which is guided by this question: How is such intimate linkage between self-specificity and temporal continuity manifested on the phenomenal level of consciousness? The global temporal continuity of the resting-state activity was associated with "inner time consciousness," and more specifically the extension of the discrete time points of the stimuli and their contents beyond themselves, to other discrete points in time. We recall that the "continuity-based hypothesis of self-specificity" postulates that higher degrees of self-specificity are associated with longer phase durations.

Taking both phenomenal time and self-specificity together, one would expect personally relevant and thus highly self-specific contents to be stretched and extended into time much more than those that remain personally irrelevant, i.e., low self-specific ones. In other words, personally relevant, self-specific objects or events have a longer time duration in our experience and thus in consciousness than non-relevant ones, i.e., non-self-specific ones. Conversely, one would expect objects or events with a longer time duration to show a higher degree of self-specificity, thus being more personally relevant.

Time and self-specificity may thus be postulated to stand in a positive relationship to each other on the phenomenal level of consciousness. The longer the subjective time duration, for example, the "width of the present" and the "duration bloc" (see Chapters 14 and 15), associated with a specific object or event, the higher possible degrees of self-specificity can possibly

be associated with the object or event itself. In contrast, the converse holds, too, with shorter subjective time durations going along with lower degrees of self-specificity, e.g., personal relevance, of the respective object or event (see left graph in Fig. 24-3).

Such intimate linkage between self-specificity and time amounts to what I describe as the "temporalization of self-specificity." The concept of "temporalization of self-specificity" describes that the self-specific stimuli are put and thus linked and integrated into the neural activity underlying the constitution of "inner time consciousness." Even more strongly, the concept of "temporalization of self-specificity" implies dependence of the stimuli's degree of self-specificity" on the degree of their integration and linkage to the underlying "inner time consciousness."

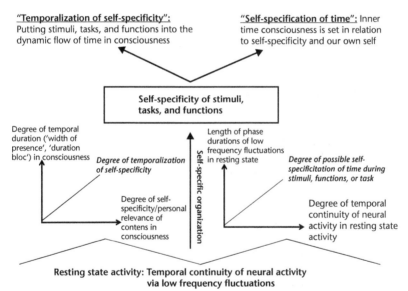

Figure 24-3 Temporal continuity and self-specificity. The figure illustrates the "continuity-based hypothesis of self-specificity." The resting-state activity provides temporal continuity via its low-frequency fluctuations and their long phase durations (lowest part). Based on that, the resting state shows self-specific organization (middle part), which, on the phenomenal level of consciousness, leads to the "temporalization of self-specificity" (upper left) and the "self-specification of time" (upper right). The degree of self-specificity assigned to stimuli is strongly dependent on the degree of temporal duration on the phenomenal level of consciousness (left graph), while, at the same time, the resting state's temporal continuity of its neural activity can impact and thus "has a strong say" in modulating the degree to which itself, e.g., the temporal continuity of own neural activity, becomes self-specified during the exposure to stimuli, tasks, and functions (right graph).

Neurophenomenal Hypothesis IB: Phenomenal and Neuronal Evidence for the "Temporalization of Self-Specificity"

How can we describe such "temporalization" of self-specificity in more detail? We experience, as said earlier, stimuli and their respective contents, functions, and tasks in terms of time and thus in a temporalized way. They are "put" into time and have therefore always already have a relationship to the different time dimensions of present, past, and future. This amounts to what I describe as "temporalization of self-specificity" (see left upper part in Figure 24-3).

The concept "temporalization of self-specificity" refers to the linkage between self-specificity and temporal continuity, which, on the phenomenal level, results in the experience of a "dynamic flow" with a "width of present" and "duration bloc" and thus phenomenal time in especially high self-specific stimuli. Since such "temporalization of self-specificity" occurs by default in every stimulus, regardless of its particular degree of self-specificity, it must be considered necessary or unavoidable.

How can we lend further support for such a concept of "temporalization of self-specificity"? Phenomenally, one can support the "temporalization of self-specificity" by the linkage between self-awareness and time. Edmund Husserl, the founder of phenomenological philosophy, suggested that the most basic and fundamental form of self-awareness, pre-reflective self-awareness, is essentially temporal. By experiencing "inner time consciousness" with the "width of present" and the "duration bloc," we experience time not only in consciousness but also in our own self. Following Husserl, this is an intrinsic linkage, such that the self and thus what he describes as pre-reflective self-awareness, cannot avoid being associated with time in our consciousness.

How is such an intrinsic linkage between self and time possible? As I pointed out earlier, I postulate that this is ultimately predisposed by the overlap in the neural processing of self-specificity and time in the neural activity in the midline regions. One could suggest that the degree of midline neural activity during "inner time consciousness," that is, subjective experience of time, predicts the degree of both the stimulus-induced activity (in midline regions) and its associated degree of self-specificity as it is experienced in time. This is a very testable hypothesis, which is currently underway in our group.

Neuro-phenomenal Hypothesis IC: "Phenomenal Continuity" versus "Psychological Continuity"

How can we describe such temporalization in further phenomenal detail? By becoming temporalized, the contents, tasks, and functions are embedded into what philosopher Barry Dainton (2008, xii–xiv) describes as "experiential continuity," the experience of a stream of consciousness. Since it concerns the phenomenal level, such "experiential continuity" may also be described as "phenomenal continuity," the term I will use in the following discussion.

What do I mean by the concept of "phenomenal continuity"? The concept of "phenomenal continuity" concerns not only stimuli and tasks, e.g., self- and non-self-specific ones, but also the various psychological functions, e.g., affective, cognitive, etc. This means that we also experience these psychological functions in a temporally continuous way. There is thus "phenomenal continuity," which, however, must be well distinguished from the concept of "psychological continuity."

The concept of psychological continuity describes the continuity of affective, sensorimotor, and cognitive functions independent of any experience. The recruitment of emotions or cognitive functions like attention may be present for some time and overlap with each other. There may thus be a chain of recruited psychological time across time, which leads to what I describe as "psychological continuity" (see also Derek Parfit (1984) on the philosophical side for the concept of psychological continuity in the context of the philosophical debate about personal identity).

How does such psychological continuity stand in relation to the "phenomenal continuity"? I postulate that psychological continuity is possible only on the basis of the preceding linkage of the various functions with the midline regions and their temporal continuity. Since the linkage to the midline regions implicates the earlier-described integration of the respective psychological function with the temporal continuity of their resting state's ongoing neural activity, "phenomenal continuity" must occur earlier and precede the "psychological continuity." One would consequently postulate the "psychological continuity" to presuppose and be based on the "phenomenal continuity."

My hypothesis about the relationship between phenomenal and psychological continuity supports the earlier assumption that, in a more general scope, the brain's neurophenomenal functions precede and are more basic than its neurosensory, neuromotor, neuroaffective, and neurocognitive functions. The latter functions occur within and thus presuppose the "phenomenal continuity" of the neurophenomenal functions, since otherwise we would probably be unable to perform any of these functions. This also implies that psychological continuity must presuppose and is possible only on the basis of phenomenal continuity in very much the same way stimulus-induced and task-related activity are possible only on the basis of the brain's resting state activity.

NEURO-PHENOMENAL HYPOTHESIS
ID: "SELF-SPECIFICATION OF TIME"

Let us turn back to the relationship between time and self-specificity. We have so far described how the global temporal continuity of the resting state's neural activity affects the stimuli (and tasks and functions) and how that interaction differs (gradually or quantitatively rather than qualitatively) between self- and non-self-specific stimuli. This lead to what we described as "temporalization of self-specificity" and "phenomenal continuity."

However, in addition to the self-specific (and non-specific) stimuli being affected by the resting state's global temporal continuity, their interaction can also go the reverse way. This means that the global temporal continuity of the resting state's neural activity may by itself also be affected by the degree of self-specificity of the respective stimuli (or tasks or functions). We are thus no longer talking about the "temporalization of self-specificity" but rather of the converse situation, which can be described as the "self-specification of time."

What do I mean by the concept of "self-specification of time"? I suggest the "self-specification of time" to be related neuronally to the degree to which the resting-state activity's temporal continuity becomes aligned with the low-frequency fluctuations and their phase durations during the exposure to specific stimuli or tasks (see right graph in Figure 24-3).

How about the phenomenal implication of the "self-specification of time"? Phenomenally, the "self-specification of time" describes that the time itself becomes affected by the degree of self-specificity: in the same way that self-specific contents become temporalized, the temporal durations themselves and thus our "inner time consciousness" become self-specified in our experience. We have consequently no other way to experience time than in terms of self-specificity and ultimately our own self (or subject; see right upper part in Figure 24-3).

Due to such "self-specification of time," we remain unable to experience time, i.e., phenomenal time, independently of the degrees of self-specificity associated with tasks, stimuli, and functions (and thus ultimately our own self). Accordingly, our experience of time is always already bound to our particular individual degree of self-specificity assigned to the respective contents. In the same way, we cannot avoid the "temporalization of self-specificity," the "self-specification of time" also occurs by default as it is ultimately based on the intimate linkage between the neural processing of temporal continuity and self-specificity in our brain's midline regions.

I therefore postulate the earlier, purely neuronal, stated "continuity-based hypothesis of self-specificity" to be manifested in a double gestalt on the phenomenal level of consciousness. Self-specificity becomes linked to temporality, which is manifested in "temporalization of self-specification," so that any content, functions, and tasks cannot help but be experienced in time. Conversely, our "inner time consciousness" also becomes self-specified, resulting in "self-specification of time"; this is manifested in the intimate relationship of our subjective time experience to the degrees of self-specificity and ultimately our own self.

NEUROPHENOMENAL HYPOTHESIS IIA: FROM SELF-SPECIFICITY TO THE SELF—"ENVIRONMENT–BRAIN UNITY"

We have so far dealt with the "easy nut" to crack, the association of self-specificity with consciousness. This nut was cracked by claiming for the "temporalization of self-specificity" and "self-specification of time." That was the easy part. How about the "hard" nut to crack?

We have left open the "hard nut" and its two halves, the linkage of self-specificity with a self and the association of the self with consciousness. This nut is a hard one to crack because it involves two highly controversial issues: the one about the definition of the self, and the one about the relationship between the self and consciousness. We will not enter here into the extensive conceptual and philosophical discussions about these issues. I will thus not enter into the metaphysical debate about the existence and reality of self and consciousness. Instead, I limit myself here to purely phenomenal issues, how we experience our self in consciousness. Hence, I aim to put forward tentative neurophenomenal hypotheses for both steps in order to understand why we experience our self in the way we do while refraining from making any metaphysical (or epistemological) claims about the self (see Appendix 4 where I discuss first steps for a future metaphysical definition of the self).

Let us start with the first half of the nut, the step from self-specificity to the self. For that, we need to go back to what we described as the environment–brain unity and point of view in Chapters 20 and 21. In a nutshell, the "environment–brain unity" described a virtual statistically and spatiotemporally based relationship between the spatial and temporal neuronal measures of the brain's intrinsic activity and the statistically based spatial and temporal distribution of the extrinsic stimuli in the environment.

By comparing and matching extrinsic stimuli and neuronal measures in a spatiotemporally and statistically based way, the "natural and social statistics" of the extrinsic stimuli are encoded into the brain's neural activity. Such encoding of the spatial and temporal differences between intrinsic activity and extrinsic stimuli was supposed to be mediated neuronally by the shifting of the low-frequency fluctuations' phase onsets in orientation to the onset of the extrinsic stimuli. This is also described as "phase alignment" or "stimulus-phase coupling" that seems to predominantly occur in low-frequency fluctuations (see Chapter 20). I postulated that such "stimulus-phase coupling" may be a central mechanisms in constituting what I described as "environment-brain unity" including its virtual and spatiotemporally- and statistically-based character.

NEUROPHENOMENAL HYPOTHESIS IIB: FROM SELF-SPECIFICITY TO THE SELF—"SELF-SPECIFICATION OF POINT OF VIEW"

How is such environment–brain unity related to consciousness? I postulated that the statistically and spatiotemporally based environment–brain unity provides a point of view. The concept of "point of view" describes a stance of the biophysical organism within the physical world. Such a stance "anchors" the organism within the physical world in a species-specific way, while at the same time predisposing the organism's possible experience and thus consciousness of that very same world (see Chapters 20 and 21 for details).

How then can we link such a spatiotemporally and statistically based point of view of the organism to the self-specific organization of its brain's resting-state activity? Neuronally, this means that we need to link the stimulus-phase coupling underlying the constitution of the point of view (see Chapter 20 for details) with the low-frequency fluctuations and their long phase durations especially in the midline regions' self-specific organization (see Chapter 22 for details). Since stimulus-phase coupling occurs predominantly in low-frequency fluctuations, there is a direct neural overlap and possibly interaction between both.

What does such possible interaction between stimulus-phase coupling and the low-frequency fluctuations' long phase durations imply for the relationship between point of view and self-specificity? It means that the point of view becomes linked and integrated with the self-specific organization and thus with self-specificity. I call such linkage and integration the "self-specification of point of view."

The concept of "self-specification of point of view" describes that the point of view that defines the biophysical organism in a species-specific way within the physical world is put into the context of the individually specific resting-state activity and its self-specific organization. The species-specific point of view is thus not only self-specified but also individualized, meaning that it is linked and integrated within the individual organism and its resting-state activity's self-specific organization (see later for more details on such individualization).

NEUROPHENOMENAL HYPOTHESIS IIC: FROM SELF-SPECIFICITY TO THE SELF— "SELF-SPECIFICATION" AS "INDIVIDUALIZATION OF THE POINT OF VIEW"

How is such "self-specification of point of view" manifested neuronally and phenomenally? I postulate that neuronally it is manifested in the relationship between the degree of stimulus-phase coupling and the phase duration of the low-frequency fluctuations. The higher the degree of stimulus-phase coupling, the more the low-frequency fluctuations are aligned to particular stimuli, and the less the midline's neural activity will deviate from its resting-state activity level. As described in Chapter 22, this is accompanied by the assignment of higher degrees of self-specificity to the stimuli and consequently with a higher degree of self-specification of the point of view.

I consequently suggest that the degree of self-specificity is directly dependent upon the degree of stimulus-phase coupling and its associated point of view. This means that higher degree of stimulus-phase coupling predispose higher degrees of possible self-specification of

the point of view. In contrast, lower degrees of stimulus-phase coupling may rather lead to low degrees of possible self-specification of the point of view (via increased deviation from the resting state and decreased assignment of self-specificity to the (then-non-aligned) stimuli (see upper graph in Fig. 24-4a).

How is the "self-specification of point of view" manifested phenomenally? By aligning the individually specific self-specific organization to the species-specific point of view, the latter becomes individualized and specifies thus the individual organism itself, rather than the organism as a particular species. The specification of an individual organism entails what conceptually is often described by the term self, an "individualized self" as I will say later (see lower part in Figure 24-4a).

How can we describe such a self? Such a self is obviously based on the organism's point of view, but it is not identical to it, because that would mean to neglect the self-specification of the point of view (and to neglect the difference between species and individual). I will argue that such self is experienced in consciousness in terms of a "sense of self." Such a "sense of self" amounts to a phenomenal concept of self and comes more or less close to the concept of "self-experience" as suggested by authors like Dainton (2008) and Zahavi (2005) who relies on the phenomenological concept of pre-reflective self-awareness (see, e.g., Zahavi 2005).

NEUROPHENOMENAL HYPOTHESIS IIIA: BODY AND ITS "PROTO-SELF" AS "SELF-SPECIFIED AND INDIVIDUALIZED POINT OF VIEW"?

How can we lend empirical support to the hypothesis of the "individualization" of the point of view as point of view–based self? Neuroscientific authors like Panksepp (1998a and b) and Damasio (1999, 2010) may want to argue that such an individualized self comes close to what they describe as "proto-self." The concept of the "proto-self" describes mainly the homeostatic regulation of the body and is therefore essentially defined by the body and its physiological features. Similar to our concept of

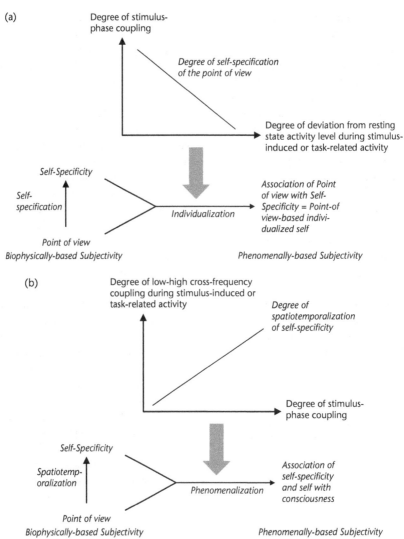

Figure 24-4a and b Bilateral interaction between self-specificity and point of view. The figure illustrates the bilateral relationship between point of view and self-specificity with self-specification of the point of view (*a*) and spatiotemporalization of self-specificity by the point of view (*b*). (*a*) The figure shows that the degree of self-specification of the point of view is dependent upon the relationship between the degree of stimulus-phase coupling and the degree of deviation from the resting-state activity during stimulus-induced activity (graph in upper part). This leads to the self-specification of the point of view and its subsequent individualization which results in a point of view–based individualized self (lower part). Such individualization makes possible the transformation of the specific-specific non-individual biophysically based subjectivity into an individually specific phenomenally based subjectivity (lowest part). (*b*) The figure shows that the degree of spatiotemporalization of self-specificity by the point of view depends on the relationship between the degree of stimulus-phase coupling and the degree of low-high cross-frequency coupling (graph in upper part). This leads to the spatiotemporalization of self-specificity by the point of view and its subsequent phenomenalization, which results in the association of self-specificity and self with consciousness and its phenomenal features (lower part). Such phenomenalization makes possible the transformation of the species-specific non-individual biophysically based subjectivity into an individually specific phenomenally based subjectivity (lowest part). The phenomenally based subjectivity can thus be considered the individualized and phenomenalized version of the biophysically based subjectivity and its associated point of view.

self, such a "proto-self" is not yet experienced in consciousness as such. This, however, is where the similarities between the two concepts of the "individualized self" and the proto-self end.

In contrast to the "proto-self," my concept of the "individualized self" cannot be limited to the confines of the body and its physiological mechanisms. Rather than being identified with the body, the self I have in mind is based on the point of view and is associated with the environment–brain unity. My concept of self is thus point of view–based rather than bodily based. As such, it is statistically and spatiotemporally based like its underlying point of view, rather than physiologically and homeostasis-based like the proto-self.

How can I lend neuronal and phenomenal support to my claim of a point-of view–based self that extends beyond the boundaries of the body and is statistically and spatiotemporally based rather than physiologically and homeostasis-based? Based on my earlier considerations, I suggest that the neuronal mechanisms may involve those that are also implicated in constituting the environment–brain unity, like low-frequency fluctuations and their stimulus-phase coupling and alignment to the environment. Furthermore, one would expect such a point of view–based self to be elicited not only by bodily stimuli, as in the case of the "proto-self," but also by other non-bodily stimuli, such as words or letters. This can indeed be supported, as will be discussed in the next sections.

Neurophenomenal Hypothesis IIIB: Experimental Testing of the Non-Individualized and Individualized Self

How can we investigate such an individualized self experimentally? One would expect two different processing steps. The first step should consist of the processing of the distinction between *somebody* and *nobody*, between a person and a non-person. This would correspond more or less to the here-suggested distinction between "point of view" and "no point of view."

If there is a point of view, there must be some kind of person independent of whether it is one's own self or some other self. In contrast, the absence of a point of view entails the absence of any kind of "person." One would consequently expect the first processing step to make this rather basic distinction independently of whether it is one's own or some other person; such person would not yet be individualized or specified by a particular person like my own self or another self. The first processing step would thus occur prior to the self-specification and individualization of the point of view. This is different in the second processing step. Here, the distinction no longer concerns the one between "person" and "no person" but rather between different particular persons like my own self versus another self. The point of view and its self are individualized now, and thus self-specified.

How can we support this distinction between a non-individualized self and an individualized self in an empirical-experimental regard? The researcher Peter Walla, who was originally born in Austria but lives now in in Australia, conducted two studies (Walla et al. 2007, 2008) where he tested both processing steps, the first one between person and non-person, and the second one between self and other during measurement of EEG and MEG. Subjects were visually presented nouns (3–9 letters long) which were combined with three different words, *a*, *my*, and *his*. The article "a" indicates a non-person in conjunction with the noun, while the pronouns "my" and "his" signify persons rather than non-persons (first processing step) as well as the distinction between self and other (second processing step).

In addition to the three different words, subjects had to make different decisions. First, subjects had to decide whether the first and last letter were in alphabetical order, which, so Walla, reflects "perceptual encoding." Or subjects had to decide whether the noun describes a living or non-living object, requiring "semantic encoding as Walla says." Finally, subjects had to think of a short, meaningful sentence that integrated the noun into a wider context, while making the decision about whether it was living and non-living; this amounted to what Walla describes as "contextual encoding."

NEUROPHENOMENAL HYPOTHESIS IIIC: EARLY AND LATE CHANGES DURING NON-INDIVIDUALIZED AND INDIVIDUALIZED SELF

What did Walla et al. (2007, 2008) observe in their results? They showed early differences at around 200–400 ms when hearing the article "a" when compared to both "my" and "his": there were different amplitudes in the event-related potentials and higher neural activity in left occipital cortex during the article "a" when compared to both "my" and "his." This suggests that these early neuronal mechanisms underlie the distinction between person and non-person which accounts for the first processing step as postulated above.

More or less the same result was also observed in another EEG study (Herbert et al. 2011) on emotional words and the same three words (*a, my, his*) where a similar time window showed analogous changes, particularly during the "a." In addition to occipital electrodes, there was also involvement of fronto-central electrodes and their underlying anterior and posterior midline regions. The observation of such early changes is further supported by other EEG studies that show a more or less similar time window for the distinction between *person* and *non-person* (see Esslen et al. 2008; Perrin et al. 2006; Zhou et al. 2010; Shi et al. 2011, as well as earlier in this chapter).

How about the distinction between "my" and "his," the second processing step? Following the results by Walla et al. (2007, 2008) and Herbert et al. (2011), this was associated with later processes at around 500–800 ms. The late positive potentials distinguished between both conditions, which anatomically were associated with neural activity in left frontal and temporal cortex.

How do the authors interpret these findings? Walla concludes that there may be two different types of self-awareness, which amounts to what he describes as "multiple aspect theory of the self." The first aspect concerns the general distinction between person and non-person, independently of whether it is one's own self or another person; such a non-individualized self concept is associated with early subconscious

processing in occipital cortex (and midline regions; see Herbert et al. 2011). This corresponds well to our first processing step, as postulated earlier. The second aspect refers to the individualized self with its distinction between self and other, which is mediated by later conscious processing in frontal and temporal cortex. That mirrors more or less what I described as the second processing step.

NEUROPHENOMENAL HYPOTHESIS IIID: PRE-STIMULUS RESTING-STATE ACTIVITY PREDICTS STIMULUS-INDUCED ACTIVITY CHANGES

How do these data stand in relation to the neurophenomenal hypotheses suggested here? For the answer, we need to be clear about what the data show and, even more importantly, what they do not show. What do the data show? They provide evidence in favor of different neuronal mechanisms for the two distinctions: between persons and non-persons and between self and non-self. Both distinctions are related to different neuronal mechanisms in temporal (early versus late) and spatial (frontal versus occipital) regards. How does that relate to my neurophenomenal hypotheses? The data provide empirical evidence in favor of my distinction between the non-self-specified and self-specified point of view that mirrors more or less the distinction between a non-individualized person and an individualized self. This is what the data show.

What do the data do not show? They leave open what happens in the very early time period, between 0 ms and 200 ms and, even more interesting, what happens prior to stimulus onset. They thus miss the preceding resting-state activity and how it is modulated by the stimulus. More specifically, the data do not show anything about low- and high-frequency ranges that are not reported. Moreover, there is no information provided in the current data about both power and phase changes like low-high frequency phase-power or phase-phase coupling. Nor are any data presented about stimulus-phase coupling prior to stimulus onset in the preceding resting-state period. Finally, no findings are given about the midline regions' resting-state activity level prior to and around stimulus onset and how their activity is modulated during both the words themselves ("a," "my," "his") and their associated nouns.

Basically, almost none of the neuronal features and mechanisms that we postulated to be relevant in our neurophenomenal hypotheses are addressed in these studies. Why? The studies by Walla and others focus almost exclusively on stimulus-induced (or task-related) activity and thus on neurocognitive functions independently of the brain's resting-state activity and its neurophenomenal functions. Since my neurophenomenal hypotheses are all based on the resting-state activity, being resting-state-based rather than stimulus-based, the data fail to provide any direct evidence for my neurophenomenal hypothesis.

That, however, does not imply that the data are irrelevant. Rather than direct evidence, they may nevertheless provide some indirect evidence. Presupposing the neuronal mechanisms associated with the resting-state activity postulated here, one would assume exactly the kind of stimulus-induced activity changes Walla and others observed. In other words, I would expect the resting-state neuronal measures to predict the kind of stimulus-induced (or task-related) changes Walla and others observed. I postulate, for instance, that the pre-stimulus low-frequency fluctuations, including their stimulus-phase coupling and their cross-frequency phase-power coupling, predict especially the early ERP-changes and their associated psychological distinction between person and non-person that Walla and others observed.

Finally, I would hypothesize that the midline regions' pre-stimulus resting-state activity level may impact the occipital regions' resting-state activity, which in turn may predetermine the range of possible stimulus-induced activity in that region, as observed by Walla. Future studies are however necessary to show direct modulation of the stimulus-induced activity by the resting state activity and its impact on the distinctions between person and non-person and self and non-self.

NEUROPHENOMENAL HYPOTHESIS IIIE: PRE-STIMULUS RESTING-STATE ACTIVITY AND ITS NEURONAL MEASURES PREDICT THE STIMULUS' POSSIBLE DEGREE OF "INDIVIDUALIZATION" AND "PHENOMENALIZATION"

Does Walla associate the distinction between person and non-person exclusively with the stimuli themselves and their related stimulus-induced activities? This would mean to presuppose a neurocognitive approach that associates the distinction between (for instance) person and non-person only with the stimuli themselves rather than with the brain.

Walla himself seems to deny such a purely neurocognitive approach, however. He focuses very much on the encoding, and distinguishes, as mentioned earlier, between "perceptual, semantic, and contextual encoding," which, as shown in the data, can be associated with early and late neural processes and different anatomical locations. Most important, he argues that the "concept of a "person' also exists as a meta-representation in the human brain and can be elicited by personal pronouns" (Walla et al. 2007, 807).

Unfortunately, he leaves open the question of what such a "meta-representation of the concept of person in the human brain" looks like and how stimuli like "personal pronouns can elicit it." This is exactly the point where his study converges with my neurophenomenal hypotheses. My neurophenomenal hypotheses postulate that the point of view and its underlying neuronal mechanisms provide a first, most general, and non-individualized version of a person. This is associated with the environment–brain unity and neuronal mechanism in the preceding resting state like stimulus-phase coupling, midline regions' resting-state activity, and low-high frequency phase-power coupling. Those neuronal mechanisms that operate in the resting state prior to any stimulus may yield and thus underlie Walla's assumption that the "person" is somehow "meta-represented in the human brain" (see Table 24-1).

I postulate the following. The non-individualized point of view is supposed to be

Table 24-1 Neural processing of the self and its relationship to consciousness in different time periods.

	Neuronal Mechanisms	Encoding into Neural Activity	Relation to Consciousness
–800–0 ms	Stimulus-phase coupling Rhythmic versus continuous mode	*Mode of brain function*: Environment-brain unity	*Principle Nonconscious*: Neuronal and biochemical processes are inaccessible
0–100 ms	Low–high frequency coupling, midline regions' deviation	*Spatiotemporal encoding*: Point of view	*Principle Consciousness*: Distinction from Principle Nonconscious
100–300 ms	ERP amplitude changes, sensory cortex and midline regions	*Perceptual encoding*: Self-specification of point of view	*Phenomenal Consciousness of environment* and subconscious of self
300–500 ms	P300 amplitude changes, sensory and frontal cortex	*Semantic encoding*: Individualization of point of view	Phenomenal consciousness of self as *pre-reflective self-awareness*
500–800ms	Late positive potentials, frontal and temporal cortex	*Contextual encoding*: Contextualization of self with other	*Access and Reflective Consciousness* of self

The table illustrates the different time periods before (–800–0 ms) and after (0–800 ms) stimulus onset (left row), the suggested and observed neuronal mechanisms (second row from the left), the suggested and postulated encoding processes (third row from the left), and the associated form of consciousness (right row). Note that the neuronal mechanisms and the type of encoding in the time periods form 150 ms to 800 ms are based on the findings and hypotheses by Walla et al. (2007, 2008) and Herbert et al. (2011), as discussed in the main text. In contrast, the neuronal mechanisms and encoding types in the preceding time periods from –800 ms to 150 ms are mainly based on my own neuronal and neurophenomenal hypothesis. The same holds for the relationship to consciousness, as illustrated in the right row where I use terms that I mainly described and defined in the second Introduction.

individualized by the resting-state activity's self-specific organization that also determines the stimuli's degree of self-specificity. This is neuronally supposed to be manifested in the degree of deviation from the resting-state activity's level in especially the midline regions. The degree of stimulus-induced deviation from the midline's resting-state activity level may find its analogue in Walla's assumption that a stimulus can elicit the brain's "meta-representation of the concept of a person" and its individualization.

Why are the here-postulated neuronal measures in the preceding resting-state activity so important? I suggest that different neuronal measures in the preceding resting-state activity, like the low-frequency fluctuations, predetermine how the subsequent stimuli can be encoded into neural activity and how they can be integrated and linked to the intrinsic activity's spatiotemporal structures. And that may ultimately predispose and determine the degree

to which the processing steps during subsequent stimulus-induced activity can take place. Metaphorically speaking, the preceding resting state is the period wherein the germs or seeds are planted for the stimuli's individualization and phenomenalization and their association with both an individualized self and consciousness.

NEUROPHENOMENAL HYPOTHESIS IIIF: SPATIOTEMPORAL ENCODING AS THE MOST BASIC, FUNDAMENTAL, AND EARLIEST FORM OF ENCODING

I postulated that the pre-stimulus resting-state activity predicts both the stimulus-induced activity changes and the degree of the stimulus' individualization and phenomenalization. This leaves open, however, the question of why and how the first one, the stimulus-induced activity changes, can mediate the second, the individualization and phenomenalization. I postulate that this is possible because both stimulus-induced activity and individualization/phenomenalization have a shared neuronal basis, the resting-state activity.

More specifically, stimulus-induced activity and individualization/phenomenalization share the spatiotemporal structure associated with the resting-state activity. As detailed especially in Chapters 4 and 5, the intrinsic activity continuously "works on its spatiotemporal structure," which therefore is dynamic and continuously changing. When encoding the stimulus into neural activity, the intrinsic activity "imposes" its spatiotemporal structure upon the extrinsic stimulus, which, I postulate, becomes thereby "individualized" and "phenomenalized." This needs to be explicated in more detail, though.

What exactly happens during this early encoding period around stimulus onset and between 0–50 ms? As argued here and in many other chapters of this book, the early period around stimulus onset and between 0 and 50/100 ms is characterized by the encoding of statistically based spatial and temporal differences into the brain's neural activity. Due to such difference-based coding, the stimuli and their discrete points in time and space become "spatialized" and "temporalized," which makes their integration and linkage to the brain's intrinsic activity and its spatiotemporal structure possible. And that in turn allows the individualization and phenomenalization of the extrinsic stimulus.

I consequently postulate that Walla's three forms of encoding—perceptual, semantic, and contextual—need to be complemented by an even more basic one, spatiotemporal encoding, as I call it. The concept of "spatiotemporal encoding" describes that the stimuli are encoded into neural activity in terms of their spatial and temporal relationships to both each other and the brain's intrinsic activity. Only by presupposing spatiotemporal encoding in the very early stages of neural processing around stimulus onset and 0–50/100 ms can the stimulus be linked to the environment–brain unity and its point of view. Such linkage does in turn predispose the self-specification of the point of view with the subsequent constitution of an individualized self and its association with consciousness.

Based on these considerations, I propose that spatiotemporal encoding is a necessary condition of both individualization and phenomenalization (see further down for a separate account on especially phenomenalization). Without such spatiotemporal encoding, neither individualization nor phenomenalization of the point of view would be possible. We would then have neither an individualized self nor consciousness. Accordingly, I consider that spatiotemporal encoding is necessary for both individualization and phenomenalization (see Fig. 24-4b).

NEUROPHENOMENAL HYPOTHESIS IVA: FROM POINT OF VIEW TO CONSCIOUSNESS—CHANGE IN SELF-SPECIFICITY BY ITS ENCOUNTER WITH THE POINT OF VIEW

Where are we now? We have so far described only the self-specification and thus individualization of the point of view and its potentially underlying neuronal mechanisms. This, however, did not yet include any reference to neuronal mechanisms that allow for the association of such a self-specified point of view with consciousness where it is manifested as the "sense of self" (which is here understood more or less similar to what has been described in philosophy as self-experience or pre-reflective self-awareness; see above as well as Appendix 4). In short, the self is now "individualized" but not yet really "phenomenalized."

We thus need to account on separate grounds for the association of such an "individualized self" with consciousness and thus for what can be described as the "phenomenalization of the self" (see later). Put differently, this means that we have so far addressed one half of the "hard nut" to crack, the step from self-specificity to the self. This has left the other half, the step from self to consciousness.

How is possible that the self as a point of view–based self (see earlier) is associated with consciousness? For that, I argue that we need to consider the reverse direction of the relationship between self-specificity and point of view. We have investigated what happens to the point of view when it interacts with self-specificity, which leads to the earlier described "self-specification of point of view." However, it is not only the point of view that changes by its encounter with self-specificity, but also the self-specificity when it interacts with the point of view.

NEUROPHENOMENAL HYPOTHESIS IVB: FROM POINT OF VIEW TO CONSCIOUSNESS— "SPATIOTEMPORALIZATION OF SELF-SPECIFICITY"

How does the linkage to the point of view impact and thus change self-specificity? Let us recall from Chapters 20 and 21. The point of view was supposed to be associated with the environment–brain unity, which is defined in a statistically and spatiotemporally based way. Being "spatiotemporally based" means that the point of view and its environment–brain unity describe certain spatiotemporal trajectories; these spatiotemporal trajectories are based on the statistically based encoding of spatial and temporal differences between the different extrinsic stimuli in the environment by the brain's intrinsic activity (see above and Chapters 20 and 21 for details).

Accordingly, the point of view and its environment–brain unity can be characterized by some kind of spatiotemporal grid or template. When interacting with the resting-state activity's self-specific organization, this spatiotemporal grid or template is imposed upon the former. The resting-state activity's self-specific organization becomes consequently "spatiotemporalized" by the statistically-based virtual spatiotemporal grid or template of the point of view and its environment–brain unity. This amounts to what I refer to as "spatiotemporalization of self-specificity."

The concept of "spatiotemporalization of self-specificity" describes the integration and linkage of the resting-state activity's self-specific organization with the statistically-based spatiotemporal grid or template of the environment–brain unity. Most importantly, this spatiotemporal grid or template shows a larger degree of spatiotemporal extension than the one of the resting-state activity's self-specific organization.

Why is there such difference in the degree of spatiotemporal extension? Due to the inclusion of the environment, the environment–brain unity

can extend its spatiotemporal grid or template to a much larger degree than the resting-state activity itself and its self-specific organization, which are confined to the spatiotemporal boundaries of the brain. Such a difference in the degree of spatiotemporal extension implies that the smaller one, the resting-state activity's self-specificity, is integrated and thus "nested" within the larger spatiotemporal grid of the environment–brain unity. This means that the self-specificity and ultimately the point of view–based self (see earlier) are linked to and integrated within the wider network of the spatiotemporal trajectories of the environment–brain unity and its point of view. That results in what I describe as the "spatiotemporalization of self-specificity".

In contrast, the converse integration of the point of view within the self-specific organization remains impossible. Why? Due to larger degree in spatiotemporal extension, the environment-brain unity cannot be integrated within the brain's intrinsic activity. The unilateral integration and thus nestedness of the intrinsic activity's self-specific organization within the point of view of the environment-brain unity occurs thus by default. The "spatiotemporalization of self-specificity" is a necessary consequence of the differences in the degree of statistically-based spatiotemporal extension between the environment-brain unity and the brain's intrinsic activity.

NEUROPHENOMENAL HYPOTHESIS IVC: FROM POINT OF VIEW TO CONSCIOUSNESS—"PHENOMENALIZATION" OF SELF AND SELF-SPECIFICITY

How does consciousness now come into the picture? The unilateral (or better, nested) spatiotemporalization, I suggest, makes possible the association of self-specificity and its point of view-based self with consciousness. This means that self-specificity including the point-of view–based self become "phenomenalized" and can thus be experienced in consciousness. The initial, purely biophysically based, subjectivity of the point of view (see Chapter 21) is now both individualized and phenomenalized; this makes possible its transformation into the subjective experience of a self, which mirrors what I described as "phenomenally based subjectivity" (see Chapter 21). In short, I consider "phenomenally based subjectivity" the individualized and phenomenalized version of biophysically based subjectivity.

How is such phenomenalization of self-specificity manifested neuronally and phenomenally? Let us start with the neuronal side of things. The stimulus-phase coupling of the environment–brain unity occurs predominantly in low-frequency fluctuations, while the stimulus-induced or task-related activity during self-specific stimuli or tasks induces higher frequency fluctuations like in the gamma range (see earlier). The better these high-frequency fluctuations are aligned and thus coupled to the low-frequency fluctuations and especially their phase onsets (which in turn are coupled to the onset of the stimuli), the better the resting-state activity's self-specific organization is spatiotemporally linked and integrated to the environment–brain unity.

I consequently hypothesize that the degree of low-high frequency coupling predicts the degree of consciousness that can be associated with the resting-state activity's self-specific organization. Higher degrees of low-high cross-frequency coupling; that is, phase-phase or phase-power coupling, will lead to a higher degree in the spatiotemporalization of self-specificity, which in turn makes its association with consciousness more likely (see upper graph in Fig. 24-4b).

Neurophenomenal Hypothesis VA: From the "Spatiotemporalization of Self-Specificity" to the "Self-Perspectival Organization" of Consciousness

How is such spatiotemporalization of the self-specific organization manifested on the phenomenal level of consciousness? I suggest that it is manifested in what the philosophers refer to as "self-perspectival organization." The concept of "self-perspectival organization" describes that consciousness, and thus our subjective experience, is centered around a subject that experiences the contents in a perspectival way in consciousness.

I now tentatively postulate that what is described as the center or self in self-perspectival organization corresponds to the self-specified and individualized point of view. The perspectival nature, in contrast, finds its analogue in the spatiotemporalization of self-specificity; the spatiotemporalization provides a spatiotemporal grid that makes possible the perspectival nature with its extension to spatiotemporally distant areas reaching far beyond one's own self and its body. Based on these considerations, I postulate that the concept of "self-perspectival organization" describes the spatiotemporal structure of our consciousness. Since it provides the underlying spatiotemporal structure, any content associated with consciousness is necessarily or unavoidably integrated and linked to that spatiotemporal structure (see Fig. 24-5a).

This means that any content in consciousness, independently of whether it originates in the environment (as during the experience or consciousness of environmental objects, events, or persons), in the body (as during bodily self-consciousness; see Blanke 2012), or in one's own brain (as during dreams), becomes necessarily associated with the spatiotemporal structure of consciousness and its self-perspectival organization. We have thus no choice other than to experience our environment, our body, and our own resting-state activity (as in dreams) as well as our own self in a spatiotemporal and thus self-perspectival way. How can we better illustrate what is meant by "self-perspectival organization"? For that, I conclude with an impressive quote by the philosopher Robert van Gulick:

> The perspectival structure of consciousness is one aspect of its overall phenomenal organization, but it is important enough to merit discussion in its own right. Insofar as the key perspective is that of the conscious self, the specific feature might be called *self-perspectuality*. Conscious experiences do not exist as isolated mental atoms, but as modes or states of a conscious self or subject (Descartes 1644, Searle 1992, though *pace* Hume 1739). A visual experience of a blue sphere is always a matter of there being some self or subject who is appeared to in that way. A sharp and stabbing pain is always a pain felt or experienced by some conscious subject. The self need not appear as an

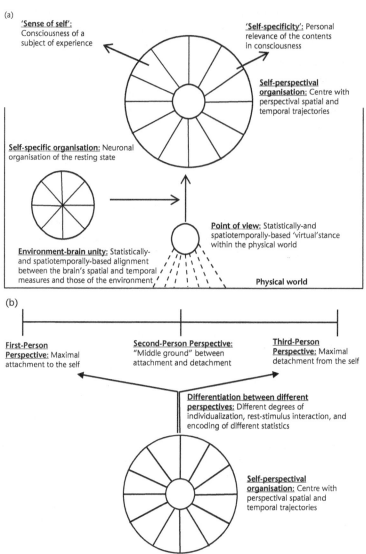

Figure 24-5a and b Relationship between point of view, self-perspectival organization, and perspectives. (*a*) Self-specificity and self-perspectival organization. The figure illustrates how the statistically and spatiotemporally based "virtual" point of view, the organism's stance within the physical world (lower part, dotted lines indicate statistically based coupling between brain and environment), provides the very basis for the constitution of self-perspectival organization (upper part). For that to be possible, the environment–brain unity and its point of view must be linked and integrated with the resting-state activity's self-specific organization (left part). Combining point of view and self-specific organization allows then the constitution of self-perspectival organization as characterized in a double way by a center and its perspectival nature, with the latter being related to spatial and temporal trajectories (as indicated by dotted lines). This double origin and characterization of self-perspectival organization is manifested in consciousness as the experience of a "sense of self" (or an "experiencing self") (upper left) and "self-specificity," i.e., personal relevance, of the contents, the "experienced contents." (*b*) Self-perspectival organization and the different perspectives. The figure illustrates that self-perspectival organization (lower part) and its underlying point of view (see figure a) are the basis for the perspectival character of all three perspectives: first-, second-, and third-person perspectives (upper part). Such differentiation of the self-perspectival organization into three different perspectives is made possible by processing different degrees of individualization, rest–stimulus interaction, and the encoding of different statistical frequency distributions (see text).

explicit element in our experiences, but as Kant (1787) noted the "I think" must at least potentially accompany each of them. The self might be taken as the perspectival point from which the world of objects is present to experience (Wittgenstein 1921). It provides not only a spatial and temporal perspective for our experience of the world but one of meaning and intelligibility as well. The intentional coherence of the experiential domain relies upon the dual interdependence between self and world: the self as perspective from which objects are known and the world as the integrated structure of objects and events whose possibilities of being experienced implicitly define the nature and location of the self (Kant 1787, Husserl 1929). Conscious organisms obviously differ in the extent to which they constitute a unified and coherent self, and they likely differ accordingly in the sort or degree of perspectival focus they embody in their respective forms of experience (Lorenz 1977). Consciousness may not require a distinct or substantial self of the traditional Cartesian sort, but at least some degree of perspectively self-like organization seems essential for the existence of anything that might count as conscious experience. Experiences seem no more able to exist without a self or subject to undergo them than could ocean waves exist without the sea through which they move. The descriptive question thus requires some account of the self-perspectival aspect of experience and the self-like organization of conscious minds on which it depends, even if the relevant account treats the self in a relatively deflationary and virtual way (Dennett 1991, 1992). (van Gulick 2011, pp. 4–5)

NEUROPHENOMENAL HYPOTHESIS VB: FROM THE ENVIRONMENT TO THE SELF—"UNITY-BASED HYPOTHESIS OF SELF-PERSPECTIVAL ORGANIZATION"

We here do not intend to venture into the philosophical debate. Instead I remain within the phenomenal realm without venturing into the metaphysical and epistemological territory of philosophy. I now suppose that what the philosophers describe as self-perspectival organization can be traced back ultimately to the environment-brain unity and its point of view and its coupling to the various temporal and

self-specific processes, the temporalization and self-specification, I described in this chapter. Due to its basis in the environment-brain unity, one may want to speak of a "unity-based hypothesis of self-perspectival organization."

The hallmark feature of the "unity-based hypothesis of self-perspectival organization" is that the self-perspectival organization is at once environmental and thus social as well as individual and thus personal. The individualization or personalization is here considered just a specification of the prior given socialization or environmentalization of the brain's intrinsic activity in the environment-brain unity (see Chapter 20 for details).

I postulate that, due to its basis in the environment-brain unity, the self-perspectival organization is intrinsically spatiotemporal. This, as demonstrated, is highly relevant for the phenomenal domain of consciousness. It would though be also interesting to see how the intrinsically spatiotemporal character of the self-perspectival organization stands to past and current philosophical or better ontological and metaphysical approaches to self and consciousness. This however is beyond the current purely neurophenomenal approach and will need to be dealt with in a future neurophilosophy.

NEUROPHENOMENAL HYPOTHESIS VC: "SPATIOTEMPORALIZATION" IS THE "COMMON CURRENCY" BETWEEN BRAIN AND CONSCIOUSNESS

We have so far described the neuronal and phenomenal pathways that supposedly lead to the self-perspectival organization of consciousness. The neuronal pathway involved the interaction between the different layers of neural organization in the brain's resting-state activity, its temporal and spatial organization, its neurosocial and -ecological organization (the environment–brain unity), and its self-specific organization. This was complemented on the phenomenal side by generating "inner time and space consciousness," "biophysically and phenomenally based subjectivity," and the sense of self in consciousness.

One could now argue that I did not really link and integrate the neuronal and phenomenal pathways. The integration between neuronal and phenomenal pathways, however, is necessary to suggest a truly neurophenomenal hypothesis. What links and integrates neuronal and phenomenal pathways in an intrinsic and thus necessary way so that the neuronal mechanisms cannot help but lead to the self-perspectival organization of consciousness by default?

This is the question of what is the common denominator, the "common currency" between neuronal and phenomenal pathways. I suggest that the "common currency" consists of the spatiotemporalization of both the brain's neural activity and the phenomenal features of consciousness. Due to its encoding in terms of spatial and temporal differences via difference-based coding, the brain's neural activity is necessarily and unavoidably spatialized and temporalized, and spans in a virtual and statistically and spatiotemporally-based way across the physical boundaries between brain, body, and environment (see also Volume I).

Such spatiotemporalization of the encoded neural activity does predispose the association of consciousness with the otherwise purely neuronal resting state and stimulus-induced activity. If so, one would expect that the brain's spatiotemporalization of its neural activity across the physical boundaries between brain, body, and environment is manifested on the phenomenal level of consciousness. I suggest that this is indeed the case, as is manifested in the self-perspectival organization of consciousness.

This, however, is only the starting point. We need to trace down the spatiotemporal features of the brain's neural activity in both our consciousness of the external environment and our consciousness of our self, our sense of self. Otherwise our hypothesis of spatiotemporalization as "common currency" between brain and consciousness remains incomplete. Finally, consciousness of contents in the external environment is characterized by *qualia*, what it is like to perceive and experience a particular content in first-person perspective (see Chapter 30 for more detailed definition). Based on the here-suggested role of spatiotemporalization, one would now suggest that qualia and their various features are by definition and thus intrinsically spatial and temporal. This, I postulate, can indeed be demonstrated, as I will discuss in full detail in Chapter 30.

How about the spatiotemporalization of the consciousness of our self, the sense of self? Previous phenomenological philosophers like Martin Heidegger did indeed attempt to describe the experience and thus consciousness of our self in spatial and temporal terms. This leads to a spatial and temporal account of our experience of our own self as the basis of our very existence, which reaches deeply into the territory of the existential-ontological domain as developed by Heidegger and his philosophy. Since my focus is on consciousness rather than the self and its existence, I here refrain from such venture.

NEUROPHENOMENAL HYPOTHESIS VIA: FROM CONSCIOUSNESS TO PERSPECTIVES—FIRST-, SECOND-, AND THIRD-PERSON PERSPECTIVE

We have discussed the step from the environment–brain unity and its associated point of view to the self-perspectival organization of consciousness and our experience of a self. This left open, however, the question of how the different perspectives—first-, second-, and third-person—are related to the here-described mechanisms and how they are generated and differentiated. This is the focus in the final sections of this chapter.

How can we briefly characterize the different perspectives? The first-person perspective (FPP) describes the subjective experience: we experience our own self, our body, and the objects and events in the environment in FPP. This is different from the mere observation of the environmental objects and events in third-person perspective (TPP). Unlike FPP, TPP remains completely detached from the self and is therefore considered "objective" rather than "subjective" like FPP.

Finally, we need to distinguish the second-person perspective (SPP), which is sandwiched between FPP and TPP. The SPP has often been associated with the introspection into one's own self in philosophy (see Northoff and Heinzel 2003). More recently though, the SPP has been related to the interaction between different selves (see Schilbach et al. 2013; Pfeiffer et al. 2013). The interaction between our own and other selves has traditionally been conceived of in a merely observational mode and thus from the outside. Pfeiffer et al. (2013) speak of an "off-line mode" of social cognition that presupposes TPP.

One may, however, also consider the interaction between different selves from the inside rather than the outside. This reflects what Pfeiffer et al. (2013) and Schilbach et al. (2013) describe as "on-line mode" of social cognition. Such an "on-line mode," as perspective from the inside of the interaction between one's own and another self, can be characterized neither by FPP nor by TPP: FPP is completely attached to the self, whereas TPP is detached from the self. This is the moment where SPP comes in: SPP is still attached to the self while also being *detached* from it when interacting with the other person's self. SPP thus describes a "middle ground" between complete attachment (as in FPP) and detachment (as in TPP) (see Northoff and Heinzel 2003; Schilbach et al. 2013).

NEUROPHENOMENAL HYPOTHESIS VIB: FROM CONSCIOUSNESS TO PERSPECTIVES—POINT OF VIEW-BASED CHARACTERIZATION OF THE DIFFERENT PERSPECTIVES

How, then, are all three perspectives—FPP, SPP, and TPP—related to the self-perspectival organization of consciousness? Current cognitive neuroscience and philosophy of mind often associate FPP with consciousness and its self-perspectival organization. TPP, in contrast, is supposed to remain completely detached from the self and thus from any self-perspectival organization and ultimately also from consciousness. One may consequently conclude that TPP lies outside consciousness.

This is to confuse FPP and self-perspectival organization, however. The contents in all three perspectives are always already associated with consciousness. All three perspectives occur on the basis of consciousness. FPP, SPP, and TPP must thus presuppose self-perspectival organization and its associated consciousness as their commonly underlying necessary condition. Without the underlying self-perspectival organization, neither FPP nor SPP and TPP and thus the perspectival differentiation altogether would remain impossible. This implies that, unlike in current philosophy of mind and cognitive neuroscience, FPP cannot be identified with self-perspectival organization and consciousness (see Fig. 24-5b).

What does this imply for the characterization of FPP, SPP, and TPP? I suggested the self-perspectival organization to be based on the point of view and its associated biophysically based subjectivity (see earlier). This means that all three perspectives are based on the point of view and are biophysically subjective. Therefore, I speak of a point of view–based characterization of FPP, SPP, and TPP. The point of view-based characterization of FPP, SPP, and TPP postulates that neither of the three perspectives would be possible without an underlying point of view. Accordingly, without a point of view and its associated biophysically based subjectivity, none of these perspectives would be possible, amounting to an "aperspectival" rather than perspectival characterization. Needless to say, neither consciousness nor any kind of self would be possible in the case of such an aperspectival characterization.

In the same way that we cannot identify FPP with the self-perspectival organization of consciousness, we cannot identify FPP with the point of view, either. The point of view is more basic than the FPP since it first and foremost makes possible the perspectival character of all three—FPP, SPP, and TPP. Such perspectival character may then be further differentiated into different perspectives like FPP, SPP, and TPP, as shall be discussed in the following section.

How can we empirically support our hypothesis of the point of view-based characterization of FPP, SPP, and TPP? If the three perspectives are indeed based on the point of view, both point of view and perspectives should be able to dissociate from each other. One may for instance have a point of view while the perspectives themselves may be deficient (the reverse, perspectives without point of view, is, however, not possible since perspectives are based on the point of view). That is for instance the case in neuropsychiatric disorders like autism, schizophrenia, and depression (see chapters 27 for details).

One may now be inclined to argue that the availability of a point of view entails especially FPP. This however is to confuse the necessary conditions of possible FPP, the point of view, with the necessary and sufficient conditions of actual FPP. As we have seen in this chapter, many processes like temporalization and self-specification are sandwiched between point of view and FPP. These processes may be deficient so that the point of view will then not be associated with the "normal" perspectives. This seems to be the case in especially schizophrenia where both temporalization (see chapter 17) and self-specification (see chapter 27) are abnormally altered. Hence, schizophrenic patients still have available a point of view upon which though a "normal" FPP is no longer built.

NEUROPHENOMENAL HYPOTHESIS VIC: FROM CONSCIOUSNESS TO PERSPECTIVES— "PERSPECTIVAL DIFFERENTIATION" BETWEEN FIRST-PERSON, SECOND-PERSON, AND THIRD-PERSON PERSPECTIVES

We emphasized that the point of view and its associated biophysically based subjectivity provide the basis and thus the necessary condition of all three: FPP, SPP, and TPP. This leaves open, however, the question of their sufficient conditions, which must address how the three different perspectives can differentiate from each other.

Let us start with the self-perspectival organization. As described earlier, the self-perspectival organization may show different degrees of individualization. I now postulate that the different perspectives correspond to different degrees of individualization and self-specification of the point of view. The higher the degree to which the point of view is self-specified and individualized, the higher the degree of FPP and the lower the degree of TPP. Conversely, a low degree of self-specification and individualization of the point of view is supposed to lead to low degrees of FPP, medium degrees of SPP, and higher degrees of TPP. FPP, SPP, and TPP are then no longer considered as qualitatively different perspectives but rather as different points on an underlying perspectival continuum.

How can we now specify the neuronal processes that may underlie the differentiation among the different perspectives? I argued that the self-perspectival organization of consciousness results from the integration of the resting state's self-specific organization and the environment–brain unity. The resting state's self-specific organization interacts with various stimuli from the brain (neuronal stimuli), which amounts to rest–rest interaction. And the resting state also interacts with stimuli from the body (interoceptive stimuli) and the environment (exteroceptive stimuli), as can be described as rest–intero and rest–extero interaction (Chapters 8 and 9, Volume I).

There is a balance among all three types of interactions, rest–rest, rest–intero, and rest–extero, as detailed in Chapters 4, 5, 8, and 9. I now postulate that the balance among the three interactions provides the basis for the predominant perspective: if rest–rest interaction dominates over rest–intero and rest–extero, the degree of FPP is rather high, while the degrees of TPP and SPP may be low (as for instance in dreams). If, in contrast, rest–extero is dominant when compared to the other two, TPP will take on a high degree at the expense of FPP and SPP. Finally, a balance between rest–intero and rest–extero may lead to high degrees of SPP at the expense of both FPP and TPP.

The degree of the three t interactions may ultimately be traced back to the encoding of the different stimuli' statistical frequency distribution by the environment–brain unity: in the case of high degrees of rest–rest interaction, the encoding of the resting-state activity's neuronal statistics predominates (see Chapters 8 and 9 for the concept of "neuronal statistics"). In contrast, high degrees of rest–intero interaction may lead to high degrees of encoding of vegetative (and social) statistics into the brain's neural activity. And finally, a high degree of rest–extero interaction implies the encoding of natural statistics to dominate the encoding of neural activity.

On a whole, I postulate that the differentiation between FPP, SPP, and TPP can be traced back to different degrees of individualization of the self-perspectival organization. This is related to different degrees of rest–rest, rest–intero, and rest–extero interaction, which in turn are based on the encoding of the balance among different statistical frequency distributions—neuronal, vegetative, social, and natural statistics—into neural activity.

How can we empirically support our hypothesis of the perspectival differentiation? I suggest that again neuropsychiatric disorders like schizophrenia and autism as well as neurological disorders like lesions may provide some indirect evidence. For instance, autism has been associated with deficits in specifically SPP while TPP and FPP seem to remain intact. This suggests possible dissociation between FPP, SPP, and TPP which hints upon different neuronal mechanisms. That, however, needs to be explored in the future.

NEUROPHENOMENAL HYPOTHESIS VID: FROM CONSCIOUSNESS TO PERSPECTIVES— "PERSPECTIVAL CONTINUUM" IS *BRAIN-BASED* RATHER THAN *COGNITION-BASED*

What does our description of the neuronal mechanisms imply for the conceptual characterization of FPP, SPP, and TPP? Since the underlying neuronal mechanisms concern different degrees and balances, FPP, SPP, and TPP cannot be distinguished from each other in an all-or-nothing, qualitative, and mutually exclusive way. Instead, there seems to be a continuum with multiple transitions between FPP, SPP, and TPP. This means that FPP, SPP, and TPP occur in different degrees at the same time, rather than occurring in an all-or-nothing and mutually exclusive way. Accordingly, the different perspectives are continuum-based rather than all-or-nothing-based.

This leads me to another feature of the different perspectives. Traditional philosophy suggested the different perspective to be based on a mind, with which FPP was especially associated. Such a mind-based view of FPP has recently been replaced by a cognition-based view. FPP is here associated with specific self- and meta-representational processes that are related to cognition and cognitive functions (see, e.g., Metzinger 2003; Churchland 2002). Cognition is then assumed to provide the very basis of the

differentiation between TPP and FPP. The traditional mind-based view is here replaced by a cognition-based view of FPP.

How does such a cognition-based view stand in relationship to the here-postulated view of the different perspectives as differentiations on an underlying perspectival continuum? Since the perspectival continuum is supposed to underlie the differentiation between the different perspectives, the perspectival continuum is not compatible with a cognition-based view. That would be to confuse the necessary condition, the perspectival continuum, with what it conditions, the perspectival differentiation between FPP, SPP, and TPP.

We consequently have to search for a basis for the perspectival continuum other than in cognition. I postulate that this basis can be found in the brain's intrinsic activity and its spatiotemporal organization. This entails a brain-based view rather than cognition- or mind-based view of the "perspectival continuum" which is well compatible with subsequent perspectival differentiation between FPP, SPP, and TPP.

NEUROMETAPHORICAL EXCURSION IA: NEURONAL EQUIPMENT OF THE BRAIN'S "LIVING ROOM"

After having discussed the complexities of the self-perspectival organization of consciousness, let me now illustrate this with a metaphorical comparison of the brain with a living room. The silent assumption is often that the stimulus encounters a practically empty and passive brain. This implies that the stimulus itself basically determines completely, that is, sufficiently, whatever happens in the brain once it enters. The brain is here tacitly supposed to be an empty, vast space of mere gray matter, which comes to life only with the entrance of the stimulus.

But this is not the case. As shown in Volume I, and the preceding chapters in this volume, the stimulus encounters a highly structured, well-organized, and extremely active brain; that is, its resting-state activity. The stimulus is just a "guest" in the brain and enters a well-structured "living room" with high ceilings, plenty of nice furniture, and a marble floor partially covered by beautiful carpets. I here focus only on the brain itself and thus compare it to the living room. In contrast, I neglect the house that is, the environment and thus the social context in which the living room, namely the brain and its intrinsic activity, are situated. Since I already focused on the social and thus environmental context of the brain in Chapters 20 and 21, I here neglect the social and environmental context of the living room, the house, in my comparison.

Let us describe the living room of the brain in further detail, as we sketched it in Volume I (see Part II). The stimulus encounters different frequency oscillations that are nested within each other. These may correspond to different streams and shadings of light within the living room which cross and overlap with each other and entail different degrees of temporal (and spatial) nestedness. Moreover, the stimulus encounters an already high resting-state activity level. This may correspond to the level of the marble floor in the living room compared to the floors in the rest of the house.

Furthermore, there are different regions and networks in the brain, like inner, middle, and outer rings, that may correspond to the different pieces of furniture at different spots in the living room. Finally, there is plenty of functional connectivity between the different regions of the brain that may be analogous to the carpets extending between and connecting the different pieces of furniture.

NEUROMETAPHORICAL EXCURSION
IB: NEUROPHENOMENAL EQUIPMENT
OF THE BRAIN'S LIVING ROOM

This is the brain's living room described in a purely neuronal way. Let us now switch perspectives from the neuronal to the phenomenal perspective on the brain's living room. We thus now view the brain's living room from the phenomenal perspective of consciousness, rather than from the neuronal perspective of the brain. There is, as was demonstrated in the previous chapters, spatiotemporal continuity (see Part V). The designer of the living room did an excellent

job by creating continuity between, for instance, the colors of the different pieces of furniture as well as between furniture and carpets. Most importantly, these color continuities let your perception slide effortlessly across space and time in the living room, amounting to a dynamic flow of spatiotemporal continuity.

Despite the different colors and pieces of furniture, everything looks unified. There is homogeneity and unity in the room. And even better, once you enter, you can immediately connect to the room and feel a part of that unity, its spatiotemporal unity. The same is true in the case of the brain. The stimulus may easily connect to the brain's resting-state activity and its spatial and temporal measures. There may consequently be a spatiotemporal unity between the environmental stimuli and your resting-state activity, an environment–brain unity, that resembles very much the unity between the different pieces of furniture, the walls, and the floor in the living room.

Now, finally, let us consider the highlight of the room: everything is centered around a heightened chair. This golden chair is the center to and from which all the trajectories of the living room lead; all furniture in the other parts of the living room is positioned in relationship to this heightened chair, which is supposed to provide the person sitting on it with a special point of view and perspective.

The room's designer intended to make you feel like a king, a monarch, and to give you a royal point of view from which you can see and observe everything. This chair and its central position in the living room corresponds well to what I described as the self-perspectival organization in consciousness, which can be traced back to the conjoining between the resting state's s self-specific organization and the brain's unity with the environment: the environment–brain unity.

NEUROMETAPHORICAL EXCURSION
IIA: STIMULI AS GUESTS IN THE LIVING
ROOM OF THE BRAIN

Now imagine yourself entering this living room for the first time. What do you do? How do you interact with the room and make yourself feel comfortable and at home? You may want to look for certain features in the room you can relate to and that remind you of your own home, while neglecting those you cannot relate to so much. The ones you can relate to will be assigned a high degree of self-specificity, thus being personally relevant to you. In contrast, the others will show a low degree of self-specificity, remaining personally irrelevant to you. The degree of personal relevance you attributed to the various features will in turn determine the degree to which you will recruit your sensory, motor, affective, cognitive and social functions.

In the same way that you are guest in the living room, the stimulus is a guest in the brain's living room, i.e., its resting-state activity. The stimulus enters the living room of the brain; that is, its resting-state activity. There the stimulus "tries" to relate to the resting-state activity and its spatial and temporal neuronal measures (i.e., low-frequency oscillations and functional connectivity) and make itself "feel" comfortable and "at home." This is what happens during rest–stimulus interaction.

There is one important difference, however. In the case of the living room, the person enters, becomes active, and changes the room; whereas in the case of the brain, it is the brain itself and more specifically its resting-state activity that becomes active by itself. The resting-state activity itself changes its own living room in order to accommodate the stimulus; thereby the resting state aims to integrate the stimulus in such way that it, the resting-state activity, needs to undergo as little change as possible.

Hence, in the case of the brain, it is the resting-state activity itself that becomes active, whereas in the case of the real living room, it is only the guest that actively makes changes. This difference, however, should not distract us from further pursuing our example.

NEUROMETAPHORICAL EXCURSION
IIB: "FEELING AT HOME AND COMFORTABLE" IN THE LIVING ROOM OF THE BRAIN

Let us go on. You are now sitting on the various chairs in the living room. You move on and wander around, try to open the door of the closet and try out the table over there. You move the curtains. And you also sit on the heightened chair in the center of the room. You feel at home, finally. You feel integrated, like a part of the room, and you sense that the room now belongs to you. You experience it as your room, and you thus say: "This is my room."

The same occurs in the case of the stimulus. The stimulus, too, wanders around in the resting-state activity of the brain. The resting-state activity tries out its different spatial and temporal neuronal measures to accommodate the stimulus and its particular spatiotemporal features. For instance, the resting-state activity tries to align its own temporal features those ones of the stimulus by, for example, phase shifting with stimulus-phase coupling via its low-frequency oscillations and its different regions' neural activities.

By recruiting its various spatial and temporal neuronal measures, the resting-state activity probes and thus tests where and how it can best integrate and align the stimulus to itself and its own living room. If the resting-state activity finds ways to integrate and align the stimulus, the resting state (and the stimulus, too) will "feel" comfortable and "at home." The elicited stimulus-induced activity will consequently not deviate much from the resting-state activity. Since the resulting stimulus-induced activity remains close to the preceding resting-state activity, with both showing low degrees of deviation from each other, the stimulus is assigned a high degree of self-specificity.

What though happens in the opposite case, when the stimulus cannot be aligned to the brain's resting-state activity? If you do not feel at home in the living room, you will move the furniture around; for instance, the heightened chair. You do not like to sit in the center of the room and be potentially observed by everybody, so you move the chair to the corner so that it no longer occupies the room anymore. Now you feel that you can breathe in the room after all.

The same again is the case in the brain's resting-state activity when it cannot align the stimulus to itself. The resting-state activity then tries to move around its neuronal furniture, meaning that it changes its regional activity pattern, functional connectivity, and low-frequency fluctuations in order to accommodate its guest, the stimulus. For instance, the brain's resting-state activity can generate high-frequency fluctuations like gamma to accommodate the stimulus' temporal features. And the resting state activity may yield substantial changes in its pattern of functional connectivity to accommodate the regional activity changes the stimulus elicits. Due to these changes in its resting-state activity, the resulting stimulus-induced activity will differ substantially from the initial resting-state activity. That goes along with the assignment of a rather low degree of self-specificity to the respective stimulus.

Neurometaphorical Excursion IIC: The Brain Associates Consciousness to the Stimuli as the Guests of its Living Room

Now let us shift from the neuronal description of the brain's living room to what it implies for a phenomenal description of consciousness and thus how you perceive and experience the living room. You love the room as it is, and sit comfortably on the heightened chair in the center. You feel like the owner of the room. You feel like the king. You thus have a strong sense of self and experience high degrees of personal relevance. The room has thus successfully integrated you which is manifested in your experience of high degrees of personal relevance of the room and its various features.

The same applies in the case of the brain. The stimuli from the environment make it easy for the resting-state activity to impose its own self-specific organization upon them. The resting-state activity consequently assigns a high degree of self-specificity to the stimuli and "feels" like a king, the "king of the stimulus and the world." Environment–brain unity and self-specific organization are well merged, resulting in a high degree of self-perspectival organization with a strong sense of self and a high degree of self-specificity, e.g., personal relevance. That is how you experience yourself sitting on the heightened chair in the middle of the room.

Now consider the opposite case. You hate the room and move the heightened chair to the corner. You do not feel at all like the owner of the room. You do not experience a strong sense of self. Nor does anything in the room, including the stupid heightened chair, bear any personal relevance to you; there is thus a rather low degree of self-specificity. You hate how the room imposes itself upon you and try to counterbalance that by imposing yourself on the room.

The same is true in the case of the brain. In this case, your brain's resting-state activity remains unable to align the phase onsets of its low-frequency fluctuations to the stimuli in the environment. This means that your brain's resting-state activity cannot impose its own spatial and temporal neuronal measures onto the stimulus. Instead of being accommodated and integrated and thereby inducing minimal deviation from the resting-state activity, the stimulus and its resulting stimulus-induced activity will differ strongly from the initial resting-state activity.

In other words, the stimulus disrupts the resting-state activity's neuronal unity between high- and low-frequency fluctuations as well as the brain's unity with the environment, the environment–brain unity. The degree of your environment–brain unity is consequently rather low. That, in turn, makes it more difficult to merge it with your resting-state activity's self-specific organization; the point of view and the self-specific organization's spatial and temporal trajectories are consequently not properly linked and integrated.

Such decreased integration and linkage lead to decreased self-perspectival organization and consequently to a decreased sense of self and decreased degrees of consciousness of the objects and events in the environment. You consequently feel detached from the room; your own self is not part of it and thus an outsider rather than an insider.

Now it is too much. You cannot stand the room any longer and leave it to preserve your sense of self. In the same way you leave the room alone when nothing works, the resting-state activity leaves the stimulus alone and does not do anything to it anymore.

At best, the stimulus is processed somehow and elicits some degree of stimulus-induced activity. However, despite inducing stimulus-induced activity in the brain, the latter's resting-state activity no longer associates consciousness with that very same stimulus. The stimulus is thus processed in an unconscious way, as we as observers say. The situation can get worse, however. In this case, the stimulus is completely disregarded by the resting-state activity and henceforth does not elicit any stimulus-induced activity at all anymore. There is thus no more processing at all. In that case, you are not only unconscious but non-conscious; and that means that your brain is no longer alive, but dead.

Open Questions

One of the major claims here is that the resting-state activity's self-specific organization predisposes and biases the subsequent stimulus-induced activity and its associated phenomenal features. This neural predisposition was, as I hypothesized, manifest in the stimulus' degree of self-specificity. For that, I gathered empirical support from recent studies on self-specific stimuli and their effects on functional connectivity, regional activation pattern, and low- and high-frequency fluctuations.

However, I left open the exact neuronal mechanisms of rest–stimulus interaction and how they transform the resting state's self-specific organization into a full-blown phenomenal state and thus consciousness. This will be the task and focus of Part VIII, where I discuss how rest–stimulus can generate qualia as a phenomenal hallmark feature of phenomenal consciousness.

Another issue almost completely neglected here is the concept of the person as well as the question for the self. Let me focus on the self and let the discussion about the concept of the person open for future philosophical/neurophilosophical exploration. I spoke of the resting state's self-specific organization and how that predisposes the

self-perspectival organization on the phenomenal level of consciousness. The term "self" has been defined in different contexts or domains like in metaphysical (Strawson 2009), phenomenal (Dainton 2008), representational-functionalistic (Metzinger 2003), phenomenological (Zahavi 2005), logical-conceptual (Bennett and Hacker 2003), and mentalistic (McGinn 1991) ways, to name just a few. These approaches concern the question for the nature of the self: What is the self?

How would this question be answered in the present context? Based on my account, I would argue that the self as we experience it, i.e., the "sense of self," consists in a statistically and spatiotemporally based "virtual" center in our experience that links and distinguishes us from the environment. On the phenomenal level of consciousness, this may then be experienced as sense of self as the "virtual" center in our experience (see, nevertheless, Appendix 4 for some discussion of the concept of the self).

Such a sense of self must be distinguished from the discussion about the existence and reality of a self independent of our experience. This pertains to the existence and reality of a self (as distinguished from mere experience) implying the metaphysical/ ontological domain rather than the phenomenal domain of experience. As they are beyond the scope of this book, I leave those discussions to the philosophers, who may find some inspiration from the view advocated here.

There is, however, much more to consciousness than self and self-perspectival organization. We experience contents in consciousness toward which our experience is directed. This reflects "directedness toward," which signifies what is usually described by the concept of *intentionality* in philosophy. How now can we account for such directedness toward contents in our experience and thus for intentionality? This will be the focus of Chapter 25.

CHAPTER 25
Resting State Activity and Preintentional Organization

Summary

So far, I have discussed the resting-state activity to show a self-specific organization and how this manifests itself during stimulus-induced activity in our experience of a sense of self and self-specificity. Thereby experience is directed toward objects or events in consciousness. This is described as "directedness toward" or "intentionality" in the philosophical debate. What are the neuronal mechanisms underlying intentionality? This is the focus in the present chapter. Recent findings show a neural activity balance between the midline network and the lateral cortical network. Both networks are anticorrelated with each other in their degree of neural activity and functional connectivity. Moreover, it has been shown that the two neural networks are associated with distinct forms of awareness: Internal awareness targeting internal contents is associated with the midline network, while external awareness directed toward external content is rather related to neural activity in the lateral network. How is such directedness toward either internal or external contents possible? I here hypothesize that the relationship between midline and lateral networks is encoded neuronally by their neural differences, thus presupposing difference-based coding on a network level. This is what I describe as the "balance-based hypothesis of contents." The balance-based hypothesis of contents concerns the designation of contents as internal or external, which I suggest depends on the neural balance between midline and lateral networks' activities. I propose that contents designated in this way can well account for the occurrence of external contents during resting-state activity as, for instance, in dreams. The designation of contents as internal or external must be distinguished from the constitution of contents. For that, I propose difference-based coding to be central in that it allows for constituting contents on the basis of encoding differences between different stimuli and their associated activities in the different neural networks. Such difference-based coding must be distinguished from stimulus-based coding that encodes the origin of stimuli from either outside (i.e., environment) or inside (i.e., body and brain) rather than encoding the differences between different stimuli. This amounts to what I describe as "difference-based hypothesis of contents," as distinguished from an "origin-based hypothesis of contents." How does such difference-based coding of contents make possible the "directedness toward" contents in consciousness? I propose the degree of neural difference between the midline-lateral network activity and the rest of the brain's activity, i.e., the other regions and networks to be essential in predisposing directedness toward and thus intentionality on a neural level. Such integration of the midline-lateral balance with the rest of the brain makes it possible to link the various contents to the point of view as constituted by the statistically and spatiotemporally based environment–brain unity (see Chapters 20 and 21 in Part VI). Such linkage between contents and point of view allows the latter, the point of view, to be directed toward the former, the contents in our experience, i.e., consciousness. I therefore postulate what I describe as "point of view–based hypothesis of directedness The "point of view–based hypothesis of directedness" postulates that contents and point of view need to be linked and integrated in order to elicit directedness toward and thus intentionality on the phenomenal level of consciousness. Accordingly, such directedness toward and hence intentionality are already predisposed by the way the resting-state activity is organized and structured, as is well reflected in the environment–brain unity and the difference-based coding of contents. Therefore I characterize the resting-state activity by what I describe as "preintentional organization." The chapter concludes with a neuroconceptual excursion into the philosophical discussion about the concept of intentionality. More specifically, I will discuss what the philosopher J. R. Searle calls "network of preintentional capacities" and how that stands in relation to the here-suggested preintentional organization of the resting state.

Key Concepts and Topics Covered

Internal and external awareness, midline network, lateral network, difference-based coding, neural balance, difference-based hypothesis, origin-based hypothesis, balance-based hypothesis, directedness toward, intentionality, preintentional, network of preintentional capacities

METHODOLOGICAL BACKGROUND
IA: *PHILOSOPHICAL* APPROACH TO INTENTIONALITY

So far I have discussed how the contents of consciousness are assigned different degrees of self-specificity (Chapter 24) and how that is predisposed by the resting state's self-specific organization (Chapter 23). How is the assignment of self-specificity to the stimuli possible? I postulated that the resting state's self-specific organization imposes itself upon the stimuli and links and associates them thereby to itself. However, despite such close linkage between stimuli and resting state on the neuronal level, we are nevertheless able to distinguish between the contents themselves on one hand, and the experience itself, i.e., consciousness, on the other. Rather than being identical with the contents themselves, our experience is directed toward the contents and about them, which philosophically has been described by the concepts "directedness" and "aboutness" as subsumed under the concept of "intentionality." This directedness and aboutness of our experience and thus its intentionality are the topic in the present chapter.

What exactly is meant by the concept of intentionality? There has been much discussion about intentionality in philosophy especially in phenomenological philosophy as established by E. Husserl. He considered the concept of intentionality that describes the "aboutness of mental states" (see F. Brentano) as central to consciousness. The more recent philosophy of mind has picked up the concept of intentionality and considers it a core nucleus of consciousness (see Siewert 2006 for an overview). This is, for instance, suggested by John Searle (2004) whose position will be discussed in more detail at the end of this chapter. However, a more detailed philosophical account of intentionality is beyond the scope of this book and is therefore left to future philosophical (and neurophilosophical) discussion.

METHODOLOGICAL BACKGROUND
IB: *NEUROSCIENTIFIC* APPROACH TO INTENTIONALITY

In addition to philosophy, neuroscience also gained a strong interest in intentionality. Based on medieval-philosophical concepts of intentionality and his own neuroscientific research, the neuroscientist Walter J. Freeman (2003, 2007, 2010) proposes intentionality to be constituted by the neuronal processes of the brain on a prepersonal level. He argues that the prepersonal level of neural activity provides a grid or matrix for the constitution of intentionality in consciousness (see the end of this chapter for more detailed discussion of his position).

Besides the account by Freeman, intentionality has also surfaced in at least four other areas of current neuroscientific research. First, intentionality is central in the neuronal mechanisms underlying action where it has been extensively investigated by Patrick Haggard (see, for instance, Filevich et al. 2012; Brass and Haggard 2010). Our actions are directed toward certain objects in the environment, thus implying intentionality. Second, intentionality is obviously central in the neuronal mechanisms underlying free will. This has first been addressed neuroscientifically by Benjamin Libet (see Libet 2004 for his summary and book). Free will is usually investigated neuroscientifically in close relationship to action and implies directedness and aboutness and thus intentionality (see Haggard 2008). Third, intentionality is also implied by intentions to, for instance, act and make decisions as it has been investigated in decoding techniques of human brain-imaging signals (see, for instance, Haynes 2011; Soon et al. 2008).

Fourth, intentionality is also implicated by the many findings on social interaction as, for instance, manifest in empathy and the kind of neurosocial interactions we described in Chapter 20. Empathy describes the resonance between two different persons' feelings, which has been related to the mirror neurons in the premotor cortex and other regions like the insula and the anterior cingulate (see Fan, Duncan, et al. 2011a). The feelings of one person are apparently directed toward the feelings of another person, with the former being about the latter, thus implying intentionality.

These various lines of research focus on the sufficient neural conditions and thus the neural correlates of intentionality during stimulus-induced activity. They leave open, however, the question of the neuronal mechanisms that make possible and thus predispose the sufficient conditions to instantiate intentionality.

METHODOLOGICAL BACKGROUND
IC: *NEUROPHENOMENAL* APPROACH TO INTENTIONALITY

How must the resting-state activity's spatial and temporal neuronal measures be organized and structured to predispose the constitution of intentionality during subsequent stimulus-induced activity? Rather than discussing the various suggestions for the neural correlates of intentionality, I here focus on the neural predisposition of intentionality.

In addition to its focus on neural predisposition (rather than neural correlate), our approach differs in yet another way from the above-mentioned neuroscientific (and many current philosophical) approaches. Neuroscientific approaches consider intentionality in a purely objective sense, as one can observe it in third-person perspective. This implies that they neglect the subjective-experiential component: they do not consider the way we

subjectively experience directedness toward content and thus intentionality in the first-person perspective of consciousness. The main target is here the subjective-experiential component of intentionality.

How can we subjectively experience directedness toward contents in our consciousness? To address this question, I focus on the resting-state activity itself and the specific spatiotemporal organization of its neural activity, rather than on stimulus-induced activity as do the above-mentioned neuroscientific approaches.

NEUROPHENOMENAL BACKGROUND IA: "EASY" AND "HARD" CASES OF INTENTIONALITY DURING *STIMULUS-INDUCED ACTIVITY*

The neurophenomenal approach aims to focus on the brain's resting-state activity and argues that it has a central role, namely a predisposing one, for making intentionality possible. How can we address and investigate the relationship between intentionality and the brain's resting-state activity? To explain that, I start with the occurrence of intentionality during both resting state and stimulus-induced activity. Intentionality concerns contents that can be either external or internal. Let us start with the external contents.

External contents are associated with the environment, like events, objects, or persons. We are exposed to exteroceptive stimuli from the environment whose associated external contents we experience in an intentional way. The stimulus-induced activity is here accompanied by intentionality toward external contents. The occurrence of intentionality and its external contents can be inferred from the presence of the external stimuli and their stimulus-induced activity. Therefore, I here speak of an "easy" case of intentionality during stimulus-induced activity.

However, things may go differently, too. Even during the exposure to exteroceptive stimuli, our intentionality may nevertheless be directed toward internal contents like our own thoughts. While reading these lines, you are exposed to exteroceptive stimuli, and your brain yields stimulus-induced activity. Despite the stimulus-induced activity, your intentionality though is not directed toward this book as external content, but rather toward your own thoughts as internal contents. This is called "mind wandering" in current psychology.

How is such directedness toward internal contents in the presence of exteroceptive stimuli and their related stimulus-induced activity possible? The occurrence of both internal contents and intentionality can no longer be inferred from the exteroceptive stimuli and their stimulus-induced activity, which would predispose only external, but not internal, contents. The explanation is thus much more difficult, for which reason I speak of a "hard" case of intentionality during stimulus-induced activity (see Table 25-1).

The stimulus-induced activity alone seems to be insufficient here to account for the occurrence of intentionality as being directed toward internal contents. We must therefore bring in some additional factor to explain, first, the internal contents themselves, and second, the intentionality toward internal rather than external contents. In order to do so, I postulate that we need to go back to the resting-state activity itself.

Neurophenomenal Background IB: "Easy" and "Hard" Cases of Intentionality During *Resting-State Activity*

In addition to intentionality during stimulus-induced activity, we also experience intentionality during the resting state itself. For instance, while you are asleep and your brain is in a resting state, you dream; and your dreams are full of contents. The contents can concern your own thoughts, which are thus internal contents. You dream about your own images and thoughts, and your dream experience is directed toward them. There is thus intentionality toward internal contents during the resting state and its absence of external stimuli. Here, the internal contents must stem somehow from the resting-state activity itself. This is the "easy" case of intentionality during resting-state activity.

Nothing, however, is easy when it comes to the brain and consciousness. Even in the absence of any external stimuli and stimulus-induced activity, we can nevertheless experience external contents. Even during dreams, we can experience directedness toward external contents. You may, for instance, hear a voice from your colleague saying to you that you should have not started reading this book. Or you may hear your spouse complaining that you did not clean the kitchen properly and spend all the time working on your papers and books. All that and much more you can experience during dreams. Another instance of the occurrence of external contents during the absence of exteroceptive stimuli are hallucinations, and especially auditory hallucinations,

Table 25-1 "Easy" and "hard" cases of intentionality during stimulus-induced and resting-state activity

	"Easy" case of Intentionality	"Hard" case of Intentionality
Stimulus-induced activity	- *Presence* of *exteroceptive* stimuli - Directedness toward *external* contents **"Usual" state**	- *Presence* of *exteroceptive* stimuli - Directedness toward *internal* contents **Mind wandering**
Resting State activity	- *Absence* of *exteroceptive* stimuli - Directedness toward *internal* contents **"Usual" state**	- *Absence* of *exteroceptive* stimuli - Directedness toward *external* contents **Dreams, Hallucinations**

The table shows the different possible constellations between intentionality and resting state and stimulus-induced activity. Intentionality, as the directedness toward contents in our experience, i.e., consciousness, may occur in both resting-state activity and stimulus-induced activity. It may be directed toward external or internal contents during stimulus-induced activity. Since the directedness toward internal contents in the presence of exteroceptive stimuli, as in mind wandering, can no longer be explained in terms of stimulus-induced activity, I here speak of a "hard" case. The same applies to the occurrence of external contents during resting-state activity with the absence of exteroceptive stimuli, as in dreams, which can be considered the "hard" case of intentionality during resting-state activity.

where one "hears" voices despite the absence of any person speaking.

This is rather puzzling, though. How can we experience external contents with our experience being directed toward them in the absence of any exteroceptive stimulus input? The external contents cannot originate from any external stimuli, because they remain absent in the resting state. We can therefore not revert to stimulus-induced activity to explain the occurrence of external contents during the resting state. I therefore speak of a "hard" case of intentionality during resting-state activity.

How can we solve especially the "hard" case of intentionality during the resting state? I will postulate that we need to go deeply into the mechanisms of how contents are constituted and especially how they are designated as internal or external. We already discussed the neuronal mechanisms of how stimuli are transformed into contents. Several neuronal mechanisms, like binding and binding-by-synchronization, were discussed and postulated to be central in transforming mere stimuli into contents. This was the focus in Chapter 18 and especially Chapter 19.

However, this left open the answer to how the resulting contents can be designated as either internal or external. The "hard" cases of intentionality during both resting state and stimulus-induced activity seem to defy direct association between contents and neural activity: one can apparently not infer internal contents from the resting-state activity, since the occurrence of internal contents during stimulus-induced activity such as in mind wandering should then remain impossible. Conversely, one cannot infer external contents from the stimulus-induced activity either, since the occurrence of external contents during resting-state activity as in dreams should then remain impossible.

The first main focus in this chapter is therefore on the neuronal mechanisms that enable the designation of contents as internal or external. Such a purely neuronal account of the designation of contents will be accompanied by a second, more neurophenomenal, focus: The question here is how those neuronal mechanisms that allow us to associate consciousness and, more

specifically, directedness toward or intentionality to the internal or external contents. Finally, I will briefly put the here-suggested neurophenomenal mechanism of intentionality into a philosophical context by comparing it with the concept of intentionality as suggested by philosopher J. R. Searle.

NEURONAL FINDINGS IA: INTERNAL AND EXTERNAL AWARENESS IN THE RESTING STATE

To investigate directedness and intentionality, I turn to the resting state again. There have been several studies on meditation (see, for instance, Lou et al. 1999; Brewer et al. 2011) and free or random thoughts (see, for instance, Doucet et al. 2012) that all show the midline regions and the default-mode network to be highly active (see also Andrews-Hanna 2012 for a recent review, as well as Andrews-Hanna et al. 2010). Since they all take place in the resting state, these studies presuppose only internal contents like thoughts in the resting state itself. That, however, leaves open whether external contents as associated with the outside world can also occur in the resting state.

This has been tested in a recent study by Vanhaudenhuyse et al. (2011), who directly compared the neuronal mechanisms underlying internal and external contents in the resting state. Vanhaudenhuyse et al. (2011) investigated a group of healthy subjects with both behavioral testing and functional magnetic resonance imaging (fMRI) in the resting state. In the behavioral task, subjects were asked to keep their eyes closed and were presented a tone around every 20 s. After each tone, subjects had to indicate their degree (0–3) of internal (inner speech, autobiographical memories, wandering thoughts) and external (perception of environmental sensory stimuli—auditory, visual, somaesthetic) contents in their awareness (as used more or less synonymously here and in the following with the term "consciousness"). This allowed them to investigate the relation, that is, switches, between internal and external contents in consciousness based on the subjects' own indication.

This behavioral task was followed by an fMRI experiment where subjects were lying in the scanner with eyes closed while not doing any-thing; thus, they were in a resting state. Again they were presented every 20 s with a cue where they had to indicate their degree (moderately, strongly) of awareness of internal and external contents. This allowed the authors to calculate which regions' neural activity was modulated in which way by awareness of either internal or external contents.

NEURONAL FINDINGS IB: NEGATIVE ANTICORRELATING RELATIONSHIP BETWEEN INTERNAL AND EXTERNAL AWARENESS IN THE RESTING STATE

What are the behavioral results? The behavioral data showed that subjects switched around every 28 s (average) between external and internal contents in their awareness. That amounts to a frequency of 0.03/0.05 Hz. This, as the authors themselves remark, corresponds well to the phase duration of the resting state's low-frequency fluctuations. The frequency of the "phenomenal switch" between internal and external contents in awareness may consecutively well reflect the frequency of the "neuronal switch" between the subsequent phases of the resting state's low-frequency fluctuations.

Furthermore, the authors correlated the different degrees of awareness of internal and external contents with each other. This yielded a negative relationship: the stronger the signs that awareness was on internal contents (i.e., speech, memories, thoughts), the less strong was the awareness of external contents (i.e., perceptions of the sensory environment) in the resting state. Such negative relationship obviously implies also the converse, namely that weaker awareness of internal contents goes along with stronger awareness of external contents (see Fig. 25-1).

How were these behavioral data related to the signal changes and thus the neural activity observed in fMRI? The two different degrees (moderately, strongly) of awareness of internal contents correlated linearly with the degree of neuronal activity in various medial/midline regions, for example, the perigenual anterior cingulate cortex, the medial prefrontal

cortex, the posterior cingulate cortex, and the parahippocampal gyrus.

In contrast, neither of these regions showed strong activity during awareness of external contents. Instead, awareness of external contents induced activity in the inferior parietal lobule and lateral prefrontal cortex in a linear way. Interestingly, awareness of internal contents did not elicit any activity here.

NEURONAL FINDINGS IC: INTRINSIC AND EXTRINSIC NEURONAL SYSTEMS

Are these results with the different and (partially) converse involvement of medial and lateral regions during awareness of internal and external contents specific for the resting state? Interestingly, analogous findings have been observed during stimulus-induced activity. Recent imaging studies showed that the awareness of external events and objects in the environment goes along with activation in a lateral fronto-parietal network and sensory regions like the visual and auditory cortex (see Boly et al. 2007a and b, 2008 for a nice review). In contrast, the awareness of internal events as, for instance, in dreaming, daydreaming, mental imagery, and mind wandering seems to recruit regions in especially the midline of the brain, the cortical midline structures being the core regions of the default-mode network (see Mason et al. 2007; Boly et al. 2007a and b, 2008; McKiernan et al. 2006; Goldberg et al. 2006; Golland et al. 2007).

Taken together, these results demonstrate that resting-state activity and stimulus-induced activity can show awareness of both internal and external contents. Both seem to be processed by different neural networks: Awareness of internal contents like one's own internal thoughts, memories, mental events, and so on, seems to be associated with neuronal activity in the anterior and posterior cortical midline structures. Awareness of external contents like events and objects in the environment, in contrast, seems to be more related to neuronal activity in lateral fronto-parietal regions.

Since they are associated with awareness of internal and external contents, both neural

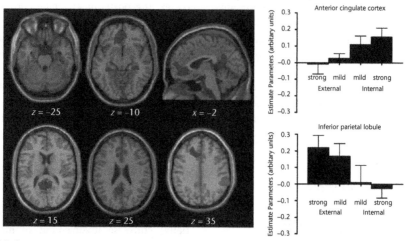

Figure 25-1 Neural activity during internal and external awareness in the resting state. Brain regions showing a correlation between BOLD signal and the intensity of internal and external awareness scores in 22 healthy volunteers. Stronger internal awareness scores correlate with increased activity in anterior cingulate/mesiofrontal, posterior cingulate/precuneal, and parahippocampal cortices (areas in dark gray). External awareness scores correlate with increased activity in bilateral inferior parietal lobule and dorsolateral prefrontal cortices (in light gray). Reprinted with permission of MIT Press, from Vanhaudenhuyse A, Demertzi A, Schabus M, Noirhomme Q, Bredart S, Boly M, Phillips C, Soddu A, Luxen A, Moonen G, Laureys S. Two distinct neuronal networks mediate the awareness of environment and of self. *J Cogn Neurosci.* 2011 Mar;23(3):570–8.

networks have also been described as *intrinsic* and *extrinsic* networks: The intrinsic network concerns mainly the midline regions that seem to be implicated strongly in awareness of internal contents. The extrinsic network, in contrast, refers to the lateral fronto-parietal regions that are apparently implicated in the processing of the awareness of external contents. Interestingly, the distinction between intrinsic and extrinsic networks and their relationship to awareness of internal and external contents seems to hold for both resting-state and stimulus-induced activity.

In addition to intrinsic and extrinsic networks operating across the divide of resting state and stimulus-induced activity, the data also strongly suggest correspondence between behavioral and neuronal levels in two regards. First, the frequency of switches between the awareness of internal and external contents including their respective durations seems to correspond on the behavioral level to the phase duration of the resting state's low-frequency oscillations. There may thus be direct correspondence between

behavioral measures, e.g., duration of awareness of contents, and neuronal measures, e.g., duration of the resting state's low-frequency fluctuations.

Second, what is observed on the behavioral level as negative correlation between awareness of internal and external contents may correspond on the neuronal level to the anticorrelation between the intrinsic, e.g., task-negative networks (e.g., default-mode network including the midline regions) and the extrinsic, e.g., task-positive network (e.g., lateral fronto-parietal network) (see Chapter 1, Volume I, for further details). These findings that the converse relationship between the awareness of internal and external contents seems to correspond to the converse relationship between intrinsic and extrinsic networks. Both neuro-behavioral correspondences shall serve in the following discussion as the starting point to develop neuronal and neurophenomenal hypotheses about the constitution of contents and how they are related to consciousness.

NEURONAL HYPOTHESIS IA: EXTERNAL CONTENTS AND THE BRAIN'S RESTING-STATE ACTIVITY

These findings raise some important questions. First, they show that awareness and phenomenal consciousness can already occur in the resting state itself. We do not need an extrinsic stimulus and consecutively stimulus-induced activity to induce experience and thus consciousness. Instead, this seems to be possible already during the resting state itself. That is well documented in the earlier-described studies as well as during phenomena like dreams and auditory hallucinations (see Chapter 26 for details). We will come back later to explore how such phenomenal consciousness can possibly be constituted during the resting state itself. For now, we will focus more on the contents themselves, how internal and external contents are constituted.

Besides the occurrence of consciousness in the resting state itself, the findings demonstrate yet another remarkable feature. Let us recall that we focused exclusively on the resting state itself. That means that the external stimulus input from the environment remains absent, meaning that the extrinsic sensory input is minimized or zero. Despite such minimization of the external stimulus' input, we nevertheless experience external contents from the environment. This is manifest in the imaginary perception of environmental stimuli (auditory, visual) in the resting state as described as the earlier reported study on the awareness of internal and external contents.

How can we experience external contents like specific objects or events in our consciousness, even though we do not receive the respective external stimulus input from the environment? Simply put, this raises the question of how such external contents come into the resting state such that subsequent consciousness during the resting-state activity itself can be directed toward external contents.

NEURONAL HYPOTHESIS IB: *PARALLEL-SEGREGATED* PROCESSING OF THE NEURAL ACTIVITIES RELATED TO STIMULI AND NETWORKS

How do the external contents of the environment come into the resting state? For that, as I claim, we need to go back to the neuronal level and more specifically the neural relationship between midline and lateral networks. We recall from the earlier described study. External contents were associated with the lateral network, while internal contents were rather related to the midline network.

How are these two neural networks related to each other? I here suggest that different models of their relationship can be conceived: parallel-segregated processing and interactive-integrative processing. Let me start with the parallel-segregated processing in this section. The model of parallel-segregated processing proposes that neural activity in midline and lateral networks is processed in a parallel and segregated way. By the term "parallel" I mean that both networks' neural activities are processed independently of each other. This means that there is no interaction between them so that they remain largely independent of each other. This is complemented by the concept of "segregated" that points out the separation between the two neural networks' neural activities. The neural activities of the two neural networks are constituted in a separate and thus segregated way.

One may now propose such parallel-segregated processing on different levels, which shall be listed briefly in the following discussion while their detailed explanation will be picked up in subsequent sections. First, parallel-segregated processing may operate on the level of stimuli with both internal and external stimuli being processed in a parallel and segregated way. Second, parallel-segregated processing may refer to the processing of neural activity on the level of neural networks, such as midline, e.g., intrinsic, and lateral, e.g., extrinsic networks.

Third, parallel-segregated processing could be proposed to apply to the level of contents, internal and external contents like internal thoughts and external events. Fourth and finally, one may associate parallel-segregated processing with the phenomenal level of consciousness describing whether it is internally or externally directed. In this and the next section I will focus on the first two levels, and I will come back to the third and fourth level in the later sections.

NEURONAL HYPOTHESIS IC: *PARALLEL-SEGREGATED* PROCESSING OF THE NEURAL ACTIVITIES RELATED TO *INTERNAL AND EXTERNAL STIMULI*

Let's start with the parallel-segregated processing of internal and external stimuli. How empirically plausible is the assumption of parallel-segregated processing between internal and external stimuli with regard to the midline and the lateral networks? Internal stimuli are those that originate in either the own body, that is, interoceptive stimuli, or the own brain, that is, neuronal stimuli (see Chapter 4 in Volume I for details), while external stimuli concern exteroceptive stimuli from the environment.

Are now internal and external stimuli processed in an independent and thus parallel way? As we have seen in previous chapters, there is plenty of interaction between internal and external and thus between interoceptive and exteroceptive stimuli going on in all parts of the brain, starting from the subcortical to the cortical regions. This makes it rather unlikely that internal and external stimuli are processed independently of each other with no interaction between them and thus in a purely parallel way.

How about segregated processing and thus separate constitution of the neural activity related to internal and external stimuli? There is strong convergence in anatomical connections between the external sensory inputs from the different sensory cortices and the interoceptive inputs from regions like the insula and subcortical regions like the periaqueductal gray (PAG). This concerns especially the anterior midline regions like the perigenual anterior cingulate cortex (PACC) and the ventromedial prefrontal cortex (VMPFC), while it also holds for the lateral cortical regions like the dorsolateral prefrontal cortex, where the exteroceptive input seems to predominate. Such anatomical convergence makes it rather unlikely that the neural activity in, for instance, the midline regions is constituted solely and exclusively on the basis of internal stimuli alone. The same holds for the lateral network's neural activity that analogously may not be traced back to external stimuli exclusively (see Fig. 25-2a).

That needs to be more detailed below with regard to the recent fMRI results. An external stimulus induces increase in signal changes, that is, an activation, in fMRI in the lateral network as, for instance, in lateral prefrontal cortex. At the same time the very same external stimulus also elicits signal changes in the midline regions like the perigenual anterior cingulate cortex and the ventromedial prefrontal cortex. More specifically, the external stimulus induces decrease in signal changes, so-called deactivation, in fMRI (see Northoff et al. 2004; and Goel and Dolan 2003, for details as well as the earlier mentioned studies).

Interestingly the same holds in the case of internal stimuli (from the body) that also induce signal changes in both midline and lateral networks but in a reverse way: here less deactivation or even activation is induced in the midline regions which goes along with lower degrees of activation in the lateral regions (see Northoff et al. 2004; Wiebking et al. 2010).

Taken together, these data suggest that the neural activities in the two networks are not processed completely independently of each other and thus in a segregated way. Why? Because then the external stimulus should not induce activity changes in the midline network in the same way as the internal stimulus should not elicit signal changes in the lateral regions. There is thus no independence between the two neural networks in their processing of internal and external stimuli. Instead, both types of stimuli seem to induce activity changes in both neural networks. (One may now want to argue that this was not the case in the study by Vanhaudenhuyse et al. 2011 as described earlier. Since the study was conducted in the resting state, it may simply be that the activity changes in the respective other networks were too small to be detected.)

NEURONAL HYPOTHESIS ID: *PARALLEL-SEGREGATED* PROCESSING AND ANTICORRELATION BETWEEN *MEDIAL AND LATERAL NETWORKS'* NEURAL ACTIVITIES

How about the segregation between the two networks? One most consistent finding is that the two networks' neural activities anticorrelate with each other. This has been demonstrated for the

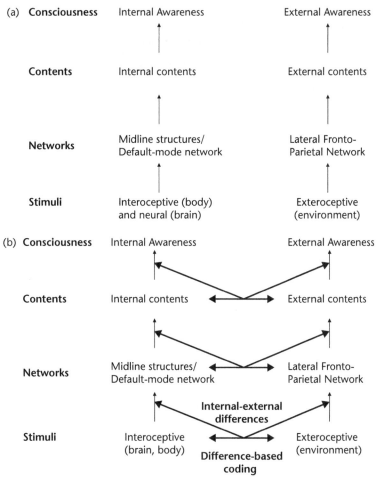

Figure 25-2a-d Relationship between midline and lateral networks. The figure shows different forms of processing between midline and lateral cortical networks (*a* and *b*) and how the two networks are related to each other (*c* and *d*). (*a*) The figure illustrates the model of parallel-integrated processing. Internal and external stimuli (lowest level) are processed in parallel and segregated in midline and lateral cortical networks (second level from bottom). This leads to internal and external contents (third level from bottom) and ultimately to internal and external awareness (highest level). (*b*) The figure illustrates the model of interactive-integrative processing. Internal and external stimuli (lowest level) are processed in difference and thus relative to each other. These differences are processed in midline and lateral cortical networks (second level from bottom) though in opposite ways. The designation of contents as internal or external is then no longer based on the origin of the stimuli but rather on the degree of difference (third level from bottom) with the same holding for internal and external awareness (highest level). (*c*) The figure illustrates the relationship between the degree of differences encoded into neural activity and the degree of anticorrelation between midline and lateral cortical networks: the larger the differences encoded into the neural activities of each network, the larger their degree of anticorrelation. (*d*) The figure illustrates the dependence of the neural activities in both midline and lateral cortical networks on the difference between intero- and exteroceptive stimuli: the stronger exteroceptive stimuli are when compared to interoceptive ones, the larger the degree of differences encoded into the neural activities of both midline and lateral networks (though in opposite, i.e., negative and positive ways), and the stronger the neural activity changes in lateral (i.e., more positive) and midline (i.e., more negative) in midline cortical networks.

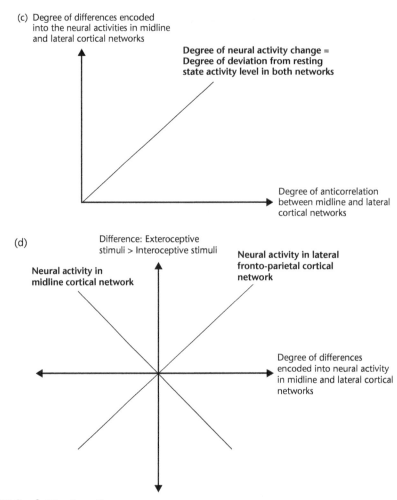

Figure 25-2a-d (Continued)

degree of stimulus-related signal changes as well as for resting state functional connectivity (see Chapter 4, Volume I, for details).

Let us start with the stimulus-related signal changes. Higher negative signal changes in the midline regions, that is, deactivation, go along with higher positive signal changes in the lateral networks, that is, activation, and vice versa (see the earlier-described study as well as Northoff et al. 2004 and Goel and Dolan 2003 for details). There is thus what we called "reciprocal modulation" (Northoff et al. 2004; Bermpohl et al. 2009) that well mirrors anticorrelation. Besides signal changes, anticorrelation also holds for functional connectivity in the resting state: higher positive values in functional connectivity within the midline network going along with more negative indices of functional connectivity in the lateral network (see, for instance, Fox et al. 2005 and Beckmann et al. 2006 as well as Chapter 4, Volume I).

Such anticorrelation between midline and lateral networks makes the assumption of segregated processing of internal and external stimuli rather unlikely, however. If the two networks' neural activities are anticorrelated, neither can constitute its neural activity separate from the respective other. That puts the assumption of segregated and more generally parallel-segregated processing between midline and lateral networks into doubt. And makes necessary the search for a different way of neural processing.

NEURONAL HYPOTHESIS IIA: *INTERACTIVE-INTEGRATIVE* PROCESSING BETWEEN THE NEURAL ACTIVITIES RELATED TO *INTERNAL AND EXTERNAL STIMULI*

We saw that the model of parallel-segregated processing is not empirically plausible on both levels stimuli and networks. We may therefore need to propose a different model. I here suggest the model of "interactive-integrative processing."". What kind of neural processing does the model of interactive-integrative processing suggest? Rather than being processed in parallel with no interaction, one may propose interaction in the neural processing between, for instance, internal and external stimuli or between midline and lateral networks. Hence, the term "interaction" is here determined by dependence of neural activity, while the term "integrative" denotes the constitution of neural activity. Neural activity may be based no longer on the specific stimulus or network alone but may rather result from the integration of different stimuli or networks. As in the case of parallel-segregated processing, the model of interactive-integrative processing may apply to both levels of stimuli and networks (see Fig. 25-2b).

Is such an interactive-integrative model empirically plausible on the level of stimuli? I already mentioned the anatomical convergence between internal and external stimulus' input in both midline and lateral networks. This is complemented on the functional level by assuming difference-based coding rather than stimulus-based coding. Simply put, stimulus-based coding means that, for instance, external stimuli are encoded into neural activity on the basis of the respective external stimulus alone. In contrast, difference-based coding describes that the single stimulus, be it internal or external, is encoded into neural activity on the basis of its relationship or difference to other stimuli, including both external and internal (see Volume I for details).

I gathered plenty of empirical evidence for difference-based coding of both internal and external stimuli in Volume II. In contrast to difference-based coding, stimulus-based coding seems to be rather empirically implausible. Neural activity is thus difference rather than stimulus based. When we associate neural activity with an internal stimulus, the observed neural activity must thus be proposed to be based on the difference and thus the integration of that particular interoceptive stimulus with the exteroceptive stimuli in its respective context.

What does such difference-based coding imply for the possible distinction between internal and external stimuli? There is no principal distinction between internal and external stimuli within the neural activity itself possible anymore. Instead of separating internal and external stimuli in neural activity, we may need to distinguish between different degrees of differences between different stimuli (including both intero- and exteroceptive stimuli) as encoded into neural activity. These differences that are encoded into neural activity presuppose the interaction and integration between internal and external stimuli, thus mirroring what I describe above as interactive-integrative processing.

NEURONAL HYPOTHESIS IIB: *INTERACTIVE-INTEGRATIVE* PROCESSING BETWEEN *MEDIAL AND LATERAL NETWORKS' NEURAL ACTIVITIES*

How about interactive-integrative processing on the network level? We already discussed the anticorrelation holding between the midline and the lateral networks. How is such anticorrelation possible? This is possible only, as I claim, if the neural activities in both networks are based on their difference rather than on each network alone. I thus propose difference-based coding to also hold on the level of networks. This needs to be explained in further detail. We recall from Volume I that I proposed difference-based coding to hold on the cellular and population level of neural activity (see Chapter 1, Volume I). This was then extended to the biochemical level (see Chapter 2) and the regional level (see Chapter 3) of neural activity. Now however I go one step further and propose difference-based coding to also hold on the level of the neural network. This means that the neural activity of, for instance, the midline network and its resting-state activity level and degree of functional connectivity are coded in direct relationship to the lateral network. What we observe as neural activity level and degree of functional connectivity in the midline regions may not stem only from the midline regions themselves. Instead, what we observe in the midline network may rather be related to the difference between the midline's actual state and that of the lateral network. In short, the midline network's neural activity may stem from its difference from the lateral network.

The same holds true, of course, for the lateral network. As the midline network, the lateral network codes its neural activity level and degree of functional connectivity in relationship and thus difference to the one of the midline network. Hence, both networks do exactly the same thing: the midline codes its neural activity in difference to the lateral one in very much the same way the lateral network codes its neural activity relative to the midline regions. If so, both networks' neural activities and functional connectivity's must be reciprocally and thus negatively related to each other. And this is exactly what one observes in the often reported anticorrelation between midline and lateral networks.

Let me reiterate the same point in a slightly different way. The two networks' neural activities are coded in direct dependence to each other. Therefore, the neural activities we observe cannot be taken as "absolute" activities of the network itself in isolation from the ones of the respective other network. Instead, both networks show "relative" activities, reflecting the networks' stand or relationship to the respective other network. How is such mutual encoding between the two networks' activities possible? I propose this to be possible only on the basis of difference-based coding between the two networks' activities. The observed pattern of "relative" activities can be explained only, if the neural activity of (for instance) the midline network is encoded relative to and thus in difference from the one of the lateral network and vice versa. Such difference-based coding on the network level must be distinguished from mere stimulus-based coding where the neural activities of each network would be encoded

in an independent and absolute rather than dependent and relative way. Unlike in the case of difference-based coding, stimulus-based coding could not account for the observation of the earlier-described "relative activities," including the anticorrelation. This leads me to suggest the following neuronal hypothesis about the relationship between difference-based coding and the anticorrelation between the two networks. I propose the degree of anticorrelation between midline and lateral networks to be dependent on the degree of their differences as they are encoded into the networks' neural activities. The larger the differences encoded into their neural activities, the larger the two networks' activities will anticorrelate with each other. In contrast, smaller differences will lead to lower degrees of anticorrelation and consequently to smaller degrees of neural activity changes in both networks (see Fig. 25-2c).

Neuronal Hypothesis
IIC: Relationship between Stimuli and Networks

How are now the two levels stimuli and networks related to each other? As the literature shows, we often tend to associate internal stimuli (and internal contents) with the midline network, while external stimuli (and contents) are usually related to the lateral network. My assumption of interactive-integrative processing on both levels, stimuli and networks, sheds a different light, however.

I suggest a direct relationship between the stimulus level and the level of network, with their relationship being mediated by difference-based coding. More specifically, I propose that the degree of differences as they are encoded into the networks' neural activities is dependent on the relationship between internal and external stimuli. The larger the input of internal stimuli relative to the external stimulus' input, the more positive the difference that is encoded into the midline's neural activity and the more negative the difference encoded into the lateral network's activity.

Obviously the converse holds if the external stimulus' input predominates over the internal stimulus' input. The larger the input of external stimuli relative to the internal stimulus' input, the more positive (or the less negative) the difference that is encoded into the lateral network's neural activity and the more negative (or less positive) the difference encoded into the midline network's activity (see Fig. 25-2d).

This is well in accordance with the earlier described reciprocal modulation and anticorrelation between midline and lateral networks. The degree of anticorrelation is consequently signified by the degree of either positive or negative difference: the larger the difference value, whether positive or negative, the larger the degree of the anticorrelation between midline and lateral networks. However, future studies are needed to lend direct support for the proposed dependence of the degree of the medial-lateral network anticorrelation on the balance between internal and external stimulus input.

How is such a difference-based linkage between stimulus and network level related to the model of interactive-integrative processing? Metaphorically speaking, one may describe the situation in the following way: The midline activity level and its (internal and external) stimulus input reflect how the midline network itself "sees" (or "perceives") its relationship to the lateral network. In contrast, the lateral activity and its (internal and external) stimulus input reflect how the lateral network, from its particular "perspective," "sees" or "perceives" itself in relation to its respective context, the midline network. If now one network "perceives" itself stronger and yields more activity (when compared to the other one), the respective other cannot but "perceive" and "see" itself as weaker (when compared to the other one). Neural activities and consecutively "strength and weakness" are thus considered in a relative and context-dependent way.

NEURONAL HYPOTHESIS IIIA: FROM DIFFERENCE-BASED CODING OF STIMULI TO INTERNAL AND EXTERNAL CONTENTS

So far, I have described interactive-integrative processing only on the level of stimuli and networks, while I left open the level of contents and

consciousness. I now want to focus on the level of contents and more specifically on the neuronal mechanisms that allow for the constitution of contents and their subsequent designation as *internal* or *external*.

Why do I distinguish between contents and stimuli? We experience contents in consciousness like objects, persons, or events. In contrast, we do not experience the single stimuli themselves that form the respective contents. The single stimulus is always integrated within a particular content in consciousness; a *phenomenal content*, as the philosophers say. The constitution of the contents themselves (independently of their association with consciousness; see later for that) will be the focus in this and the next sections.

We already touched upon the issue of contents in previous chapters. For instance, the constitution of contents was discussed in the context of the binding problem that describes how different stimuli are tied and linked together into one object or event, for example, the content (see Chapter 18). In addition to the constitution of content, we also distinguished the *selection* of contents, meaning which of the constituted contents are selected for consciousness to become phenomenal contents. We proposed the selection of contents to be dependent upon the regional distribution of pre-stimulus resting-state activity levels (see Chapter 19).

However, we left open the question of the exact neuronal mechanisms underlying the constitution of contents. We just proposed that different stimuli are tied and linked together without showing the neuronal mechanisms underlying such linkage. This is the focus in the present section. The often rather tacit assumption is that the internal contents of consciousness can be traced back to internal stimuli from the own body and the brain. In contrast, the external contents of consciousness are tacitly presupposed to be related to external stimuli from the environment.

This, however, is not empirically plausible given the earlier-discussed interactive-integrative processing between internal and external stimuli. Instead of being traced back to internal stimuli alone, internal contents may need to be traced back to the difference between internal and external stimuli. And the same holds true for external contents that must be based on the difference between external and internal stimuli, rather than on the external stimuli alone. This is rather puzzling, however. The constitution of both internal and external contents is based on the difference between internal and external stimuli, rather than on the respective stimuli alone. Since both stimuli are no longer processed separately, distinction between internal and external stimuli should remain impossible. One would then assume that there is only the *type* of content, difference-based content, which then can be neither internal nor external. This, however, contradicts our conceptual distinction as well as our phenomenal experience, wherein we are quite able to distinguish between internal and external contents.

NEURONAL HYPOTHESIS
IIIB: "*DIFFERENCE*-BASED HYPOTHESIS OF CONTENTS" VERSUS "*ORIGIN*-BASED HYPOTHESIS OF CONTENTS"

How can we distinguish between internal and external contents at all? For that answer, one may go back to the different coding strategies I discussed above. Difference-based coding claims that the brain encodes differences between stimuli, rather than single stimuli, including their origins, being encoded into neural activity. This contrasts with stimulus-based coding where the single stimulus and thus its origin are supposed to be encoded into neural activity (see Volume I for details).

Let us put difference-based coding into the context of the constitution of contents out of stimuli. In the case of internal contents, one would propose the internal stimuli to be relatively stronger than the external ones, while in the case of external contents, external stimuli may predominate over internal stimuli. The difference between internal and external contents amounts, then, to different balances in the relationship between internal and external stimuli; as described earlier, contents are then encoded into neural activity in a difference-based rather than origin-based

way. Conceptually, one may then more properly speak of external(-internal) contents and internal(-external) contents (from which for the sake of simplicity I refrain). This is what I describe as the "difference-based hypothesis of contents" (see Fig. 25-3a).

The difference-based hypothesis of contents proposes that the constitution of contents in consciousness is based on the encoding of difference between different stimuli into neural activity rather than on the single stimuli themselves. This means that the origin that signifies the single stimuli, e.g., whether their origin is internal in one's own body/brain or external in the environment, is no longer as relevant in the constitution of contents. Instead, what matters is the difference between different stimuli, regardless of their origin.

The "difference-based hypothesis of contents" determines what matters for the brain's encoding of stimuli and their respective contents into its neural activity. Rather than the stimuli themselves and their respective origins, it is the difference between different stimuli across their different origins in either body/brain or environment that matters for the brain's encoding and generation of neural activity. Most important, the "difference-based hypothesis of contents" implies the rejection of what may be called the "origin-based hypothesis of contents." In that case, the brain would "care" very much about the origin of the stimuli and would then encode the single stimuli, including their origins, into its neural activity. This presupposes stimulus-based coding (rather than difference-based coding).

The "origin-based hypothesis of contents," however, contradicts both how the brain encodes its neural activity (see Volume I) and our phenomenal experience. Accordingly, to put it simply, all the brain seems to "care" about is the degree of differences between different stimuli it has to process and accommodate. In contrast, the brain does not seem "care" so much about where these differences and the underlying stimuli come from, e.g., from either brain, body, or environment. This though makes the "origin-based hypothesis of contents" rather implausible in empirical regard.

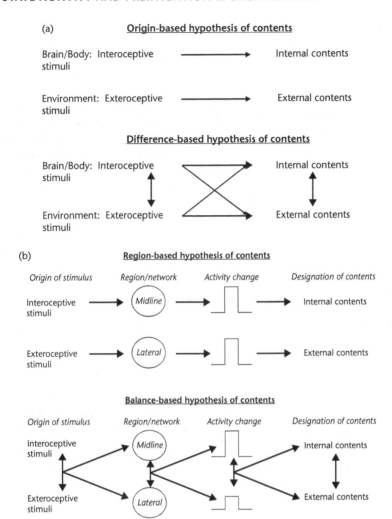

Figure 25-3a and b Constitution and designation of content. The figure shows different features in the constitution of contents, whether they are processed on the basis of their origin (*a*) or networks (*b*). (*a*) The figure illustrates two alternative hypotheses in the constitution of contents being either origin based (*upper part*) or difference based (*lower part*). In the origin-based processing (*upper part*), contents are designated as internal or external as based on the origin of intero- and exteroceptive stimuli in either brain/body (interoceptive) or environment (exteroceptive). This is different in the difference-based hypotheses (*lower part*). Here contents are based on the difference between intero- and exteroceptive stimuli rather than on their respective origins in either body/brain or environment. The designation of contents as internal or external no longer depends on the origin of the underlying stimuli but rather on the degree of their difference. (*b*) The figure illustrates two alternative hypotheses in the neural processing of contents being either region/network based (*upper part*) or balance based (*lower part*). In the region/network-based processing (*upper part*), internal and external contents can be traced back to the degree of activity in their respectively underlying network, that is, midline and lateral, whose activity depends on the degree of intero- and exteroceptive stimulus input. Strong interoceptive stimulus input strongly activates the midline network and that, in turn, leads to internal contents. The same holds for the lateral network with regard to exteroceptive stimuli and external contents. The balance-based hypothesis (*lower part*) proposes that the degree of neural activity in midline and lateral networks is based on the difference between intero- and exteroceptive stimuli. The difference between the two networks does, in turn, determine the designation of contents as either internal or external. Hence, the designation of contents is here no longer based on the neural activity in a particular network or region but rather on their neural balance.

Neuronal Hypothesis IIIc: *"Balance Hypothesis of Contents"* versus *"Region/Network*-Based Hypothesis of Contents"

How is such constitution of contents related to the midline and lateral networks, which, as the earlier-described findings demonstrate, seem to be central? Internal contents seem to be more related to the midline network, while external contents are rather associated with the lateral network. Do we therefore need to propose that the difference-based coding on the level of stimuli is neurally associated with exclusively one network, the midline or the lateral network? If that holds, one would propose that difference-based coding of internal contents is associated with the midline network, whereas difference-based coding of external contents is related to the lateral network.

However, such exclusive association of the two networks with the two contents, internal and external, is not in accordance with their interactive-integrative processing. Earlier I proposed difference-based coding between the two networks to hold. This means that the neural activity in, for instance, the midline network results from the integral and thus the difference between the actual midline's activity level and the one in the lateral network. The converse also holds for the lateral network whose activity level is determined in difference to the one in the midline network.

What does this imply for the contents associated with the neural activity in the two networks? The neural processing of contents in the two networks may very much depend on their balance rather than on the activity in each of the two networks and their respective regions. Whether a content is designated as internal or external may not so much depend on the neural activity and functional connectivity within the midline network alone but rather on its balance to the lateral network.

The neural balance between midline and lateral networks rather than the activity of each network alone may therefore be the determining factor in whether a content is designated as internal or external. This amounts to what I describe as the "balance hypothesis of contents." The balance-based hypothesis of contents describes the designation of contents as internal or external to be dependent upon the neural balance between different networks, the midline and the lateral network.

How would a possible alternative thesis look like? The alternative thesis to the "balance hypothesis of contents" would be that the designation of contents as internal or external may be dependent upon the neural activity in only one particular network. For instance, internal contents would then be related to the midline network alone, while external contents would be associated exclusively with the lateral (and the sensory) network(s). Instead of their relative activity level to each other being central, the absolute level of activity in each network would determine the respective content. This would amount to what may be called a "region/network-based hypothesis of contents" (see Fig. 25-3b).

Neuronal Hypothesis IIId: *"Difference*-Based Hypothesis of Contents" Provides the *Basis or Fundament* for the "*Balance* Hypothesis of Contents"

Which hypothesis is now more empirically plausible? We earlier described the anticorrelation between midline and lateral networks. And interestingly, such anticorrelation was not only observed on the neuronal level but also on the behavioral level with a switch between internal and external contents. The stronger and the more often the internal contents occurred, the weaker and less often the external contents were present.

Accordingly, the anticorrelation on the neural level (between the two networks) seems to accompany an anticorrelation on the level of contents. Since anticorrelation can be observed on both the neural level of networks and the behavioral level of contents, one would propose the designation of contents to depend on the balance between the two neural networks rather than on one of the networks alone. This speaks strongly in favor of the "balance-based hypothesis of contents" rather than the "region/network-based hypothesis of contents."

Earlier, we proposed the "difference-based hypothesis of contents" that proposes contents to be related to the difference between different stimuli, regardless of their origin, rather than to single stimuli and their specific origin. What, then, is the difference between the "difference-based hypothesis of contents" and the here-postulated "balance-based hypothesis of contents"? The difference-based hypothesis of contents concerns stimuli and how they are constituted into contents. In contrast, the balance-based hypothesis of contents is more related to the contents themselves and how they are designated as either internal or external.

In sum, the "difference-based hypothesis of contents" is about the neuronal mechanisms underlying the constitution of contents (out of stimuli). In contrast, the "balance-based hypothesis" targets the neuronal mechanisms involved in the designation of contents (as internal or external). Despite their differences, both hypotheses obviously built on each other with the balance-based hypothesis of contents standing on the shoulders of the difference-based hypothesis of contents.

NEURONAL HYPOTHESIS IVA: "EASY" AND "HARD" CASES OF CONTENTS IN THE *RESTING STATE*

How can we now differentiate between internal and external contents? Rather than distinguishing them on the basis of either internal or external stimuli and their different origins, we associated them with different degrees of differences between internal and external stimuli. This is what the difference-based hypothesis of contents tells us. And we can also distinguish them on the basis of the neural balance between midline and lateral networks rather than associating them with one particular region or network. That is suggested by the balance-based hypothesis of contents.

How, then, does such a distinction between internal and external contents relate to the neuronal distinction between resting-state activity and stimulus-induced activity? Usually, internal contents are associated with resting-state activity, while stimulus-induced activity is related

to external contents. That, however, is put into doubt by the occurrence of external contents during resting-state activity as observed in the earlier described study on internal and external awareness in the resting state.

The association of external contents with stimulus-induced activity is equally put into doubt by the occurrence of external contents from the environment in, for instance, dreams during the absence of external stimuli. When we sleep, our brain is supposedly at rest, encountering a minimum (if not complete absence) of external stimuli from the environment. Despite the absence or minimum of external stimuli from the environment, we nevertheless experience external contents in our consciousness when dreaming.

Even more puzzling is the case of auditory hallucination in schizophrenia. These patients hear concrete voices in the absence of any auditory stimulus input. How is that possible? This is the "hard" case of contents (and ultimately of intentionality; see earlier) that describes the presence of external contents in the absence of external stimuli, such as during the resting state.

Such a "hard" case needs to be distinguished from an "easy" case of contents (and ultimately intentionality; see earlier) that refers to the presence of internal contents in the presence of internal stimuli in the resting state. How can we explain the "hard" case of contents? This is the focus in the following neuronal hypotheses.

NEURONAL HYPOTHESIS IVB: *"ORIGIN*-BASED HYPOTHESIS OF CONTENTS" *CANNOT* ACCOUNT FOR THE "HARD" CASE IN THE *RESTING STATE*

Let us go back to our hypotheses, and more specifically, to what we earlier described as the "origin-based hypothesis of contents." The "origin-based hypothesis of contents" describes that the constitution of contents is based on the origin of the respectively implicated stimuli, i.e., whether they originate from brain/body or environment. This "origin-based hypothesis of contents" was contrasted with a "difference-based hypothesis of contents" where contents were proposed to result from the differences between different stimuli (regardless of their origin), rather than to the single stimuli and their respective origins.

How do "origin- and difference-based hypotheses of contents" stand in relation to the neural distinction between resting state and stimulus-induced activity? Let us starts with the "origin-based hypothesis of contents." An origin-based hypothesis of contents can well account for the occurrence of internal contents in the resting state: internal input from body and brain is still present in the resting state and may therefore account for the occurrence of internal contents. This occurrence of internal contents during the brain's resting-state activity can thus be easily accounted for; therefore, I speak of an "easy" case.

How about the occurrence of external contents in the resting state, such as during dreams and auditory hallucinations? In that case the "origin-based hypothesis of contents" may run into serious problems: if external contents were constituted on the basis of external stimuli alone and their origin in the environment, the latter's absence in the resting state should go along with complete absence of external contents during rest.

That, however, is not the case, as was documented by the above-mentioned study and the examples of dreams and auditory hallucinations. Hence, the origin-based hypothesis of contents fails to account for the occurrence of external contents in the resting state. Since the occurrence of external contents during the resting-state activity cannot be as easily explained by the "origin-based hypothesis of contents" as the occurrence of internal contents, one may speak here of a "hard case."

NEURONAL HYPOTHESIS IVC: *"DIFFERENCE-BASED HYPOTHESIS OF CONTENTS" CAN ACCOUNT FOR THE "HARD" CASE IN THE RESTING STATE*

How about the difference-based hypothesis of contents? We recall that the "difference-based hypothesis of contents" proposes contents in general, and thus also internal contents in the resting state, to be based on the encoding of the difference between internal and external stimuli. In the case of internal stimuli, they are relatively stronger and predominate over the external ones. That is when we experience internal contents in the resting state as, for instance, random thoughts. This is the "easy case" of the resting state, as described above.

How about the "hard case" that concerns the occurrence of external contents in the resting state where external stimuli are absent? This leads us to the question of how external contents can be yielded on the basis of the encoding of differences in the resting state. I would propose the following: The stimulus input from body and brain during the resting state may become weaker, that is, relatively weaker when compared to the stimulus input from the environment, so that their balance or relationship changes.

The change in their relationship or balance may now take on a negative score, signifying that the balance is shifted toward the stimulus input from the environment. This means that the respective content is designated as external rather than internal—the subsequent experience and thus intentionality will consequently be directed toward external contents in the resting state. I consequently propose the occurrence of external contents in the resting state to stem from changes in the stimulus input from body and brain, i.e., from interoceptive and neural stimuli, rather than from the occurrence of stimuli in the environment, i.e., exteroceptive stimuli. This is a testable hypothesis that can be investigated in the future in, for instance, auditory hallucinations and dreams.

Awaiting further empirical support, the "difference-based hypothesis of contents" and its sibling, the "balance-hypothesis of contents" can well account for the occurrence of external contents in the resting state, which I considered the "hard case." This gives the "difference-based hypothesis of contents" an advantage over the "origin-based hypothesis of contents" that cannot account for the "hard case," i.e., the occurrence of external contents in the resting state (see Fig. 25-4a).

I proposed difference-based coding between internal and external stimulus input to hold during the resting state, which entailed the "difference-based hypothesis of content." This presupposes the occurrence of external stimulus input in the resting state. That sounds paradoxical, however, since the resting state is usually characterized by the absence of external stimulus input.

Why is the external stimulus input so important? Without external stimulus input, difference-based coding would become impossible: there would be no external stimulus

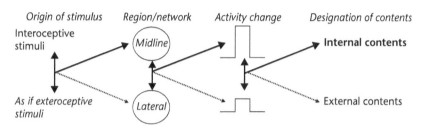

(a)   'Easy case': Constitution of <u>internal</u> contents (free or random thoughts)

'Hard case': Constitution of <u>external</u> contents (dreams, hallucinations)

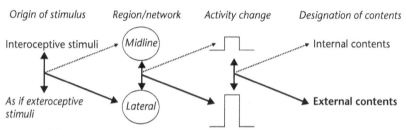

Figure 25-4a and b "Easy" and "hard" cases. The figure shows "easy" and "hard" cases in the constitution of internal and external contents in the resting-state (*a*) and stimulus-induced activity (*b*). (*a*) *Upper part*: "Easy case": Constitution of *internal* contents (free or random thoughts) during *resting state activity. Lower part*: "Hard case: Constitution of external contents (dreams, hallucinations) during *resting state activity.* The figure illustrates the constitution of external and internal contents in the resting state. Based on the difference- and balance-based hypothesis, both internal and external contents can be constituted in the resting state. The explanation of internal contents like free or random thoughts is the "easy case," while external contents are harder to account for, thus being the "hard case" (as in dreams or hallucinations). The figure illustrates that the two types of contents reflect different differences between intero- and exteroceptive stimuli and different balances between midline and lateral networks' activities. The degree of differences and balances determines whether the content will be designated as either internal or external. (*b*) *Upper part*: "Easy case": Constitution of *external* contents (perception) during *stimulus-induced activity. Lower part*: "Hard case": Constitution of *external* contents (mind wandering) during *stimulus-induced activity.* The figure illustrates the constitution of external and internal contents during stimulus-induced activity. Based on the difference- and balance-based hypothesis, both internal and external contents can be constituted during stimulus-induced activity. The explanation of external contents as in perception is the "easy case," while internal contents are harder to account for, thus being the "hard case" (as in mind wandering). The figure illustrates that the two types of contents reflect different differences between intero- and exteroceptive stimuli and different balances between midline and lateral networks' activities. The degree of differences and balances determines whether the content will be designated as either internal or external.

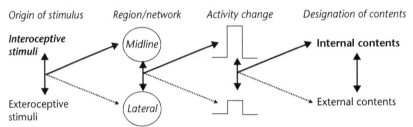

Figure 25-4a and b (Continued)

input against which the internal stimuli could be compared in order to yield spatial and temporal differences between different stimuli for the encoding of neural activity, as postulated by difference-based coding. Difference-based coding would then become impossible, which also would make the "difference-based hypothesis of contents" futile, at least in the case of the resting state.

Accordingly, if we nevertheless want to apply the "difference-based hypothesis of contents" to the resting state, we need to search for some kind of external stimulus input, or at least an analogue of it, into the brain's resting-state activity. This shall be the focus in this section. Let us start with the resting state itself.

The concept of the "resting state" is a purely operational definition that is used to operationalize the brain's intrinsic activity in experimental paradigms (see Chapter 4, Volume I). As such, it implies nothing about the presence or absence of particular stimuli. And, indeed, as discussed in Chapters 4 through 6, there is exteroceptive stimulus input already in the resting state, since even during eyes closed as in sleep, the other four sensory modalities (auditory, olfactory, gustatory, tactile) are still "open" and processing

external stimuli from the environment. Such continuous sensory input may, for instance, be relevant in the constitution of external contents, especially during dreams in sleep (see Chapter 26 for details).

In addition, we have to consider the situation of the sensory cortices during the resting state. We have to remind ourselves that the sensory cortices also show high activity in the resting state itself, which, most importantly, undergoes continuous change. There are thus changes in the neural activity level of the sensory cortices, even during the resting state itself. And it is these changes in the sensory cortices' resting-state activity level against which the internal stimuli, i.e., those from one's own body and the own brain, and their underlying regional activities are set and computed.

This implies that difference-based coding is possible even in the resting state: what is encoded and computed here amounts to the neural difference between the regions' resting state activities that are associated with the respective internal and external stimulus inputs. This makes it possible for contents to still be constituted on the basis of the encoded differences between the different regions/networks activities that are usually associated with internal and external stimuli inputs. Contents can thus still be constituted so that the "difference-based hypothesis of contents" can be applied, even in the resting state.

NEURONAL HYPOTHESIS IVE: DREAMS AND AUDITORY HALLUCINATIONS REFLECT *DIFFERENT PATHWAYS* IN THE CONSTITUTION OF *EXTERNAL CONTENTS* IN THE *RESTING STATE*

Let us give a concrete example: auditory hallucinations in schizophrenia. These patients hear voices when there is no external auditory stimulus input. Recent evidence suggests that this may be related to increased activity changes in the resting state itself, in especially the auditory cortex (see Northoff and Qin 2011; see also Chapters 17, 22 and 27 for a more detailed discussion of schizophrenia). The degree of change in the resting-state activity itself may here be as large as what is usually associated with external stimulus input. This suggests that the degree of activity change may "signal" an external stimulus, even though there is no such external stimulus present, so that the patients experience external voices, the auditory hallucinations.

Why does the degree of activity "signal" an external stimulus? Since the same degree of auditory cortical activity change is usually associated with exteroceptive auditory input, such change to an increased resting-state activity in the auditory cortex may be associated with what conceptually can be described by the term "as-if exteroceptive stimuli" or "as-if external stimuli" (see Chapter 26 for definition of the concept of "as-if-exteroceptive stimuli"). That must be distinguished from the "real" exteroceptive or external stimuli. We will discuss later in Chapter 26 on dreams the exact details of such confusion between "real" and "as if" exteroceptive stimuli (see also Northoff 2011, chapter 8).

What does the presence of such "as-if-exteroceptive stimuli" imply for the "difference-based hypothesis of contents"? It means that the internal stimuli and their respective regional activities can still be set against external stimuli, i.e., the "as-if-exteroceptive stimuli" as associated with the increased resting-state activity in their respective sensory cortices.

This high resting-state activity and the "high" "as-if-exteroceptive stimuli" input imply that the difference between internal and external stimuli is shifted toward the latter and becomes therefore negative (if one presupposes internal – external as the main computation). This means, though, that the external contents or better the "as-if-external contents" predominate over the internal ones, which is exactly the case in auditory hallucinations (see Chapters 22 and 27 for more details on schizophrenia).

More generally, this means that both internal and external contents can still be constituted on the basis of differences between different stimuli, regardless of their origin as either internal, external or as-if-external. Since contents are constituted on the basis of the differences between internal and external (or as-if-external) stimulus input, changes in the balance between internal and external input can contribute to the occurrence of external contents in the resting state. This suggests that multiple pathways can be taken to constitute external contents in the resting state.

One may propose decreases in the internal stimulus input from the body to be central for the occurrence of external contents in dreams (see earlier, as well as Chapter 26). Conversely, abnormal increases in external stimulus input, or better, "as-if-exteroceptive stimulus input," may also change the difference and thereby shift the balance between internal and external stimulus input toward the latter, the external stimulus input. This may lead to the predominance and subsequent occurrence of external contents (or better, as-if-contents) during the resting state as in auditory hallucinations.

NEURONAL HYPOTHESIS VA: "EASY" AND "HARD" CASES OF CONTENT DURING *STIMULUS-INDUCED ACTIVITY*

We have so far discussed only the occurrence of internal and external contents during resting-state activity. How about stimulus-induced activity? Stimulus-induced activity is usually associated with external contents in consciousness, such as in perception of the environment. Due to the association of the external stimuli with stimulus-induced activity, such external content can be easily explained in terms of stimulus-induced activity. It can therefore be considered the "easy" case of content during stimulus-induced activity (see Chapter 18, as well as Chapter 10 in Volume I).

How about internal contents during stimulus-induced activity? Here we are confronted with the "hard" case of stimulus-induced activity. This is the case in mind wandering, where, despite the presence of external stimuli, the attention slips toward internal contents (see below for details). Why is this a "hard" case? The predominance of external stimulus input during stimulus-induced activity should lead to the constitution of external rather than internal contents in consciousness.

In short, one would expect external contents rather than internal contents in the presence of external stimuli. This, however, is not the case in, for instance, mind wandering. Mind wandering describes slips of the mind from externally oriented tasks to the own thoughts (see Chapter 26 for more details). Hence, mind wandering implies a shift from external to internal contents during the presence of external stimuli (see Chapter 26 for more details on mind wandering).

How is such a shift from external to internal contents during the presence of external stimuli, as in mind wandering, possible? If contents are constituted on the basis of the origin of the stimuli in either brain, body or environment, as postulated by the "origin-based hypothesis of contents" (see earlier), one would propose the occurrence of external stimuli to go along with external rather than internal contents. This means that, if the "origin-based hypothesis of contents" were true, mind wandering as the occurrence of internal contents during external stimuli should remain impossible.

Neuronal Hypothesis VB: "*Difference*-based Hypothesis of Contents" *can* account for "Mind Wandering" as the "Hard" Case during *Stimulus-Induced Activity*

Alternatively to the "origin-based hypothesis of contents," one may propose a "difference-based hypothesis of contents" that postulates contents to be constituted on the basis of differences between internal external stimuli, rather than on the stimuli themselves. How does the "difference-based hypothesis of contents" account for mind wandering and its occurrence of internal contents in the presence of external stimuli? One may propose that the balance or difference between internal and external stimulus input shifts towards the internal stimulus input during mind wandering so that the internal stimulus input becomes relatively stronger than and predominate over the external stimulus input.

As in the case of the occurrence of external contents in the resting state (see earlier), the balance or difference between internal and external stimulus input can be changed in different ways, with multiple pathways leading to internal contents: either the external stimulus input decreases, which means that the internal stimulus input becomes relatively stronger, so that the computation "internal versus external" becoming positive. Or, alternatively, the internal stimulus input suddenly predominates due to increased interoceptive input from the body (or the neural input from the brain itself and its intrinsic or spontaneous state). This seems to be the case in mind wandering, where the external stimulus input remains constant (see Fig. 25-4b).

The "difference-based hypothesis of content" can account for the occurrence of internal contents during the presence of external stimulus input, as in mind wandering. As in the case of the occurrence of external contents in the resting state (see earlier), there are multiple pathways by which internal contents can be constituted and predominate over external contents during stimulus-induced activity.

This provides specific hypotheses that are very amenable to future experimental testing. In particular, future empirical results need to account for what I here described as "hard cases"; these include the occurrence of internal contents during the presence of external stimuli and their associated stimulus-induced activity as in mind wandering, as well as the occurrence of external contents during the absence of external stimuli in the resting state as in dreams.

Accordingly, both mind wandering and dreams seem to be well suitable to serve as paradigms to further illustrate our "difference-based hypothesis of contents" and its underlying neuronal mechanism. Since the detailed description of both mind wandering and dreams is beyond the scope of this chapter, I will devote the entirety of Chapter 26 to the discussion of both cases in full detail. This will provide additional empirical support in favor of the "difference-based hypothesis of contents," while it will discard further the "origin-based hypothesis of contents."

Neurophenomenal Hypothesis
IA: DIFFERENCE-BASED CODING MEDIATES THE ENCODING OF THE RELATIONSHIP BETWEEN THE *MIDLINE-LATERAL BALANCE* AND THE *BRAIN AS WHOLE* INTO NEURAL ACTIVITY

So far, I have considered only stimuli, networks, and contents. None of them is intrinsically related to phenomenal features by itself and thus consciousness, however. We must therefore move on from the level of contents to the phenomenal level of consciousness. How is it possible that the contents designated as internal or external are associated with the phenomenal state, e.g., consciousness and how, e.g., in which gestalt, does such association features in our experience?

More specifically, we need to investigate how it is possible for us to experience the contents in an intentional way in consciousness and thus in the gestalt of "directedness toward." We thus raise the question how intentionality, as the directedness toward content, is constituted on the phenomenal level of consciousness. For that, we need to go back first to the neuronal side of things.

We recall that the neural balance between midline and lateral networks was central in designating contents as internal or external. That, however, neglected the rest of the brain, e.g., its other regions and networks. The lateral and midline networks do not act alone and thus in isolation but rather in conjunction with the other networks and regions in the brain. These include the various subcortical regions as well as, the other cortical networks like the sensorimotor network and the salience network (see Menon 2011) as they can be distinguished already in the resting state itself (see Chapter 4,

Volume I). Most important, all these regions and neural networks show intrinsic activity and thus resting-state activity.

How, then, does the midline-lateral network interact with the regions and networks of the whole brain? As discussed earlier, difference-based coding is supposed to hold on the network level as well (see earlier); this means that the neural activity in the one network is determined on the basis of its relationship to or difference from the respective other (and vice versa). The activity balance between midline and lateral networks may consequently depend on their difference to the other cortical and subcortical networks in the brain as whole.

In the same way as the neural activity in both midline and lateral networks is generated by encoding their (spatial and temporal) differences, the midline-lateral networks' balance is encoded in relationship to and thus difference from the activity in the rest of the brain as a whole. Difference-based coding is thus supposed to also hold for the encoding of neural balances across the whole brain into the brain's neural activity during both resting state and stimulus-induced activity.

Neurophenomenal Hypothesis
IB: THE *MIDLINE-LATERAL BALANCE* IS LINKED AND INTEGRATED WITH THE RESTING STATE'S *"ENVIRONMENT–BRAIN UNITY"*

This is the neuronal side of things. What does it imply for the phenomenal level of consciousness in general and, more specifically, for its association with contents in particular? Let us recall the characterization of the resting-state activity as described in Volume I and so far here in Volume II. The resting-state activity in the whole brain was characterized by a particular spatiotemporal structure of its neural activity, as it was introduced in Part II in Volume I.

I detailed the resting-state activity's spatiotemporal structure by specific features here in Volume II: this included spatiotemporal continuity (Part V), spatiotemporal unity (Part VI), and self-specific organization (see Chapters 23 and 24 in this part). Since they are proposed to predispose consciousness, i.e., being necessary conditions of the possibility of its phenomenal features, I characterized the spatiotemporal structures of the resting state's neural activity as *prephenomenal* rather than non-phenomenal or phenomenal.

What does the prephenomenal characterization of the resting-state activity imply for the midline-lateral network's balance and its dependence upon the whole brain's regions/networks? One would propose the midline-lateral balance to interact with the spatiotemporal structures of the resting state's neural activity and thus with its prephenomenal features. This means that the contents themselves and their designation as internal or external by the midline-lateral network's balance will be linked and integrated with the resting state and the spatiotemporal structure of its neural activity.

NEUROPHENOMENAL HYPOTHESIS IC: THE INTERNAL AND EXTERNAL *CONTENTS* ARE LINKED AND INTEGRATED WITH THE RESTING STATE'S "ENVIRONMENT–BRAIN UNITY" AND ITS *POINT OF VIEW*

What does the integration between midline-lateral network and environment–brain unity imply for the contents designated as internal or external by the midline-lateral network's balance? I want to focus on especially the interaction of the midline-lateral network's balance with the spatiotemporal unity and more specifically the "environment–brain unity" of the resting state (see Chapters 20 and 21). Empirical evidence suggests that the resting-state activity aligns its own spatial and temporal features to the ones of the external stimuli in the environment in a statistically based way. This led me speak of a virtual statistically and spatiotemporally based "environment–brain unity" (see Chapter 20).

How, then, is this environment–brain unity related to the phenomenal features of consciousness? While being purely statistical by itself, this "environment–brain unity" is supposed to provide the very basis of what philosophers like Thomas Nagel describe as "point of view" (see Chapter 21). Simply put, a "point of view" anchors us in the rest of the physical world in

a virtual, e.g., statistically and spatiotemporally based way. This, in turn, makes it possible for us to experience the world from the point of view in a self-perspectival way (see Chapter 24 for the concept of "self-perspectival organization").

How now does the alleged environment–brain unity and its point of view relate to the contents as associated with the midline-lateral balance? I propose that the midline-lateral network's balance is neurally processed and thus encoded in spatial and temporal difference from the neural activity in the whole brain and its various regions and networks. The contents as associated with the midline-lateral network's balance are consequently, that is, necessary and unavoidably, related and linked to the resting state's environment–brain unity and its point of view. Since the latter, i.e., the environment–brain unity and its point of view, predispose consciousness and are therefore prephenomenal, the contents themselves are now predisposed to become associated with consciousness and its various phenomenal features.

Therefore I propose that the neural difference or balance between midline-lateral networks and the whole brain's regions/networks enables the linkage and integration of contents to the environment–brain unity and its associated point of view. Since the latter, the point of view, predisposes consciousness, such linkage is supposed to make possible the association of contents with consciousness. What are the exact neurophenomenal mechanisms that enable the association of contents with consciousness? This is the focus in the next sections.

NEUROPHENOMENAL HYPOTHESIS IIA: SPATIOTEMPORALLY BASED *"UNILATERAL DIRECTEDNESS"* IN THE NEURAL ACTIVITIES BETWEEN *WHOLE BRAIN* AND *MIDLINE-LATERAL NETWORKS*

We have focused so far on the relationship between the midline-lateral network and the whole brain's neural activity. Most important, I argued that the encoding of their relationship or difference into neural activity is central in linking point of view and content, which in turn predisposes the association of the contents with consciousness. Why does the encoding of the relationship between midline-lateral network and whole brain's neural activity predisposes the association of contents with consciousness? For the answer, we need to go into detail about the spatiotemporal features associated with both the brain's neural activity and the phenomenal features of consciousness. Let us start with the neuronal side of things.

Based on their difference-based coding (see earlier), one would propose that the midline-lateral network's balance becomes integrated and thus nested into the neural activity of the whole brain's regions/networks. What exactly happens during their integration? *Integration* means that the spatial and temporal differences between the neural activity in the midline-lateral network and the whole brain's neural activity are encoded into neural activity. Since the whole brain occupies a much larger spatial and temporal range than the midline-lateral network, the degree of spatiotemporal extension of the neural activity related to the whole brain is much larger than the one of the mid-lateral network.

Due to the large degree of spatiotemporal extension or range of the whole brain's neural activity compared to that of the midline-lateral network, one would propose a positive difference (when subtracting the latter from the former). This value cannot become negative, because that would mean we would attribute larger degrees of spatiotemporal extension of neural activity to the midline-lateral network than to the whole brain's neural activity. That is impossible, however, so their difference value is unavoidably and thus necessarily positive by default.

To put it differently, the larger spatial and temporal range or extension of the neural activity in the whole brain's regions/networks compared to that of the midline-lateral networks prevents the former from being integrated into the latter. There is thus a spatiotemporally based unilateral directedness in the neural activities between the whole brain's regions/networks and the midline-lateral networks on the neuronal level. This applies to both resting state and stimulus-induced activity, which both have to encounter the need to integrate the continuous activity changes in both the midline-lateral network and the whole brain.

What does such spatiotemporally based "unilateral directedness" on the neuronal level imply for the phenomenal level of consciousness? This will be the focus in the next section.

NEUROPHENOMENAL HYPOTHESIS IIB: SPATIOTEMPORALLY BASED *"UNILATERAL DIRECTEDNESS"* BETWEEN *POINT OF VIEW* AND *CONTENT*

What does such spatiotemporally based unilateral directedness between the whole brain's neural activity and that of the midline-lateral network imply for the relationship between point of view and content? We recall from the previous sections that we associated the whole brain's neural activity with the point of view (and the environment–brain unity), while the midline-lateral network is related to contents and their designation as internal or external.

What does the spatiotemporal difference between the midline-lateral network's and the whole brain's neural activities imply for how point of view and content can be linked and integrated to each other? The linkage between content and point of view implies the interaction between two different statistically and difference-based spatiotemporal frameworks. Both spatiotemporal frameworks differ in their spatial and temporal extension or range: the spatiotemporal framework of the point of view is larger and more extended than the one associated with the contents.

This means, however, that a complete merge and fusion between point of view and content into one common, virtual statistically based, spatiotemporal framework is impossible. Instead, the larger spatiotemporal framework of the point of view can only embed, nest, and integrate the smaller one of the content within itself. In other words, the smaller spatiotemporal framework of the contents becomes nested within the larger one related to the point of view.

In contrast, the reverse scenario, nesting of the larger spatiotemporal framework of the point of view within the smaller one of the contents, remains impossible (see Fig. 25-5a). There is thus what one may describe as "spatiotemporally based unilateral directedness" from the

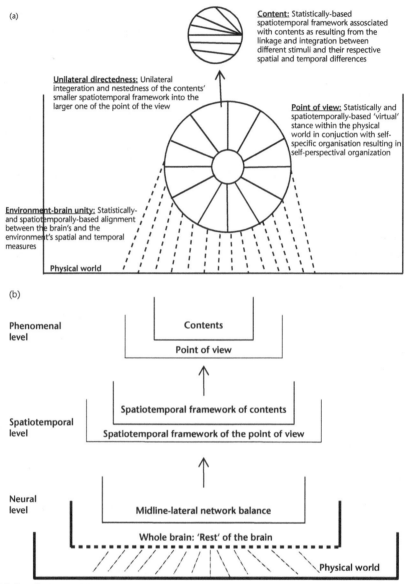

Figure 25-5a-d "Point of view–based hypothesis of directedness." The figure shows distinct aspects of the "point of view–based hypothesis of directedness," including the relationship between point of view and contents (*a*); the nested organization on neuronal, spatiotemporal, and phenomenal levels (*b*); and the dependence of such directedness on neural (*c*), and spatiotemporal (*d*) differences. The lower part of the figure shows the statistically and spatiotemporally based "virtual" environmental–brain unity with the consequent constitution of a point of view as the organism's stance within the physical world. The point of view is spatiotemporal, as illustrated by the spatial and temporal trajectories. The contents also show a certain spatiotemporal structure as based on the difference- and statistically based integration and linkage between different stimuli; this is again indicated by the lines within the circle symbolizing spatial and temporal trajectories (upper part). However, the spatiotemporal framework of the content is much smaller, i.e., less extended in time and space, than the one of the point view and its associated self-perspectival organization. Therefore, the content is integrated or nested within the point of view, with the latter being directed towards the former; hence the one-way arrow from the point of view to the contents; while the reverse directedness from content to point of view remains impossible. (*b*)

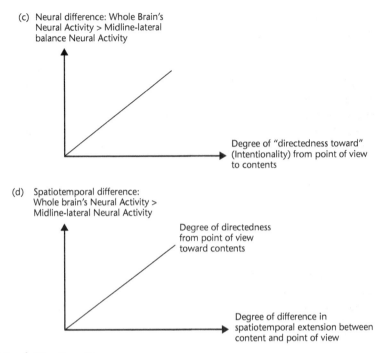

Figure 25-5a-d (Continued)

The figure illustrates the nestedness on neuronal (lower), spatiotemporal (middle), and phenomenal (upper) levels. Lower part: The midline-lateral networks and their balance are nested within the whole brain's regions/networks, which in turn are nested within the physical world via its statistically and spatiotemporally based environment–brain unity (as indicated by the dotted lines). Middle part: The point of view and its associated self-perspectival organization provide a large spatiotemporal framework that is more extended than the one associated with the content, with the latter therefore being nested within the former. Upper part: The point of view is directed toward contents, which are thus nested within the former. In contrast, the converse, that is, directedness from contents to the point of view, remains impossible. (*c*) The figure illustrates the dependence of directedness of the point of view toward contents on the degree of neural differences: the larger the neural differences between midline-lateral networks and the whole brain's neural activity, the larger the degree of directedness of the point of view toward contents. (*d*) The figure shows how the neural differences between the whole brain's neural activity and the midline-lateral balance is related to spatiotemporal differences between point of view and contents, which in turn determines the degree of directedness of the point of view toward contents: the larger the neural differences between midline-lateral networks and the whole brain's neural activity, the larger the associated spatiotemporal differences, and the larger the degree of directedness of the point of view toward contents.

point of view toward the contents, with the contents being nested within the point of view (see Feinberg 2009, 2010, 2012; as well as Northoff et al. 2011a, for the concept of nestedness). In contrast, the reverse scenario, "spatiotemporally based unilateral directedness from contents to point of view, with nesting of the point of view within the contents remains impossible.

Let us illustrate the situation in further detail. The here-sketched scenario is more or less analogous to that of the famous Russian dolls. There, too, the smaller dolls can only be "integrated" within the larger ones, while the reverse scenario, integration of the larger dolls within smaller ones, remains impossible. The integration is thus unilateral, showing spatiotemporally based "unilateral directedness or nestedness" from point of view to content (see Figure 25-5b)

In sum, I postulate that the relationship between point of view and content can be determined in spatiotemporal terms and more specifically by "spatiotemporally based unilateral directedness." This, as I suggest, predisposes what phenomenally is described as "directedness toward," or intentionality, which shall be detailed in the next sections.

NEUROPHENOMENAL HYPOTHESIS IIC: "POINT OF VIEW–BASED HYPOTHESIS OF DIRECTEDNESS"

The consideration of the earlier-discussed spatiotemporal differences leads me to propose what I describe as the "point of view–based hypothesis of directedness." The point of view–based hypothesis of directedness proposes the directedness toward, and thus intentionality, to be dependent upon the point of view and its degree of spatiotemporal difference to the respective content. This, however, needs to be explained on both neuronal and phenomenal levels.

Let me start with the neuronal level. The point of view–based hypothesis of directedness proposes the directedness toward (and ultimately intentionality on the phenomenal level of consciousness) to be dependent upon the neural differences between the midline-lateral networks and the rest of the brain's networks during both resting state and stimulus-induced activity. The larger and more positive the neural differences in the spatial and temporal measures between the whole brain and the midline-lateral network, the larger the degree of directedness toward from point of view to content; that is, intentionality. In contrast, smaller and less positive neural differences will be associated with smaller degrees of directedness toward (and thus intentionality) (see Fig. 25-5c).

Since, as stated earlier, the networks' neural activities constitute a statistically based spatiotemporal framework, the point of view–based hypothesis of directedness must be formulated on the spatiotemporal level, too. The point of view–based hypothesis of directedness proposes the directedness toward and ultimately intentionality to be dependent upon the differences in the degree and scope of temporal and spatial extension associated with the earlier described networks.

Intentionality is consequently considered in spatiotemporal terms and can therefore be characterized by the degree of spatiotemporal extension (see below for details). The larger and more positive their spatiotemporal differences, the larger the degree of directedness toward (and thus intentionality). In contrast, smaller and less positive spatiotemporal differences will lead to smaller degrees of directedness toward (and thus intentionality) (see Fig. 25-5d).

NEUROPHENOMENAL HYPOTHESIS IID: THE BRAIN'S RESTING-STATE ACTIVITY SHOWS A "PREINTENTIONAL ORGANIZATION"

What does the "point of view hypothesis of directedness" imply for the characterization of the brain's resting-state activity? Due to the encoding of neural activity in terms of spatial and temporal differences between the whole brain's neural activity and that of the midline-lateral network, the brain and its resting-state activity show a spatiotemporal organization that predisposes them to constitute intentionality. Such spatiotemporal organization may be described by the term "preintentional organization," which by itself is not yet phenomenal but predisposes the constitution of intentionality during the actual realization of consciousness. Therefore, the resting-state activity's preintentional organization may be characterized as prephenomenal.

How can we illustrate the situation in a more metaphorical way? For that, let us return to our example of the Russian dolls and put it into the phenomenal context of intentionality. The smaller Russian doll is put into the next larger one and so forth, in the same way that contents are put into the large spatiotemporal extension of the point of view and its environment–brain unity. In contrast, the converse, putting the larger ones within the smaller ones, remains impossible because of their difference in the degree of spatiotemporal extension, so that the point of view cannot be put into the contents.

Most importantly, the unilateral directedness is already predisposed by the mere size of the different dolls even if they al lie side by side on the table. There is thus a predisposition for unilateral directedness from the larger dolls to the smaller dolls, in the same way the resting state's neuronal organization predisposes that subsequent directedness is targeted from the point of view to the contents rather than from contents to point of view.

In sum, the "point of view–based hypothesis of directedness" suggests that the larger spatiotemporal extension of the point of view predisposes the unilateral nestedness and thus the directedness from point of view toward contents. Metaphorically put, the preintentional organization of the brain's resting-state activity is the germ or seed of the basic predisposition for any subsequent intentionality as "directedness toward" in consciousness. How does that seed need to grow to flourish into the full-blown plant of intentionality? That will be discussed in the next sections.

NEUROPHENOMENAL HYPOTHESIS IIIA: PHENOMENAL AND NEURAL NECESSITY FOR THE SPATIOTEMPORAL CHARACTERIZATION OF INTENTIONALITY

The "point of view–based hypothesis of directedness" states the necessary conditions of possible intentionality in consciousness. These necessary conditions include the neural condition, the balance between the whole brain's neural activity and the midline-lateral network; and spatiotemporal conditions, the different degrees in spatiotemporal extension of point of view and content. This characterizes intentionality in spatiotemporal terms, with the "directedness toward" being specified as the unilateral directedness from a spatiotemporally more extended point of view to spatiotemporally less extended contents.

Most importantly, I postulate that such spatiotemporal characterization of intentionality is a necessary or unavoidable feature of intentionality. Why? If point of view and content were determined in non-spatiotemporal terms, independently of their degrees of spatiotemporal extension, the unilateral "directedness toward" from the point of view to contents with the subsequent experience of intentionality in consciousness would be altogether impossible. There is thus what one may describe as

a *phenomenal* (and, even stronger, *conceptual*) necessity to characterize intentionality in spatiotemporal terms.

In addition to such a phenomenal necessity, there is also an empirical, or better, neural, necessity. How is such neural necessity supported by the empirical data? I suggested that the relationship between the whole brain's neural activity and the midline-lateral network is encoded into neural activity in terms of spatial and temporal differences, thus presupposing difference-based coding (rather than stimulus-based coding). I determined difference-based coding as the brain's encoding strategy to encode and generate any kind of neural activity in the brain (see Volume I).

What does such difference-based coding imply for the neural activity of the brain as whole? Thhe brain cannot avoid encoding the relationship between the whole brain's neural activity and the midline-lateral network in terms of spatial and temporal differences. Since such encoding leads unavoidably and necessarily to different degrees of spatiotemporal extension between point of view and contents, there is an empirical or *neural* necessity to characterize intentionality in spatiotemporal terms.

NEUROPHENOMENAL HYPOTHESIS IIIB: INTENTIONALITY IS INTRINSICALLY SPATIOTEMPORAL AND BRAIN-BASED IN (AT LEAST) THE NATURAL WORLD

Taking both phenomenal and neural necessity together implies that intentionality is intrinsically spatiotemporal. There is no non-spatiotemporal form of intentionality. Accordingly, we cannot even imagine a non-spatiotemporal form of intentionality to hold true in our actual natural world (while this does not exclude the conceivability of non-spatiotemporal intentionality in a logically possible world as it is usually presupposed by philosophers).

Why can we not even imagine a non-spatiotemporal form of intentionality in our natural world? Being part of the natural world, our brain encodes its neural activity in a way, namely, by difference-based coding, that makes any such non-spatiotemporal form of intentionality impossible from the very beginning; that is, by default. If, in contrast, our brain was encoding its neural activity in terms of stimulus-based coding, there would no longer be a need for such spatiotemporal characterization. That, however, would make intentionality, at least in the form in which we associate it with consciousness, altogether impossible.

This means that intentionality as we can conceive of it in our natural world is not only spatiotemporally based but also brain-based (rather than either brain-reductive or mind-based; see later in this chapter as well as Appendix 3 in Volume I). Accordingly, our brain and its particular encoding strategy make necessary and unavoidable, and thus predispose, intentionality in an intrinsically spatiotemporal form. Since any thought and imagination is based on our brain and its encoding strategy, we remain in principle unable even to imagine a non-spatiotemporal form of intentionality in at least our actual natural world. Therefore, at least in our natural world (of neuroscience as distinguished from the logical world of philosophy), intentionality cannot be thought of or imagined otherwise than in an intrinsically spatiotemporal way.

Neurophenomenal Hypothesis IIIC: Spatiotemporal versus Cognitive Approaches to Intentionality

The intrinsically spatiotemporal and brain-based character of intentionality is neglected in cognitive (and affective and sensorimotor) approaches to intentionality in current neuroscience and philosophy (see the beginning of this section as well as Slaby and Stephan 2008; Metzinger 2003; and the very many cognitive models of intentionality in current "philosophy of mind"). They start from the content itself and isolate it from any kind of spatiotemporal characterization.

Why do the cognitive approaches start with the content itself and neglect its spatiotemporal character? Cognitive (and affective and sensorimotor) approaches start with stimulus-induced activity as it is associated with the neural processing of contents. This, however, neglects the need of the brain to link and integrate the neural processing of contents and their associated

stimulus-induced activity with the brain's own intrinsic activity. Accordingly, their disregard of the brain's intrinsic activity entails that they overlook its spatiotemporal structure and organization and how that is imposed upon any kind of content during subsequent stimulus-induced activity. In other terms, the neurocognitive approaches remain "blind" to the spatiotemporal structure of the contents they aim to explain in purely cognitive terms. We have to better understand, though, how and why the neurocognitive approaches neglect the spatiotemporal structure of the contents. The double neglect of both the brain's intrinsic activity and its spatiotemporal structure entails that the environment–brain unity and its point of view are neglected in neurocognitive (and neuroaffective and sensorimotor) approaches. This in turn makes it impossible to account for a point of view and to establish its spatiotemporal relationship with contents in the gestalt of a spatiotemporally based unilateral directedness from point of view to contents.

If, however, neither point of view nor its spatiotemporal relationship to contents is considered, intentionality as the directedness from point of view to contents remains altogether mysterious and becomes inexplicable. This however is different in the here suggested spatiotemporal approach to intentionality that implies a neurophenomenal approach and must therefore must be distinguished from neurocognitive (and neuroaffective and neurosensory) approaches

Neurophenomenal Hypothesis IIID: Intentionality Is Intrinsically Subjective (in a Biophysically Based Way)

How do the neurocognitive (and neuroaffective and sensorimotor) approaches account for intentionality? They argue that the constitution of "directedness toward" content is an integral part of the respective cognitive, affective, or sensorimotor functions themselves. That, however, neglects the basically subjective character of intentionality, the experience of directedness toward contents in consciousness. Intentionality is then considered in a purely objective way, while remaining devoid of all its subjective features, including its association with consciousness.

I argue that such "objective intentionality" remains impossible because intentionality and its spatiotemporal characterization implies a basic form of subjectivity, biophysically based subjectivity as it is associated with the point of view (see Chapter 21). Understood in this way, intentionality cannot help but be (biophysically based) subjective which makes possible and thus predisposes its association with consciousness. More radically, I postulate that, without its basically subjective character, intentionality would simply remain impossible. Accordingly, intentionality is not only intrinsically spatiotemporal and brain-based but also intrinsically subjective (in a biophysically based way).

Let us return one final time to the example of the Russian dolls. Neurocognitive approaches take the last doll, the smallest, as their starting point, while disregarding all the other dolls, the larger ones. They then wonder how it is possible that the smaller doll shows some hints of being integrated and nested spatiotemporally into larger dolls as is manifested in intentionality. That remains mysterious as long as one does not consider the larger dolls themselves, the point of view and its larger spatiotemporal extension and their constitution by the brain's intrinsic activity.

CONCEPTUAL BACKGROUND IA: SEARLE'S CONCEPT OF INTENTIONALITY AND ITS INTERNAL GENERATION AND ASPECTUAL NATURE

How can we further characterize the concept of "intentionality"? The notion of intentionality stems from medieval philosophy and has been reintroduced in the twentieth century by Franz Brentano. He described intentionality as the capacity of the mind to "refer" to or be "directed" to objects that exist solely in the mind while remaining absent in the environment. The objects can thus be characterized by "mental or intentional inexistence." The exact characterization of such mental or intentional inexistence of the objects in intentionality remains unclear, however.

While there are plenty of different meanings and definitions of the concept of intentionality in past and current philosophy (see Siewert 2006), I here want to focus on the definition provided by the well-known current philosopher John R. Searle. Searle is a famous philosopher who teaches at the University of California–Berkeley; he has made major contributions to different fields in philosophy, among them philosophy of mind.

Searle (2004) describes intentionality as the "mental directedness or mental aboutness" (see also Siewert 2006 for a good overview) that refers to "that property of many mental states and events by which they are directed or about or of objects and states of affairs in the world" (Searle 1983, 1). Hence, a mental state is about or directed toward an object or event in the external world even when the object or event is by itself not physically present within the environment.

The content of the mental state is thus a content that is experienced as if it is "located" in the outer world, the external environment, even though its underlying neural activity is generated in the inside world, the own brain. Due to its internal generation, Searle characterizes the intentional content as internal to the intentional state itself, rather than as external as coming from the outside, that is, the external environment. In short, the intentional content is internal rather than external.

Besides being internal to the intentional state, the intentional content is also aspectual, meaning that it is always under a certain aspect, thereby excluding others and thus showing what Searle (2004, 117) calls "aspectual shapes." For instance, intentionality might represent an object as the Morning Star rather than as the Evening Star, even though both refer (physically) to one and the same object (Searle 2004, 117). The same physical star is thus referred to in the intentional state under a certain aspect, e.g., as a star in the morning rather than as a star in the evening.

CONCEPTUAL BACKGROUND IB: SEARLE'S ASSUMPTION OF THE MATCHING AND FIT BETWEEN MIND AND WORLD

Searle considers intentionality to result from the matching between the contents in the world and those in the mind. Such matching can go in both directions, from world to mind and from mind to world. Let us start with the direction from the mind to the world as it is, for instance, the case in beliefs. In beliefs, the world is supposed to be represented in the belief and more specifically in its contents. The belief and other mental states like perception, convictions, hypotheses, and so on are thus proposed to fit (or do not fit) the world—Searle (2004, 118) calls this "direction of fit" as "mind-to-world direction of fit."

The reverse scenario in, for instance, desires or intentions may also be possible, however. In that case, the content of the mental state is not supposed to fit the content in the world but rather the other way around: the content in the world is supposed to fit the content in the mental state, entailing "world-to-mind direction of fit," rather than "mind-to-world direction of fit." Both mind-to-world direction of fit and world-to-mind direction of fit are only extreme poles on a continuum. Following Searle, one may also show states where there is equal balance between the contents of the mind and those of the world. This is, for instance, the case when saying, "I am glad the sun is shining" entailing "null direction of fit between the world's and the mind's content." In sum, put in an extremely abbreviated way, Searle characterizes the concept of intentionality and its respective contents by three features: internal generation of contents, the aspectual nature of contents, and the fit between mind's and world's contents.

Neuroconceptual Hypothesis
IA: DIFFERENCE-BASED CODING MEDIATES THE INTERNAL GENERATION OF CONTENTS

How can we now relate the three features Searle attributed to intentionality and its contents to the earlier discussed neurophenomenal hypotheses? Let us start with the internal generation of the contents of intentionality. We recall our difference-based hypothesis of contents. Rather than being related to the origin of stimuli, contents are constituted on the basis of differences between different stimuli. While the origin of the stimuli can indeed lie in the environment, thus being external, the contents themselves are constituted within the brain itself. That constitution of contents by the brain is based upon the differences between different stimuli as they are encoded into neural activity.

How does such difference-based coding in the constitution of content stand in relation to Searle's assumption of the internal generation of contents? Superficially considered, Searle seems to be essentially correct when he says that the contents are internally generated. They are generated within the brain itself no matter whether the respective contents originate externally in the environment or internally in body and brain.

Since the constitution of both internal and external contents is based on the differences between different stimuli as they are processed in the brain's neural activity, all contents are generated inside the brain itself. Hence, Searle seems to be correct indeed when he proposes that contents come from the inside of the brain and are thus internally generated. Such supposedly internal generation distinguishes the contents of intentionality from stimuli that can be generated either internally (within the brain and the body) or externally (within the environment).

Neuroconceptual Hypothesis
IB: BRAIN-*BASED* VERSUS BRAIN-*REDUCTIVE* CONCEPTS OF INTENTIONALITY

We need to be more careful here, however. I proposed that contents are generated internally in brain. This means that their constitution touches upon the brain's statistically and spatiotemporally based interface with the environment, the environment–brain unity. This allows the contents to be linked to a particular point of view within the world, and that, in turn, is necessary for the contents to be linked to intentionality and thus to become intentional contents. More specifically, the linkage between content and point of view was supposed to be necessary to constitute directedness toward and thus intentionality. Hence, directedness toward and intentionality are ultimately based on the statistically and spatiotemporally based environment–brain unity.

The implication of the environment–brain unity in the constitution of contents undermines Searle's characterization of intentionality as purely internal, however. The environment–brain unity can by itself neither be characterized as purely internal nor as purely external. Instead of being described as internal or external, the environment-unity can best be characterized as truly *relational*. If this is so, anything that is based on the environment–brain unity, like the constitution of intentional contents, cannot be characterized as purely internal and thus as "located" exclusively within the brain itself. This implies that we cannot reduce intentionality and its contents to the brain itself, which excludes a brain-reductive concept of intentionality.

Accordingly, while acknowledging the brain itself and its intrinsic activity, we also need to consider its relationship to the environment, the environment–brain unity. Intentionality can thus neither be "located" within the brain itself nor reduced to it and its neural activity. That implies that we need to develop a brain-based rather than brain-reductive (or even mind-based) concept of intentionality (see also Appendix 3 for the distinction between brain-based and brain-reductive concepts).

How does the distinction between brain-reductive and brain-based accounts of intentional contents stand in relation to Searle's assumption of the internal generation of contents? Searle is right in that contents are generated internally rather than externally to the mind. It is the mind itself that generates the content, rather than the contents' being generated in the world. The contents are internal to both the mind and its intentionality.

How, then, can we relate Searle's mind-based account of the internal generation of content to the brain? We can preserve his assumption of the internal generation of contents. However, rather than being generated internally to some mind, the contents are now generated internally to the brain and its neural activity. The mind-based account of the internal generation of intentional contents would then be replaced by a brain-reductive account. That, however, as indicated earlier, entails the neglect of the intrinsic relationship of the brain's neural activity with the environment, the environment–brain unity. The consideration o the environment–brain unity implies a brain-based rather than a brain-reductive approach. Therefore, the concept of the internal generation

of intentional contents does not necessarily imply a brain-reductive approach, as many authors on the philosophical side, including Searle, would probably opt for. Instead, the assumption of the internal generation of intentional contents is very compatible with a brain-based approach as distinguished from a brain-reductive approach.

Even stronger, I claim that such brain-based approach is necessary in order to preserve the intentional nature of the contents. Contents can only become intentional contents when they are brain-based, whereas this would remain impossible if they were brain-reductive. A brain-reductive approach could at best account for the contents themselves, while it would leave open the question of their intentional nature and thus the intentional contents.

NEUROCONCEPTUAL HYPOTHESIS IC: "RELATIONAL" VERSUS "ISOLATED" CONCEPTS OF INTENTIONAL CONTENTS

What does the brain-based rather than brain-reductive nature of the concept of intentionality imply for the "location" of the contents? Rather than in the brain itself (or some kind of mind) the contents may better be "located" right in-between the external environment and the internal brain, thus being intrinsically relational (see also Northoff 2011). We may therefore need to develop a more conceptually refined account of intentionality and its intentional contents that goes beyond the internal-external dichotomy.

This amounts to what I describe as the "relational" concept of intentional contents. The "relational" concept of intentional contents associates the contents with a particular relationship, the statistically and spatiotemporally based relationship between environment and brain. This implies that the intentional contents can be "located" neither in the brain itself nor in the environment (or some kind of "mind"). Either case would amount to an "isolated" concept of intentional contents wherein they are detached (and thus isolated) from either the environment/world or the brain/mind.

Such a relational nature of intentionality is well compatible with its aspectual character as described by Searle. As I discussed earlier, intentionality is possible only on the basis of the linkage of the contents to a specific point of view as associated with the respective environment–brain unity. Otherwise, that is, if there were no such linkage between point of view and content, directedness toward and thus intentionality would remain impossible.

I now propose that the necessity of the linkage of intentionality to a point of view and its spatiotemporal features accounts for its aspectual nature as described by Searle. Due to the linkage of the content to a particular point of view, that content can only be experienced in terms of specific aspects, while leaving out others, thus accounting for the aspectual nature of intentional contents. Hence, what Searle describes as the "aspectual nature of intentional contents" is proposed to correspond well to my assumption of a necessary linkage between content and point of view as core features in constituting directedness toward and ultimately intentionality.

This means that the intrinsically spatiotemporal character of intentionality predisposes and thus makes necessary what Searle describes as the "aspectual nature of intentional contents." Only on the basis of their spatiotemporal characterization can intentional contents become aspectual. This means that the aspectual nature of intentional contents is made necessary by the intrinsically spatiotemporal and thus relational character of intentional contents. If, in contrast, intentional contents were not spatiotemporal anymore and thus isolated rather than relational, they could not be aspectual in the way Searle states. The contents would then be non-aspectual. This implies, however, that the content would also be no longer intentional, but mere contents stripped off their intentionality. In short, intentional contents would remain impossible if they were no longer intrinsically spatiotemporal and aspectual.

Neuroconceptual Hypothesis ID: Searle's Mind-Based "Bi-Directional Fit Between Mind and World" Can Be Rephrased as Brain-Based "Bi-Directional Fit Between Environment–Brain Unity and Environmental Stimuli"

Finally, Searle's assumption of a matching between the mind's contents and the ones of the world superficially seems to correspond to what I described as the balance between internal and external contents. If the external contents predominate over the internal contents, one may speak of "mind-to-world direction of fit," while in the case of internal contents predominating, one may rather propose the reverse direction, world-to-mind direction of fit (see Fig. 25-6a).

However, we again need to be careful here. The point Searle addresses is a deeper one. Rather than concerning only the balance between internal and external contents, he aims to examine the direction in the adaptation between the mind's and the world's contents: either the mind's contents adapts to the ones of the world or the world's contents are supposed to adapt to the mind's contents.

How is such a bilateral fit between the mind's and the world's contents possible? I tentatively propose that empirically, this balance may be related to the neural balance between resting-state activity and stimulus-induced activity. If the resting-state activity predominates over the stimulus-induced activity, "world-to-mind direction of fit" may be more prominent. In contrast, in the reverse case of stimulus-induced activity being stronger than resting-state activity, the pendulum may be shifted more toward a "mind-to-world direction of fit." There is thus a continuum rather than an all-or-nothing alternative between both directions of fit. As Searle himself says, there is a continuum between both fits, which on the empirical side I propose to correspond to the neuronal continuum between resting state and stimulus-induced activity.

I therefore postulate that the "bi-directional fit between mind and world" as postulated by Searle on the mental level corresponds on the neuronal side to the "bi-directional fit between resting state and stimulus-induced activity." Searle suggests that mind and world can be matched and fitted together in both directions—mind to world and world to mind, Analogously, resting state and stimulus-induced activity are matched and fitted together in both ways, rest to stimulus leading to rest–stimulus interaction, and stimulus to rest entailing stimulus–rest interaction (see Chapter 11).

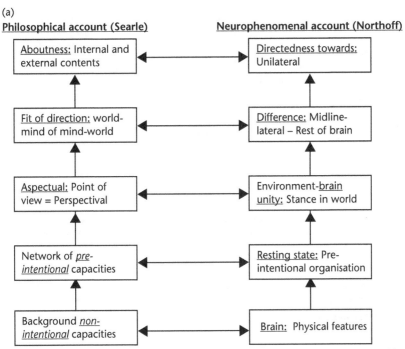

Figure 25-6 Brain and intentionality. (*a*) The figure shows the relationship between Searle's concept of intentionality and specific neuronal mechanisms of the brain, and how the brain relates to the environment (*a*), and what that implies for the characterization of the brain (*b*). (*a*) Comparison between philosophical and neurophenomenal accounts of intentionality. The figure shows the comparison between a philosophical account of intentionality (by Searle; left part) and the here-suggested neurophenomenal account (right part).On the left, one can see the progression from non-intentional background capacities over pre-intentional capacities to intentionality, as suggested by the philosopher Searle. On the right, I plotted the corresponding neuro-phenomenal hypothesis. Lowest part: What Searle calls "non-intentional background capacities" may correspond to the brain's basic biophysical-computational spectrum. That is strictly non-intentional by itself. Lowest part: Searle's concept of pre-intentional capacities may correspond to what I described as the resting state's pre-intentional organization. Second from lowest: Searle characterizes intentionality by its "aspectual nature," as he says. This is related on the neurophenomenal side to the constitution of an environment–brain unity and its associated point of view. Third from lowest: Searle proposes a "fit of direction" between world and mind in intentionality whether the mind appropriates and enslaves the world, as in desires, or conversely, as in belief. This, I propose, is related to neural differences as computed between midline-lateral networks and the rest of the brain's regions/networks. Top: Searle characterizes intentionality by "aboutness"; mental states are about contents whether they are internal or external. I propose that such aboutness corresponds to the directedness towards from the point of view to the contents, which I associate with spatiotemporal differences between both. (*b*) The figure illustrates the characterization of the brain in the context of intentionality. Left: On the left the brain is depicted as a merely physical brain that is part of the physical world (circle). Here the characterization of the brain is purely physical, empirical, and completely non-intentional which comes close to what Searle describes as "background non-intentional capacities." Middle: Here the brain encodes its neural activity, which makes possible the generation of a virtual statistically and spatiotemporally based continuity or unity between environment and brain, the environment–brain unity, which is associated with what philosophically is described as a point of view. This is indicated by the dotted lines from the brain to the physical world. The brain can here be characterized biophysically, in a neurotranscendental way, and by what Searle describes as "network of preintentional capacities." Right: Here the brain encodes the contents from the world (as illustrated by the red arrows from the physical world to the brain) and processes them via its various functions. The characterization of the brain here is her presupposed as psychological, neuroempirical, and phenomenal.

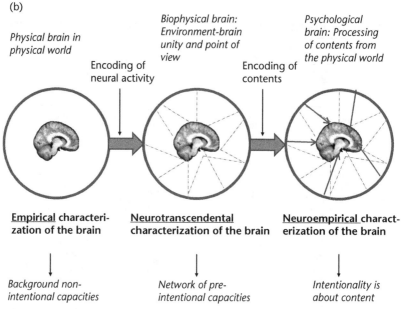

Figure 25-6 (Continued)

How do the two "fits," Searle's mental fit and my neuronal fit, converge and integrate? I claim that the brain's resting-state activity entails the linkage to the world in the gestalt of the environment–brain unity. The fit between resting state and stimulus-induced activity is then no longer a brain-reductive fit between two different forms of neural activity, resting state and stimulus-induced activity that take place exclusively within the brain itself. Instead, it is a brain-based fit between an extrinsic stimulus at a particular discrete point in physical time and space of the environment on the one hand and the brain's intrinsic activity that spans virtually and statistically across the divide of brain, body, and environment on the other.

How does that relate to Searle's account? The brain and the virtual and statistically based extension of its intrinsic activity to the environment, the environment–brain unity, make the assumption of a "mind" superfluous. All that the concept of mind is supposed to account for, the basic subjectivity and its association with consciousness (and other mental features like self and free will), can be taken over by the

environment–brain unity and its biophysically based subjectivity (see Chapter 21). Searle's concept of a "bi-directional fit between mind and world" can consequently be rephrased as the "bi-directional fit between the brain's intrinsic activity and the world's extrinsic stimuli," and more specifically as the "bi-directional fit between environment–brain unity and environmental stimuli."

CONCEPTUAL BACKGROUND II: SEARLE'S CONCEPTS OF THE "NETWORK OF PREINTENTIONAL CAPACITIES" AND THE "BACKGROUND OF NONINTENTIONAL CAPACITIES"

How is intentionality constituted? Searle (2004, 121–122) proposes what he calls the "background of nonintentional capacities." Such a background of nonintentional capacities may, however, be preintentional as he himself speaks of a "network of preintentional capacities": The "preintentional capacities" refer to a set of abilities that are dispositions and different ways of coping with the world. This, in turn, may be based upon our innate biological capacities and our life experiences (see Searle 2004, 131). He, however, does not specify this meeting or convergence point between biology and intentionality.

Other authors like Ralph Pred and Walter Freeman use analogous concepts like "preperceptual intentionality" (see Pred 2005, 98, as well as Freeman 2007, 2011 for analogous concepts). The manifestation of intentionality prior to the occurrence of any specific object or event is also thematized by Rowlands (2010, chapters 7 and 8). He characterizes our experience by a "noneliminable intentional core" with intentionality describing the "directedness toward the world" (Rowland 2010, 187).

Most important, Rowland proposes this noneliminable intentional core to occur prior to the constitution of any contents of intentionality and represents an intrinsic and thus defining (rather than extrinsic) feature of intentionality (which probably comes conceptually close to what W. J. Freeman [2003, 2010] means when he describes intentionality as "intrinsic"). This leads Rowland to consider such prior "non-eliminable intentional core" as transcendental that describes "what allows something to appear as object of consciousness" (Rowland 2010, 179) (see also appendix 3 in this Volume as well as Northoff 2011, chapters 1 and 2 for the notion of "neurotranscendental").

Neuroconceptual hypothesis
IIA: NEUROPHENOMENAL APPROACH TO THE "NETWORK OF PREINTENTIONAL CAPACITIES"

How can we now relate what Searle calls "preintentional capacities" to the neuronal context of the brain? I earlier characterized the resting state by "preintentional organization" that proposed the resting state's spatiotemporal organization to predispose directedness toward and thus intentionality. One may now propose that what Searle (and Rowland, Pred, and Freeman) describes as "network of preintentional capacities" (to use Searle's term) may well correspond on the conceptual level to what I referred to on the empirical level as the resting state's preintentional organization.

But let us be more specific. What exactly do the different terms in network of preintentional capacities mean within the empirical context of the brain? There is, of course, the term "network." That is an easy one. It refers to the midline and lateral networks and how they are related to the other networks in the rest of the brain.

What are now the "capacities" associated with these networks? The capacities concern the constitution of contents on the basis of differences between internal and external stimuli as proposed in my earlier-described difference-based hypothesis of contents. In addition, the "capacities" also concern the designation of contents as internal or external on the basis of the neural balance between midline and lateral networks as stated in my balance-based hypothesis of contents (see earlier).

Most important, the capacities concern the constitution of a point of view as based on the environment–brain unity (see earlier). This is supposed to be possible on the basis of the spatial and temporal alignment of the resting state's neural measures to the environmental stimuli. However, all the different "capacities" described so far are by themselves not yet sufficient to constitute directedness toward and thus intentionality.

Something additional must be suggested, though. This, as I proposed, is that both contents and point of view must be linked in order to sufficiently constitute intentionality. Such linkage is, I propose, associated with the neural integration and thus the spatiotemporally based neural difference between midline-lateral balance and the whole brain's neural activity. I therefore propose that the environment–brain unity and its associated point of view are indispensable, necessary, and predisposing conditions for constituting intentionality.

This is the reason why I described the resting state by a "preintentional organization" (see earlier). That may correspond on the conceptual side to what Rowland describes as the "noneliminable intentional core." And it also meshes nicely with his description of this "noneliminable intentional core" as transcendental, that is, "what allows something to appear as object of consciousness" (Rowland 2010, 179).

NEUROCONCEPTUAL HYPOTHESIS IIB: ROWLAND'S CONCEPT OF THE "NONELIMINABLE INTENTIONAL CORE" CORRESPONDS TO THE RESTING-STATE ACTIVITY'S "PREINTENTIONAL ORGANIZATION"

How is Rowland's transcendental characterization of his concept of the "noneliminable intentional core" related to my concept of the resting state's "preintentional organization"? I here complement Rowland's account by assuming that such a "non-eliminable intentional core" is not merely transcendental but, being based on the resting state's "preintentional organization," rather neurotranscendental (see also Appendix 3 here, as well as chapters 1 and 2 in Northoff 2011).

The concept of "neurotranscendental" denotes that certain empirical mechanisms of the brain, like the spatiotemporal organization of its resting state's neural activity, have a transcendental (or better neurotranscendental) role in that they make necessary or unavoidable the possible constitution of intentionality in particular and consciousness in general. In other words, these alleged neuronal mechanisms predispose possible intentionality and consciousness; they thus concern what I described as "principal consciousness" in the second Introduction as distinguished from actual consciousness. Such a neurotranscendental role must be distinguished from an empirical or neuroempirical role whose mechanisms would be necessary and/or sufficient conditions of actual (rather than possible) intentionality and consciousness.

How can we further specify the neurotranscendental role or characterization of the resting-state activity's "preintentional organization"? It is based on the statistically and spatial-temporally based unity between brain and environment, the environment–brain unity. To be more precise, one may speak of "neurosocial activity" here (as discussed in full detail in Chapter 20), which signifies both the environment and the brain. I now propose the intrinsically neurosocial environment–brain unity to take on a transcendental, that is, neurotranscendental, role by predisposing the possibility of intentionality in particular and consciousness in general. The resting-state activity's preintentional organization may thus correspond on the empirical side to Rowland's concept of the "noneliminable intentional core."

NEUROCONCEPTUAL HYPOTHESIS IIC: SEARLE'S DISTINCTION BETWEEN "NETWORK OF PREINTENTIONAL CAPACITIES" AND "BACKGROUND OF NONINTENTIONAL CAPACITIES" CORRESPONDS TO THE DISTINCTION BETWEEN THE BRAIN'S NEURAL ACTIVITY AND THE BRAIN'S PHYSICAL FEATURES

What about the concepts of "preintentional" and "nonintentional" in Searle's account? Searle himself does not seem to make major distinctions between "preintentional" as in "network of preintentional capacities" and "nonintentional" as in "background of nonintentional capacities." In contrast, I argue that we need to make a principal distinction between "preintentional" and "nonintentional."

The concept of background of nonintentional capacities refers to the brain's physical equipment that remains completely nonintentional by itself (rather than being preintentional). If so, the brain's physical equipment neither shows any intentionality by itself, i.e., being phenomenal, nor any predisposition for the constitution of directedness toward and intentionality, i.e., being prephenomenal. This changes, however, once the brain's biophysical equipment is used in a particular way when it generates neural activity and encodes it in a particular way. The step from the brain's physical equipment to its biophysical use is thus the central one. And it is here at the intersection between the physical equipment and its biophysical use where the brain's encoding strategy—how it encodes and thus generates its neural activity—comes into play.

I determined the brain's encoding strategy by difference-based coding and distinguished it from stimulus-based coding. Difference-based coding is supposed to be the necessary condition of possible consciousness in general and intentionality in particular. That, I suppose, is possible by encoding spatial and temporal differences into the brain's intrinsic activity, which thereby constitutes a statistically based spatiotemporal structure that virtually spans across the physical boundaries of brain, body, and environment.

What does this characterization of difference-based coding imply for what Searle describes as "network of preintentional capacities"? I postulate that difference-based coding and the resting-state activity's spatiotemporal structure including its virtual statistically-based spatiotemporal extension across the boundaries of brain, body, and environment are related to the "network of preintentional capacities."

The "network of preintentional capacities" is consequently associated with the brain's biophysical use of its intrinsic activity. The virtual statistically-based and spatiotemporal "network of preintentional capacities" must consequently be distinguished from the "background of nonintentional capacities" as they are related to the brain's merely physical equipment prior to its encoding and generation of any neural activity.

NEUROCONCEPTUAL HYPOTHESIS IIIA: NEUROTRANSCENDENTAL CHARACTERIZATION OF THE BRAIN

How is all this related to Searle and his concepts? Let us briefly recapitulate from the preceding section. The existence of the brain's physical equipment as being non-intentional by itself corresponds to what Searle describes conceptually as "background of nonintentional capacities,." This is complemented by his concept of "network of preintentional capacities," which may then refer to a specific way of encoding neural activity, difference- rather than stimulus-based coding, on the ground of the brain's biophysical equipment. That makes possible the subsequent constitution of the resting state's preintentional organization (see earlier). Accordingly, to neglect their distinction or to use both concepts, "background of nonintentional capacities" and "network of preintentional capacities," in an interchangeable way would be to confuse the brain's physical equipment with the brain's neural code, that is, difference-based coding that the brain itself applies to transform its own physical equipment into neural activity.

We need to be even more radical, however. To neglect the difference between the brain's physical equipment and its biophysical use with the application of particular neural code is to confuse not only the brain's "nonintentional background capacities" and its "preintentional capacities," but also the brain's empirical and neurotranscendental characterizations. The brain's physical features characterize the brain in purely empirical regard and bear no relationship at all to intentionality and consciousness; therefore, the brain's physical features are purely non-intentional and non-phenomenal by themselves and must thus be characterized as merely empirical (see Fig. 25-6b).

The situation is different, however, once one considers the neural code the brain itself applies to encode and generate its own neural activity. By preferring difference- over stimulus-based coding, the brain's (non-intentional and non-phenomenal) physical features are transformed into a kind of neural activity that predisposes the possible constitution of intentionality and consciousness. The brain's intrinsic activity in particular and its neural activity in general are thus preintentional and prephenomenal, rather than nonintentional and nonphenomenal. This means that the brain's encoding strategy, i.e., difference-based coding, characterizes the brain no longer in a purely empirical way but rather takes on a transcendental, or better, neurotranscendental, role.

NEUROCONCEPTUAL HYPOTHESIS IIIB: THREEFOLD CHARACTERIZATION OF THE BRAIN AS EMPIRICAL, NEUROTRANSCENDENTAL, AND NEUROEMPIRICAL

The neurotranscendental role of the brain's encoding strategy consists in that it predisposes possible consciousness, that is, "principal consciousness" as distinguished from "principal nonconsciousness" (see second Introduction). In contrast, additional neuronal mechanisms are required to actually realize and implement consciousness, as distinguished from the unconscious (see second Introduction). These additional neuronal mechanisms thus take on a neuroempirical rather than neurotranscendental role with regard to consciousness.

Accordingly, to disregard the difference between the brain's encoding strategy and the additional neuronal mechanisms is not only to neglect neuronal differences but also to confuse different characterizations of the brain, neurotranscendental and neuroempirical. The brain itself therefore seems to force us to distinguish among three different levels—empirical, neurotranscendental, and neuroempirical—in the characterization of the brain. I thus postulate a threefold characterization of the brain in conceptual regard as it shall be explicated in the following.

The empirical level concerns the merely physical features of the brain, as they differ between different species. Such an empirical characterization occurs prior to and independently of any neural activity. This is different in the neurotranscendental characterization. The neurotranscendental level is about the brain's neural code and how it encodes and generates its own neural activity; the neurotranscendental characterization thus focuses on how the brain uses its own physical features and transforms them into neural activity.

Finally, the neuroempirical level concerns the neuronal mechanisms and the different functions of the brain: sensory, motor, affective, cognitive, and social. The neuroempirical level thus describes the way the brain uses and transforms its neural activity to generate the various functions. This is the predominant approach these days to both brain and consciousness.

Why is all that important? The neuroscientists (and current neurophilosophers) may want to argue that this is "pure theory" and therefore irrelevant to understanding how the brain works and brings forth consciousness. We had better refrain from such dangerous theoretical speculation and focus only on the neuroempirical level. This is suggested, for instance, in the current neurosensory, neuromotor, neuroaffective, neurocognitive, and neurosocial (and also neurophilosophical) approaches to the brain and consciousness.

This, however, would mean giving up our experimental access to investigate consciousness and its relationship to the brain. To experimentally access consciousness, we need to consider the brain not only on the neuroempirical level, but also on the neurotranscendental level. We therefore need to shift our focus from the various functions of the brain to its neural activity and how the brain encodes its neural activity. Only if we shift from a "theory of brain function" to a "theory of brain activity," as suggested in Volume I, can we get a grip on consciousness. This means that neurotranscendental and neuroempirical approaches to the brain must work closely together to reveal the brain-based nature of consciousness in general and intentionality in particular.

Open Questions

One issue left open was how the directedness toward and the resting state's preintentional organization are associated with a phenomenal state and thus converted into full-blown intentionality on the level of consciousness. This, I propose, is dependent on the specific way neural activity changes in either the resting state or, during stimulus-induced activity, how it interacts with the resting-state activity level.

Accordingly, the kind and degree of rest–stimulus interaction is central in determining how much the resting state's prephenomenal structures, including its self-specific and preintentional organization, will be carried over and transferred to the newly resulting neural activity level, the stimulus-induced activity. And that, in turn, is important for their association with a phenomenal state and thus consciousness. This will be the focus in Chapters 28 through 30 in this volume.

First, however, we need to gather more empirical evidence in favor of the resting state's preintentional organization. For that, I turn to the examples of dreams and mind wandering. Dreams occur in the resting state and thus in the absence of external stimulus input. They nevertheless show external contents. The converse holds in the case of mind wandering. Mind wandering describes mind slips to internal contents in the presence of external stimuli. Hence, both mind wandering and dreams can be considered paradigmatic examples to lend further support to the resting state's preintentional organization. This will be the focus in the next chapter.

CHAPTER 26
Neurophenomenal Evidence—Dreams and Mind Wandering

Summary

So far, I have proposed the resting state to show preintentional organization. If that assumption holds, one would already expect directedness toward external contents to be manifest in the resting state during the absence of external stimuli. This is, for instance, the case in dreams. At the same time, however, there may also be directedness toward internal contents during external stimuli and their respective stimulus-induced activity. This is the case in mind wandering. Therefore, I here discuss the examples of dreams and mind wandering in neuronal and phenomenal detail to test whether they lend further evidence to my neurophenomenal hypotheses developed in Chapter 25. Dreams occur in the resting state and can be characterized by phenomenal consciousness that can be directed toward both internal and external contents. Neuronally, one can observe hyperactivity in the midline regions, while the lateral regions are rather hypoactive during dreams. This lends empirical support to the assumption that the neural balance between midline and lateral networks is central for predisposing the balance between internal and external contents including the directedness toward contents in consciousness. Most important, the example of dreams lends additional support to the assumption that directedness toward external contents and thus intentionality can occur already in the resting state itself. This implies that the constitution of external contents in consciousness does not necessarily depend on the presence of external stimuli from the environment and their respectively associated stimulus-induced activities. Hence the example of dreams lends empirical support to the assumption that the coding of the degree of differences between different stimuli rather than the origin of the stimuli is central in making possible "directedness toward" and ultimately intentionality. Accordingly, I propose "directedness toward" and intentionality to be difference based rather than origin based. In addition, the example of dreams also carries phenomenal implications. The fact that external contents can be experienced already during the resting state itself in an intentional way, i.e., implying "directedness toward," lends also support to the assumption of some kind of pre-intentional organization in the resting-state activity itself that therefore may be characterized as prephenomenal. This, however, leaves open the question of whether the same neuronal mechanisms also operate during stimulus-induced activity. For that, I turn to the example of mind wandering. Mind wandering describes the slips into the own internal thoughts during the stimulation with specific external stimuli. Neuronally, strong activity in the midline regions has been observed, which seems to be abnormally balanced with the neural activity in lateral regions. Moreover, the findings indicate that the less the stimulus-induced activity deviates from the resting-state activity, the greater the degree of mind wandering. The degree of neural activity change that can be elicited by external stimuli is consequently reduced during mind wandering. This suggest that the neural balance between midline and lateral networks and its impact on designating contents as either internal or external operates across the divide between resting-state and stimulus-induced activity. This makes possible the occurrence of internal contents during external stimuli and their respective stimulus-induced activity in mind wandering. Taking all this together, I conclude the examples of dreams and mind wandering to lend further empirical, that is, neuronal and phenomenal, support to my neurophenomenal hypotheses about the constitution of contents and the resting state's pre-intentional organization as suggested in Chapter 25.

Key Concepts and Topics Covered

Dreams, perceptions, internal and external awareness, midline and lateral networks, spontaneous activity, difference-based coding, self-specific organization, preintentional organization, difference-based coding, neural balance

NEUROEMPIRICAL BACKGROUND

IA: DREAMS AND MIND WANDERING
AS "HARD" CASES OF RESTING STATE
AND STIMULUS-INDUCED ACTIVITY

I characterized the resting-state activity by a preintentional organization as manifested in directedness toward content; this was supposed to be manifested in the degree of the midline-lateral networks' integration within the whole brain regions and networks and the spatiotemporal organization of their resting state (see Chapter 25). In contrast, I associated the designation of contents as either internal or external to be predisposed by the neural balance between midline and lateral networks.

How we can garner further empirical evidence that these neuronal mechanisms do indeed predispose intentionality on the phenomenal level of consciousness? For the answer to that, I will next discuss the examples of dreams and mind wandering in this chapter.

Why do I take dreams and mind wandering, rather than other examples like meditation (see, for instance, Brewer et al. 2011; Lou et al. 1999) and free or random thoughts (see Doucet et al. 2012; see also Andrews-Hanna 2012 for a recent review)? I described dreams and mind wandering as the "hard cases" of resting state and stimulus-induced activity. Dreams raise the question how external content and intentionality can occur in the absence of any specific external stimuli and their associated contents, as in the night when sleeping. Dreams as the presence of external contents in the absence of external stimuli can therefore be described as the "hard"

case of the resting state in the preceding chapter (see Chapter 25).

This is different from mind wandering. "Mind wandering" describes the slippage into internal contents during the presence of external contents (see below for a more exact definition). This raises the question of how it is possible that our mind slips into internal contents like our own thoughts during the simultaneous presence of external contents. Mind wandering was therefore described as the "hard" case of stimulus-induced activity (see Chapter 25).

Taken together, this means that the explanation of dreams and mind wandering can lend further support to our assumption of the resting-state activity's preintentional organization and its relation to internal and external contents. Therefore, I focus on dreams and mind wandering in the following discussion.

NEUROEMPIRICAL BACKGROUND IB: WHAT

DREAMS CAN TELL US ABOUT THE
RESTING-STATE ACTIVITY'S PREINTENTIONAL
ORGANIZATION AND ITS CONTENTS

Let us start with dreams. Dreams occur in the resting state of the brain, more specifically during the night when we sleep, and are not exposed to specific exteroceptive stimuli. Despite the minimization or even absence of exteroceptive stimulus input from the environment, there is often intense visual and/or auditory imagery in dreams. Though sleeping, the dreamer perceives and experiences the objects, persons, and events as if he were awake, thus being deluded about his own state and the origin of his experiences. While pertaining somehow to reality, the objects, events, and persons occurring during the dream often include bizarre distortions of objects, persons, and events. Dreams can consequently be characterized by vivid perceptions of scenario-like structures as a simulacrum of the world, thereby integrating highly disparate images and themes into a seamless scenario (see, for instance, Hobson 2009 804, for a nice description of dream perception in a painting from Salvador Dali).

Accordingly, put into the framework of intentionality, dreams can be considered an example of directedness toward external (and internal) objects in the absence of external stimulus input. The question is, of course, how it is possible to experience external contents in consciousness while there is no input from external stimuli. Dreams may therefore question the neuronal mechanisms underlying the constitution of contents and their subsequent designation as internal or external.

NEURONAL FINDINGS IA: RESTING-STATE ACTIVITY IN DREAMS

What are the neuronal underpinnings of dreams? Let's start with a special focus on the resting-state activity. Empirically, there is indeed abundant support that the brain's resting-state activity is high in both the awake state and especially in those sleep stages where dreaming occurs abundantly, for example, rapid eye movement (REM) sleep. In contrast, the brain's resting-state activity is rather low in sleep stages where dreams seem to remain absent or occur less frequently as, for example, in non-REM sleep.[1]

The high resting-state activity has led Hobson (2009, 808–9; see also Hobson and Friston 2012) to propose that dreams result from self-activation of the brain. More specifically, the brainstem with the pons as generator may extend and spread its activation to the forebrain (see also Solms 1995, 1997, 2000, who argues against the brainstem theory and regards the basal forebrain to be central). Let's be more specific with regard to the regions showing high resting-state activity in dreams. Resting-state activity in the pontine tegmentum, the amygdala, the hippocampus, the occipital cortex, the mediobasal prefrontal cortex, the anterior commissure, the parietal operculum, the midline thalamus, the deep frontal white matter, and the anterior cingulate cortex has been found to be increased in REM sleep when compared to the waking state (see Hobson 2009, 810, Honson and Friston 2012 as well as Wehrle et al. 2007 and Walker 2009a and b). In contrast, other regions like the dorsolateral prefrontal cortex and the posterior cingulate show rather decreased resting-state activity in REM sleep/dreams.

The observation of different levels of resting-state activity across different brain regions suggests that there must be some rest–rest interaction ongoing in dreams. Most important, due to the different resting-state activity levels in the different regions, such rest–rest interaction across the different brain regions must be different in dreams from the ones in the waking state. If there are such different kinds of rest–rest interaction across different regions, one would expect differences in the degrees of resting state functional connectivity between the different regions in the dreaming and the waking state.

This is indeed supported by empirical evidence. For instance, Kaufmann et al. (2006) observed increased functional connectivity of several cortical and subcortical core (e.g., median) regions with the hypothalamus in the dreaming state when compared to the waking state. Such differential functional connectivity patterns could be indicative of different kinds of rest–rest interactions in the dreaming state.

The observation of changes in resting-state functional connectivity during dreaming is further supported by the results from the group around Tononi. As described extensively in Chapters 15 and 16, REM sleep, which is usually associated with dreams, shows increased functional connectivity when compared to non-REM sleep, where dreams occur less often. Accordingly, there seems to be empirical support for different functional connectivity patterns in dreams that are indicative of a different kind of rest–rest interaction (see Walker 2009 for a recent review, as well as Larson-Prior et al. 2009).

NEURONAL FINDINGS IB: RESTING-STATE AND STIMULUS-INDUCED ACTIVITY IN DREAMS

Can rest–rest interaction account for the occurrence of perceptions in dreams? How can the vivid perceptions about objects, persons, or events in the environment, for example, the imagery and hallucinations be generated in dreams despite the absence of exteroceptive stimuli from the environment?

Let us go back to the sensory cortex. Hobson (2009, 809; see also Hobson and Friston 2012) postulates that there is what he calls "input-output gating" in REM sleep/dreams: He suggests that the sensory cortex and the motor cortex are actively suppressed and thus shut down during dreams. Such shutting-down of the sensory cortex makes it impossible for exteroceptive stimuli to enter the brain and interact with its intrinsic activity—the brain is consequently kept "offline" as he says (Hobson 2009, 809). What about the motor cortex? The neural activity in the motor cortex is also suppressed, so that now motor stimuli cannot get out of the brain and generate some kind of movement and action. Since stimuli can neither get into the brain nor get out of the brain, the brain is "locked in" and shut off from the environment.

How can we lend further empirical support for such a shutdown of the sensory cortex during dreams? Wehrle et al. (2005, 2007) investigated auditory stimulation during phasic and tonic REM sleep and non-REM sleep with especially the former being associated with dreams. Using fMRI, they observed significantly decreased activity change, for example, increased deactivation, in the auditory cortex during auditory stimulation in phasic REM sleep as associated with dreams. The same group reported a similar finding in an earlier study that showed increased deactivation in visual and auditory cortex also in non-REM sleep, indicating decreased activity (Czisch et al. 2004; Kaufmann et al. 2006; see also Walker 2009).

Taken together, these findings indicate altered, for example, decreased reactivity to exteroceptive stimuli in sensory cortex as in visual and auditory cortex, which reflects reduced stimulus-induced activity. This is indeed indicative of decreased neural reactivity of the sensory cortex to exteroceptive stimuli during dreams.

Hence, the resting-state activity in the sensory cortex must have changed in certain, yet unknown ways such as it no longer allows the exteroceptive stimuli to elicit changes in its activity level; that is, stimulus-induced activity. These yet-unknown changes in the resting state's neural features consequently lead to decreased neuronal reactivity of the sensory cortex to exteroceptive stimuli. This in turn shuts off the brain from the environment and leads consequently to what may be described as the "locked-in syndrome" of the brain.

NEUROPHENOMENAL HYPOTHESIS IA: DIFFERENCE-BASED CODING MEDIATES THE CARRYOVER AND TRANSFER OF THE RESTING STATE'S PREPHENOMENAL STRUCTURES TO THE STIMULUS AND ITS ASSOCIATION WITH CONSCIOUSNESS IN THE *AWAKE STATE*

How can we account for the vivid perceptions in the gestalt of imagery and hallucinations in dreams in the neuronal context of the brain? This raises two issues: How is it possible that there is phenomenal consciousness in dreams despite being in a pure resting state? And how can the dreamer perceive something at all in his dreams, that is, real objects, events, and so on, while there is no exteroceptive stimulus input at all? Let me start with the first issue, the question for phenomenal consciousness in the resting state, while I will deal with the second issue in the next section.

My main hypothesis is as follows. I hypothesize that the same neuronal mechanisms are at work in dreams during rest–rest interaction as in the awake and conscious state during rest–stimulus interaction and its subsequent stimulus-induced activity. How is that possible? For that the answer, let us recall briefly from Volume I.

We characterized perception by the interaction of an exteroceptive stimulus with the brain's intrinsic activity, its resting-state activity, and designated this with the term *rest–stimulus interaction* (see Volume I, Chapter 11). This led to the assumption of difference-based coding as distinguished from stimulus-based coding: the brain's neural activity encodes the difference of the exteroceptive stimulus to the brain's resting-state activity rather than the former, the stimulus, being coded by itself independent of the brain's intrinsic activity (which would imply stimulus- rather than difference-based coding).

What is encoded into the neural activity during the brain's encounter with the stimulus is therefore its difference from the brain's intrinsic activity. By encoding that difference, the intrinsic activity and its various prephenomenal structures can be carried over and transferred to the stimulus itself and its subsequent stimulus-induced activity (see Part VIII for more details). Such a carryover and transfer enables the association of the stimulus and its stimulus-induced activity with the features of the resting state's prephenomenal structures.

In other words, the stimulus becomes integrated within and linked to the spatiotemporal continuity, unity, and organization of the resting state's neural activity (see previous chapters). That, in turn, makes it possible to associate consciousness and its phenomenal features to the stimulus and its stimulus-induced activity (see Part VIII for more details of these processes).

NEUROPHENOMENAL HYPOTHESIS IB: ENCODING OF LARGE DIFFERENCES DURING REST–REST INTERACTION MEDIATES THE ASSOCIATION OF ACTIVITY CHANGES WITH CONSCIOUSNESS *IN DREAMS* AND THEIR VIVID PERCEPTIONS

How is all this related to the occurrence of the vivid perceptions in dreams? I now hypothesize that the very same neuronal mechanism of carryover and transfer is also at work in the perceptions of dreams. How is this possible?

One may at first be puzzled because there is one essential difference between the awake state and the dream state: the awake state can be characterized by exteroceptive input, which remains absent in the dream state. One must consequently propose that rest–stimulus interaction also remains absent in dreams. This seems to imply that the carryover and transfer of the resting-state activity's prephenomenal structures to the newly resulting activity level, the stimulus-induced activity, also remains absent. If so, any kind of phenomenal feature and thus consciousness should also remain absent.

How is it possible, however, to assign a phenomenal feature and thus consciousness to the imaginary and hallucinatory objects, events, or persons during the dreaming state, even in the absence of any kind of exteroceptive stimulus?

For that answer, we may need to go back to difference-based coding. What matters most for the brain is the amount or degree of neural differences that it needs to encode into its neural activity. Whether these neural differences are elicited by exteroceptive stimuli or within the resting-state activity itself does not matter. The brain encodes the neural difference into its neural activity, and it does not care so much about the origin of that neural difference or whether it can be traced back to an exteroceptive stimulus or not (See Chapter 25 for details).

This means that the brain "treats" a large difference that is elicited within the resting-state activity itself in very much the same way as it processes the same amount of neural difference elicited by an exteroceptive stimulus. What does this imply for the carryover and transfer of the resting state's prephenomenal structures to the newly resulting activity level? It entails that the resting-state activity's prephenomenal structures are carried over and transferred to the newly resulting activity level independently of whether the neural differences are elicited by either the stimulus or the resting-state activity itself.

Accordingly, what matters for the carryover and transfer is the amount or degree of neural difference, while the origin of that neural difference does not matter at all. I now hypothesize that the encoded neural differences during the resting-state activity itself, i.e., rest–rest interaction, are sufficiently large during REM-sleep and dreams. If that is so, one would expect larger activity changes during REM-sleep than in non-REM sleep. This is indeed supported by the data, since, unlike in non-REM sleep, rest–rest interactions seem to be larger in REM sleep, as described earlier.

One could consequently propose that the neural differences encoded into neural activity during the REM sleep's resting-state activity may be large enough to induce the carryover and transfer of the resting-state activity's prephenomenal structures to the newly resulting resting-state activity level. Due to the carryover and transfer of the resting state's prephenomenal structures, the newly resulting resting-state activity can be associated with consciousness and its various phenomenal features (see Part VIII for detailed neuronal mechanisms). This is manifested in the vivid perceptions, e.g., the imagery and hallucinations, in dreams.

NEUROPHENOMENAL HYPOTHESIS IC: PGO-WAVES AND K-COMPLEXES SIGNIFY THE ENCODING OF LARGE NEURAL DIFFERENCES *DURING DREAMS*

How can we lend more empirical support for the encoding of larger neural differences during rest–rest interaction in dreams? One may want to see the findings of reduced stimulus-induced activity as indirect support. Stimulus-induced activity may be reduced because resting-state activity, that is, rest–rest interaction, is too large so that there, figuratively speaking, is "no room anymore" for the stimulus to induce changes in the resting-state activity. This is supported by the aforementioned findings of decreased reactivity of the sensory cortex's resting state to exteroceptive stimuli.

However, one would like to have more direct empirical support for the processing of larger neural differences in the resting state itself. More direct empirical support for the processing of increased neural differences in the resting state itself can, for instance, be found in what is referred to as *cortical desynchronization*. "Cortical desynchronization" describes that neural activities in the different regions and networks are not synchronized and thus not coordinated and adjusted to each other.

Can we measure cortical desynchronization? There are different electrophysiological measures of cortical desynchronization: these may be indicative of increased rest–rest interaction, which supposedly reflects the processing of abnormally large neural differences in the resting-state activity during dreams. One neuronal measure of cortical descynchronization that indicates the processing of abnormally large differences are ponto-geniculo-occipital (PGO) waves, which are spontaneous waves of neural activity change that spread from the subcortical regions, e.g., the pons and the lateral geniculate to the occipital cortex, and occur specifically during dreams. Another electrophysiological measure of increased resting rest–rest interaction and hence of cortical desynchronization is what is described as low K-complexes and delta waves (see Czisch et al. 2004).There thus seems to be indeed some empirical evidence for the assumption of increased rest–rest interaction with the subsequent processing of larger neural differences in the dreaming state.

What does the increase in rest–rest interaction with the encoding of larger neural differences in the resting-state activity during dreams imply for their subsequent association with consciousness and its phenomenal features? I suggest the following neurophenomenal hypothesis.

I propose that the degree of neural differences processed during rest–rest interaction, as manifested in the afore-mentioned measures of cortical desynchronization like PGO waves, low K-complex, and delta waves, is directly and proportionally related to the degree of phenomenal consciousness during the dreaming state (see Hobson and Friston 2012, who associate the PGO waves with free energy in the brain that is not bound or tied to any particular neural event): the stronger the degree of cortical desynchronization (and the higher the degree of the respective neural measures), the stronger the degree of phenomenal consciousness the dreamer will experience (see Fig. 26-1a).

NEUROPHENOMENAL HYPOTHESIS IIA: MIDLINE-LATERAL BALANCE MEDIATES THE BALANCE BETWEEN INTERNAL AND EXTERNAL CONTENTS *IN DREAMS*

Now we can turn our focus to the second issue. How do the objects, events, and persons enter the dreams despite the fact that there are no exteroceptive stimuli at all? The only way for the objects, events, and persons to enter the perceptions during dreams is through the resting state itself.

The external contents in the phenomenal consciousness during dreams, though distorted, can only come from the resting state itself, because there are no major exteroceptive stimuli input anymore (except some basic intero- and exteroceptive stimuli) and a shutdown of the sensory cortex (see earlier) during dreams. We are consequently referred to the resting state itself in our search for the origin of the external contents during dreams. .

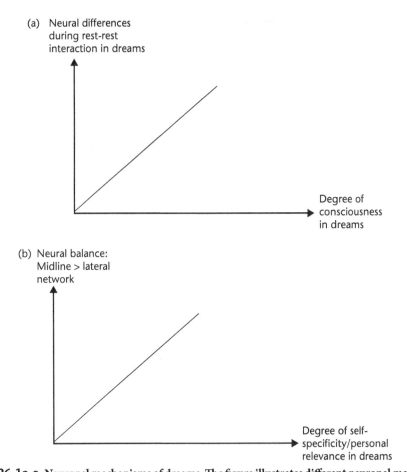

Figure 26-1a-e Neuronal mechanisms of dreams. The figure illustrates different neuronal mechanisms in dreams (*a*, *b*, *d*, and *e*) and compares dreams to perceptions in the awake state (*c*). (*a*) The figure shows the relationship between rest–rest interaction and the degree of consciousness in dreams. The more rest–rest interaction (with subsequently higher degrees of neural differences in the resting state itself) during dreams, the higher the degree of consciousness associated with the dreaming. (*b*) The figure shows the relationship between the midline-lateral cortical balance and the degree of self-specificity in dreams. The more the neural balance between midline and lateral networks is tilted toward the former, the higher the degree of self-specificity of the contents occurring during dreams. (*c*) The figure compares the constitution of perceptions in the awake state and the dreaming state. The absence of the stimulus in the dreaming state is compensated for by the large neural differences during rest–rest interaction. Due to the subsequently triggered carryover and transfer of the resting state's intentional organization to the newly resulting neural activity, this will be associated with phenomenal consciousness as manifest in perception of objects and events. Thereby the latter are based on previous objects and events as encoded in the resting state by stimulus–rest interaction in the awake state. I describe these events and objects thus as "as-if events and objects" (see Northoff 2011 for details) in order to distinguish them from the real objects and events experienced in the awake state. (*d*) The figure shows the relationship between the deviation of resting-state activity levels and the deviation of contents. The more both resting-state activity levels in awake and dreaming state deviate from each other, the more their respective contents in consciousness, e.g., during dream and awake state, will differ from each other. (*e*) The figure shows the relationship between the subcortical-cortical neural difference and the degree of directedness in dreams. The more the midline-lateral networks differ (e.g., showing higher degrees of neural differences) from the whole brain's regions/networks, including its subcortical regions, the higher the degree of directedness from a point of view toward contents in the dreaming state.

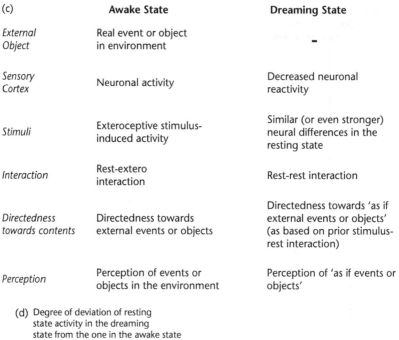

(c)	Awake State	Dreaming State
External Object	Real event or object in environment	-
Sensory Cortex	Neuronal activity	Decreased neuronal reactivity
Stimuli	Exteroceptive stimulus-induced activity	Similar (or even stronger) neural differences in the resting state
Interaction	Rest-extero interaction	Rest-rest interaction
Directedness towards contents	Directedness towards external events or objects	Directedness towards 'as if external events or objects' (as based on prior stimulus-rest interaction)
Perception	Perception of events or objects in the environment	Perception of 'as if events or objects'

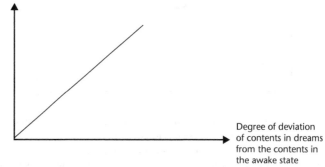

(d) Degree of deviation of resting state activity in the dreaming state from the one in the awake state

Degree of deviation of contents in dreams from the contents in the awake state

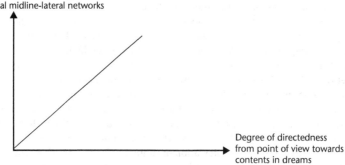

(e) Degree of neural difference between subcortical regions and cortical midline-lateral networks

Degree of directedness from point of view towards contents in dreams

Figure 26-1a-e (Continued)

How, then, can the resting state itself and its rest–rest interactions provide the neural basis for the objects, persons, and events in our perceptions during dreams? Let us recall from Chapter 25. There I distinguished between midline and lateral networks. Strong activity in the midline network was associated with a shift toward internal contents in consciousness, while activity in the lateral network led to stronger external contents in consciousness. This was summarized in what I described as the "balance hypothesis of contents" that proposed the neural balance between midline and lateral networks to be central in designating contents as internal or external.

How does the "balance hypothesis of contents" apply to dreams? The earlier-described findings show that, during dreams, the midline regions, e.g., the limbic-anterior midline regions, show extremely high activity that is even higher than in the awake resting state. In contrast, the lateral cortical regions' resting-state activity is rather hypoactive during dreams. That means that the resting state's neural balance between midline and lateral networks is shifted toward the midline regions in the dreaming state.

What does the shift in the neural balance toward the midline network imply for the designation of contents in dreams? Since the shift of the neural balance toward the midline network is associated with designating contents as internal, one would expect increased internal contents in dreams. In contrast, external contents may be less in dreams compared to those in the awake state where the neural balance between midline and lateral networks seems to be more even and less unilateral.

One may therefore hypothesize the following: The less the neural balance between midline and lateral networks is shifted toward the midline network, the more external contents are perceived and thus experienced in dreams. In contrast, stronger shifts of the neural balance between midline ad lateral networks toward the midline network may lead to the perception and experience of less external contents and a higher number of internal contents in dreams.

NEUROPHENOMENAL HYPOTHESIS IIB: MIDLINE-LATERAL BALANCE MEDIATES THE DEGREE OF SELF-SPECIFICITY OF CONTENTS *IN DREAMS*

The shift of the neural balance toward the midline network has yet another important implication. We recall from Chapters 23 and 24 that the midline network is apparently instrumental in assigning self-specificity to stimuli and contents.

If now the midline-lateral balance shifts toward the midline network in dreams, one would expect assignment of increased self-specificity to the contents (independently of whether they are designated as internal or external). That should be manifest in increased personal meaning and significance in relation to the internal and external contents, for example, the objects, events, and persons perceived and experienced in dreams (see Fig. 26-1b).

This leads me to postulate the following hypothesis: the larger the shift of the neural balance toward the midline network, the larger the degree of self-specificity and consequently the more personal meaning is associated with the internal and external contents as perceived and experienced in dreams. Interestingly, the assumption of self-specificity and personal meaning in dreams harks back to Sigmund Freud, who, roughly 100 years ago, postulated that hidden personal meanings are associated with the objects, events, and persons experienced and perceived during dreams (see Northoff 2011, chapter 7 for details).

NEUROPHENOMENAL HYPOTHESIS IIIA: STIMULUS–REST INTERACTION ENCODES CONTENTS INTO THE BRAIN'S RESTING-STATE ACTIVITY IN THE *AWAKE STATE*

So far, I have discussed the occurrence of internal and external contents in dreams and their assignment of high degrees of self-specificity. Now the question is how the brain is able to constitute external contents in the resting state, despite the fact that any exteroceptive stimulus input is (more or less) absent. One step in this direction was already indicated in the previous chapter.

I proposed that the constitution of external (and internal) contents is not based on the stimuli themselves and their particular origin as being either intero- or exteroceptive. Instead, what matters for the designation of contents as either internal or external is the direction of the neural differences encoded into neural activity; whereas, the origin of the origin of the underlying stimuli as either intero- or exteroceptive simply does ultimately not matter. This, however, is only the first step.

The second step is that the differences encoded into neural activity must be associated with specific persons, objects, or events accounting for the external (or internal) contents. How is such an association of the neural differences with specific objects, person, or events, and thus internal or external contents, possible? This raises the question of how the neural differences encoded in the resting-state activity and its rest–rest interaction are associated with specific objects, events, or persons as internal or external contents in dreams.

How do the objects, persons, or events come into the resting-state activity during dreams where they surface as internal or external contents? For the answer, I turn to stimulus–rest interaction. We provided empirical evidence for stimulus–rest interaction in Chapter 11 in Volume I. More specifically, we saw that the preceding stimuli impact the neuronal activity in the subsequent resting state by modulating its level, functional connectivity, and/or low-frequency fluctuations.

To put it metaphorically, the intero- and exteroceptive stimuli "leave their traces" in the resting-state activity, which therefore must encode some information about the respectively associated objects, persons, and events in its neural activity in the awake state.

NEUROPHENOMENAL HYPOTHESIS IIIB: REST–REST INTERACTION MODULATES THE ENCODED CONTENTS IN THE RESTING STATE AND MAKES POSSIBLE THEIR *BIZARRE APPEARANCE IN DREAMS*

What does such encoding of information about previous objects, persons, or events into the resting-state activity during the awake state imply for dreams? We showed earlier that the resting-state activity seems to show increased rest–rest interaction with larger neural differences during dreams. For instance, the midline-lateral balance and the balance between cortical and subcortical regions (with the latter being emphasized by Hobson; see earlier) seem to shift during dreams, compared to the awake state.

The increased rest–rest interaction may therefore alter not only the level of the newly resulting resting-state activity (see earlier) but also the information that is encoded into the very same resting-state activity. This means that the objects, events, and persons encoded into the resting-state activity will be modified in an abnormal way. That in turn may account for the perception and experience of the often strange and bizarre objects, events, and persons as internal or external contents in dreams (see Fig. 26-1c).

This leads me to the following neurophenomenal hypothesis. I propose the degree of deviation of the internal and external contents during dreams from those perceived and experienced in the awake state to be directly dependent upon and thus proportional to the degree of difference between the resting-state activity in the awake state and in the dream state. The more the resting-state activity during dreams deviates from the activity in the awake state, the more likely it is that the persons, objects, and events, and thus the internal or external contents in dreams, will differ from the ones in the awake state. If, in contrast, the neural difference between the two resting states' levels and features is rather small, the internal and external contents between awake and dream state may not differ as much (see Fig. 26-1d).

NEUROPHENOMENAL HYPOTHESIS IIIC: DEPENDENCE OF ACTUAL REST–REST INTERACTION ON PRIOR STIMULUS–REST INTERACTION MEDIATES THE *RESEMBLANCE BETWEEN CONTENTS IN DREAMS AND THE AWAKE STATE*

We have so far only talked about deviation of the contents in dreams from those in the awake state. How about their similarity or resemblance?

Often the contents in dreams are related to the persons, events, and objects we experience in the preceding awake states. This is supported by a recent study from Kahan and LaBerge (2011), who report remarkable similarity in the sensory and cognitive qualities between dreaming and waking experiences.

How is such resemblance between dream and awake contents possible? This is, I propose, made possible by the fact that the association of neural differences in the resting-state activity with specific objects, persons, and contents is based on previous stimulus–rest interaction in the preceding awake states. The reliance of the resting state's neural activity and its contents during dreams on the resting state in the preceding awake state makes it almost necessary for the contents in dreams to show a close relationship to the experiences of that person in the preceding awake state.

Despite the earlier-reported deviation and distortion of the contents during dreams, that very same distortion and deviation cannot avoid to be based on the contents that are already encoded into the resting-state activity via prior stimulus–rest interaction in the awake state. Even if the dream contents' distortion and deviation is strong, there will nevertheless always be some, even if small, degree of resemblance to the contents in the awake state and thus to the person itself. This has already been well described by Sigmund Freud.

NEUROPHENOMENAL HYPOTHESIS IVA: NEURAL DIFFERENCES BETWEEN MIDLINE-LATERAL NETWORKS AND THE REST OF THE BRAIN MEDIATE INTENTIONALITY IN THE *AWAKE STATE*

We have discussed the constitution of contents and their designation as either internal or external in dreams. I suggested the contents to show a high degree of self-specificity and argued that their origin may stem from previous stimulus–rest interactions in previous awake states. This covers plenty of ground, but leaves one final issue open: namely, how the contents can be associated with intentionality as manifested in the experience of "directedness toward."

For that answer, we may want to return briefly to Chapter 25, where I proposed the "point of view–based hypothesis of directedness. It stated that the contents must be associated with the point of view in order for intentionality in the gestalt of "directedness toward" to be constituted.

Once the contents are linked to the point of view, the latter becomes directed toward the contents, which leads to what is described as *directedness toward* or *intentionality* (see Chapter 26). Neuronally, I proposed the association of the point of view with content to be related to the balance between midline-lateral networks and the whole brain's regions/networks (which includes the other cortical regions and the subcortical regions).

NEUROPHENOMENAL HYPOTHESIS IVB: LARGE NEURAL DIFFERENCES BETWEEN MIDLINE-LATERAL NETWORKS AND THE REST OF THE BRAIN MEDIATE INTENTIONALITY *IN DREAMS*

How does that hypothesis about intentionality in general stand up to the empirical findings in the more specific case of dreams? We remember that Hobson does indeed propose abnormal spread of neural activity from the subcortical regions to the cortical networks in dreams.

This means that the midline-lateral network is integrated within and linked to the other cortical networks and its subcortical regions in the rest of the brain. Such integration even if differing from the awake state may then link and connect contents and point of view with the consequent constitution of directedness toward and thus intentionality. This leads me to the following neurophenomenal hypothesis.

I propose that the degree of directedness toward and thus the intentionality in dreams is directly dependent upon and therefore proportional to the neural balance between midline-lateral networks and the whole brain's regions/networks, including its subcortical regions. The smaller the neural difference between midline-lateral networks and the whole brain's regions/networks, including its subcortical regions, the lower the degree of directedness toward and thus intentionality the respective subject experiences during the perception and experience of the contents in its dreams. This, I suggest, seems to be the case in non-REM sleep, where there is no perception and experience and thus no consciousness.

In contrast, higher degrees of neural differences between midline-lateral networks and the whole brain's regions/networks, including its subcortical regions, should accompany higher degrees of directedness toward and intentionality in dreams. This, I propose, should be the case in REM-sleep and thus during dreams. That is indeed consistent with the earlier-reported findings of increased rest–rest interaction and the processing of larger neural differences during REM-sleep (see Fig. 26-1e).

Our assumption is especially consistent with the observation of large subcortical changes in resting-state activity during dreams, as suggested by Hobson. Why is this so? Large changes in subcortical activity may also change and possibly increase their difference from the midline-lateral networks. And, as hypothesized, such an increase in the neural difference between midline-lateral networks and the whole brain's regions/networks, including the subcortical regions, should increase the degree of directedness and thus intentionality. This is exactly what one observes during dreams in REM-sleep (when compared to non-REM sleep).

NEUROEMPIRICAL BACKGROUND II: WHAT MIND WANDERING CAN TELL US ABOUT THE RESTING-STATE ACTIVITY'S PREINTENTIONAL ORGANIZATION AND ITS CONTENTS

I have demonstrated that external contents can be constituted and be associated with phenomenal consciousness in the absence of exteroceptive stimuli, that is, in the resting state. This was exemplified by the example of dreams. I now turn to internal contents. These can occur in the resting state itself as, for instance, during free or random thoughts (see Doucet et al. 2012) as well as in meditation (though internal contents may be minimized during meditation) (see Brewer et al. 2011), which both strongly recruit the midline regions and the default-mode network (see Andrews-Hanna et al. 2011).

The occurrence of internal contents in the resting-state activity is the easy case. It becomes more difficult to explain the occurrence of internal contents during the presence of external stimuli and their associated stimulus-induced activity. How is it possible that internal contents occur despite the presence of exteroceptive stimuli? I described those instances as the "hard cases" of stimulus-induced activity, such as in mind wandering. This will be the focus in the following sections.

"Mind wandering" is defined as the shift of attention from a specific target or task in the external environment to the own internal thoughts (see Smallwood and Schooler 2006; Gruberger et al. 2011; Smallwood et al. 2008a and b). The assumption is that internal or random thoughts are continuously ongoing in both the resting state and stimulus-induced state. Usually the demands of, for instance, cognitive tasks let the subjects attention shift toward the external task rather than the ongoing internal thoughts.

One, however, may slip back into attending the own internal thoughts more than the external cognitive tasks. This attention slip is called mind wandering, meaning that the mind wanders away from the external cognitive task and its external contents to the internal contents of the own thoughts. That means, as it is relevant here in the present context, mind wandering shows the predominance of internal contents during the presence of exteroceptive stimuli as in stimulus-induced activity.

NEURONAL FINDINGS IIA: MIND WANDERING AND MIDLINE REGIONS

How can we characterize mind wandering in further psychological detail? Smallwood and Schooler (2006, 953–957; see also Schooler et al. 2011) emphasize that mind wandering is often initiated by a personally relevant goal, meaning that attention is very sensitive to self- or goal-relevant information. If the internal thoughts show such a personally or self-relevant goal, the cognitive functions and their executive control of the external cognitive task may become usurped or hijacked by the more personally relevant goal of the internal thoughts. The importance of self-relevance is also documented in the contents of the internal thoughts during mind wandering. The mind wandering's contents often reflect current concerns of the person associated with its current or past life, including personal comforts and problems.

How about the neuroanatomical regions implicated in mind wandering (see Gruberger et al. 2011 for a recent review)? Mason et al. (2007) investigated subjects in functional magnetic resonance imaging (fMRI) while they performed a working memory task that was either novel or practiced before. They compared both novel and practiced working memory tasks with a baseline (i.e., fixation cross—they subtracted the working memory conditions from the baseline) to reveal those regions showing high activity during the resting state.

As expected, this yielded the typical regions of the DMN with especially the anterior and posterior cingulate cortex, the precuneus, the insula, the medial prefrontal cortex, and the lateral parietal cortex. The authors then compared practiced versus novel working memory versions The practiced version showed a higher degree of stimulus-independent thoughts, that is, mind wandering, when compared to the novel one, while neuronally the novel version elicited significantly stronger signal changes, for example, negative BOLD responses (NBRs), than the practiced version.

What does this imply for the novel version? The novel version thus induced stronger deviation from the resting-state activity level than the practiced version. Conversely, the practiced version showed decreased deviation from the resting state, which is indicative of increased stimulus-independent thoughts (as observed behaviorally) and thus mind wandering (when compared to the novel version). Interestingly this pattern holds for all midline regions of especially those of the inner (anterior and posterior cingulate) ring.

Even more important, signal changes in the anterior and posterior cingulate cortex and the insula also correlated with the degree of mind wandering as measured by an independent scale, the daydreaming scale from the Imaginal Process Inventory (IPI). The less the task-related signal changes deviated from the resting state in the midline regions, the higher the degree of mind wandering reported by the subjects (see Fig. 26-2a).

NEURONAL FINDINGS IIB: REGIONAL ACTIVITY PATTERN DURING MIND WANDERING

How can we further substantiate the neuronal findings in mind wandering? Another fMRI study by Christoff et al. (2009) let subjects perform a Go/No-Go task and evaluate from time to time whether their attention was focused on the task ("on-task periods") or something else ("off-task periods") and whether they were aware that their attention was focused. The analysis focused on the 10-second periods preceding the evaluations ("thought probes") that were divided according to whether the subjects were focused on the task ("on-task") or not ("off-task").

How about the results? The off-task periods showed significantly stronger signal changes (when compared to the on-task periods) in the various regions of the DMN, the anterior and posterior cingulate cortex, the medial prefrontal cortex, and the temporo-parietal junction, as well as in the insula. In addition, lateral cortical regions like the dorsolateral prefrontal cortex were also observed to be active during the off-task periods (see Fig. 26-2b).

The involvement of the DMN and lateral cortical regions was further confirmed when comparing the periods before subjects made mistakes in the Go/No-Go task with those where they gave the correct answer. Comparison of both periods again yielded signal changes in more or less the same DMN and lateral cortical regions as described earlier. The assumption here is that mistakes may be due to increased mind wandering, which corresponds well to the involvement of the DMN and midline regions.

Finally, based on the answers to the second question, i.e., whether they were aware that their attention was focused, the authors compared those mind-wandering periods where subjects were unaware ("without meta-awareness") with those where they indicated to be aware ("with meta-awareness"). Mind wandering without meta-awareness showed significantly stronger signal changes in the regions reported earlier, e.g., DMN and lateral cortical regions, when compared to mind wandering with meta-awareness.

Taken together, mind wandering can be understood as the manifestation of the balance between internal and external contents during stimulus-induced activity. The data suggest that this balance between internal and external content seems to be related to a neural activity pattern across both midline and lateral regions

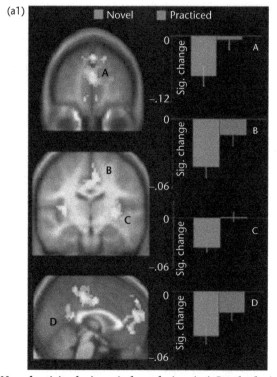

Figure 26-2a and b Neural activity during mind wandering. (*a1*) Graphs depict regions of the default network exhibiting significantly greater activity during practiced blocks (darker gray) relative to novel blocks (lighter gray) at a threshold of $P < 0.001$, number of voxels (k) = 10. Mean activity was computed for each participant by averaging the signal in regions within 10 mm of the peak, across the duration of the entire block. Graphs depict the mean signal change across all participants. (A) Left (L.) mPFC (BA 9; –6, 54, 22); (B) cingulate (BA 24; 0, –7, 36); (C) Right (R.) insula (45, –26, 4); and (D) L. posterior cingulate (BA 23/31; –9, –39, 27). Activity is plotted on the average high-resolution anatomical image and displayed per neurological convention (left hemisphere is depicted on the left). (*a2*) Graphs depict regions that exhibited a significant positive relation, $r(14) > 0.50$, $P < 0.05$, between the frequency of mind-wandering and the change in BOLD signal observed when people performed practiced relative to novel blocks. Participants' BOLD difference scores (practiced – novel) are plotted against their standardized IPI daydreaming score. BOLD signal values for the two blocks were computed for each participant by averaging the signal in regions within 10 mm of the peak, from 4 TRs (10 s) until 10 TRs (22.5 s) after the block onset. (A) B. mPFC (BA 10; –6, 51, –9; $k = 25$); (B) B. precuneus and p. cingulate (BA 31, 7; –3, –45, 37; $k = 72$); (C) R. cingulate (BA 31; 7, –21, 51; $k = 73$); (D) L. insula (BA 13; –36, –16, 17; $k = 10$); (E) R. insula (BA 13; 47, 0, 4; $k = 13$). Activity is plotted on the average high-resolution anatomical image and displayed in neurological convention (left hemisphere is depicted on the left). (*b*) Activations preceding reports of mind wandering (intervals prior to off-task versus on-task probes). Upward arrows, default network regions; downward arrows, executive network regions. Regions of activation included: (A) dorsal ACC (BA 32), (B) ventral ACC (BA 24/32), (C) precuneus (BA 7), (D) bilateral temporoparietal junction (BA 39), and (E) bilateral DLPFC (BA 9). Height threshold $P < 0.005$, extent threshold $k < 5$ voxels.

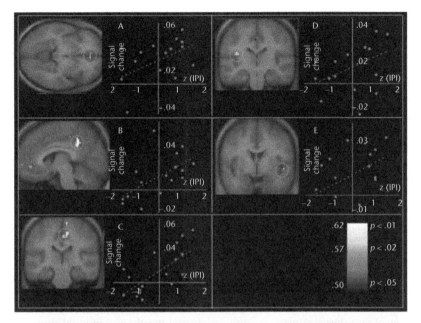

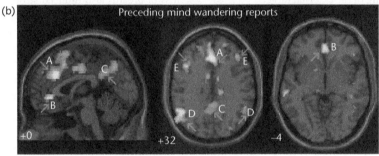

Figure 26-2a and b (Continued)

(see also Gruberger et al. 2011 for a recent review). This can also be accompanied by what is described as meta-awareness, the awareness of the own internal thoughts as mind wandering (see also Schooler et al. 2011).

NEURONAL FINDINGS IIC: EXTERNALLY ORIENTED ATTENTION AND MIND WANDERING

The study by Christoff described mind wandering and its underlying neural activity pattern during the performance of an external task. This demonstrated clearly that mind wandering interferes with the processing of the external stimuli and the respectively associated tasks. How exactly does such interference work? This is the focus in the present section.

Smallwood, Beach, et al. (2008a) conducted an EEG study where subjects had to perform a sustained attention task. They had to respond to frequent nontargets (digit 0–9) while they were instructed to withhold responses to infrequent targets (letter x). When subjects withhold a behavioral response to the frequent nontargets, mind wandering was proposed to occur; this was behaviorally corroborated by the subjects' reports of having intense internal thoughts when withholding the response.

Electrophysiologically, the focus was on the P300, which is an event-related potential and has been clearly shown to be related to the attention and cognitive processing of external stimuli. Interestingly, the P300 was reduced in all those nontarget trials where subjects showed mind wandering as measured either behaviorally (i.e., withhold response) or subjectively (i.e., subjective thought probes). Moreover, subjective and behavioral measures of mind wandering were correlated with the degree of the P300 amplitude: The higher the number of withheld responses (during frequent non-targets) and the more internal thoughts were reported, the more reduced the amplitude of the P300. This means that the psychological shift of attention from the external target to the internal thoughts was accompanied by the reduction of the P300 associated with the attention to and thus the cognitive processing of the external target.

What do these EEG results tell us about the neuronal basis of mind wandering? The study tells us that the balance between internal and external contents is shifted toward the internal pole, as is well indicated by the increased internal thoughts, the increased number of withheld responses, and the reduced P300 amplitude during mind wandering. The results demonstrate the neural and behavioral mechanisms that underlie the shift in the focus of attention from the external to the internal contents. In contrast, the results leave open the question of what neural mechanisms underlie the internal thought itself.

Neuronal findings IID: Internal thoughts and mind wandering

Another EEG study on mind wandering was conducted by Braboszcz and Delorme (2011). Subjects had to keep their eyes closed and to attend their breath cycles by counting them (1–10). Subjects were asked to indicate by a right-hand button when they became aware that they lost track of their breath count, indicating episodes of mind wandering. All this happened while tones were played in the background (to which subjects had not to respond) in the sense of an auditory oddball paradigm with 80%

similar stimuli (500 Hz) and 20% deviating stimuli (1000 Hz).

The authors analyzed all the time periods in their EEG when subjects indicated they had lost track of their breath count. In these periods of loss of breath, the power in the delta- (2–3.5 Hz) and theta- (4–7 Hz) frequency bands was significantly enhanced when compared to the episodes without mind wandering, that is, when subjects were able to focus on their breath. These changes in power frequencies were observed throughout the whole cortex with the delta changes being strongest in fronto-central regions and the theta changes being most prominent in occipital and parietal regions.

How about the impact of the auditory stimuli that were presented in the background? The auditory stimuli that were presented during the episodes of mind wandering episodes (e.g., loss of breath) also induced stronger delta- and theta-frequency power increases when compared to their occurrence during the breath focus. How about the higher-frequency ranges? In contrast to the lower-frequency bands (delta, theta), the power of higher frequencies like alpha (9–11 Hz) and beta (15–30 Hz) was significantly reduced during the mind wandering when compared to the breath focus.

Taken together, the results suggest that mind wandering may be accompanied by a shift from higher to lower frequencies. External stimuli and their cognitive processing seem to shift the power toward higher frequencies (alpha, beta) while internal thoughts and thus mind wandering are associated rather with power shifts toward lower frequencies (delta, theta) (see also Schooler et al. 2011 for a recent review; they also speak of "perceptual decoupling" in this context).

One may consequently propose speculatively that internal thoughts in particular, and possibly external contents in general, are more related to low-frequency oscillations whereas cognitive processing of external stimuli instantiates higher frequency oscillations. Hence, it may be the balance between high- and low-frequency oscillations that sustains the balance between internally and externally oriented attention and thus between internal and external contents.

NEUROPHENOMENAL HYPOTHESIS VA: DEVIATION FROM RESTING STATE ACTIVITY MEDIATES THE OCCURRENCE OF INTERNAL CONTENTS DURING MIND WANDERING

What do mind wandering and the neuronal findings tell us about our neurophenomenal hypotheses about internal and external contents and their directedness toward, e.g., intentionality in our experience? First and foremost, they tell us that the balance between midline and lateral networks seems to be central in mind wandering, rather than the midline network alone. This is evidenced by the findings by Christoff et al. (2009), who showed involvement of both midline and lateral cortical regions in the episodes during mind wandering as earlier described (see also the review by Gruberger et al. 2011).

How does the assumption of such a neural balance between midline and lateral cortical regions stand in relation to the findings by Mason et al. (2007), who showed sole involvement of the midline regions during mind wandering? One may be inclined to propose that the findings by Mason et al. (2007) show the opposite, namely, that the midline network alone is essential. However, when looking into the details of Mason's study, it becomes clear that regions outside the midline network were not considered at all for the correlation analysis between neural and behavioral data. Therefore, the Mason study cannot be taken as support for the assumption that mind wandering depends on the midline network alone independent of the lateral network.

What does the here-proposed neural balance between midline and lateral networks imply for the distinction between internal and external contents? Mind wandering reflects internal contents and thus internal directedness, while perception is related to external contents and thus external directedness. As Cristoff herself proposes, internal and external contents seem to be balanced with each other, and their balance apparently corresponds to the neural balance between midline and lateral networks. This therefore supports to my "balance-based hypothesis of contents" (see Chapter 25). It proposes the neural balance between midline and lateral network to be central in designating contents as either internal or external.

The earlier-described EEG results from the interaction between externally oriented attention and mind wandering reveal yet another point. The closer the neural activity is to the resting state with regard to, for instance, its low-frequency oscillations, the more likely internal contents will predominate over external contents; and the more likely that the subsequent consciousness will be directed toward internal rather than external contents.

At the same time, the neural activity related to external stimuli—as signified by, for instance, the electrophysiological potential of the P300—will decrease, as demonstrated in the aforementioned findings. Such a reduction in the underlying neuronal measures signifies decreased processing of the external content, which makes it more likely for the neural processing underlying internal contents to become predominant (see Fig. 26-3a).

NEUROPHENOMENAL HYPOTHESIS VB: INTERNAL AND EXTERNAL CONTENTS COMPETE FOR SELF-SPECIFICITY DURING MIND WANDERING

The neural mechanisms underlying the shift toward internal contents seem to strongly implicate the midline regions. In the preceding chapters, these midline regions were associated with the processing of self-specificity. Since the neural activity shifts during mind wandering toward the midline regions, one would propose higher degrees of self-specificity to be attributed to the internal thoughts in particular and the internal contents in general. This means that the contents in mind wandering are not only designated as internal but are also assigned a high degree of self-specificity (see Fig. 26-3b). That is well reflected in the phenomenology with personally relevant contents triggering episodes of mind wandering (see earlier for description).

One may go even one step further and raise the following question: Why and how is the neural shift from the lateral toward the midline regions and the subsequent shift from external to internal contents instantiated? If the resting-state

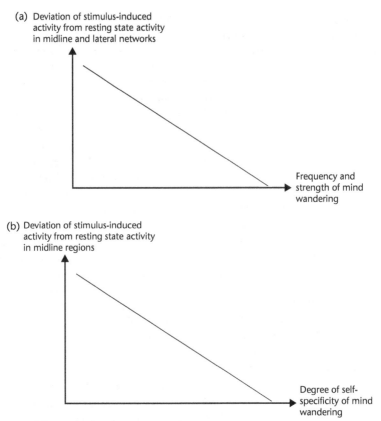

Figure 26-3a and b Neuronal mechanisms of mind wandering. The figure illustrates different neuronal mechanisms in mind wandering: how it is dependent on the resting-state activity (*a*) and how that modulates self-specificity in mind wandering (*b*). (*a*) The figure shows the relationship between the deviation of stimulus-induced activity from the resting-state activity level in midline and lateral networks and the degree of mind wandering. The less the stimulus-induced activity in midline and lateral networks deviates from the resting-state activity, the stronger the possible degree of mind wandering even during stimulus-induced activity. (*b*) The figure shows the relationship between the deviation of stimulus-induced activity in midline regions from their resting-state activity level and the degree of self-specificity of mind wandering. The less the stimulus-induced activity in the midline regions deviates from the resting state, the higher the degree of self-specificity assigned to the contents in mind wandering. Figure 26-2a reprinted with permission of *Science*, from Mason MF, Norton MI, Van Horn JD, Wegner DM, Grafton ST, Macrae CN. Wandering minds: the default network and stimulus-independent thought. *Science*. 2007 Jan 19;315(5810):393–5. Figure 26-2b reprinted with permission from Christoff K, Gordon AM, Smallwood J, Smith R, Schooler JW. Experience sampling during fMRI reveals default network and executive system contributions to mind wandering. *Proc Natl Acad Sci USA*. 2009 May 26;106(21):8719–24.

activity does indeed show a self-specific organization, as suggested in earlier chapters, one may propose that the resting state exerts a strong impact on the processing of the stimuli related to both internal and external contents: the better the extrinsic stimuli can align to the intrinsic

resting-state activity and its self-specific organization, the more the stimuli's their underlying neural activity, e.g., midline or lateral, will predominate the respective other one.

The shift from external to internal contents may thus be due to the fact that the stimuli underlying the internal contents simply elicit a higher degree of self-specificity than the ones associated with external contents. This implies that the competition between internal and external contents may then be rephrased as "competition between different degrees of self-specificity." This in turn may be traced back to the degree to which the underlying stimuli can relate to the resting state's self-specific organization.

NEUROPHENOMENAL HYPOTHESIS VC: NEURAL BALANCE BETWEEN MIDLINE AND LATERAL NETWORKS MEDIATES THE BALANCE BETWEEN EXTERNAL AND INTERNAL CONTENTS DURING MIND WANDERING

How is it possible that internal contents are constituted in consciousness during the presence of external stimuli as in mind wandering? This pertains to the "hard" case of stimulus-induced activity (see the preceding chapter): How is it possible that the external stimuli are neglected in mind wandering and replaced by the internal contents? Such a "hard case" must be distinguished from an "easy case" that describes the occurrence of external contents during the presence of external stimuli, as in perception. In the following discussion, my interest is in the "hard case," since the "easy case" is easy to explain whereas the explanation of the "hard case" is not as obvious.

Let us recall from the earlier chapter where I proposed the neural balance between midline and lateral networks to be central in designating contents as either internal or external. The more that neural balance shifts toward the midline regions, the more likely the internal contents will predominate over the external contents. Thereby, as in the case of dreams, it does not matter whether the neural activity is characterized as resting-state activity or stimulus-induced activity.

Accordingly, all the brain itself "cares" about is the degree of difference between midline and lateral networks it has to process, regardless of whether this difference can be traced back to stimulus-induced activity or to the resting state itself, that is, rest–rest interaction. I consequently proposed the designation of contents as either internal or external to be based on the processing of neural differences between midline and lateral networks rather than on the origin of stimuli.

In other words, neural activity operates on the level of neural differences between different stimuli rather than on the level of the single stimuli and their respective origins. By encoding the difference between different stimuli rather than the single stimuli themselves into neural activity, contents are constituted and thereby distinguished from the mere stimuli. This is reflected in what I described as "difference-based hypothesis of contents" in the preceding chapter.

How does the "difference-based hypothesis of contents" relate to the association of the contents with consciousness? We experience contents, whether internal or external, in the gestalt of "directedness toward," which in philosophy is described by the term *intentionality*: Our experience is directed from a particular point of view toward the respective content. In the case of mind wandering, our experience shifts its "directedness toward" from external to internal contents. In other words, the phenomenal balance between internal and external contents shifts from the latter to the former in mind wandering.

NEUROPHENOMENAL HYPOTHESIS VIA: NEURAL BALANCE BETWEEN MIDLINE-LATERAL NETWORK AND THE REST OF THE BRAIN MEDIATES THE PHENOMENAL BALANCE BETWEEN DIRECTEDNESS TOWARD INTERNAL AND EXTERNAL CONTENTS DURING MIND WANDERING

How, then, is such a phenomenal balance related to the earlier-described neural balance between midline and lateral regions as described in mind wandering? For that answer, we need to tackle two questions: first, how contents can be associated with consciousness at all, and second, how the phenomenal balance can shift from external to internal contents in mind wandering.

Let us tackle the first question, the association of the contents in mind wandering with consciousness. Let us recall from Chapter 25 what I called the "point of view–based hypothesis of directedness." This hypothesis stated that the directedness toward either internal or external contents is related to the linkage and connection between contents and point of view. This was to be mediated by the neural balance between midline-lateral networks and the rest of the brain. I showed this mechanism to operate in the case of dreams during resting-state activity. And I now propose the same neuronal mechanisms to also be at work during mind wandering.

More specifically, the study by Christoff demonstrates neural activity changes in basically the whole brain, including midline and lateral networks as well as other cortical networks and subcortical regions. This strongly supports the assumption that mind wandering is related to the integration of the midline-lateral balance within the whole brain's regions/networks. I consequently propose that this integration between midline-lateral networks and the whole brain's regions/networks is related to the association of the contents with the point of view during mind wandering.

What does this imply for intentionality? This association between content and point of view, in turn, makes possible the constitution of "directedness toward" and thus intentionality. More generally, it means that the contents, whether internal or external, are associated with a phenomenal state and thus consciousness.

How about the second question, the one of the phenomenal balance between internal and external contents in the "directedness toward" and thus intentionality of consciousness? I proposed the designation of contents as either internal or external to be dependent upon the neural differences between midline and lateral networks (see earlier). If this neural balance between midline-lateral networks is now associated with a phenomenal state, i.e., consciousness, it will be transformed into a phenomenal balance in consciousness.

More specifically, the neural balance between midline and lateral networks and their associated balance between internal and external contents will surface on the phenomenal level of consciousness in the balance between

directedness toward internal and external content. Accordingly, the neural balance is transformed into a phenomenal balance between internal and external "directedness toward" on the basis of the balance between internal and external contents.

NEUROPHENOMENAL HYPOTHESIS VIB: NEURAL AND PHENOMENAL BALANCES OPERATE ACROSS RESTING STATE AND STIMULUS-INDUCED ACTIVITY

What does the example of mind wandering tell us about the phenomenal balance between internal and external directedness toward in consciousness? It tells us that this phenomenal balance is present and operates during both stimulus-induced and resting-state activity: The example of mind wandering shows that the phenomenal balance can be tilted towards internal directedness even during stimulus-induced activity, which is possible only if the phenomenal balance (and the underlying neural balance) still operates.

In contrast, the example of dreams, with their directedness toward both internal and external contents, tells us that the phenomenal balance between internal and external "directedness toward" also operates during the resting state itself. In other words, like the neural balance and the one between internal and external contents, the phenomenal balance also operates across the divide between resting state and stimulus-induced activity (see Fig. 26-4).

Taken together, both neural and phenomenal balances operate across the divide of resting-state and stimulus-induced activity. This is what the examples of mind wandering and dreams can tell us. Only by assuming the operation of both neural and phenomenal balances across the rest–stimulus divide can the directedness toward internal contents in mind wandering and toward external contents in dreams be accounted for. In contrast, the opposite, a clear-cut separation between resting-state and stimulus-induced activity with the consequent assumption of an internal-external divide, would remain unable to account for the

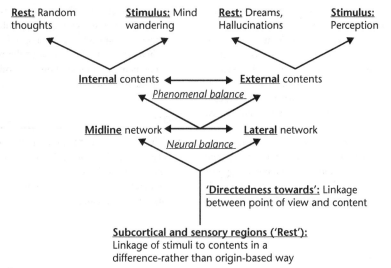

Figure 26-4 Neural balance and phenomenal balance. The figure illustrates the relationship between the neural balance (between midline and lateral networks) and the phenomenal balance (between directedness toward internal and external contents in consciousness). (*Lower*) Subcortical and sensory cortical regions process stimuli from brain, body, and environment in orientation on their differences rather than their origin. This allows for the constitution of contents. The neural differences corresponding to specific contents are conveyed to the midline and lateral cortical networks. By that, the contents are linked to a point of view as stemming from the environment–brain unity (not shown here). This linkage allows for the constitution of directedness of a point of view toward contents in consciousness. (*Middle*) Depending on the neural balance between the two networks, the neural differences and their corresponding contents are designated as either internal or external independent of the origin of their initially underlying stimuli. Since the midline-lateral network is already integrated with the whole brain's regions/networks ("rest of the brain"), the contents, whether designated as internal or external, are associated with a phenomenal state, e.g., consciousness. The contents thus resurface on the phenomenal level in the gestalt of "directedness toward" either internal or external contents in our experience. (*Upper*) Both neural and phenomenal balance operate across the divide of resting state and stimulus-induced activity; this means that both directedness towards both internal and external contents can be manifested in both resting state ("rest") and stimulus-induced activity ("stimulus"), for which the respective examples are given in the upper level.

kind of contents we experience in dreams and mind wandering.

Open Questions

First, the future empirical investigation of my neurophenomenal claims necessitates the development of novel neuronal and phenomenal measures. Neuronally, one would like to develop measures for the ratio or relationship between midline and lateral activity and thus some measure of patterns of activity across different regions. Furthermore, one would like to obtain measures for the ratio between midline-lateral networks and the whole brain's regions/networks.

Their neural differences need to be operationalized, too. In the case of dreams, one would also like to see indexes of spontaneous activity that subsume the electrophysiological measures available so far into one homogenous variable. The need for novel tools extends to the phenomenal level. Phenomenally, measures of the degrees of both self-specificity and intentionality are required. This may, for instance, lead to better quantification of the perceptions in dreams.

Second, I here considered both dreams and mind wandering in a rather narrow sense, leaving out many issues and features that would require separate explanations (see Northoff 2011 for dreams).

I here took them only as paradigmatic examples of the proposed mechanisms on both neural and phenomenal levels, for example, neural balance between midline and lateral networks as well as phenomenal balance between internal and external "directedness toward." As such, they can provide empirical, that is, neuronal and phenomenal support, to my neurophenomenal claims voiced in Chapter 25.

We should be aware that such empirical support can only be indirect, making separate investigations for more direct empirical support necessary. This will be the task for future studies. Another source of empirical support can be neuropsychiatric disorders like schizophrenia and depression. These go along with changes in their intentionality and self-specificity and may therefore support our case of the resting state's preintentional organization. This will be the focus in the next chapter.

NOTE

1. I here neglected to mention that dreams can also occur in non-REM sleep stages, where they seem to be less accessible for subsequent remembrance and report than dreams associated with REM sleep (see Mancia 2006, 90–91).

CHAPTER 27
Neuropsychiatric Evidence—Schizophrenia and Depression

Summary

In the preceding chapters, I proposed the carry-over and transfer of the resting state's self-specific and preintentional organization to predispose self-perspectival organization and intentionality on the phenomenal level of consciousness. Now the question is how we can gather further empirical support in favor of the resting state's self-specific and preintentional organization and its predisposing role for consciousness. In short, I am now seeking further empirical support to my neurophenomenal hypotheses in an indirect way, via the disruption of the suggested neurophenomenal mechanisms. I therefore turn to neuropsychiatric disorders like schizophrenia and depression. Schizophrenia can be characterized by a basic disturbance of the self wherein the person's own self and the environment are experienced in an altered way with abnormal degrees of self-specificity. Recent imaging studies demonstrated resting-state activity abnormalities in schizophrenia with abnormal functional connectivity and low-frequency fluctuations in especially the midline regions. This is complemented by observations of abnormal neural activity in the same network during self-specific stimuli. Taking both clinical self-abnormalities and the abnormal resting-state activity findings into account, I propose the example of schizophrenia to lend neurophenomenal support to the assumption of a self-specific organization in the resting-state activity and its predisposition of self-perspectival organization on the phenomenal level of consciousness.

How about depression? The preceding chapters (Chapters 25 and 26) argued that the reciprocal neural balance between midline and lateral networks may be central for the directedness toward internal and external contents and thus intentionality. This led me to propose a preintentional organization in the resting-state activity. Depression shows resting-state activity abnormalities with hyperactivity in the midline network and hypoactivity in the lateral network. Such a midline-lateral imbalance implies imbalance between self-specific and preintentional organization during the resting-state activity, which predisposes what on the phenomenal level can be described as "self-focus" and "decreased environment focus." The concept of "increased self-focus" points out that the phenomenal consciousness is directed more strongly toward one's own self rather than the environment, e.g., decreased environment-focus. Together with the resting-state activity abnormalities and their midline-lateral shift, such an abnormal balance between increased self-focus and decreased environment-focus is indicative of an abnormal preintentional organization in the resting-state activity itself; this makes possible and thus predisposes the depressed patients' abnormal directedness toward internal contents on the phenomenal level of consciousness. Hence, the example of depression supports my neurophenomenal claim of a preintentional organization in the resting-state activity and its predisposition of the directedness toward either internal or external contents on the phenomenal level of consciousness.

Key Concepts and Topics Covered

Schizophrenia, basic disturbance of self, self-specificity, self-specific organization, resting-state activity, self-affection, depression, midline-lateral networks, increased self-focus, decreased environment focus, neural balance, phenomenal balance

Neuroempirical Background IA: Empirical Support for the Resting-State Activity's Self-Specific and Preintentional Organization

I characterized the resting-state activity by "self-specific organization" (Chapter 23) and "preintentional organization" (Chapter 25). The self-specific organization means that the neuronal activity of the resting-state activity, i.e., its temporal and spatial features, is organized and structured around the relevance or specificity for the respective person or organism. While the concept of the preintentional organization points out that the resting state's neural activity predisposes the directedness from a point of view toward either internal or external content, i.e., intentionality.

Due to these characterizations, I proposed the resting-state activity to predispose consciousness and its phenomenal features like self-specificity and intentionality (see Chapters 24 and 25). The assumption of the resting state's self-specific and preintentional organization was then further supported by considering the examples of dreams and mind wandering (Chapter 26). The specific kinds of phenomena observed in both dreams and mind wandering were supposed to be possible only on the basis of assuming some kind of neural predispositions in the resting-state activity itself and more specifically its self-specific and preintentional organization.

How can we now gather additional empirical support for the resting-state activity's self-specific and preintentional organization beyond dreams and mind wandering? One possible way is a rather indirect one: by investigating the impact of abnormal changes in the resting state on experience and phenomenal consciousness.

Following my hypothesis, abnormalities in the resting-state activity should impair its self-specific and/or preintentional organization; these resting-state activity impairments should then also be carried over and transferred to the subsequent stimulus-induced activity during either intero- or exteroceptive stimuli. This means that the various kinds of stimuli and their respective internal or external contents should then be assigned abnormal degrees of self-specificity and intentionality and

consequently be experienced in an abnormal way in phenomenal consciousness.

Neuroempirical Background IB: Schizophrenia and Depression

I propose such a scenario to indeed hold in neuropsychiatric disorders like schizophrenia and depression. Schizophrenia can be characterized by major abnormalities in the experience of self and more specifically by the assignment of abnormal degrees of self-specificity. Depression, in contrast, shows abnormal intentionality, with patients being no longer able to properly direct their experience and thus consciousness toward external contents in the environment, with the directedness toward internal contents predominating.

The question is now whether the phenomenal abnormalities in both schizophrenia and depression can indeed be traced back to an abnormal resting-state activity with alterations in its self-specific and preintentional organization. If so, the examples of schizophrenia and depression would lend empirical support to my neurophenomenal hypothesis of the carryover and transfer of the resting state's self-specific and preintentional organization to the resulting stimulus-induced activity and its associated phenomenal state, e.g., consciousness.

In the following I will first focus on schizophrenia and self-specificity, while in the second part of this chapter depression will be discussed. Thereby the intention is not to give a full-blown review of the different findings in schizophrenia and depression in the various domains of research, ranging from molecular to genetic to psychopathological abnormalities, which would be beyond the scope of this book.

Instead, I here focus mainly on functional brain imaging results concerning resting-state activity and self-specificity, while leaving out and thus neglecting other areas like the imaging of affective, sensory, and cognitive functions in these disorders (but see Chapter 22 for more details about sensory abnormalities in schizophrenia as well as Chapter 17 for biochemical abnormalities in GABA and glutamate in depression and schizophrenia).

Why do I leave out the bulk of findings in these disorders? My main focus is not so much on depression and schizophrenia themselves but rather on their support of my assumption of the resting-state activity's self-specific and preintentional organization. More generally, by revealing the impact of resting-state activity abnormalities on consciousness in schizophrenia and depression, I characterize them, not only as what may be described as "resting state disorders" (Northoff et al. 2011; Northoff and Qin 2011; Northoff 2013), but also as disorders of the organization or form of consciousness (see second Introduction as well as Northoff 2013). As such, they must be distinguished from disorders of the level, degree, or state of consciousness like vegetative state, as it will be discussed in part VIII (see also Northoff 2013).

NEURONAL FINDINGS IA: RESTING-STATE ACTIVITY IN SCHIZOPHRENIA

Various studies investigated recently the default-mode network (DMN) in schizophrenia (see Kuhn and Gallinat (2013, for a recent review). Recent imaging studies in schizophrenia reported abnormal resting-state activity and functional connectivity in the anterior cortical midline structures (aCMS).

One study (Whitfield-Gabrieli et al. 2009) demonstrated that the aCMS (and posterior CMS like the posterior cingulate cortex [PCC]/precuneus) show decreased task-induced deactivation (TID) during a working memory task. This was observed in both schizophrenic patients and their relatives when compared to healthy subjects. Such TID is indicative of decreased task-related suppression and possibly increased resting-state activity. In addition to reduced TID, the very same schizophrenic subjects also showed increased functional connectivity of the aCMS with other posterior regions of the CMS, such as the PCC. Both functional hyperconnectivity and decreased TID correlated negatively with each other. The more task-related suppression as manifested in TID is decreased, the more the degree of functional connectivity increases. Finally, both decreased TID and increased functional connectivity in aCMS correlated with psychopathology, that is, predominantly positive symptoms like

auditory hallucinations and delusions as measured with the PANS scale.

The observation of reduced task-related suppression is further supported by other studies. Decreased TID in aCMS was also observed in an earlier study that investigated working memory (Pomarol-Clotet et al. 2008a and b). Similar to the study described earlier, they let subjects perform a working memory task and observed abnormally decreased TID in aCMS in schizophrenic patients when compared to healthy subjects. They also observed abnormally reduced task-related activation in the right dorsolateral prefrontal cortex in schizophrenic patients. Another study (Mannell et al. 2010) also reported abnormal TID in aCMS as well as abnormal functional connectivity from aCMS and posterior CMS to the insula in schizophrenic patients (see also Calhoun et al. 2008; Park et al. 2009; Jafri et al. 2008; Williamson 2007). In addition to TID and functional connectivity, another abnormal measure of resting-state activity is the temporal features, more specifically fluctuations or oscillations in certain temporal frequencies. For instance, Hoptman et al. (2010) demonstrated that low-frequency fluctuations in the resting state were increased in the aCMS (and the parahippocampal gyrus) in schizophrenic patients, while they were decreased in other regions like the insula. Abnormally increased low-frequency oscillations (<0.06 Hz) in the aCMS (and posterior CMS regions and the auditory network) and their correlation with positive symptom severity were also observed in another study on schizophrenic patients (Rotarska-Jagiela et al. 2010).

NEURONAL FINDINGS IB: SELF-SPECIFICITY IN SCHIZOPHRENIA

This concerns alterations in the resting-state activity. How about changes during stimulus-induced activity and their relation to self-specificity?

A recent imaging study by Holt et al. (2011) showed that abnormal anterior-to-posterior midline connectivity is related to self-specificity. They investigated schizophrenic patients during a word task where subjects had to judge trait adjectives according to their degree of self-specificity (and also two other tasks: other-reflection, i.e., relation of that word to another person) and perception-reflection (i.e., word printed in uppercase or lowercase letters).

How about their results? Schizophrenic patients showed significantly elevated activity in posterior midline regions like the mid- and posterior cingulate cortex during self-reflection. In contrast, signal changes in the anterior midline regions like the medial prefrontal cortex were significantly reduced when compared to healthy subjects. Finally, functional connectivity was abnormally elevated from the posterior to the anterior midline regions during the processing of the self-specific stimuli in schizophrenic patients. Analogous results of altered midline activity with a imbalance between anterior and posterior midline regions are also observed in other studies on self-specificity in schizophrenia (see Taylor et al. 2007; Menon et al. 2011).

Taken together, these results demonstrate abnormal resting-state activity in especially the anterior and posterior midline network in schizophrenia (see Kuhn and Gallinat 2013 for a recent meta-analysis). The very same network also shows alterations in the balance between anterior and posterior midline regions when probing for self-specific stimuli.

How are the resting state abnormalities related to those observed during self-specificity? Unfortunately, studies testing the linkage between resting-state abnormalities and self-specific stimuli remain to be conducted in schizophrenia. This would be needed to support the argument of the carryover and transfer of the resting state's self-specific organization onto subsequent stimulus-induced activity and the associated phenomenal state of consciousness.

NEUROPHENOMENAL HYPOTHESIS IA: "BASIC DISTURBANCE OF THE SELF" IN SCHIZOPHRENIA

In contrast to the somehow sparse neuronal evidence, there is plenty of phenomenal evidence of schizophrenic patients' suffering from an abnormality in self-specificity in their experience. For instance, schizophrenic patients often abnormally experience non-self-related external contents in the environment as being closely related to their self; this is described as the "delusion of

reference." And in even more extreme cases, they can experience their self as the self of another person when they, for instance, take on the identity of Jesus or Buddha in their experience.

How can we explain that? I propose that this is possible only when we assume that an already abnormal self-specific organization in the resting-state activity is carried over and transferred onto the subsequent stimulus-induced activity and its associated phenomenal states.

How can we now link more closely the clinical abnormalities in the experience of self in schizophrenia with the observed resting-state activity changes? I have shown empirical evidence for resting-state activity abnormalities in schizophrenia. Now I turn to the phenomenal side; I will first go briefly into the history of schizophrenia and will then, in the next section, give a more detailed phenomenal account and how that relates to the neuronal changes.

Early German-speaking psychiatrists like E. Kraepelin and E. Bleuler at the beginning of the twentieth century proposed abnormality of the self to be basic in schizophrenia. Unlike in our times, these early psychiatrists had to rely on nothing but clinical observation, since no brain imaging tools had been developed yet. Based on that, they proposed an abnormal change of the self to be fundamental in schizophrenia. More specifically, German psychiatrist Emil Kraepelin (1913, 668) characterized schizophrenia as "the peculiar destruction of the inner coherence of the personality" with a "disunity of consciousness" ("orchestra without a conductor").

His Swiss colleague Eugen Bleuler (1911, 58; 1916) also pointed out that schizophrenia is a "disorder of the personality by splitting, dissociation" where the "I is never completely intact." A contemporary of Bleuler and Kraepelin, Berze (1914) even referred to schizophrenia as "basic alteration of self-consciousness." Yet another psychiatrist (and philosopher) Karl Jaspers (1963, 581) also noticed "incoherence, dissociation, fragmenting of consciousness, intrapsychic ataxia, weakness of apperception, insufficiency of psychic activity and disturbance of association, etc." to be basic as unifying "central factors" in schizophrenia.

NEUROPHENOMENAL HYPOTHESIS IB: "BASIC DISTURBANCE OF THE SELF" AND THE RESTING-STATE ACTIVITY'S SELF-SPECIFIC ORGANIZATION

How does that relate to our assumptions made earlier? I suggest that what the early psychiatrists described as "the peculiar destruction of the inner coherence of the personality" or "basic alteration of self-consciousness" may correspond to what here refer to the changes in the resting state's self-specific organization. Let me spell this out in further detail.

Following the early psychiatrists' descriptions, the basic disturbance in the self is supposed to impact all other subsequent functions (cognitive, affective, etc.) and domains of the personality. This is well reflected in the neuropsychological findings in schizophrenia that report weaker or stronger abnormalities in basically all psychological functions, e.g., cognitive, affective, social, sensory, and motor.

Analogously, I propose the resting state's self-specific organization to also affect any subsequent stimulus-induced activity and consequently all functions, including sensory, motor, affective, and cognitive functions (as it seems indeed to be the case in cognitive, affective, sensory, and motor functions). In the same way that the basic disturbance of the self is present everywhere and affects all its various functions, the resting state, metaphorically speaking, "has its hands" in all kinds of neural processing related to different stimuli, tasks, and their respectively associated functions. In short, schizophrenia may be characterized by an overall presence of the "basic disturbance of the self."

How is such overall presence of the "basic disturbance of the self" possible? It must indeed be very basic. I do understand the term *basic* here in the same way as, for instance, the resting state is "basic" to any kind of subsequent stimulus-induced activity. This meaning of *basic* in the context of the resting state is possible only when assuming that the resting state is in some way carried over and transferred to the subsequent stimulus and its associated contents and functions.

Analogously, I now propose that what the early psychiatrists described as the "basic disturbance of the self" is carried over and transferred to every domain of the subject's mental life, e.g., the phenomenal features of consciousness and the various task-related functions, such as cognitive, affective, etc. Hence, I suggest that the "basic disturbance of the self" is carried over and transferred to the subsequent phenomenal states and subsequent functions in very much the same way as the resting state's abnormal self-specific organization is carried over and transferred to the subsequent stimulus-induced activity and its associated functions.

Where, however, do the "basic disturbance of the self" and the supposedly underlying abnormal self-specific organization in the resting state come from? I propose the resting state's abnormal self-specific organization to be ultimately traced back to an abnormal encoding of the environmental stimuli's statistical frequency distribution by the resting state's neural activity as discussed in Chapter 20. This, in turn, leads to an abnormal "environment brain unity," which then affects and abnormally modulates the resting state's self-specific organization (see Fig. 27-1). That is what I discussed in more detail in the previous part, in Chapter 22.

Why do I attribute such importance to the abnormal self-specific organization of the resting state? I propose the resting state and its abnormal self-specific organization to be carried over and transferred to subsequent stimulus-induced activity and its association with a phenomenal state of consciousness. If so, one would propose the resting state's abnormal self-specific organization to predispose and ultimately lead to abnormal experience of both self and environment on the phenomenal level of consciousness. This will be the focus of the next section.

NEUROPHENOMENAL HYPOTHESIS IC: EXPERIENCE OF AN ABNORMAL SELF IN SCHIZOPHRENIA

How is the resting-state activity's abnormal self-specific organization manifested phenomenally in stimulus-induced activity? The early psychiatrists' descriptions of a disrupted self are complemented by current phenomenological accounts that focus predominantly on the

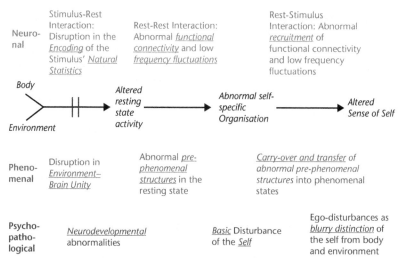

Figure 27-1 Basic disturbance of the self in schizophrenia. The figure shows different stages in the constitution of an altered sense of self in schizophrenia. I propose the encoding of stimuli and their natural statistics to be abnormal in schizophrenia during stimulus–rest interaction. That leads to abnormal resting-state activity with abnormal prephenomenal structures. The abnormal prephenomenal structures in the resting state will then affect subsequent rest–rest interaction, which leads to abnormal self-specific organization in the resting state. Any encounter with stimuli during rest–stimulus interaction will be affected by that which results in the consequent experience of an abnormal sense of self. I indicated three levels, neuronal (*upper*), phenomenal (*middle low*), and psychopathological (*lower*). I propose that the neuronal mechanisms (described earlier) correspond to the respective phenomenal and psychopathological features.

experience of one's own self in relation to the world. Danish psychiatrist Josef Parnas (Parnas et al. 2001; Parnas 2003) describes what he calls "presence" as being altered in schizophrenia: The experience of the world and its objects is not accompanied by the tacit or automatic experience of a self anymore, e.g., a pre-reflective self-awareness.

Let me elaborate on this point. One's own self, the self that experiences the experience of the world, is no longer included in that very experience of the world. This is well illustrated in the following quote from Parnas:

> The prominent feature of altered presence in the pre-onset stages of schizophrenia is disturbed ipseity, a disturbance in which the sense of self no longer saturates the experience. For instance, the sense of mineness of experience may become subtly affected: one of our patients reported that this feeling of his experience as his own experience only "appeared a split-second delayed." (Parnas 2003, 225)

How can we further illustrate the abnormal experience of the self in schizophrenia? The patients remain unable to refer to themselves in their experience of the world. It is as if the experience of the world is no longer their own experience of their own self. Instead, their experience may belong to and be experienced by someone else, but it is no longer their own self who makes and experiences those experiences.

Due to the absence (as opposed to presence) of one's own self in their experience of the world, patients with schizophrenia become detached, alienated, and estranged from their own experience. Such detachment of the experiences from their own self makes it impossible for them to experience their experiences as subjective and thus as belonging to their own self. The experiencing self is consequently no longer affected by its own experiences, which Sass (2003) describes as "disorder of self-affectivity": one's own self is no longer experienced as one's own self and, most importantly, is no longer experienced as the vital center and source of one's own experiences, actions, perceptions, thoughts, and so on.

This reflects what Sass (2003) calls the "diminished self-affection," meaning that the self is no longer affected by its own experiences. If, however, the self is not affected anymore by its own experience, one's own self is experienced as standing apart and thus detached from the objects and the events in the world that are experienced. A gulf, a phenomenological distance as Parnas says (2003, 225), opens up between world and self. The objects and events of the world no longer make intuitive sense and are thus not meaningful anymore to the experiencing subject. One's own self becomes thus almost objective and mechanical in its experience and perception of the world.

NEUROPHENOMENAL HYPOTHESIS IIA: ABNORMAL SELF-SPECIFIC AND SELF-PERSPECTIVAL ORGANIZATION IN SCHIZOPHRENIA

How do these phenomenal descriptions relate to the here-postulated neuronal mechanisms? I propose that the phenomenal abnormalities of the self in schizophrenia reflect an abnormal self-specific organization in the resting-state activity as it is carried over and transferred to subsequent stimulus-induced activity. This is in accordance with the earlier described neuronal results of an abnormal resting state and abnormal neural activity during self-specific stimuli.

Let me be more specific. Due to the resting-state activity abnormalities, the stimuli cannot be properly integrated into the resting-state activity's prephenomenal self-specific organization. The lack of the stimuli's integration into the resting state's self-specific organization makes it impossible for the resting state to assign any kind of degree of self-specificity to the stimuli themselves during stimulus-induced activity. Such decreased or lacking assignment of self-specificity to the stimuli is then manifested on the phenomenal level of consciousness in what is described as decreases in both self-affection and sense of *mineness* and *belongingness* (see Part VIII for the description of these phenomenal features). This amounts to exactly the way Parnas and others characterize experience in schizophrenia, which may therefore mirror an abnormal self-perspectival organization on the phenomenal level of consciousness (see Chapter 22 for the concept of self-perspectival organization).

How about phenomenal consciousness itself? Unlike patients in a vegetative state, schizophrenic patients still show phenomenal consciousness whose level or state thus remains intact. Something else, however, is no longer intact in the consciousness of these patients; namely, what I referred as the *form* or *organization* (as a third dimension of consciousness; see Northoff 2013) in the second Introduction; this shall be specified below. I therefore propose that the occurrence of abnormal contents and an abnormal self in phenomenal consciousness in schizophrenia can ultimately be traced back to their resting-state activity's abnormal self-specific and preintentional organization and its subsequent carryover and transfer to any kind of stimulus-induced activity and its associated phenomenal state, i.e., consciousness.

More specifically, I consider the main problem in schizophrenia to lie in the resting-state activity itself, whose abnormal changes are then carried over and transferred to any subsequent neural activity. Any kind of stimulus-induced activity and the respectively associated experiences; that is, phenomenal consciousness, then cannot avoid being affected by the abnormalities in the resting-state activity's self-specific organization.

NEUROPHENOMENAL HYPOTHESIS IIB: "DISORDERS OF FORM OF CONSCIOUSNESS" VERSUS "DISORDERS OF LEVEL OF CONSCIOUSNESS"

How can we distinguish the case of schizophrenia from the case of the vegetative state? Vegetative patients show loss of consciousness; their state or level of consciousness is reduced, if not completely absent. The case of schizophrenia must be distinguished from vegetative patients who do not show any phenomenal consciousness. In contrast to schizophrenia, where the resting state itself is abnormal, I propose the process of carryover and transfer to be affected by itself in vegetative state, as I will discuss in further detail in Part VIII.

Accordingly, we need to distinguish between "what" is carried over and transferred and "how" this occurs. The "what" is altered in schizophrenia, while the "how" is disturbed in the vegetative state. As we can see, both lead to radically different consequences for phenomenal consciousness. This also pertains to the distinction between form and level/state of consciousness as discussed in the second Introduction. The form or organization of consciousness concerns the "what" and thus the resting-state activity and its prephenomenal structures. The "what" is affected and thus abnormal in schizophrenia and depression. Neuropsychiatric disorders like schizophrenia and depression can thus be described as "disorders of the form of consciousness" (Northoff 2013).

In contrast, the vegetative state may more concern how the resting-state activity and its prephenomenal structures are carried over and transferred to subsequent stimulus-induced activity. This will be described in further detail in the next chapter. Rather than referring to the form of consciousness, the "how" refers to the state of consciousness, the level of consciousness, which, I propose, is related to the degree of carryover and transfer. This is deficient in the vegetative state and other disorders of consciousness.

Vegetative state and other disorders of consciousness can therefore be regarded as "disorders of the state or level of consciousness." As such, they must be distinguished from neuropsychiatric disorders (like schizophrenia and depression) that are rather "disorders of the form of consciousness" (Northoff 2013). Before focusing on the "how" of the carryover and transfer in Part VIII, let me give another example of how an abnormal "what" can affect phenomenal consciousness. For that, I turn to the example of depression.

NEURONAL FINDINGS IIA: RESTING-STATE ACTIVITY IN MIDLINE AND LATERAL NETWORKS IN DEPRESSION

We have so far discussed schizophrenia to lend neurophenomenal support to the self-organization of the resting state. In addition

to the self-specific organization, we also characterized the resting state by a preintentional organization that predisposes "directedness toward" and thus intentionality on the phenomenal level of consciousness.

How can we lend further neurophenomenal support for the resting state's preintentional organization? For the answer, I turn to the example of depression. Major depressive disorder (MDD) is a psychiatric disorder that is characterized by extremely negative emotions, suicidal thoughts, hopelessness, diffuse bodily symptoms, lack of pleasure, that is, anhedonia, ruminations, and enhanced stress sensitivity (see Hasler and Northoff 2011 as well as Northoff et al. 2011 for a recent overview and Kuhn and Gallinat 2013).

What are the neuronal underpinnings of MDD? Let me first describe the findings of altered resting-state activity in MDD (Alcaro et al., 2010; Mayberg, 2002; Price and Drevets, 2010;). We here are able to only briefly highlight the main findings and conclusions from these various reviews and then relate them to functional networks as delineated in normal-healthy brains (see Northoff et al. 2011; Hassler and Northoff 2011 for recent reviews).

Alcaro et al. (2010) conducted a meta-analysis of all imaging studies in human MDD that had focused on resting-state activity. This yielded resting state hyperactive regions in the perigenual anterior cingulate cortex (PACC), the ventromedial prefrontal cortex (VMPFC), thalamic regions like the dorsomedial thalamus and the pulvinar, pallidum/putamen and midbrain regions like the ventral tegmental area, substantia nigra, the tectum, and the periaqueductal gray (PAG). In contrast, resting-state activity was hypoactive and thus reduced in the dorsolateral prefrontal cortex (DLPFC), the PCC, and adjacent precuneus/cuneus (Alcaro et al. 2010).

These results are well in accordance with other meta-analyses (see Fitzgerald et al. 2006, 2007; Price and Drevets 2010; Savitz and Drevets 2009a and b). Also, Price and Drevets (2010) and Savitz and Drevets (2009a and b) emphasized the role of the hippocampus, parahippocampus, and the amygdala where resting-state hyperactivity was also evident in MDD. Interestingly, the very same regions and the PACC also show structural abnormalities with reduced gray matter volume in imaging studies and reduced cell count markers of cellular function in postmortem studies (see Price and Drevets 2010; Savitz and Drevets 2009a and b).

Involvement of these regions in MDD is further corroborated by the investigation of resting-state activity in animal models of MDD. Reviewing evidence for resting-state hyperactivity in various animal models yielded diverse participating brain regions—the anterior cingulate cortex, the central and basolateral nuclei of the amygdala, the bed nucleus of the stria terminalis, the dorsal raphe, the habenula, the hippocampus, the hypothalamus, the nucleus accumbens, the PAG, the DMT, the nucleus of the solitary tract, and the piriform and prelimbic cortex (Alcaro et al., 2010). In contrast, evidence of hypoactive resting-state activity in animal models remains sparse with no clear results (Alcaro et al. 2010).

Taken together, these findings indicate abnormally high resting-state activity being either hyper- or hypoactive in extended subcortical and cortical midline regions of the brain. This has led authors like Phillips (2003) Mayberg (2002, 2009), and Drevets (see Price and Drevets 2010; and Savitz and Drevets 2009a, 2009b) to propose dysfunction in the limbic system in depression or more specifically in the "limbic-cortico-striato-pallido-thalamic circuit" with reciprocal interactions between medial prefrontal and limbic regions being crucial (Price and Drevets 2010a).

NEURONAL FINDINGS IIB: RESTING-STATE ACTIVITY IMBALANCE BETWEEN INNER AND OUTER RINGS IN DEPRESSION

How do these findings fit into the delineated anatomical characterization of the healthy brain as characterized by inner, middle, and outer rings (see Chapter 4, Volume I)? We recall from Volume I that there is strong evidence for a threefold anatomical organization that links subcortical and cortical regions, as distinguished from the usual medial-lateral and subcortical-cortical dichotomies. The inner ring covers the subcortical and cortical regions that are directly adjacent to the ventricle and the corpus callosum. In

contrast, regions of the outer ring include those at the outer surface of the cortex and the outermost part of the subcortical regions. Finally, the middle ring's regions are those that are in between the ones of the inner and the outer ring.

How does this threefold anatomical organization relate to the resting-state findings in depression? What was conceptualized as inner and middle rings at the cortical level, the paralimbic areas and the cortical midline structures, generally show hyperactivity during resting state in MDD. In contrast, the regions of the outer ring, like the lateral prefrontal cortex, seem to show hypoactivity in the resting state in MDD (see Fig. 27-2a).

Resting-state activity in MDD may therefore be characterized by an imbalance between subcortical-cortical inner/middle and lateral rings. More specifically, the inner and middle rings' regions seem to be hyperactive in the resting state. In contrast, subcortical and especially cortical regions of the lateral-cognitive ring, like the lateral prefrontal cortex and the sensory-motor cortices, seem to show hypoactivity in the resting state (see also Northoff et al. 2011).

NEUROPHENOMENAL HYPOTHESIS IIIA: "INCREASED SELF-FOCUS" IN DEPRESSION

The aforementioned findings indicate imbalance in the resting-state activity between inner/middle and outer rings. More specifically, they show that resting-state activity in the anterior portions of the inner ring and also to some degree in the middle ring is abnormally elevated, while the outer ring's resting-state activity is decreased. This means that there is a imbalance in the resting-state activity in depression along the aforementioned inner-to-outer and anterior-to-posterior gradients.

I now propose the neural balance between the three anatomical rings and their corresponding functional connectivity to be central in constituting the prephenomenal balance between self-specific and preintentional organization in the resting state. Why? For the answer, we need to go into more detail about how contents are constituted and how that surfaces on the phenomenal level.

We recall from the previous chapters that the neural balance between midline and lateral networks is central in designating contents as internal or external as well as in constituting the directedness toward contents. Since the neuronal balance between the three anatomical rings is altered in depression, one would expect a shift toward increased internal contents and decreased external contents. This indeed is the case and surfaces on the phenomenal level, as I describe in the following.

(a1) MDD > CO (rest)

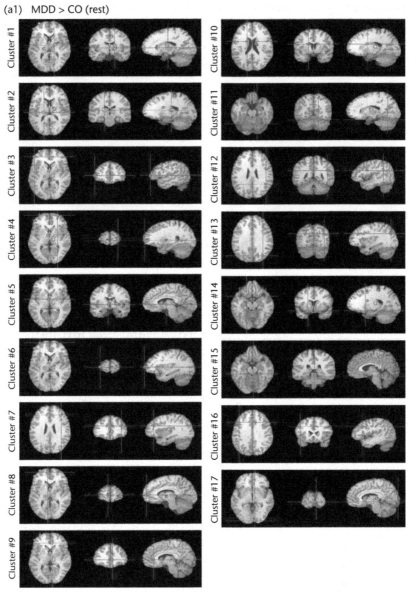

Figure 27-2a Neural and phenomenal abnormalities in depression. Abnormal resting-state activity in the three subcortical-cortical rings (inner, middle, outer) in depression. (*a1*) Resting state hyperactivity in humans revealed by ALE analysis [MDD > Co]. MDD = major depressive disorder; Co = controls. (*a2*) Resting state hypoactivity in humans revealed by ALE analysis [Co > MDD]. MDD = major depressive disorder; Co = controls. Reprinted with permission of Elsevier, from Alcaro A, Panksepp J, Witczak J, Hayes DJ, Northoff G. Is subcortical-cortical midline activity in depression mediated by glutamate and GABA? A cross-species translational approach. *Neurosci Biobehav Rev.* 2010 Mar;34(4):592–605.

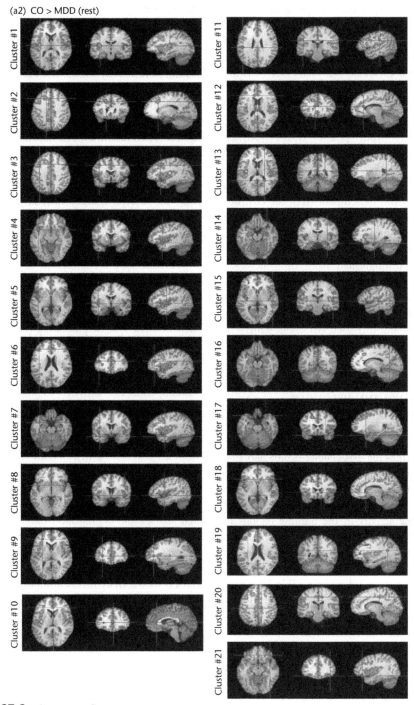

(a2) CO > MDD (rest)

Cluster #1, Cluster #2, Cluster #3, Cluster #4, Cluster #5, Cluster #6, Cluster #7, Cluster #8, Cluster #9, Cluster #10, Cluster #11, Cluster #12, Cluster #13, Cluster #14, Cluster #15, Cluster #16, Cluster #17, Cluster #18, Cluster #19, Cluster #20, Cluster #21

Figure 27-2a (Continued)

Phenomenally, a core symptom in MDD is the extremely increased focus on one's own self. All thoughts and feelings are circulating around one's own self, one's own person, which we described as increased self-focus (see Northoff 2007; Northoff et al. 2011; see also Lemogne et al. 2012, who distinguishes such increased self-focus as associated with phasic VMPFC hyperactivity from phasic DMPFC-activity, which, he supposes, mediates cognitive elaboration of the self).

Most important, such increased self-focus goes along with detachment from the environment, that is, from the persons, objects, and events, with the patients feeling disconnected. We described this as "decreased environment focus," as distinguished from the "increased self-focus" (see Northoff et al. 2011). How is the phenomenal shift in the focus from the environment to the self, that is, decreased environment focus and increased self-focus, generated on the neuronal level? For that, we turn to the resting-state activity in MDD.

NEUROPHENOMENAL HYPOTHESIS IIIB: RESTING-STATE HYPERACTIVITY MEDIATES AN "INCREASED SELF-FOCUS" IN DEPRESSION

We recall from the first chapter in this part that the midline regions, and especially those of the anterior inner ring, are related to self-specificity. One would consequently expect elevated resting-state activity in the midline regions to lead to increased self-specificity and hence to abnormally increased personal concerns in patients with MDD during both resting-state and stimulus-induced activity. This is indeed supported by recent empirical data.

Grimm et al. (2009, 2011) from our group (and others like Lemogne et al. 2009a and b, 2010, 2012, who additionally, distinguish between phasic and tonic activity) observed behaviorally significantly increased scores for self-specificity with regard to especially negative emotional pictures. Neuronally this went along with decreased signal changes during self-specific stimuli in anterior cortical midline regions compared to baseline, e.g., resting state. Such a decrease in signal changes supposedly reflects the abnormally high resting-state activity and its associated assignment of abnormally increased self-specificity to stimuli. If so, one would propose abnormal self-specific organization in the resting-state activity itself. The assumption of an increased self-focus on the phenomenal level in MDD with increased self-specificity on the neuronal (and behavioral) level is further supported by the observation of the following correlation. We observed that the increased behavioral scores of self-specificity were predicted by the decreased stimulus-induced activity in especially the anterior midline structures: the lower the stimulus-induced activity when compared to baseline, the higher the degree of self-specificity attributed to the stimuli. One may consequently hypothesize that the increased self-specificity as observed behaviorally stems from the abnormally increased resting-state activity in the midline regions and their apparently increased self-specific processing (Grimm et al. 2009, 2011).

What do these findings imply in neurophenomenal regard? We observed decreased stimulus-induced activity in the anterior midline regions, while at the same time the stimuli were assigned increased degrees of self-specificity. How is it possible that decreased stimulus-induced activity goes along with increased self-specificity? I propose that this is due to the carryover and transfer of the increased resting-state activity and its abnormal self-specific organization onto subsequent stimulus-induced activity and the respectively associated stimuli.

Let me be more specific. The increased resting-state activity makes it impossible for the stimulus to induce major activity changes, hence the decreased stimulus-induced activity Since the resting-state activity is not much changed, its associated self-specific organization is strongly carried over and transferred to the subsequent stimulus-induced activity and the associated stimulus. The stimulus is consequently assigned an abnormally high degree of self-specificity, which, on the phenomenal level, leads to a centering of experience, and thus consciousness around one's own self, as described in the concept of the increased self-focus.

Neuronal Findings IIIA: Abnormal Exteroceptive Processing in Depression

We have focused on the resting state's self-specific organization and how it is altered in MDD where it leads to the increased self-focus. This, however, leaves open the matter of the resting state's preintentional organization. How about the resting state's preintentional organization in depression? For that answer, we need to consider how interoceptive from one's own body and especially exteroceptive stimuli from the environment are processed in MDD.

Patients with MDD often suffer from generalized bodily symptoms like heart pounding, increased breathing (with yawning), and multiple-diffuse bodily aches. This seems to go along with abnormally increased awareness of their own bodily processes (body perception), including sensitivity to stress and autonomic-vegetative changes as demonstrated in a recent work (Wiebking et al., 2010). Such an increased focus on one's own experience, e.g., consciousness, may be described by the term "increased body focus" (Northoff et al. 2011).

In addition to the behavioral markers, the study by Wiebking et al. (2010) also investigated the neuronal activity during exteroceptive and interoceptive awareness (tone and heartbeat counting) in relation to the brain's resting-state activity. Interoceptive stimuli by themselves (e.g., the heartbeat) induced a "normal" degree of brain signal changes (activation) in the bilateral anterior insula[1] in depressed patients when considered relative to the preceding resting-state activity levels. This suggests that there is no abnormality in interoceptive stimulus processing itself in depression.

In contrast to stimulus-induced activity during interoceptive stimuli (e.g., counting one's own heartbeat), we observed abnormally reduced activity during exteroceptive stimuli (e.g., counting tones). More specifically, exteroceptive stimuli induced decreased stimulus-induced activity in the insula in depressed patients when compared to healthy subjects.

This let us further question whether such reduced activity is related either to the exteroceptive stimulus itself or rather to abnormal resting-state activity levels in the insula. The latter was indeed the case, as we observed increased resting-state activity in the insula itself, which consequently led to decreased stimulus-induced activity during specifically exteroceptive stimuli. The observation of increased resting-state activity in the insula is well in line with the earlier-described resting-state hyperactivity in the inner ring, the core-paralimbic system to which the insula belongs.

To test for changes in exteroceptively related stimulus-induced activity by itself, we then calculated the exteroceptively related stimulus-induced activity relative to the preceding resting-state activity level. Interestingly, the initially observed difference between healthy and depressed patients in "absolute," for example, resting-state-independent, signal changes during exteroceptive stimuli disappeared when calculating them in such "relative" way, i.e., in dependence on the preceding resting-state activity level.

Accordingly, when including the preceding resting-state activity level in our analysis, there were no differences anymore in signal changes during exteroceptive processing between healthy and depressed subjects. This suggests that the observed signal differences during exteroceptive stimuli must be due to the resting-state activity itself, rather than to the exteroceptive stimuli themselves.

Neuronal Findings IIIB: Interoceptive Processing and "Increased Body-Focus" in Depression

In contrast to the exteroceptive stimuli, no differences between healthy and depressed subjects were evident in interoceptive stimuli in both relative (e.g., in dependence on the resting state) and absolute (e.g., independently of the resting state) signal changes. There thus seems to be a difference in how the resting state processes intero- and exteroceptive stimuli in depression.

More specifically, this difference between interoceptive and exteroceptive stimuli with regard to relative and absolute signal changes suggests differential interaction of both kinds of stimuli with resting-state activity: The interaction between resting state and exteroceptive stimuli may be reduced. Alternatively, the interoceptive stimuli's interaction with the resting state may be increased. Unfortunately, the two possibilities cannot be differentiated on the basis of our findings.

However, what is clear is that there is unbalanced activity between intero- and exteroceptive stimulus processing, including their respective interaction with the resting-state activity level. This means that the findings suggest abnormal differential reactivity or sensitivity of the resting-state activity to extero- and interoceptive stimuli in depression. That, though, remains subject to future investigation of changes in interoceptive and exteroceptive stimulus-processing in depression.

How are these abnormalities in intero- and exteroceptive stimulus-processing related to the subjective experience of a person's own body and the environment? The study by Wiebking et al. (2010) also investigated psychological measures of body perception, employing the Body Perception Questionnaire (BPQ). The BPQ scores were significantly increased in depressed patients which is indicative of increased bodily awareness. Most interestingly, unlike in healthy subjects, the increased BPQ scores no longer correlated with the signal changes during both the resting-state itself and the ones related to the exteroceptive condition. Both resting-state and exteroceptively-induced activity thus seem to be decoupled from the abnormally increased subjective experience of one's own body as measured with the BPQ.

What do these findings mean on the phenomenal level of experience? The observed dissociation or decoupling between neuronal and subjective-experiential measures suggests that depressed patients are no longer able to properly modulate their degree of neuronal activity in a fine-grained way in dependence on different degrees of subjective experience. Their experience seems to be "stuck" in its focus on their own body: The patients remain apparently unable to properly down-modulate their perception and awareness of their own body and to shift attention from the body to the environment.

This may explain the many somatic features that characterize MDD who often complain of experiencing various bodily symptoms that have no "objective" basis and remain thus purely subjective. In other words, their resting-state activity and exteroceptively-induced activity are no longer flexible enough to generate different degrees of experience of their own body. Instead, the depressed patients' neuronal activity and consequently their subjective experience is stuck, unable to be shifted at all, which phenomenally results in what I earlier described as "increased body focus."

NEUROPHENOMENAL HYPOTHESIS IVA: REST-EXTERO INTERACTION MEDIATES A "DECREASED ENVIRONMENT-FOCUS" IN DEPRESSION

What do these findings tell us about the resting state and its prephenomenal features? The findings in depression are indicative of an imbalance in the neural processing between interoceptive and exteroceptive stimuli, with only the latter but not the former inducing abnormal decreases in neural activity (when compared to healthy subjects).

Such reduced exteroceptively induced activity may consequently lead to relatively increased neural processing of interoceptive processing and rest–intero interaction when compared to the apparently reduced exteroceptive processing and rest–extero interaction. This implies an abnormal shift in neural activity toward interoceptive processing, which, on the phenomenal level, may then be manifested in the increased bodily awareness and subsequent concerns with undesired bodily symptoms, e. g,. the increased body focus.

Meanwhile, the decreased exteroceptive processing may be accompanied by reduced awareness of and concern with environmental changes, especially positive events that could beneficially impact depression (see Fig. 27-2b). The experience and therefore consciousness is thus predominated by self and body, whereas it leaves no room for experiencing the environment, from which the patients feel consequently disconnected and detached. One may therefore speak phenomenally not only of an increased

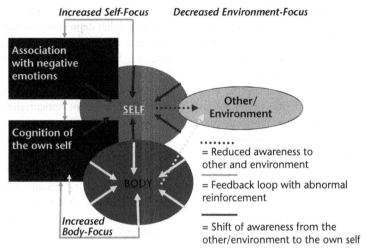

Figure 27-2b Neural and phenomenal abnormalities in depression. The figure shows the relationship between the directedness toward internal or external contents in phenomenal consciousness in depression. Phenomenal consciousness can be directed either externally, toward external contents in the environment, or internally, toward either internal contents like one's own self or the body. In depression, there is increased directedness toward internal contents, e.g., one's own self and the body (increased self- and body-focus), while the directedness toward external contents in the environment is decreased (decreased environment-focus). The increased self- and body-foci are symbolized by larger circles and inward arrows; the decreased relationship of both self and body to the environment is illustrated by thinned arrows. The consequences of the increased self-focus for subsequent psychological functions are indicated on the far left, leading to increased association with negative emotions and increased cognitions of the person's own self.

self-focus and an increased bodily –focus, but also of a decreased environment focus (see also Northoff et al. 2011).

Why, though, are rest–extero interaction and external awareness reduced when compared to rest–intero interaction and internal (i.e., bodily and self-) awareness? Recall that I proposed the increased self-focus and increased self-specificity during stimulus-induced activity to be traced back to the increased resting-state activity and the anterior regions of the inner ring, the midline network. At the same time, however, the resting state data also showed decreased resting-state activity in the lateral regions of the outer ring (see earlier).

How, then, is such decreased resting-state activity in the outer ring, the lateral regions, manifested in the resting state's prephenomenal organization and the phenomenal experience associated with stimulus-induced activity during exteroceptive stimuli? We already know

that stimulus-induced activity is reduced during exteroceptive stimuli, which supposedly may be mediated by decreased rest–extero interaction. That, in turn, may phenomenally go along with decreased external awareness, which I described by the term "decreased environment focus." Now the question arises of how both decreased stimulus-induced activity in lateral regions and the decreased environment focus are related to the abnormally low resting-state activity in the very same regions.

NEUROPHENOMENAL HYPOTHESIS IVB: "SELF-PERSPECTIVAL–INTENTIONAL IMBALANCE" IN DEPRESSION

In Chapter 25, we proposed preintentional organization of the resting state that we supposed to be associated with the neural balance between midline and lateral networks in the resting state. If now this neural balance is abnormally shifted toward the midline regions at the expense of the lateral regions, as it seems to be the case in depression (see earlier), the associated prephenomenal balance will also shift. More specifically, the resting-state activity's prephenomenal balance will shift toward its self-specific organization and away from its preintentional organization. That means that any subsequent phenomenal consciousness is predisposed and biased toward increased self-specificity while at the same time going along with decreased external directedness, e.g., intentionality.

In short, one would propose an imbalance between self-specificity and intentionality. Such an imbalance between self-specificity and intentionality corresponds exactly to what one observes clinically in depression. The resting-state activity's abnormally strong self-specific organization is manifest in increased self-specificity which goes along with increased directedness toward internal contents that is one's own self and one's own body.

However nothing comes or free. The increased directedness toward internal contents comes at the expense of external contents toward which the patients are directed in a reduced way. Accordingly, the directedness toward internal contents (like own self and body) is increased whereas the directedness toward external contents (like events, persons, or objects the environment) is reduced.

How is such imbalance in the directedness toward external and internal content manifested on the phenomenal level of experience? I propose that the imbalance in directedness is reflected in phenomenal imbalance between increased self-focus and a decreased environment focus in these patients (see earlier). I propose that such phenomenal imbalance is possible only if the resting state's preintentional organization is unbalanced toward internal contents, which I suggest to correspond to the abnormal neural balance between midline and lateral networks, that is, between inner/middle and outer rings.

Neurophenomenal Hypothesis IVC: Neural Balance and Phenomenal Balance in Depression

What can we learn from the example of depression for our assumption of the relationship between neural and phenomenal balances? Let's start with what depression can tell us in a purely neuronal regard. The example of depression provides further empirical support for the neural balance between midline and lateral regions in the resting state. And that this neural balance is indeed reciprocal or anticorrelating since otherwise the midline increases in the resting-state activity would not accompany concurrent resting-state activity decreases in lateral regions. Accordingly, depression lends further support to the reciprocal neural balance between midline and lateral regions during the resting state itself.

Moreover, the example of depression also tells us that the resting-state activity abnormalities are apparently carried forth and transferred to the subsequent stimulus-induced activity and thereby strongly impact the latter. This is possible only via rest–stimulus interaction, which, due to the abnormally high resting-state activity, itself becomes abnormal in depression, as is manifested in the earlier-described findings of abnormal stimulus-induced activity. That is what depression can tell us neuronally.

What can depression tell us about our phenomenal and more specifically neurophenomenal assumptions? Depression can tell us that the resting-state activity's neural balance between midline and lateral activity may indeed be associated with a prephenomenal balance between self-specific and preintentional organization. Only by presupposing some kind of prephenomenal balance (or imbalance) between self-specific and preintentional organization in the resting-state activity itself, can the latter's neural imbalance between midline and lateral networks possibly lead to the imbalance between an increased self-focus and a decreased environment-focus as phenomenal hallmarks of depression.

Accordingly, the example of depression tells us that some kind of self-specific and preintentional organization must be encoded into the resting-state activity. Most important, the resting-state activity's abnormal imbalance between self-specific and preintentional organization predisposes the subsequent stimulus-induced activity to be associated with an imbalance between internal and external directedness on the phenomenal level of consciousness.

The consciousness of depressed patients is consequently characterized by abnormally increased directedness toward internal contents as is manifested in the increased self-focus. This, however, comes at a price, in which is decreased directedness toward external contents—the decreased environment-focus. I thus propose the phenomenal imbalance between internal and external directedness to be predisposed by the resting-state activity's prephenomenal imbalance (between self-specific and preintentional organization) and its neural imbalance (between midline and lateral networks).

Open Questions

I here considered schizophrenia in a very narrow sense. I focused only on neural abnormalities in the resting-state activity and stimulus-induced activity only during self-specific stimuli, while I left out the various findings on affective, motor, and cognitive abnormalities. Why? I propose the affective and cognitive functions to build on the resting-state activity and its prephenomenal organization (see Chapter 24 for details). Hence, if the resting-state activity and its neurophenomenal functions are abnormal in themselves, any subsequent sensory, motor, affective, and cognitive functions are also abnormal, which is exactly what can be observed in schizophrenia.

Why, then, did I not investigate the interaction between resting-state activity and affective or cognitive functions? The main focus here was on the neurophenomenal functions and thus on consciousness. More specifically, I investigated the neurophenomenal mechanisms that I propose to underlie the generation of the phenomenal features of consciousness. These in turn, e.g., consciousness, provide the very framework within which affective, sensorimotor, and cognitive functions are generated.

In other words, I consider the neurophenomenal functions associated with consciousness to provide the fundament or basis on and within which sensorimotor, affective, and cognitive functions occur—hence my focus on the neurophenomenal abnormalities in schizophrenia and my neglect of its neuroaffective and neurocognitive abnormalities. However, future studies may target how the here-described abnormalities in the resting-state activity and its neurophenomenal functions are manifested in the various neuroaffective and neurocognitive functions in schizophrenia.

Furthermore, I left out molecular and genetic abnormalities and thus the cellular and subcellular levels of schizophrenia and depression. There are numerous findings in both disorders on these levels. Future investigation may therefore want to see how the here discussed neurophenomenal functions on a regional level relate to the cellular and subcellular levels of neural activity.

One possible bridge, as indicated especially in Volume I, would be difference-based coding, which I would propose to hold on all the different levels, from the cellular, to the population, to the regional, and to the network level. What will be needed in the future is to link these different levels of difference-based coding to the prephenomenal features of the resting-state activity as discussed here.

NOTE

1. The abnormalities in depression are not confined to the insula, but also seen in typical exteroceptive regions like the visual cortex (see Keedwell et al. 2010; Desseilles et al. 2009; Golomb et al. 2009), which observation further supports our assumption of abnormalities in exteroceptive stimulus processing in depression.

PART VIII
Spatiotemporal Quality and Consciousness

Where are we now? I extensively discussed the resting state itself and how its neural activity is structured in spatial and temporal regard. For that, I focused especially on the resting state's functional connectivity and low- and high-frequency fluctuations. That let me suggest specific spatiotemporal structures in the resting state like spatiotemporal continuity (Part V), different forms of unity (Part VI), and self-specific and preintentional organization (Part VII).

Most important, I proposed these spatiotemporal structures of the resting state to predispose and thus make possible the association of any subsequent changes in neural activity with consciousness, including its various phenomenal features. I therefore characterized the resting-state activity's spatiotemporal structures as prephenomenal.

How can we further describe the prephenomenal structures of the resting state activity? The resting-state activity's spatiotemporal structures are proposed to predispose consciousness, thus being a necessary condition of its possibility. At the same time, they are not yet phenomenal by themselves. Therefore, I characterized the resting-state activity's spatiotemporal structures as prephenomenal rather than being either nonphenomenal or phenomenal. As such, they may be considered necessary though not sufficient neural conditions of possible (rather than actual) consciousness. I hence characterized them as neural predispositions of consciousness (NPC). This, however, leaves open the sufficient neural conditions of actual consciousness, namely as consciousness is actually realized; these neural conditions are subsumed under the umbrella term of the neural correlates of consciousness (NCC), which I have neglected almost completely so far. Therefore, this last part of these two volumes will focus on the NCC.

How can we investigate the sufficient neural conditions of actual consciousness? One would propose that both necessary and sufficient conditions must work in conjunction in order to instantiate consciousness. The resting-state activity and its prephenomenal structures must thus interact in specific ways with the stimulus in order for the latter to become associated with consciousness.

Rather than on stimulus-induced activity itself, in isolation of the resting-state activity, we therefore have to focus on the interaction between resting-state activity and stimulus and thus on what I described as rest–stimulus interaction. My subsequent assumption is that rest–stimulus interaction and its neuronal mechanisms are central in providing the transition from the resting state's prephenomenal structures to the full-blown phenomenal state of consciousness. Accordingly, we have to discuss the neuronal mechanisms underlying rest–stimulus interaction in order to get a grip on the NCC.

What exactly occurs on the phenomenal side during rest–stimulus interaction? I here propose *qualia* (e.g., individual instances of subjective, conscious experience) as central, which are usually considered the phenomenal hallmark of consciousness. The concept of *qualia* describes the "what it is like" of experience: its subjective and qualitative features that signify consciousness. To explain and account for consciousness in a neurophenomenal way, we have to investigate qualia, including their phenomenal features in relation to the neuronal mechanisms of rest–stimulus interaction. This is the aim and focus of the present part.

How about the different dimensions of consciousness? We recall from the second Introduction that the current literature distinguishes between content and level or state of consciousness. To this I added a third dimension—form, structure, or organization of consciousness (see the second Introduction for details). Let us briefly describe these three dimensions: contents, level, and form, in further detail.

The *contents* concern the objects and events we experience in consciousness; therefore, the philosophers speak here of *phenomenal contents*. We have touched upon the neuronal mechanisms underlying phenomenal contents in various places in this book. For instance, I discussed the constitution of contents on the basis of difference-based coding (see Chapter 25), while the selection of contents was related to the level of resting-state activity in different regions (see Chapter 19). Finally, the designation of contents as either internal or external was proposed to be mediated by the neural balance between midline and lateral networks (see Chapter 25).

How about the *form* of consciousness? The concept of "form" describes the organization and structure of the contents in space and time on the phenomenal level of consciousness. I proposed the resting-state activity's different spatiotemporal structures to provide the neural predisposition for the organization or form of consciousness. I consequently propose the phenomenal organization or form of consciousness to be characterized by spatiotemporal continuity, spatiotemporal unity, and self-specific and intentional organization. This was extensively discussed in Parts V–VII when focusing on the resting state's prephenomenal structures and how they are manifest on the phenomenal level of consciousness.

That, however, leaves open the neuronal mechanisms underlying the level or degree of consciousness. I here propose this question to be closely related to the one of the sufficient neural conditions of consciousness, i.e., the NCC. This is the focus of this part.

Thereby, we will also see how all three features, contents, form, and level/degree of consciousness, are closely related to and thus interdependent on each other. In other words, form, organization, and level/degree converge in what is phenomenally described as qualia. To exemplify this, I will take the loss of consciousness in the vegetative state (VS) as a paradigmatic example to develop specific neurophenomenal hypotheses about qualia in particular and consciousness in general.

GENERAL OVERVIEW

Chapter 28 focuses on the relevance of the resting state for consciousness. More specifically, based on resting-state findings in VS, I propose the degree of rest–rest interaction to be central in triggering and instantiating consciousness. Thereby, the position of the resting state's neural operation relative to its own underlying biophysical-computational spectrum may be central. The more closely the resting state operates toward its either maximal or minimal biophysical limits, the less likely it is that consciousness can be instantiated.

That leads me to propose what I refer to as the "biophysical spectrum hypothesis of consciousness," which describes the relationship between the range of biophysical-computational features and the actual occurrence of consciousness. This will be complemented by showing how the resting state and its actual "position" within its respective biophysical-computational spectra impact and modulate the degree of spatial and temporal differences that can be encoded into neural activity, i.e., difference-based coding. This results in the "difference-based coding hypothesis of consciousness" (see also first

Introduction) that suggests a close and intricate relationship between the degree of differences encoded into neural activity and the level or state of consciousness.

Chapter 29 moves on from the resting state to rest–stimulus interaction. I here discuss the most recent findings during cognitive and self-specific stimulation in patients with VS. Based on these findings, I suggest abnormal neural dissociation between resting-state and stimulus-induced activity in VS. This lets me hypothesize that rest–stimulus interaction is central for generating consciousness in general.

More specifically, I propose the degrees of both nonlinearity and GABAergic-mediated neural inhibition during rest–stimulus interaction to predict the degree of qualia and thus consciousness. This amounts to what I describe as the "nonlinearity hypothesis of consciousness" that points out the central role of supposedly GABA-ergic-mediated non-linearity during rest–stimulus interaction for the instantiation of consciousness.

Chapter 30 addresses the question why and how qualia show phenomenal features like nonstructural homogeneity, transparency, and *ipseity* (individual identity; selfhood). Both nonlinearity and GABAergic-mediated neural inhibition are proposed to make possible the carryover and transfer of the resting state's prephenomenal structures to the stimulus and its associated stimulus-induced activity. Such carryover and transfer are supposed to impact both resting state and stimulus-induced activity in one sweep that is central for associating consciousness to the stimulus-induced activity: the carryover and transfer make possible the association of stimulus-induced activity with the phenomenal features of qualia by changing and modulating the resting-state activity and its prephenomenal features.

The resting state's prephenomenal structures are thus transformed into a phenomenal state; that is, consciousness. This is what I call the "transfer hypothesis," which suggests that the phenomenal features of qualia like nonstructural homogeneity, transparency, and ipseity result from the carryover and transfer of the resting

state's prephenomenal structures to the stimulus during rest–stimulus interaction.

Chapter 31 focuses the attention on a set of regions in the brain that have been rather neglected so far: subcortical regions and their relevance for consciousness. Based on their anatomical-structural features, I propose difference-based coding to be present in subcortical regions in very much the same way as in cortical regions. One would then propose that phenomenal qualia and thus consciousness can also be elicited just on the basis of the subcortical regions alone.

This is supported by the central relevance of subcortical regions in affect and emotions and hence in affective consciousness as described by Jaak Panksepp. Finally, patients with no cortex serve as an example to illustrate the possibility of consciousness on the basis of the subcortical regions themselves. I consequently consider the subcortical regions to be sufficient neural conditions of consciousness, albeit in a spatially and temporally restricted way.

We have focused so far mainly on consciousness of the environment, whereas we neglected our experience, i.e., consciousness, of our own body, which is often described as *interoceptive awareness*; this will be discussed in Chapter 32. Recent findings show the insula specifically to be associated with interoceptive awareness. How is the neural processing of the body's interoceptive stimuli associated with a phenomenal state and thus qualia? I propose the same principles of rest–stimulus interaction like difference-based coding, nonlinearity, and GABAergic-mediated neural inhibition to hold in the insula too.

Rest–intero interaction in this sense allows for the carryover and transfer of the resting state's prephenomenal structures to the interoceptive stimulus, which in turn makes possible the interoceptive stimulus' association with qualia and thus consciousness. The chapter concludes with a brief neurotheoretical remark about the concepts of interoception and perception that touch upon the more conceptual characterization of consciousness by embodiment and embeddedness.

CHAPTER 28
Resting-State Activity and Qualia

Summary

After having discussed the role of the rest-ing state and its prephenomenal structures, we now move on to how they are manifested on the phenomenal level of consciousness. Qualia are considered the phenomenal hallmarks of consciousness that describe the subjective and qualitative features, the "what it is like" of expe-rience and thus consciousness. I here take the loss of consciousness in the pathological disor-der of the vegetative state (VS) as a paradigm to investigate the neuronal mechanisms underlying qualia in particular and consciousness in general. For that, I first focus on the various resting-state abnormalities reported in the recent literature. They show decreased functional and effective connectivity as well as decreased or even absent higher-frequency oscillations in the resting state in VS. Moreover, the results show decreased neu-ronal reactivity or propensity of the resting state to changes in its neural activity. How is it possible that the resting-state activity is less sensitive and reactive to changes in its neural activity in VS? I propose that the resting state in VS operates close to its minimal biophysical-computational limits which decreases its reactivity or propen-sity for neural activity changes. I consequently suggest what I describe as the "biophysical spec-trum hypothesis of consciousness": the "bio-physical spectrum hypothesis of consciousness." It proposes the degree of consciousness to be directly dependent upon the actual "position" of the resting-state activity within and thus in rela-tion to its underlying biophysical-computational spectrum. Thereby I propose the degree of global metabolism and thus energy supply to the brain as central. Since global energy supply and metabolism are greatly reduced in VS patients, the actual "position" of their resting-state activ-ity tends to be "located" at the lower or minimal end of the biophysical-computational spectrum of these patients' brains. Why is a high degree of global energy and metabolism necessary for consciousness? Better and higher degrees of global metabolism make possible higher degrees of changes in the resting-state activity and consequently its encoding of neural activity in terms of spatial and temporal difference; that is, difference-based coding. And the higher the degree of difference-based coding, the higher the actual degree of consciousness. This leads me to propose what I describe as the "difference-based coding hypothesis of consciousness" (DHC): The DHC claims that the degree of conscious-ness is directly dependent upon the degree of difference-based coding. The degree of differ-ences encoded into neural activity on the basis of difference-based coding may therefore be regarded as a sufficient condition and thus neu-ral correlate of consciousness (NCC). Since "difference-based coding" describes the encod-ing of temporal and spatial differences between difference stimuli into neural activity, one would propose qualia to be based on differences between different stimuli and thus to be inher-ently spatial and temporal in phenomenal regard.

Key Concepts and Topics Covered

Vegetative state, qualia, consciousness, rest-ing state, difference-based coding, biophysical spectrum hypothesis of consciousness, vegeta-tive state, neuronal reactivity, rest–rest interac-tion, global metabolism, difference-based coding hypothesis of consciousness

NEUROEMPIRICAL BACKGROUND IA: QUALIA SIGNIFY CONSCIOUSNESS

So far, we have discussed how the resting-state activity is structured and organized in spatial and temporal terms. This led us to propose spatiotemporal continuity, neuronal and statistically based unity, and self-specific and preintentional organization of the resting state's neuronal activity. Since the resting-state activity's spatiotemporal structures were suggested to predispose the phenomenal states of consciousness, we characterized them as prephenomenal. To put it slightly differently, the resting-state activity's spatiotemporal structures are necessary but not sufficient neural conditions of possible consciousness and thus what I describe as neural predispositions of consciousness (NPC) (see first Introduction). We now though want to move on, and reveal the neural mechanisms that underlie the manifestation of actual consciousness itself, that is, its actual realization. This is the question for the sufficient neural conditions of actual consciousness, the neural correlates of consciousness (NCC).

What exactly do the sufficient conditions, the neural correlates, instantiate on the phenomenal side of consciousness itself? Consciousness is supposed to be manifest in what is called "qualia." Tentatively put, qualia describe the subjective and qualitative aspects of our experience, the "what it is like." This is, for instance, manifested in our experience of the redness of the color red or the painfulness of pain (see Chapter 30 for a more extensive definition of *qualia*). How, then, can we search for such qualitative and subjective features in the neuronal states of the brain? This is where the difficulty starts. All we can observe in the brain are neuronal states in a quantitative and objective way. There is no "subjective" component, let alone the qualitative-phenomenal feeling, visible in the brain, implying that we cannot, for instance, see the chocolate itself as you taste it. In short, qualia, being purely subjective, cannot be observed in the rather objective neuronal activity of the brain.

The search for the underlying neuronal mechanisms of qualia is therefore regarded as one of the hardest nuts to crack. This is well expressed in the following quote by Francis Crick and Christoph Koch (2003), who pioneered the neuroscientific research in consciousness:

> The most difficult aspect of consciousness is the so-called hard problem of qualia—the redness of

red, the painfulness of pain, and so on. No one has produced any plausible explanation as to how the experience of the redness of red could arise from the actions of the brain. It appears fruitless to approach this problem head-on. (Crick and Koch 2003, 119)

NEUROEMPIRICAL BACKGROUND IB: INDIRECT APPROACH TO QUALIA THROUGH THEIR LOSS IN VEGETATIVE STATE

How can we tackle the search for the neuronal mechanisms of qualia and thus the NCC? I here pursue an indirect approach to consciousness. What happens in the brain when qualia and thus consciousness are lost? This leads me to what is described as the "disorders of consciousness," which include anesthesia, vegetative state, and non-REM sleep.

One of the most prominent disorders of consciousness is the vegetative state (VS). In a vegetative state, patients seem to lose their ability to experience anything at all, indicating a loss of qualia and of consciousness in general. Investigating the neuronal changes in VS may consequently give us an indirect clue about which neuronal mechanisms are central and sufficient to induce qualia and thus consciousness. However, we must be more specific. VS is a disorder of consciousness that concerns the level, state, or degree of consciousness as it is strongly diminished in these patients. Hence, when investigating the neuronal mechanisms underlying VS, we focus on the neural correlates of the *level* of consciousness.

As outlined in the introduction, such focus on the neural correlates of the *level* of consciousness must be distinguished from searching for the neural correlates of the *contents* of consciousness and the neural correlates of the *form* or organization of consciousness. We already touched upon the neural correlates of the *contents* of consciousness when revealing the neuronal mechanisms of the selection, constitution, and designation of contents (see Chapter 19, and especially Chapter 25). In contrast to the neural correlates of the contents of consciousness, however, we left open the search for the neural correlates of the *level* and the *form* of consciousness.

This is the focus in the present Part. More specifically, Chapter 30 will discuss the neural correlates of the *form* of consciousness. In contrast, the present chapter centers on the neural correlates of the *level* of consciousness, which will be complemented by linking the neural correlates of *levels* and *contents* of consciousness in Chapter 29.

NEUROEMPIRICAL BACKGROUND IC: CLINICAL SYMPTOMS IN VEGETATIVE STATE

Now we are finally ready to tackle VS itself. For that, we will want to get to know Steven Laureys. A prominent Belgian neuroscientist, Laureys is a medical doctor and neuroscientist who investigates patients who, due to brain damage and lesion, lost their consciousness and suffer from VS. These patients have their eyes open but do not show any signs of conscious behavior and reaction. This pertains to the outside world, one may want to add, since their inner world may still be preserved, as suggested by some recent results, as will be described later in Chapter 29. Clinically, patients suffering from VS are to be distinguished from patients in a coma, who do not even open their eyes anymore, and patients with brain death. On the other end of the spectrum, VS must be distinguished from minimally conscious state (MCS) patients, who show some signs of consciousness. Finally, patients with locked-in syndrome (LIS) show preserved consciousness but are "locked into" their bodies, unable to communicate with the outside world.

Steven Laureys and another scientist from Cambridge, England, Adrian Owen (see Chapter 29 for details), were instrumental in introducing functional imaging to these patients to explore their neuronal changes. This included stimulation with different kinds of cognitive stimuli, self-specific stimuli, and affective-emotional stimuli, as well as investigations of these patients' resting-state activity. I here focus in this chapter on the latter, the resting-state activity in VS, while the results on the various kinds of stimulus-induced activity will be discussed in Chapter 29.

NEURONAL FINDINGS IA: *FUNCTIONAL CONNECTIVITY IN THE RESTING STATE IN THE VEGETATIVE STATE*

There have been plenty of studies on VS during both resting-state and stimulus-induced activity using positron emission tomography (PET), functional magnetic resonance imaging (fMRI), and electroencephalography (EEG; see Laureys and Schiff 2012, especially Tables 1–3, for a recent excellent overview of all studies in VS). It would be beyond the scope of this chapter to discuss all studies in detail, hence my focus on the ones that appear to be the most relevant in the present context.

I here focus in particular on the spatial and temporal measures of the resting state's neural activity in VS, functional connectivity and low-frequency fluctuations, because of their presumed central role in consciousness (see the preceding parts), while I reserve the results on the global metabolism in VS as measured with PET for later sections.

A 2010 study by the group around Steven Laureys (Vanhaudenhuyse et al. 2010) investigated functional connectivity in the resting state using fMRI. They included healthy subjects as well as four VS patients, five coma patients, four MCS patients, and one LIS patient (see Huang et al. 2013, for another recent study on resting state functional connectivity in VS).

Taking healthy subjects and all patients together, the default-mode network (DMN) could be well reproduced. Strong functional connectivity was observed in the neural network between anterior midline regions (perigenual anterior cingulate cortex, ventromedial prefrontal cortex, subgenual anterior cingulate cortex, and dorsomedial prefrontal cortex), posterior midline regions (posterior cingulate cortex [PCC], precuneus, and retrosplenial cortex), medial temporal (hippocampus and parahippocampus), and the bilateral temporo-parietal junction. Thereby the posterior midline regions like the PCC and the precuneus showed the strongest functional connectivity indices in all groups compared to that in the other regions.

How is the functional connectivity of the DMN related to consciousness? For that, Vanhaudenhuyse et al. (2010) grouped their different subjects according to their degree of consciousness. This revealed the following pattern: functional connectivity was highest in the DMN (and the thalamus and the brainstem) in healthy subjects. The one LIS patient exhibited almost similar degrees of functional connectivity as the healthy subjects. In contrast, the MCS patients showed lower degrees of functional connectivity, which were still considerably higher than the ones in VS. VS patients' degree of functional connectivity was, in turn, higher than the one in the coma patients.

These results suggest the degree of consciousness to be directly dependent upon the degree of functional connectivity in the DMN. This was further confirmed in a subsequent correlation analyses where the degree of functional connectivity was correlated with the degree of consciousness as measured by the Coma Recovery Scale–Revised (CRS-R). The higher the degree of functional connectivity between the various regions in the DMN, the higher the degree of consciousness obtained on the CRS-R in the various subjects (see Fig. 28-1).

These data clearly demonstrate severe alterations; that is, reduction in resting state functional connectivity throughout the whole brain in VS, including the brainstem, thalamus, and especially the midline structures as the core nucleus of the DMN. This is further supported by other studies showing similar reductions in resting-state functional connectivity in VS (see Cauda et al. 2009; Silva et al. 2010; Boly et al. 2009; Huang et al. 2013; Laureys and Schiff 2012). Interestingly, a single brain-dead patient did not show any long-distance functional connectivity at all. Correlations were found here only locally, without any anticorrelation between DMN (as task negative) and more lateral regions (as task positive) (Boly et al. 2009).

In addition to the DMN, the thalamus seems to have an essential role in resting-state functional connectivity. VS patients show decreased functional connectivity between the thalamus and anterior and posterior medial and lateral cortical regions (see Boly et al. 2009; Vanhaudenhuyse et al. 2010; Zhou et al. 2011; Huang et al. 2013). The central role of the

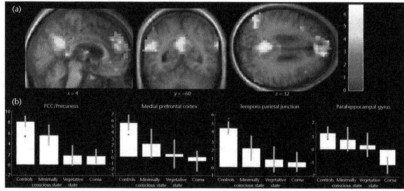

Figure 28-1 Functional connectivity in vegetative state. Default network connectivity correlates with the level of consciousness, ranging from healthy controls, to minimally conscious, vegetative then comatose patients. (A) Areas showing a linear correlation between default network connectivity and consciousness. Results are thresholded for display at uncorrected $P < 0.05$ and rendered on the mean T_1 structural image of the patients. (B) Mean Z-scores and 90% confidence interval for default network connectivity in PCC/precuneus, temporo-parietal junction, medial prefrontal cortex, and parahippocampal gyrus across patient populations. Locked-in syndrome patient Z-scores are displayed for illustrative purposes as an additional circles overlaid on control population data. Reprinted with permission of Oxford University Press, from Vanhaudenhuyse A, Noirhomme Q, Tshibanda LJ, Bruno MA, Boveroux P, Schnakers C, Soddu A, Perlbarg V, Ledoux D, Brichant JF, Moonen G, Maquet P, Greicius MD, Laureys S, Boly M. Default network connectivity reflects the level of consciousness in noncommunicative brain-damaged patients. *Brain.* 2010 Jan;133(Pt 1):161–71.

thalamus is further supported by the observation that electrical stimulation in the thalamus induced recovery of consciousness in one VS patient (see Schiff 2009, 2010).

Neuronal Findings IB: *EFFECTIVE CONNECTIVITY IN THE RESTING STATE IN THE VEGETATIVE STATE*

The earlier-described studies investigated functional connectivity in the resting state in VS. What remains unclear, however, is whether that functional connectivity really mediates causal interaction between the connected regions. The different regions' neural activities may just be correlated with each other, thus showing functional connectivity without really causally impacting each other. We therefore have to investigate whether the reduced functional connectivity in VS is no longer as causally efficient anymore, thus addressing what is described as "effective connectivity" (see Chapter 5 for the discussion of both concepts—functional and effective connectivity).

How can one investigate effective connectivity? For that, one may want to causally impact one region's neural activity and measures its impact on other regions' neural activities. That is possible by combining transcranial magnetic stimulation (TMS) that causally impacts one regions, with EEG that can record the effects of that causal impact on other regions. The group around the Italian researcher Guilio Tononi, who is based in the United States, combined TMS and EEG in five patients with VS, five patients with MCS, and two patients with LIS (Rosanova et al. 2012). An additional five patients were investigated several times in different stages of their improvement, VS, MCS, and a fully conscious state (only three patients in the latter).

Magnetic impulses (every 200–230 ms = 0.4–0.5 Hz; intensity of 140 V/m to 200 V/m) were applied via TMS on right and left medial frontal (superior frontal gyrus) and parietal (superior parietal gyrus) cortex to probe these regions' neural activity changes in the resting state. The neural effects and especially the temporal and spatial spread and propagation of such local magnetic stimulation were measured with the simultaneous high-density, 60-channel EEG. This design allowed for probing effective connectivity, the causal interaction between the neural activities of different regions, rather than their mere temporal correlation, that is, functional connectivity.

What about the results? The VS patients showed a simple positive-negative EEG response that remained local, short, and did not change at all. This contrasted with the MCS patients, where the TMS impulse triggered a more complex EEG response that spread both spatially and temporally and also changed over time. The pattern in MCS resembled more closely the one in the two LIS patients than the one in VS patients (see Fig. 28-2a).

A similar pattern was observed in the longitudinal investigation in the five patients who were investigated several times Their response pattern became more complex and thus spatially and temporally more propagated in the three patients who recovered from VS over MCS to the fully conscious state. In contrast, such more-extended spatial and temporal propagation as well as a more complex response pattern could not be observed in the two patients who remained in VS (Fig. 28-2b).

Taken together, these results clearly demonstrate the breakdown of global, that is, transregional, functional (i.e., mere temporal correlation), and effective (i.e., causal interaction) connectivity in VS. Especially the functional and effective connectivity in the midline regions as the core of the DMN seems to be altered. Less technically put, neural activity seems to remain simple, local, and short in VS compared to that in the conscious states, where it is more complex, global, and longer. The resting-state activity in VS thus seems to show decreased neural reactivity or propensity for spatial and temporal changes with increased degrees of extension and complexity in the patterns of neural activity.

Neuronal Findings
IIA: ELECTROPHYSIOLOGICAL ACTIVITY IN THE RESTING-STATE IN THE VEGETATIVE STATE

So far, I have described only the spatial features of the resting state, while more or less neglecting

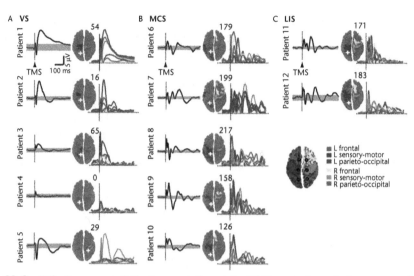

Figure 28-2a Effective connectivity in vegetative state. TMS-evoked cortical responses in Group I patients. A group of five vegetative state (VS, A), five minimally conscious state (MCS, B), and two patients with locked-in syndrome (LIS, C) underwent one TMS/EEG session after seven days of repeated evaluations by means of the CRS-R. For each patient, the averaged TMS-evoked potentials recorded at one electrode under the stimulator (the trace) and the respective significance threshold (upper and lower boundaries of the bands; bootstrap statistics, $P < 0.01$) are shown. The sources involved by maximum cortical currents (10 most active sources) during the significant post-stimulus period of the global mean field power are plotted on the cortical surface and coded according to their location in six anatomical macro-areas as indicated in the legend; the number of detected sources is indicated at the *top right* of each map. The time-series (traces) represent TMS-evoked cortical currents recorded from an array of six sources (the circles on the cortical map in the legend) located ~2 cm lateral to the midline, one for each macro-area. The white crosses mark the sites of stimulation. For all patients, the responses to the left parietal cortex stimulation are shown, except for one patient (Patient 5) in whom a significant response could only be detected in the right hemisphere. EEG positivity is upward. L = left; R = right. Reprinted with permission of Oxford University Press, from Rosanova M, Gosseries O, Casarotto S, Boly M, Casali AG, Bruno MA, Mariotti M, Boveroux P, Tononi G, Laureys S, Massimini M. Recovery of cortical effective connectivity and recovery of consciousness in vegetative patients. *Brain.* 2012 Jan 6. *135*(Pt 4), 1308–1320.

its temporal features. These shall be the focus of the present section, where I will mainly present findings from EEG studies (see also Laureys and Schiff 2012, for an overview).

In addition to the stimulation with TMS, the earlier study by Rosanova et al. (2012) also measured spontaneous EEG in the resting state in their patients. Interestingly, the patients converting from MCS into a fully conscious state did show an increase in the power of higher-frequency oscillations like alpha and beta. In contrast, the power of high-frequency oscillations in the resting state remained rather low, if not absent, in all VS and MCS patients,

including those who did not convert to a fully conscious state (see Fig. 28-2c).

This is in accordance with findings from other groups. Using EEG, Fingelkurts et al. (2011) investigated VS and MCS patients during the resting state (for 30 min) with eyes closed (as closed manually by hand). They then analyzed the spectral pattern, its diversity and variability, as well as the probability (and power) of the neural activity fluctuations in the different frequency bands.

VS and MCS patients who died within 6 months after the EEG recording showed a significantly lower degree of diversity and variability

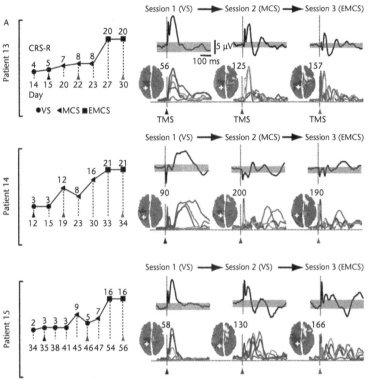

Figure 28-2b Effective connectivity in vegetative state. Clinical evaluation and TMS-evoked cortical responses in Group II patients. CRS-R total scores are plotted for the patients who were studied longitudinally (Group II) and eventually emerged from a minimally conscious state (EMCS, A) or remained in a vegetative state (VS, B); the first assessment (Session 1) was carried out 48 hours after withdrawal of sedation, as patients exited from coma. The symbols indicate the associated clinical diagnosis (filled circles = vegetative state; filled triangles = minimally conscious state; filled squares = emergence from minimally conscious state). Colored arrow tips mark the days when TMS/EEG recordings were performed and the time of TMS delivery. For every patient and measurement, averaged potentials triggered by TMS (vertical dashed lines) of parietal cortex and recorded from the electrode under the stimulator are shown. The corresponding spread and the time-course of the cortical currents evoked by TMS is measured. The sources involved by maximum neuronal currents during the significant post-stimulus period are plotted on the cortical surface and color-coded according to their location in six anatomical macro-areas (Fig. 28-1); the number of detected sources is indicated at the top right of each map. The time-series represent TMS-evoked cortical currents recorded from an array of six sources (see their locations in Fig. 28-1) located ~2 cm lateral to the midline, one for each macro-area. The white crosses mark the sites of stimulation; in each patient, the left parietal cortex was stimulated when patients entered a vegetative state from coma (Session 1), soon after transition to a minimally conscious state or at least 30 days of permanence in a vegetative state (Session 2) and after emergence from a minimally conscious state (Session 3), when subjects recovered functional communication. EEG positivity is upward. Reprinted with permission of Oxford University Press, from Rosanova M, Gosseries O, Casarotto S, Boly M, Casali AG, Bruno MA, Mariotti M, Boveroux P, Tononi G, Laureys S, Massimini M. Recovery of cortical effective connectivity and recovery of consciousness in vegetative patients. *Brain.* 2012 Jan 6. *135*(Pt 4), 1308–1320.

in their spectral patterns compared to that in those who survived after 6 months. The same group of patients also exhibited significantly higher probability values of lower-frequency oscillations, that is, delta and slow-theta waves.

In contrast, higher-frequency oscillations showed decreased probability of higher frequencies, that is, fast-theta and alpha, compared to that in the patients who survived after 6 months. Like the findings reported earlier, these results

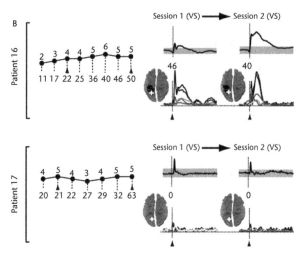

Figure 28-2b (Continued)

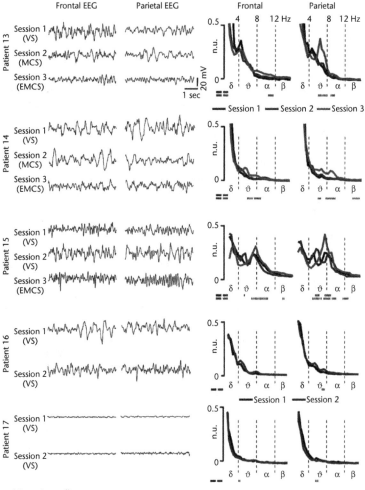

Figure 28-2c (Continued)

further underline the absence or decrease of high-frequency oscillations in VS.

NEURONAL FINDINGS IIB: FREQUENCY FLUCTUATIONS IN THE RESTING STATE IN THE VEGETATIVE STATE

Can the degree of electrophysiological activity, including high-frequency oscillations, distinguish between different levels of consciousness? The same group (Fingelkurts et al. 2011) investigated the same sample of patients with regard to their distinction between VS and MCS. For that, they focused on microstates that can be defined as transiently synchronized neural activities across different neuronal assemblies (as operationalized in EEG by the correlation between different local electrodes' signals). They investigated the spatial and temporal extent of the various microstates (see also Lehmann et al. 1998; Lehmann 2010; Lehmann and Michel 2010) as well as the relationship, that is, synchronization, between the various microstates.

The microstates themselves were smaller, more unstable, and temporally shorter in especially VS and to some degree also in MCS compared to that in healthy subjects. Resting-state EEG (during eyes closed) showed decreased operational synchrony, that is, extent and strength, between the different microstates. The degree of neural synchrony, or *operational synchrony* as the authors call it, was smallest in VS and largest in healthy subjects while MCS showed values intermediate between both groups. These abnormalities in microstates and neural synchrony hint again at decreased spatial and temporal spread of neural activity in VS.

Another EEG study investigated five VS and five MCS patients during sleep (Landsness et al. 2011). Can these patients modulate their electrophysiological pattern of resting-state activity during sleep in the same way healthy subjects do? Behaviorally the five VS patients showed normal patterns of sleep with alternating periods of eyes open and closed.

In contrast, they did not exhibit the "normal" electrophysiological pattern. It was impossible to distinguish REM sleep and non-REM sleep stages in the EEG, even though behaviorally both sleep stages could be distinguished from each other by eyes open and closed. Let's be more specific. While eyes closed went along with the some degree of the typical slowing of activity into slow frequency bands, that is, delta and theta, the difference between eyes open and closed remained nevertheless insignificant.

This indicates a lack of slow waves in VS. Such a lack of slow waves is also in accordance with the observation that there was no homeostatic decline of slow-wave activity throughout the whole night in VS. Finally, the spindle activity characteristic of non-REM sleep in healthy subjects was not observed at all in VS (see Chapter 15 for neuronal details about non-REM sleep).

In contrast to the VS patients, the five MCS patients did show a distinction between REM sleep and non-REM sleep in their EEG. There was significant increase of slow-wave activity in non-REM sleep and homeostatic decline over the night. Therefore, unlike in VS, the neuronal reactivity to neuronal change as between non-REM and REM sleep seems to be preserved to some degree in MCS.

How about the even lower-frequency fluctuations in VS like the ones smaller than 0.01? An fMRI study by our group (Huang et al. 2013) focused on the amplitude of the low-frequency fluctuations (<0.01 Hz) in the resting state in 11 VS patients. Compared to the healthy subjects, VS patients showed significantly lower amplitudes, that is, power, in the low-frequency fluctuations (i.e., slow 4 and

Figure 28-2c Effective connectivity in vegetative state. EEG spectra show evident changes from minimally conscious state (MCS) to emergence from minimally conscious state (EMCS) but not from vegetative state (VS) to minimally conscious state. Spontaneous EEG traces (5 s) and EEG spectra (calculated on 2 min; average of 5 s epochs) are shown for the five subjects who underwent longitudinal recording sessions (Group II); in these patients, changes in the EEG spectrum were assessed statistically by means of a two-tailed paired *t*-test. The dotted lines at the bottom of each plot indicate the frequency bins that show statistically significant differences of power (*t*-test, $P < 0.01$). EEG positivity is upward. n.u. = normalized units.

5) in especially the anterior (e.g., perigenual anterior cingulate cortex) and posterior (i.e., PCC/precuneus) midline regions. Though these are apparently the first results on low-frequency fluctuations in VS, they suggest both low- and high-frequency fluctuations to be deficient in VS.

Taken together, these results demonstrate decreased power in high-frequency oscillations like alpha, beta, and gamma in the resting state in VS. In addition to the high-frequency oscillations, lower ones in the slow domain lower than 0.01 Hz seem to also be deficient in their power in VS. Moreover, the results on the frequency oscillations demonstrate again the decreased spatial and temporal spread of neural activity and the resting state's reduced reactivity or propensity for changes in neural activity in VS.

NEURONAL HYPOTHESIS IA: REDUCED REST–REST INTERACTION IN THE VEGETATIVE STATE

The findings show decreased neuronal activity in the resting state in VS. The functional and effective connectivity remains more local and is thus less globally extended to other more distant regions. In addition to the less extended functional connectivity, high-frequency oscillations are reduced in VS while low-frequency fluctuations seem to be more or less preserved.

Most important, especially the results of the TMS-EEG investigation and the sleep study demonstrate reduced propensity of the resting-state activity for changes in the degree of its spatial and temporal neural activity patterns. Neural activity in the resting state is simply not as reactive anymore and can consequently no longer trigger more complex spatial and temporal patterns to propagate changes in neural activity (either within the resting state itself, or as elicited by stimuli).

The changes in the resting-state activity itself and its decreased propensity for spatial and temporal changes are indicative of reduced rest–rest interaction. There seems to be less neural activity change going on in the resting state itself entailing reduced interaction between different regions and frequencies in the resting state itself. This is suggested by the decreased functional connectivity, the decreased complexity of the response pattern, the absence of high-frequency

oscillations, and the decreased spatiotemporal spread and propagation of neural activity. Such reduced rest–rest interaction may signify the decreased neuronal reactivity or propensity of the resting state for spatial and temporal changes.

To put it metaphorically, the level of spatial and temporal noise and fuzz in the resting state signifying rest–rest interaction seems to be significantly reduced in VS. The resting state is, metaphorically speaking, more silent in VS. There is only one lonely child silently playing in the room of the brain's resting state in VS as compared to the loud chatter of the 20 children playing in the room of the resting state in the healthy brain.

NEURONAL HYPOTHESIS IB: SUBCORTICAL VERSUS SUBCORTICAL-CORTICAL MECHANISMS OF REDUCED REST–REST INTERACTION IN THE VEGETATIVE STATE

Why is there decreased rest–rest interaction in VS? We currently do not know. Based on their results from sleep in VS, Landsness et al. (2011) propose two possible mechanisms. One possibility is that there is a primary lesion in the brainstem itself, in the ascending arousal system, that is relevant for activating the brain. VS would then be regarded primarily a subcortical disorder by itself. This is supported by the clinical observation of the occurrence of coma and VS in patients with lesions in the pons, the brainstem and its various nuclei, including the raphe nucleus, the tegmental nucleus, the parabrachial nucleus, and the locus coeruleus (see Parvizi and Damasio 2001, 2003; and see Chapter 31 herein for a more extensive discussion of the role of subcortical regions in consciousness).

Alternatively, VS patients may suffer from a disruption in the transfer from subcortical to cortical regions via the thalamus as it may be related to structural or functional disconnection between subcortical and cortical regions. VS may then be regarded a subcortical-cortical disconnection syndrome rather than a primary subcortical disorder (see, for instance, Panksepp et al. 2007 as well as Schiff 2009, 2010 arguing in this direction; see also Chapter 31 for more details of the disconnection hypothesis).

This is supported by concurrent observations of thalamic and anterior and posterior cortical midline resting-state abnormalities in VS as described earlier. This hypothesis is further supported by the observation that deep brain stimulation in the central thalamus led to recovery with conversion to full consciousness in one patient who was in MCS for 6 years (see Schiff et al. 2007; see also Brown et al. 2010). Analogous subcortical-cortical disconnection may also occur in other states where consciousness is reduced as, for instance, in NREM sleep (see Chapters 14 and 15) and in anesthesia (see Chapters 15 and 16; as well as Mhuircheartaigh et al. 2010).

How does such structural-functional disconnection between subcortical and cortical regions occur? It may occur either on structural or functional grounds. As Rosanova et al. (2012) mention in their discussion, preserved structural subcortical-cortical connectivity may nevertheless go along with changes in functional connectivity. The deficits in functional connectivity may then be due to alterations in physiological processes like the excitation-inhibition balance or network instability or bi-stability (Schiff 2010). (I here leave out the structural alterations in VS; see Laureys and Schiff 2012 for an overview.)

The issue of subcortical versus subcortical-cortical is currently not yet decided. What is clear, however, is that either characterization of VS—as subcortical disorder or as subcortical-cortical disconnection syndrome—can well account for the actual changes in the resting-state activity itself. This, however, leaves open question of what neuronal mechanisms underlie the resting-state activity's reduced propensity to change.

NEURONAL HYPOTHESIS IC: ORIGIN OF THE RESTING-STATE ACTIVITY'S REDUCED PROPENSITY TO CHANGE

What about the reduced propensity of the resting-state activity for spatial and temporal changes? The decreased changes in neuronal measures like functional and effective connectivity and high-frequency oscillations may result from the resting state's reduced neuronal reactivity or propensity to change its activity level and pattern. In that case, these neuronal measures signify the reduced neuronal reactivity or

propensity to change in the resting state's neural activity. They can thus be considered a *sufficient* neural condition; that is, a neural correlate of actual consciousness. In contrast, they do not explain why there is such reduced propensity or reactivity and therefore cannot be considered a *necessary* non-sufficient neural condition, i.e., a neural predisposition of possible consciousness.

More specifically, it remains unclear which neuronal measures make the resting state's activity less sensitive and reactive to possible spatial and temporal changes. For that, I claim, we need to go back to the brain itself and its biophysical-computational equipment that determines the possible range of neural activity in the resting state. This will be the focus of the following sections.

NEURONAL HYPOTHESIS IIA: "BIOPHYSICAL-COMPUTATIONAL SPECTRUM" AND THE THRESHOLD OF THE RESTING-STATE ACTIVITY

Why is the resting state's neural reactivity or propensity to change diminished in VS? For that answer we may need to return briefly to the first volume. As we recall from Part IV in Volume I, the resting-state activity level was proposed to be central in setting the threshold for the induction of any subsequent neural activity during either rest–rest (Chapter 6) or rest–stimulus interaction (Chapter 11).

There we suggested that the resting-state activity provides a "spatiotemporal window of opportunity" for any kind of neural processing including activity changes. By modulating its own level, the resting-state activity can make subsequent changes in its level of neural activity either more or less likely, and thereby, metaphorically speaking, it "opens or closes its own spatiotemporal window (to itself and to the extrinsic stimuli) in different degrees." More technically put, the resting-state activity level itself provides a threshold that determines the degree of its possible change during its subsequent encounter with either extrinsic stimuli or intrinsic changes in the resting-state activity itself.

How, however, is the threshold that the resting-state activity provides generated and modulated by itself? The resting-state activity's threshold was itself supposed to be related to and thus traced back to the brain's biophysical-computational properties: the closer the resting-state activity level operates to its maximal and minimal biophysical-computational limits, the higher the threshold for the induction of activity changes during subsequent rest–rest or rest–stimulus interaction (see Chapter 11).

The "position" of the actual resting-state activity level relative to the spectrum of its underlying biophysical-computational properties defines the level of the threshold (and the degree of openness of its own "spatiotemporal window of opportunity") it applies to and exerts on subsequent activity changes. If the "position" of the resting-state activity level is in the middle of the biophysical-computational spectrum, between its minimal and maximal ends, the resting-state activity's threshold may be set in a way that is ideal to induce a possible high degree of activity changes. In contrast, the threshold may be set much higher for possible activity changes when the resting-state activity operates closer to either the minimal or maximal end of its biophysical-computational spectrum.

I consequently propose that the threshold the resting-state activity itself provides for subsequent activity change is directly dependent upon the actual position of the level of the resting state's operation relative to the brain's biophysical–computational spectrum. The resting state's operation close to both minimal and maximal ends of the brain's biophysical-computational spectrum elevates its threshold for subsequent activity change. This entails an inverted U-curve in the relationship between the resting state's position within its underlying biophysical-computational spectrum on the one hand and its propensity for change on the other (see Fig. 28-3a).

Neuronal Hypothesis
IIB: Metabolism and the Threshold of the Resting-State Activity

How now can we acquire experimental measures direct or indirect of the resting state's actual "position" within its biophysical-computational spectrum? Following Shulman (2012) and his investigations of the brain's baseline metabolism

and energy supply, I propose the degree of resting-state metabolism and consequently its energy supply to be such a measure (see first Introduction and Chapters 15 and 16).

Why is the resting state metabolism such an important measure? The baseline metabolism in the resting state supplies the brain with energy, which is necessary in order for it to change its neural activity. The degree of metabolism and the energy supply of the resting state may thus set the threshold for possible activity changes. If, for instance, metabolism and energy supply are decreased, the resting state's threshold for possible change may rise and consequent make activity change more difficult and thus less likely. Such a rise in the threshold makes neural activity changes sparse in order to avoid wasting the precious, highly reduced energy resources.

This means that the various spatial and temporal measures as discussed so far may be less prone to change, either when induced spontaneously or by stimuli. I consequently propose the degree of changes in the various spatial and temporal measures of the resting-state activity like functional connectivity and high- and low-frequency fluctuations to be directly dependent on the degree of the global metabolism (this is well evidenced by the work from R. G. Shulman, as described in Part II in Volume I).

Neuronal Hypothesis IIC: Vegetative State as "Neuroenergetic Disorder"

How is all this related to the reduced reactivity or propensity of the resting-state activity in VS? The metabolism and energy supply are postulated to set the threshold of the resting-state activity for subsequent activity change. One would consequently expect the decreased propensity of the resting state for activity change in VS to be related to reduced global metabolism and thus decreased energy supply. Interestingly, there is indeed empirical support for that.

Using positron emission tomography (PET), an early study by Rudolf et al. (1999, 2002) demonstrated the global metabolism in 24 unmedicated VS patients to be highly and significantly reduced throughout the whole brain (only sparing the cerebellum). A general overview of all

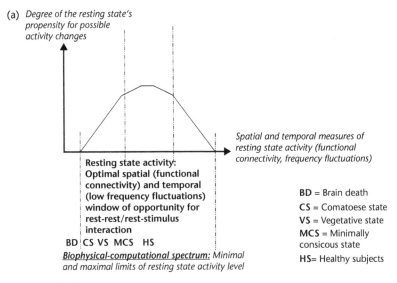

(a) *Degree of the resting state's propensity for possible activity changes*

Spatial and temporal measures of resting state activity (functional connectivity, frequency fluctuations)

Resting state activity:
Optimal spatial (functional
connectivity) and temporal
(low frequency fluctuations)
window of opportunity for
rest-rest/rest-stimulus
interaction

BD ⋮CS VS MCS   HS

Biophysical-computational spectrum: Minimal
and maximal limits of resting state activity level

BD = Brain death
CS = Comatoese state
VS = Vegetative state
MCS = Minimally conscious state
HS= Healthy subjects

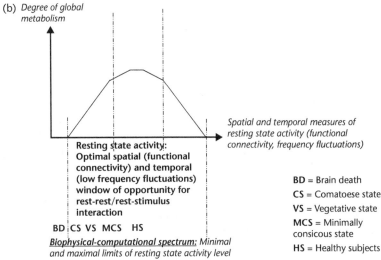

(b) *Degree of global metabolism*

Spatial and temporal measures of resting state activity (functional connectivity, frequency fluctuations)

Resting state activity:
Optimal spatial (functional
connectivity) and temporal
(low frequency fluctuations)
window of opportunity for
rest-rest/rest-stimulus
interaction

BD ⋮CS VS MCS   HS

Biophysical-computational spectrum: Minimal
and maximal limits of resting state activity level

BD = Brain death
CS = Comatoese state
VS = Vegetative state
MCS = Minimally conscious state
HS = Healthy subjects

Figure 28-3a-c Biophysical spectrum hypothesis of consciousness. The figure demonstrates the proposed relationship between the minimal and maximal biophysical-computational limits (downward dotted lines) of the resting state's spatial and temporal measures (on the x-axis) and the resting state's other neuronal, metabolic, and phenomenal variables (on the y-axis) like reactivity or propensity for activity change (*a*), global metabolism (*b*), and consciousness (*c*). I propose the brain's biophysical-computational spectrum (x-axis) to provide the resting state with an optimal spatiotemporal window of opportunity (upward dotted lines) for activity changes during subsequent rest–rest and rest–stimulus interaction. That is closely related to the neural reactivity or propensity for changes in neural activity (*a*), global metabolism (*b*), and consciousness (*c*). The more the resting state operates within the optimal and thus middle range of the brain's biophysical-computational spectrum and thus within its optimal spatiotemporal window of opportunity, the higher the resting state's neural reactivity or propensity for subsequent activity changes (*a*), the higher the degree of global metabolism (*b*), and the higher the degree of consciousness (*c*). Conversely, the more closely the resting state operates to the brain's minimal or maximal biophysical-computational limits, the more likely the degree of the different neuronal, metabolic and phenomenal variables of the resting state will decrease. There is thus an inverted U-shape in the relationship between resting state and the various measures compared to that in the brain's biophysical-computational spectrum. This is where I propose brain death (BD), vegetative state (VS), comatose state (CS), and minimally conscious state (MCS) to be "located," as indicated in the lower part of the figure. HS = healthy subject.

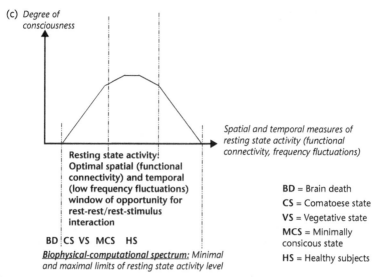

Figure 28-3a-c (Continued)

PET results (see Table 1 in Laureys and Schiff 2012; as well as Heiss 2012, and Hyder et al. 2013) demonstrates highly reduced overall global metabolism with a 25%–60% overall decrease in VS compared to that in healthy subjects.

Let us further describe these results on reduced metabolism and energy supply in VS. The regional metabolic deficits are particularly pronounced in the thalamus and the cortical midline regions (see also Monti et al. 2010; Schiff 2009, 2010; Heiss 2012; and Hyder et al. 2013, for reviews). Improvement from VS to MCS seems to reverse the decrease in metabolism with gradual recovery of the metabolism especially in posterior midline regions like the medial parietal cortex and the PCC (see Laureys and Schiff 2012; Heiss 2012; Hyder et al. 2013).

What does such reduction in the global overall metabolism with a special focus in thalamus and cortical midline regions imply for the neural operation of the resting state in VS? The decrease in global metabolism implies a decrease in global energy supply for the induction of neural activity. The decrease in energy supply makes it less likely that the neurons will undergo active hypopolarization and consequently become excited and change its activity level. Instead, the neurons' activity level may become hyperpolarized with reduced firing

rates, as in the brainstem, the thalamus, and the midbrain including the pons.

If, however, the firing rates of the subcortical regions are reduced, the cortex gets less input and is thus deafferentiated from the subcortical regions. This will ultimately lead to what is described as the "subcortical-cortical disconnection syndrome" (see earlier) with reductions in the firing levels of both subcortical and cortical regions. What do such reductions in firing rates and neural activity levels imply for the neuronal reactivity or propensity for possible activity change? If firing rates and the neural activity level are too low, they may be more resistant to change. Why? Any change in activity costs energy and requires therefore metabolic supply, which is sparse and reduced. To avoid any waste and use of the reduced energy supply, the neurons may be kept in a hyperpolarized state with low neural activity levels.

Such lower firing rates of the neurons with their subsequent hyperpolarization make it more difficult to elicit any changes in the neurons' activity levels; this signifies an elevated threshold for possible activity change. The reduced resting-state activity and its reduced propensity for activity change in VS may therefore ultimately be the result of reduced metabolic supply. VS may consequently be considered a neuroenergetic or neurometabolic disorder, rather than a purely neuronal disorder.

Neuronal Hypothesis IID: "Biophysical-Computational Spectrum" and the Level or State of Consciousness

The reduced energy supply has two major consequences: (i) it leads to a reduction of activity levels in the resting state itself; and by that means, (ii) it elevates the resting state's threshold for any subsequent activity change.

This leads me to postulate the following neurometabolic hypothesis: the lower the degree of global metabolism, the less energy the resting-state activity receives, the lower its activity level, and the higher its threshold for subsequent activity changes. I thus propose that the resting-state activity's level and propensity for change during either rest–rest or rest–stimulus interaction is directly dependent upon the degree of global metabolism and energy supply (see Fig. 28-3b).

How does all that relate to the data in VS described above? I showed that VS can be characterized by reduced global metabolism and energy supply. If my hypothesis is correct, reduced metabolism and energy supply should lead to a reduced activity level in the resting state itself, for instance, in its functional connectivity and the low-frequency fluctuations. This, as reported above, is exactly what has been observed in the recent data. In addition, one would expect reduced neural reactivity or propensity of the resting state for subsequent activity changes during either the resting state itself or stimulus-induced activity. This, again, is exactly what the data show, as described earlier.

Why, however, does the reduced metabolic and energy supply of the resting state in VS elevate the thresholds for subsequent activity change? I proposed the position of the resting-state activity's operation relative to the brain's biophysical-computational spectrum to be central in determining the level of the resting state's threshold for activity change.

What does this imply for VS in particular? I suggest the following hypothesis: I propose that, due to the decreased metabolic and energetic supply, the resting state operates close to the minimal end of the brain's biophysical-computational spectrum. And, as suggested earlier, this leads to abnormal elevation of the resting-state activity's threshold for subsequent activity changes, which is manifested on the neural level as reduced reactivity or propensity for activity changes. I consequently postulate the resting state's reduced reactivity or propensity for activity changes in VS to be directly dependent upon the degree to which the resting state operates close to the minimal end of the brain's biophysical-computational spectrum. The same, I propose, holds in the other disorders of consciousness like anesthesia and non-REM sleep (see Chapters 15 and 16 for more extensive discussion).

What does this imply for consciousness in general? The possible level or state of consciousness may be directly dependent upon the resting-state activity's threshold, which predisposes the possible degree of change in the resting state's activity level. As mentioned before, the resting-state activity's threshold is by itself determined by its own position relative to the brain's biophysical-computational spectrum (see earlier). The possible level or state of consciousness is consequently determined indirectly by the actual resting state's position relative to its underlying biophysical-computational spectrum.

This leads me to suggest the following hypothesis about the level or state of consciousness. I postulate that the highest level or state of consciousness is possible when the resting-state activity operates in the middle of rather than toward the minimal and maximal ends of the brain's underlying biophysical-computational spectrum. This leads me to what I describe as the "biophysical spectrum hypothesis of consciousness."

Neuronal Hypothesis IIE: "Biophysical Spectrum Hypothesis of Consciousness"

What do I mean by the "biophysical spectrum hypothesis of consciousness"? It proposes the actual position of the resting state's level relative to the brain's underlying biophysical-computational spectrum to be directly related to the possible degree of consciousness.

The more and closer the resting state operates toward its minimal or maximal biophysical-computational limits, the higher the resting state's threshold for subsequent activity change is set. And the higher the threshold, the more reduced the resting state's propensity for subsequent activity changes, resulting in decreased rest–rest and rest–stimulus interaction. This in turn makes the association of consciousness with the respective neural activities less likely (see Fig. 28-3c).

Accordingly, the "biophysical spectrum hypothesis of consciousness" proposes that the resting-state activity's position within and thus relative to the brain's biophysical spectrum determines its propensity and thus reactivity for possible change in its level of neural activity. Since the degree of activity change is central in determining the level or state of consciousness (see Chapter 29 for details), the resting-state activity's position relative to the brain's biophysical-computational spectrum is directly relevant for consciousness.

Metaphorically speaking, the "biophysical position" of the resting-state activity's operation may signify the possible range of "neural opportunities" the resting-state activity itself can provide for subsequent neural activity changes during either rest–rest or rest–stimulus interaction. A "position" in the middle of its biophysical-computational spectrum may provide the resting state with a greater range of neural opportunities for subsequent neural activity changes than a "position" closer to the biophysical-computational spectrum's minimal or maximal ends.

Since these "neural opportunities" can be traced back to the resting-state activity's spatial and temporal features, that is, its frequency oscillations and functional connectivity, I here speak of a "spatiotemporal window of opportunity" (see also Chapters 11 and 12 for details). I propose the resting-state activity's "spatiotemporal window of opportunity" for possible neural activity changes to be the largest in the middle of its biophysical spectrum. In contrast, the resting-state activity's "spatiotemporal window of opportunity" becomes smaller when the resting-state activity's operation tilts toward either the minimal or maximal end of its biophysical-computational spectrum.

How now does the resting-state activity's "spatiotemporal window of opportunity" relate to VS and thus to consciousness? The healthy subjects' resting-state activity operates in the medium or middle range of its biophysical-computational spectrum, thereby providing the largest "spatiotemporal window of opportunity."

In contrast, the resting-state activity's operation in VS may be shifted more toward the minimal end of its biophysical-computational spectrum with the MCS patients being halfway between healthy and vegetative subjects. The resting-state activity's "spatiotemporal window of opportunity" is consequently smaller in MCS compared to that in healthy subjects, while it is still larger than the one in VS. Finally, the resting-state activity's biophysical-computational minimal limits seem to be almost reached in coma and ultimately to be touched in brain death, where the "spatiotemporal window of opportunity" is closed completely.

NEUROMETAPHORICAL EXCURSION
I: WINDOWS AND LIGHT

I propose that the extent or degree of the resting-state activity's spatiotemporal window of opportunity is closely related to the level of consciousness. How can we illustrate that in a more comprehensive way? For that, I will make some metaphorical comparisons to an analogous imaginary scenario of a house owner: If the resting state's spatiotemporal window of opportunity is completely closed, one is brain-dead.

That compares metaphorically to an imaginary situation where the owner of an apartment literally closes the window and turns off all lights because of an energy shortage; the apartment is consequently completely dark. Analogously, the brain itself, and more specifically its resting state, closes its window to any possible activity change because of its lacking energy supply. This results in brain death.

Now let us imagine a slightly different scenario. If the resting-state activity's spatiotemporal window is open slightly, some dim light comes in, meaning some minimal activity change in the resting state is still possible. One is then in a coma. Now the resting state's spatiotemporal window is opened a little further, meaning that more light comes in, with a larger degree of activity changes in the resting state being possible.. One reverts to VS.

Imagine opening the window further. Now the spatiotemporal window of the resting state is almost half opened, so that more light and an even larger degree of activity changes come into the room of the brain. One is on the way toward the healthy state of consciousness by stopping in between, at what is described as MCS.

This, however, is only half of the story—the path from the minimal end of the brain's biophysical-computational spectrum toward its middle can be described as the path from brain death via coma, VS, and MCS to the healthy state. How about the other half of the path, from the middle to its maximal end?

Here we can only speculate. Approaching the maximal end of the biophysical-computational spectrum implies that the resting state's spatiotemporal window of opportunity is opened almost completely. Metaphorically, one is then "blinded" by the light coming through the widely opened window while at the same time showing "too much" of consciousness, that is, *hyperconsciousness* as one may want to say.

How would such hyperconscious be manifested neuronally? One would expect abnormally increased activity changes in the resting state itself, e.g., during rest–rest interaction. This should be manifested in increased functional and effective connectivity and high-frequency fluctuations in the resting state. That may, for instance, be the case in schizophrenia, which can indeed be characterized by the here sketched neuronal and phenomenal changes (see Chapters 22 and 27 for details). However, my assumption that the resting state in schizophrenia operates at the maximal end of the brain's biophysical-computational spectrum must be considered rather tentative and speculative at this point in time.

NEURONAL HYPOTHESIS IIIA: CONTINUUM BETWEEN DIFFERENCE- AND STIMULUS-BASED CODING

I proposed a central role for global metabolism and energy supply in setting the resting state's threshold for activity changes as elicited either during the resting state itself or by stimuli. The energy supply that comes with the metabolism must therefore enable the resting-state activity to perform certain neural operations which otherwise, i.e., without energy supply, it would remain unable to do. What though does the energy supply enable the resting-state activity to do that it cannot do otherwise? And how is that related to consciousness?

Recall from Volume I (see Part II) that we characterized the resting-state activity as encoding its neural activity in terms of spatial and temporal differences (see Chapters 4–6). More specifically, the temporal and spatial differences between the same or different (neuronal) stimuli across their respective different discrete points in physical time and space are encoded into the resting-state activity. And what applies to the extrinsic stimuli holds also for the encoding of the different regions activities within the brain itself: they are also encoded into neural activity on the basis of their temporal and spatial differences across their different discrete points in physical time and space.

Such encoding of neural activity in terms of temporal and spatial differences was described as difference-based coding. Difference-based coding must be distinguished from stimulus-based coding. Here the stimuli or the regions' neural activities themselves and their respective discrete points in physical time and space are encoded into the neural activity of the resting state.

Why is that important? I proposed the brain to operate on the basis of difference-based coding rather than stimulus-based coding, though there is a continuum between both forms of coding. Usually, in the healthy brain, the degree of difference-based coding is high, whereas the degree of stimulus-based coding is rather low. In other words, difference-based coding predominates over stimulus-based coding (see Chapter 11).

NEURONAL HYPOTHESIS IIIB: DIFFERENCE-BASED CODING REQUIRES HIGH DEGREES OF METABOLISM AND ENERGY

How, then, is difference-based coding related to the global metabolism and its energy supply?

Very simple: encoding of temporal and spatial differences during either rest–rest or rest–stimulus interaction requires energy. Hence, if there is sufficient energy as in the healthy brain, one would expect a high degree of difference-based coding, while the degree of stimulus-based coding will remain rather low.

How is such predominance of difference-based coding manifest in neural activity? Due to the encoding of spatial and temporal differences, one would expect the stimulus-induced activity to extend beyond its actual discrete point in physical time and space. In other words, the neural activity may spatially and temporally spread and propagate to more distant discrete points in physical time and space and thus to other regions and networks in the brain. This is exactly what the earlier described TMS-EEG study by Rosanova et al. (2012) shows in healthy awake subjects and MCS patients (see earlier) as well as in REM sleep (see Chapters 15 and 16).

The situation changes, however, once the energy supply is reduced. Reduction in energy may decrease the ability to encode neural activity in terms of spatial and temporal differences, thus decreasing the degree of difference-based coding, while at the same time the degree of stimulus-based coding will increase.

I thus propose decreased degrees of difference-based coding and increased degrees of stimulus-based coding in VS. The degree of difference-based coding may thus be directly related to the degree (or level or state) of consciousness, as I will explicate in the following section.

Neuronal Hypothesis IIIC: Reduced Energy Leads to Decreased Difference-Based Coding in Vegetative State

How is such increased degree of stimulus-based coding as suggested in VS manifest in neural activity? One would expect neural activity to stay spatially more local and temporally shorter and more transient as related to the stimulus' discrete position in time and space. This is exactly what the previously described TMS-EEG study by Rosanova et al. (2012) demonstrates in VS patients, which, in the same way, is also present in anesthesia and non-REM sleep (see Chapters 15 and 16).

Furthermore, a recent EEG study in 6 VS and 11 MCS patients by Cavinato et al. (2011) shows that many VS and all MCS patients can elicit the P300 when listening to their own names. However, the duration of the P300 was the shortest in VS, longer in MCS, and the longest in healthy subjects. Moreover, healthy and MCS subjects were able to modulate the latency and thus the duration of their P300, which lasted longer with increasing stimulus complexity (by presenting their own name versus a sine-wave tone and a familiar name). This was not the case, however, in VS patients, who remained unable to modulate the duration of their P300 in response to increasing stimulus complexity.

The presence of the P300 in VS was also confirmed in an earlier study by Perrin et al. (2006), who let subjects listen to their own names while being recording on the EEG. They also observed the P300 to be present in MCS and VS patients. The only difference from healthy subjects was that the latency and thus the onset of the P300 was delayed.

Why are the VS patients able to elicit a P300 while they remain unable to modulate it or to properly time it in its onset? I propose that the induction of P300 is related to the encoding of the stimulus itself and its discrete point in physical time and space into neural activity. There is thus stimulus-based coding that is proposed to account for the induction of the P300.

However, the P300 is shorter in its duration (and delayed in its onset) because the neural activity is no longer based on the encoding of temporal differences between different stimuli and their respective different discrete points in time. Instead, it is rather based on the encoding of the single stimuli's discrete points in time and space, which obviously entails shorter duration in the resulting neural activity, the P300.

If now, due to increasing stimulus complexity, larger temporal differences may need to be encoded into neural activity, the VS patients remain unable to do. Why? Their encoding is based on stimulus- rather than difference-based coding, which makes it impossible for them to encode any temporal differences between different stimuli and their respective discrete points in time. This means that the duration of the encoded neural activity, like in the P300, cannot be modulated anymore by more complex stimuli which would requires to encode more complex temporal differences; the inability to encode more complex temporal differences may neuronally be manifested in the reported lack of modulation in the P300's duration during increase in stimulus complexity.

One may now want to argue that such an increased degree of stimulus-based coding is not at all related to consciousness but that it is cognitively (i.e., attentionally) but not phenomenally relevant. But this is not in line with the findings.

However, the findings show that, unlike VS, MCS patients show a longer duration in the P300, and they are also able to increase the duration of their P300 during increase in stimulus complexity. And despite being much better than the VS patients, the MCS patients nevertheless were not completely identical to the healthy subjects. This strongly suggests gradation in the duration and modulation of the P300 in orientation to the different levels of consciousness (and subsequently recruitment of attentional resources) associated with VS, MCS, and healthy state.

Neuronal Hypothesis IIID: Reduced Difference-Based Coding is Coupled to Decreased Functional Connectivity

What are the exact neuronal mechanisms underlying such a decrease in the degree of difference-based coding? The earlier-proposed hyperpolarization of the neurons with the reductions in both firing rates and global neural activity decreases their propensity or reactivity to the encoding of temporal and spatial differences. Let us sketch the scenario briefly starting from the above described lack of energy supply. The energy and thus the metabolic supply may still be sufficient to encode the stimulus itself and its discrete point in time and space. In contrast, the amount of available energy may no longer be sufficient to encode the extrinsic stimulus' spatial and temporal difference from the next stimulus into the brain's neural activity.

How is this lack of energy supply manifested in the encoding of neural activity in

terms of difference-based coding? I propose that, due to the lack of available energy, the resting-state activity's neuronal spatial and temporal measures, like functional connectivity and low-frequency fluctuations, are no longer able to properly encode spatial and temporal differences into their neural activity.

This needs to be detailed. Let us start with the functional connectivity and see how its changes affect the encoding of neural activity; namely, difference-based coding. The observed decrease in functional connectivity on the cortical and subcortical level in VS may make it more difficult for these patients' brains to encode spatial and temporal differences into neural activity. The more the functional connectivity between different regions is reduced, the less globalized and the more localized the neural activity in VS (and all other states showing reduction of consciousness).

Such increased localization of neural activity may make it more difficult, if not impossible, to encode especially larger spatial (and temporal) differences between different stimuli and their respective regions into neural activity (see Chapter 16 for details). The degree of difference-based coding in spatial terms may thus be reduced along with an increase in the degree of stimulus-based coding.

Neuronal Hypothesis IIIE: Abnormal Phases in Low and High-Frequency Fluctuations are Coupled to Reduced Difference-Based Coding

The same principle applies on the temporal side, where the changes in the resting-state activity's low-frequency fluctuations may also impact the encoding of neural activity and thus difference-based coding. The reduced degrees in the power of the high- and low-frequency fluctuations in the resting-state activity in VS may decrease the sensitivity of the time spans; for example, the phase durations, to link and integrate and thus to encode different stimuli at different discrete points in physical time within one phase duration (see Chapters 14 and 15 for details).

If however, due to the reduced power in VS, the stimuli can no longer be linked and integrated within one phase duration, they will instead be encoded separately within the same phase duration and thus in a stimulus- rather than difference-based way. This means that the different stimuli will be encoded in a parallel and segregated way even within the same phase duration rather than being linked and integrated. That obviously decreases the degree of difference-based coding, while increasing the degree of stimulus-based coding.

We should be careful with the latter point, however, since all investigations in VS have focused so far only on power change. To further support my hypothesis of reduced degrees of difference-based coding in VS, one would need to investigate the phases of the resting-state activity's low-frequency fluctuations, including cross-frequency phase-phase and phase-power coupling. One would propose the reduced degrees of difference-based coding in VS to be dependent upon the potentially lower degree of phase shifting and cross-frequency phase-phase and phase-power coupling in the resting-state activity.

What leads me to make this proposal? The latter neuronal mechanisms that is, the phase coupling of the resting-state activity's low and high-frequency fluctuations allow the brain to constitute a higher degree of temporal continuity in the resting state's neural activity. This, as discussed in Chapters 13 through 15, is essential for the subsequent encoding of a high degree of spatial and temporal differences into neural activity, which in turn predisposes the possible degree of the level of consciousness. This leads me to propose what I describe as the "difference-based coding hypothesis of consciousness" in the next section.

NEUROPHENOMENAL HYPOTHESIS IA: "DIFFERENCE-BASED CODING HYPOTHESIS OF CONSCIOUSNESS" (DHC)

I have described the resting-state activity itself and characterized it by the threshold it sets for its own subsequent activity changes and the "position" of its operation relative to the brain's biophysical-computational spectrum. Moreover, I proposed metabolic and energetic

supply to be central in the neural operation of the resting-state activity and more specifically in determining its degree of difference-based coding relative to stimulus-based coding.

However, none of these features necessarily implies consciousness so far. Neither of the discussed neuronal mechanisms make necessary and unavoidable the association of the purely neural activity with the phenomenal features of consciousness. Hence, I so far discussed only neuronal hypotheses, while I left out neurophenomenal hypotheses. The latter shall be the focus in this and the following sections.

Based on earlier described neuronal hypotheses, I suggest what I describe as the "difference-based coding hypothesis of consciousness" (or DHC; see also the first Introduction for discussion of the DHC as one subset of the more general "coding hypothesis of consciousness" [CHC]). The DHC proposes the possible degree or level of consciousness to be directly dependent upon the degree of difference-based coding during rest–rest and rest–stimulus interaction. The higher the degree of difference-based coding and consequently the lower the degree of stimulus-based coding during rest–rest and rest–stimulus interaction, the higher the possible degree or level of consciousness the respective neural activity change can be associated with.

How can we explain the "difference-based coding hypothesis of consciousness" in further detail? I propose the level or state of consciousness to be directly dependent upon the degree of difference-based coding during either resting-state or stimulus-induced activity. Larger degrees of difference-based coding make possible the encoding of larger spatial and temporal differences (between different discrete points in physical time and space) into neural activity. And the larger the encoded spatial and temporal differences, the higher the level or state of consciousness that can possibly be associated with the newly resulting neural activity (see Fig. 28-4a).

I consequently postulate that the level or state of consciousness is directly dependent upon the degree of spatial and temporal differences that are encoded into neural activity. Since the extrinsic stimuli are more likely to elicit higher

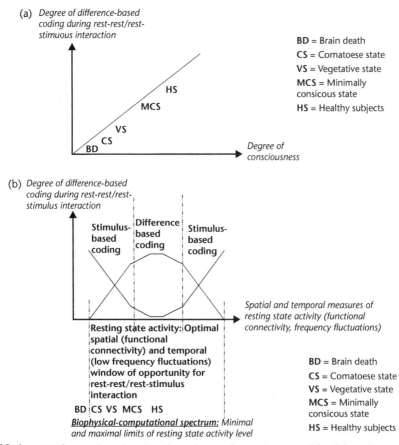

Figure 28-4a-c Difference-based coding hypothesis of consciousness. The figure demonstrates distinct aspects of the "difference-based coding hypothesis of consciousness" concerning its relationship to difference-based coding (*a*), the biophysical-computational spectrum (*b*), and qualia (*c*). (*a*) The figure shows the relationship between the degree of difference-based coding and the degree of consciousness. The higher the degree of difference-based coding during rest–rest or rest–stimulus interaction, the higher the degree of consciousness. I thus propose low degrees of difference-based coding to hold in vegetative state. (*b*) The figure demonstrates how the relationship between difference-based coding and consciousness is related to the brain's biophysical-computational spectrum: The more the resting state's neural activity operates within the optimal spatiotemporal window of the brain's biophysical-computational spectrum, the higher the possible degree of consciousness. If, in contrast, the resting-state activity operates close to both the minimal or maximal limits of the brain's biophysical-computational spectrum, the more the degree of difference-based coding will decrease; this in turn is supposed to reduce the level or state of consciousness that can be associated with the newly resulting neural activity level. This implies an inverted U-shape curve, as is visible in the figure. (*c*) The figure shows how the statistically based encoding of the temporal and spatial differences between the different stimuli's discrete points in time and space leads to the spatiotemporally based qualia. *Lowest level:* Stimuli occurring at different discrete points in time and space. *Middle level:* Encoding of the temporal and spatial differences between the different stimuli into neural activity as distinguished from the encoding of the stimuli and their respective discrete points in physical time and space by themselves. *Upper level:* Spatiotemporal extension of qualia across different discrete points in time and space in orientation on the difference-based encoding of the spatial and temporal differences between the stimuli's different discrete points in physical time and space. Each triangle indicates one specific quale with the dotted lines indicating its statistically and spatiotemporally based "virtual" nature. *Abbreviations:* BD, brain death; CS, comatose state; HS, healthy subject; MCS, minimally conscious state; VS, vegetative state.

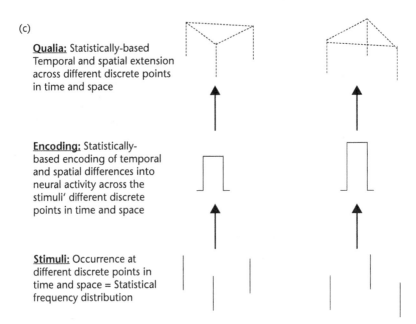

(c)

Qualia: Statistically-based Temporal and spatial extension across different discrete points in time and space

Encoding: Statistically-based encoding of temporal and spatial differences into neural activity across the stimuli' different discrete points in time and space

Stimuli: Occurrence at different discrete points in time and space = Statistical frequency distribution

Figure 28-4a-c (Continued)

degrees of spatial and temporal differences during rest–stimulus interaction compared to that during mere rest–rest interaction, the likelihood of a higher level or state of consciousness is much higher during stimulus-induced activity compared to that in the resting-state activity itself.

Neurophenomenal Hypothesis IB: "Difference-Based Coding Hypothesis of Consciousness" and the "Biophysical Spectrum Hypothesis of Consciousness"

How is the "difference-based coding hypothesis of consciousness" related to the "biophysical spectrum hypothesis of consciousness"? I proposed the degree of global metabolism and thus the energy supply to be central in determining the resting state's "position" relative to the brain's biophysical-computational spectrum (see earlier). The more metabolism, the more likely the resting state's operation may be "located" in the middle of the biophysical-computational spectrum.

At the same time, the metabolism and the energy supply were supposed to be relevant in predisposing the degree of possible

difference-based coding; higher degrees of energy supply are supposed to accompany higher degrees of difference-based coding and the consequent encoding of larger spatial and temporal differences into neural activity. And, as already said before, the larger the encoded differences, the higher the level of consciousness that can possibly be assigned to the newly resulting neural activity.

Taken together, the degree of metabolism and energetic supply determines both the "position" of the resting state's operation relative to the brain's biophysical-computational spectrum and its degree of difference-based coding. Now let us put both together.

The higher the global metabolism and energy supply, the more likely it is that the resting-state activity will operate in the middle of the brain's biophysical-computational spectrum, and the higher the degree of difference-based coding. And since higher degrees of difference-based coding make more likely the encoding of larger spatial and temporal differences into neural activity and ultimately higher levels of consciousness, one can draw a line directly from the brain's biophysical-computational spectrum over the resting-state activity's possible degree of difference-based coding to the level or state of consciousness.

How about VS? The data clearly show reduced global metabolism and energy supply in VS, as described earlier. That shifts the resting-state activity's operation toward the minimal end of the brain's biophysical-computational spectrum. This in turn decreases the degree of difference-based coding, while increasing the degree of stimulus-based coding. If, however, the degree of difference-based coding is decreased, the likelihood of encoding larger spatial and temporal differences into neural activity during either rest–rest or rest–stimulus interaction is reduced, too. The encoding of reduced spatial and temporal differences into neural activity, however, decreases the probability of associating a higher level or state of consciousness with the newly resulting activity level during either stimulus-induced or resting-state activity.

Accordingly, I propose that increased degrees of stimulus-based coding lead to decreased degrees in the level or state of consciousness, as I suggested to be the case in VS (and other disorders of consciousness) as detailed earlier. This is well in accordance with the empirical findings of decreased spatial and temporal spread and propagation of neural activity in VS and other disorders of consciousness (see Fig. 28-4b).

NEUROPHENOMENAL HYPOTHESIS IIA: *DEGREE OF ENCODED DIFFERENCES* AS THE NEURAL *CORRELATE* OF THE *LEVEL* OF CONSCIOUSNESS

One may now want to raise two objections. First, we did not really tackle the *sufficient* neural conditions of consciousness and thus the NCC. Instead, we remained within the realm of the necessary neural conditions and thus neural predispositions of consciousness (NPC) when focusing on the resting-state activity itself. And secondly, we did not really address the question of qualia as the phenomenal hallmarks of consciousness, but discussed only consciousness in general.

Let me start with the first issue, that of NCC versus NPC. Yes, we indeed focused again on the resting-state activity itself and therefore seemingly on the NPC rather than the NCC. That is what is similar to the preceding parts. There,

however, we did not draw a direct relationship between the resting-state activity itself and the degree or level of actual consciousness. We only considered the resting-state activity itself as necessary and predisposing for possible consciousness, while assuming that something else must happen in addition in order for consciousness to be actually realized and become manifest. Hence, we did not propose a direct one-to-one relationship between the neuronal measures of the resting state and the degree or level of consciousness in Parts V–VII.

This is different in the present Part. Here we did indeed draw a direct relationship between specific neuronal measures of the resting state itself and the degree or level of (actual) consciousness. More specifically, I proposed the resting state's neural reactivity or propensity for activity change to be directly related to the degree of consciousness. The higher the resting state's neural reactivity or propensity for activity change, the higher the degree or level of actual consciousness can be generated. How is this effect of the resting state activity on the level of consciousness mediated? I suggest that the resting state's neuronal reactivity or propensity for activity change is directly related to difference-based coding during rest–rest and/or rest–stimulus interaction which in turn is supposed to predict the level of consciousness.

What does this imply for our search for the NCC? One may consider the degree of spatial and temporal differences that are (or can be) encoded into neural activity via difference-based coding a sufficient neural condition of consciousness. If sufficiently large spatial and temporal differences are encoded during rest–rest or rest–stimulus interaction, the newly resulting neural activity level is associated with a high level or state of consciousness.

For that, I claim, no additional factor besides the encoding of sufficiently large spatial and temporal differences is needed. In other words, I propose the resting-state activity's degree of difference-based coding and the subsequent encoding of sufficiently large spatial and temporal differences into neural activity during rest–rest or rest–stimulus interaction to be a sufficient neural condition of the level or state of consciousness and thus a level-based NCC.

NEUROPHENOMENAL HYPOTHESIS IIB: DIFFERENCE-BASED CODING AS THE STATISTICALLY-BASED ENCODING OF SPATIAL AND TEMPORAL DIFFERENCES

How are the spatial and temporal differences, as encoded into neural activity via difference-based coding, related to qualia? Qualia are considered the phenomenal hallmarks of consciousness. Both terms, *consciousness* and *qualia*, are often even used interchangeably (see Chapter 30 for details). As indicated, qualia describe the subjective and qualitative aspects of our experience as they are manifested in, for instance the experience of redness of the color red.

Based on the earlier considerations, I now propose qualia to be directly dependent upon the degree of the spatial and temporal differences as they are (or can be) encoded into neural activity via difference-based coding. The larger the spatial and temporal differences that are encoded into neural activity via difference-based coding, the larger the degree of qualia and thus the more subjective and qualitative aspects are associated with the newly resulting neural activity level during either the resting state or stimulus-induced activity (see Fig. 28-4c).

How can we specify this hypothesis of the relationship between difference-based coding and qualia? Difference-based coding makes possible the encoding of temporal and spatial differences into neural activity. What do the spatial and temporal differences themselves signify? As we recall, especially from Volume I, the spatial and temporal differences signify the statistical frequency distributions of the respective stimuli or neural activities across different discrete points in physical time and space; that is, their "natural statistics" (and social, vegetative, and neuronal statistics; see Chapters 1, 8, and 9 in Volume I).

NEUROPHENOMENAL HYPOTHESIS IIC: STATISTICAL AND SPATIOTEMPORAL CHARACTERIZATION OF QUALIA

What does my hypothesis imply for the characterization of qualia? I proposed the degree of qualia to be directly dependent upon the degree of spatial and temporal differences that are encoded into neural activity. If the degrees of spatial and temporal differences are themselves dependent upon the statistical frequency distributions of either the stimuli or the resting-state activity that are their natural and neuronal statistics, one would characterize qualia as both spatiotemporally and statistically based.

Qualia as spatiotemporally and statistically based are then ultimately based and predisposed by the brain's particular encoding strategy, difference-based coding as statistically based encoding strategy (see Volume I for details). This means that if the brain were encoding its neural activity in a different way as for instance in a physically based way as in stimulus-based coding, qualia would no longer be spatiotemporally and statistically based. And, to put it even more strongly, qualia would then no longer be possible at all (at least in our actual natural world with is particular brain and its specific encoding strategy). This means that consciousness in general and qualia in particular are dependent on and thus predisposed by the brain's particular encoding strategy.

That reflects what I described as the "encoding hypothesis of consciousness" (EHC) as the second subset of the "coding hypothesis of consciousness" (CHC) besides the "difference-based coding hypothesis of consciousness" (DHC; see earlier and first Introduction). These, however, are more conceptual and philosophical issues that we will come back to at the end of Chapter 30. Before that, though, we need to know more about the sufficient neural conditions of consciousness, the neural correlates of consciousness. We will therefore shift our focus from the resting-state activity itself to stimulus-induced activity, more specifically to rest–stimulus interaction. This is the focus in Chapter 29.

NEUROMETAPHORICAL EXCURSION IIA: PARTY OF THE RESTING STATE

How do we imagine the resting state in VS? Let us invoke yet another fictive scenario'. You are at a party in New York in a friend's private one-bedroom apartment. The party is hosted to celebrate the last hours of the apartment before the building will be demolished to make space for a new glass tower by Donald Trump.

Let's jump into the midst of the party. Some of the people stand around a little table in one corner. Others are assembled close to the wall on the left, where a nice painting is hanging. Another group of people can be found on and beside the sofa in one of the corners. The majority of peoples sit on chairs around the big round table in the middle of the room.

And, as usual at parties, there is plenty of exchange not only among the people within each group, that is, local interactions, but also between the different groups, with people walking across the room between the different groups; that is, global interactions. That can be easily compared to the brain and its resting state. The brain is the apartment, while the party corresponds to the resting-state activity. The different groups of people can be compared to the different regions in the brain, which interact locally within each region or group as well as globally between the different groups of people; that is, the different regions. There is thus rest–rest interaction in the apartment of the brain.

How about the furniture, the painting, the little table, the sofa, and the big round table in the middle? The furniture structures the apartment and the room and it is a part of its inventory.

Analogously, I propose the resting-state activity's spatiotemporal structure to structure and organize the room of the brain. And in the same way there are different kinds of furniture, there are different spatiotemporal structures (via functional connectivity and frequency oscillations) in the room of the brain, that is, spatiotemporal continuity, the different forms of unity, and self-specific and preintentional organization (see Parts V–VIII).

Extending our fictive comparison, one may now be inclined to propose that the brain and its resting state are partying. The resting state is a continuously ongoing party. This is manifest neuronally in rest–rest interaction and its functional connectivity, high- and low-frequency fluctuations, and its reactivity and variability across time and space.

Phenomenally, the resting state's ongoing party is manifested in your thoughts' wandering back and forth between the party's guests and your own very private concerns reflecting your distraction and thus what is described as "mind wandering" (see Part VIII). And even when you go home and sleep, you may still dream about the party, so that even during sleep, your resting state seems to prefer to party rather than to rest.

NEUROMETAPHORICAL EXCURSION
IIB: END OF THE RESTING STATE'S PARTY

However, your brain's resting state party is over when you are in a vegetative state. The guests are gone and the apartment's room is empty. Literally empty. Not only devoid of people and thus of local and global interactions across time and space within the brain. Everything is silent, including the resting state's prephenomenal spatiotemporal structures, which are "frozen" due to lack of energy supply in very much the same way the light bulbs do not provide light because of a lack of power supply. The fewer people and the less furniture, the emptier the room, and the more closely the room operates at its minimal limits of functioning as a room.

The same is true in the case of the brain. The less rest–rest interaction and the less spatiotemporal structure, the emptier and more silent the resting state, and the more closely the brain's resting state operates close to its own minimal biophysical-computational limits. And the closer the room of the brain comes to its minimal biophysical-computational limits, the less likely it is that it can "host a party" and thus changes in its neural activity such as in its functional connectivity and low- and high-frequency fluctuations.

Put slightly differently, the brain's resting state is then less likely able to host its party for the various guests; that is, the stimuli coming from either the brain itself (the neuronal stimuli), the body (interoceptive stimuli), or the environment (exteroceptive stimuli) which can no longer induce changes in the resting state's activity during rest–rest and rest–stimulus interaction.

How do we have to imagine the resting state in the vegetative state? You remember: This was the last party before the apartment was to be demolished. The party was almost over with only a few people left. That is when you were probably still minimally conscious. Now the few people left started taking out the furniture, piece by piece. That is when you slipped into a vegetative state. Finally, the light was turned off in the room. No electricity at all anymore. No power supply at all. The same is true in the case of the brain. The brain's global metabolism and thus its energy supply thin out almost completely. It becomes dark in the brain. You slip gradually into a coma.

Let us extend our fictive scenario to its most extreme limits. The apartment is now completely dark. All windows are closed. No light at all. No power supply, no energy anymore. Nothing moves about anymore. You cannot see anything and cannot hold on to anything in the room. You leave. Nothing but darkness and silence. The apartment is ready for demolishing. Just like the brain. The stimuli cannot attach themselves to anything in the brain's resting state because the latter lacks any kind of spatiotemporal structure.

Metaphorically speaking, the stimuli thus "fell through" the brain: they did not induce anything anymore. Nothing is happening during either the resting state itself or during its exposure to stimuli. No guests are admitted to the room of the brain, which is completely empty and thus devoid of anything. There is nothing but silence, darkness, and emptiness in the room of the brain. Your brain is dead.

Open Questions

The first question concerns the exact details of the range of the biophysical-computational spectrum. While there are some data about the resting-state activity in VS, no data are currently available about the absolute values of the minimal and maximal ends of the brain's possible biophysical-computational spectrum. To lend further empirical support to my biophysical spectrum hypothesis, one would need to determine the various neuronal measures of the resting state (like functional connectivity and low-frequency fluctuations) relative to the absolute minima and maxima of the brain's biophysical-computational spectrum.

One may then determine an index that could be described as the "resting state's actual biophysical-computational spectrum." I hypothesize that this index will predict the degree of the level or state of consciousness and thus qualia that can possibly be associated with any neural activity change during either rest–rest or rest–stimulus interaction.

The second question concerns both neuronal and phenomenal features. We have to specify the neuronal mechanisms that enable the instantiation of consciousness. More specifically, we need to investigate in much more detail how the resting state interacts with stimuli so that the latter can be associated with consciousness. This will be the focus of Chapter 29. However, neuronal specification on the side of rest–stimulus interaction needs to go along with a more detailed and specific account of the phenomenal features on the side of consciousness: so far, I spoke of qualia in general without specifying their different phenomenal features. This will be the focus in Chapter 30.

CHAPTER 29
Rest–Stimulus Interaction and Qualia

Summary

After having discussed the direct relationship of the resting-state activity to consciousness, I now turn to stimulus-induced activity. More specifically, I aim to investigate how the purely neuronal stimulus-induced activity can become associated with consciousness and its phenomenal features. For that, I again rely on the loss of consciousness in the vegetative state (VS) as a paradigmatic example. Recent studies during cognitive stimulation show neural activity changes in VS regions, for instance, during visual and motor imagery tasks. Moreover, imaging studies using self-specific stimuli like one's own name or self-referential tasks show neural activity changes, including proper neuronal differentiation in predominantly the cortical midline regions in VS. Most interestingly, the degree of neural activity changes elicited by self-specific stimuli is directly related to the degree of consciousness. How is it possible for the VS patients to elicit almost proper stimulus-induced activity without associating the stimulus with subjective experience and phenomenal features; that is, consciousness? I propose that such neuronal-phenomenal dissociation between stimulus-induced activity and consciousness can ultimately be traced back to the purely neuronal dissociation between resting-state activity and stimulus-induced activity. In order to understand the loss of the phenomenal state, i.e., consciousness, in VS, we therefore need to go back to the neuronal mechanisms underlying the stimuli's interaction with the resting-state activity; that is, rest–stimulus interaction. As demonstrated in Volume I (see Chapters 2, 11, and 12), rest–stimulus interaction can be characterized as nonlinear and nonadditive, implying interactive and integrative processing between resting-state activity and stimulus. I now propose the degree of nonlinearity during rest–stimulus interaction to be directly related to the degree of consciousness. This is what I describe as the "nonlinearity hypothesis of consciousness." How is such nonlinearity mediated on the neuronal level? GABA-ergic-mediated neural inhibition seems to be central here. Interestingly, findings in VS indicate global decrease in GABA-A receptors, suggesting a major deficit in GABA-ergic-mediated neural inhibition. Such deficit in GABA-ergic-mediated neural inhibition may make it impossible for the brain in VS to generate proper spatial and temporal differences during the encoding of stimuli (and activity changes in general) into neural activity. Instead of spatial and temporal differences, the stimuli's different discrete points in physical time and space are encoded into neural activity, entailing a high degree of stimulus-based coding and a rather low degree of difference-based coding. That, however, makes the association of the newly resulting stimulus-induced activity with consciousness impossible and therefore leads to the loss of consciousness, as observed in VS.

Key Concepts and Topics Covered

Qualia, rest–stimulus interaction, vegetative state, self-specific stimuli, imagination, cognitive tasks, self-specificity, self-referential tasks, consciousness, nonlinearity, GABA-ergic-mediated neural inhibition, GABA, glutamate, neural differences

NEUROEMPIRICAL BACKGROUND: IS CONSCIOUSNESS BASED ON COGNITION?

I demonstrated in the last chapter how the resting-state activity is directly related to consciousness. More specifically, I proposed the resting-state activity's neural propensity for activity changes and the degree of spatial and temporal differences encoded via difference-based coding during rest–rest (and rest–stimulus) interaction to predict the level or state of consciousness. I consequently regarded the degree of spatial and temporal differences encoded via difference-based coding during rest–rest interaction as a sufficient neural condition and thus as a neural correlate of the level or state of consciousness (NCC).

In contrast to the detailed of the resting-state activity itself in the previous chapter, we left open the nature of the stimulus-induced activity and its relationship to consciousness. What exactly must happen during rest–stimulus interaction in order to associate the resulting stimulus-induced activity with consciousness? This is the focus in the present chapter. As in the previous chapter, I again take the loss of consciousness in the vegetative state (VS) as a paradigm.

Various imaging studies have been conducted during passive sensory stimulation, using mostly auditory, somatosensory, and visual stimuli (see table 2 in Laureys and Schiff 2012 for an overview). Most of these studies show somehow preserved activation in auditory and visual cortex in VS, though on a lower level compared to that in minimally conscious state (MCS) and healthy subjects. More specifically, MCS patients show a more widespread activation and higher degrees of long-range functional connectivity in midline regions and lateral fronto-parietal cortex than in VS patients.

These earlier sensory-based studies have recently been complemented by more active cognitive tasks (see later) and emotions (see Chapter 31 for details). This is especially relevant since consciousness has often been associated with higher-order cognitive functions like imagination, memory, executive functions, attentions, and so on (see first Introduction and Appendix 1 for an overview). Therefore, loss of consciousness in VS, for instance, was tacitly assumed to be associated with loss of cognitive functions, including their "willful modulation" by the subject itself (see Hohwy 2012 for a nice overview of the different functions of consciousness in vegetative state; see focus here mainly on the purely phenomenal aspects).

Based on these findings one may want to raise the following question: Is consciousness based on cognitive functions and thus cognition-based? I will first discuss various findings from recent studies in VS. This will lead me to reject the hypothesis that consciousness, that is, phenomenal consciousness, is based on cognitive function and thus cognition-based. Instead, consciousness is based on the phenomenal functions of the brain as I already suggested in the introduction and will now be further explicated.

NEURONAL FINDINGS IA: COGNITIVE TASKS INDUCE REGION-SPECIFIC NEURAL ACTIVITY IN THE VEGETATIVE STATE

As we all know only too well, life is full of surprises. And why should that be different in the case of the brain? Let us turn, therefore, to Adrian Owen. Adrian Owen is a researcher who is interested in consciousness; he especially focuses on the absence of consciousness in VS. Back in Cambridge, England, he investigated one patient with VS during different imagery tasks. This yielded some rather amazing results, as I will describe (see Owen et al. 2006).

What did Arian Owen do? He scanned a VS patient in fMRI and let him perform specific cognitive tasks. While lying in the scanner, the VS patient was instructed to perform motor and visual imagery tasks (Owen et al. 2006): the patient was asked to imagine playing tennis. Surprisingly this yielded neural activity in the supplementary motor area in the VS patients. This region is related to movements as one imagines or executes them when playing tennis either mentally or physically. Most interestingly, the same region was activated in more or less the same way in healthy subjects. Hence, the VS patient was apparently able to perform a cognitive task as complex as imagining playing tennis. However, one cannot exclude that the observed neural activity is less based on the task itself but generated rather by pure chance.

To exclude such a possibility, Owen conducted the imaging during yet another task, a spatial navigation task, where the patient was asked to imagine visiting and walking around in the rooms of her house. As in the first task, neural activity changes were again induced— this time in other regions like the parahippocampal gyrus and the parietal cortex regions that are closely associated with spatial cognition as required by the task. The very same regions were also recruited in healthy subjects during the same task with regard to their own house or apartment.

Taken together, the results indicate that the VS patient was apparently quite able to perform a cognitive task like seeing visual and motor imagery. Most importantly, the VS patient was very able to differentiate between both tasks in the underlying neural activity patterns (see Fig. 29-1).

The results were recently replicated in a larger sample by Monti et al. (2010). Analogous paradigms were here conducted in a larger group of 54 patients, of whom 23 were diagnosed with VS and 31 with MCS (Monti et al. 2010). They had to perform the same tasks, imagining playing tennis and imagining walking from room to room in their own house. Five patients (four VS, one MCS) were indeed able to willfully modulate their neural activity during the tasks in a proper way: imagining playing tennis led to activation in the supplementary motor area (SMA) in all five patients, a region typically associated with either physical or imaginary movements.

In contrast, imagining walking in their own house induced neural activity changes in the parahippocampal gyrus in three VS and one MCS patients. These neural patterns were again similar to those in the healthy control subjects. Since then, other investigations of cognitive tasks requiring task-related efforts and willful modulation have been conducted in VS and MCS, with

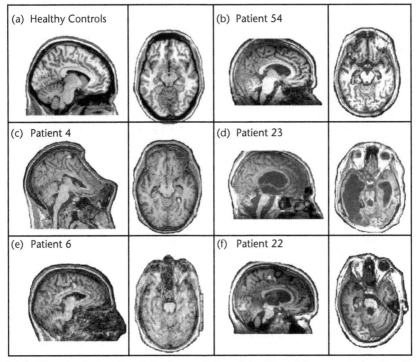

Figure 29-1 Stimulus-induced activity in vegetative state. Mental-imagery tasks. Functional MRI scans show activations associated with the motor imagery as compared with spatial imagery tasks (light colour) and the spatial imagery as compared with motor imagery tasks (darker colour). These scans were obtained from a group of healthy control subjects and five patients with traumatic brain injury. Reprinted with permission from Monti MM, Vanhaudenhuyse A, Coleman MR, Boly M, Pickard JD, Tshibanda L, Owen AM, Laureys S. Willful modulation of brain activity in disorders of consciousness. *N Engl J Med.* 2010 Feb 18;362(7):579–89.

all showing some preserved neural activity in the respective regions in these patients (see table 3 in Laureys and Schiff 2012 for an overview).

NEURONAL FINDINGS IB: CAN THE PRESENCE OF CONSCIOUSNESS BE INFERRED FROM THE PRESENCE OF STIMULUS-INDUCED (OR TASK-RELATED) ACTIVITY?

What do these results tell us about VS in particular and consciousness in general? The presence of stimulus-induced activity lets many neuroscientists and philosophers propose that consciousness must be present, too. Otherwise, subjects would be unable to perform the cognitive tasks and elicit stimulus-induced activity. They thus infer the presence of consciousness from the presence of stimulus-induced and task-related activity.

Therefore, a subset of VS patients is these days described as showing "wakefulness," which is further specified as either "responsive" or "unresponsive" (Laureys and Schiff 2012). However, other investigators have disputed and thus opposed this inference of the presence of consciousness from the observation of stimulus-induced and task-related activity in these patients (see Hohwy 2012; Bernat 2010; Panksepp et al. 2007; Nachev and Hacker 2010; and Monti et al. 2010, for discussion).

The opponents argue that the presence of a certain type of neuronal activity itself does not imply anything about the presence or absence of consciousness. Or, they put forward a more behavioral argument stating that the presence or absence of consciousness can only be decided on behavioral grounds, i.e., by the presence or absence of particular behavioral signs, rather than on purely neuronal grounds. We will not follow this discussion at this point in detail; we will come back to it, however, when discussing the relationship between cognition and consciousness in later sections.

Are the VS patients conscious? We do not know at this point, because the VS patients themselves are unable to tell us. What we do know for sure is that the VS patient investigated initially by Owen has regained consciousness since. And we know that these patients seem to show stimulus-induced or task-related activity. That is what we know at this point in time.

In contrast, we do not know whether such stimulus-induced activity that is purely neuronal by itself is accompanied by consciousness and its phenomenal features. More poignantly, we still do not know whether stimulus-induced or task-related activity necessarily or unavoidably entails its own association with consciousness and its phenomenal features.

NEURONAL FINDINGS IIA: ELECTROPHYSIOLOGICAL RESPONSE TO PATIENT'S OWN NAME IN THE VEGETATIVE STATE

We discussed so far how the brain in VS reacts to cognitive tasks. This, however, neglected self-specific stimuli, which, as shown in Chapters 23 and 24, seem to relate in a special way to the brain's intrinsic activity. The application of self-specific stimuli may therefore be of high interest in VS. How are self-specific stimuli like one's own name processed in the absence of consciousness and thus in VS?

One can present one's own name in an auditory way and record the related changes in neural activity by electrophysiological measures like electroencephalography (EEG). Do the VS patients show neural activity changes in response to their own names in the same way as they do during cognitive tasks as described earlier? A single case study investigated an MCS patient in EEG during stimulation with emotional stimuli (crying infant) and self-related stimuli (own name). They observed an almost "normal" activation pattern in the patient. The P300, a specific event-related component in EEG associated with cognitive processing, was well preserved while listening to especially the subject's own name (see Laureys, Perrin, et al. 2004).

A study by Perrin et al. (2005) (see also Perrin et al. 2006) observed the same during auditory evoked potentials in response to the subjects' own names in VS and MCS patients. The P300 was more or less preserved in all MCS patients and present in three of five VS patients. Only the onset or latency of the P300 was significantly delayed in MCS and VS patients compared to that in the healthy subjects.

Another study, by Schnakers et al. (2008), included 22 VS/MCS patients. Schnakers et al. demonstrated that subject's own name induced higher activity in another, later, more cognitive electrophysiological potential, the P300, compared to that in reaction to another person's name. This was stronger in an active (counting of names) than in a passive (mere perception without counting) mode. The difference between active and passive modes was observed only in MCS patients (14), while VS patients did not show any such difference. They were thus apparently unable to properly differentiate between the active and passive condition on a neuronal level.

Fellinger et al. (2011) also conducted an EEG study during one's own and unknown names that were presented in active and passive modes. Overall, the patients (13 MCS, 8 VS) showed stronger lower frequencies (delta, theta) and weaker higher frequencies (alpha, beta) than healthy subjects during hearing both their own and unknown names. Finally, frontal theta (at Fz) especially when hearing their own name was higher in the patients than the healthy subjects.

The pattern was different when the researchers compared active and passive modes of presentation. Healthy subjects showed stronger frontal theta power during the active mode compared to that in the passive mode. This was different in the patients. Like the earlier-mentioned study, the patients could not well differentiate between the two modes, i.e., active and passive, and also showed a delayed onset in frontal theta power compared to that in healthy subjects.

NEURONAL FINDINGS IIB: PREATTENTIVE PROCESSING OF ONE'S OWN NAME IN THE VEGETATIVE STATE

Probing another electrophysiological component in EEG, Pengmin Qin, from China, who is now in our group, investigated the same patients with EEG and focused on a specific electrophysiological potential, the MisMatch Negativity (MMN) (Qin et al. 2008; see also Chapter 7 in Volume I as well as Chapter 22 for more details on the MMN).

The MMN taps into preattentive auditory sensory processing (at around 125–250 ms) by comparing the electrophysiological responses to the same repeating stimuli with the one during one deviant stimulus (see Chapters 7 and 22 for detailed discussion of the MMN in the context of difference-based coding). To test for self-specificity in the MMN, Pengmin Qin determined the deviant stimulus as one's own name, while a non-self-specific name served as repeating stimulus.

The data show that Pengmin Qin's experimental design was well suited to eliciting an MMN during hearing their own name in all healthy subjects and in the seven patients (two coma, three VS, two MCS). Surprisingly there was no major difference in amplitude and latency in MMN between healthy subjects and the patients. In addition to the MMN, an earlier potential at around 100 ms (i.e., N100) could also be elicited in the seven patients and in two more patients. Interestingly, all the patients who reverted to MCS after 3 months showed an MMN and an N100. In contrast, no MMN (and N100) was observed in those VS patients who did not revert to MCS (see also Boly et al. 2011 for recent, more or less similar results on the MMN in VS).

What do these and other electrophysiological findings (see Cavinato et al. 2011, as described in chapter 28; as well as Laureys and Schiff 2012, for an overview of all studies) tell us about the stimulus-induced activity in VS and its relationship to consciousness? They demonstrate that self-specific stimuli can easily elicit neural activity changes in the brain of VS patients. The brain of these patients and thus their resting-state activity seem to be still reactive to stimuli like hearing one's own name. Accordingly, the electrophysiological results concerning self-specific stimuli are very compatible with the ones during cognitive tasks that, as described earlier, also showed preserved stimulus-induced activity in VS.

NEURONAL FINDINGS IIC: NEURAL ACTIVITY IN MIDLINE REGIONS DURING SELF-SPECIFIC STIMULI PREDICTS THE DEGREE OF CONSCIOUSNESS IN THE VEGETATIVE STATE

To investigate the functional anatomy, we turn from EEG and its electrophysiological measures to fMRI, which has a much better spatial resolution.

We recall from Chapters 23 and 24 that the cortical midline regions seem to have a special role in processing self-specific stimuli. This raises the question of whether the VS patients and their midline regions' neural activity are still reactive to self-specific stimuli. There have indeed been two studies that tested for self-specificity in VS patients as conducted by our group.

Pengmin Qin from our group (Qin et al. 2010) auditorily presented one's own name to seven VS and four MCS patients while they were lying in the scanner (fMRI). He first mapped the relevant regions in healthy subjects by comparing one's own name to familiar and unfamiliar, that is, unknown, names. This yielded activity changes in various midline structures like the supragenual anterior cingulate cortex (sACC), dorsal anterior cingulate cortex (dACC), SMA, superior temporal gyrus (STG), posterior cingulate cortex (PCC), and bilateral insula.

What happens in these midline regions in VS and MCS during auditory presentation of one's own name? All patients were able to induce activity changes though to different degrees. The MCS patients showed higher neural activity in sACC, dACC, PCC, and SMA compared to that in the VS patients. This clearly suggests that these patients' midline regions are still somewhat reactive, meaning that they can induce neural activity changes during self-specific stimuli.

How is the midline activity during one's own name related to consciousness? Pengmin Qin observed significant correlation between the consciousness scores (as measured with the Coma Recovery Scale–Revised; CRS-R) and the degree of neural activity in the dACC. The higher the signal change in the dACC during the auditory presentation of one's own name, the higher the degree of consciousness the patients exhibited. Those patients with VS showing the highest signal changes were the ones who were most likely to revert to MCS 3 months later (see Fig. 29-2a).

One may now want to argue that one cannot be completely sure whether subjects really listened to their own name. The name was presented in a merely passive way requiring no active effort by the subjects to listen so that subjects may have simply not even listened to the name. One can therefore not exclude the neural activity change to stem from sources other than

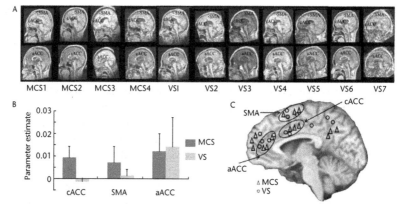

Figure 29-2a Neural activity during passive self-specific stimuli and prediction of consciousness in vegetative state. Patient fMRI results. (A) ROIs defined for cACC, SMA, and aACC (caudal anterior cingulate cortex, supplementary motor area, affective anterior cingulate cortex) in the patients with disorders of consciousness (DOC). (B) Parameter estimates for the VS and MCS patients respectively in the three regions of interest (ROI's) (mean ± S.E.). (C) Schematic representation of the midline structures activated during subject's own name in a familiar voice (SON-FV) in the patients. Those activated areas (labeled with points) in the same circle were regarded as the activations in the same anatomical localization. Reprinted with permission of Wiley Blackwell, from Qin P, Di H, Liu Y, Yu S, Gong Q, Duncan N, Weng X, Laureys S, Northoff G. Anterior cingulate activity and the self in disorders of consciousness. *Hum Brain Mapp.* 2010 Dec;31(12):1993–2002.

their own name. Hence, one would need an active task where subjects have to actively relate the stimulus to themselves, that is, their own self.

NEURONAL FINDINGS IID: ACTIVE SELF-REFERENTIAL TASK LEADS TO DECREASED SELF–NON-SELF DIFFERENTIATION OF MIDLINE NEURAL ACTIVITY IN THE VEGETATIVE STATE

This is exactly what a subsequent fMRI study of ours in VS by Huang et al. (2013) did. Instead of letting subjects merely passively listen to their own name, they now had to perform an active self-referential task wherein they had to refer to themselves, i.e., their own self. Two types of questions, autobiographical and common-sense, were presented in the auditory mode. The autobiographical questions asked for real facts in subjects' lives as obtained from their relatives.

This required subjects to actively refer the question to their own self, thus being a self-referential task. The control condition consisted of common-sense questions as non-self-referential, where subjects were asked for basic facts like whether one minute is 60 seconds. Instead of giving a real response via button click (as it is impossible in these patients), the subjects were asked to answer (mentally not behaviorally) with "yes" or "no."

Huang first compared autobiographical and common-sense questions in healthy subjects. As expected, this yielded significant signal changes in the midline regions, including the anterior regions like the perigenual anterior cingulate cortex (PACC) (extending to ventromedial prefrontal cortex [VMPFC]) and posterior regions like the PCC.

What did the brains in the VS patients now show in the very same regions? They showed signal changes in these regions that were reduced compared to those in healthy subjects. More specifically, while the VS patients were able to somehow differentiate between the two questions in their neural activity, the degree of neural differentiation remained much lower (see Fig. 29-2b).

How are these signal changes now related to consciousness? As in the study by Pengmin Qin, a significant correlation in anterior midline regions was observed. The midline regions' activity, the PACC the dorsal anterior cingulate cortex (dACC), and the PCC correlated with the

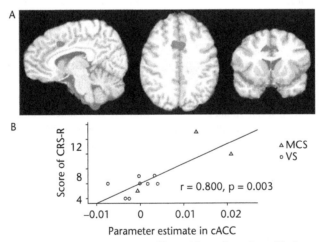

Figure 29-2b Neural activity during active self-specific task and prediction of consciousness in vegetative state. Correlation between neural activity in cACC (caudal anterior cingulate cortex) and consciousness. (A) The cACC as a ROI defined from Experiment 1, which was used as the template to obtain the cACC location for each patient. (B) Correlations between the parameter estimates in cACC and the CRS-R (Consciousness Recovery Scale-Revised) scores at the time of fMRI. Reprinted with permission of Wiley Blackwell, from Qin P, Di H, Liu Y, Yu S, Gong Q, Duncan N, Weng X, Laureys S, Northoff G. Anterior cingulate activity and the self in disorders of consciousness. *Hum Brain Mapp.* 2010 Dec;31(12):1993–2002.

degree of consciousness (as measured with the CRS-R scale).

How is the exact relationship between neural activity in these regions and the level of consciousness? The better the signal changes in these regions differentiated neuronally between self- and non-self-referential conditions, the higher levels of consciousness patients exhibited. Accordingly, as in the earlier-described study, we here observed a direct relationship between the degree of neuronal self–non-self differentiation and the level of consciousness in anterior and posterior midline regions.

NEURONAL FINDINGS IIE: RESTING-STATE ACTIVITY IN MIDLINE REGIONS PREDICTS STIMULUS-INDUCED ACTIVITY DURING SELF-REFERENTIAL TASK IN THE VEGETATIVE STATE

How about the resting-state activity in the same patients? As described in Chapter 28, vegetative patients show strong alterations in the resting-state activity. One wants to know now whether the diminished responses to self-specific stimuli are related to changes in the resting state in the very same regions.

For that, Huang et al. (2013) also investigated functional connectivity and low-frequency fluctuations in exactly those regions that showed diminished signal differentiation during the self-referential task. As in the previous studies (see Chapter 28 for details), the VS patients showed significantly reduced functional connectivity from the PACC to the PCC in the resting state. In addition, the power of particular ranges or bands in the low-frequency fluctuations was significantly lower in the PACC and the PCC in VS compared to that in healthy subjects.

Given that we investigated exactly the same regions during both resting state and task, this strongly suggests that the resting-state abnormalities in these regions are somehow related to the earlier described changes during the self-referential task. This was further supported by correlation analysis: The higher the degree of low-frequency fluctuations in the resting state of the midline regions, the better the stimulus-induced neuronal differentiation between self- and non-self-referential conditions.

Taken together, these findings demonstrate that VS patients not only can induce neural activity changes in their brain in response to merely passively presented self-specific stimuli. VS patients are apparently also able to actively refer to themselves and thus to engage by referring stimuli or questions to their own self, as required in the self-referential task. Thereby the anterior and posterior midline regions, like the anterior cingulate and its distinct parts (i.e., PACC, dACC, PCC), are recruited and seem to be of special significance for associated consciousness to the stimulus-induced or task-related activity.

NEURONAL HYPOTHESIS IA: "NEURONAL-PHENOMENAL *DISSOCIATION*"

What do these findings tell us? First and foremost they tell us that something must be "right" in the VS patients' brains. Otherwise they would not be able to induce neural activity changes during either cognitive or self-referential tasks. Nor would they be able to differentiate between the different tasks as, for instance, between motor (e.g., tennis playing) and visual (e.g., house navigation) imagery or between self- and non-self-referential stimuli.

These data suggest that what is "right" in VS concerns the induction of stimulus-induced and task-related activity and its relationship to specific tasks or stimuli. This was the easy part. Now comes the hard part. Something must also be "wrong" in the VS patients' brain. Even though they are quite able to induce stimulus-induced activity, they nevertheless seem to suffer from loss of consciousness, thus being vegetative.

More specifically, the stimulus-induced activity is apparently no longer associated with consciousness. There is thus what one may describe as a *dissociation* between stimulus-induced activity and consciousness. In contrast to the healthy brain, stimulus-induced activity in VS is no longer associated with consciousness. The purely neuronal stimulus-induced or task-related activity is thus dissociated from the phenomenal state of consciousness; one may therefore speak of "neuronal-phenomenal dissociation."

What exactly do I mean by the concept of "neuronal-phenomenal dissociation"? It means that neuronal and phenomenal states can no longer be characterized by co-occurrence. Even though there is neuronal activity like (more or less) proper stimulus-induced activity as in VS, it is no longer associated with a phenomenal state and thus consciousness. The stimulus-induced activity is consequently detached or dissociated from consciousness and its phenomenal features. This implies what I describe as neuronal-phenomenal dissociation (see later for a more detailed definition).

Neuronal Hypothesis
IB: "NEURONAL-PHENOMENAL *INFERENCE*"

One may now want to argue that such "neuronal-phenomenal dissociation" does not apply for those patients who are actively able to perform cognitive and self-referential tasks as described earlier. Does the presence of neuronal activity during the active cognitive and self-referential tasks signify the presence of consciousness? Such an inference, from the presence of stimulus-induced or task-related activity to the presence of consciousness, seems to be suggested by the most recent introduction of the terms "responsive" and "unresponsive wakefulness" to describe VS (see Schiff and Laureys 2012).

What does the concept of "responsive and unresponsive wakefulness" mean? The terms "responsive" and "unresponsive" indicate whether these subjects show stimulus-induced or task-related activity in response to certain stimuli or tasks. The term "wakefulness" suggests the presence of an awake and somehow conscious state that is assumed to be necessary for performing the task. The presence of a phenomenal state; that is, consciousness as wakefulness, is here inferred from the presence of the purely neuronal stimulus-induced or task-related activity. Such inference from the presence of a neuronal state to the presence of consciousness and its phenomenal features can be described as the "neuronal-phenomenal inference."

Such a neuronal-phenomenal inference is problematic, however, for several reasons, both empirical and conceptual. Let us focus here on the empirical side of things (while I leave aside the conceptual-logical reasons). As Laureyes and Schiff (2012) themselves remark, the absence of neuronal activity in response to task-specific instructions may occur for several reasons (as, for instance, technological dependence). Therefore, the absence of neural activity cannot be taken as a marker for the absence of consciousness.

How about the reverse, the presence of task-specific neural activity indicating the presence of consciousness? Does task-specific neuronal activity require and thus presuppose consciousness? If so, these patients must be assumed to be conscious indeed and may therefore suffer from what Laureys and Schiff (2012) describe as "functional locked-in-syndrome." But one needs to be careful here.

Subjects remaining unconscious may show more or less the same activity pattern during the same kind of tasks. We perform plenty of tasks daily in a rather unconscious mode, meaning that we do not "experience" these tasks. We are thus both responsive and wakeful, but not conscious, with regard to these tasks. This means that responsiveness and wakefulness, including their underlying stimulus-induced or task-related activities, do not imply anything by themselves about the presence or absence of consciousness and its phenomenal features.

Neuronal Hypothesis
IC: "NEURONAL-*PHENOMENAL* INFERENCE" VERSUS "NEURONAL-*COGNITIVE* INFERENCE"

Let me be clear what exactly I mean here by the concept of "consciousness and its phenomenal features." The phenomenal features I am targeting here, are the "phenomenal features" in a strict sense, including "inner time and space consciousness," phenomenal unity, self-perspectival and intentional organization, and qualia. These phenomenal features must be distinguished from other, more cognitive features of consciousness like willful modulation, attention, awareness, and access to contents, which I do not debate here (see Hohwy 2012, for an overview).

This implies a strict distinction between phenomenal and cognitive functions of the brain. The observed results with the neural activity during cognitive tasks suggest that the cognitive functions are somehow preserved in VS. One may thus reason from the presence of neural activity to the presence of the cognitive functions, making a so-called "neuronal-cognitive inference." That does not imply anything about the phenomenal functions themselves, however. To infer phenomenal features and consciousness from the observed neural activity is to confuse cognitive and phenomenal functions of the brain. Accordingly, the results allow for a "neuronal-cognitive inference" but not for a "neuronal-phenomenal inference."

Why do the proponents of the description of VS as "responsive or unresponsive wakefulness" nevertheless confuse these two inferences: the "neuronal-cognitive inference" and the "neuronal-phenomenal inference"? The tacit supposition here is that consciousness is based on cognitive functions and their associated stimulus-induced or task-related activity. This amounts to a cognition- and stimulus-based view of consciousness.

That, however, as we can see, does not really account for the data in VS. Here, the presence of stimulus-induced activity during cognitive tasks is accompanied by the absence of consciousness. This implies dissociation between the "neuronal-cognitive inference" and the "neuronal-phenomenal inference," with only the former, not the latter, being valid. Most important, the rejection of the "neuronal-phenomenal inference" forces us to develop a different account of consciousness, one that is not based on cognitive functions and stimulus-induced activity but rather on phenomenal functions and resting-state activity.

Neuronal Hypothesis IIa: From "Neuronal-Phenomenal Dissociation" to "Neuronal-Neuronal Dissociation"

How about empirical reality? Empirical reality tells us that stimulus-induced and/or task-related activity is present in VS patients, while consciousness seems to be absent. How is such a dissociation between neuronal activity and phenomenal features possible? Let us briefly recapitulate what is clear and what is not in VS.

What is clear is that there is neuronal activity in VS and MCS patients in response to passive sensory stimuli and active cognitive tasks. That is a consistent finding, as described earlier.

Their neural activity, the observed task-related activity, is still associated with particular psychological functions like imagining, navigation, self-referencing and so on (see earlier). This suggests that there is apparently no dissociation between stimulus-induced activity and cognitive functions. There is no "neuronal-cognitive dissociation" in VS, as can be observed in depression or schizophrenia (see Chapters 22 and 27).

In addition, it is also clear that the VS patients show changes in their consciousness in that they are not able to properly associate their otherwise purely neuronal stimulus-induced or task-related activity with consciousness and its phenomenal features. They can no longer experience their own cognitive (and sensory, motor, affective, cognitive, and social) functions in a subjective way, in first-person perspective, as being indicative of consciousness. They thus show a phenomenal deficit, if one wants to say so. One may consequently postulate a dissociation between the neuronal activity during cognitive tasks and the phenomenal features of consciousness. As already indicated, I therefore speak of a "neuronal-phenomenal dissociation," in VS.

How can we further substantiate the concept of the "neuronal-phenomenal dissociation"? The observation of dissociation between two different states or functions usually implies that there must be two different underlying neuronal mechanisms. These two neuronal mechanisms may now dissociate from each other in VS, with one being intact and the other deficient.

What are the two neuronal mechanisms in question? There is the neuronal mechanism that enables the generation of stimulus-induced or task-related activity. And there is the neuronal mechanism that allows to associate the otherwise purely neuronal stimulus-induced or task-related activity with consciousness and its phenomenal features. What does this imply for the neuronal-phenomenal dissociation in VS? The neuronal-phenomenal dissociation suggests that the neuronal mechanisms for generating the neural activity during cognitive tasks are still more or less intact in VS. In contrast, the neuronal mechanisms related to the phenomenal features of consciousness seem to be deficient in VS (see Fig. 29-3).

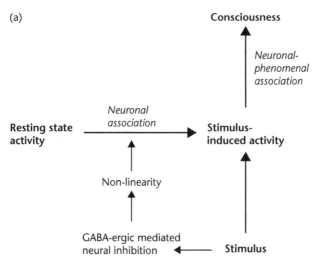

Figure 29-3a-e Rest–stimulus interaction and consciousness. The figure demonstrates the relationship between the neuronal mechanisms of rest–stimulus interaction and consciousness. (*a*) The figure concerns the healthy brain and shows the central role of GABA-ergic-mediated neural inhibition and nonlinearity in the interaction between resting state and stimulus (*left lower part*). There is thus direct nonlinear interaction between resting-state activity and stimulus, mutually changing each other, which results in what one may describe as a "neuronal association." Such a "neuronal association" between resting-state activity and stimulus allows in turn for the newly resulting activity, the stimulus-induced or task-related activity, to be associated with consciousness (*right middle and upper part*). This is what I describe as the "neuronal-phenomenal association." (*b*) The same processes as in Figure 29-3a are now depicted in the case of the vegetative state. The stimulus still induces stimulus-induced activity (*right lower part*). However, it no longer connects to GABA-ergic-mediated neural inhibition (due to possible lack of GABA-A receptors), which in turn makes nonlinear rest–stimulus interaction impossible (*left lower part*). This is indicated by the dotted lines. That results in "neuronal dissociation" between resting-state activity and stimulus-induced activity in vegetative state. The resulting stimulus-induced or task-related activity is thus no longer affected by the resting state and can therefore not be associated anymore with consciousness, as indicated by the dotted line (*right upper part*). There is thus what I describe as neuronal-phenomenal dissociation with the consequent loss of consciousness in vegetative state. (*c*) The figure shows the relationship between nonlinearity during rest–rest or rest–stimulus interaction (y-axis) and the degree of consciousness (x-axis). The more nonlinear the interaction between the stimulus and the resting state (or within the resting state itself), the higher the degree of consciousness associated with the respective change in neural activity. I propose the degree of nonlinearity to be lowest in coma, slightly higher in vegetative state, and almost normalized in minimal conscious state. (*d*) The figure shows the relationship between nonlinearity (x-axis) and GABA-ergic-mediated neural inhibition (y-axis) during rest–rest or rest–stimulus interaction and how they relate to the degree of consciousness. The stronger GABA-ergic-mediated neural inhibition, the more nonlinear the interaction between the stimulus and the resting state (or within the resting state itself), and the higher the degree of consciousness that is associated with the respective change in neural activity. I propose the degree of GABA-ergic-mediated neural inhibition to be lowest in coma, slightly higher in vegetative state, and almost normalized in minimal conscious state. (*e*) The figure shows the relationship between the degree of differences coded in difference-based coding (x-axis) and GABA-ergic-mediated neural inhibition (y-axis) during rest–rest or rest–stimulus interaction and how they relate to the degree of consciousness. The stronger the GABA-ergic-mediated neural inhibition, the more nonlinear the interaction between the stimulus and the resting state (or within the resting state itself), and the higher the degree of consciousness associated with the respective change in neural activity. I propose the degree of GABA-ergic-mediated neural inhibition to be lowest in coma, slightly higher in vegetative state, and almost normalized in minimal conscious state. *Abbreviations*: BD, brain death; CS, comatose state; HS, healthy subject; MCS, minimally conscious state; VS, vegetative state.

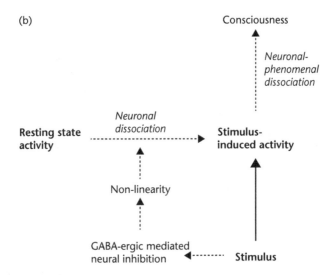

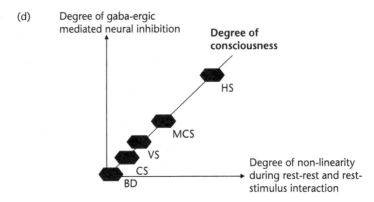

BD = Brain death; CS = Comatose state; VS = Vegetative state;
MCS = Minimal conscious state; HS = Healthy subjects

Figure 29-3a-e (Continued)

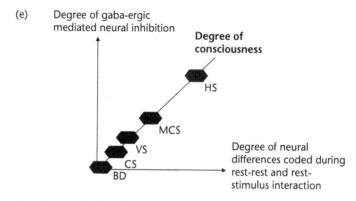

BD = Brain death; CS = Comatose state; VS = Vegetative state;
MCS = Minimal conscious state; HS = Healthy subjects

Figure 29-3a-e (Continued)

The postulated neuronal-phenomenal dissociation in VS can be traced back to the dissociation between two different neuronal mechanisms: one for generating neural activity (during for instance cognitive functions), and the other for the association of that neural activity with the phenomenal features of consciousness. One can therefore specify the alleged "neuronal-phenomenal dissociation" by what I refer to as "neuronal-neuronal dissociation." What do I mean by "neuronal-neuronal dissociation"? This will be the focus in the next section.

NEURONAL HYPOTHESIS IIB: FROM "NEURONAL-NEURONAL DISSOCIATION" TO "REST–STIMULUS DISSOCIATION"

Exactly what kind of neuronal mechanism are we looking for? The neuronal mechanism in question must allow for the association of a phenomenal state with the purely neuronal stimulus-induced or task-related activity.

At the same time, however, the neuronal mechanism in question must be different from the ones underlying the generation of stimulus-induced or task-related activity by itself. Why? The neuronal mechanisms underlying the generation of the stimulus-induced or task-related activity by itself must be more or less preserved in VS, allowing them to show "normal" stimulus-induced activity. We must

therefore search for a neuronal mechanism that lies beneath or beyond the stimulus-induced activity or task-related itself.

How can we better illustrate the situation? Metaphorically speaking, there must be an additional factor coming in besides the stimulus or task itself. And this additional factor must be crucial for associating the purely neuronal stimulus/task and its stimulus-induced or task-related activity with the phenomenal state of consciousness.

What is this additional factor? Let's look at what happens prior to the stimulus-induced activity. The stimulus must interact with the resting-state activity in order to elicit stimulus-induced activity. Such rest–stimulus interaction shows special features like nonlinear interaction via GABA-ergic-mediated neural inhibition, as we will see in further detail in the next section. I now propose that proper rest–stimulus interaction is central for associating the otherwise purely neuronal stimulus-induced or task-related activity with a phenomenal state and thus consciousness.

If, in contrast, rest–stimulus interaction is abnormal, that is, decreased, the resulting stimulus-induced or task-related activity will no longer be associated with consciousness anymore. There may thus be "neuronal-neuronal dissociation" between resting-state activity and stimulus-induced activity in VS. Such neuronal dissociation may, in turn, be central for the loss of consciousness in VS. Since it concerns the coupling between resting-state and stimulus-induced activity, I describe such neuronal-neuronal dissociation also as "rest–stimulus dissociation" (see Fig. 29-3).

Taken all together, I propose three different concepts of dissociation in VS. First, stimulus-induced or task-related activity dissociates from the phenomenal features of consciousness, implying what I describe as "neuronal-phenomenal dissociation." I trace such neuronal-phenomenal dissociation back to the decoupling of the neuronal mechanisms underlying stimulus-induced or task-related activity from those related to associating that neural activity with consciousness. I therefore spoke of "neuronal-neuronal dissociation."

I now postulate that the neuronal-neuronal dissociation can be traced back to the decoupling between resting-state activity and stimulus-induced activity. For that reason I speak of "rest–stimulus dissociation"; this concept can be regarded as the empirical specification of the more general concepts of "neuronal-phenomenal dissociation" and "neuronal-neuronal dissociation."

NEURONAL HYPOTHESIS IIIA: NONLINEARITY DURING REST–STIMULUS INTERACTION

I proposed proper rest–stimulus interaction to be central in allowing for the association of stimulus-induced or task-related activity with consciousness and its phenomenal features. We therefore want to detail the neuronal mechanisms underlying rest–stimulus interaction. For that, we have to go back briefly to Volume I and more specifically to Chapters 11 and 12.

Rest–stimulus interaction was characterized by nonlinear and nonadditive interaction. What does that mean? The resting state shows a certain level of neural activity. The stimulus (or task) elicits neural activity changes on the basis of the resting state's level of neural activity. The question is now what exactly the stimulus (or task) must do in order to interact properly with the resting-state activity as to associate the resulting stimulus-induced or task-related activity with consciousness.

Let us sketch some hypothetical scenarios. The stimulus or task could, for instance, elicit

changes in neural activity that remain independent of the resting-state activity level. Each stimulus or task may have its specific degree of neural activity change in the brain independent of the latter's resting-state activity level. The resulting stimulus-induced activity would then consist of the mere addition between the resting-state activity level and the changes related to the stimulus itself. There would then be linear and additive rest–stimulus interaction; resting-state activity and stimulus-induced activity would then be processed largely in parallel and segregated from each other.

However, one could also imagine another way for stimulus-induced (or task-related) and resting-state-related activity to interact. In that case, the stimulus or task would impinge upon the resting state itself and change the spatial and temporal structure of its neural activity. In that case both stimuli/task and resting state would change implying direct and mutual interaction.

Such mutual interaction would obviously change both the resting-state activity, for example, its level and some of its yet unknown features, and the degree of stimulus-induced (or task-related) activity the stimulus (or task) can possibly elicit (as compared to when it would not interact with the resting state). Unlike in the earlier-described case of parallel operation, one would then no longer be able to clearly distinguish between resting-state activity on one hand and stimulus-induced or task-related activity on the other.

NEURONAL HYPOTHESIS IIIB: "NONLINEARITY HYPOTHESIS OF CONSCIOUSNESS"

How does such nonlinear rest–stimulus interaction affect the resulting stimulus-induced or task-related activity? The resulting stimulus-induced or task-related activity could be higher or lower compared to that in the one the stimulus or task alone would elicit if it were not interacting with the resting state. There is thus what one can describe as a nonlinear and nonadditive rest–stimulus interaction.

This shows that resting state and stimulus-induced (or task-related) activity are closely intertwined and integrated. There is thus interactive and integrative rather than parallel and segregated processing between resting-state activity and stimulus-induced (or task-related) activity.

As discussed in Volume I (see Chapters 11 and 12) as well as here in Volume II (see Chapter 19), there is strong empirical evidence for nonlinear and nonadditive rest–stimulus interaction in healthy subjects. The resulting stimulus-induced or task-related activity can thus not be explained without considering the preceding resting-state activity level. Due to nonlinearity, the resulting stimulus-induced or task-related activity must be considered the result of specific rest–stimulus interaction with fusion, merger, or integration between resting state and stimulus-induced (or task-related) activity.

How is the nonlinearity during rest–stimulus interaction related to consciousness? This leads me to propose what I call the "nonlinearity hypothesis of consciousness" (see Fig. 29-3c). The nonlinearity hypothesis of consciousness proposes the degree of consciousness to be directly dependent upon the degree of nonlinearity during any kind of neural activity change, be it rest–stimulus interaction (as in the awake state) or rest–rest interaction (as in the dreaming state; see Chapter 26).

More specifically, the nonlinearity hypothesis of consciousness claims for the following relationship. The higher the degree of nonlinearity during changes in neural activity levels as, for instance, during rest–stimulus (or rest–rest) interaction, the higher the degree or level of consciousness that can be associated with the newly resulting level of neural activity, that is, stimulus-induced or task-related activity.

Neuronal Hypothesis IIIC: "Nonlinearity Hypothesis of Consciousness" and the Global Neuronal Workspace Theory

How can we further specify the kind of nonlinearity we are looking for to determine proper rest–stimulus interaction? The here-described nonlinearity in rest–stimulus interaction must be distinguished from the kind of nonlinearity Dehaene proposes as a core component in his global neuronal workspace (GNW) theory of consciousness (see Chapter 19 for details).

Simply put, the GNW theory proposes later changes (at around 300 ms) in the fronto-parietal-temporal network to be nonlinear, thereby gating the access for stimuli or tasks to consciousness. This is based on a study by Cul et al. (2007). They demonstrated that the nonlinear increase in visibility of contents matched with the nonlinear increase in late (>275 ms) electrophysiological events, including the P300, as related to the spread of neural activity in fronto-parietal-temporal networks.

How does such late nonlinearity stand up to the here proposed nonlinear rest–stimulus interaction? I propose rest–stimulus interaction to occur early right after the onset of the stimulus; this implies that I would associate the nonlinearity during rest–stimulus interaction with early rather than late changes. This is supported by the demonstration of early changes in EEG in VS like the N100 (occurring at 100 ms after stimulus onset) and the MMN that occurs at around 125–150 ms (see the studies described earlier). These early changes may then lead to the later changes in VS as, for instance, observed in the P300 (see earlier).

In addition, the GNW focuses on the nonlinear changes occurring in the fronto-parietal-temporal network as a result of their top-down modulation of posterior occipito-temporo pathways. The nonlinear interaction may thus be associated with a region-to-region interaction. This is different in our case. Here the nonlinearity is supposed to be related to rest–stimulus interaction in any kind of region and is therefore not limited to the fronto-parietal network as in the GNW.

Moreover, the nonlinear rest–stimulus interaction is not about region-to-region interaction as in the GNW. Instead, it is about the basic mechanisms underlying the interaction of any kind of resting-state activity in the whole brain with any kind of stimuli or tasks. As such, non-linear rest–stimulus interaction concerns any stimulus (or spontaneous activity change) that "wants to elicit" changes in the resting-state activity itself in whatever region of the brain, including both lower-order sensory and higher-order cognitive regions, in order to become processed in the brain by yielding stimulus-induced or task-related activity.

Neuronal Hypothesis IIID: "Experience-Based Approach to Consciousness" versus "Cognition-Based Approach to Consciousness"

How can we support our neurophenomenal approach and its emphasis on non-linear rest–stimulus interaction in a most basic way by the empirical data? We recall that sensory stimulation leads to neural activity changes in the auditory and visual cortex in VS (see earlier), but nevertheless it is not accompanied by consciousness.

I thus propose abnormal, that is, linear rather than nonlinear, rest–stimulus interaction in VS to already occur in the sensory cortex as well as in every other region of the brain. Hence, unlike the GNW, I do not limit nonlinearity to a specific region or network. The nonlinearity here serves for the stimulus to access the brain's resting-state activity and the different layers of its spatiotemporal structures. Such access must occur in a nonlinear way in order to associate the stimulus and its purely neuronal stimulus-induced activity with consciousness and its phenomenal features.

This is different in the GNW. Nonlinearity in the context of the GNW is supposed to account for the access to contents in consciousness and thus for access consciousness (see Chapter 19 for details). That obviously differs from my neurophenomenal hypothesis. Here, nonlinearity serves to access (and thus make possible and constitute) experience itself rather than merely accessing the already constituted contents of experience. My neurophenomenal approach thus focus on phenomenal consciousness rather than access consciousness as the GNW (see Chapter 18 and 19). Due to that difference, the GNW must ultimately remain "blind" to the experience itself whose phenomenal features and subjective nature it cannot explain. In contrast, the GNW can explain the contents of experience and our access to the contents.

My purely neurophenomenal approach targets only the phenomenal features and thus phenomenal consciousness; it is focused on experience itself. In contrast, it does not target the contents of consciousness, including their processing in the various cognitive features like attention, awareness, reporting, access, and so on (see Hohwy 2012 for an overview). One can thus characterize the neurophenomenal approach as an "experience-based approach to consciousness" that presupposes phenomenal consciousness (see Chapters 18 and 19).

This is different in the GNW. The GNW bases its hypothesis of consciousness on the ability of the subjects to report their experience. Since that presupposes access to one's own experience, which requires cognitive processing, the GNW presupposes a "cognition-based approach to consciousness" that implies access consciousness, if not higher-order forms of consciousness like reflective consciousness.

Neuronal Hypothesis IVA: GABA-ergic-Mediated Nonlinearity and Consciousness

What are the exact neuronal mechanisms underlying the occurrence of nonlinearity during rest–stimulus-interaction? Following Buzsaki (2006), GABA exerts inhibitory effects via inhibitory interneurons and thereby introduces nonlinearity into neural activity.

How does GABA inject nonlinearity into neural activity? The number of inhibitory interneurons is relative higher than the number of excitatory pyramidal cells. This has important consequences. While the inhibitory interneurons need to be excited by pyramidal cells and their glutamate, the consequently resulting degree of GABA-ergic-mediated neural inhibition is much higher compared to that in the initial degree of glutamatergic-mediated neural excitation.

Accordingly, the neural balance is tilted toward neural inhibition. Why? The number of inhibitory interneurons that are excited by the pyramidal cells is higher than the number of pyramidal cells that are excited (see Chapter 2 for details). The degree of neural inhibition is consequently higher relative to the initial degree of neural excitation. That, in turn, makes possible a nonlinear change in the level of neural activity and results consequently in what we observe as stimulus-induced or task-related activity (see Chapters 2, 6, and 12 in Volume I for details).

Based on the close relationship between GABA-ergic-mediated neural inhibition and nonlinearity, one may propose the following. The degree of consciousness may be directly dependent upon the degree of change in GABA-ergic-mediated neural inhibition during any kind of neural activity change, that is, rest–rest or rest–stimulus interaction.

The higher the degree of GABA-ergic-mediated neural inhibition changes during neural activity changes, the more likely the newly resulting activity level will change in a nonlinear way and the more likely it will be associated with a higher degree of consciousness. Accordingly, I propose a central role for GABA-ergic-mediated neural inhibition in mediating nonlinearity during rest–stimulus interaction and the subsequent association of its purely neuronal neural activity with consciousness (see Fig. 29-3d).

NEURONAL HYPOTHESIS IVB: DECREASE OF GABA-ERGIC-MEDIATED NONLINEARITY IN THE VEGETATIVE STATE

How can we support this hypothesis by empirical data? If my hypothesis of GABA-ergic-mediated nonlinearity during rest–stimulus interaction holds, and if that in turn predicts the degree of consciousness, one would expect the VS patients to show abnormally low GABA. This seems to be indeed the case, as VS patients show strong abnormalities in GABA.

One early study (see Rudolf et al. 2000) investigated the density of GABA-A receptors in nine benzodiazepine-free VS patients using 11-C-Flumazenil positron emission tomography (PET). Compared to healthy subjects, the VS patients showed an overall global reduction of GABA-A receptor density in all cortical regions while sparing the cerebellum. In contrast to such global reduction, no specific focal or regional differences in GABA-A receptor density could be detected in VS patients (see Rudolf et al. 2000 and Heiss 2012 for a recent overview).

Interestingly, the reduction in GABA-A receptor density went along with a reduction in overall glucose metabolism in the same patients (see Rudolf et al. 1999, 2002). While this suggests correspondence between global GABA deficits

and global metabolism, their direct relationship remains unclear (see also Shulman 2012, Hyder et al. 2013).

Besides such direct empirical support for the central role of GABA in consciousness, more indirect support comes from single case reports. Single case reports demonstrated therapeutic efficacy of GABA-A receptor agonists like Zolpidem (i.e., orally) or Baclofen (i.e., intrathecal) in reverting patients with VS back to MCS or full-blown consciousness (see Clauss 2010 for an excellent summary as well as Laureys and Schiff 2012).

NEURONAL HYPOTHESIS IVC: "DORMANT" STATE OF GABA-A RECEPTORS AND THE "PARADOXICAL" EFFECTS OF BENZODIAZEPINES IN THE VEGETATIVE STATE

Such an increase in the level of consciousness in VS by GABA-A receptor agonists seems to be almost paradoxical, however, when compared to their effects in healthy subjects. Applied to healthy subjects, GABA-A receptor antagonists decrease (rather than increase) the level of consciousness by sedating them. Higher doses of GABA-A receptor antagonists can even lead to complete loss of consciousness in healthy subjects, as in anesthesia.

How is it possible that the same substance leads to the loss of consciousness in healthy subjects and the recovery of consciousness in VS? Clauss (2010) proposes that the low energy and metabolic supply in VS may induce a state of "neurodormancy" in the GABA-A receptors: the GABA-A receptors are "dormant" in VS to avoid neural inhibition with further reduction of neural activity. Most important, such a "dormant" state changes the sensitivity and affinity of the GABA-A receptors in an abnormal way: their activation by GABA-A receptor agonistic drugs now leads to neural excitation (rather than neural inhibition) and consequently to an increase (rather than decrease) in both neural activity and the level of consciousness.

The GABA-A receptors may also change the configuration of their subunits (i.e., alpha, beta, gamma) possibly due to altered gene expression in the presence of low metabolism. Such an "abnormal" state of the GABA-A receptors may then mediate the "abnormal" therapeutic effects of GABA-ergic drugs in some (not all) VS patients on their level of consciousness.

I thus propose that the GABA-ergic drugs like Zolpidem may reinstate the ability of GABA-A receptors to exert their nonlinear effects on neural activity changes during rest–stimulus (or rest–rest) interaction. By stimulating GABA-A receptors, nonlinear effects are reintroduced into neural activity: I suppose that this make possible the association of the newly resulting neural activity with consciousness.

This may be different in healthy subjects. In contrast to VS, the use of high doses of GABA-ergic drugs in the healthy subject may increase the GABA-ergic-mediated neural inhibition to an abnormal degree. Such increased neural inhibition makes any neural activity changes including the exertion of nonlinear effects impossible and therefore ultimately results in the loss of consciousness as in anesthesia (see also Chapter 17 for the impact of GABA and glutamate on consciousness).

In addition to GABA-ergic drugs, other drugs are also used to induce anesthesia; these include dopaminergic drugs like L-dopa or bromocriptine as well as glutamatergic (dopaminergic) drugs like amantadine, which have also been shown to be therapeutically effective in single VS patients (see Clauss 2010 as well as Laureys and Schiff 2012; see also Changeux and Lou 2011 for the biochemical modulation of consciousness). This is not a surprise since both dopamine and glutamine are closely related and linked to GABA.

NEUROPHENOMENAL HYPOTHESIS IA: LOSS OF GABA-ERGIC-MEDIATED NONLINEARITY PREDICTS THE DEGREE OF "REST–STIMULUS DISSOCIATION" IN THE VEGETATIVE STATE

How can the apparent deficit in GABA-A receptors in VS contribute to the loss of consciousness in these patients? The stimulus or task may still elicit glutamatergic excitation, which may account for the observed stimulus-induced or task-related activity.

However, such glutamatergic-mediated excitation may no longer be coupled to GABA-ergic-mediated neural inhibition because of the lack of GABA-A receptors. Hence, even if the stimulus elicits glutamatergic-mediated neural excitation, it can no longer excite and thus recruit GABA-ergic-mediated neural inhibition. The proportion and thus the balance between glutamatergic-mediated neural excitation and GABA-ergic-mediated neural inhibition can consequently no longer become as asymmetric, that is, tilted toward neural inhibition, as in healthy subjects.

If, however, GABA-ergic-mediated neural inhibition no longer exceeds glutamatergic-mediated neural excitation, the possible degree of nonlinearity is reduced during rest–stimulus interaction, while the degree of linearity during rest–stimulus interaction increases. Resting-state activity and stimulus are thus no longer processed in an interactive and integrative way but rather largely parallel and segregated. The stimulus can still elicit changes in neural activity, these however remain largely independent of and thus parallel and segregated to the resting-state activity (see Chapter 11 in Volume I for details).

How is that related to the loss of consciousness in VS? The lack of GABA-ergic-mediated neural inhibition may considerably increase the degree of neuronal dissociation between resting-state activity and stimulus-induced (or task-related) activity. There is thus increased rest–stimulus dissociation, as I described earlier.

Increased rest-stimulus dissociation leads, in turn, to a decoupling of the neuronal mechanisms underlying stimulus-induced or task-related activity from the neuronal mechanisms that are related to the latter's association with consciousness. There is thus a "neuronal-neuronal dissociation." That, however, decreases the likelihood of associating the resulting stimulus-induced (or task-related) activity with consciousness, entailing neuronal-phenomenal dissociation.

In sum, I propose neuronal-phenomenal dissociation in VS to be dependent upon neuronal-neuronal dissociation, that is, "rest–stimulus dissociation," which, in turn, may be traced back to the loss of GABA-ergic-mediated neural inhibition during rest–stimulus (and rest–rest) interaction.

NEUROPHENOMENAL HYPOTHESIS IB: THE DEGREE OF GABA-ERGIC-MEDIATED ENCODED SPATIAL AND TEMPORAL DIFFERENCES DURING REST–STIMULUS INTERACTION PREDICTS THE DEGREE OF THE LEVEL OF CONSCIOUSNESS

So far, I have explained the neuronal mechanisms underlying rest–stimulus interaction and demonstrated how they are related to consciousness. What remained unclear, however, is why GABA-ergic-mediated nonlinearity is central for the association of the newly resulting activity level with particularly qualia as the phenomenal hallmark of consciousness (see Chapter 28).

What exactly happens during GABA-ergic-mediated neural inhibition? GABA exerts disproportionately strong neural inhibition compared to that in glutamatergic-mediated neural excitation. By that, GABA introduces and enlarges the neural difference between the preceding level of neural activity, the resting state, and the newly resulting activity level, as, for instance, the stimulus-induced (or task-related) activity. This means that the interaction between the resting-state activity and the stimulus is encoded in terms of GABA-ergic-mediated neural differences. That makes possible difference-based coding as distinguished from stimulus-based coding where the single stimulus itself independent of the resting-state activity level is encoded into neural activity (see Chapters 2, 6, and 12 in Volume I for details on the relationship between GABA and difference-based coding).

Let us describe the relationship between GABA and difference-based coding in further detail. Due to it inhibitory impact, stronger degrees of GABA-ergic-mediated neural inhibition will lead to the encoding of larger neural differences during rest–rest or rest–stimulus interaction. Following Chapter 28, I now propose the degree of the level of consciousness to be directly dependent upon the degree of spatial and temporal differences as they are encoded into neural activity during rest–rest or rest–stimulus interaction.

The larger the GABA-ergic-mediated neural inhibition and nonlinearity during any change in neural activity, the larger the degree of the spatial and temporal differences that are (or can be) encoded into neural activity, and the higher the degree in the level or state of consciousness that can be associated with the newly resulting activity level, that is, stimulus-induced or task-related activity (or a new resting-state activity level) (see Fig. 29-3e).

NEUROPHENOMENAL HYPOTHESIS IC: LOSS OF GABA-ERGIC-MEDIATED DIFFERENCE-BASED CODING LEADS TO THE LOSS OF CONSCIOUSNESS IN THE VEGETATIVE STATE

What about VS? Due to the apparent decrease in GABA-ergic-mediated neural inhibition, neural activity changes related to stimuli or tasks may no longer be encoded relative to the resting-state activity in VS patients' brains. Instead, the stimuli may be encoded in isolation and thus independent of the resting-state activity; this implies a high degree of stimulus-based coding rather than difference-based coding.

A higher degree of stimulus-based coding, however, makes it less likely for GABA-ergic-mediated nonlinear interaction to occur during rest–stimulus interaction. That in turn decreases the likelihood for the association of the newly resulting activity, i.e., stimulus-induced or task-related activity, with consciousness and its phenomenal features. One would consequently propose that stimulus-induced or task-related activity is present, whereas consciousness, due to the lack of GABA-ergic-mediated nonlinear interaction, may be absent. Interestingly, this is exactly what the data show (see also Chapter 28): presence of stimulus-induced or task-related activity, absence of consciousness. However, while explaining the neuronal mechanisms that supposedly allow to associate the stimulus-induced or task-related activity with the level or state of consciousness in general, we remained unclear about qualia in particular as the phenomenal hallmark of consciousness.

Why does the here-described association of stimulus-induced or task-related activity with consciousness generate qualia, including their various phenomenal and qualitative features; that is, the "what it is like"? This is the question of the neuronal mechanisms that underlie the various phenomenal features of qualia in particular. I propose the resting-state activity itself and more specifically the different layers of its spatiotemporal organization to be central. Since that leads us deeply into the phenomenal territory of qualia, I discuss the details of such neurophenomenal linkage in the next chapter.

NEUROMETAPHORICAL EXCURSION IA: BORING PARTY WITH NO "REAL COMMUNICATION" AMONG PARTY GUESTS

How can we better explain and illustrate what exactly happens during rest–stimulus interaction so that the newly resulting stimulus-induced activity is associated with consciousness and its phenomenal features? You recall your imaginary visit to a party in New York in Chapter 28. Now let us go back to New York and that party.

Imagine you are in a gloomy mood, troubled by nagging thoughts about your latest book. You stand in a group of people but cannot really connect with them. Though touching on themes usually relevant to you, the conversation does not reach you. You remain isolated and do not really interact with the group. Your thoughts continue and do not make room for the ones associated with the other people's conversation.

That means that your mood also remains the same; it is not being affected at all by the jovial mood of the other party guests. This corresponds to the situation of mere linear and additive interaction between resting state and stimulus, with both remaining more or less unchanged during their mutual encounter. You somehow notice the other peoples' conversation, but they do not touch and affect you in any way—the stimulus induces stimulus-induced activity, which, however, does not interact with the resting-state activity.

Let us now imagine the following scenario. Some guests have already arrived. They stand and sit in two different groups in the room. While there is much communication within each group, there is also plenty of interaction between the two groups. People run back and forth so that there is constant new mingling and change. Why? Because both groups' people all work in the same tower in the same business—insurance for private houses—with the only difference being the companies where they are employed.

Now another group of people enters the room. They are put off by all the talk about the latest insurance deals. All being professional philosophers, they have no idea about insurance. They thus do not connect at all with the other two groups: no interaction, let alone any integration. Instead, they go to the other end of the room and talk among themselves about the metaphysics of houses (rather than about house insurance). And thereby they almost completely neglect the other two groups, the insurance people.

NEUROMETAPHORICAL EXCURSION IB: THE "REAL PARTY" OF THE BRAIN

How can we compare this to VS? The insurance people and their two groups correspond to the resting state, while their lively communication stands for rest–rest interaction. The group of philosophers, the newly arriving people, can be compared to the stimulus entering the brain and its resting state. And in the same way the professional background of the philosophers did not match at all with the ones already being there, the insurance people, the new stimulus' statistical structure does not match at all with the one of the resting-state activity.

There is consequently not much exchange between the insurance people, that is, the resting state, and the philosophers, that is, the stimulus. Instead, both operate largely in parallel and segregated from each other in different parts of the room. Analogously, the stimulus in VS does not really interact and integrate at all with the resting-state activity. Resting state and stimulus-induced activity do operate consequently in parallel and are segregated, showing, if at all, merely linear and additive interaction. This is the situation in VS.

Let us describe the scenario in further detail. There is plenty of local interaction in the different parts of the rooms within each group, while there is no global interaction across the different parts of the room and the different groups. Hence, there is not much difference between each group meeting at their respective workplace or at the party. The people, insurance managers and philosophers, do what they usually do anyway, talking among themselves without much contact with the world outside of their respective professions. In other words, the party is not a "real" party, which would imply real interaction among all the people, independent of their respective professional backgrounds.

The situation is analogous in VS. The stimulus does what it does anyway; it elicits stimulus-induced activity in very much the same way as the philosophers and insurance people do what they do anyway, talking about insurance or philosophy. That corresponds well to the local interactions within the different parts of the rooms, as observed during the party. Such local interaction is, however, no longer accompanied by global interaction as manifest in the spatial and temporal spread and propagation of neural activity; this corresponds well to the lacking global interaction between the different groups across the whole room.

What is the consequence of such a lack of global interaction? The party is not a "real" party and is therefore not much different from any workplace meeting. The same now happens in VS. The stimulus-induced activity is similarly not "real" because it is no longer associated with consciousness. In the same way the guests are at a party but do not behave like that, the stimulus elicits stimulus-induced activity that does not properly "behave" because it no longer interacts with the resting-state activity in order to triggers its association with consciousness.

Accordingly, the stimulus-induced activity is in itself thus not principally different from the one elicited by any other stimulus in the healthy brain. However, despite the apparent similarity on the surface, the stimulus-induced activity can no longer take part in a "real" party of the brain, because the brain cannot associate its own stimulus-induced activity with consciousness anymore.

Neurometaphorical Excursion IC: "Coincidental Presence" versus "Real Communication"

What do we learn from this? One should not confuse stimulus-induced activity and consciousness. As described above, both are supposedly entertained by different neuronal mechanisms. To infer the presence of consciousness from the presence of stimulus-induced or task-related activity is to confuse their different underlying neuronal mechanisms. This is why any kind of "neuronal-phenomenal inference" does not work. The example of VS tells us exactly that, that the neuronal mechanisms underlying stimulus-induced or task-related activity and those related to the latter's association with consciousness different, they are two different ballgames.

That is exactly what we can also learn from our party. To suggest that interaction took place between the insurance managers and the philosophers from their mere concurrent presence in the same room at the same party is to confuse their "coincidental presence" with "real communication." In the same way stimulus-induced and resting-state activity are concurrently present in VS, both groups of people, insurance and philosophers, are present in the same room at the same time. That, however, does not yet imply that they really talk to and communicate with each other.

Hence, to infer the presence of interaction from their mere concurrent presence in one and the same room is to false positively identify "real communication" and "coincidental presence" between different people. The different groups of people are merely coincidentally present in one and the same room but do not really interact and communicate with each other. In the same way, both stimulus-induced and resting-state activity are coincidentally present in VS without really interacting and communicating with each other.

What does the difference between "real interaction" and "coincidental presence" imply for the party itself? Interaction among people makes a party a "real" party. The same is true in the case of the brain. The proper kind of rest–stimulus interaction and the consequent association of stimulus-induced activity with consciousness make the party of the brain a "real" party. Therefore, rest–stimulus interaction makes the party of the brain a "real" party which we will be able to enjoy fully; namely, on the basis of our consciousness.

VS patients, in contrast, are no longer able to enjoy the party of their brain due the absence of proper rest–stimulus interaction. Most important, the example of VS reminds and tells us how important our brain's "real" party with "real interaction," rather than mere "coincidental presence," is for us and our very human life and existence. No life is worth living without consciousness and our brain's "real" party. In short, no life without party and interaction.

Open Questions

The first question pertains to the exact mechanisms of rest–stimulus interaction. The concept of nonlinear and nonadditive interaction is basically a negative concept. It describes only what does not happen during rest–stimulus interaction: resting-state-related activity and stimulus-related activity do not interact in a linear and additive way.

In contrast, the concept of nonlinear and nonadditive interaction does not describe what exactly must happen during rest–stimulus interaction in order for it to yield nonlinear and nonadditive effects. Future investigations will therefore want to apply some nonlinear tools for statistical analyses of, for instance, rest–stimulus interaction, which would then also provide a way to test our hypotheses of absent nonlinearity during rest–stimulus interaction in VS.

The characterization of nonlinearity by GABA-ergic-mediated neural inhibition provides a first, though insufficient, step in this direction. We need to know, for instance, the exact neuronal features in the resting state itself that allow the stimulus to impinge upon the resting state in order to merge and fuse with it. At the same time, the stimulus forces the resting-state activity to change its level of activity (and most likely other yet-unknown neuronal features, too) that may be essential for its impact on stimulus-induced activity.

The more detailed characterization of the nonlinear and nonadditive rest–stimulus interaction may then also shed a better light on how and why the stimulus and its stimulus-induced activity can (or cannot) be associated with consciousness. The better insight into the nonlinear mechanisms may then also open the door for us to investigate our hypothesis of the transfer and carryover of the resting state's prephenomenal structures to the resulting stimulus-induced or task-related activity.

This will make the transition from the prephenomenal structures of the resting state to the phenomenal realm of the stimulus-induced activity clearer. More specifically, one would like to know how the resting state's prephenomenal structures surface and are manifested in the phenomenal features of qualia during stimulus-induced activity. That will be the focus in the next chapter.

CHAPTER 30
Neuronal Transfer and Qualia

Summary

So far, I have discussed how the neuronal mechanisms underlying the resting-state activity itself (Chapter 28) and rest–stimulus interaction (Chapter 29) constitute qualia and thus consciousness. However, I left unresolved how it is possible for them to constitute the specific phenomenal features associated with the concept of qualia. This is the focus in the present chapter. I propose what I call the "transfer hypothesis of qualia." The transfer hypothesis of qualia suggests that the various phenomenal features of qualia can be traced back to the spatiotemporal structures constituted by the neuronal activity in the resting state. This means that the resting-state activity's spatiotemporal structures like spatiotemporal continuity, spatiotemporal unity, and self-specific and preintentional organization are manifest in the phenomenal features of qualia. That is possible only if they are carried over and transferred to the stimulus itself and its underlying stimulus-induced (or task-related) activity. Based on such carryover and transfer, I here suggest the following neurophenomenal relationships: (1) the spatial and temporal coincidence of the stimulus with the spatial and temporal features of the resting-state activity may correspond on the phenomenal side to what has been described as *nonstructural homogeneity*; (2) the degree of spatial and temporal differences encoded into neural activity during rest–stimulus interaction may be related to what is expressed phenomenally by the terms *availability* and *transparency* of particular contents in qualia; (3) the degree to which the stimulus (or task) and its particular statistical structure can be coupled to the resting-state activity's low-frequency fluctuations may correspond on the phenomenal side to what is referred as *ipseity*, which connotes the presence of a point of view with a spatiotemporal field in consciousness. Taking all these together, one may want to characterize qualia as a "final common neurophenomenal pathway" during the interaction between the brain's intrinsic resting-state activity and the extrinsic stimuli (or tasks) from body and environment.

Key Concepts and Topics Covered

Qualia, rest–stimulus interaction, phenomenal features of qualia, ipseity, transparency, nonstructural homogeneity, nonlinearity, difference-based coding, subjectivity, environment–brain unity

NEUROEMPIRICAL BACKGROUND IA: NEURAL *PREDISPOSITIONS* AND NEURAL *CORRELATES* OF THE *CONTENTS* OF CONSCIOUSNESS

We have come a long way. We have covered many different territories, starting from the brain's intrinsic activity over extrinsic stimuli, to stimulus-induced or task-related activity and its association with consciousness. This gave us plenty of insights into different neuronal mechanisms that were postulated to be necessary for possible consciousness and sufficient for actual consciousness. In other words, we determined the neural predispositions and neural correlates (which also include the neural prerequisites) of consciousness (see the second Introduction for this distinction).

As outlined in the second Introduction (see also Northoff 2013), consciousness is far from being homogenous, however. Consciousness comes in different dimensions, including content, level, and form. The *contents* concern the objects, persons, or events of which we are conscious. The *level* or *state* of consciousness refers to the degree of arousal, while the *form* of consciousness describes the spatiotemporal organization of the contents in subjective experience (see the second Introduction for details).

What are the neural predispositions and neural correlates of the contents, level, and form of consciousness? Let us start with the content of consciousness, which was mainly discussed in Chapters 18 and 19. The low-frequency fluctuations of the intrinsic activity and their phase-power and phase-phase coupling to the high-frequency fluctuations constitute what I described as "prephenomenal unity" in the neural activity of the resting state. Such "prephenomenal unity" predisposes the resting-state activity to link and integrate the different stimuli and their respective stimulus-induced activities into a unified content as we experience them in consciousness. The low-frequency fluctuations and their phase-power and phase-phase coupling to the high-frequency fluctuations can therefore be considered the necessary neural conditions of possible contents in consciousness and thus as their neural predispositions (see Chapter 18 for details, and see Table 30-1).

How about the neural correlates of the contents of consciousness? The high-frequency fluctuations in the gamma range are particularly important in binding the different actual stimuli into one coherent and unified content in terms of a "phenomenal unity" in consciousness (see Chapter 19). This linkage between different stimuli into one unified content has been described as "binding," which neuronally is mediated by cortical synchronization in the gamma range; that is, binding-by-synchronization (see Chapter 19). Therefore, binding and binding-by-synchronization in the gamma range can be considered neural correlates of the contents of consciousness.

We have to be careful, however, not to confuse the contents of consciousness with consciousness itself. The neuronal mechanisms described in Chapters 18 and 19 concern neural predispositions and correlates of the contents themselves and how they are constituted. In contrast, the described neuronal mechanisms do not account by themselves for the association of these contents with the actual state or level of consciousness. For that, we have to search for yet other neuronal mechanisms underlying the level or state of consciousness, which will be the focus in the next section.

Table 30-1 Neural predispositions and correlates of the three dimensions of consciousness (level, form, content)

	Neural predisposition	Neural correlate
Content	*Phase durations* of *low* frequency fluctuations and their *phase-power/phase-phase coupling* with *high* frequency fluctuations in the resting state	*Gamma* frequency fluctuations and their modulation of *"binding"* and *"binding-by-synchronization"* during rest-stimulus interaction
Level	Degree of *spatial and temporal differences* that can *possibly* be encoded into neural activity as thresholded by the resting state	Degree of *spatial and temporal differences* that are *actually* encoded into neural activity during rest-stimulus interaction
Form	Different layers of the *intrinsic* activity's *spatiotemporal organization and structure* in the resting state	Degree of *transfer* of the *intrinsic* activity's *spatiotemporal organization* and structure to the *extrinsic* stimulus during rest-stimulus interaction

The table illustrates the different neuronal mechanisms that are supposed to serve as neural predispositions and neural correlates of the three different dimensions of consciousness, content, level, and form. The neural predispositions and correlates of contents of consciousness were mainly discussed in Chapters 18 and 19. The neural predispositions and correlates of the level of consciousness were the focus in Chapters 28 and 29 and discussed in the context of the vegetative state. Finally, the neural predispositions of the form of consciousness were discussed throughout Parts V to VII. The neural correlates of the form of consciousness and how they link to qualia as the phenomenal correlates of the form of consciousness are the focus in this chapter.

Neuroempirical Background IB: *Possible* Degree of Encoded Differences as Neural *Predisposition* of the *Level* of Consciousness

Chapters 28 and 29 investigated various neuronal mechanisms that allow for the association of consciousness with stimulus-induced or task-related activity in the brain. I postulated three different hypotheses of consciousness: the "biophysical spectrum of consciousness," the "nonlinearity hypothesis of consciousness," and the "difference-based coding hypothesis of consciousness." Let us quickly review them in order to link them to qualia and their phenomenal features.

The "biophysical-computational spectrum hypothesis of consciousness" describes that the position of the brain's actual neural operation relative to its underlying biophysical-computational spectrum predisposes its possible degree of difference-based coding; the degree of difference-based coding in turn predicts the possible degree of the level or state of consciousness that can be associated with the brain's neural activity (see Chapter 28). The more the brain's neural operations are "located" in the middle of its own underlying biophysical-computational spectrum, the higher the possible degree of difference-based coding, and the higher the possible level or state of consciousness that can be associated with the otherwise purely neuronal resting state and stimulus-induced activity.

The "biophysical-computational spectrum hypothesis of consciousness" is connected to another hypothesis. The "nonlinearity hypothesis of consciousness" points out the central relevance of GABAergic-mediated neural inhibition and its introduction of nonlinearity during rest–stimulus (or rest–rest) interaction (see Chapter 29). The higher the degree of gaba-ergic-mediated nonlinearity during rest–stimulus (or rest–rest) interaction, the more likely it is that the newly resulting purely neuronal activity level, i.e., stimulus-induced or task-related activity, will be associated with consciousness and its phenomenal features.

Why does the introduction of GABAergic-mediated nonlinearity during rest–stimulus interaction lead to the association of consciousness with the otherwise purely neuronal stimulus-induced or resting-state activity? GABA-ergic-mediated neural inhibition increases the degree of spatial and temporal differences that can possibly be encoded into neural activity, which makes it likelier that the changes in neural activity will become associated with consciousness.

Taken together, both hypotheses—"biophysical spectrum of consciousness" and "nonlinearity hypothesis of consciousness"—concern neuronal mechanisms that determine how the brain itself can manipulate its own neural activity by setting the range for the degree of the spatial and temporal differences that can possibly be encoded into its own neural activity.

Since I suppose the degree of the encoded spatial and temporal differences to be central especially for the level or state of consciousness, the brain itself has a "strong say" in whether its own neural activity can possibly be associated with consciousness. Therefore, I consider both the "biophysical spectrum of consciousness" and the "nonlinearity hypothesis of consciousness" to describe the necessary neural conditions of the possible level or state of consciousness. Accordingly, both hypotheses concern what I refer to as "neural predispositions of the level of consciousness" (NPC) (see second Introduction).

Neuroempirical Background IC: Degree of *Actually* Encoded Differences as Neural *Correlate* of the *Level* of Consciousness

The "nonlinearity hypothesis of consciousness" shares with the "biophysical-computational spectrum hypothesis of consciousness" the focus on the encoding of spatial and temporal differences into neural activity. Both hypotheses target neural mechanisms that determine how the brain itself can actively manipulate and thus predispose the degree of spatial and temporal differences that it can possibly encode into its own neural activity.

Accordingly, both hypotheses converge into difference-based coding, and more specifically, the degree of spatial and temporal differences that are actually encoded into neural activity. The degree of the actually encoded temporal and spatial differences can consequently be considered the final common neural pathway into which both the brain's actual position (relative to its biophysical-computational spectrum) and its possible degree of nonlinearity (via GABA-ergic-mediated inhibition) converge.

Based on these considerations, I suggested the "difference-based coding hypothesis of consciousness" (see Chapters 28 and 29). The "difference-based coding hypothesis of consciousness" postulates that the degree of spatial and temporal difference that are (or can be) encoded into neural activity determines the actual degree of the level or state of consciousness. The degree of the actually encoded spatial and temporal differences can thus be regarded as a sufficient neural condition of the level or state of consciousness and thus as a neural correlate of the level of consciousness (NCC).

How are the three hypotheses related to each other? All three hypotheses go hand in hand by targeting either the possible or the actual degree of the encoded spatial and temporal differences via difference-based coding. The "difference-based coding hypothesis of consciousness" as the neural correlate of consciousness stands consequently on the shoulders of the neural predispositions of consciousness, the "biophysical spectrum hypothesis of consciousness," and the "nonlinearity hypothesis of consciousness."

NEURONAL HYPOTHESIS IA: DIFFERENT LAYERS OF THE INTRINSIC ACTIVITY'S *SPATIOTEMPORAL STRUCTURE* AS NEURAL *PREDISPOSITION* OF THE *FORM* OF CONSCIOUSNESS

Where does this leave us? So far, I have I determined the neural predispositions and the neural correlates of the level or state of consciousness (see Chapters 28 and 29 for details). This complemented my account of the contents of consciousness, whose neural predispositions and neural correlates I discussed in Chapters 18 and 19. That, however, leaves open the question of the neural predispositions and neural correlates of the third dimension of consciousness, the *form* of consciousness (see the second Introduction for details, as well as Northoff 2013).

The concept of the "form" of consciousness refers to how the contents in consciousness are structured and organized in spatial and temporal terms (see the second Introduction as well as Northoff 2013 for details). What are the neuronal mechanisms underlying the form of consciousness? For that the answer, I delved deeply into the brain's intrinsic activity, its resting-state activity, and described how its neural activity is structured and organized in different layers. These included the spatiotemporal continuity (Part V), spatiotemporal unity (Part VI), and self-specific and pre-intentional organization (Part VII) of the resting state's neural activity.

Most important, these different layers in the structure and organization of the brain's intrinsic activity were suggested to make possible and thus predispose how the contents of consciousness are structured and organized in spatial and temporal terms. The spatiotemporal continuity of the brain's intrinsic activity was postulated to predispose "inner time and space consciousness," the spatiotemporal unity predisposes the unity of consciousness, and the self-specific and preintentional organization predisposes the self-perspectival and intentional organization of consciousness.

What exactly did I do here? I described the neural mechanisms that are necessary to make possible a certain spatial and temporal organization of the contents in consciousness. Therefore, I consider the different layers of the intrinsic activity's spatiotemporal organization and structure as the neural predisposition of the form of consciousness. More specifically, the spatiotemporal continuity and unity of the brain's intrinsic activity, as well as its self-specific and preintentional organization, must be considered neural predispositions of consciousness.

NEURONAL HYPOTHESIS IB: *QUALIA* AS THE *PHENOMENAL CORRELATE* OF THE *FORM* OF CONSCIOUSNESS

This leaves open, however, the question of what are the sufficient neural conditions and thus the neural correlates of the form of consciousness. The focus in this chapter is on the neural correlates of the form of consciousness, as distinguished from its neural predispositions.

What are the neuronal mechanisms that are sufficient to actually realize and implement (rather than predispose) the form in consciousness? I will postulate that the brain's intrinsic activity and the extrinsic stimuli from the environment must interact in a certain way in order to enable the carryover and transfer of the different layers of the intrinsic activity's spatiotemporal structure and organization to the extrinsic stimulus. Let me explicate this carryover and transfer in a first try. By linking and integrating the extrinsic stimulus to the spatiotemporal structure and organization of the brain's intrinsic activity, the contents associated with the stimulus can be spatially and temporally structured and organized which in turn allows to associate consciousness to them. Therefore, I postulate that the neuronal transfer of the intrinsic activity's spatiotemporal organization and structure to the extrinsic stimulus during rest–stimulus interaction is a sufficient neural condition, and thus neural correlate, of the form of consciousness. Rather than on rest–stimulus interaction itself (see Chapters 11 and 29), I will therefore focus in this chapter on the transfer itself.

How is this transfer of the intrinsic activity's spatiotemporal structure and organization manifested on the phenomenal level of consciousness? This concerns the question of the phenomenal correlates of what I described as the "form of consciousness." I postulate that what I described empirically as the form of consciousness is manifested on the phenomenal level of consciousness in the gestalt of qualia.

What are qualia? *Qualia* refer to the "what it is like" of our experience (see later in this chapter, as well as the second Introduction) and can therefore be characterized by both qualitative and phenomenal features (see later). I now postulate that the qualitative features of qualia are closely related to the form of consciousness. There is a spatiotemporal continuity and unity to qualia in our subjective experience. Moreover qualia are self-perspectival and intentional. Accordingly, the different layers of the intrinsic activity's spatiotemporal organization and structure seem to converge in qualia.

Qualia can therefore be considered the sufficient phenomenal condition and thus a phenomenal correlate of what I described empirically as the form of consciousness. How, then, are the earlier-suggested neuronal carryover and transfer during rest–stimulus interaction related to the qualia as the phenomenal correlates of the form of consciousness? This is the guiding question in this chapter.

NEURONAL HYPOTHESIS IC: *"NEURONAL TRANSFER"* OF THE INTRINSIC ACTIVITY'S *SPATIOTEMPORAL STRUCTURES* TO THE *EXTRINSIC STIMULUS*

What are the neuronal mechanisms that are sufficient to realize and implement qualia as the phenomenal correlate of the form of consciousness? This is the question of the neural correlates of qualia and thus the form of consciousness.

Qualia are usually associated with a particular stimulus and its content. We experience the content in a subjective way from the first-person perspective, which, say the philosophers, can be characterized by "What it is like," which signifies the qualitative and phenomenal feature of qualia. In order to become associated with qualia, the stimulus must undergo some changes. First, it must be transformed into content, as we discussed, especially in Chapters 18 and 19. Secondly, that content must be associated with consciousness in general and qualia in particular. This is the focus in the present chapter.

What exactly happens to the extrinsic stimulus when it "wants to be processed" in the brain? The stimulus must encounter the brain's intrinsic activity and the different layers of its spatiotemporal structures. This means that the extrinsic stimulus must be linked and integrated to the intrinsic activity in order to be processed by the brain. There is therefore what I described as rest–stimulus interaction. The exact neuronal mechanisms of rest–stimulus interaction were discussed in Chapters 11 (in Volume I) and 29. This, however, left open what such rest–stimulus interaction implies for the phenomenal features of consciousness and thus for qualia.

What do the merger and integration between intrinsic activity and extrinsic stimulus during rest–stimulus interaction imply for the extrinsic stimulus itself? The stimulus' merger, fusion, and integration with the brain's resting-state activity make it possible for the latter's spatiotemporal structures to be carried over and transferred to the former, the stimulus and its associated contents.

What do I mean by "carryover and transfer"? Let us first describe the "carryover and transfer" in metaphorical terms. Metaphorically put, the stimulus "gets something additional" from the resting-state activity that "goes beyond" the stimulus itself and its features (see also Chapter 19). That "something additional" provides the stimulus (or task) with something that is not included in the stimulus (or task) itself.

NEURONAL HYPOTHESIS ID: *"NEURONAL TRANSFER"* AS THE NEURAL *CORRELATE* OF *QUALIA* AS THE *FORM* OF CONSCIOUSNESS

What exactly is this "something additional" the stimulus gets during rest–stimulus interaction? I postulate that this "something additional" consists of the different layers of the intrinsic activity's spatiotemporal structures. The linkage and integration to the spatiotemporal structures of the brain's intrinsic activity strongly affect and modulate the stimulus itself.

The stimulus is now integrated and embedded into the spatiotemporal continuity, the spatiotemporal unity, and the self-specific and preintentional organization of the resting state's neural activity. This means that the stimulus becomes spatially and temporally structured and organized. I now postulate that this spatial and temporal structure accounts for the various qualitative and phenomenal features of qualia on the phenomenal level of consciousness, as I will demonstrate below.

Based on these considerations, I propose what I describe as the "transfer hypothesis of qualia." The "transfer hypothesis of qualia" proposes the degree of qualia (and thus consciousness; see later for their conceptual relation) to be directly dependent upon the degree of transfer and carryover of the resting-state activity's spatiotemporal structures to the stimulus and its associated stimulus-induced activity. The better

the stimulus can be integrated and merged with the resting-state activity, the higher the degree of transfer and carryover of the latter's spatiotemporal structures to the stimulus, and the higher the degree of qualia (and thus consciousness) that can be associated with the resulting stimulus-induced (or task-related) activity (see Fig. 30-1a).

NEUROMETAPHORICAL EXCURSION IA: MERGER BETWEEN HIGHWAYS RESULTS IN QUALIA

How can we better illustrate exactly what happens during the encounter between intrinsic activity and extrinsic stimuli and how that leads to the association of the resulting stimulus-induced activity with consciousness? For that I briefly invoke another metaphorical comparison.

One may want to compare the merger, fusion, and integration between resting state and stimulus to the merging of two different highways. Imagine two highways, with each having four lanes. This makes a total of eight lanes. These eight lanes are now merged into five lanes in the new highway. The various cars riding on each highway must thus spatially (i.e., the lanes they are riding in) and temporally (i.e., their speed) reorganize and "restructure" themselves to make it into the new highway and its five lanes. After the merger and fusion of the two highways, one can consequently no longer distinguish the cars coming from one highway and those from the other.

In the same way that the new highway with the five lanes is the final common highway for the other two highways, the resulting stimulus-induced activity is the final common neuronal pathway for both stimulus and resting state (that is, like the different lanes of the highway, come into the brain from different directions). The more and better the two "highways" called *stimulus* and *resting state* merge, fuse, and integrate, the higher the degree of their unification into one unified highway.

In the case of the brain, this unified highway is described as *stimulus-induced* (or *task-related*) activity, while on the phenomenal level of consciousness, one may rather speak of *qualia* to signify such unified highway. Qualia can thus

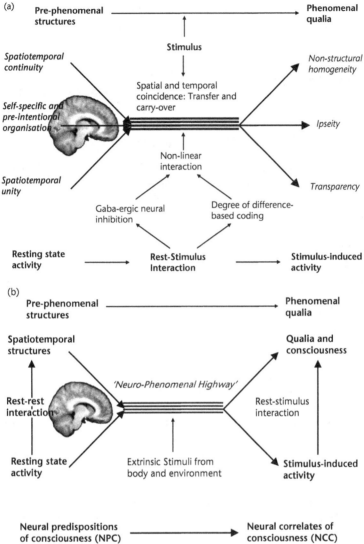

Figure 30-1a and b "Transfer hypothesis" of qualia. The figure demonstrates the various aspects of the "transfer hypothesis of qualia," like the carryover and transfer of the resting state's prephenomenal structures (*a*), and the "neurophenomenal highway" (*b*). (*a*) The figure depicts in the upper part how the resting state's prephenomenal spatiotemporal structures (*left upper part*) are carried over and transferred (*middle upper part*) to the phenomenal level and thus the phenomenal features of qualia (*right upper part*) during rest–stimulus interaction (*lower part*). I propose that, in order for such transfer and carryover to be possible, rest–stimulus interaction must be nonlinear as mediated by GABA-ergic neural inhibition and difference-based coding (*lower middle part*), which makes possible their statistically based matching between resting-state activity and stimulus with regard to spatial and temporal coincidence. I thus suggest that the purely neuronal rest–stimulus interaction makes possible the carryover and transfer of the resting state's prephenomenal spatiotemporal structure to a phenomenal state with qualia. More specifically, I hypothesize the resting-state activity's spatiotemporal continuity to correspond on the phenomenal side to nonstructural homogeneity, self-specific and preintentional organization may correspond to ipseity, and spatiotemporal unity may be equivalent to transparency. (*b*) The figure illustrates basically the same, now indicating that the carryover and transfer link the neural predispositions and the neural correlates of consciousness (*lower part*). The convergence and integration between intrinsic activity and extrinsic stimulus is described as a common functional final pathway, or better, as a "neurophenomenal highway."

be considered the "final common phenomenal pathway" of consciousness.

NEUROMETAPHORICAL EXCURSION
IB: HIGHWAYS FOR CARS AND QUALIA

How does the assumption of qualia as the "final common phenomenal pathway" relate to our example of the highways? In the same way that the two highways' eight lanes merge into one highway with five lanes, the resting-state activity's various spatiotemporal structures are merged into one phenomenal feature called qualia. The different cars and their drivers need to spatially and temporally reorganize themselves in order to enter the five lanes of the new highway.

Analogously, the resting-state activity's spatiotemporal structures resurface (see the neuroconceptual account at the end of this chapter for the more detailed conceptual account of the concept of "resurfacing") in a slightly different spatiotemporal arrangement in the resulting phenomenal state as signified by qualia. Qualia are consequently nothing but the merged highway of consciousness, its "final common phenomenal pathway," that results from a "neurophenomenal highway" where the different highways called intrinsic resting-state activity and extrinsic stimuli/tasks are in the process of converging, fusing, integrating, and merging (see Fig. 30-1b).

Imagine now yet another scenario. The two highways and their four lanes each are not really merged with each other. Instead, all the lanes of the two highways are simply continued and run parallel. This results in one highway with eight lanes. What do the drivers from each highway do? Unlike in the first case, they do not change anything in their spatial and temporal position; that is, speed-wise and lane-wise, but simply continue in the same lane as they did before.

This corresponds to the case when resting-state activity and stimulus-induced activity are processed in merely a parallel and segregated way. Although you as a driver may appreciate such processing in the case of the highway, you as a person may no longer be able to experience such appreciation in the case of parallel and segregated processing between stimuli and the resting state

activity in the brain. Why? You would lose consciousness and fall into a vegetative state and ultimately into a coma (see Chapter 29).

NEUROPHENOMENAL HYPOTHESIS IA:
"NEURAL OVERLAP AND COINCIDENCE" BETWEEN INTRINSIC RESTING-STATE ACTIVITY AND EXTRINSIC STIMULI DURING REST–STIMULUS INTERACTION

How does the transfer of the different layers of the intrinsic activity's spatiotemporal structures during rest–stimulus interaction lead to qualia? After having postulated a particular neuronal mechanism—that is, neuronal transfer during rest–stimulus interaction—we now need to explain why and how such a neuronal transfer realizes and implements the various phenomenal and qualitative features of qualia. I will focus here on three such features: the non-structural homogeneity, transparency, and ipseity of qualia (see below for exact definitions). Let us start with the first feature, non-structural homogeneity.

How exactly does the stimulus interact with the resting-state activity so that both can merge and fuse with each other? One central principle of rest–stimulus interaction is spatial and temporal coincidence (see Chapters 10 and 11 in Volume I for details). Spatial and temporal coincidence describe that the spatial and temporal patterns of the resting state may overlap and thus coincide with the ones of the stimulus. There is thus neural overlap and coincidence between resting state and stimulus.

What exactly does such neural overlap and coincidence mean? The resting-state activity is characterized by temporal features like its low-frequency fluctuations that exhibit, for instance, certain durations in their fluctuating phases. In addition, the resting-state activity is also characterized by functional connectivity that spans across the spatial and temporal differences between the different regions' neural activities within the brain.

How are these spatial and temporal features of the resting-state activity now related to the ones of the stimuli? The stimuli exhibit spatial features in their occurrence across different discrete points in space. For instance, stimulus a occurs at point *x*, while stimulus *b* appears at point *y*. The same on the temporal side: the temporal distances between the distinct discrete points in time *w* and *v* at which the same stimulus *f* occurs two times may be central for the coding of the subsequent neural activity. This presupposes difference-based coding. "Difference-based coding" describes that the temporal and spatial differences between different discrete points in physical time and space are encoded into neural activity rather than the discrete points in physical time and space themselves (see Part I in Volume I).

In other words, the neural activity encodes the stimuli's temporal and spatial differences across different discrete points in time and space (i.e., their statistical frequency distributions) rather than the stimuli themselves, including their discrete points in time and space. This has major implications not only for rest–stimulus interaction itself, but also for the phenomenal features of qualia, as we will see below.

NEUROPHENOMENAL HYPOTHESIS IB: "STATISTICALLY BASED HOMOGENEITY" BETWEEN INTRINSIC RESTING-STATE ACTIVITY AND EXTRINSIC STIMULI DURING REST–STIMULUS INTERACTION

What does the postulated "neural overlap and coincidence" between resting-state activity and stimuli during rest–stimulus interaction imply for the stimuli themselves? The better the stimuli match and thus coincide in the statistical distribution of their spatial and temporal features with the statistics of the spatial and temporal features of the resting-state activity, the more easily the latter can encode the former. And the better the stimuli are encoded by the resting-state activity, the better both can fuse, merge, and integrate, which in turn makes possible higher degrees of nonlinearity during rest–stimulus interaction.

Rest–stimulus interaction and its nonlinearity may consequently be characterized as a statistically based matching process where two different statistical distributions, the one from the stimulus and the one from the resting state, are matched and compared with each other. Such statistically based matching processes make

possible what I earlier described as the "neural overlap and coincidence" between intrinsic resting-state activity and extrinsic stimuli.

Such statistically based matching between the statistical frequency distributions of resting-state activity and stimuli has important implications, especially for the stimuli themselves. If they match well with each other, the extrinsic stimulus and its discrete point in time and space become indistinguishable from the intrinsic resting-state activity's spatial and temporal structures in the newly resulting neural activity. This may result in what one may want to describe as "statistically based homogeneity" in the neural activity between stimulus and resting state signifying neural overlap and coincidence.

We have to be careful though. The here-postulated "statistically based homogeneity" of neural activity during rest–stimulus interaction must be distinguished from the case when the stimulus is not matched at all with the resting-state activity's spatial and temporal features. What is encoded into the newly resulting neural activity is then no longer the "neural overlap and coincidence" between extrinsic stimuli and intrinsic resting-state activity, but rather the single physical stimuli by themselves, at their particular discrete points in time and space. Since the newly resulting activity is then mainly based on the physical features of the single stimuli themselves, one may want to speak of a "physically based heterogeneity" rather than "statistically based homogeneity" of neural activity during rest–stimulus interaction.

NEUROPHENOMENAL HYPOTHESIS IC: PHENOMENAL CHARACTERIZATION OF THE "NONSTRUCTURAL HOMOGENEITY" OF QUALIA

How is such "statistically based homogeneity" of neural activity during rest–stimulus interaction manifested on the phenomenal level of qualia? For that the answer, I turn to "nonstructural homogeneity," which is considered one central phenomenal feature of qualia.

Nonstructural homogeneity" or "wholeness" describes that segregation and distinction of experience and thus of qualia into different parts and elements remains impossible (Gadenne 1996, 26–28). This is proposed to account for what phenomenally is described by the terms of simplicity and monadicity/atomicity and spatial and temporal homogeneity of qualia (Levine 1983, 357–359; 1990, 478; 1993, see also Northoff and Heinzel 2003).

Besides nonstructural homogeneity, the "feeling of direct contact" is often considered as another phenomenal feature of qualia. The phenomenal concept of feeling of direct contact describes the experience of being in direct contact to the content in consciousness. That is further detailed in other phenomenal terms like "feeling of completeness," "lucidity," "immediateness," and "phenomenal certainty" as phenomenal features of qualia (see Metzinger 1995, 25–27, Northoff and Heinzel 2003). The concept of "lucidity" describes the direct givenness of the event, which is experienced as direct part of the world itself (rather than being part of the subject itself). "Immediateness" points out that the event is experienced without any further mediation, while "phenomenal certainty" signifies the experience of an absolute conviction about the event or object in question.

NEUROPHENOMENAL HYPOTHESIS ID: "STATISTICALLY BASED HOMOGENEITY" DURING REST–STIMULUS INTERACTION "RESURFACES" IN THE "NONSTRUCTURAL HOMOGENEITY" ON THE PHENOMENAL LEVEL OF QUALIA

How are these phenomenal features of qualia related to the earlier suggested statistically based homogeneity of neural activity during rest–stimulus interaction? I propose that the phenomenal features of nonstructural homogeneity and feeling of direct contact are directly related to the "statistically based homogeneity" of neural activity during rest–stimulus interaction.

This means that the resting state's degree of spatial and temporal coincidence with the statistical frequency distribution of the stimulus may be central in allowing not only for homogeneity on the level of neural activity, i.e., statistically based homogeneity, but also for homogeneity on the phenomenal level, i.e., non-structural

homogeneity. I thus suggest that the "statistically based homogeneity" on the neuronal level resurfaces (see the neuroconceptual account at the end of this chapter for a more detailed account of the concept of "resurface") on the phenomenal level in "non-structural homogeneity."

I propose the following relationship: the more the stimuli's spatial and temporal features coincide statistically with those of the resting-state activity's neuronal spatial and temporal measures, the likelier it is that the stimulus will appear as "homogeneous and nonstructural" on the phenomenal level of qualia (see Fig. 30-2a).

Furthermore, the more the stimulus and its statistical frequency distribution are integrated, fused, and merged with the resting-state activity's statistical frequency distribution (of its spatial and temporal measures), the likelier it is that the extrinsic stimulus will be associated with a feeling of direct contact.

Why? The better the extrinsic stimulus merges, integrates, and fuses with the intrinsic resting-state activity, the closer it is to us and ourselves, including our brain, which phenomenally may be manifested in the "feeling of direct contact." The "feeling of direct contact" on the phenomenal level may thus be traced back neuronally to the merger, integration, and fusion between the extrinsic stimulus from the environment and the intrinsic resting-state activity in the brain.

If my neurophenomenal hypothesis is correct, one would expect both "non-structural homogeneity" and the "feeling of direct contact" to be absent in vegetative state (VS). Due to the earlier-described abnormalities in their resting-state activity, rest–stimulus interaction can no longer generate "statistically based homogeneity" but rather yields only "physically based heterogeneity." That makes "nonstructural homogeneity" and the "feeling of direct contact" on the phenomenal level of consciousness impossible; these are then replaced by what may be described as "structural heterogeneity" and "lack of direct contact."

NEUROPHENOMENAL HYPOTHESIS IE: QUALIA ARE INTRINSICALLY SPATIOTEMPORAL

Let us return to the healthy brain and go into more neurophenomenal detail. How are such

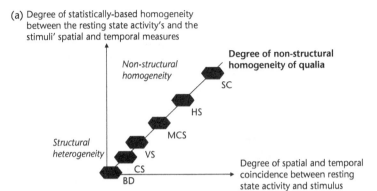

(a) Degree of statistically-based homogeneity between the resting state activity's and the stimuli' spatial and temporal measures

Non-structural homogeneity

Degree of non-structural homogeneity of qualia

SC

HS

MCS

Structural heterogeneity

VS

CS

BD

Degree of spatial and temporal coincidence between resting state activity and stimulus

Figure 30-2a-d Neurophenomenal hypotheses of qualia. The figure demonstrates the relationship between specific neuronal mechanisms during resting-state and stimulus-induced activity and the distinct phenomenal features of qualia. (*a*) The figure shows the dependence of the phenomenal feature of non-structural homogeneity on the degree of statistically based matching between resting-state activity (y-axis) and stimulus and their degree of spatial and temporal coincidence (x-axis). The better resting-state activity and stimuli, for example, their respective spatial and temporal measures, statistically match with each other, the higher their degree of statistically based spatial and temporal coincidence, and the higher the subsequent degree of nonstructural homogeneity in qualia. Obviously I propose coma and vegetative state to be at the lower end of this curve with too low nonstructural homogeneity, while schizophrenia may range at the upper end showing too much nonstructural homogeneity (when compared to healthy subjects). (*b*) The figure shows the dependence of the phenomenal feature of transparency and its phenomenal opposite, opacity, on the degree of differences coded during rest–rest and rest–stimulus interaction (y-axis) and the unavailability of the single stimulus' discrete point in time and space in neural activity (x-axis). The larger the degree of difference-based coding during rest–rest or rest–stimulus interaction, the higher the degree of unavailability of the single stimulus' discrete point in time and space in neural activity, and the higher the degree of transparency in phenomenal qualia, while the converse holds for the phenomenal opposite, opacity. Obviously I propose coma and vegetative state to be at the lower end of this curve with too low transparency, while schizophrenia may range at the upper end showing too much transparency (when compared to healthy subjects). (*c*) The figure symbolically illustrates how the phenomenal feature of ipseity describing "phenomenally based subjectivity" (see later for details) (*upper part*) is based on the point of view and its "biophysically based subjectivity" (*middle part*). That, in turn, is supposed to be traced back to the statistically and spatiotemporally based alignment (dotted lines) between the environment's and the resting state's spatial and temporal measures (*lower part*). That anchors the brain and its species-specific biophysical-computational spectrum within the rest of the physical world (very bottom). Due to such spatiotemporally and statistically based point of view, the respective organism shows a biophysically based subjectivity that provides him with a stance within the physical world (*middle left*). The stimulus needs to be aligned to the environment–brain unity and its point of view, while at the same time it must interact in specific ways, for example, nonlinear, with the resting state. If both conditions (i.e., the two arrows in middle left) are met, the point of view will resurface on the phenomenal level in the gestalt of qualia and more specifically in ipseity as their phenomenal hallmark feature (*upper part*). The point of view becomes thus experienced in consciousness, which I describe as "phenomenally based subjectivity. " (*d*) The figure shows the dependence of the phenomenal feature of ipseity on the degree of neural alignment of the stimuli to the resting state's statistically and spatiotemporally based unity with the environment, the environment–brain unity. The more the stimulus is linked and thus aligned to the resting state's spatiotemporally and statistically based unity with the environment, the environment–brain unity, the higher the alignment of the stimulus to the latter's point of view as stance within the physical world, and the higher the subsequent degree of ipseity on the phenomenal level of qualia. Obviously I propose coma and vegetative state to be at the lower end of this curve with too low ipseity, while schizophrenia may range at the upper end, showing too much ipseity (when compared to healthy subjects). *Abbreviations:* BD, brain death; CS, comatose state; HS, healthy subject; MCS, minimally conscious state; SC, schizophrenia; VS, vegetative state.

(b) Degree of spatial and temporal differences encoded during rest-stimulus interaction

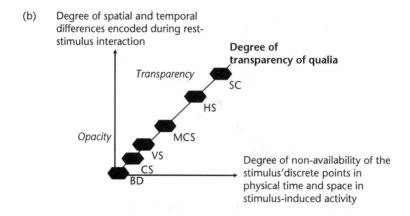

(c)

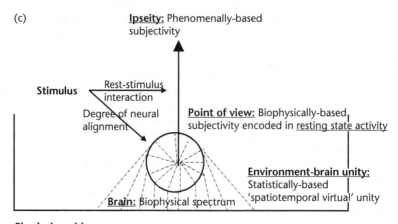

(d) Degree of the stimulus' linkage to the resting state activity's statistically-based spatiotemporal unity with the environment

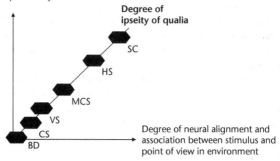

Figure 30-2a-d (Continued)

nonstructural homogeneity and feeling of direct contact related to the neuronal activity of the resting-state activity and its prephenomenal structures? Nonstructural homogeneity and feeling of direct contact are based on the stimulus' integration and merging with the resting-state activity's spatial and temporal measures.

These, as we have seen in Part V, constitute what I described as the 'spatiotemporal continuity' of neuronal activity in the resting state. The integration and merger of the extrinsic stimulus with the intrinsic resting-state activity consequently implies the integration and merger of the stimulus' discrete position in space and time with the resting state's spatiotemporal continuity. This allows for replacing the heterogeneity of the stimulus and its discrete position in physical time and space by the spatial and temporal homogeneity of the resting-state activity's spatiotemporal continuity. The resting-state activity's spatiotemporal continuity is thus transferred and carried over to the stimulus; the stimulus and its single discrete point in time and space are thus integrated embedded into the temporal continuity of the resting state's neural activity. Such integration and embedding is, I suggest, manifested on the phenomenal level in the "nonstructural homogeneity" of qualia.

What does this imply for the characterization of qualia? Due to the integration into the resting-state activity's spatiotemporal structures, qualia must be characterized as intrinsically spatial and temporal. The intrinsically spatial and temporal nature of qualia is well reflected in their phenomenal characterization by what has been described as "spatial and temporal homogeneity" (Levine 1983, 357–359; 1990, 478; 1993, see also Northoff and Heinzel 2003).The phenomenal concept of "spatial and temporal homogeneity" describes that qualia are temporally and spatially unified and thus homogeneous, rather than including different discrete and segregated points in physical time and space.

Qualia may consequently be characterized by a specific spatiotemporal constellation and arrangement on the phenomenal level of consciousness (see also Tononi 2008, who speaks of "qualia space," though in a slightly different context). Such "spatial and temporal homogeneity" of qualia can, I propose, ultimately be traced back to the resting-state activity's spatiotemporal continuity and the degree of its transfer and carryover to the extrinsic stimuli during rest–stimulus interaction.

I therefore characterize qualia as spatiotemporal, and even more strongly state that they are intrinsically spatiotemporal by default. This means that qualia would remain impossible if they were not spatiotemporal. There would be no qualia in the absence of the spatiotemporal structure of the brain's intrinsic resting-state activity and its neuronal transfer to the extrinsic stimulus during rest–stimulus interaction.

Why are qualia intrinsically spatiotemporal? The underlying neuronal mechanisms make it necessary and unavoidable for qualia to be spatiotemporal. Therefore, qualia are by definition and thus intrinsically spatiotemporal. This, though, holds true only in the actual natural world, where we and our brain are located. In contrast, it leaves open the possibility of non-spatiotemporal qualia in a purely logical world. That, though, is not a concern for the neuroscientist and neurophilosopher, but only for the philosopher.

NEUROPHENOMENAL HYPOTHESIS IIA: "NEURONAL BALANCE" BETWEEN "AVAILABILITY" AND "UNAVAILABILITY" OF STIMULI DURING STIMULUS-INDUCED ACTIVITY

What kind of neural coding does such a statistically based matching process between resting-state activity and stimulus imply? What is matched here with each other is nothing but spatial and temporal differences: the stimulus' spatial difference between the points x and y is matched with the spatial differences in the brain's resting state as, for instance, is signified by its functional connectivity. And the stimulus' temporal differences between the points w and v are matched with the temporal differences in the resting state's neural activity as, for instance, is manifested in the phase durations of the resting-state activity's low-frequency fluctuations.

What is encoded into neural activity is thus not the stimuli themselves and their different discrete positions in physical time and space. This would suggest stimulus-based coding. Instead, the spatial and temporal differences between the different stimuli and their respective different discrete points in time and space are encoded into neural activity. This amounts to what I describe as difference-based coding (see Volume I for details).

What does such difference-based coding imply for the single stimulus itself? The single stimulus' discrete position in physical time and space is lost by itself when it is coded in difference to other stimuli's discrete positions in time and space. The only way the single stimulus' discrete position in time and space remains available is in the gestalt of a spatial and temporal difference as encoded into neural activity, while the stimulus' discrete position in time and space as such is by itself no longer available.

The brain's application of difference-based coding to its neural processing of stimuli thus goes along with a loss and a gain. The gain is that different stimuli can be processed in one neural activity as based on their spatial and temporal differences. This is a quite economical coding strategy since, by encoding several stimuli in one sweep of neural activity, the precious metabolic and energetic resources are used in a maximally efficient way (see Chapters 1 and 2 as well as Chapters 28 and 29 for further discussion of the metabolic side of things; see also Hyder et al. 2012).

Such a gain is accompanied by a loss, however. The loss consists of the single discrete positions in physical time and space as associated with the single stimuli themselves. Temporal and spatial differences between different stimuli are well available, while the single discrete positions in time and space remain (more or less) unavailable.

There is thus a neuronal balance between availability and unavailability of the stimuli's discrete positions in physical time and space during stimulus-induced activity. I suppose that ultimately the neural balance between the single stimulus' availability and unavailability

can be traced back to the balance between stimulus- and difference-based coding (see Chapter 28): Higher degrees of stimulus-based coding lead to higher degrees of availability of the single stimulus itself, whereas higher degrees of difference-based coding increase the degree of the single stimuli's degrees of unavailability.

NEUROPHENOMENAL HYPOTHESIS IIB: "NEURONAL BALANCE" BETWEEN "AVAILABILITY" AND "UNAVAILABILITY" OF STIMULI DURING STIMULUS-INDUCED ACTIVITY "RESURFACES" IN THE PHENOMENAL BALANCE BETWEEN TRANSPARENCY AND OPACITY OF CONTENTS DURING QUALIA

How is such a balance between neural availability and unavailability manifest on the phenomenal level of qualia? The unavailability of the stimulus and its single discrete point in time and space is described as "transparency" on the phenomenal level of consciousness. Let us first define the concept of "transparency."

Following philosopher Thomas Metzinger (2003, 163; 1995, 25–27), "transparency" is the quality of something that we can "see through"; we "see through" the contents of consciousness without seeing their underlying properties, like the vehicle that carries the content (see the original definition by G. E. Moore 1903; quoted in Metzinger 2003, 163). For instance, we see the bird flying by, but we do not see the window: "We don't see the window, but only the bird flying by" (Metzinger 2003, 169). There is thus some missing information in our consciousness, e.g., the information of the window is missing in our experience of the bird flying by. Therefore, transparency can be considered as "synonymous to a missing of information" (Metzinger 2003, 175).

What is the phenomenal opposite to transparency? Metzinger yields here the term "opacity." In contrast to transparency, information is no longer missing in the case of opacity. We then see the window, which may cloud our view of seeing the bird flying by. That may, for instance, be the case if the window is extremely dirty. Information about the window is here no longer unavailable but available, leading to stronger degrees of opacity at the expense of transparency. There is thus a phenomenal balance between transparency and opacity in qualia that, following Metzinger, may be related to the balance between unavailable and available.

How is this phenomenal balance between transparency and opacity related to the earlier postulated neuronal balance between the unavailability and availability of the single stimulus in neural activity? I propose the phenomenal balance between transparency and opacity in qualia to be dependent upon the neuronal balance between unavailability and availability of the stimuli's discrete positions in time and space in the associated stimulus-induced activity.

The higher the degree of unavailability of the single stimuli's discrete positions in time and space in neural activity, i.e., stimulus-induced activity, the higher degrees of transparency that can be associated with the stimuli on the phenomenal level of the qualia, and the lower the degrees of opacity. In short, the phenomenal balance may be directly dependent upon the neuronal balance (see Fig. 30-2b).

NEUROPHENOMENAL HYPOTHESIS IIC: ABNORMAL "NEURONAL BALANCE" MEDIATES "PHENOMENAL IMBALANCE" IN VEGETATIVE STATE AND SCHIZOPHRENIA

The scenario can also take place in a reverse way. Higher degrees of neuronal availability of the stimuli's discrete positions in time and space in stimulus-induced activity may then go along with higher degrees of opacity and lower degrees of transparency on the phenomenal level. This is what I propose to be the case in VS.

Due to their decreased degrees of difference-based coding and consequently increased degrees of stimulus-based coding, the different stimuli's discrete positions in time and space are better and more precisely available in neural activity, e.g., stimulus-induced (or task-related) activity. Such increased neuronal availability of the single stimulus by itself, however, shifts the phenomenal balance toward extreme degrees of opacity at the expense of transparency. There may thus be

extremely high degrees of opacity but low degrees of transparency in VS.

What can we learn from VS? Too much neuronal availability of the single stimuli's discrete positions in time and space is not good, since it may lead to the loss of transparency on the phenomenal level of experience. If our brain and its resting-state activity yield too much information about the single stimulus, leading to high degrees of neuronal availability, we seem to remain unable to really enjoy and thus experience such increased availability on a phenomenal level and thus in our consciousness.

However, too much nonavailability of the single stimuli's discrete positions in time and space in not good, either. In this case, we will miss too much information and will not look only through the vehicle, i.e., the window but also through the content itself, i.e., the bird flying by. We then might look through the contents themselves directly into the world and the universe as a whole. Phenomenally, we then show abnormally increased transparency in our qualia, while the degree of opacity will be rather low. What is usually associated phenomenally with the experience of specific contents within the world, the "feeling of direct contact" and non-structural homogeneity, is then related to the world as a whole and the universe as such.

That is, I tentatively propose, the case in schizophrenia, where patients do indeed often experience a "feeling of direct contact" and "non-structural homogeneity" with the world as a whole or the universe. This is often described as "self-transcendence," as is manifested in feeling unified with the world and the universe while being detached and apparently "looking through" its particular contents (see Chapters 22 and 27 as well as chapters 11 and 12 in Northoff 2011 for more details on schizophrenia).

NEUROPHENOMENAL HYPOTHESIS IID: COGNITION- VERSUS CODING-BASED ACCOUNTS OF TRANSPARENCY

Where does the transparency on the phenomenal level of consciousness come from? Metzinger proposes that transparency and opacity are a matter of attention, that is, attentional unavailability: "Phenomenal opacity is simply the degree of attentional availability of earlier processing stages, and the degree depends on how adaptive it was to make these earlier processing stages globally available" (Metzinger 2003, 175). Transparency is here related to (the degree of) attention that is a cognitive function. This presupposes a cognition-based view of transparency and its twin sibling opacity.

However, this differs from my account. Rather than invoking a special cognitive ability or inability like attention to allow for the stimuli's transparency in qualia, I propose their neural coding in terms of spatial and temporal differences into neural activity to be central. The higher the degree of difference-based coding on the neuronal level, the higher the degree of transparency on the phenomenal level of consciousness. In contrast, higher degrees of stimulus-based coding (going along with lower degrees of difference-based coding) are proposed to lead to lower levels of transparency and higher degrees of opacity on the phenomenal level.

I thus suggest a coding-based account of transparency as distinguished from the more cognition-based account by Metzinger. Let us specify my coding-based account of transparency. I propose the stimulus' degree of transparency to depend directly on the degree of difference-based coding of neural activity changes during rest–stimulus interaction. The higher the degree of difference-based coding of the spatial and temporal differences between resting state and stimuli during rest–stimulus interaction, the likelier it is that the stimulus and resting state will be integrated, linked, and merged, and the likelier it is that the stimulus will become unavailable, invisible, and thus "transparent" on the phenomenal level of experience.

By encoding the stimuli's spatial and temporal differences into the spatial and temporal measures of the resting-state activity, the stimuli become also integrated and merged with the resting state's spatiotemporal ongoing continuity and unity of its neuronal activity. The stimulus thus blends in and merges with the statistically based spatiotemporal continuity and unity of the resting state's neural activity. And the better both merge, the higher the degree of the subsequent transparency of the stimulus relative to the resting state and its spatiotemporal continuity and unity.

NEUROPHENOMENAL HYPOTHESIS IIE: "SPATIOTEMPORAL TRANSPARENCY" AS A "NEUROPHENOMENAL BRIDGE CONCEPT"

Finally, one may want to make a more conceptual remark. Metzinger speaks of "phenomenal transparency" and distinguishes it from other forms of transparency: "Epistemic transparency" concerns missed conceptual and propositional information, "semantic transparency" describes missing information in extensional contexts, and "referential transparency" refers to missing information in the context of media as used in the theory of telecommunication (Metzinger, 2003, 170, 339–340, 436; but see Tye 1995, 136; and also Legrand 2005, 8, for slightly different definitions of transparency that, unlike the here-suggested phenomenal determination, refer more to introspection and representation).

Without discussing these different concepts of transparency, I would like to add yet another one to this list: the concept of "spatiotemporal transparency" and its opposite, "spatiotemporal opacity." The concept of "spatiotemporal transparency" describes the availability or unavailability of spatial and temporal information and more specifically information about single discrete points in time and space.

The more information about single discrete points in physical time and space that is available, the higher the degree of subsequent spatiotemporal opacity and the lower the degree of spatiotemporal transparency. In contrast, the reverse holds if less information about single discrete points in physical time and space is available, which then increases the degree of spatiotemporal transparency.

Why do I introduce yet another concept of transparency, that of spatiotemporal transparency? Because I propose it to be central in understanding the implications of difference-based coding for the phenomenal level of qualia and thus what Metzinger describes as "phenomenal transparency."

In other words, my coding-based account of phenomenal transparency makes necessary the introduction of a concept that mediates between the neuronally encoded spatial and temporal differences on one hand, and the phenomenal concept of transparency in the context of qualia on the other. The novel concept of spatiotemporal transparency does not belong to either the phenomenal or neuronal level and can therefore be regarded as a "neurophenomenal bridge concept." In the same way one cannot get from one side of the river to the other without a bridge, we will not be able to bridge the gap between the neuronally encoded spatial and temporal differences on one hand and the phenomenal level of transparency on the other. For that we need a bridge, and that bridge is provided by the concept of spatiotemporal transparency.

NEUROPHENOMENAL HYPOTHESIS IIIA: "ENVIRONMENT–BRAIN UNITY" AND POINT OF VIEW

There is more to qualia, however, than the so-far-discussed phenomenal features of non-structural homogeneity, transparency, and feeling of direct contact. One of the main phenomenal features of qualia is a point of view, a stance from which the experience and its contents are experienced. Such a stance or point of view is often described by the concept of *ipseity* in the context of qualia. Ipseity is considered a phenomenal hallmark of qualia, and therefore is the focus in the next sections.

First, let us go back to the neuronal side of things. The stimulus does not only encounter the resting state itself and the spatiotemporal continuity and unity of its neural activity. In addition, the stimulus also encounters the resting state's statistically based spatiotemporal unity with the environment, the "environment–brain unity." We recall from Chapter 20 that the concept of environment–brain unity describes a spatiotemporal, statistically based, and thus "virtual" unity between the stimuli's occurrences in (the physical time and space of) the environment and the spatial and temporal neuronal measures of the resting state.

How is such environment–brain unity constituted? We proposed that such environment–brain unity is constituted by the degree of neural alignment of the resting state's spatial and temporal neuronal measures (like low-frequency fluctuations and functional connectivity) to the statistically based spatial and temporal features of the stimulus. For instance, based on the empirical data (as described in Chapter 20), the phase durations of the resting state's low-frequency oscillations may couple and thus align themselves to the onset of the stimuli in the environment. Such neural alignment is obviously particularly likely when the stimuli are presented in a rhythmic way in the environment, while the neural alignment is much more difficult when the stimuli are presented in a nonrhythmic way (see Chapter 20 for details).

The constitution of such spatiotemporal 'and statistically based environment–brain unity makes it possible for the respective organism to take a "stance" within the world. The organism occupies a particular spatiotemporal position, which, due to its statistically based nature, must be regarded as "virtual" (rather than being "physically real"). I described such a spatiotemporal, statistically based, and "virtual" position within the world by the concept of "point of view." The point of view describes the stance we as humans take within the world, and it is from these that we can approach the world and its various contents (see Chapter 22 for details; also see Fig. 30-2c).

NEUROPHENOMENAL HYPOTHESIS IIIB: STIMULI MUST BE LINKED TO THE "POINT OF VIEW" AND ITS "BIOPHYSICALLY BASED SUBJECTIVITY" IN ORDER TO BE PROCESSED IN THE BRAIN

Most important, the concept of the point of view also refers to the stance from which we subsequently experience that very same world and its various contents in our consciousness. That let me characterize such a point of view by the concept of "biophysically based subjectivity." (see Chapter 21).

The concept of biophysically based subjectivity describes the spatiotemporal stance of humans within the physical world on the basis of our brain's species-specific biophysical equipment. I propose such biophysically based subjectivity and its underlying neural mechanisms to provide a necessary, non-sufficient bio-physical (and neural) condition of possible consciousness, e.g., a neural predisposition of consciousness (NPC).

As such, biophysically based subjectivity must be distinguished from the concept of "phenomenally based subjectivity" that refers to the subjective nature of consciousness, that is, the manifestation of subjectivity in phenomenal states (see Chapter 21 for details). "Phenomenally based subjectivity" is a phenomenal concept that can be considered a sufficient condition and thus a phenomenal correlate of consciousness; its underlying neuronal mechanism may thus signify the sufficient neural condition of actual consciousness, i.e., the neural correlate of consciousness (NCC).

What does this imply for the environment–brain unity? The environment–brain unity signifies (and constitutes) what I described as "biophysically based subjectivity." This means that the environment–brain unity can be understood as a statistically based "virtual" spatiotemporal field that spans across the physical boundaries between brain, body and environment. As such the environment–brain unity allows the organism to take a "stance" within that world, i.e., a point of view signifying its biophysically based subjectivity. In other words, environment–brain unity, point of view, and biophysically based subjectivity go hand in hand, with all three co-occurring and being dependent upon each other.

What now happens when the environment–brain unity encounters specific stimuli? If the environment–brain unity encounters a stimulus, that stimulus is related and integrated into this spatiotemporal field and its point of view. To put it more strongly, for the stimulus to be processed at all, it must be related to the statistically based virtual spatiotemporal field of the environment–brain unity and hence to its associated point of view. Otherwise, the stimulus will not be processed at all. Accordingly, the linkage of the stimuli to the point of view (of the underlying environment–brain unity) is a necessary condition for the stimuli to be processed at all. This has major implications for the phenomenal level, as we will discuss in the following section.

NEUROPHENOMENAL HYPOTHESIS IIIC: THE "POINT OF VIEW" OF THE "ENVIRONMENT–BRAIN UNITY" RESURFACES IN THE IPSEITY AND THE SPATIOTEMPORAL ORGANIZATION IN QUALIA

How is this relationship of the stimulus to the environment–brain unity's spatiotemporal field and point of view manifested on the phenomenal level of consciousness? I propose that it is closely related to what the philosophers call "ipseity." What is ipseity? "Ipseity" is well defined by Kircher and David (2003, 448):

> Let us first consider what philosophers mean by *ipseity*. The I in every experience (qualia, raw feelings) is implicitly and prereflectively present in the *field of awareness and is crucial to the whole structure. The I is not yet a "pole" but more a field, through which all experiences pass.* This basic self does not arise from any inferential reflection or introspection, because it is not a relation, but an intrinsic property of qualia. When I have a perception of pain, this perception is simultaneously a tacit self-awareness, because my act of perception is given to me in the first-person perspective, *from my point of view and only in my field of awareness. This basic dimension of subjecthood, ipseity, is a medium in which all experience,* including more explicit and thematic reflection, is rendered possible and takes place. (Kircher and David 2003, 448; *emphasis mine*)

How does this characterization of ipseity relate to the above-described environment–brain unity" and its associated point of view? Kircher and David do speak of a "field of awareness and [it] is crucial to the whole structure. The I is not yet a 'pole' but more a field, through which all experiences pass."

What they here describe as a "field" and "structure" may correspond well to the spatiotemporal and statistically based field spanning "virtually" between the environment and the brain's resting state, the environment–brain unity. Every stimulus encounters this spatiotemporal field, the environment–brain unity, and needs to pass "through" it in very much the same way as Kircher and David describe.

Kircher and David also seem to associate such a "field" with a point of view as reflected in the following part of their quote: "from my point of view and only in my field of awareness. This basic dimension of subjecthood, ipseity, is a medium in which all experience." What they here describe as point of view corresponds well to what I earlier characterized as point of view, for example, its underlying environment–brain unity and its relation to the rest of the physical world.

What exactly is a point of view? The point of view is a stance that anchors us in the physical world. At the same time, the point of view provides us with a perspective from which we can experience that very same world, thus being a "basic dimension of subjecthood," as Kircher and David say, or "biophysically based subjectivity" as I conceptualize it. Most important, a point of view in this sense, i.e., as biophysically based subjectivity, is by itself not yet experienced as such and therefore cannot be considered a phenomenal concept; instead, it reflects a prephenomenal concept that describes a neural predisposition rather than a neural correlate of consciousness as stated earlier.

How, though, is such a prephenomenal point of view manifested on the phenomenal level of consciousness? I now suppose that a point of view in such biophysical sense is manifested on the phenomenal level of consciousness in the gestalt of ipseity, which signifies what I described earlier as "phenomenally based subjectivity" (see Fig. 30-2c).

NEUROPHENOMENAL HYPOTHESIS
IIID: "NEURAL ALIGNMENT" OF THE STIMULUS TO THE "ENVIRONMENT–BRAIN UNITY" PREDICTS THE DEGREE OF IPSEITY IN QUALIA

On the basis of these correspondences, I suggest the following hypothesis. I propose the degree of ipseity to depend directly on the degree to which the stimulus is related to and thus aligned with the environment–brain unity; that is, its spatiotemporal field and its associated point of view.

The more the stimulus is aligned to, for instance, the resting state's low-frequency fluctuations and their already established alignment to the spatial and temporal features of the environment, the likelier it is that the stimulus will be associated with the environment–brain unity's

spatiotemporal field and point of view. And that, in turn, makes it more likely to associate a higher degree of specifically ipseity with the stimulus on the phenomenal level in the resulting qualia (see Fig. 30-2d).

I consequently propose that the stimulus needs to be linked, fused, integrated, and merged with the environment–brain unity. The better the stimulus and its spatial and temporal features link, fuse, and merge with the virtual statistically based spatiotemporal field of the environment–brain unity, the likelier it is that the stimulus can be assigned a high degree of ipseity in subsequent consciousness.

Why is this integration between environment–brain unity and stimulus so important? Because it makes possible the stimulus' association or alignment with the point of view as related to the environment–brain unity and its spatiotemporal field. Metaphorically speaking, the stimulus' alignment to the point of view anchors the stimulus in the rest of the physical world, while, at the same time, giving the particular person a particular perspective or stance from which he can experience that very same stimulus as part of the physical world.

NEUROPHENOMENAL HYPOTHESIS
IIIE: DISSOCIATION BETWEEN "BIOPHYSICALLY BASED SUBJECTIVITY" AND "PHENOMENALLY BASED SUBJECTIVITY" IN THE VEGETATIVE STATE

What about VS? I propose such alignment of the stimulus to the environment–brain unity (and its associated point of view) to no longer take place in VS. The stimuli are still processed yielding stimulus-induced activity, as is well observed in the data described in the preceding chapters. However, due to the lack of proper rest–stimulus interaction, the stimulus and its spatial and temporal features are no longer aligned to the spatiotemporal field of the environment–brain unity and its associated point of view.

If, however, the stimulus is no longer linked to the environment–brain unity, the stimulus can no longer be related to the point of view (as associated with the environment–brain unity). That, though, makes impossible (or better, prevents) the possible association of the stimulus with the subject itself so that there is no longer any experience of ipseity on the phenomenal level of consciousness.

Let me put this differently. The biophysically based subjectivity reflecting the environment–brain unity and its point of view can no longer be carried over and transferred to the stimulus in VS. This makes impossible the stimulus' association with ipseity and thus qualia on the phenomenal level as manifestations of phenomenally based subjectivity. I consequently propose a dissociation between biophysically and phenomenally based subjectivity in VS: The biophysically based subjectivity is still preserved by itself. However, due to the lack of proper rest–stimulus interaction, that biophysically based subjectivity can no longer be properly carried over and transformed to the phenomenal level and its "phenomenally based subjectivity."

Since "phenomenally based subjectivity" is specific to the individual, the VS patients and their brain's neural activity lack the individualization that is necessary to transform the non-individual biophysically based subjectivity into an individually specific phenomenally based subjectivity. The "phenomenally based subjectivity" thus gets lost in VS patients, which we diagnose as the absence of qualia in particular and consciousness in general.

NEUROCONCEPTUAL REMARK IA: NEURAL PREDISPOSITIONS AND NEURAL CORRELATES OF QUALIA

I suggested that the rest–stimulus interaction and its underlying neuronal mechanisms like the "neuronal transfer" can be considered the neural correlates of qualia. Metaphorically speaking, the extrinsic stimulus (or a major activity change in the resting-state activity itself, as during dreams) is "needed" to "activate," or better, "awaken," the "dormant" resting-state activity's spatiotemporal structures and "bring them to life"; that is, consciousness. All that is possible, however, only on the basis of the resting-state activity itself and more specifically its spatiotemporal structures.

Consider the case of VS. Due to lack of energy supply, the resting-state activity's spatiotemporal structures are "frozen" and no longer

active by themselves. Stimulus-induced activity is still possible, as we can see in VS patients (see Chapter 29). But it is no longer based on true rest–stimulus interaction with the neuronal transfer of the intrinsic resting-state activity's spatiotemporal structure to the extrinsic stimulus (see Chapter 29 for detailed mechanisms). For that, the price is high: the loss of qualia and consciousness.

This makes it clear that qualia are ultimately based on the resting-state activity and its spatiotemporal structure. If there are no active spatiotemporal structures in the resting-state activity, their neuronal transfer to the stimulus during subsequent rest–stimulus interaction is impossible.

Accordingly, the resting-state activity's spatiotemporal structure can be regarded the neural predisposition of qualia, while their neuronal transfer to the stimulus during rest–stimulus interaction is the neural correlate of qualia. Metaphorically speaking, qualia (in particular and consciousness in general) must be considered the result of a *pas de deux* between the intrinsic activity's spatiotemporal structure and the extrinsic stimulus.

NEUROCONCEPTUAL REMARK IB: "RESTING STATE-*BASED* APPROACH TO QUALIA" VERSUS "RESTING STATE-*REDUCTIVE* APPROACH TO QUALIA"

My account presupposes that qualia are based on the brain's intrinsic activity and its spatiotemporal structure. Without the brain's intrinsic activity and its spatiotemporal structure, qualia would be impossible. However, at the same time, the brain's intrinsic activity and its spatiotemporal structure are not sufficient by themselves to realize and implement qualia—for which either an extrinsic stimulus or major activity changes (as in dreams) are needed.

Based on these considerations, one can characterize my approach as a "resting state-based approach to qualia." The concept of a "resting state-based approach to qualia" describes that the brain's resting-state activity is necessary for and thus predisposes qualia, while not being sufficient for them. Furthermore, the concept of the "resting state-based approach to qualia" does not imply that the resting-state activity itself is the basis of qualia. Instead, it is the spatiotemporal structure and its different layers of the neural activity in the resting state that provide the basis and thus the necessary condition for qualia.

Why is the difference between resting state activity and its spatiotemporal structure important? Both seem to dissociate from each other in VS. This entails that the resting state activity itself and its spatiotemporal structure must be entertained by different underlying neuronal mechanisms. Therefore, when I talk of a "resting state-based approach to qualia," I mean that the resting-state activity's spatiotemporal structure, rather than the resting-state activity itself (independently of its spatiotemporal structure), provides the neural basis or predisposition for qualia.

In addition, the concept of "resting state-based approach to qualia" does not imply that the resting-state activity itself can sufficiently account for qualia. My "resting state-*based* approach to qualia" must thus be distinguished from a "resting state-*reductive* approach to qualia." Such "resting state-reductive approach to qualia" seems to be implied in the account of He and Raichle (2009), who consider the resting-state activity the sufficient condition of and thus as neural correlate of qualia and consciousness (see Chapter 14 for a detailed discussion of their position).

NEUROCONCEPTUAL REMARK IC: *"RESTING STATE*-BASED APPROACH TO QUALIA" VERSUS *"STIMULUS*-BASED APPROACH TO QUALIA"

My "resting state-based approach to qualia" in this sense has to be also distinguished from a "*stimulus*-based approach to qualia." Unlike the "*resting state* approach to qualia," a "stimulus-based approach to qualia" considers the stimulus-induced activity by itself to be both the necessary and the sufficient neural condition of qualia. Qualia are here exclusively associated with the extrinsic stimulus and its stimulus-induced activity, while the brain's intrinsic resting-state activity, let alone its spatiotemporal structure, are completely neglected. This seems to be the case in most current neuroscientific accounts of qualia (see, for instance,

Orpwood 1994, 2007, 2010; Feinberg 2009, 2011; Tononi 2004, 2008).

Why is the distinction between "resting state and stimulus-based approaches to qualia" so important? By considering the stimulus itself and its stimulus-induced activity as sufficient to induce qualia, the proponents of a "stimulus-based approach to qualia" must focus on the neural processing of the stimulus in the brain. This leads them to search for qualia in the various functions of the brain—sensory, motor, affective, cognitive, and social—as has been postulated by various authors in both neuroscience and philosophy (see Panksepp 1998a and b; Graziano, M. S., & Kastner, S. (2011); Prinz 2012; Dahaene and Changeux 2011; Koch 2004; see also the first Introduction and Appendix 1 herein for a more extensive list and discussion). Therefore, a "stimulus-based approach to qualia" leads invariably to a neurosensory, neuromotor, neuroaffective, neurocognitive, or neurosocial approach to qualia.

This, however, is the point where the problem starts. The neurosensory, neuromotor, neuroaffective, neurocognitive, or neurosocial approaches to qualia, and thus "stimulus-based approaches to qualia" in general, can provide neuronal hypotheses about qualia. However, they leave unexplained why and how these neuronal mechanisms are associated with qualia rather than with non-qualia. This means that these approaches fail to show the necessity of qualia: why stimuli and their stimulus-induced activity are necessarily and unavoidably associated with qualia by default. In other words, there remains a gap between the neuronal mechanisms of the brain on the one hand and the phenomenal features of qualia on the other in "stimulus-based approaches to qualia," an "explanatory gap" as it is called in current philosophy of mind.

NEUROCONCEPTUAL REMARK IIA: *"STATISTICALLY-* AND *SPATIOTEMPORALLY-* BASED QUALIA" VERSUS *"PHYSICALLY-* AND *NON-SPATIOTEMPORALLY-* BASED QUALIA"

What exactly does the concept of the "explanatory gap" mean? Most generally (and without going into conceptual details as discussed in philosophy), the concept of the "explanatory gap" describes a principal difference between neuronal and phenomenal features in our explanation of consciousness in general and qualia in particular.

What inclines the philosopher to speak of an "explanatory gap"? There is nothing in our explanations of the brain's neuronal mechanisms that implies and entails and thus make necessary or unavoidable the occurrence of the phenomenal features of qualia (and consciousness in general). The philosophers stress necessity as distinguished from contingency. *Necessity* means that the neuronal mechanisms in question cannot occur without the phenomenal feature in question, meaning non-qualia in our case. The occurrence of qualia as phenomenal features is consequently supposed to be necessarily implied by the neuronal mechanisms: qualia can then be inferred from the neuronal mechanisms in the same way we can infer from the concept of *bachelor* a non-married person.

How does my neurophenomenal hypothesis of qualia stand in relation to such an "explanatory gap" between neuronal mechanisms and phenomenal features? This is the question of whether the here-suggested neuronal mechanisms necessarily imply and entail the occurrence of the phenomenal feature of qualia. For that the answer, let us consider what exactly I did in my various neurophenomenal hypotheses, as explicated earlier.

I suggested that the brain encodes the extrinsic stimuli (and its own intrinsic resting-state activity changes) in terms of their statistical frequency distributions and thus in a statistically based way. Such statistically based encoding strategy must be distinguished from a physically based encoding strategy that encodes the single stimuli's physical features by themselves, rather than their statistical frequency distributions into neural activity (see Volume I for the details of the difference between statistically and physically based encoding strategies).

How is such statistically based encoding of the brain's neural activity related to the phenomenal features of qualia? The statistically based encoding strategy of the brain allows it to encode spatiotemporal differences, which more or less reflect the spatiotemporal structure of the stimuli. This means that the brain's encoding strategy "spatiotemporalizes" the extrinsic stimuli during their interaction with the brain's intrinsic activity and its own spatiotemporal structure.

I now postulate that such "spatiotemporalization" of the extrinsic stimuli by their encoding into neural activity during rest–stimulus interaction makes necessary and unavoidable their association with the phenomenal features of qualia. I demonstrated this for different phenomenal and qualitative features of qualia: "non-structural homogeneity," "transparency," and "ipseity." The statistically based "spatiotemporalization" of the stimuli can thus not avoid becoming manifest or "resurfacing" (as I said earlier) in the "non-structural homogeneity," the "transparency," and the "ipseity" of qualia.

What does this "spatiotemporalization" imply for the characterization of qualia? The phenomenal features of qualia must be characterized as intrinsically statistical and spatiotemporal. This means that I here opt for a statistically and spatiotemporally based account of qualia, as distinguished from a physically and non-spatiotemporally based account of qualia. I postulate that physically and non-spatiotemporally based qualia remain impossible, at least in the actual natural world of our brain and its particular encoding strategy. In contrast, I leave open to future philosophical discussion whether such physically and non-spatiotemporally based qualia are conceivable in at least a purely logical world.

NEUROCONCEPTUAL REMARK IIB: *HOW* THE *"RESTING* STATE-BASED APPROACH TO QUALIA" CAN *AVOID* THE "EXPLANATORY GAP"

What does such a statistically and spatiotemporally based account of qualia imply for the "explanatory gap"? I postulate that the statistically rather than physically based encoding strategy of the brain's neural activity makes necessary or unavoidable the association of the resulting stimulus-induced activity with the phenomenal features of qualia.

This means that my statistically and spatiotemporally based account of qualia can avoid the problem of the '"explanatory gap" altogether by choosing the "right" starting point. Due to the choice of the "right" starting points, the brain's encoding strategy and the spatiotemporal structure of its intrinsic activity, the question of the "explanatory gap" cannot even be raised

anymore. This is exactly what I suggested in my "resting state-based approach to qualia," which therefore is not prone to the problem of the "explanatory gap." (see Fig. 30-3a).

If, in contrast, one presupposes a physically based encoding strategy as the "stimulus-based

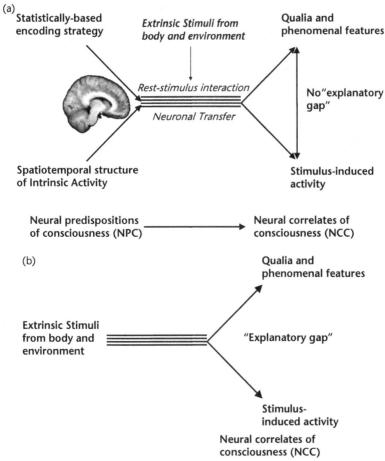

Figure 30-3a and b "Explanatory gap" in "resting state-based approach to qualia" (a) and "stimulus-based approach to qualia" (b). (a) The figure illustrates on the left the brain and two of its intrinsic features, the statistically based encoding strategy and the spatiotemporal structures of its intrinsic activity. These predispose the phenomenal features of qualia (lower part). During the rest–stimulus interaction with the extrinsic stimuli, the intrinsic activity's spatiotemporal structures are carried over and transferred to the resulting stimulus-induced activity (middle and right) which is then necessarily and unavoidably associated with qualia and their phenomenal features. The question of the explanatory gap between neuronal mechanisms and phenomenal features therefore cannot even be raised anymore. (b) This is different in the case of "stimulus-based approaches to qualia." Here, the brain itself and its intrinsic features, the encoding strategy and the spatiotemporal structure, are neglected. Instead, the starting point here is the stimulus-induced activity itself. The association of the purely neuronal stimulus-induced activity with the phenomenal features of qualia remains then unclear and purely contingent, as is illustrated by the disrupted arrows between qualia and stimulus-induced activity. There is thus an explanatory gap between neuronal mechanisms and phenomenal features.

approaches to qualia," the necessary linkage between the brain's neural activity and the phenomenal features of qualia is disrupted and becomes purely contingent. The presupposition of a physically based encoding strategy leads to a physically and non-spatiotemporally based account of qualia. That, however, I postulate, will unavoidably and thus necessarily raise the question of the "explanatory gap." This is the case in the current "stimulus-based approaches to qualia" in both neuroscience and philosophy. That, however, needs to be explained in further detail, which is the focus in the next section.

NEUROCONCEPTUAL REMARK IIC: *WHY* THE *"STIMULUS*-BASED APPROACH TO QUALIA" LEADS *NECESSARILY* TO THE "EXPLANATORY GAP"

Why do "stimulus-based approaches to qualia" lead to the "explanatory gap"? I postulate that the "stimulus-based approach to qualia" does necessarily imply the "explanatory gap" between neuronal mechanisms and phenomenal features. Conceptually, "stimulus-based approaches to qualia" do usually not distinguish between neural predispositions and neural correlates of consciousness. This makes it impossible for them to distinguish between *necessary* conditions of possible qualia and (necessary and) *sufficient* conditions of actual qualia. Such conceptual neglect is accompanied by an empirical neglect, that consists in the exclusive focus on stimulus-induced activity at the expense of the brain's intrinsic activity and its spatiotemporal structures.

Taking both conceptual and empirical neglect together means that the proponents of a "stimulus-based approach to qualia" associate qualia with stimulus-induced activity exclusively. That, however, limits and restricts them to stimulus-induced activity that, unlike the brain's intrinsic activity and its prephenomenal structures, does not predispose and nor imply anything about phenomenal feature. In other words, the stimulus-induced activity remains completely non-phenomenal by itself when considered in isolation from the resting-state activity and its prephenomenal structures.

Due to their exclusive focus on stimulus-induced activity as the neural correlate of qualia, the advocates of a "stimulus-based approach to qualia" "lose sight of" the phenomenal features of qualia right at the beginning when choosing stimulus-induced activity rather than resting-state activity as starting point. As hard as the proponents of a "stimulus-based approach to qualia" try to subsequently explain qualia and their phenomenal features in terms of the various sensory, motor, affective, cognitive, or social functions, they will not be able to do so.

Metaphorically speaking, the advocates of a "stimulus-based approach to qualia" remain unable to bring back the initially lost predisposition of the phenomenal features of qualia due to their initial neglect of the brain's resting-state activity and its spatiotemporal structures. The relationship between neuronal mechanisms and phenomenal features must consequently remain contingent, rather than necessary. This means, however, that the proponents of a stimulus-based approach to qualia cannot avoid raising the question of the explanatory gap by default (see Fig. 30-3b).

Open Questions

The first question pertains to the exact neuronal mechanisms of how rest–stimulus interaction mediates the distinct phenomenal features of qualia. Future research may want to specify the presumed neuronal-phenomenal link in much more neuronal and phenomenal detail than we did here.

For that, we first need to better understand the neuronal mechanisms of rest–stimulus interaction, and secondly, need to be more detailed about the phenomenal features of qualia. For that, one may also want to draw on other neuropsychiatric disorders like schizophrenia or depression, from which one can learn much about how an altered resting state impacts the various phenomenal features of qualia.

One would also need to develop measures to quantify the distinct phenomenal features of qualia. More specifically, one may want to investigate the phenomenal characteristics of qualia with regard to their spatial and temporal features. I propose that the different phenomenal features of qualia like non-structural homogeneity, feeling of direct contact, ipseity, and transparency (and others) reflect different constellations of spatial and temporal features on a phenomenal level. This provides the phenomenal prelude for the neurophenomenal fugue; namely, the hypothesis that the distinct spatiotemporal features on the phenomenal level of qualia may correspond to different spatiotemporal constellations of the various neuronal measures during rest–stimulus interaction.

Methodologically, this assumption implies a mutual exchange between neuronal and phenomenal investigation. Both neuronal and phenomenal investigations of (neuronal and phenomenal) spatiotemporal constellations may enrich and complement each other. By considering the spatiotemporal constellations on the neuronal level, the phenomenal level may specify its spatiotemporal description of qualia and its phenomenal features. Conversely, the neuronal level may benefit from detailing the spatiotemporal constellations on the phenomenal level by using the latter as a roadmap and guidance for what to look for in the brain's intrinsic activity and its spatial and temporal neuronal measures.

One strong spatiotemporal candidate from the neuronal side would, for instance, be the entrainment between high- and low-frequency fluctuations: different temporal constellations between high- and low-frequency fluctuations' phases may correspond to different spatial and temporal features on the phenomenal level of qualia. This, however, is a speculative hypothesis at this point. Another candidate on the neuronal side would be sparse coding. In Volume I, I showed that GABA and neural inhibition predispose the degree of sparse coding during rest–stimulus interaction.

If so, one would propose that the generation of qualia and their phenomenal features also depends on the degree of temporal and spatial sparsening of neural activity during rest–stimulus interaction. If so, the degree of sparse coding during rest–stimulus interaction should predict the degree of the phenomenal features of qualia and thus of consciousness in general.

On the phenomenal side, one may have missed the discussion of the transfer of the resting state's self-specific and preintentional organization in this chapter. Qualia are also self-specific and intentional. I propose that both phenomenal features can be traced back to the resting state's self-specific and preintentional organization (see Chapters 23–25).

I already demonstrated how the resting state's self-specific and preintentional organization are converted and transferred onto the phenomenal level and thus to the stimulus and its associated stimulus-induced activity. I therefore refrained from their discussion in the context of qualia in this part.

Finally, one may want to argue that I so far considered mainly cortical regions. Does this mean that subcortical regions have no relevance at all for consciousness? This will be the focus of the next chapter. I also neglected the consciousness of one's own body in my focus on the consciousness of the environment. Therefore, I will devote yet another chapter specifically to consciousness of one's own body; that is, interoceptive awareness, as it shall be discussed in the final chapter. This will tie in with the more theoretical assumptions of consciousness being embodied and embedded.

CHAPTER 31
Subcortical Regions and Qualia

Summary

Thus far, I have demonstrated how the resting-state activity and rest–stimulus interaction are central in yielding qualia. I predominantly focused on cortical regions, while leaving subcortical regions more or less aside. The present chapter therefore focuses on subcortical regions and how they are related to consciousness. First, I discuss the structural anatomy and the various connections in the subcortical regions. Reasoning from the structural anatomy, I hypothesize that neural activity in subcortical regions is encoded into neural activity in terms of spatial and temporal differences between different stimuli, rather than by encoding the different discrete points of the stimuli in physical time and space by themselves. In short, I postulate difference-based coding rather than stimulus-based coding to operate in subcortical regions. Based on recent work by Merker and Panksepp, one would postulate the constitution of a statistically based spatiotemporal structure in subcortical resting-state activity in very much the same way I discussed it for the cortical regions. That implies the assumption of prephenomenal structures with spatiotemporal continuity, unity, and self-specific and preintentional organization in the resting-state activity of subcortical regions. Since I suggest prephenomenal structures to predispose consciousness, one would expect phenomenal states and thus consciousness to be associated with neural activity in the subcortical regions. Even in the absence of the cortex as a whole, one would therefore postulate consciousness to be present, albeit in a rather limited spatial and temporal way. This is evidenced by findings from patients suffering from decortication, where only the subcortical regions are left. Since the subcortical regions are strongly implicated in the neural of processing affect and emotions, one would postulate their phenomenal output, qualia, to be strongly affective. Based on the work by especially Jaak Panksepp (and others), I therefore postulate qualia to be intrinsically affective, thus speaking of "affective qualia": Subcortical regions are unavoidably implicated in any kind of neural processing on the cortical level. Therefore, any kind of qualia cannot avoid including some kind of affective component at their very core. The chapter concludes with a neurophenomenal remark about the relationship between qualia, affect, and subjectivity. The affective or emotional component of qualia is postulated to account for what phenomenally is often described as "feeling" or "qualitative feel" during the subjective experience of qualia.

Key Concepts and Topics Covered

Subcortical regions, difference-based coding, spatiotemporal structure, prephenomenal structures, self-specific organization, consciousness, qualia, affective qualia, decortication, spatiotemporal extension, vegetative state, qualitative feel, subjectivity

NEUROEMPIRICAL BACKGROUND
IA: SUBCORTICAL REGIONS
AND CONSCIOUSNESS

The focus in current neuroscientific research on consciousness is clearly on cortical regions. Consciousness is often considered a higher-order cognitive function that therefore is associated predominantly with cortical regions like the prefrontal cortex. This is the main and predominant view on consciousness in current neuroscience as well as in philosophy (see Appendix 1). Most research on consciousness has consequently focused on cortical regions as it is also reflected in the various examples I discussed throughout both volumes.

In contrast, subcortical regions and their vegetative-interoceptive and affective functions are often postulated to have no substantial role in yielding consciousness. However, accounts of consciousness by, for instance, Jaak Panksepp (1998a and b) and Antonio Damasio (1999a and b, 2010, Vandekerckhove and Panksepp 2009) deny that. They consider subcortical regions and their associated functions like affect and interoception as highly relevant for yielding consciousness. Therefore, the focus in this chapter is on affect and consciousness, while Chapter 32 targets interoception. Where have we encountered subcortical regions in this two-volume book? The only point where subcortical regions were explicitly thematized was when I discussed the threefold organization with inner, middle, and outer rings that, I hypothesized, stretch from subcortical to cortical regions (see Chapter 4 in Volume I).

Briefly, we distinguished on purely anatomical grounds three distinct subcortical-cortical rings: the inner one around the first to fourth ventricles, the outer one on the outer surface of the brain, and the middle one sandwiched between inner and outer rings. Based on the inner ring's anatomy in conjunction with recent functional imaging data, I postulated a subcortical-cortical midline system as anatomical and functional unity (see Northoff et al. 2011; Northoff et al. 2010 Northoff and Panksepp 2008; Panksepp and Northoff 2009). The purpose of this chapter is now to go beyond the purely neuronal account of especially the subcortical midline regions and to point out their neurophenomenal relevance for consciousness.

NEUROEMPIRICAL BACKGROUND IB: AFFECT AND CONSCIOUSNESS

One subcortical exception to the rule of cortical predominance in current accounts of consciousness is the thalamus: The thalamus is considered a central node in relaying information back to the cortex via its re-entrant connections; the thalamus's reentrant connections have been postulated by Edelman and Tononi to be the neural correlate of consciousness (see Tononi and Edelman 2000; see the discussion of Tononi's Information Integration Theory in Appendix 1). Moreover, the thalamus surfaces in the context of the vegetative state (VS). Based on successful electrode stimulation in the thalamus in one VS patient, Schiff (2009, 2010) considers VS to be a subcortical-cortical disconnection syndrome (see Chapter 28 for details).

However, the subcortical regions are not limited to the thalamus but include a variety of other regions (see later) whose neuronal processing may also be highly relevant to generate consciousness (see, for instance, Merker 2005, 2007; Panksepp 1998a and b, 2007; and Damasio 1999a and b, 2010; see also Parvizi and Damasio 2001). Functionally especially the various subcortical midline regions (see later and Chapter 4 for details) have mostly been associated with affect and emotion (see Panksepp 1998a and b, 2011; Damasio 1999a and b, 2010).

In the following I therefore want to shed some light on these other subcortical regions and how they are related to affect and ultimately consciousness. My account can, however, only be limited focusing on the relevance of subcortical regions for consciousness, while leaving out many other anatomical and functional details of the subcortical regions as well as a detailed account of affect and emotion by themselves.

NEURONAL FINDINGS IA: ANATOMY AND FUNCTIONS OF SUBCORTICAL REGIONS

Let's start with a rough sketch of the subcortical anatomy (see Parvizi and Damasio 2001, for an excellent account). Anatomically, the subcortical regions include lower brainstem regions. These concern the nuclei for the cranial nerves, including the regulation of the autonomous nervous system that controls the body's vegetative function (like heart rate and breathing rate). And there are also the locus coerulus, the raphe nucleus, the ventral tegmental area (VTA), and the nucleus basalis of Meynert; these are the originating structures of neuromodulatory transmitters like adrenalin/noradrenaline, serotonin, dopamine, and acetylcholine. These structures send efferences to all cortical regions and impact thereby their neuronal activity.

The raphe nucleus sends efferences to the PACC in the anterior cortical midline terminating there on especially GABAergic interneurons (see Northoff et al. 2011 for details). This means that serotonin (and the other neuromodulators too) has direct access to cortical regions and can modulate their neuronal activity according to their own actual subcortical state. This may, for instance, be highly relevant in depression where altered serotoninergic subcortical-cortical midline modulation (in the inner subcortical-cortical ring) may be a central factor in the pathogenesis of this disorder (see Chapter 27; Northoff et al. 2011).

In addition to the lower brainstem regions, there are brainstem regions that are situated at a higher level and are closely connected to the motor regions of the basal ganglia (see later). These upper brain stem regions include the superior and inferior colliculi, the tectum, and the periaqueductal gray (PAG). The superior colliculus (SC) seems to be a nodal point. The SC receives afferent connections from different sensory modalities, including visual, auditory, and olfactory. It may therefore be central in integrating different senses. At the same time it is also closely related to motor regions like the basal ganglia, allowing for sensorimotor integration (Merker 2007).

How about the PAG? The PAG receives afferences from both the environments' exteroceptive inputs and one's own body's interoceptive inputs (as afferent connections from the hypothalamus and lower brainstem regions). And the PAG is closely connected to the basal ganglia and their processing of motor-related signals (see later; also see Fig. 31-1a). As such, the PAG may be a hub or nodal point between intero- and exteroceptive sensory inputs on the one hand and the motor system of the basal ganglia on the other (Panksepp 1998a and b, 2003a and b, 2007).

Both PAG and SC are closely and directly connected with the basal ganglia, the prime subcortical motor regions. The basal ganglia contain a set of regions that include the internal and external globus pallidus; the striatum, including the ventral striatum/nucleus accumbens, putamen, and the caudate; the substantia nigra/ventral tegmental area; and the subthalamic nucleus. These regions are well known to be central for generating motor programs with the subsequent generation of movements. This is, for instance, disturbed in a motor disorder like Parkinson's disease; dopaminergic deficits in the substantia nigra and the striatum yield motor symptoms like akinesia (inability to move), rigidity (increased muscle tone), and tremor.

NEURONAL FINDINGS IB: SUBCORTICAL INPUTS AND OUTPUTS

The complex input and output pattern of the PAG and SC suggests their central role in integrating and converting different kinds of stimuli. Merker (2007, 70–72), for instance, postulates the SC and the PAG to be involved in target selection (SC), action selection (i.e., basal ganglia), and the motivational state, that is, PAG. He describes this as the "selection triangle" and "triangular dependency." It is triangular because sensory-exteroceptive and vegetative-interoceptive inputs converge here with motor outputs. Functionally this links and brings together target, action, and motivation.

In addition to the basal ganglia, the PAG and the SC are closely connected to the thalamus, a set of different nuclei located just beneath the cortex. The outputs of these nuclei converge predominantly on one thalamic nucleus in the midline, the dorsomedial thalamus (DMT). The DMT then relays back to the cortex and is therefore a central part of the cortico-thalamic-cortical loops as the prime example of a re-entrant connection (see earlier).

Merker (2007, 75–77) postulates a particular structure, the zona incerta, that lies between the PAG/SC and the thalamic nuclei, to be central in mediating between subcortical sensory and motor regions. Interestingly, the zona incerta seems to be predominantly inhibitory in that it contains mainly GABAergic neurons so that inhibition and disinhibition must be postulated to be central here.

Recent imaging studies in the resting state in humans further support the subcortical regions' dense connections in functional regard, that is,

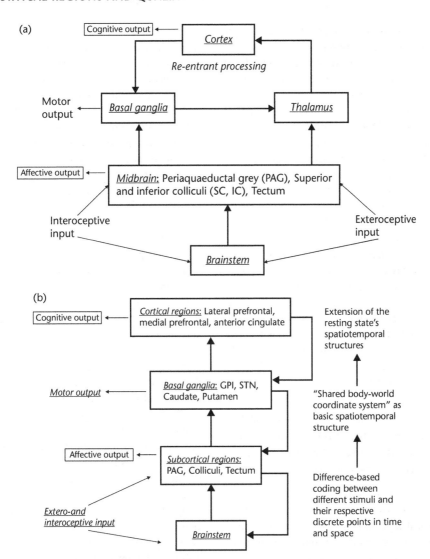

Figure 31-1a and b Difference-based coding in subcortical regions. The figures illustrate the organization of the relationship between the different subcortical regions and their link to the cortex (*a*) and how that predisposes them to difference-based coding and the constitution of a statistically based virtual spatiotemporal structure (*b*). (*a*) The brainstem and the midbrain receive multiple interoceptive and exteroceptive inputs from body and environment (*lower part*), which are conveyed to the basal ganglia and the thalamus (*middle part*). These are then transmitted to the cortex, which relays them back to the thalamus and the basal ganglia, amounting to re-entrant processing of neural activity and the associated information. (*b*) The figure specifies the previous one with regard to difference-based coding and the constitution of a spatiotemporal structure (*right part*). All regions receive multiple inputs, neuronal, interoceptive and exteroceptive, which, as I postulate, predispose them for difference- rather than stimulus-based coding. Difference-based coding does, in turn, predispose the constitution of a statistically based virtual spatiotemporal structure across the distinct stimuli from brain, body, and environment that the subcortical regions receive. What Bjoern Merker (2007) described as a "shared body-world coordinate system" corresponds well to the subcortical regions' constitution of a very basic statistically based spatiotemporal structure across the divide between brain, body, and environment as it is already constituted by the subcortical regions themselves.

functional connectivity. Cole et al. (2010), for instance, investigated human subjects in fMRI during the resting state. They determined global brain connectivity as an index of resting-state functional connectivity. In addition to various cortical midline regions, subcortical midline regions like the DMT, the basal ganglia, and the midbrain (and hippocampus and amygdala) showed particularly high indices of global brain connectivity (see also Tomasi and Volkov 2011). Hence, the earlier described dense and multiconvergent structural connectivity seems to translate into analogously dense functional connectivity in the resting state.

Taken together, this brief (and admittedly rather sketchy and incomplete) account of subcortical regions already suggests that these regions are highly structured and closely connected with each other. Thereby they seem to make possible for both extero- and interoceptive inputs to converge onto motor outputs and linking them in a triangular way, as pointed out by Merker especially (2007).

NEURONAL HYPOTHESIS IA: DIFFERENCE-BASED CODING CONSTITUTES A STATISTICALLY BASED VIRTUAL SPATIAL STRUCTURE IN THE NEURAL ACTIVITY OF SUBCORTICAL REGIONS

What does this anatomical and functional connectivity pattern imply for the encoding of the subcortical region's neural activity? The neural activity in the subcortical midline regions must stem from the integration between intero- and exteroceptive inputs that encounter the neuronal inputs from the resting-state activity itself.

More specifically, subcortical neural activity must be based on the earlier described "trilateral interaction" between intero- and exteroceptive and neuronal stimuli. The resulting neural activity must thus be based on the difference between the different stimuli rather than the actual stimuli themselves; that is, in isolation and independently of each other. If so, one would hypothesize difference-based coding rather than stimulus-based coding to encode neural activity in subcortical regions.

How can we specify difference-based coding in these subcortical regions? Based on its

connectivity pattern, Merker (2007) postulates that especially the SC is central in yielding what he describes as a "shared spatial coordinate system" between the inputs from the world (exteroceptive input), the body (interoceptive input), and the motivation/brain (neuronal input). How is the constitution of such a shared spatial coordinate system possible? I postulate this to be possible on the basis of difference-based coding. The SC integrates and encodes the different inputs, including their spatial and temporal features, in direct relationship to or difference from each other; this presupposes difference-based coding (rather than stimulus-based coding).

Let us specify how exactly difference-based coding operates in subcortical regions. Difference-based coding implies that the statistical frequency distribution of the different inputs, for example, intero—and exteroceptive and neuronal, is encoded into neuronal activity. This means that the different stimuli's spatial and temporal differences, rather than their single discrete points in physical time and space, are encoded into subcortical neural activity.

Such encoding of spatial and temporal differences into neural activity makes possible the constitution of a statistically based spatial structure across the different discrete points in physical time and space as associated with the single intero- and exteroceptive stimuli from body and environment. Such statistically based spatial (and temporal) structure may then "virtually" span across the different discrete points in the physical space of brain, body, and environment.

How is the subcortical regions' spatial structure constituted? Certainly during stimulus-induced activity, when specific exteroceptive stimuli are processed. However, there is continuous interoceptive input form the body, even in the resting state. One would consequently expect the statistically based spatial structure, especially in subcortical regions, to be already constituted during the resting state itself.

If that is so, one would expect continuous and high resting-state activity to occur in the subcortical regions. Empirically, there is indeed evidence for high neural activity already in the resting state itself as manifested in rest–rest interaction. This is suggested by the subcortical regions' high resting-state metabolism (which is especially high in the PAG) and resting-state functional connectivity, which is also spontaneously changing across time (see Fig. 31-1b).

NEURONAL HYPOTHESIS IB: DIFFERENCE-BASED CODING CONSTITUTES A STATISTICALLY BASED VIRTUAL TEMPORAL STRUCTURE IN THE NEURAL ACTIVITY OF SUBCORTICAL REGIONS

How about the temporal domain? Difference-based coding may not only hold in spatial but also in temporal regard. Unfortunately, as to my knowledge, there are not many investigations available about low-frequency fluctuations in subcortical regions in humans. Therefore, I have to speculatively postulate the following.

The temporal input structure of intero- and exteroceptive input may differ from each other. Interoceptive input is continuously and regularly provided as, for instance, the heart beat that occurs every second without any interruption. This, in contrast, is different in the case of exteroceptive input, which is more irregular and arrhythmic and therefore shows a different, more discontinuous and irregular temporal structure. If intero- and exteroceptive inputs are now linked and encoded into neural activity in orientation to their temporal (and spatial) differences, their different discrete temporal points s must also be integrated, thereby yielding a certain temporal structure. Analogous to the "shared spatial coordinate system" (see earlier), one may therefore also speak of a "shared temporal coordinate system."

Such a "shared temporal coordinate system" can reflect the integration and merger between the different temporal features of the different involved stimuli, continuous in the case of interoceptive stimuli, and discontinuous for exteroceptive stimuli. The merger and integration between different temporal features is possible on the basis of difference-based coding (in the temporal domain), which in turn provides the very ground for establishing some of "virtual" statistically based temporal structure of the neural activity in the subcortical regions.

Another component in constituting such a shared temporal coordinate system may be the temporal extension of the subcortical regions' neuronal activity by neuropeptides. Based on his own empirical investigation, Panksepp (1998a and b, 2007, 2011) postulates that the various subcortical neuropeptides (oxytocin, morphine, substance P, etc.) temporally extend the subcortical regions' neuronal activity as induced by the stimuli and their different discrete points in physical time.

This may thus extend the temporal differences that are encoded into subcortical neural activity even further. In conjunction with difference-based coding, the neuropeptides may consequently allow for the transition from a merely temporally discrete neural activity to a temporally more continuous pattern of neuronal activity.

NEURONAL HYPOTHESIS IC: THE STATISTICALLY BASED VIRTUAL SPATIOTEMPORAL STRUCTURE IN SUBCORTICAL NEURAL ACTIVITY CONSTITUTES A "SHARED BODY-WORLD COORDINATE SYSTEM"

The convergence between different inputs and outputs predisposes the subcortical regions to difference- rather than stimulus-based coding. This also makes it possible for the subcortical regions to constitute a statistically based virtual spatiotemporal structure in their resting-state activity in very much the same way as we already discussed at length for cortical regions in previous parts and chapters.

What Bjoern Merker describes as a "shared body-world coordinate system" may then very well correspond to what I here designate as the "spatiotemporal structure" of the resting state's neural activity. This spatiotemporal structure spans in a statistically based and thus "virtual" way across the different discrete points in physical time and space as associated with the different inputs from brain, body, and environment.

Accordingly, brain, body, and environment may be intrinsically integrated and linked in a virtual statistically based way by the spatiotemporal structure of the subcortical regions' neural activity. This means that any specific stimulus, intero- or exteroceptive, must encounter the subcortical regions and their statistically based virtual spatiotemporal structure. This, as we will discuss in the following sections, predisposes the possible association of the resulting stimulus-induced activity with consciousness.

NEURONAL FINDINGS IIA: SUBCORTICAL REGIONS IN THE VEGETATIVE STATE

So far, I have demonstrated the anatomical organization and structure of the subcortical regions. I also postulated this structure to be constituted on the basis of difference-based coding rather than stimulus-based coding. This, however, remains within the purely neuronal context of the brain. What does this imply for the role of subcortical regions in the phenomenal context of consciousness?

Let us recall from the previous chapters and parts that I considered the degree of difference-based coding to be directly related to the degree or level of consciousness (see Chapter 28): The higher the degree of difference-based coding (and the lower the degree of stimulus-based coding), the higher the level of consciousness that can possibly be associated with the respective stimuli.

One would consequently postulate that difference-based coding in subcortical regions should also affect the level of consciousness. If so, one would expect lesions in the brainstem and/or the midbrain to lead to coma and vegetative state. This is exactly what can be observed. A retrospective analysis of 47 patients with brainstem stroke showed nine of them to be in coma suffering from lesions in the raphe nucleus, the locus coeruleus, parabrachial nucleus, and the tegmental nucleus (see Parvizi and Damasio 2003).

These data provide neuroanatomical evidence, which is always rather indirect. Is there also some more direct empirical support from functional brain imaging for the role of subcortical regions in consciousness? Functional imaging of subcortical regions is more difficult that of cortical regions. Moreover, pure sensory or cognitive paradigms predominantly involve cortical regions rather than subcortical ones. One exception is affective function that implicates subcortical regions as associated with affect and emotions (see Panksepp 1998a and b, 2011).

How about patients in vegetative state? Do these patients' subcortical regions show stimulus-induced activity during affective stimuli in the same way as their cortical regions (see Chapter 29) do during sensory and cognitive tasks? There are indeed a couple of imaging studies during the presentation of affective stimuli in vegetative state (VS) that shall be reported in the following.

NEURONAL FINDINGS IIB: AFFECT AND EMOTIONS IN THE VEGETATIVE STATE

In Germany, Simon Eickhoff et al. (2008) investigated a 41-year-old woman with bilateral midbrain damage in functional MRI while being in VS. They used visual (flicker), auditory (non-emotional words), and tactile (brushing with a sponge) stimuli to investigate neural activity during sensory processing.

This led to robust neural activity changes in auditory cortex during auditory stimuli, visual cortex during visual stimulation, and somatosensory cortex during tactile stimuli. Since the paradigm used words, auditory stimulation also yielded activity changes in regions typically associated with the processing of language and words, Broca's and Wernicke's regions. Taken together, these results show more or less intact neural activity during sensory-related stimulus-induced activity in primary sensory regions during different kinds of sensory processing.

In addition to the sensory stimulation, Eickhoff et al. (2008) also conducted a second fMRI investigation in the same patient. This time they used speech stimuli, for example, verbal utterances: These speech stimuli were recorded from the patient's two children (6- and 8-year- old girls), two close female friends, and a female student who was unknown to the patient: children, friends, a stranger. Each of the three conditions was presented once in an emotional and directly addressing way ("Hello, I am so and so...") and once in an unemotional and non-addressing way.

Presentation of these stimuli in fMRI yielded significant activity changes in the left amygdala and the right anterior superior temporal sulcus. In both regions, emotional conditions yielded stronger signal changes than non-emotional conditions. This holds true especially for the left amygdala across all three speakers (i.e., children, friends, strangers). Most important, however, the emotional voices of one's own children induced the strongest signal changes, especially in the left amygdala, while the stranger's voice was associated with the lowest activity, and reactions to the friends' voice ranged between both (see Fig. 31-2).

Analogous results during emotional stimulation could also be observed by another study of patients in a minimally conscious state (MCS). Using functional magnetic resonance imaging (fMRI), Zhu et al. (2009) used emotional pictures from the international affective pictures (IAPS)

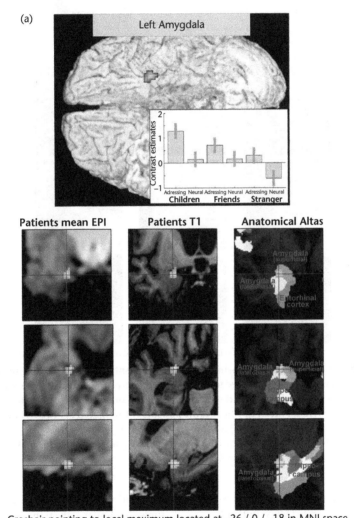

(a)

Left Amygdala

Patients mean EPI   Patients T1   Anatomical Altas

Croshair pointing to local maximum located at –26 / 0 / –18 in MNI space

Figure 31-2a Subcortical activity during personally relevant emotional stimuli in vegetative state. Stronger response during speech directed to the patient compared to neutral phrases, as well as a significant speaker effect, were detected in the left amygdala (as localized by comparison with the patients' individual mean EPI image, the patients' T1 weighted MPRAGE images, and an anatomical atlas). Reprinted with permission, from Eickhoff SB, Dafotakis M, Grefkes C, Stöcker T, Shah NJ, Schnitzler A, Zilles K, Siebler M. FMRI reveals cognitive and emotional processing in a long-term comatose patient. *Exp Neurol.* 2008;214:240–46.

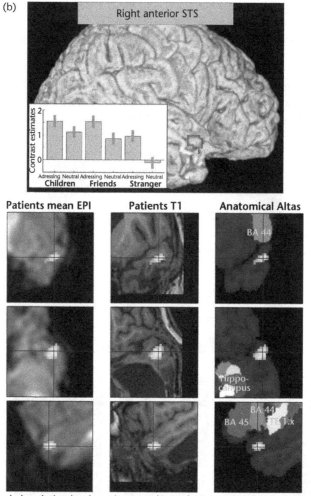

Croshair pointing local maximum to located at –56 / 12 / –18 in MNI space

Figure 31-2b **Subcortical activity during personally relevant emotional stimuli in vegetative state.** Stronger response during speech directed to the patient compared to neutral phrases, as well as a significant speaker effect were also detected in the superior temporal sulcus (STS) (again shown in comparison with the patients' individual mean EPI image, the patients' T1 weighted MPRAGE images, and an anatomical atlas). Reprinted with permission, from Eickhoff SB, Dafotakis M, Grefkes C, Stöcker T, Shah NJ, Schnitzler A, Zilles K, Siebler M. FMRI reveals cognitive and emotional processing in a long-term comatose patient. *Exp Neurol.* 2008;214:240–46.

to stimulate neural activity in nine patients in a minimally conscious state (MCS) in fMRI.

They also distinguished between intimate familiar pictures and high- or low-stimulating emotional pictures. This yielded robust signal changes in visual networks, including the visual cortex, the temporal cortex, the prefrontal cortex, and the orbitofrontal gyrus. Though the amount of activity change was lower than in

the healthy subjects, MCS patients nevertheless showed a similar activation pattern. Importantly, this was strongest especially during the intimate familiar pictures, as shown in six cases; this is in line with the results from the single case study that also showed the strongest activity during familiar emotional stimuli.

Taken together, these findings demonstrate that vegetative patients do indeed still show stimulus-induced activity in subcortical regions during emotional stimulation that is strongest if the respective emotions are related to the subjects themselves; that is, personally relevant or self-specific. In contrast to such neuronal activity, the very same patients do not seem to exhibit the corresponding behavior, affect, and phenomenal state; that is, affective qualia or emotional feelings (see, however, Panksepp et al. 2007, who deny that). Hence, there seems to be dissociation between neuronal activity on the one hand and behavior and affective qualia on the other in these patients; one may therefore want to speak of neurobehavioral and neurophenomenal dissociation.

NEURONAL FINDINGS IIIA: SUBCORTICAL REGIONS AND AFFECT

After having characterized subcortical regions neuronally, that is, by difference-based coding, and functionally; that is, by affect and emotions, we now need to specify their role in phenomenal terms. In a first step, we characterize the subcortical regions by affect and emotions, which then serves as a stepping stone for the second step, their association with phenomenal states and thus consciousness.

Let me introduce Jaak Panksepp. Jaak Panksepp is originally from the Baltic states. His parents left during the Soviet Russian occupation, and Jaak grew up in the United States. There he underwent neuroscience training, which at the time was still very much dominated by behaviorism, which argues for the understanding of psychological functions as mere input–output and stimulus–response relationships.

Jaak Panksepp, however, did not like the behaviorism at all. It simply did not correspond to what he observed in the animals he studied. From early on, he therefore postulated animals to have a self and show consciousness, and thus to show subjective experience that cannot be subsumed under mere input–output and stimulus–response relationships. He postulated that animals, to a certain degree, show consciousness in very much the same way as we humans do, with contents, however, that are species-specific.

One example he detected is that rats play and show "laughter" as manifested in 40 Hz oscillations in the brain's neural activity. He conducted many neurobehavioral experiments and wrote a famous book, *Affective Neuroscience*, which (re) introduced emotion and affect as major topics into current neuroscience. And, even more important, he became a close friend of mine, finding common interest in a more basic precognitive sense of self (see later for details).

NEURONAL HYPOTHESIS IIIB: DIFFERENT TYPES OF AFFECT ARE ASSOCIATED WITH DIFFERENT SUBCORTICAL REGIONS

Panksepp (1998a and b, 2011) associates *affect* (or *emotions*, as used synonymously in the following) with the neural processing in the subcortical regions. More specifically, he associates different kinds of basic or primary affects like SEEKING (see Volume I, Chapter 8, for details), FEAR, RAGE, PANIC, CARE, PLAY, and LUST (see Panksepp 1998a and b, 2011, for details). He associated these different affects with different subcortical networks and regions based on his animal studies.

Apart from these specific affects, Panksepp (1998a and b, 2007) distinguishes among three basic types of affects. "Sensory affects" are affects in relation to particular exteroceptive stimuli from the environment. "Homeostatic affects" are the affects that are based on interoceptive stimuli from the body. Finally, there are what Panksepp describes as "emotional affects," which reflect the arousal/motivation of the brain's intrinsic instinctual systems and thus the brain's intrinsic activity, its resting state and neuronal stimuli (see Chapter 7, Volume I, for details).

How is it possible to distinguish among the three different kinds of affects? I postulate that the three different kinds of affects, sensory, homeostatic, and emotional, reflect predominant changes in one of the three different stimuli, intero- and exteroceptive and neuronal, relative to each other. Let me detail this for each type of affect. "Sensory affects" may be predominated by strong changes in exteroceptive stimuli, while interoceptive and neuronal stimuli changes are lower and consequently exert less impact on the relative change in their balance.

This is different in "homoeostatic affects." Interoceptive stimuli may undergo major change and consequently exert the strongest influence on their balance with exteroceptive and neuronal stimuli in "homeostatic affects." Exteroceptive and neuronal stimuli may here show less and thus a lower degree of change when compared to the changes in interoceptive stimuli from the body.

Finally, "emotional affect" may signal major change in the neuronal stimuli from the brain's intrinsic activity itself. This is the case, for instance, in rest–rest interaction and possibly also in stimulus–rest interaction, while intero- and exteroceptive stimuli remain more or less constant. How are these different affects and their underlying neural differences related to consciousness and, more specifically, to qualia? This will be our focus in the next section.

NEUROPHENOMENAL HYPOTHESIS IA: DIFFERENCE-BASED CODING IN SUBCORTICAL REGIONS MEDIATES AFFECTIVE QUALIA

What does the difference-based coding in subcortical regions and its relationship to the different affects tell us about qualia, and especially affective qualia? Unlike the behavioral (and cognitive) neuroscientists, Panksepp postulates an experience, a basic emotional feeling, to always go along with these different affects (that is why he capitalizes the terms for the specific affects as seen earlier). He speaks of a "raw affective feeling" that implies "affective qualia" that signify the experience of, for instance, "fearness" during fear, anxiousness during anxiety, etc. (see later for more details).

How is the generation of such subjective experience in the gestalt of affective qualia possible? I demonstrated earlier strong evidence for difference-based coding in subcortical regions. I also showed that the three basic types of affect, sensory, homeostatic, and emotional, are constituted on the basis of difference-based coding. Such difference-based coding, as we may remember, is also supposed to be a sufficient neural condition and thus a neural correlate of consciousness (see Chapters 28 and 29).

This led me to formulate what I described as the "difference-based coding hypothesis of consciousness" (see Chapter 28). The "difference-based coding hypothesis of consciousness" postulates the degree of the level of consciousness to be directly dependent on the degree of difference-based coding: The higher the degree of difference-based coding, the higher the level of consciousness that can be assigned to changes in neural activity, such as during rest–rest or rest–stimulus interaction.

How, then, is the difference-based coding hypothesis of consciousness related to subcortical regions and affective qualia? Difference-based coding implies interactive and integrative coding between the different stimuli in terms of their statistically based spatial and temporal differences, which may, for instance, differ among the three different basic affects described earlier. I therefore postulate that different-based coding in subcortical regions mediates affective qualia.

NEUROPHENOMENAL HYPOTHESIS IB: STIMULUS-BASED CODING IN SUBCORTICAL REGIONS LEADS TO NEUROBEHAVIORAL AND NEUROPHENOMENAL DISSOCIATION IN VEGETATIVE STATE

How would stimulus-based coding be manifested in subcortical regions? In the case of stimulus-based coding there would be parallel and segregated coding rather than interactive and integrative coding. Each type of affect would then be related exclusively to one particular stimulus type: interoceptive (from body), exteroceptive (from environment), or neuronal (from brain) stimuli.

This, however, I postulate, would no longer result in any kind of behavior, nor any affect including affective qualia. That is well exemplified by the above-described results from the VS patients who still show stimulus-induced activity but no longer any behavior, affect, or qualia related to the affect processed in the neural activity. VS patient thus seem to show a high degree of stimulus-based coding and a low degree of difference-based coding in subcortical regions. Such a high degree of stimulus-based coding still yields stimulus-induced activity, as observed in the data (see above).

However, there is an association of that neural activity with both behavioral and phenomenal features, like the subjective experience of affect, or emotional feeling. There is thus a dissociation between the presence of the purely neuronal stimulus-induced activity related to affect on one hand, and the absence of its behavioral and phenomenal manifestation on the other.

As indicated above, I therefore speak of *neuronal behavioral* and *neuronal phenomenal dissociation* in VS. Since the degree of stimulus-based coding may be abnormally high in VS, I consider VS a "coding disorder," wherein the "wrong" neural code is applied to encode changes into neural activity in both subcortical and cortical regions (see Chapter 29 for details). This distinguishes my hypothesis from alternative and more region- or network-based ones that consider VS to be a subcortical disorder or a subcortical–cortical disconnection syndrome (see Panksepp et al. 2007; Schiff 2009, 2010).

NEUROPHENOMENAL HYPOTHESIS IC: STATISTICALLY BASED SPATIOTEMPORAL CONTINUITY BETWEEN BRAIN, BODY, AND ENVIRONMENT PREDISPOSES BOTH BEHAVIOR AND QUALIA

How is it possible that the presence of stimulus-based coding can accompany the absence of behavior, affect, and qualia in VS?

For behavior, affect, and qualia to be generated, the differences between the different stimuli and their respective different discrete points in time and space must be encoded into neural activity. The resulting neural activity thus needs to span across the different discrete points in physical time and space as associated with the different stimuli from brain, body, and environment. That, in turn, makes possible the generation of behavior, affect, and qualia, with all three reflecting a certain degree of temporal and spatial continuity across different discrete points in physical time and space in brain, body, and environment.

What does this mean for the relationship between stimulus-induced activity and consciousness? Stimulus-induced activity in subcortical regions is by itself not sufficient to induce behavior, affect, and qualia. In addition to the stimuli eliciting neural activity changes, e.g.,

stimulus-induced activity, the stimuli must also be encoded in a specific way into the brain's resting-state activity. If only the stimulus itself and its discrete point in physical time and space are coded, the resulting neural activity will not be able to generate behavior, affect, and qualia.

The neural activity will then not show any spatial and temporal continuity across the different stimuli and their respective origins in brain, body, and environment. If, however, there is no virtual statistically based spatiotemporal continuity of neural activity across the divide of brain, body, and environment, neither behavior nor affect, let alone qualia, can be anymore associated with the otherwise purely neuronal stimulus-induced activity. Accordingly, bridging the divide between brain, body, and environment by a statistically based virtual spatiotemporal continuity is essential for associating the respective stimulus-induced activity with qualia and thus consciousness.

NEURONAL FINDINGS IVA: DECORTICATION AND CONSCIOUSNESS

We showed the possible absence of consciousness in the presence of stimulus-induced activity in subcortical regions in VS. How about the presence of consciousness related to exclusively the subcortical regions themselves? Bjoern Merker (2007, 78ff) investigated human children who, due to a birth defect, do not have a cortex, but only subcortical regions. This is called hydranencephaly. Do these children have consciousness?

He observed that these children are very much alert and awake and are very responsive to their surroundings. They even show emotional or orienting reactions to their environmental events, such as sounds or visual stimuli, and indicate an experience of pleasure by smiling and laughing. They also show preferences for certain people, events, and familiarity with regard to toys, tunes, and videos. Moreover, the children sometimes yield behavioral initiatives, though sparse. Interestingly, while they did not retain any parts of their auditory cortex, they nevertheless showed some preservation of their auditory sense, being able to listen and hear.

Based on his observations, Merker (2007) concludes that these patients integrate environmental events, motivation/emotions, and actions. Following him, they thus exhibit some degree of trilateral interaction between motivation (e.g., neuronal stimuli), target (e.g., sensory stimuli), and action (e.g., motor stimuli) (see earlier). That is, I say, indicative of difference-based coding (as distinguished from mere stimulus-based coding). Such difference-based coding, even if of low degree, is indispensable for generating some degree of spatiotemporal continuity even if extremely limited in its spatial and temporal scope (see later for details).

Moreover, the fact that these subjects have clear preferences in their behavior (see earlier) suggests that they must have some limited degree of self-specific organization, including a very basic and existential sense of self (see later for details). Finally,, however limited, they do show some behavioral initiatives, which suggest a basic intentionality and hence preintentional organization.

Despite their decortication, therefore, these patients nevertheless show some signs of consciousness that signifies the resting state's various prephenomenal structures on the phenomenal level. This strongly suggests that the resting state's neural activity in subcortical regions shows some spatiotemporal structure in its neural activity, which I presuppose as indispensable for the association of neural activity changes with consciousness.

NEURONAL FINDINGS IVB: EPILEPSY AND CONSCIOUSNESS

The case of decortication shows the presence of consciousness in the absence of cortical regions. How about the reverse case with the absence of consciousness in the presence of altered subcortical regions? I already considered the case of brainstem lesions leading to VS and coma (see Parvizi and Damasio 2003).

Another example is epilepsy. Epilepsy describes seizures with different types, with the most well known being the tonic-clonic grand mal seizures as related to the temporal lobe, the hippocampus. Most important, the epileptic seizures go along with a loss of consciousness.

Giving only a very brief and less detailed account, recent investigations demonstrated major abnormalities, that is, reductions, in the functional connectivity of the anterior and posterior midline regions in the resting-state activity in epilepsy (see Kay et al. 2013, as well as Bagshaw and Cavenna 2012, for a recent overview)). This can be observed in different kinds of epilepsy and may therefore be related to the loss of consciousness (see Danielson et al. 2011).

How is that possible? Most often epileptic seizures start in one cortical region as, for instance, the hippocampus that becomes hyperactive and shows abnormally synchronized neural activity. Following the "network inhibition hypothesis" by Blumenfeld (see Danielson et al. 2011), such hyperactivity in one region or network leads to the inhibition of the neural activity in yet another region or network with subsequent deactivation in the same regions/networks. .

More specifically, the hyperactivity in the hippocampus during tonic-clonic grand mal seizures may inhibit the neural activity in the subcortical regions (see Danielson et al. 2011). The decreased subcortical activity in brainstem and midbrain may then lead to reduced excitation of the arousal and motivation associated with the thalamus, the upper brainstem, and the basal forebrain. That, in turn, may induce widespread deactivation in cortical midline regions and the lateral frontoparietal network. Hence, cortical activity is reduced via subcortical inhibition.

Temporal lobe seizures going along with a loss of consciousness may thus be characterized by subcortical inhibition of cortical activity. In contrast, the seizures that do not accompany loss of consciousness do not show such widespread subcortical inhibition. Instead, neural hyperactivity remains more local and restricted to the temporal lobe without affecting the subcortical (and consequently the cortical) regions. Hence, they spare the cortical midline regions, where neural activity remains more or less normal.

Taken together, the case of epilepsy demonstrates the central role of subcortical regions for consciousness. Unlike in decortication, however, the case of epilepsy does not lend empirical support to the assumption that subcortical regions are by themselves sufficient for consciousness. Instead, the example of epilepsy demonstrates that subcortical regions are necessary for consciousness.

NEUROPHENOMENAL HYPOTHESIS IIA: SUBCORTICAL REGIONS SHOW SPATIOTEMPORAL CONTINUITY IN THEIR NEURAL ACTIVITY

What exactly happens in the above-described patients without cortex? In the case of the cortex and its cortical regions, I postulated the transfer of the resting state's prephenomenal structures onto the stimulus and its associated stimulus-induced activity to be central. By that, I mean that the stimulus becomes integrated and merged with the resting state's prephenomenal structures, which makes possible its association with qualia and its phenomenal features (see Chapter 30 for details).

I now postulate exactly the same to happen in the case of subcortical regions. I demonstrated evidence for difference-based coding of neural activity in subcortical regions. That makes possible the constitution of spatiotemporal structure by the subcortical resting-state activity, and more specifically of spatiotemporal continuity in its neural activity.

Such spatiotemporal continuity is statistically based and spans virtually across the divide of the brain's neuronal stimuli, the body's interoceptive stimuli, and the environment's exteroceptive stimuli.

This is nicely reflected in Merker's (2007) description of subcortical neural activity by concepts like a "shared body-world coordinate system," the "simulated nature of our body and world," or a "synthetic reality space." Such spatiotemporal continuity in subcortical neural activity may, however, be rather limited in its degree of spatial and temporal extension. Why? I postulated the encoding of sufficiently large spatial and temporal differences, i.e., difference-based coding, to be essential in constituting spatiotemporal continuity in neural activity and to associate it with consciousness (see above and Part V).

What does this mean for the subcortical regions? The limited spatial and temporal extension of the subcortical regions implies the encoding of rather small temporal and spatial differences into the neural activity of subcortical regions, compared to that in the much larger and more extended cortex. There may be difference-based coding in subcortical regions, as stated above; but the degree of spatial and temporal differences that can be encoded into neural activity may be rather small in subcortical regions due to their limited spatial and temporal extension. This shall be further explicated in the following section.

NEUROPHENOMENAL HYPOTHESIS IIB: DEGREE OF EXTENSION IN PHYSICAL SPACE AND TIME IN SUBCORTICAL AND CORTICAL REGIONS PREDICTS THE DEGREE OF SPATIOTEMPORAL CONTINUITY IN THEIR NEURAL ACTIVITY

Why are the encoded temporal and spatial differences rather small in the case of subcortical regions? The degree of temporal and spatial differences that can possibly be encoded into neural activity may be closely related to the temporal and spatial extension of their neural environment; that is, cortical and subcortical regions.

The more spatially and temporally extended the neural environment, the more the resulting neural activity can spread and propagate in spatial and temporal regard, and the larger the spatial and temporal differences that can be encoded into neural activity. This may, for instance, be manifest in the extent of long-range functional connectivity and the ranges of frequency fluctuations. The range of the frequency fluctuations may be strongly dependent upon the spatial extend and thus the physical space of the neural environment with lower-frequency ranges requiring larger spatial extension than higher frequencies (see Chapters 5 and 10 for details).

The same holds true for functional connectivity in the spatial dimension; the larger the physical space of the neural environment, the wider the possible range of functional connectivity among different regions/networks. And the larger the range of frequencies and the wider the range of functional connectivity, the larger the spatial and temporal differences that can possibly be encoded into neural activity via difference-based coding. Accordingly, a spatially and temporally more extended neural environment like the cortex allows for the encoding of larger spatiotemporal differences into neural activity.

If, in contrast, the neural environment is spatially and temporally more restricted and limited, the resulting neural activity can no longer spatially and temporally spread and propagated as much. This may be manifested in limited long-range functional connectivity and decreased (especially lower) ranges of different frequency fluctuations (with, e.g., the lower-frequency ranges remaining absent). The temporal and spatial differences that can then be encoded into neural activity remain consequently rather small.

How does the claim about spatiotemporal extension apply to the subcortical regions? The subcortical regions can be regarded as an instance of a neural environment with a rather small extension in physical time and space. This means that the degree of spatial and temporal differences the subcortical regions can possibly encode into their neural activity remains rather small compared to that of the much more extensive cortex. The subcortical neural activity's degree of spatiotemporal extension and continuity may be thus smaller and less extended than that of the cortex (see Fig. 31-3a).

Neurophenomenal Hypothesis IIC: Spatiotemporal Extension of Subcortical Regions and Qualia

This leads me to suggest the following rather tentative hypothesis. The main difference between subcortical and cortical regions' neural processing may consist of the degrees of spatial and temporal differences they can possibly encode into their neural activity.

The more extended space and time of the cortical regions may allow for increased spatial and temporal extension of their neural activity with the encoding of larger spatiotemporal differences into neural activity compared to that of the subcortical regions. The resulting spatiotemporal continuity of the resting state's neural activity is consequently more extended, both spatially and temporally, in cortical regions than in subcortical regions.

What does this imply for the resting-state activity's spatiotemporal structures and ultimately for qualia and consciousness? It means that, for instance, the degree of global spatiotemporal continuity is much more limited spatially and temporally in subcortical than in cortical regions. And it implies that the spatial extension and the temporal duration of the resting-state activity's prephenomenal unity and environment–brain unity are much more limited in subcortical regions. If considered separately (which is impossible in empirical reality), the subcortical regions' spatiotemporal structure may thus be spatiotemporally much more restricted and limited, and thus less complex and structured, compared to the one of the cortex (Fig. 31-3b).

Since the resting-state activity's spatiotemporal structures are carried over and transferred to the stimulus, the spatial and temporal scope of the phenomenal level and thus the resulting qualia and consciousness in general will also be rather limited. The degree of spatial and temporal scope of the qualia may thus be extremely small and narrow.

This is well reflected in the description of the patients without cortex (see earlier). They seem to show some degree of consciousness, albeit in an extremely limited and highly restricted way in both regards, spatially and temporally. In other words, even neural activity in subcortical regions may still be associated with qualia, which, however, are spatially and temporally extremely restricted and limited.

Neuronal Findings VA: Subcortical Regions and the Self

How about the third prephenomenal structure—the self-specific and preintentional organization? Jaak Panksepp postulates that the subcortical structures mediate a basic sense of self, a SELF, as he capitalizes it (see below, as well as Northoff and Panksepp 2008; Panksepp and Northoff 2009). Such a SELF is a basic neuropsychic mechanism located in the subcortical regions, more specifically the midbrain, the subcortical midline structure (SC, PAG; see also Merker 2005, 2007), and the limbic structures.

What does this more basic form of self look like? Jaak Panksepp (1998a and b, 2003a and b; see also Northoff and Panksepp 2008; and Panksepp and Northoff 2009) postulates that the self is already constituted in the neural activity on the subcortical level. He considers the self to be a "Simple Egotype Life Form" ("SELF"). Such a biologically basic sense of self can be subjectively experienced in consciousness, where it may be manifested phenomenally in what can be

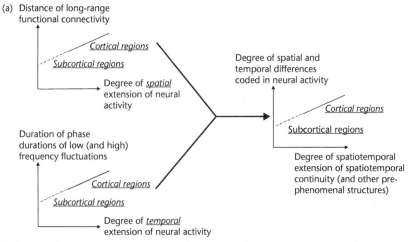

Figure 31-3a and b Comparison between subcortical and cortical regions. The figure compares subcortical and cortical regions with regard to the spatiotemporal extension of their neural activity (*a*) and their degrees in difference-based coding in relation to the brain's underlying biophysical-computational spectrum (*b*). (*a*) The figure describes the degree of spatial (i.e., functional connectivity) (*left upper*) and temporal (i.e., range of low- and high-frequency fluctuations) (*left lower*) measures of neural activity, as well as their degree of spatial and temporal extension across different discrete points in time and space (see graphs on the left). The wider-reaching the functional connectivity and the longer the phase durations in the frequency fluctuations, the higher the amount of neural activity that can be extended across different discrete points in time and space (*left part of figure*). Due to their larger spatial and temporal extension, the degree of spatial and temporal extension of the neural activity is obviously much higher in cortical regions than in subcortical ones with the latter being indicated by a dotted line. The difference in spatiotemporal extension should be neurally mirrored in the degree of spatial and temporal differences coded in neural activity (graph in the right part of the figure). The larger the spatial and temporal differences coded in neural activity, the more the spatiotemporal continuity of neural activity can extend across time and space. (*b*) The figure describes the degree of difference-based coding in subcortical and cortical regions in relation to the brain's underlying biophysical-computational spectrum (*left part*) and the degree of consciousness (*right part*). *Left part*: The x-axis describes the brain's biophysical-computational spectrum with its species-specific maximal and minimal spatiotemporal limits (dotted lines pointing downward toward the bottom) with an optimal range, the optimal spatiotemporal window, for inducing maximal neural activity changes during rest–rest or rest–stimulus interaction (dotted lines pointing upward toward the top). Within the optimal spatiotemporal window for the resting state, maximally large differences (y-axis) and thus neural activity changes can be encoded into neural activity. Thereby the degree of spatiotemporal difference that can be encoded into neural activity is much larger in cortical regions (*upper curve*) than in subcortical regions (*lower curve*). This leads to an inverted u-shape curve when compared to the maximal and minimal limits of the brain's biophysical spectrum. When considering only the increase in the differences encoded within the range of the optimal spatiotemporal window (*upper part with graph*), one yields the following relationship with a linear curve as plotted in the graph on the right. The larger the spatiotemporal differences encoded into neural activity (y-axis), the larger and stronger the degree of the spatiotemporal extension of consciousness (x-axis). This holds much stronger for cortical than subcortical regions, with the latter being indicated by the dotted line.

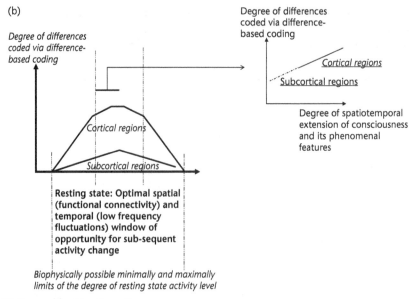

Figure 31-3a and b (Continued)

described as "unreflective, existential feeling of I-ness" (Panksepp 2003a and b, 200–201).

Panksepp's concept of SELF comes somehow close to Damasio's concept of a "protoself" that is supposed to allow for homeostatic regulation of the body by the brain and its subcortical regions (brainstem and hypothalamus as well as the insular cortex; see Damasio 1999a and b, 2010; Parvizi and Damasio 2001; also see Chapter 24 herein for a detailed discussion of Damasio's concept of the protoself). Both concepts, Panksepp's SELF and Damasio's protoself, must be distinguished from a more cognitive and cortical self that refers rather to a "reflective, cognitive feeling of me-ness." (See also Chapter 24 and Appendix 4 for a discussion of the concept of self).

How is such a basic concept of self possible? I postulate the subcortical regions to show some degree of self-specific organization (see Chapter 23 for details). Such self-specific organization in the subcortical regions' neuronal processing may account for a first and very basic assignment of self-specificity to stimuli (and ultimately for a very basic sense of self). During rest–stimulus interaction, the subcortical pre-phenomenal self-specific organization may be assigned to the respective stimuli and thereby

induce a basic "unreflective, existential feeling of I-ness" that accompanies all our perceptions, cognitions, and feelings, and so on.

Interestingly, Merker (2005, 105) goes even as far to postulate that this basic sense of self, as entertained by the subcortical regions' neural activity, corresponds to what German philosopher Immanuel Kant described as "synthetic unity of apperception," and his successor Arthur Schopenhauer as "pure subject of knowing" (see Appendix 3 for a brief discussion of the relationship between my neurophenomenal hypotheses and Kant's philosophy; see also Northoff 2011, chapters 1 and 2, as well as Northoff 2012). There is thus an interesting convergence between philosophical approaches and neuroscientific hypotheses, as suggested here. However, to further explicate such neurophilosophical convergence is beyond the scope of this book and must therefore be left to other books.

Neuronal findings VB: Subcortical regions mediate the degree of self-specificity of extrinsic stimuli

Let us come back to the empirical data. Is there any evidence from humans that the subcortical regions are indeed already involved in processing self-specificity? Unlike most current imaging studies on the self, our own studies did not apply a cognitive task, that is, judgement, but let subjects rather merely perceive the stimuli without requiring any task. This minimizes task-related effects like stimulus judgement or evaluation (see Northoff et al. 2009; Schneider et al. 2008).

We indeed observed subcortical activity in the PAG, the tectum, the SC, the DMT, the amygdala, the ventral striatum, and even the ventral tegmental area. These regions' neural activity differentiated well between self- and non-self-specific emotional or rewarding stimuli (see de Greck et al. 2008; Enzi et al. 2009; Schneider et al. 2008; Northoff et al. 2009). Furthermore, we also observed parametric dependence of the stimuli's degree of self-specificity on the degree of neural activity in these regions. The higher the neural activity in the subcortical regions, the higher the degree of self-specificity assigned to the respective emotional or rewarding stimuli. These results lend empirical evidence to the involvement of the subcortical regions in processing self-specificity.

In addition to the subcortical midline regions, various cortical midline regions like the PACC, the VMPFC, the DMPFC, and the PCC and precuneus were also implicated. Hence, neural activity in the subcortical-cortical midline system seems to be central in processing self-specificity and its assignment to stimuli (see Northoff and Panksepp 2008; Panksepp and Northoff 2009; see Chapter 23 herein for details). If this is so, one would postulate the midline regions' resting-state activity to exhibit what we earlier described as *self-specific organization*, the organization of neural activity around the needs, demands, and relevance of stimuli for the respective organism.

Therefore, there is some tentative evidence for self-specific organization in the subcortical regions' resting-state activity. This, in turn, makes possible the participation of subcortical regions in assigning self-specificity to stimuli. Phenomenally, such self-specific organization may be manifested in a basic existential and non-reflective experience or feeling of an *I* or sense of self, which may already be associated with neural

activity in the subcortical regions themselves, e.g., independently of the neural activity in the cortex.

NEUROPHENOMENAL HYPOTHESIS IIIA: "PRIMARY OR ANOETIC CONSCIOUSNESS" REFLECTS "RAW EXPERIENCE"

Thus far, I have focused on characterizing the subcortical regions and how they are related to qualia and thus consciousness. This bears some important implications for the description and characterization of qualia in general. Qualia in the context of the subcortical regions were characterized as affective; I therefore spoke of *affective qualia*.

Such affective qualia are not limited to the subcortical regions, though. Since subcortical regions are directly or indirectly involved in shaping neural activity of the cortex, even qualia predominantly related to cortical activity always already implicate the affective dimension. In other words, any kind of qualia may not be able to avoid the implication of the affective component, affective qualia, to some degree. postulate

Let us see what the neuroscientists say about this proclaimed association between affect and qualia. Panksepp (2007, 2011) associates affect with primary consciousness, as distinguished from secondary and tertiary consciousness. Before explaining *primary* or *anoetic consciousness* in further detail, let us briefly describe the concepts of secondary and tertiary consciousness.

The concept of *secondary consciousness* refers to cognitive consciousness and related cognitive functions, including learning, attention, memory, etc. As such, secondary consciousness involves knowledge about the world and can therefore be described as *noetic consciousness*. Finally, *tertiary consciousness* describes thoughts about one's own thoughts and feelings and may therefore be characterized by knowledge about one's own self *as* self; this is described as *reflective* and *autonoetic consciousness*.

What is *primary* or *anoetic consciousness*? Following Panksepp, primary consciousness concerns affect and feelings, which can also be described as anoetic consciousness. Anoetic consciousness may phenomenally be manifested in what is described as "raw experience" or "raw emotional feelings" that do not involve any explicit knowledge about the world or the self as such. Hence, primary consciousness can be characterized as *anoetic* and *affective*.

Such anoetic or primary consciousness is pre-reflective, which means that it does not yet involve any reflection, including propositional and conceptual contents. Instead, it refers rather to what William James (1890) described as the "free water of consciousness"; as "free water that flows around" (see also Vandekerckhove and Panksepp 2009, 1019). Panksepp suggest that such anoetic or primary consciousness is largely affective, which signifies the most basic emotional feelings: "raw affective feelings or experiences." As such, anoetic or primary consciousness concerns mainly automatic and unexperienced processing in the brain's neural activity that is not yet associated with a particular object or content (see also Vandekerckhove and Panksepp 2009).

NEUROPHENOMENAL HYPOTHESIS IIIB: STIMULUS-PHASE COUPLING MEDIATES "RAW EXPERIENCE"

How can such primary or anoetic consciousness be further characterized in both neuronal and phenomenal regards? Let us start with the neuronal side of things. I suggest that such primary or anoetic consciousness is related to neuronal mechanisms underlying the environment–brain unity like the stimulus-phase coupling of the low-frequency fluctuations (see Chapter 20). "Stimulus-phase coupling" describes the shifting and linkage of the brain's intrinsic activity and its low-frequency fluctuations' phase onsets to the onset of the extrinsic stimuli (see Chapter 20).

Usually, stimulus-phase coupling and the associated statistically based environment–brain unity are superseded by the constitution of contents and the subsequent neuronal unity of low-high cross-frequency coupling (see Chapters 18 and 19). If associated subsequently with consciousness, the contents will dominate our experience, which, following Panksepp, results in noetic/secondary and autonoetic/tertiary consciousness (Vandekerckhove and Panksepp 2009). If, however, the contents do not dominate consciousness, the environment–brain unity itself may surface and dominate in consciousness.

I consequently propose that what Panksepp describes as "primary or anoetic consciousness" is neuronally related to the environment–brain unity and its underlying neuronal mechanisms, like stimulus-phase coupling. The stronger the degree of stimulus-phase coupling, the stronger the degree of the environment–brain unity, which in conjunction with decreased stimulus input and constitution of contents may shift the environment–brain unity itself into the focus of our consciousness. This is the moment where, I claim, we experience what Panksepp describes as "raw experience," which usually, in the presence of content, recedes and remains in the background or the fringes of our consciousness.

NEUROPHENOMENAL HYPOTHESIS IIIC: "EXISTENTIAL FEELINGS" ARE A "SPATIOTEMPORAL GRID BETWEEN BRAIN, BODY, AND ENVIRONMENT"

How about a more precise phenomenal characterization? What Panksepp calls "raw experiences" may come close to what others describe as "existential feelings." The concept of "existential feeling" is a term that is associated with the phenomenological tradition of philosophy and goes back to Martin Heidegger (see Ratcliffe 2005; Slaby and Stephan 2008, who also distinguish among different levels of "existential feelings," which shall not be pursued here in detail).

The term "existential feelings" is a phenomenal concept that describes the experience and feeling of one's own existence, one's own body and one's relationship to and standing in the world. As indicated by the term itself, these existential feelings concern the existence itself rather than specific contents; they are about the experience of one's own existence and one's relationship to the world independently of any specific contents.

How can we now relate such "existential feelings" on the phenomenal level to their potentially underlying neuronal mechanisms—stimulus-phase coupling and its associated environment–brain unity? We recall that the environment–brain unity was not only statistically based but also spatiotemporally based (see Chapter 20 for details). Due to the encoding of the spatial and temporal differences between the brain's intrinsic activity and the extrinsic stimuli, the resulting neural activity can be characterized by a statistically and spatiotemporally based virtual continuity between brain and environment (and body; see Chapter 20). Metaphorically speaking, there seems to be an "invisible spatiotemporal grid or template spanning between brain and environment."

I now postulate that the experience of the existential feelings (or the "raw experiences," as Panksepp would say) reflects this "invisible spatiotemporal grid or template spanning between brain and environment." This corresponds well to the observation that these existential feelings signify "the basis of the ways that a person relates to the world" and do therefore "disclose our standing in the world" (see Slaby and Stephan 2008, 511).

NEUROPHENOMENAL HYPOTHESIS IIID: EXISTENTIAL FEELINGS ARE THE EXPERIENCE OF THE ENVIRONMENT–BRAIN UNITY AND ITS ASSOCIATED POINT OF VIEW

What exactly do the existential feelings disclose? They "disclose" the degree and extension of the "invisible spatiotemporal grid or template spanning between brain and environment" and thus the degree to which our self and its existence are integrated and linked in the environment.

I consequently suggest the following neurophenomenal relationship. The stronger the degree of stimulus-phase coupling, the more extended the statistically based spatiotemporal grid or template between brain and environment, and the stronger the possible degree of the existential feelings (or raw experiences). Since there are different possible spatiotemporal constellations between environment and brain, one may assume different kinds of existential feelings, which is indeed the case (see Slaby and Stephan 2008).

In sum, I suggest that existential feelings can be characterized in spatiotemporal terms and are therefore based on the relationship between brain and environment. The existential feelings

reflect, then, the experience of the environment–brain unity itself and its associated point of view (see Chapter 20). The point of view may be considered the very basis of our existence, or better, our existence by itself, independent of any particular content.

How can we provide empirical evidence for such a daring hypothesis? The subcortical regions are already associated with the self, as described earlier. I now postulate that this basic self comes close to what I described as the "point of view," itself which is not yet superseded by contents as they are predominantly mediated by cortical regions. The down-modulation of neural activity in the cortical regions may lay bare the subcortical regions and the point of view itself independent of its association with contents. This may be the moment where one experiences what philosophers described as "existential feelings."

NEUROCONCEPTUAL REMARK IA: NEUROAFFECTIVE APPROACH TO QUALIA

The previous neurophenomenal hypothesis suggested a close relationship between qualia and affect, with existential feelings (or raw experiences) being the first and most fundamental manifestation of consciousness. Are qualia thus intrinsically affective? Panksepp and philosopher Alfred North Whitehead seem to succumb to such a claim of the intrinsic affective nature of qualia.

Panksepp postulates that affective qualia "lie" directly at the interface between neuronal and phenomenal states, that is, where both are transformed into each other. This is well reflected in Panksepp's characterization of affect at the border between brain and mind: "the nature of affect lies at the very core of the mind-matter dilemma" (see Panksepp 2011, 1; see also Damasio 2010).

Following Panksepp, affective qualia are the point where mere neuronal processing is transformed into a phenomenal state and thus experience; how such a transformation is possible, and by what kind of neuronal mechanisms it is mediated are left unresolved in his account, however. He says, though, that such affective qualia are manifested on the phenomenal level in what is described as "feeling" or "qualitative feel" (Searle 2004) as one phenomenal hallmarks of qualia (see Chapter 30 for the other phenomenal features of qualia).

By linking affect and qualia, the feeling signifying the former—that is, affect—is transferred and carried over to the latter, the qualia. Qualia are consequently associated with a "feeling": resulting in the "qualitative feel." Hence, affect may be a central feature of qualia that therefore may be characterized as affective at their very core. However, the reverse also holds. Qualia are transferred to the affect and emotions. Affect and emotions are consequently and unavoidably associated with experience and thus some kind of feeling, a "basic emotional feeling," that signifies consciousness (see also Northoff 2012b on emotional consciousness).

A philosopher who also postulated the prime importance of feelings, affect, and emotions for consciousness was Alfred North Whitehead (1929–1979). He speaks of a "basic affective tone" that underlies all our consciousness: "the basis of experience is emotional." He regards emotions as the "subjective form" of consciousness (see also the illuminating discussion of Whitehead in Pred 2005, pp. 121ff). (I must, however, leave it to future neurophilosophical investigation to elaborate on and tighten the link between my account and Whitehead's).

How do both accounts stand in relation to each other? Though coming from the almost opposite starting points of brain and consciousness, Panksepp and Whitehead nevertheless share the assumption that qualia and thus consciousness are intrinsically affective. Panksepp comes to the central role of affect in consciousness by tracing cortical activity to its very neural basis in subcortical regions. And from there, he concludes that any affect includes experience and thus consciousness; that is, emotional feeling.

How about Whitehead? In contrast to Panksepp, Whitehead starts with consciousness, which he traces back down to its very basic affective roots. That leads him to suggest that affect and emotions are the basis upon which any consciousness stands. He therefore postulates the core or basis of qualia and thus consciousness to be affective.

NEUROCONCEPTUAL REMARK IB: NEUROAFFECTIVE VERSUS NEUROPHENOMENAL APPROACHES TO QUALIA

Are qualia and thus consciousness intrinsically affective? Is affect an intrinsic and therefore defining feature of qualia and consciousness? The accounts by Panksepp and Whitehead seem to suggest that a neuroaffective approach can indeed account for qualia. Does this mean that the here-suggested neurophenomenal approach to qualia needs to be replaced by a neuroaffective one?

We should be careful, though. I postulate that qualia are closely linked to affect, with both often coming together. This, however, does not prove that affect is an intrinsic or defining feature of qualia. A defining and thus intrinsic feature of qualia is subjectivity and its determination by a point of view (see Chapter 30 for details). If there is no association of the stimulus with a point of view and thus subjectivity, any kind of qualia, whether they are more or less affective, remain impossible. The point of view and thus subjectivity are therefore defining and consequently intrinsic features of qualia. Without them, qualia would remain impossible. Qualia are the subjective and qualitative features of our experience. This, as I postulated, is only possible if they are associated with a point of view and thus subjectivity. Qualia are thus intrinsically subjective.

How is such subjectivity related to affect? The subjectivity and hence qualia are now first and foremost manifested in affect and emotions. But they are also manifested in our perceptions, in our cognitions, and in all of our behavior. And there may also be many instances where qualia do not go along with affect, as for instance in perceptual qualia. Accordingly, unlike subjectivity, affect cannot be considered a defining and therefore intrinsic feature of qualia. Instead affect remains extrinsic rather than intrinsic to qualia (see Fig. 31-4).

To define qualia by affect would be to confuse a defining feature— one that constitutes qualia as such, like the point of view and its subjectivity—with their manifestation in different functions, like affect, cognitive functions, etc. More

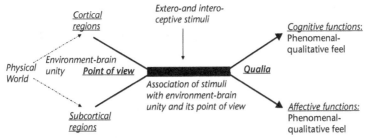

Figure 31-4 Regions, functions, and qualia. The figure shows the relationship between the environment–brain unity (*left part*) and the manifestation of qualia in different functions (*right part*). *Left part*: The resting state from both cortical and subcortical regions aligns its neuronal spatial and temporal measures to the stimuli's onsets and occurrence in the physical world. This is indicated by dotted lines, and leads to a statistically and spatiotemporally based virtual environment–brain unity. The environment–brain unity provides a stance for the organism within the rest of the physical world and thus a point of view from which he can experience the world (and himself as part of that world). Such point of view allows for the perception and experience of the world and its different contents from that particular stance. *Middle and right part*: When the resting state encounters specific interoceptive or exteroceptive stimuli, these have to be linked and associated with the environment–brain unity and its particular point of view. This, in turn, leads to the constitution of qualia, which are then manifest in all the different function as, for instance, in cognitive and affective functions (as examples while neglecting others like sensorimotor, vegetative, and social functions). Hence, the manifestation and occurrence of qualia; that is, their phenomenal-qualitative feel, is not dependent upon particular regions, subcortical or cortical, nor on specific functions, affective, cognitive, or otherwise, but rather on how well the stimulus is linked and aligned to the environment–brain unity and its associated point of view, which is related to the whole brain and its statistically and spatiotemporally based relationship to the environment in its resting-state activity.

generally put, one should not confuse phenomenal and psychological functions, and thus the neurophenomenal account of qualia, with a neuroaffective one.

NEUROCONCEPTUAL REMARK

IC: NEUROPHENOMENAL FUNCTIONS OF THE BRAIN

Why do I put so much emphasis on the distinction between neurophenomenal and neuroaffective approaches to qualia? I postulate that once one associates qualia with a particular function, like neuroaffective function, one runs into major problems when explaining why and how qualia can also occur in relation with other functions like sensory quale, motor quale, cognitive quale, and so on. This is different in the case of the neurophenomenal approach, however.

I consider the brain's neurophenomenal functions to be more basic and fundamental than its neuroaffective, neurocognitive, neurosensory,

and neuromotor functions. Due to their fundamental nature as signified by their association with the brain's intrinsic activity, the neurophenomenal functions permeate and infiltrate any subsequent function and their associated stimulus-induced activity. This means that any function and any regions' neural activity can possibly be associated with qualia and thus consciousness. Metaphorically speaking, the different functions occur "on the basis of the neurophenomenal functions" and consequently "within the space or field of consciousness."

Taking all this together, I postulate that qualia can in principle be associated with the neural processing of all regions, networks, and their respectively associated functions, including sensorimotor, affective, and cognitive functions. This includes both subcortical and cortical regions and networks, while on the functional side, it concerns emotional and affective functions as well as cognitive, sensory, and motor functions, and so on. One may consequently want to speak of *affective* qualia, *cognitive* qualia, *sensory* qualia, and so on.

Based on these considerations, I postulate that the brain exhibits neurophenomenal functions that can be related to its intrinsic activity and its different layers of spatiotemporal structures. I suggest that the intrinsic activity constitutes different neurophenomenal functions like spatiotemporal continuity and unity as well as self-specific and preintentional organization (see Parts V–VII).

Moreover, the subsequent interaction of the intrinsic activity with the extrinsic activity, rest–stimulus interaction, is central for the brain's neurophenomenal functions as manifested in qualia (see Chapter 29). This, however, is the point where the brain's neurophenomenal functions stop; and where the other functions of the brain—sensory, motor, affective, cognitive, and social—start, as they are associated with stimulus-induced or task-related activity.

Open Questions

The first open question concerns the relationship between qualia and feeling. The concept of *feeling* is usually used in the context of affect and emotion, such as, for instance, emotional feeling (see Northoff 2008, 2012). However, it is also used in the context of qualia, where it describes a certain feeling, a "qualitative feeling," as is often signified by "what it is like." The question is how much these two descriptions of the concept of feeling (and I am sure many others, too) converge and diverge from each other. This is not only a conceptual exercise but also a phenomenal and ultimately a neuronal one which I leave, however, for others to discuss and explore in the future.

Another question concerns whether there is consciousness in nonhuman animals. Animals display complex behavioral pattern, show social perception and behavior, and possess a sophisticated nervous system, including subcortical regions (see also Edelman and Seth 2009;; as well as Panksepp 1998a and b, 2007). Can we infer from that they show consciousness? In addition to the kind of behavior and the organization of their brain, I would here suggest a third criterion that consists in the presence of the "right" kind of neural coding, namely difference-based coding rather than stimulus-based coding.

Even if the nervous system is complex and shows an elaborated cortex, this may by itself not be sufficient to yield consciousness. For that, the complex cortex must be operated on by difference-based coding rather than stimulus-based coding. If, in contrast, stimulus-based coding prevails, the respective animal will not show consciousness despite its elaborated cortex, as I would postulate. Hence, the presence or absence of difference-based coding as distinguished from stimulus-based coding may be taken as criterion (being most likely sufficient) to indicate the presence or absence of consciousness in different species. Moreover, following my account from Chapter 28, I would postulate the degree of difference-based coding (and its balance with stimulus-based coding) to correspond to the degree of consciousness present in the respective species.

Another question concerns the involvement of interoceptive stimuli in subcortical regions. The subcortical regions receive major interoceptive input from the body in especially its regions in the inner ring adjacent to the ventricles. These interoceptive inputs are then conveyed onto the cortical level, where the insula plays a major role. This raises the question of whether and how the insula mediates the association of phenomenal states with interoceptive stimuli and thus the body in general. For the answer to that, however, one needs to shift the focus from the consciousness of the environment to the consciousness of one's own body. This will be the focus of the next and final chapter.

CHAPTER 32
Body and Qualia

Summary

How are the resting-state activity's prephenomenal structures transformed into a full-blown phenomenal state during stimulus-induced activity? The central stimuli input are interoceptive stimuli from the body, which continuously feed into the brain's resting-state activity. Phenomenally, such continuous interoceptive input is manifested in our consciousness of the body, which more or less is almost always present in the background or the foreground of any consciousness. How is the continuous interoceptive input transformed into qualia and thus consciousness of the body? For the answer to that, I discuss recent results from functional imaging that show how the insula and other regions like the sensorimotor cortex are recruited during interoceptive awareness. Based on both neuronal and phenomenal data, I suppose that difference-based coding between intero- and exteroceptive stimuli is central in yielding consciousness of the body, which is often described as "interoceptive awareness." Additional data show the involvement of the brain's resting-state activity in yielding interoceptive awareness and full-blown phenomenal consciousness of one's own body; that is, body qualia. Moreover, the data indicate that the degree of neural activity during interoceptive awareness is dependent upon the concentration of GABA in the same region. This leads me to suggest nonlinear and GABA-ergic-mediated rest–stimulus interaction in the insula during interoceptive stimulus processing. Finally, the data show that the insula is closely connected to the midline regions. This makes it likely that the resting-state activity's prephenomenal structures like the self-specific and preintentional organization are transferred and carried over onto subsequent stimulus-induced activity as related to interoceptive stimuli. That, in turn, makes possible the association of the interoceptive stimulus-induced activity with qualia and thus consciousness. The chapter concludes with a neuroconceptual remark about interoception and perception that must be considered in a relational way rather than as isolated from both body and environment. I therefore propose qualia in particular and consciousness in general to be intrinsically relational and thus necessarily embodied and embedded; that is, by default.

Key Concepts and Topics Covered

Interoceptive awareness, insula, difference-based coding, predictive coding, somatosensory cortex, body perception and awareness, interoceptive stimuli, nonlinearity, GABA, rest–stimulus interaction, relational concept of interoception

NEUROEMPIRICAL BACKGROUND
IA: INTEROCEPTIVE STIMULI AND THE BRAIN

I showed in the previous parts that exteroceptive stimuli are central in triggering the carryover and transfer of the prephenomenal structures from the resting state to subsequent stimulus-induced activity. This puts the focus on what I describe as "rest–extero interaction," the interaction between resting-state activity and exteroceptive stimuli, which results in what we as outside observers describe as "stimulus-induced activity."

However, besides the exteroceptive stimuli, the brain and its resting state also receive continuous interoceptive input from one's own body. Very much like exteroceptive stimuli, this interoceptive input also needs to interact with the brain's resting-state activity in order to be processed. This yields what I describe as rest–intero interaction, the interaction between resting-state activity and interoceptive stimuli.

Analogous to exteroceptive stimuli, such rest–intero interaction may also affect the resting state itself by triggering the carry-over and transfer of its prephenomenal structures onto the stimulus and its associated stimulus-induced activity. Such carryover and transfer may associate the stimulus-induced activity with a phenomenal state, e.g., qualia and thus consciousness, which is manifested in the phenomenal consciousness or awareness (both terms are used synonymously here) of one's own body.

Even more important, due to the continuous interoceptive input from one's own body, the alleged rest–intero interaction is continuously ongoing. Since the brain is always already connected to the body, its resting-state activity is closely intertwined with the continuous interoceptive input from its body. That means that the body's interoceptive input to the brain's resting state and thus rest–intero interaction are always already present when the less continuous (and thus more discontinuous) exteroceptive stimulus arrives.

Let us briefly summarize our encounter with interoceptive stimuli so far. While I focussed predominantly on exteroceptive stimuli here in Volume II, interoceptive stimuli were touched upon at numerous occasions in Volume I. The first encounter with interoceptive stimuli occurred in Volume I, Chapter 4, in the context of the spatial characterization of the brain's resting state. Based on their predominant input, I distinguished an "interoceptive baseline" in the inner ring's regions (i.e., the regions centering around the ventricles) from an "exteroceptive baseline" in the outer ring's regions (i.e., the regions at the outer surface of the brain). I thus proposed distinct neuroanatomical structures for predominant rest–intero and rest–extero interaction.

This was further extended when considering interoceptive stimuli in relation to exteroceptive stimuli from the environment. Such intero–extero interaction was shown to be central, for instance, in reward, in Volume I, Chapter 8. At the same time, however, it was made clear that the resting state itself may also play a central role here so that the alleged bilateral intero–extero interaction turned out to be a trilateral one, rest–intero–extero.

NEUROEMPIRICAL BACKGROUND IB: BODY AND CONSCIOUSNESS

This short review tells us that interoceptive stimuli are central in the neural processing of the brain. Due to the interoceptive input from our continuously present body, any exteroceptive stimulus will encounter not only the brain's resting-state activity but also interoceptive stimuli from one's own body. The postulated rest–extero interaction may thus turn out to be a trilateral interaction of the exteroceptive stimulus with the interoceptive stimuli and the resting-state activity's neuronal stimuli, amounting to rest–intero–extero interaction.

Let us describe the same process in different terms. Due to the continuous influx of the interoceptive stimuli from the body, our brain's resting-state activity, as well as its neural processing of exteroceptive stimuli, cannot avoid interoceptive stimuli in any stage of their neural processing. This means that, neuronally, any rest–rest and rest–extero interactions are always already confounded by the continuous interoceptive input from the body, implying rest–intero and rest–intero–extero interaction by default.

Phenomenally, such continuous rest–intero and rest–intero–extero interactions imply that the body is always already part of the content our consciousness toward which it is directed. Even if one's own body is not the main content of consciousness, it nevertheless may be part of the background of, for instance, our consciousness of the objects, persons, and events in the environment. Accordingly, due to the continuous rest–intero interaction, the body is always already part of our consciousness, being either in the background of other contents, or the content itself; that is, bodily consciousness.

The present chapter focuses on the neurophenomenal mechanisms of how the interoceptive input from one's own body becomes associated with consciousness and its phenomenal features. In addition to the subcortical regions, as discussed in the previous chapter, interoceptive stimuli are also strongly processed in the cortex and more specifically by the insula as key region. The focus in this chapter is therefore on the insula and its role in interoceptive processing and consciousness of one's own body.

Before going into empirical details about the insula, let me briefly point out the territory I will *not* cover here. I only focus on the insula and interoceptive processing— I will not discuss the many studies on interoceptive processing in taste and food in the context of reward. Moreover, I here focus on the body only in terms of interoceptive processing in the insula, while leaving out the neural processing of the body and its parts in other regions as investigated in the context of agency, ownership, body self-consciousness, and body image (see, for instance, Blanke 2012; Vignemont 2011; and Longo et al. 2009). Finally, I also neglect the role of the insula in emotional feeling (see Craig 2009a and b, 2011) and time perception (see Wittmann et al. 2011; van Wassenhoeve et al. 2011; Craig 2009, 2011; also see Appendix 2 and Chapter 14 for more details). This is so because my focus is here mostly on how the insula mediates interoceptive awareness in relation to exteroceptive awareness.

NEURONAL FINDINGS IA: INTEROCEPTIVE AWARENESS AND THE INSULA

What exactly is going on during the neural processing of interoceptive stimuli? Recent imaging studies using functional magnetic resonance imaging (fMRI) investigated neural activity during interoceptive stimulus processing. For that, different ways were used: evocation of blood pressure changes during isometric and mental tasks, heartbeat changes and perception, anticipatory skin conductance during gambling, and heart rate modulation during presentation of emotional faces (Critchley 2005, for a review; Pollatos et al. 2005a and b, 2007a and b; Craig 2002, 2003, 2004).

These studies observed neural activity changes in the right (and also in part in the left) insula, the anterior cingulate cortex extending from supragenual to dorsal regions (SACC/DACC), and the amygdala. This led to the assumption that specifically the insula and the SACC/DACC integrally represent autonomic and visceral

responses. The autonomic and visceral inputs to the insula are supposed to be transferred from the spinal cord through the midbrain, the hypothalamus, and the thalamocortical pathway to the right insular cortex (Craig 2002, 2003, 2004, 2010a and b; Critchley 2005).

Hugo Critchley is one of the pioneers in the functional imaging of interoceptive processing and awareness. He is a scientist from London, where he worked for a long time and explored how the body affects the brain. We have to consider the background of how functional brain imaging developed. The strongest focus in functional imaging for a long time was on higher order cognitive functions like attention and memory.

These cognitive functions are still often deemed to be central for consciousness to occur. Yes, they are. Certainly so. But they may not be as central for phenomenal consciousness but rather for the awareness or consciousness of phenomenal consciousness, that is, access or reflective consciousness (see Part VI for details). If so, the cognitive account leaves open the question of the neuronal mechanisms underlying phenomenal consciousness of both environment and body.

Critchley now shifted our consciousness to the body when investigating the neuronal mechanisms underlying interoceptive awareness: the awareness or experience of any changes in the vegetative and thus interoceptive state of one's own body. Therein, the insula turned out to be essential. This was no big surprise. And that is mainly due to the work by Bud Craig. Working in the sandy desert in Arizona, Craig planted colorful trees of knowledge in the neuronal desert surrounding the insula. Based on purely neuroanatomical investigations, he proposed the insula to be essential in specifically interoceptive awareness. He thus draws a link from mere interoceptive stimulus processing to their awareness and thus consciousness.

Let us now shed some light on the empirical data. Critchley et al. (2004) let subjects evaluate whether one's own heart beat was synchronous or asynchronous with an auditory feedback. Subjects had to count either one's own heartbeat or the tone. This allowed him to compare interoceptively and exteroceptively directed awareness.

What about the results? Interoceptive awareness to one's own heartbeat increased neural activity in the right insula, the SACC/DACC, the thalamus, and the somatomotor cortex. In contrast, exteroceptive awareness to the tone decreased and thus suppressed neural activity in the very same region (see Fig. 32-1). These results have been confirmed in subsequent studies by Critchley himself and others (Critchley 2005; Pollatos et al. 2006, 2007; Wiebking et al. 2010, 2011).

Based on these results, these regions are proposed to be involved in re-presenting the autonomic and visceral state of the body, thereby yielding interoceptive awareness. Craig (2002, 2003, 2004, 2009) proposes specifically the right insula and the SACC/DACC to be crucially involved in generating interoceptive awareness.

NEURONAL FINDINGS IB: ANATOMY OF THE INSULA

The anterior insula receives autonomic and visceral afferences from lower centers (see earlier) and "re-represents" the interoceptive body state in an integrated way by converging the different inputs from the different parts of the body; this is possible by encoding the different inputs relative to each other in terms of their spatiotemporal differences, i.e., difference-based coding. Linking the insula to the SACC/DACC, such re-representation may then be associated with consciousness, i.e., the awareness of the interoceptive state of one's own body, which in turn may yield qualia of one's own body, i.e., bodily qualia.

How can we characterize the insula in further detail? Anatomically, the insula is considered part of the inner ring that includes the regions directly adjacent to the first to fourth ventricles. Let us recall: Following Mesulam and Feinberg, one can distinguish anatomically between three radial-concentric subcortical-cortical rings (see Volume I, Chapter 4, for details).

The inner ring contains the subcortical core-paracore regions and cortically the paralimbic regions that include the anterior and posterior cingulate cortex as well as the insula. Due to its proximity to the ventricle and their predominant interoceptive input, the authors (Nieuwenhuys, Mesulam, and Feinberg) argue that the inner ring is predominantly involved in processing interoceptive stimuli and the homeostasis of the body.

This distinguishes the inner ring from the outer ring (i.e., lateral subcortical and cortical and sensorimotor cortical regions) that is more dominated by exteroceptive stimulus processing. Finally, the middle ring includes the medial subcortical and cortical regions and is considered to be more integrative by linking the intero- and exteroceptive stimuli from inner and outer rings.

Due to their different predominant inputs, I associated the three rings with different baselines and thus differences in their resting state (see Chapter 4, Volume I). Showing strong, continuous interoceptive input, the inner ring was characterized by an "interoceptive baseline," while the outer ring receives predominant rather discontinuous exteroceptive input leading to an "exteroceptive baseline." The middle ring receives no direct intero- or exteroceptive input so that the brain's intrinsic stimuli, that is, neuronal stimuli, are strongest here, resulting in what I described as a "neural baseline" (see Chapter 4 in Volume I for details).

What does this threefold anatomical organization imply for the insula? The insula is part of the inner ring and may therefore be predominated by strong and continuous interoceptive input. One needs to further distinguish, however, between different parts of the insula (Craig 2002, 2003, 2009, 2010a and b).

The posterior part of the insula receives afferences from neural systems mediating body temperature, muscular sensations, visceral inputs, and arousal. These inputs are mediated by the posterior insula's strong connections with subcortical systems like the PAG, the parabrachial nucleus, and the ventromedial thalamic nucleus. The posterior part of the insula also receives plenty of exteroceptive input as, for instance, from auditory, visual, gustatory, olfactory, and somatosensory cortex. This connectivity is in accordance with imaging data showing

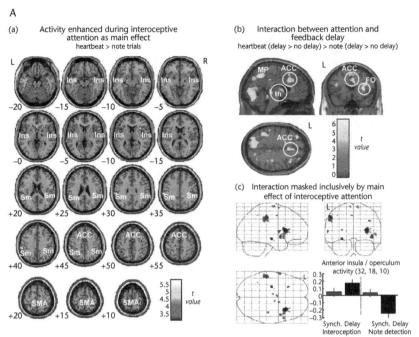

Figure 32-1 Neural activity during interoceptive awareness. (*A*) Activity relating to interoceptive attention (second-level random-effects analysis of 17 subjects, P < 0.02 corrected). (a) Main effect of interoceptive attention. Regional enhancement of brain activity during HEART trials, requiring interoceptive attention, compared to control NOTE trials. Group activity is plotted on horizontal sections of a normalized template brain to illustrate activation in bilateral anterior insula (Ins), lateral somatomotor and adjacent parietal cortices (Sm), anterior cingulate (ACC) and supplementary motor cortices (SMA). Also indicated are right (R) and left (L), and height (mm) of each of axial slice. (*B*) Activity reflecting interaction between feedback delay relative to heartbeat and interoceptive focus. Group activity is plotted on orthogonal sections of a template image to illustrate opercular (FO), anterior cingulate (ACC), medial parietal (MP) and thalamic activity (th) associated with contextual processing of feedback relative to interoceptive information [P < 0.02, corrected). Left (L) is indicated on coronal and axial sections. (c) Glass brain projection of activity identified in group analyses of both the main effect of interoceptive attention, and in interaction between interoceptive attention and feedback delay. An inclusive mask of the main effect (P < 0.02, corrected was used to constrain analysis of the interaction. The peak conjoint activity in right anterior insula/opercular cortex is marked, and the parameter estimates (with 90% confidence intervals) plotted. In this figure, and subsequent plots of neuorimaging data, units are given in arbitrary units adjusted for confounding effects. For fMRI data, units are proportional to percentage signal change. Interoceptive effects are represented by the bars on the left, with synchronous trial effects in dark and delayed trial effects in gray.(*B*) Functional neural correlates of interoceptive sensitivity. (a) Activity in right anterior insula/opercular activity correlated with performance accuracy on the heartbeat detection task in an analysis that modeled both interoceptive and exteroceptive task performance separately. The anatomical location is mapped on orthogonal sections of a template brain, with coordinates in mm from anterior commissure. (b) Activity within right insular/opercular cortex during interoceptive trials is plotted against interoceptive accuracy (relative to exteroceptive accuracy, to control for non-specific detection difficulty in the noisy scanning environment). The Pearson correlation coefficient (/?) is given in the plot. (c) Subject scores on the Hamilton Anxiety Scale (HAMA) are plotted against relative interoceptive awareness to illustrate the correlation in these subjects between sensitivity to bodily responses and subjective emotional experience, particularly of negative emotions. (d) Activity in right anterior insula/opercular activity during interoception also correlated with anxiety score, suggesting emotional feelings states are supported by explicit interoceptive representations within right insula cortex. Reprinted with permission of Nature Publishing Group, from Critchley HD, Wiens S, Rotshtein P, Ohman A, Dolan RJ. Neural systems supporting interoceptive awareness. *Nat Neurosci.* 2004 Feb;7(2):189–95.

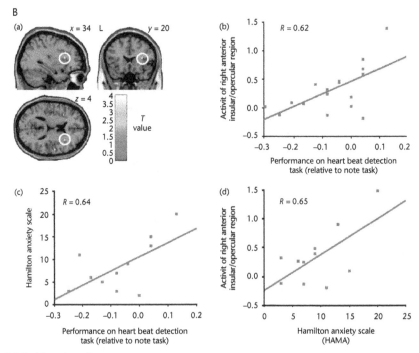

Figure 32-1 (Continued)

---

involvement of the posterior insula during pre-dominantly cognitive and sensory tasks (see also Lamm and Singer 2010).

What about the middle and anterior insula? The anterior part of the insula (AI) is more connected to the anterior cortical midline regions and the subcortical-limbic regions. The AI is consecutively recruited strongly during tasks involving interoception and interoceptive awareness as demonstrated earlier. Histologically, the anterior part of the AI is more granular while the posterior part is rather dysgranular (see also Lamm and Singer 2010); the middle part is just halfway between anterior and posterior parts.

NEURONAL FINDINGS IC: FUNCTION OF THE INSULA

Functionally, the various inputs into the posterior insula are proposed to be re-represented in the middle part of the insula and then again *re*-re-represented in the anterior insula (AI). What such re-representation and *re*-re-representation means exactly and how it

is neurally mediated remain unclear, however, at this time.

This may be especially important given the fact that the AI is the part of the insula that is most often observed to be activated in the earlier described imaging studies on interoceptive awareness of one's own heart beat. In contrast, interoceptive awareness of one's own breathing, for instance, may lead to the activation of posterior and middle parts of the insula rather than its anterior parts (Farb et al. 2012).

Another feature of the insula and especially the AI is its coactivation with the SACC/DACC (and the sensorimotor cortex and the thalamus) across different tasks and stimuli. The earlier described studies on interoceptive awareness (see Medford and Critchley 2010; Craig 2009, 2010a and b) as well as various studies on emotional feelings (Critchley et al. 2005; Lamm and Singer 2010), empathy (Yan et al. 2011; Lamm and Singer 2010), pain (Medford and Critchley 2010), and aversion (Craig 2009; Hayes and Northoff 2011, 2012) show conjoint recruitment of both the AI and the SACC/DACC.

Such co-activation between the two regions has led Craig (2009) to propose a direct and fast connection between the AI and the SACC/DACC. Such direct and fast connections may, in part, be subserved by the van Economo neurons (VEN). The VEN are specific large spindle-shaped neurons in layer 5 and, most important, they show a uniquely high density or concentration in the AI and the SACC/DACC. They are present in humans, while they do not seem to be present in many other nonhuman species.

NEURONAL HYPOTHESIS IA: DIFFERENCE-BASED CODING IN THE INSULA

I said that the insula and especially the AI is active during interoceptive awareness. Does the insula therefore process exclusively interoceptive stimuli? This contrasts with the structural and functional connectivity pattern of the insula that receives many afferences not only from vegetative and visceral origins but also from the five exteroceptive senses and their respective cortical and subcortical regions. There thus seems to be what can be described as "intero-extero convergence" in the insula.

What is the function of such intero-exteroceptive convergence in the insula? Rather than processing interoceptive stimuli in isolation and independently of exteroceptive ones, such intero-exteroceptive convergence predisposes the insula to process both types of stimuli relative to each other (see also Farb et al. 2013 for recent empirical support). More specifically, interoceptive stimulus processing seems to interact with the incoming exteroceptive ones. The highly continuous and rhythmic interoceptive input from the body may be matched and compared with the more discontinuous and arrhythmic exteroceptive input from the environment.

Such intero-extero matching implies that the neural activity changes in the insula must stem from the matching and thus the differences between intero- and exteroceptive stimuli and their respective statistical frequency distributions. Accordingly, neural activity in the insula is proposed to result not from interoceptive stimuli alone but rather from their statistically

based spatiotemporal difference to exteroceptive stimuli as processed in the same region.

What does such neural processing imply for the coding of neural activity in the insula? I hypothesize that, analogous to other regions such as the sensory cortex (see Volume I, Part I), neural activity changes in the insula are computed and encoded in terms of differences. More specifically, I propose that the spatial and temporal differences between intero- and exteroceptive stimuli are encoded into the neural activity changes we observe in the insula.

Such difference-based coding between intero- and exteroceptive stimuli must be distinguished from stimulus-based coding, where both intero- and exteroceptive stimuli, including their respective discrete points in physical time and space, are encoded independently and thus isolated from each other. Accordingly, I propose the insula to be characterized by difference- rather than stimulus-based coding (see Part I in Volume I for details).

NEURONAL HYPOTHESIS IB: DIFFERENCE-BASED CODING VERSUS PREDICTIVE CODING IN THE INSULA

The assumption of difference-based coding in the insula seems to be compatible with its recent characterization by predictive coding (see Volume I, Part III, for details). Bossard (2010; see also Seth et al. 2011 for a related assumption of predictive coding holding in the insula) proposes neural activity in the insula to reflect the generation of a prediction error.

The insula generates an interoceptive input that reflects the anticipation of a particular interoceptive state of the body, the predicted input (or the empirical prior). This predicted input is then matched and compared with the actual interoceptive input, thereby yielding the prediction error, whose amount then determines the degree of change in neural activity in the insula. In short, neural activity changes in the insula are proposed to directly correspond to the degree of the prediction error.

How does that stand in relation to my hypothesis of difference-based coding in the insula? Since it is based on the difference between predicted and actual interoceptive input, the prediction error reflects a special instance of difference-based coding (see also part III in Volume I). What remains unclear in predictive coding is how the insula generates the predicted interoceptive input (see also Volume I, Chapters 8 and 9, for this point in general).

This is the moment where the earlier described intero-exteroceptive convergence comes into play. As based on the insula's connectivity structure (see earlier), there is continuous intero- and exteroceptive input with the predominating interoceptive stimuli being processed relative to the exteroceptive ones. There is thus continuous intero-extero interaction going on in the insula. Such continuous intero-extero interaction may account for the generation of what Bossard describes as predicted "interoceptive input."

The "predicted interoceptive input" is then no longer exclusively interoceptive but rather signifies intero-extero convergence and thus the spatial and temporal differences between intero- and exteroceptive stimuli. Therefore, the predicted interoceptive input is not as purely interoceptive as is suggested by the term "predicted interoceptive input."

Moreover, the predicted interoceptive input does not predict an interoceptive state independent of the exteroceptive context but rather relative to the respective exteroceptive and thus environmental situation. Hence, both the predicted interoceptive input and the subsequent prediction error are not as purely interoceptive as proposed. They rather reflect specific intero-exteroceptive constellations, which presupposes difference-based coding rather than stimulus-based coding.

NEURONAL HYPOTHESIS
IC: INTERO-EXTEROCEPTIVE CONVERGENCE IN THE INSULA

One may want to argue, however, that the assumption of such intero-extero convergence and difference-based coding in the insula is not consistent with the imaging data described earlier. They show clearly that the interoceptive input alone induces changes in insula neural activity, thus remaining seemingly independent of the alleged predicted intero-exteroceptive convergence. This

suggests stimulus- rather than difference-based coding in the insula. Do the empirical findings on interoceptive awareness therefore contradict my hypothesis of difference-based coding in the insula? To address this question, we may want to investigate the experimental paradigms applied in these studies in further detail. All paradigms did not investigate interoceptive stimuli alone in complete isolation from exteroceptive stimuli. Critchley et al. (2004), for instance, investigated heart beat perception in relation to auditory tones as exteroceptive stimuli (see also Pollatos et al. 2005a and b, 2007a and b).

Neural activity changes proposed to be specific for interoceptive awareness thus reflect a relation or dynamic balance between intero- and exteroceptive awareness, rather than mirroring isolated interoceptive stimuli alone that supposedly remain independent of exteroceptive stimuli. This, however, is possible only if assuming difference- rather than stimulus-based coding of interoceptive stimuli relative to exteroceptive stimuli. Finally, the assumption of difference-based coding is also compatible with the characterization of the insula by Critchley. Critchley (2005, 162) proposes that the "right insula maps bodily arousal states" and "it does so contextually," which therefore "represents an integration of external emotional information with peripheral states of arousal" (Critchley et al. 2005, 759).

What Critchley calls "integration of external emotional information with peripheral states of arousal" may then correspond to what I here describe as difference-based coding of interoceptive stimuli in relative and thus in difference from exteroceptive stimuli (as distinguished from stimulus-based coding). While what is phenomenally described as interoceptive awareness with one's own body being the predominant content in consciousness may then be neurally traced back to difference-based coding with the encoding of interoceptive stimuli relative to (and thus in difference from) exteroceptive stimuli.

NEURONAL FINDINGS IIA: INSULA LESION AND INTEROCEPTIVE AWARENESS

We proposed difference-based coding to hold in the insula. That, however, only concerns the neuronal relevance while it leaves open whether difference-based coding is also relevant for phenomenal consciousness, that is, interoceptive awareness. For the answer to that, we now turn to a study that investigated the effect of an insula lesion on interoceptive awareness.

Khalsa et al. (2009) investigated a patient with bilateral lesions in the insula and the SACC. If these regions and their conjoint activation are indeed necessary and crucial for interoceptive awareness, this patient should show no awareness of his own bodily functions. Testing for interoceptive awareness, they injected a beta-adrenergic drug (Isoproterenol) to increase the heart rate and asked the patient to report the cardiac sensations he felt.

Like the healthy control group, the patient showed dose-dependent increases in the heart rate. More specifically, the patient's report about the felt and perceived cardiac sensation were the same as and thus very comparable with those of the healthy subject control group. The only (minor) difference was that the patient's interoceptive awareness was slightly delayed and thus slower when compared to the healthy subjects.

The authors then tested a second hypothesis. Most imaging studies on interoceptive awareness show activation not only of the insula and the SACC, but also of the somatosensory cortex (Khalsa et al. 2009 as well as earlier). Is the somatosensory cortex thus crucial and necessary for interoceptive awareness?

The authors tested this hypothesis in their lesioned patient by applying a local anesthetic, lidocaine, to the skin covering each participant's area of maximal heartbeat sensation (as reported before during the prior challenge). This was to exclude somatosensory exteroceptive stimuli and thus the somatosensory cortex (which processes these stimuli) in order to test the role of the somatosensory cortex in interoceptive awareness.

Neuronal Findings IIB: Insula and Somatosensory Cortex

How did the exclusion of the somatosensory stimuli from the skin affect the patient's interoceptive awareness? The patient again demonstrated normal heart rate increases. However, his awareness of his cardiac sensations was now significantly impaired, meaning he failed to experience any changes in his heartbeat sensations. This distinguished him from healthy subjects who did not suffer from any impairment in their cardiac sensations during the local anesthetic (see Fig. 32-2).

What do these findings tell us about the neural processes mediating interoceptive processing and awareness? As the authors themselves remark, the first finding, the patient's normal interoceptive awareness, suggests that the insula and the SACC are by themselves independent of other regions (like the somatosensory cortex) not necessary for interoceptive awareness. Otherwise, the patient should have shown impairments in his cardiac sensations directly related to the bilateral lesion of his insula.

The second finding tells us that interoceptive processing and awareness seem to be mediated by both the insula/SACC and somatosensory cortex. When disrupting both regions, the patient's interoceptive awareness was severely impaired. This contrasted with the healthy subjects who still showed interoceptive awareness even when their somatosensory input was blocked. Hence, the patient's interoceptive awareness was maintained as long as his somatosensory input was preserved, which was apparently able to compensate for his lesioned insula.

Neurophenomenal Hypothesis IA: Failure of Difference-Based Coding in Double Lesion in Insula and Somatosensory Cortex Disrupts Interoceptive Awareness

Do these findings support my hypothesis of difference-based coding and its behavioral relevance? What exactly happened in the patient's insula during the two experiments? Due to the lesion in the insula, intero-exteroceptive differences can apparently no longer be properly processed in the insula itself. In contrast, the patient still seems to be able to process his body's interoceptive stimuli relative to and thus differently exteroceptive stimuli processed in other regions like the somatosensory cortex.

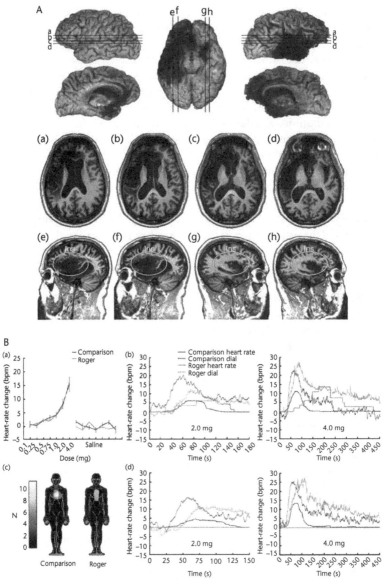

Figure 32-2 Effects of insula lesion on interoceptive awareness. (*A*) Brain damage in Roger. (a–h) Top, extent of damage (dark-black) on magnetic resonance imaging views of lateral (upper left and right), ventral (middle) and mesial (lower left and right) cerebrum. Bottom, axial (a–d) and sagittal (e–h) slices, with corresponding slice locations displayed at top. Ins, insula. (*B*) Heart rate response and on-line subjective dial ratings of interoceptive awareness changes induced by isoproterenol. (a) Roger and 11 healthy age-matched male comparison participants exhibited equivalent dose-dependent heart rate increases. (b) Time course of heart rate response and dial ratings. Roger and the healthy participants appropriately demonstrated dose-dependent changes in interoceptive awareness. Bolus infusions occurred at time 0. (c) Overlap map showing the region of maximal heartbeat sensation, corresponding to the area of topical anesthetic application. (d) Time course of heart rate response and dial ratings after anesthetic application. Roger no longer demonstrated appropriate changes in interoceptive awareness, even at the two highest doses. Comparison participants' interoceptive awareness was unaffected. All comparison data depict means. Error bars represent SEM. *N* indicates number of participants. Reprinted with permission of Nature Publishing Group, from Khalsa SS, Rudrauf D, Feinstein JS, Tranel D. The pathways of interoceptive awareness. *Nat Neurosci.* 2009 Dec;12(12):1494–6.

Instead of using his lesioned insula for processing the intero-extero difference, the patient now recruits his still-intact somatosensory cortex. This enables him to still behaviorally monitor and thus become interoceptively aware of the heart rate changes induced by the beta-adrenergic substance. Since the computation of the interoceptive stimuli relative and thus in difference to the somatosensory inputs in somatosensory cortex may no longer be as (spatially) direct as in the case of the insula, there may be a slight (temporal) delay in his interoceptive awareness, as was observed in the data.

What happens, however, in the patient when his somatosensory cortex is blocked? He no longer receives exteroceptive and thus somatosensory input from the region around his heart. The continuous interoceptive input can consecutively no longer be compared and matched with the exteroceptive input from the same spot, which prevents the generation of neural differences and hence the neural processing of further intero-extero convergences. This means that the interoceptive stimuli can no longer be set and processed relative to and differently from exteroceptive stimuli in either the insula or the somatosensory cortex. The data show that such a double blockade of both insula and somatosensory cortex severely impaired his interoceptive awareness.

Let us put the same idea in different terms. Once both insula and somatosensory cortex were blocked, the patient's brain remained unable to associate the interoceptive stimuli with a phenomenal state, e.g., interoceptive awareness. I propose that such absence of interoceptive awareness is due to the inability to process interoceptive stimuli relative to and in difference from exteroceptive ones in terms of difference-based coding.

Once difference-based coding is replaced by stimulus-based coding, as in the case of the double insula and somatosensory cortical lesion, the interoceptive stimulus-induced activity can no longer be associated with consciousness and its phenomenal features. Accordingly, this case study provides empirical support in favor of the necessity of difference-based coding for consciousness, i.e., interoceptive awareness.

NEUROPHENOMENAL HYPOTHESIS IB: ENCODING OF SPATIAL AND TEMPORAL DIFFERENCES BETWEEN INSULA AND SOMATOSENSORY CORTEX MEDIATES INTEROCEPTIVE AWARENESS

What about the healthy subjects' normally functioning interoceptive awareness during the somatosensory blockade? I presume this case to be the mirror image of the patient's insula lesion. In the case of healthy subjects, the exteroceptive input is blocked, leading to lack of neural activity changes in his somatosensory cortex. In the same way as the patient's lesioned insula lacks neural activity changes, the healthy subjects' somatosensory cortex can now longer generate neural activity changes anymore because of the lack of somatosensory input.

Unlike the patient, however, the healthy subjects still show normal interoceptive awareness. How is that possible? This is because their insula is functioning, which enables them to still generate intero-exteroceptive differences in the insula itself. Hence, the healthy subjects rely here on the same neuronal mechanisms, difference-based coding in the respective other non-impaired regions while the patients can rely on their somatosensory cortex as long as it is pharmacologically manipulated. Only when the neural activity of both regions is blocked, as in the patient's blockade of somatosensory input, severe phenomenal impairment with the absence of interoceptive awareness can be observed.

What does this case tell us about intero-exteroceptive interaction with regard to the phenomenal relevance of difference-based coding? The case demonstrates nicely that what is phenomenally relevant is not the neural coding and processing of the intero- or exteroceptive stimuli themselves alone and independently of each other. This is evidenced by the fact that the patient still shows interoceptive awareness despite his impairment in interoceptive stimulus processing in the insula and the SACC.

What is instead phenomenally relevant is his ability to still encode and yield intero-exteroceptive differences, no matter where, in either the insula or the somatosensory cortex. This is supported by the fact that the cardiac sensations are only impaired once the patient's somatosensory input is blocked, which makes the generation of intero-extero differences altogether impossible. Accordingly, I consider the encoding of spatial and temporal differences into neural activity as necessary condition of the possible association of stimulus-induced activity with consciousness, independently of where in the brain the differences are encoded and generated.

NEUROMETAPHORICAL EXCURSION
I: DOORS AND DIFFERENCES

Let us compare the situation to a small house with two exit doors. Usually, both doors function well, so that you can exit at any time. You usually take exit door number A, while door B is rarely used.

Now imagine that door A is blocked. It simply does not open. No matter how hard you push, it remains stubbornly blocked. What do you do? You look for the other door, door B, to exit. That may take a little longer, however, because door B is at the opposite end. However, as long as it functions (meaning it opens), you do not care. You will exit through door B. This is the situation for the insula lesioned patient as long as his somatosensory cortex is still functioning.

Now, suddenly, door B is blocked, too. There is no way for you to get out; you are stuck. You can neither exit through door A nor via door B. This is the situation when the exteroceptive input is blocked in the insula-lesioned patient so that he cannot revert to his somatosensory cortex to yield intero-extero differences and consecutively interoceptive awareness. Instead, he is stuck and has no way of getting out of the house to the environment and thus, analogously, to associate the stimulus with qualia and thus consciousness.

Finally, there is the situation where door B is blocked while door A is still open. Do you care? No, because you can always exit through door A. You may not even know that door B is blocked. Why care? That is the situation for the healthy subjects when their exteroceptive input and thus their somatosensory cortex is blocked.

NEURONAL FINDINGS IIIA: DOES GABA
MEDIATE REST–STIMULUS INTERACTION
IN THE INSULA?

These results suggest difference-based coding to hold in the insula and its central role in constituting interoceptive awareness, that is, consciousness of the body. How though is it possible for mere interoceptive stimulus processing in the insula to become associated with qualia and thus consciousness? Let us recall some of the neuronal mechanisms underlying rest-stimulus interaction as discussed in Chapters 29 and 30.

Rest–stimulus interaction was characterized by nonlinearity and GABA-ergic-mediated neural inhibition as central neuronal mechanisms. Nonlinearity and GABA-ergic-mediated neural inhibition were supposed to allow for the transfer and carryover of the resting state's prephenomenal structures to the subsequent stimulus-induced activity as associated with the stimulus itself. This is what I described as the "nonlinearity hypothesis of consciousness" (see Chapter 29). And that, in turn, makes it possible to associate qualia and thus consciousness with the stimulus. That amounts to what I referred to as the "transfer hypothesis of consciousness" (see Chapter 30).

I now claim the very same neuronal mechanisms for all neural activity changes—whether they are induced by exteroceptive stimuli, interoceptive stimuli, or neuronal stimuli during rest–rest, rest–extero, or rest–intero interaction. What is important is not so much the origin of the stimuli but rather the degrees of their nonlinear and GABA-ergic-mediated neural inhibition during their interaction with the resting state. Accordingly, I propose the very same neuronal mechanisms to apply to interoceptive stimuli and the insula, too.

If so, one would expect rest–intero interaction in the insula to be nonlinear and mediated specifically by GABA. Although there is currently no direct support for nonlinearity during rest–intero interaction in the insula, there is some initial support for GABA-ergic-modulation of its neural activity. This shall be the focus in the next section.

NEURONAL FINDINGS IIIB: GABA IN
THE INSULA MEDIATES INTEROCEPTIVE
AWARENESS

Christine Wiebking from our group has investigated the insula in several studies during interoceptive awareness (Wiebking et al. 2010, 2011,

2012, 2013). Most recently, she combined the fMRI with the magneto-resonance spectroscopy (MRS), which allows the measurement of the concentrations of GABA and glutamate in the insula. Her aim was to relate the signal changes as observed in the insula during interoceptive awareness to the concentration of GABA and glutamate in the same region.

In a first step, she conducted the earlier described task for interoceptive awareness in fMRI. Subjects had to become aware of their own heartbeat, which was compared against the awareness of a continuously presented tone. As expected, this led to larger signal changes in the anterior insula and other regions like the DACC and the thalamus during interoceptive awareness when compared to its exteroceptive counterpart.

In addition to the two conditions, intero- and exteroceptive awareness, she also included a longer resting-state condition, baseline condition, where subjects just saw a fixation cross. She then calculated the signal changes during intero- and exteroceptive awareness relative to this baseline condition. This was done in order to measure the neural changes the stimulus induced relative to the resting state. Hence, the obtained signal changes reflect the interaction between resting state and intero- and exteroceptive awareness rather than mirroring the latter independently of the former.

The same subjects also underwent MRS to measure their levels of GABA and glutamate in the resting state in the insula and a control region, the perigenual anterior cingulate cortex (PACC). This served to correlate the signal changes in the insula with the concentrations of GABA and glutamate.

Neuronal Findings IIIC: GABA Mediates Rest–Intero Interaction in the Insula

What did these correlations in the insula show? The signal changes relative to the baseline as induced by interoceptive awareness correlated significantly with the concentration of GABA in the same region; that is, the insula. The higher the concentration of GABA in the insula, the more signal changes relative to baseline were elicited by interoceptive awareness in the same region.

GABA thus mediates the degree to which the stimulus-induced activity deviates from the preceding resting-state activity level. In contrast, such correlation was not observed with exteroceptive related signal changes (during exteroceptive awareness) whose signal changes did not correlate with the level of GABA (see Fig. 32-3).

How about glutamate? The concentration of glutamate in the insula correlated significantly with that of GABA in the insula. This is no surprise, since GABA and glutamate are closely related and linked. One would have expected now that glutamate also correlates with the signal changes elicited by interoceptive awareness.

This, however, was not the case. The concentration of glutamate did not correlate at all with the signal changes elicited during either intero- or exteroceptive awareness. Hence, the transition from resting-state activity to stimulus-induced activity in the insula, specifically during interoceptive stimuli, was specifically modulated by GABA but not by glutamate.

Finally, one may want to ask whether the correlation with GABA was regionally specific for the insula. For the answer to that, Christine Wiebking made same analyses in the PACC. Interestingly, GABA in the PACC did not correlate with the signal changes elicited during interoceptive awareness, but rather with those related to exteroceptive awareness. This was further confirmed by a combined PET-fMRI study where the density of GABA-A receptors in PACC predicted the signal changes specifically during exteroceptive awareness, but not those related to interoceptive awareness (see Wiebking et al. 2012).

Taken together, the findings demonstrate the modulation of interoceptively induced neural activity in the insula by GABA rather than glutamate. This was specifically related to interoceptive awareness as distinguished from exteroceptive awareness. Although further studies are warranted in the future, these results suggest GABA-ergic modulation of neural activity in the insula during interoceptive awareness.

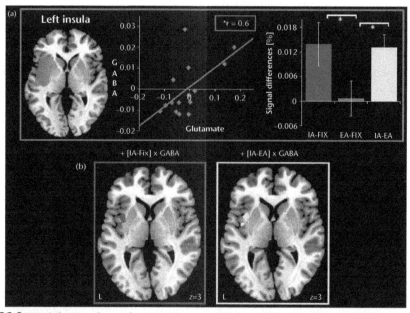

Figure 32-3 Modulation of neural activity in the insula by GABA. (*a*) GABA and glutamate concentrations have been measured in the left insula (in [*a*], MRS box in green on the left side). These values show a positive relationship when correlating their residuals, that means these values are corrected for gray matter volume in the area of interest (middle part of [*a*]) (*$p \leq$.05, r = .6, n = 15 subjects). Note that all data lay within a range of mean value ± 2.5 SD. Excluding the most positive GABA value, although not fulfilling outlier criteria, the correlation gets stronger ($p \leq$ .01, r = .8, n = 14 subjects). Bar diagrams on the right side of (*a*) show the signal differences (mean ± SEM, n = 15 subjects) of the left insula MRS box for IA-Fix (IA = interoceptive awareness; Fix = fixation cross), EA-Fix (EA= exteroceptive awareness) orange bar), and IA-EA. Signal changes between EA and Fix show the smallest difference, which differs to both other signal differences (* *p* < .05). No differences can be seen between IA-Fix and IA-EA. (*b*) Whole-brain regressions, inclusively masked with the MRS box, show positive relationships between GABA and IA-Fixas well as IA-EA. Note that the amount of gray matter in the MRS box has been included as a regressor of no interest. Regressions are set to the same threshold (*p* <.005 uncorrected, *k* > 25) and to the same horizontal plane (*z* = 3).

NEUROPHENOMENAL HYPOTHESIS IIA: GABA-ERGIC-MEDIATED NONLINEARITY LEADS TO THE ASSOCIATION OF STIMULUS-INDUCED ACTIVITY IN THE INSULA WITH INTEROCEPTIVE AWARENESS

What do these findings imply for the association of interoceptive stimuli with qualia and thus consciousness? Let us start again with the neuronal realm of the brain.

The concentration of glutamate correlated with the one of GABA, while only the latter correlated with the stimulus-induced activity as related to either intero- or exteroceptive stimuli. This is very much in line with the observation that glutamate is necessary to activate GABA-ergic-mediated interneurons, which then inhibit the glutamatergic-mediated pyramidal neurons.

Due to this suppression of glutamate-ergic neurons by the inhibitory GABA, the degree of the resulting stimulus-induced activity may then be much more strongly determined by GABA than by glutamate (see Chapter 2 in Volume I). This is very well in accordance with the described findings.

What does the correlation between GABA and glutamate mean? The correlation between GABA and glutamate may indicate the need of the interneurons to get excited by glutamatergic-mediated pyramidal cells. In contrast, the correlation of GABA with the signal changes may reflect the strong impact of GABA on the degree of stimulus-induced activity. Glutamate, in contrast, has no impact here anymore, as is signified by the missing correlation.

Accordingly, glutamate may be necessary to kick off stimulus-induced activity and GABA, while GABA may be central in eliciting and determining the degree of stimulus-induced activity. This implies a temporal hypothesis about the successive actions of glutamate and GABA, which may be worth investigating with EEG in the future.

Why, however, does the GABA-ergic-mediated rest–stimulus interaction lead to the association of consciousness with the resulting stimulus-induced activity? As discussed in Chapters 2, 6, 12, and 29, GABA-ergic-mediated neural inhibition introduces nonlinearity into the neural processing. The reported correlation of the baseline-dependent signal changes in the insula with the concentration of GABA may indicate nonlinear effects during rest–intero interaction in, for instance, the insula (or the somatosensory cortex). I am well aware that this is a rather tentative and indirect hypothesis that requires further experimental support in the future.

What do these neuronal mechanisms imply for the association of the interoceptive stimuli with qualia? Based on the "nonlinearity hypothesis of consciousness" (see Chapter 29), I propose the introduction of nonlinearity via GABA into rest–stimulus interaction in, for instance, the insula to make possible the association of the interoceptive stimulus and its related stimulus-induced activity with qualia. I consequently hypothesize the degree of interoceptive awareness to be directly dependent upon the degree of nonlinearity and GABA-ergic-mediated neural inhibition during rest–intero interaction in the insula.

Neurophenomenal Hypothesis IIB: Neuronal Transfer and Carryover of the Intrinsic Activity's Spatiotemporal Structures to the Extrinsic Interoceptive Stimulus

How is it possible that nonlinearity and GABA-ergic-mediated neural inhibition allow for the association of the interoceptive stimulus with qualia and thus consciousness? They are able to do so because they allow the carryover and transfer of the resting-state activity's spatiotemporal structures to the newly resulting stimulus-induced activity and the stimulus itself. This was proposed in what I described as the "transfer hypothesis of consciousness" in Chapter 30. The same mechanism may now apply to the insula and interoceptive stimulus processing, which are proposed to also go along with the neuronal transfer and carryover of the resting-state activity spatiotemporal structures.

I proposed that especially the midline regions are central in constituting the resting-state activity's spatiotemporal structures, more specifically its self-specific and preintentional organization (see Part VII for details). For the insula to associate its stimulus-induced activity during interoceptive stimuli with qualia, the insula's neural activity should therefore be related to the one of the midline networks.

There are indeed recent investigations that support the close relation between insula and midline network, as shall be described in the following. A recent study by Sridharan et al. (2008) investigated different paradigms (visual oddball attention, resting state, auditory event segmentation task) in fMRI and focused on the functional relationship of the insula to task-positive (lateral cortical regions mirroring the exteroceptive baseline) and task-negative (default-mode network regions mirroring the neural baseline) regions.

Using chronometric analysis techniques, they observed the insula and the SACC to be activated earlier than both task-positive and task-negative regions. Neural activity changes during both tasks showed earlier activation in the insula and the SACC, while activation in task-positive regions and deactivation in task-negative regions occurred later and was thus delayed.

The crucial role of especially the insula is further supported by analysis of functional connectivity using Granger causality analysis (Sridharan et al. 2008). This allows for determining the functional connectivity that is directed from the insula to other regions, that is, outflow connections, or whether the functional connectivity is directed from another region to the insula, that is, inflow connections.

The authors observed that the insula had causal outflow connections to basically all regions included in the task-positive and task-negative networks. In contrast to the major outflow connections to task-positive and task-negative regions, the inflow connections, e.g., the connections showing input of the insula from other regions, was rather low when compared to its outflow connections. The authors of the study conclude that such functional connectivity pattern, taken together with the specific time pattern of early activation, indicates a critical role of the insula in switching neural activity between task-positive and task-negative networks.

Most important, the data show close connection of the insula to both the midline and the lateral networks. By being activated earlier and showing outflow connections to both networks, the insula may have a special role in modulating the neural balance between midline and lateral networks. This may make possible the carryover and transfer of these networks' resting states self-specific and preintentional organization to the insula and the respective interoceptive stimuli. And that, as detailed in Chapter 30, allows for the association of the interoceptive stimulus not only with self-specificity and intentionality, but also with qualia and thus consciousness as it is phenomenally manifested in body consciousness (see Fig. 32-4).

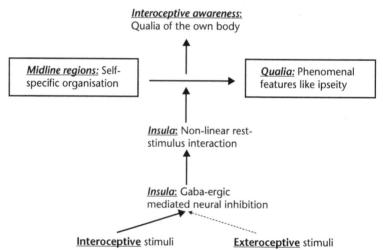

Figure 32-4 Neural mechanisms of interoceptive awareness. The figure shows a schematic and tentative illustration of possible mechanisms of interoceptive awareness. There are two main axes, horizontal and vertical. *Horizontal axis*: The horizontal axis describes on the left the resting-state activity with here the midline regions and their self-specific organization exemplified (*middle left*). During the encounter with the stimulus, the midline regions' self-specific organization is transferred and carried over to the resulting stimulus-induced activity where it is manifested in the gestalt of qualia and their phenomenal features like ipseity (*middle right*). *Vertical axis*: The brain receives continuous intero- and exteroceptive stimulus' input with either the one or the other stronger (stronger: fat arrow; weaker: dotted arrow). The predominant strong interoceptive input leads to activation in the insula via recruitment of GABA-ergic-mediated neural inhibition. That, in turn, may make possible nonlinear rest–stimulus interaction in the insula. This may also lead to interaction of the stimulus with the other regions' resting-state activity, including the midline regions (*center of the middle part*). On the basis of such nonlinear rest–stimulus interaction, the resting state's prephenomenal spatiotemporal structures like the self-specific organization are then transferred and conveyed to the stimulus-induced activity in regions like the insula. That makes possible the association of the interoceptive stimulus with qualia and thus consciousness, leading to interoceptive awareness with qualia of the body (*upper middle part*).

Neuroconceptual Remark
1A: Redefinition of Interoception

Due to their continuous input from the body, the interoceptive stimuli are always already somehow implicated in any neural processing of the brain's resting-state activity. This implies that the body is always somehow present in the contents of consciousness even if these targets predominantly concern events, objects, or persons in the environment. Neuronally that is due to the fact that any exteroceptive stimuli must be processed not only relative to the resting-state activity itself, but also in difference from the continuously present interoceptive stimuli in that very same resting-state activity.

The continuous interoceptive input into the brain's intrinsic activity may be manifested on the phenomenal level in the continuous presence of the body in our consciousness as either the target content by itself, i.e., body consciousness, or in the background of our consciousness of the environment. Such continuous presence of the body in whatever content of consciousness is often described conceptually as *embodiment*. Recent philosophical accounts consider the continuous presence of the body and thus embodiment to be central for consciousness.

One important implication of our assumption of difference-based coding concerns the definition of the concept of *interoception*. Traditionally, the concept of "interoception" describes stimuli originating in the body as distinct from those originating in the environment, the exteroceptive stimuli. But here I have demonstrated that interoceptive stimuli are processed relative to, that is, differently from, exteroceptive stimuli, and that this difference determines and encodes subsequent neural activity changes.

Hence, the encoding of stimuli into neural activity is not so much based on an origin of the stimulus in either body or environment as in intero- and exteroceptive stimuli; rather, it is based on the degree of statistically based spatial and temporal differences between different stimuli, such as between intero- and exteroceptive stimuli. There is therefore what I described here as difference-based coding rather than stimulus-based coding. Such difference-based

coding implies that the conceptual distinction between intero- and exteroception may be less clear than it is usually proposed to be on an empirical, or neuronal level. This is the conclusion Khalsa et al. (2009) came to on the basis of their results in their patient with the insula and the SACC lesions (see above for details). They regard their results that both insula and somatosensory cortex are participating in interoceptive awareness as a "challenge to the classic definition of interoception."

To constitute and generate interoceptive awareness, the brain apparently uses information from "anywhere and everywhere," including exteroceptive inputs from the skin closely related to the origin of the interoceptive stimuli. Following them, this requires a "redefinition" that no longer focuses "on the intrinsic nature of sensory pathways" but rather on the "source of stimulation in the body."

Neuroconceptual Remark 1B: Relational Definition of *Interoception*

What does this imply for the neural processing of interoception? There are no intrinsically interoceptive regions and pathways in the brain. Any processing of interoceptive stimuli apparently cannot avoid always already including exteroceptive stimuli as manifested in difference-based coding. The case described by Khalsa et al. (2009) illustrates nicely that exactly such difference-based coding is necessary to yield interoceptive awareness and thus consciousness. My hypothesis of difference-based coding thus undermines the concept of interoception as origin based and well segregated from that of exteroception. There is no pure and isolated interoception in the same way as there is no pure and isolated exteroception either.

Instead, interoception cannot be segregated and isolated from exteroception; both are mutually dependent on each other. Things are even more complicated, however. In addition, interoception can also not be isolated from the brain's intrinsic activity, its resting state and hence its prephenomenal structures.

Due to the continuous interoceptive input, there is continuous rest–intero interaction going on. This implies that body and brain, that is, interoceptive and neural stimuli, cannot be as segregated and isolated from each other as intero- and exteroceptive stimuli: for example, body and environment. This further undermines the traditional definition of interoception as origin-based and isolated from all other stimuli with a different origin.

How can we now develop and put forward an empirically more plausible concept of interoception? Presupposing difference-based coding, the term *interoception* describes a specific relationship to exteroception and thus a particular neural balance between both stimuli and, more generally, between body and environment. Furthermore, the concept of interoception refers to a specific relationship of the body's interoceptive stimuli to the brain and its intrinsic activity, e.g., neural stimuli.

Accordingly, the concept of interoception concerns the relationship of interoceptive stimuli from the body to exteroceptive stimuli from the environment and the neuronal stimuli from the brain. Interoception is thus intrinsically relational and thereby constitutes an intrinsic, i.e., necessary and unavoidable relationship between brain, body, and environment.

NEUROCONCEPTUAL REMARK IC: RELATIONAL DEFINITION OF *EXTERO*CEPTION

The same obviously applies to the concept of exteroception, which must be regarded as equally relational as interoception. And it also applies to the brain's intrinsic activity that, due to its continuous interaction with intero- and exteroceptive stimuli, must also be considered intrinsically relational.

The intrinsically relational character of interoception, exteroception, and the brain's intrinsic activity is also manifested on the phenomenal level in the continuous presence and intertwining of their respective ingredients in consciousness. The body as being traced back to interoceptive stimuli is always already present in whatever content of consciousness, no matter whether the body is the target (body consciousness) or not (as shown above). Furthermore, the events, objects, and persons

from the environment as related to the exteroceptive stimuli are also present in consciousness, either as direct targets or as background during body consciousness (see Figs. 32-5a and 32-5b).

I therefore determine the concepts of intero- and exteroception to be intrinsically relational. This means that interoceptive stimuli cannot avoid being processed relative to and thus differently from exteroceptive and neuronal stimuli, which, in a converse way, also applies to the latter two. There is thus no "pure interoception" as isolated and segregated from "exteroception." Such necessary and unavoidable intertwining is also manifested on the phenomenal level, where body, environmental contents, and internal thoughts related to the resting state are always already linked and intertwined. I suggest that this is mediated neuronally by the encoding of spatial and temporal differences among all three stimuli into neural activity.

NEUROCONCEPTUAL REMARK IIA: QUALIA ARE INTRINSICALLY RELATIONAL

What do the intrinsically relational concepts of interoception and exteroception imply for qualia and thus consciousness? Since they are supposed to be based on difference-based coding as their neural correlate (see Chapter 28 for details), qualia and consciousness must be considered intrinsically relational, too.

The absence of difference-based coding and its replacement by stimulus-based coding would make qualia and consciousness not only non-relational and thus isolated, but even worse, they would then be simply impossible. The relational character of qualia must therefore be considered an intrinsic and thus defining feature of qualia. This holds for the natural world, within which our brain and particular encoding strategy, namely, difference-based coding, are "located." Whether isolated qualia as distinguished from relational qualia are possible in at least the logical world remains subject to future philosophical discussion.

How can we further illustrate the intrinsic nature of the relational character of qualia? Let

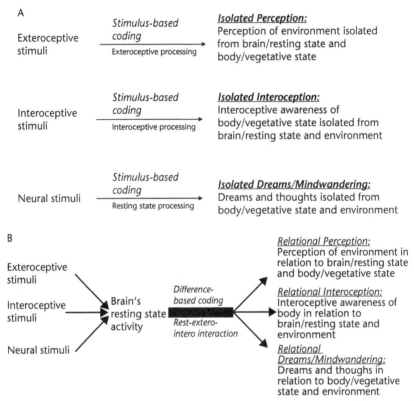

Figure 32-5 Concepts of perception and interoception. The figure shows how difference coding strategies, stimulus-based coding (*a*) and difference-based coding (*b*), entail different concepts of perception, interoception, and dreams/mind wandering. (*a*) In the case of stimulus-based coding, the different stimuli, intero- and exteroceptive and neural, are processed in a parallel and segregated way (*left and middle part*). This entails isolated concepts of perception, interoception, and dreams/mind wandering, meaning that they are isolated from the respective other stimuli and their origins in brain, body, and environment (*right part*). (*b*) This is different in the case of difference-based coding. Here the different stimuli, intero- and exteroceptive and neural (*left part*), are processed in difference and thus relative to each other as indicated by the big common line in the middle of the figure. Thereby all stimuli are processed and encoded against the brain's resting-state activity that therefore serves as common reference for the different stimuli (*middle part of the figure*). This entails relational rather than isolated concepts of interoception, perception, and dreams/mind wandering that are thus intrinsically related by default to the respective other stimuli and their origins in brain, body, and environment (*right part*).

us imagine the opposite scenario. If there were isolation presupposing stimulus- rather than difference-based coding, qualia and thus consciousness would be impossible. There would simply be no qualia and consciousness.

Isolated qualia are impossible (in atleast our natural world). We have seen this in the vegetative state, where the patients seem to show abnormally increased degrees of stimulus-based coding and abnormally decreased degrees of difference-based coding. Since stimulus-based coding and isolation leads to the absence of qualia, the relational character of qualia must be regarded an intrinsic feature that defines qualia *as* qualia. Accordingly, I propose qualia and consciousness to be intrinsically relational.

What exactly do I mean by the term "relational"? Thus far, I have described the term "relational" in a purely operational way, by the neural processing of interoceptive stimuli relative to and thus in difference from neuronal and exteroceptive stimuli (and vice versa). This implies, on a more general level, that brain, body, and environment cannot help but be linked and related to each other in neural activity (in a statistically based and thus "virtual" way).

This means that, as demonstrated above, qualia and consciousness are supposed to result from this statistically and spatiotemporal based "virtual" linkage between brain, body, and environment. Qualia are thus intrinsically relational; this implies that qualia would be impossible without such statistically and spatiotemporal based "virtual" linkage between brain, body, and environment.

Neuroconceptual Remark IIB: Qualia are Intrinsically Embedded

Qualia and consciousness can be regarded the result of the neuronal processes underlying the statistically and spatiotemporally based "virtual" linkage between brain, body, and environment. They are thus intrinsically, i.e., necessarily and unavoidably, embodied and embedded. Accordingly what is conceptually described as embodiment, embeddedness, and extension (in the context of the extended mind as discussed in philosophy) may be regarded an intrinsic, i.e., unavoidable and necessary, feature of qualia and consciousness without which neither would remain impossible.

I postulated that qualia are necessarily and thus intrinsically embodied and embedded. This implies that disembodied and disembedded qualia and consciousness remain simply impossible. If there is no body nor an environment (or their functional equivalents), qualia and consciousness remain absent and thus impossible. The relational nature is thus an intrinsic feature of qualia.

Most important, the concept of the relational qualia proposes the extension of the qualia between brain, body, and environment to be statistically based. This implies that qualia are based on temporal and spatial differences, thus being difference based rather than stimulus-based. This means that if our brain were applying a different code to encode its own neural activity, such as stimulus- rather than difference-based coding, qualia would remain impossible.

What, then, are qualia? Qualia are the result or output of the brain's constitution of a statistically and spatiotemporally based virtual structure between brain, body, and environment. This means that qualia are intrinsically spatiotemporal, which makes possible their relational character when spanning virtually and statistically across the physical boundaries between brain, body, and environment. In short, qualia are intrinsically statistical and spatiotemporal.

This is a thesis with strong ramifications. If qualia were not statistical and spatiotemporal and consequently embedded, there would be no qualia at all and consciousness would therefore remain impossible. At least in our very human world, the natural world, as the philosophers call it. In contrast, we must leave open whether our characterization of qualia as embedded, spatiotemporal, and statistical, also applies to a purely logical world where the laws of our natural world do not hold. To answer this question is however beyond our current neurophenomenal account that is limited to the natural world while leaving the logical world to the philosophers.

Open Questions

The first main question concerns the experimental testing of the interaction between resting-state activity and interoceptive stimuli, that is, rest–intero interaction. To properly test and lend empirical support to the here proposed rest–intero interaction, one would need to experimentally vary both resting state and interoceptive stimuli as independent variables.

However, since there is continuous interoceptive input into the brain's resting-state activity, it may be impossible to vary and operationalize the former independent of the latter and vice versa. One would thus propose any change in the one to be automatically accompanied by changes in the respective other.

That makes it impossible to treat both resting state and interoceptive input as independent variables. Hence, the intrinsic linkage between neural and interoceptive stimuli and thus between brain and body sets experimental constraints, which may turn out to be impossible to surpass.

I also neglected the central role of the insula in yielding emotional feeling and bodily self processing (see, for instance, Northoff 2008a and c, 2012c; Craig 2002, 2003, 2009, 2010a and b, 2011), which I have to leave open here. Moreover, recent accounts suggested involvement of the insula in yielding subjective time perception and thus inner time consciousness (see, for instance, Wittmann et al. 2010; Craig 2009, 2011; van Wassenhove et al. 2011; Seth et al. 2011). For the latter I refer to Part V and especially Appendix 2, where I further discuss the recent assumption of the insula being closely related to consciousness, perception, and cognition of time.

I here neglected very much the sensorimotor system and its role in constituting the embodiment of consciousness. Instead, I rather focused on the brain's resting-state activity and how it aligns with the environment, resulting in the "environment–brain unity." One may propose analogous mechanisms to be at work in the alignment of the resting state with the interoceptive stimuli from the body.

One may then conceptually speak of a "body–brain unity," which may account for the embodiment of consciousness. It may be interesting in the future to investigate the neuronal differences between the "environment–brain unity" and the "body–brain unity," including their implications for the phenomenal and conceptual realms of consciousness.

Finally, my relational concept of qualia is necessary and intrinsically extended, meaning that it reaches out beyond brain and body to the environment. As such, qualia can be regarded the output of what Silberstein and Chemero (2012) describe as "extended phenomenological-cognitive systems" (see also Rowlands 2010).

For that, as Silberstein and Chemero themselves as well as Rowland emphasize, no representation is necessary. While my concept of relational qualia does not imply any form of representation either, it nevertheless goes beyond the concepts of the extended mind and the embedded/extended consciousness by characterizing qualia in particular and consciousness in general in spatiotemporal rather than representational terms.

EPILOGUE: KEYHOLES IN THE BRAIN'S DOOR TO CONSCIOUSNESS

Consciousness is generally considered one of the last mysteries of our time. Much has been revealed by science over the centuries: physics and chemistry unlocked the mysteries of earth and world; biology, meanwhile, most recently found the key to life on earth: DNA as discovered by Francis Crick and James Watson. These, though, still left closed the door to consciousness.

Why is consciousness so important? Consciousness is not just life, but much more. Consciousness turns life into an experience, the experience of life. After having experienced how life was unlocked, Francis Crick searched for the key to unlock the door to that very same experience itself, to consciousness. What is the key to unlock the mystery of consciousness? Long ago philosophers thought the key was found in a mind: a mind different from both body and brain, a mind purely mental. Now we know better. It is rather the brain and its neuronal states that are the door to consciousness. This is what we have learned from the loss of consciousness in disorders of consciousness such as the vegetative state or other abnormal forms of consciousness, as they occur in neuropsychiatric disorders like depression and schizophrenia.

Why do these clinical observations suggest that the brain rather than the mind underlies consciousness? Because all of these patients show severe abnormalities in their brains' function and neuronal states. The brain, then, rather than the mind, is the door to consciousness. That is what we know at this point in time. Now let's turn to the much more interesting question.

What don't we know? We neither know the kind of key we need to unlock the "door" to the brain—in other words, we do not know the neuronal mechanisms that make consciousness possible and thus predispose it. Nor do we know where the keyhole in the door, the brain, can be found. Let's start with the key. The key of the brain is supposed to open the brain's door to consciousness and is therefore associated with specific neuronal mechanisms, namely those that are supposed to underlie consciousness. Several candidates have been suggested as the key to consciousness. Various neuronal mechanisms have been proposed as being reflected in the neural correlates of consciousness (NCC): neuronal synchronization, re-entrant circuits, information integration, global workspace, global metabolism, slow cortical potentials, cognitive functions like attention and working memory, affective functions as in emotions, and sensorimotor functions pertaining to the body. These suggestions provide highly valuable insight into the brain's neuronal mechanisms, but none of these have implied consciousness in a necessary and unavoidable way. In other words, none of these neuronal keys have yet fully opened the door to consciousness.

What can we do? We can either look for other "keys", or shift our focus to the keyhole itself. Rather than looking for other keys, I have here searched for the keyhole itself. What is the "keyhole" in the case of the brain? The keyhole is an intrinsic feature of the door. Analogously, the brain's keyhole must consist of some intrinsic feature that defines the brain *as* brain. In other words, in the same way the door would not be a door without the keyhole, the brain could no longer be defined as "brain" without the intrinsic feature in question.

In contrast to the key, the keyhole itself has attracted little attention in either neuroscience or philosophy. Therefore, my focus in Volumes I and II has been on the brain's intrinsic features, its keyholes, rather than its extrinsic features, the keys. I identified two such intrinsic features of the brain in Volume I, its resting-state activity and its encoding strategy.

The brain can be characterized by high resting-state activity, that is, intrinsic activity, that shows continuous and dynamic changes in the brain's resting state reflecting what I described as "rest–rest interaction." I thought such rest–rest interaction to constitute a statistically based, virtual spatiotemporal structure: an organization of its neuronal activity in spatial and temporal terms that ranges across the different regions and their different frequency fluctuations. This was what I discussed in Volume I. The resting-state activity's spatiotemporal structure was then further specified in Volume II. I demonstrated how the resting-state activity constitutes spatiotemporal continuity of neuronal activity across different discrete points in physical time and space (see Part V). That made possible the organizing and structuring of the brain's intrinsic activity in terms of spatiotemporal unity (see Part VI) and a self-specific and preintentional organization (see Part VII) of its neuronal activity.

How is all this related to consciousness? Some of the phenomenal features of consciousness seem to already "lie" in a dormant, prephenomenal version in the brain's intrinsic activity's spatiotemporal structures, though not in exactly the same gestalt. Consciousness shows a "stream of consciousness," a dynamic flow of time (and space) that seems to resemble the resting state's spatiotemporal continuity of its neural activity. And there is a phenomenal unity in consciousness that is apparently related to the brain's spatiotemporal unity.

Finally, self-perspectival organization and intentionality in consciousness seem to be predetermined by the resting state's self-specific and preintentional organization of its neural activity. Taken together, these various yet "dormant" prephenomenal features reflect different ways that the brain's resting state structures and organizes its own neuronal activity in spatiotemporal terms during both resting state and stimulus-induced activity.

How can we "awaken" the resting state's "dormant," purely neuronal, prephenomenal spatiotemporal structure to full-blown consciousness with its phenomenal features? The brain's intrinsic activity—that is, the resting-state activity and its prephenomenal spatiotemporal structures—are confronted by the continuous "shellfire" of extrinsic stimuli from body and environment. This is where the second intrinsic feature of the brain comes in. The brain applies a particular encoding strategy by means of which it generates and encodes its own neural activity; this concerns any kind of neural activity, including the brain's intrinsic activity, its resting-state activity, and its more extrinsic stimulus-induced activity. What exactly is the brain's encoding strategy? Encoding describes how the brain generates its own neural activity in response to changes as induced by for instance stimuli from either body or environment. I now suggest that the brain encodes its neural activity in terms of difference-based coding. Difference-based coding describes the encoding of spatial and temporal differences between different stimuli (across their different discrete points in physical time and space) relative to the actual resting-state activity level. This distinguishes it from stimulus-based coding, where the stimuli's single discrete points in physical time and space are encoded by themselves into neural activity independently of both other extrinsic stimuli and the brain's intrinsic activity.

Why did I spend so much time on the brain's encoding strategy in both volumes? I propose that the brain's encoding strategy, namely, difference-based coding, is relevant for both brain and consciousness. Applying a particular encoding strategy to generate its own neural activity makes it possible for the brain to actively impact, i.e., to structure and organize the changes in its own neural activity as triggered either by the extrinsic stimulus or by the dynamic changes in the resting state itself. The impact of the extrinsic stimuli is especially thereby contained, so that they "can no longer do whatever they want" in the brain and its intrinsic activity. Since it constrains the processing of extrinsic stimuli, the brain's encoding strategy is of high neuronal relevance for the brain itself.

Why, though, is such difference-based coding relevant to consciousness, and thus also phenomenally relevant? Difference-based coding makes possible the direct interaction of the extrinsic stimuli with the brain's intrinsic activity and its prephenomenal spatiotemporal structures. Such rest–stimulus interaction seems to be characterized by nonlinearity as it is apparently mediated by GABA-ergic-mediated neural inhibition (see chapters 2, 6, 12, 17, and 32).

This is not only neuronally but also phenomenally relevant. Due to such GABA-ergic-mediated nonlinearity, the resulting stimulus-induced activity is no longer a mere addition with a superposition of the stimulus-related changes onto the resting-state activity. Instead, the intrinsic resting-state activity itself and some of its yet-unknown neuronal and biochemical features also change during its encounter with the extrinsic stimulus. This change, I postulated, must be sufficiently large and be encoded in terms of spatial and temporal differences into the newly resulting stimulus-induced activity.

How is such rest–stimulus interaction now related to consciousness? This is very simple. If the extrinsic stimulus induces the "right" kind of changes, namely, non-linear changes in the hitherto "dormant" intrinsic activity of the brain, the latter "wakes up," "opens up," and thereby transfers and carries its prephenomenal spatiotemporal structures over to the extrinsic stimulus and its associated stimulus-induced activity. This makes possible the association of the extrinsic stimulus and its otherwise purely neuronal stimulus-induced activity with consciousness and its phenomenal features (see chapters 28–30 in Volume II).

What, then, is consciousness? The answer is very simple. Taken in an empirical perspective, consciousness ultimately comes down to a statistically-based matching or fitting process between the spatiotemporal features of the extrinsic stimulus and those of the brain's intrinsic activity: If both fit and match well, the extrinsic stimulus and its otherwise purely neuronal stimulus-induced activity are associated with consciousness, its various phenomenal features and their essentially subjective nature. If, in contrast, extrinsic stimulus and the brain's intrinsic activity do not fit well, the stimulus will be processed at best in an unconscious, or at worse in a non-conscious, mode (or not at all) and thus not be associated at all with consciousness.

Where does this leave us? The relation between the brain's intrinsic activity and the extrinsic stimuli may very much resemble the relationship between keyhole and key: both must fit and match with each other to associate the extrinsic stimulus with consciousness, and thus to open the door, that is, the brain, to consciousness. While most current approaches looked at different keys—the neuronal mechanisms related to the extrinsic stimuli—I here focused on the keyhole itself, i.e., the brain's intrinsic features. Let us continue our final round of questioning. Why did I shift my focus from the brain's extrinsic stimulus-induced activity to its intrinsic features and thus from key to keyhole to unlock the brain's door to consciousness? Because the brain's keyhole, its intrinsic features, can tell us what the key (i.e., the neuronal mechanisms related to the extrinsic stimuli) must look like in order to open the brain's door to consciousness.

Are the brain's resting-state activity and its encoding strategy really the keyholes of the brain, the intrinsic features that define the brain *as* brain? We currently do not know. Even worse, we also do not know how the extrinsic stimuli from body and environment, the keys, must interact with the brain's keyhole, its intrinsic activity, in order to open the brain's door to consciousness. All I can do at this point in time is to develop empirically, phenomenally, and conceptually plausible hypotheses about the relationship between neuronal and phenomenal features. This has resulted in what I describe as "neurophenomenal hypotheses."

My neurophenomenal hypotheses are now open for general discussion. They can be subjected to intense experimental testing and detailed conceptual and phenomenal scrutiny.

This will reveal whether they can stand the tests of being subjected to trial and error. Even if my neurophenomenal hypotheses will produce more error than success, they have nevertheless served their purpose: we would then know at least where not to look and could consequently search elsewhere for other intrinsic features in the brain, for yet other keyholes in the brain's door to consciousness.

We will start again and try fitting and matching our suggestions for other intrinsic features within the brain itself. These, very much like my suggestions of the brain's intrinsic activity and its encoding strategy, can be subjected to rigorous experimental testing. We will then impatiently observe whether the brain unlocks its door to consciousness and "awakens" the "dormant" spatiotemporal structures of its intrinsic activity; this in turn will enable the brain to associate its otherwise purely changes in its intrinsic activity with full-blown consciousness and its phenomenal features.

That is not too bad, after all. Most important, that is exactly the way the brain itself seems to work. Our brain continuously tries out whether the various keys it receives from the outside, the extrinsic stimuli, fit and match its own keyhole on the inside, its intrinsic activity. In the case of a good fit or match, the brain's door is unlocked. The result is that which we, as outside observers, call *consciousness*. In case of a bad fit or match, the brain's door remains closed to consciousness. That is unfortunately the current state of affairs with regard to our knowledge about the relationship between the brain and consciousness.

APPENDIX 1: BRAIN AND CONSCIOUSNESS

Here I suggest a neurophenomenal approach to investigating consciousness. Such a neurophenomenal approach must be distinguished from the various other approaches taken in current neuroscience and philosophy to study consciousness. I here give an overview of the different methodological strategies and compare them with my neurophenomenal approach, which will lead to a more detailed characterization of the latter.

METHODOLOGICAL BACKGROUND—DIFFERENT APPROACHES

I want to briefly compare my neurophenomenal approach with other approaches to consciousness without going into much detail. There are plenty of different approaches to consciousness that target consciousness from either the side of the brain or the side of consciousness. I already discussed many of the major neuroscientific approaches in full detail in the different chapters and parts. I want to point out here some more general aspects of competing approaches to consciousness and how they stand in relation to my neurophenomenal approach without going into neuroscientific detail.

Before getting started, one needs to be clear how to distinguish the different approaches in the study of consciousness in the current, rather jungle-like landscape. I here favor a threefold distinction among conceptual, global, and functional approaches. Conceptual approaches are those that start with the definition of the concept

of consciousness by pointing out its conceptual and/or metaphysical features. They most often originate in philosophy or neurophilosophy and will therefore be discussed as the third major approach at the end of this appendix.

Global approaches, in contrast, start with the brain when assuming the function of the whole brain rather than specific regions and their associated functions to be central for consciousness. Finally, functional approaches assume specific functions of the brain like cognitive, affective, or sensorimotor function and their associated regions and networks in the brain to be essential for consciousness. I will start with the latter, the functional approaches, and then continue to the global approaches and will end with the conceptual approaches (see Fig. A1-1).

FUNCTIONAL APPROACHES TO CONSCIOUSNESS IA—COGNITIVE APPROACHES

Let me shed a light on the functional approaches. One of the most popular functional approaches is the reference to cognitive functions. Working memory (see, for instance, LeDoux 2002) and especially attention have been considered prime candidates to mediate consciousness. Attention has often been associated with top-down modulation from prefrontal-parietal networks to lower regions like the sensory cortex (as, for instance, the visual cortex); these top-down modulations have been assumed by many as being central for consciousness (see Lamme and

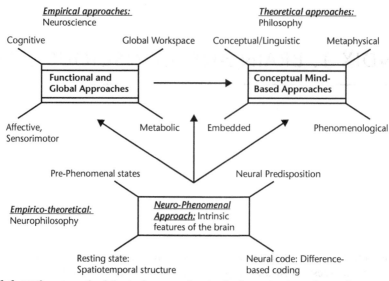

Figure A1-1 Different methodological approaches in the investigation of consciousness. The figure shows different approaches to consciousness relying on empirical strategies as in neuroscience (*upper left*), or theoretical methods as in philosophy (*upper right*). Neuroscience approaches consciousness either via specific functions like cognitive, sensorimotor, or affective functions, and their corresponding regions/networks; or it assumes a more global role of the brain as a whole as manifested in metabolic theories and the global workspace theory. This contrasts with philosophical approaches that are more conceptual, drawing on metaphysics and conceptual or phenomenological approaches. Both philosophical and neuroscientific approaches are mainly concerned with the correlates of consciousness, while the neurophenomenal approach (*lower part*) is more interested in the neural predispositions of consciousness as supposedly manifested in the resting state's prephenomenal structures. This is possible by focusing on the brain's intrinsic features as manifest in its resting state's spatiotemporal structure and its neural code; that is, difference-based coding as distinguished from stimulus-based coding. That makes a combined empirico-theoretical approach necessary, which may be subsumed under the discipline of neurophilosophy.

Roelfsema 2000, van Gaal and Lamme 2011, Lamme 2006).

However, there has been much discussion about the concept of attention itself. What is attention— Is it a process or mechanisms rather than a causal entity that as such can yield consciousness (Anderson 2011)? Even more important, there has been much debate whether consciousness may in fact be dissociable from attention (see, for instance, Graziano and Kastner 2011). Van Boxtel et al. (2010a and b) reviewed the literature and showed that attention can occur without consciousness, meaning that the former is not sufficient for consciousness. And that, reversely, consciousness can occur without attention, meaning that attention is not necessary for consciousness either. Though tentative, this suggests

different segregated neuronal mechanisms and processes for attention and consciousness.

How does that stand in relation to my neurophenomenal approach? I would propose the here sketched neuronal mechanisms underlying consciousness to occur prior to and thus preceding the ones related to cognitive functions like attention. Consciousness, as I understand it here, is supposed to be based on and predisposed by neuronal functions related to the resting state. Since they predispose phenomenal consciousness, these neuronal mechanisms can be characterized as prephenomenal rather than either nonphenomenal or phenomenal.

Most important, the here suggested prephenomenal neuronal mechanisms of consciousness must be distinguished from the ones related to cognitive functions like attention. I propose these neurocognitive functions to occur later and thus after those predisposing and manifesting consciousness. The neurocognitive mechanisms build on the ones underlying consciousness, i.e., the neurophenomenal mechanisms.

Why do I suggest that cognitive functions occur on the basis of the phenomenal functions and thus consciousness? Because any cognitive functions occurs within the prephenomenal and phenomenal space of possible consciousness. The neuronal mechanisms underlying cognitive functions like attention and others must consequently be characterized as postphenomenal rather than prephenomenal or phenomenal. I therefore consider the here-suggested neurophenomenal mechanisms to be more basic and fundamental than the neurocognitive mechanisms.

More specifically, I propose that all neurocognitive mechanisms presuppose the kind of neurophenomenal processes and mechanisms I here described, especially in Parts V–VI, when focusing on the resting state's constitution of its prephenomenal structures. These neuro-prephenomenal functions, if one wants to say so, can then serve as the starting point for any kind of subsequent stimulus-induced and/or task-related activity as associated with the different kinds of cognitive (and other psychological) functions.

What does such a neurophenomenal approach imply for the relationship between consciousness and cognitive functions? I would expect analogous dissociation between consciousness and other cognitive functions, as seems to be the case with regard to consciousness and attention. Or otherwise put, the here-described neuro-prephenomenal (and neurophenomenal) functions may constitutionally precede the various neurocognitive functions.

The assumption of neurophenomenal (or better: neuroprephenomenal) functions preceding the various neurocognitive functions implies that my neurophenomenal approach cannot be considered a subset of its more theoretical--philosophical sibling of cognitive approaches, the representational approach, either. In a nutshell, the representational approaches propose consciousness to result from some representational or metarepresentational processes sustained by cognitive functions like working memory, attention, executive functions, and so on. Such a representational approach has been considered in both neuroscience (see, for instance, Lau 2008, Lau and Rosenthal 2011) and philosophy (see, for instance, D. Rosenthal and P. Carruthers).

FUNCTIONAL APPROACHES TO CONSCIOUSNESS IB—AFFECTIVE APPROACHES

Another approach, the affective approach, targets affective functions and emotions rather than cognitive functions. This is well reflected in J. Panksepp's (2007, 1998a and b) approach (see Chapter 31 for more extensive discussion). He considers affective consciousness to be primary and basic for any subsequent higher order and more cognitive forms of consciousness, that is, secondary and tertiary consciousness (see also Damasio 1999a and b, 2010, who seems to pursue not a purely affective approach but rather a hybrid affective-cognitive approach).

Panksepp's account of primary or affective consciousness is certainly closer to the kind of neuronal processes targeted here, that is, the brain's resting-state activity, than the ones investigated in the cognitive approaches. This is, for instance, behaviorally reflected in his concept of seeking that seems to reflect the behavioral manifestation of the resting-state activity (see Chapter 8, Volume I). However, I argue that we need to go even one step further back than Panksepp does. We need to investigate those neuronal processes that first and foremost make possible the generation of affect and emotions and hence affective consciousness. Panksepp explains in a most convincing manner the physiological and neuronal mechanisms leading to the constitution of a particular function, affect. In contrast, he does not explain why that function is necessarily associated with consciousness.

For that, as I claim, we need to investigate the brain's intrinsic features, its resting state and its neural code, independent of and prior to any functions like affect, sensorimotor and cognitive. That is why I focused so much on these basic processes independent of any particular function. These more basic neuro-prephenomenal processes are, admittedly, manifested in the various functions—cognitive, affective, or sensorimotor—that provide our first door of access to the former. One should be careful, however, not to confound the neurophenomenal mechanisms themselves with their manifestation in cognitive, affective, and sensorimotor functions. That would be to confuse cause and effect and thus to false-positively associate consciousness with cognitive, affective, or sensorimotor functions.

Let us put this in a more metaphorical way to better illustrate the situation. To locate consciousness in the functions themselves, whether cognitive, affective, or sensorimotor, would be to confuse the door and the hallway you have to go through to reach the door: in the same way that you have to go through the hallway to reach the door, any cognitive, affective, or sensorimotor function has to "go through" the brain's intrinsic features, its neural code and resting state, to be constituted as such. I claim that this constitution process makes unavoidably the association of cognitive, affective, and sensorimotor functions with consciousness (see Chapter 31).

Despite these shortcomings, I nevertheless suggest that Panksepp's approach is much closer to the here suggested neurophenomenal approach than the cognitive approaches. Why? That is so because the cognitive approaches seem to target rather reflective or access consciousness (see also Kouider et al. 2010 and Lau 2008, 2010) than phenomenal consciousness (see also Block 1995, 2005). In contrast, Panksepp targets right away phenomenal consciousness, which is very much in line with the neurophenomenal approach taken here. The neurophenomenal approach, however, extends this focus to target principal consciousness as distinguished from principal non-consciousness when focusing on the neural predispositions of possible phenomenal consciousness (see second Introduction).

FUNCTIONAL APPROACHES TO CONSCIOUSNESS IC—SENSORIMOTOR APPROACHES

My neurophenomenal approach must also be distinguished from the neurophenomenological approach (see later), which, on its empirical side, strongly emphasizes the sensorimotor-based nature of consciousness (see Thompson 2007; Varela 1997). One may thus speak here of a "sensorimotor approach to consciousness" (see, for instance, Thompson 2007; Hurley 1998; Noe 2004; Cristoff et al. 2011; Legrand 2007a and b).

Let us first disentangle the terms "neurophenomenal" and "neurophenomenological." Though the terms "neurophenomenological" and "neurophenomenal" seem to be very close, the two approaches must nevertheless be distinguished from each other. They make different presuppositions about both theoretical-conceptual background and the empirical approach to the brain; let us start with the latter. Empirically, the neurophenomenological approach claims for sensorimotor functions to be central in linking the brain to the environment and to thereby constitute subjectivity and consciousness (see Christoff et al. 2011 for a recent account).

In contrast, as explained earlier, my neurophenomenal approach does not consider any specific function whether affective, sensorimotor, or cognitive, to be a necessary and predisposing condition of consciousness. This is so because my neurophenomenal approach focuses on those neuronal processes and mechanisms that must precede the constitution and differentiation of these different functions. Metaphorically speaking, the neurophenomenal approach focuses on the very ground itself, the brain's intrinsic activity, upon which different columns, the different functions, are erected. In contrast, the neurophenomenological approach focuses on one of these columns, the sensorimotor functions.

The focus on sensorimotor functions in the neurophenomenological approach implies the emphasis of embodiment in the constitution of consciousness. While sensorimotor functions certainly have a central role in expressing and manifesting consciousness, I nevertheless consider them on an equal footing as affective and cognitive function. Like the latter, sensorimotor stimuli "have to go through" the brain's intrinsic features, its resting state and neural code, in order to be constituted. And that process predisposes them to become aligned with the phenomenal features of consciousness. This means, however, that sensorimotor functions are not principally different from affective and cognitive functions when it comes to consciousness since they all are postphenomenal rather than prephenomenal (see earlier).

Theoretically and philosophically, the neurophenomenological approach relies on the phenomenological philosophy by Husserl that claims consciousness to be structured in certain ways. The neurophenomenological variant of the phenomenological approach takes the latter's characterization of consciousness as a starting point and seeks corresponding neuronal mechanisms of the structures discussed in philosophy. Since it takes consciousness and the mind as starting point, the phenomenological approach and its empirical sibling, the neurophenomenological approach, can be characterized methodologically as consciousness-based and mind-based.

This is different in the neurophenomenal approach. Rather than consciousness as described in phenomenology, I take the brain and its intrinsic features, that is, its resting state and its coding strategy, as the starting point for the subsequent search of the neuronal mechanism underlying the phenomenal features of consciousness. My methodological strategy thus starts with the brain itself and its prephenomenal predispositions, rather than taking consciousness itself and the mind as starting point. Hence, my approach reverses the traditional approach that takes consciousness and mind as independent variables and the brain and its neuronal mechanisms as dependent variables.

In other words, the brain, and more specifically its intrinsic features as the neural predispositions of consciousness, come first, i.e., as independent variable, while the phenomenal features of consciousness are considered secondary, e.g., as dependent variable, in my methodological strategy. I thus pursue a (prephenomenal) predisposition-based approach rather than a consciousness-based approach. And I opt for a brain-based rather than a mind-based approach.

GLOBAL APPROACHES TO CONSCIOUSNESS
I—METABOLIC APPROACH

Besides the here-sketched functional, e.g., cognitive, affective, and sensorimotor approaches to consciousness, one may pursue a global approach to the brain. The global approach considers the whole brain, rather than specific regions or networks associated with specific functions as central for consciousness to occur. One such global approach can be described as a "metabolic approach" to consciousness, as suggested by Shulman (2012). While I already discussed the role of the brain's metabolism in extensive detail in especially Part VIII in the context of the vegetative state, I here want to outline only its main points.

Rather than associating consciousness with particular functions and brain regions, Shulman suggests to base consciousness on the global metabolism of the whole brain, its energy metabolism and how it transforms into neural activity (see also Introduction). Hence, consciousness is here approached no longer in either behavioral or functional regards but rather in metabolic-energetic terms (see introduction as well as Part V for details).

This is very close to my approach taken here that emphasizes the brain's resting-state activity as a starting point for which obviously its energetic metabolism is of central importance. However, my neurophenomenal approach goes beyond that by aiming to account for the specific neuronal processes and mechanisms that predispose the transformation of the brain's purely neuronal states into the phenomenal states of consciousness. The metabolic approach provides an excellent starting point and background for my neurophenomenal approach. I then seek the kind of neural processes in the resting state that predispose the transformation of the latter's neuronal states into the phenomenal states of consciousness.

The difference between the metabolic and the neurophenomenal approaches is also reflected in the dimensions of consciousness that are targeted. The metabolic approach targets only the level or state of consciousness. As such, it is indeed very basic and predisposing for consciousness, as pointed out in especially Part VIII (see Chapter 28). In contrast to the level or state, the metabolic approach neglects the form of consciousness, the organization of its contents, almost completely. This, the form of consciousness, is addressed and emphasized strongly in the neurophenomenal approach. More specifically, the neurophenomenal approach aims to link the metabolic characterization of the level or state of consciousness to the neuronal mechanisms

underlying the form (or organization or structure) of consciousness.

GLOBAL APPROACHES TO CONSCIOUSNESS IIA— GLOBAL WORKSPACE OF NEURAL ACTIVITY

The global workspace theory by Baars (2005) is
a theory about the cognitive architecture that is
necessary to constitute consciousness (see also
Baars and Franklin 2007 as well as the excellent
review papers by Dehaene and Changeux 2011;
Dehaene et al. 2006). Conscious states evoke
widespread activity in and synchronization (as,
for instance, gamma oscillations) across various
regions, including many cortical and subcortical
regions, while unconscious states can be characterized by a spatially more restricted and limited
neural activity. This leads to the assumption that
consciousness may require access to and integration between the neural activities of different
regions and networks that then signify what is
called a global workspace.

The function of consciousness is to provide
global access with the consequent integration
and coordination between different functions
that are associated with the different regions and
networks (see Baars 2005, 51–52). Within this
global workspace, Baars (2005, 49–51) distinguishes between "content systems" and "context
systems": content systems are those that mediate
specific contents like the visual ventral stream,
while context systems provide the context and
must be associated with fronto-parietal regions.

How are "content system" and "context system" related to each other? The context system
is supposed to "observe" the content system.
For such observation to be possible, one must
propose some kind of observer, a self, more
specifically. Baars et al. (2003) therefore speak
of an "observing self," which they consequently
associate with the brain's resting-state activity in
fronto-parietal networks.

GLOBAL APPROACHES TO CONSCIOUSNESS IIB—GLOBAL WORKSPACE VERSUS SPATIOTEMPORAL CONTINUITY

Is my concept of the neurophenomenal approach
compatible with Baars's assumption of a global

workspace? First, both theories presuppose different starting points. The global workspace
theory presupposes a predominantly cognitive
starting point when consciousness is associated
with cognitive functions and their global distribution across different regions and networks.
Based on my earlier account, the global workspace approach and its emphasis on cognitive
functions can be characterized as a postphenomenal approach, one that presupposes the
neuronal mechanisms underlying access to phenomenal consciousness.

In contrast, the concept of the neurophenomenal approach is less cognitive and emphasizes
prephenomenal rather than the postphenomenal features of neuronal activity. Why? The
differences in the methodological strategies, pre-
versus postphenomenal, may be largely due to
the difference between cognitive functions and
the brain's intrinsic activity as starting points.
However, despite these methodological differences, both the global workspace theory and the
neurophenomenal approach share and converge
in their reference to the neuronal context of the
brain, its functional architecture and design.
That implies that both approaches require neuronal processing to occur throughout the whole
brain for consciousness to become manifest.

This is well manifested in the neurophenomenal approach when I spoke of global spatial and
temporal continuity of the resting state's neural
activity (see Part V). By extending its neural
activity in a temporally and spatially continuous way across different regions and time durations, the resting state activity itself may provide
some kind of global workspace in (more or less)
the same way as the global workspace theory
presupposes it on the cognitive level of neural
processing.

The main difference between the global workspace advocated in both approaches, then, is that
the resting state's spatiotemporal continuity of its
neural activity is more basic and not yet either
phenomenal or cognitive by itself. This is different in the global workspace theory that claims for
a cognitive global workspace. I would now claim
that the latter is based and thus dependent upon
the former: the better the resting-state activity's
prephenomenal spatiotemporal continuity is

developed, the more easily and more successfully the global workspace during subsequent cognition can be generated and recruited. I thus argue that the degree of cognitive function and ability is, in part, dependent upon the resting state's global workspace in terms of the spatiotemporal continuity of its neural activity.

One should be careful, however, One principal difference between global workspace theory and my neurophenomenal approach concerns the distinction between content and context. While the global workspace theory assumes different neuronal systems to account for content and context, the neurophenomenal approach denies the relevance of that distinction. This is so because the neurophenomenal approach presupposes difference-based coding: what the global workspace calls context is supposed to be always already encoded into any kind of neuronal activity underlying the contents. Difference-based coding assumes that any neural activity coding content is possible only on the basis of coding content in relation to the respective contexts, for example, difference. This makes the distinction between content and context superfluous in the case of difference-based coding in particular and in my neurophenomenal approach in general.[1]

GLOBAL APPROACHES TO CONSCIOUSNESS IIC—NEURAL CORRELATES OF CONSCIOUSNESS VERSUS NEURAL PREDISPOSITION OF CONSCIOUSNESS

How is it possible that the concepts of the global workspace and the neurophenomenal approach differ so much despite showing certain convergences? This may be related to a different focus in the kind of conditions with regard to consciousness they seek to explain. The global workspace theory aims to explain the minimally sufficient cognitive and neural conditions of the contents of consciousness and can therefore be considered an example of the neural correlates of consciousness (NCC).

This is different in the case of my neurophenomenal approach. The here suggested neurophenomenal approach neither targets the sufficient neural conditions nor the contents of consciousness. Instead, it aims to account for the necessary rather than the sufficient neural

conditions of consciousness. As such, it does not target the neuronal mechanisms of specific contents in consciousness, but rather how neuronal states can in principle be transformed into phenomenal states independent of and prior to their association with particular contents.

In short, the neurophenomenal approach targets the neural predisposition of consciousness (NPC), the necessary neural conditions of possible consciousness, rather than the NCC. This also makes clear that it is important to consider conceptual differences in order to better understand the empirical differences between both approaches, the neurophenomenal approach and the global workspace.

The distinction between NCC and NPC also implies another difference concerning their respective targets. The global workspace theory targets the NCC and thus the difference between unconsciousness and consciousness. This contrasts with the neurophenomenal approach that focuses on the distinction between non-consciousness and unconsciousness/consciousness (e.g., principal consciousness) rather than the distinction between unconsciousness and consciousness.

The neurophenomenal approach consequently aims to reveal the neural predispositions of what I called "principal consciousness" (see second Introduction). "Principal consciousness" describes the states that have the possibility to become conscious; the term thus includes the distinction between consciousness and unconsciousness and distinguishes it from non-consciousness, that is, "non–principal consciousness." Hence, the global workspace theory and my neurophenomenal approach can be distinguished by different targets with regard to consciousness.

Finally, both approaches, the neurophenomenal one and the global workspace theory, target different features of consciousness. The global workspace theory targets contents of consciousness and how we can access them; it thus focuses on the neuronal mechanisms that open the door of consciousness to let the contents enter (see the excellent review by Dehaene and Changeux 2011).

This is different in the neurophenomenal approach. Here, the focus is on the organization of consciousness, the form of consciousness, and the level or state of consciousness, while contents, their constitution, selection, and designation, are regarded to naturally evolve from these processes (see Chapters 19 and 25). In short, my focus is not so much on the contents of consciousness and how we can access them, but rather on the form/organization and level or state of consciousness.

GLOBAL APPROACHES TO CONSCIOUSNESS IIIA: INTEGRATED INFORMATION THEORY

Various suggestions for neuronal mechanisms have been made for the neural correlates of consciousness (see Tononi and Koch 2008 for a recent overview). One suggestion came from G. Edelman (1993, 2003, 2005), who assumed re-entrant circuits in general and thalamo-cortical circuits in particular to be crucial in consciousness.

However, there is nothing specific about re-entrant thalamo-cortical circuits since all regions, even primary sensory regions, receive re-entrant feedback. Feedback or re-entrant circuits are all over the brain so that there is nothing special about them which would make them sufficiently specific and distinct as to account for consciousness. Consciousness could, for instance, be equally related to both feed-forward and feedback circuits. This sheds some doubt, however, upon the specificity of re-entrant connections for consciousness.

Another suggestion is tonic or sustained neural activity as distinguished from phasic neural activity. This suggestion is supposed to account for the temporal duration of consciousness; however, phasic activity may also be crucially involved in generating consciousness states, thus putting the specificity of sustained activity into doubt. Gamma oscillations in particular and neural synchrony in general have been associated with consciousness as has been discussed more in Chapter 18. However, there may be plenty of gamma oscillation and neural synchrony going on in the brain without any trace of consciousness being induced (see Part VI for details). Hence, as re-entrant circuits and sustained activity, gamma oscillations and neural synchronization may turn out to be unspecific when it comes to consciousness.

What neuronal mechanisms must then be considered as specific for consciousness? Tononi (2004, 2008) suggests that the amount of information integrated is specific for consciousness. Consciousness can be characterized by an integration of an extremely high amount of information in our experience. He therefore claims that "the level of consciousness of a physical system is related to the repertoire of causal states (information) available to the system as a whole (integration)" (Tononi and Koch 2008, 253). He calls this the information integration theory (IIT).

How is the integration of information related to neurobiological mechanisms? Based on his own investigation in, for instance, sleep (see above), he argues that information is integrated by thalamo-cortical re-entrant circuits; if they are disrupted as in non-REM sleep, anesthesia, or vegetative state, the degree of consciousness is also impaired. The thalamo-cortical re-entrant circuits may thus account for information integration, and that in turn may be central for generating consciousness, as is claimed by the IIT, which shall be discussed in more detail below.

GLOBAL APPROACHES TO CONSCIOUSNESS IIIB: INTEGRATION OF INFORMATION VERSUS NEURAL CODING

How does the IIT stand in relation to my own approach, and more specifically to the neural coding hypothesis of consciousness (CHC)? As outlined in the introduction, the CHC argues that difference-based coding is central and thus a necessary condition, that is, a neural predisposition of possible consciousness. For instance, the spatial amplification and condensation of neural differences across the whole brain are central in constituting local and global spatial continuity of the resting state's neural activity as the neural predisposition of "inner space consciousness" (as one may want to say in analogy to Husserl's inner time consciousness; see Chapter 14).

How does that compare to the IIT? I will argue in the following that the IIT and the CHC are not contradictory but rather complementary in various domains, empirical, conceptual, and methodological. Let's start with the empirical domain.

I argued that the effective connectivity as pointed out by Tononi and his IIT needs to be complemented by an account of those processes that transform functional into effective connectivity (see Chapter 16). I therefore argued for the need to consider those neuronal processes that generate the effectiveness of effective connectivity; those neuronal processes were characterized by the amplification of neural differences via difference-based coding and their subsequent condensation via nonlinear and nonadditive interaction. Tononi's focus on functional connectivity (as mere correlation) between regions is thus complemented by a focus on those neuronal processes that make such connectivity effective (as causal impact between regions). More generally, this means that my more process-based approach nicely complements and converges with the more region and network- (or connectivity-) based approach of Tononi.

The same holds true with regard to the frequency fluctuations (see Chapters 13–15). Tononi considers different frequencies, low- and high-frequency fluctuations, while he leaves open how their exact relation is generated. That is where I hypothesize difference-based coding in the temporal domain to be at work in that it codes the temporal differences between different low-frequency fluctuations, thereby yielding what I described as "temporal nestedness." It is thus the degree of temporal nestedness and ultimately the degree of difference-based coding that is supposed to enable and predispose the constitution of global spatial and temporal continuity of neural activity. That in turn is supposed to be central for inner time and space consciousness (see Part V).

The difference in empirical focus, regions/networks/connectivity versus process and coding, can be nicely illustrated by a metaphor of the moving car and the gas pedal. Tononi looks mainly at the gas pedal, the motor, and the tires when the car does not move. He thus focuses on the ingredients themselves and checks them all separately. While I focus on the processes that must go on in order to transform the gas pedal push into a moving car. My neurophenomenal approach thus aims to reveal the processes that must operate across the various ingredients in order to make the car move as a whole.

GLOBAL APPROACHES TO CONSCIOUSNESS IIIC: CORRELATES OF CONTENTS VERSUS CODING AS PREDISPOSITION

The difference in the empirical focus is accompanied by a more conceptual difference. Tononi regards his IIT as a theory about the NCC that aims to reveal the sufficient neural conditions of the contents of consciousness. He thus considers integration of information as a sufficient condition to induce consciousness and its specific contents.

This is different in my CHC. The CHC is a hypothesis about the neural predisposition of consciousness (see first introduction and Chapter 14); as such, it focuses therefore on the necessary, that is, enabling, rather than the sufficient, that is, executing, conditions of (phenomenal) consciousness. Most important, such a shift from neural correlates to predispositions accompanies a shift from contents to organization and structure of the resting state's neural activity, as they are necessary to predispose (rather than manifest) consciousness.

Let me briefly summarize before continuing. The IIT is about the sufficient neural conditions and the contents of consciousness mirroring what is currently described as the NCC. The CHC, in contrast, concerns the necessary conditions and the kind of neural code that is necessary to enable consciousness, reflecting therefore what I call the NPC. Since they concern different target features (content versus code) and distinct neural conditions (necessary/predispositions versus sufficient/correlate), IIT and CHC must be assumed to be complementary rather than being contradictory.

What would be necessary in the future, however, is to investigate how my account of difference-based coding in both domains spatial and temporal is related to the amount of information integration. My hypothesis is that increased degrees of difference-based coding, that is, increased amplification and condensation of functional connectivity and frequency fluctuations, may go along with increased integration of information; this remains to be investigated in the future.

Global Approaches to Consciousness
IIID: Mind- and Model-Based Approach
Versus Brain- and Code-Based Approach

Besides their empirical and conceptual complementarity, IIT and CHC do pursue complementary approaches methodologically. The IIT has two starting points, the phenomenal concepts like qualia or wholeness/unity of information in consciousness and the mathematical models of information. These two starting points serve to make predictions for the supposedly underlying neuronal mechanisms. One may consequently characterize the methodological strategy of the IIT as a mapping of the phenomenal and mathematical level onto the neuronal level of the brain.

Due to such mapping and starting point, the IIT may be described as a model- and mind-based approach to consciousness. It is model based because it starts from a mathematical model that serves to develop predictions for the brain's neural operations. And it is mind based (at least in conceptual regard, which does not imply an ontological basis for the concept of mind) because it takes phenomenal concepts like qualia and unity as a starting point to search for corresponding neuronal mechanisms (see Fig. A1-2a).

Such a mind- and model-based approach of the IIT must be distinguished from the methodological approach presupposed in the CHC. Unlike the IIT, the CHC does not start with a mathematical model but rather with the search for a coding mechanism in the brain (which, however, needs to be mathematized in the future; see later). This is well reflected in the fact that the CHC includes two subhypotheses, the

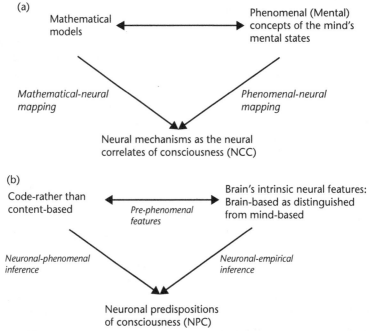

Figure A1-2a and b Comparison between the information integration theory (IIT) and the neurophenomenal approach. (*a*) This figure depicts the IIT that starts with mathematical and phenomenological models and reasons from there to the neural correlates of consciousness (NCC). This is different in the coding hypothesis of consciousness (CHC) as visualized in (*b*). Here, the brain's intrinsic features, its resting-state activity and its neural code, are the starting points. These serve to develop what I describe as "prephenomenal structures" that are considered neural predispositions of possible consciousness. The phenomenal features of consciousness are then inferred and matched with the neural code and the brain's intrinsic features.

encoding hypothesis of consciousness (EHC) and the difference-based coding hypothesis of consciousness (DHC) (see introduction). The CHC thus presupposes a code-based approach rather than a model-based approach as the IIT (see A1-2b).

Furthermore, the CHC does not take the phenomenal concepts themselves as a starting point as it is the case in the IIT. Instead, the CHC takes the brain itself, including its intrinsic features like its resting-state activity and coding strategy, as a starting point. From the intrinsic features of the brain itself, the CHC aims to infer the neural predispositions of consciousness and thus what I describe as the resting state's prephenomenal features like spatial and temporal continuity, as in Part V.

The inference from phenomenal to neuronal features, as presupposed in the IIT, is thus reversed here by inferring from the intrinsic neuronal features of the brain to the phenomenal features of consciousness. In other words, the phenomenal-neuronal mapping of the IIT is replaced in the CHC by neuronal-phenomenal inference as the main methodological strategy. This entails that the methodological strategy taken by the CHC is not only code based but also brain based rather than mind based as in the IIT.

Is the model- and mind-based approach of the IIT compatible with the code- and brain-based approach of the CHC? The strength of the IIT, its description of mathematical models, is the weakness of the CHC that yet lacks any kind of mathematization. This, however, needs to be specified in the future with regard to the particular neural code postulated here, for example, difference-based coding. One may then, for instance, see how much the mathematical description of difference-based coding might benefit (and eventually also take over) from the mathematical models applied by Tononi.

Conceptual Approaches to Consciousness IA—Mind-Based Approaches

So far, I have discussed various empirical approaches to consciousness and how they stand in relation to my neurophenomenal approach.

Now I briefly want to touch on some conceptual approaches that focus more on conceptual issues than empirical issues and are naturally discussed in philosophy rather than in neuroscience.

The concept of mind is presupposed in the metaphysical approach to consciousness that considers consciousness as a central feature of the mind. The metaphysical approach questions how the mind is related to the brain, thus raising metaphysical issues about existence and reality as discussed in philosophy of mind. The reference to the mind is also central in conceptual approaches to consciousness that focus on the meaning and use of the concept of consciousness in our language as used in daily practice, philosophy, and neuroscience (see Bennett and Hacker 2003). And we will also see the presupposition of the concept of mind in the embodied and extended mind approaches.

What do these different approaches, the metaphysical, the conceptual, and the extended mind approach, share? Despite their differences, they all take the concept of mind as the starting point (independent of whether they reduce it to the brain). They can consequently be characterized as *mind-based* approaches. As such, they must be distinguished from a *brain-based* approach that, for instance, starts with the brain itself and its intrinsic features as my neurophenomenal approach claims to do.

Most important, the here-presupposed brain-based approach needs to be distinguished from a *brain-reductive* approach. A brain-based approach takes the brain as the methodological starting point and aims from there to go on to the phenomenal features of consciousness. I therefore speak of *neurophenomenal hypotheses*.

This is different in a brain-reductive approach. In such case the phenomenal features of consciousness are no longer considered by themselves and are instead reduced to the brain and its neuronal mechanisms. Instead of starting from the brain to the phenomenal features of consciousness as the brain-based approach does, the brain-reductive approach proceeds in the reverse way, when mapping the phenomenal features of consciousness onto the brain's neuronal features, The brain-reductive approach may thus turn out to be a hidden mind-based approach where the concept of mind serves as negative foil or template for any subsequent consideration of the brain itself.

CONCEPTUAL APPROACHES TO CONSCIOUSNESS IB—EXTENDED MIND-BASED APPROACHES

My neurophenomenal approach raises the question of how it stands in relation to the concept of the "extended mind," the "embodied mind," or the "embedded mind" (see chapter 3 in Rowlands 2010 for their conceptual distinction). In a nutshell, an "embedded approach" assumes the mind and its mental states to be no longer "located" in the mind and ultimately being represented within the brain itself. Instead, the mind is to be "located" beyond the brain itself by being constituted in conjunction with body and environment.

Mental states are consequently neither represented in the brain itself nor is the brain regarded as the underlying sufficient cause of them. Instead, the concepts of representation and causality are discarded and replaced by "replacement and constitution theses" (see Shapiro 2011, 4ff; see later) that consider the relevance of body and environment in constituting and representing mental states. For that to be possible, we need to adapt and change our mental concepts to account for the constitutional role of body and environment ("conceptualization thesis" following Shapiro 2011). One consequence is, for instance, that mental states can no longer be regarded as either being internal in mind/brain or external in the environment with this dichotomy thus collapsing and becoming inappropriate.

How does the concept of the embodied and extended mind (I leave out the concepts of enacted and embedded mind; see chapter 3 in Rowland 2010) stand in relation to my neurophenomenal approach? First, the concepts of the embodied and extended mind are about the mind, whereas my approach is about the brain. This also implies that, second, the approach presupposed in the embodied and extended mind is predominantly conceptual.

Such a predominantly conceptual approach contrasts with my neurophenomenal approach, which is primarily empirical rather than conceptual (with conceptual implications being only secondary). Accordingly, the embodied and extended mind approach is more conceptual and thus philosophical, while my neurophenomenal hypothesis is rather empirical and predominantly neuroscientific (which, though, carries major implications for the conceptual side of things).

Third, the embodied and extended mind approach is a reaction against standard cognitive science that ultimately reduces the mind to the brain. This contrasts with my neurophenomenal approach, which is a reaction against what one may call "standard neuroscience" that tends to view the brain in constitutive isolation from body and environment with the latter only secondarily modulating the brain and its neuronal states.

How can we resolve these differences? The differences entail different remedies. Rowland (2010, 83–84) suggests the concept of an "amalgamated mind" that links the concepts of the embodied and extended mind into one unifying concept. The concept of the amalgamated mind describes that cognitive and thus mental processes depend constitutively on neural, bodily, and environmental processes and their respective structures.

CONCEPTUAL APPROACHES TO CONSCIOUSNESS IC—"AMALGAMATED MIND" VERSUS "AMALGAMATED BRAIN"

Taken into account the here-presupposed context of the brain, one may want to speak conceptually of an "amalgamated brain": The brain's neuronal activity must be assumed to reflect an amalgam of neuronal and intero- and exteroceptive stimuli (see Volume I). Most important, the different stimuli, including their different origins, may no longer be clearly distinguishable from each other in the brain's neuronal states because of difference-based coding (see Chapter 25 for details). Using Rowland's term, the different stimuli are thus *amalgamated* which I suppose to be possible on the grounds of specific neuronal mechanisms.

Following the lines of Volume I, such amalgamation between the different stimuli is highly plausible in empirical regard as demonstrated by the continuous interaction between all three stimuli (intero, extero, neuronal) in rest–stimulus and stimulus–rest interaction. And it is also manifest in the brain's specific way of coding these interactions by relying mainly on difference-based coding rather than stimulus-based coding.

I therefore tentatively propose that such amalgamation of the different stimuli may well correspond on the empirical side that is, in the neuroscientific context of the brain, to what Rowland describes conceptually as the "amalgamated mind" in the more philosophical context of the mind.

Accordingly, Rowland's concept of the amalgamated mind may well be complementary to the kind of neuronal mechanisms, that is, the brain's intrinsic features, which may ultimately amount to what could be described as the "amalgamated brain." If so, Rowland's concept of the "amalgamated mind" may be considered the conceptual analogue on the philosophical side to the here-suggested concept of an "amalgamated brain" within the empirical context of neuroscience.

NOTE

1. Where does the distinction between content and context come from? The concept of the neurophenomenal approach would argue that this distinction is more related to the observer than the brain itself; it is thus what I call an observer-based rather than a brain-based distinction (see Appendix 4 in Volume I). This contrasts with the concept of the global workspace that seems to propose the brain-based nature of this distinction when it associates context and content with different neural systems.

APPENDIX 2: BRAIN AND TIME

I considered the constitution of temporal continuity in the resting state to be central (see Chapters 13–15). This raises the question of how my neurophenomenal account of time compares to some other neuroscientific theories of time, which shall be briefly discussed in this appendix. In addition, I aim to point out how my neurophenomenal account of time relates to physical time as investigated in physics as well as to the perception and cognition of time as researched in psychology and neuroscience.

Neuroempirical Remark Ia: Temporality versus Perception and Cognition of Time

Dan Lloyd (2002; 2011, 1 and 3) distinguishes between perception and cognition of time on one hand, and what he calls "temporality" on the other. The perception and cognition of time refers to our ability to implicitly and explicitly perceive and think about ("cognize") time. This can be tested, for instance, in time-dependent tasks like temporal order and temporal simultaneity judgements, duration estimation, and reproduction tasks. In these cases, time is the target variable and becomes a stimulus in itself, as defined by a specific and discrete position in time and space. Such (implicit and) explicit perception and cognition of time has been studied extensively in recent cognitive neuroscience (see Poeppel 2009; Wittmann 2011; Wittmann 2009, 2011; Wittmann et al., 2010a and b; Wittmann and van Wasserhove 2009).

The (implicit and) explicit perception and cognition of time must be distinguished from "temporality," which is based on phenomenological or subjective experiential accounts of time as developed by William James and Edmund Husserl. What is "temporality"? The concept of "temporality" describes the flow of time in which every stimulus, including the temporal stimulus that is (implicitly or) explicitly perceived and cognized, is integrated and linked. Temporality in this sense refers to the temporal structure of our consciousness upon which any kind of subsequent (implicit or explicit) perception and cognition of time stand and are based.

William James described such temporality by his metaphors of the "stream of consciousness" and the "precious present." The concept of the "precious present" describes a brief temporal window where past and future converge into the present, a co-presence of past, present, and future. Such integration of past and future into the present moment was called by Husserl "retention" and "protention" (see Chapters 14 and 15). Both "protention" and "retention" can be characterized by the merger and integration between different discrete points in (physical) time; the past and future discrete points in (physical) time are linked in one "present moment," the "precious present" as James called it.

Most importantly, such a merger and linkage between different discrete points in time provides the temporal template or grid upon which any subsequent (implicit or explicit) perception and cognition of time is based. For instance, the perception and cognition of a particular time interval that is to be estimated in time-perception tasks is possible only by comparing the duration with those of the underlying temporal grid or template that signifies what James called the "stream of consciousness."

Only on the basis of such a temporal grid or template are perception and cognition of time possible; otherwise, none of the contents, like the time duration to be estimated in a time-judgement task, could be associated with consciousness at all, and thus be perceived or "cognized." This is what James meant when he was talking about a "stream of consciousness": In the same way as the water in a river is indispensable for any kind of boat or other things to float upon or flow in the river, the perception and cognition of time (and other contents in time) necessarily presuppose some kind of underlying temporal grid or template, a "temporal stream" as the "stream of consciousness."

Analogous to the concept of temporality, one may also speak of "spatiality." Spatiality may similarly describe the merger and integration of different discrete points in space into one "moment in space"; this basic spatiality may then provide the spatial template or grid for any subsequent (implicit or explicit) perception and cognition of space and contents in space.

Neuroempirical Remark IB: Constitution of Phenomenal Time

How can we characterize the concepts of temporality and spatiality in further detail? Both concepts presuppose the phenomenal context of subjective experience; namely, how we subjectively experience time and space in consciousness. One may therefore want to speak of phenomenal time and space. Time and space are here considered in the gestalt of a grid or template that ranges across different discrete points in time and space. Such phenomenal context must be distinguished from a purely objective and thus physical context where time and space are considered in terms of different discrete points in time and space. One may rather speak here of physical time (Lloyd 2011; Fingelkurts et al. 2010).

What is the difference between phenomenal and physical time? The main difference between physical and phenomenal time pertains to the relationship between different discrete points in time. Physical time distinguishes and separates between different discrete points in time. This results in temporal heterogeneity, discreteness, and ultimately discontinuity. In contrast, phenomenal time links and integrates the different discrete points in time and space into a spatial and temporal homogeneity and continuity where they can no longer be distinguished and separated from each other. This makes any temporal discreteness impossible.

How does the difference between phenomenal and physical time stand in relation to the brain and its neuronal mechanisms? I hypothesized here that low-frequency fluctuations are central in yielding phenomenal space and time (see Chapters 13–15). Does this mean that the brain can be characterized by phenomenal rather than physical time/space? Yes and No. Let's start with the No. The brain itself is ultimately a physical organ and cannot therefore by itself be characterized by phenomenal time and space. Hence, to characterize the brain itself by phenomenal time and space (as, for instance, Fingelkurts et al. 2010, 217ff seem to suggest) would be to confuse the neuronal, that is, physical, context of the brain and the phenomenal context of consciousness.

We would thus be confronted with what conceptually (logically) may be described as *false-positive phenomenal-neuronal inference*, a phenomenal-neuronal fallacy: in this case, one infers directly from the structure of the phenomenal features of consciousness to deduce the neuronal features of the brain. This is the case, for instance, when claiming there is isomorphism between phenomenal and neuronal features (see, for instance, Fingelkurts et al. 2010 for such isomorphism on the neuroscientific side).

However, the *No* (including the rejection of phenomenal-neuronal isomorphism) is not as clear as one would like it to be. This is so because one could answer the same question also with a Yes. Yes, the brain can be characterized by phenomenal space and time. Though the Yes is only partial since the brain's neuronal mechanisms are only a necessary but not sufficient condition of phenomenal time and space. Let us be more specific. I considered low-frequency fluctuations and continuous changes in the brain's resting-state activity to be necessary neural conditions of consciousness and thus as neural predispositions of possible phenomenal time.

NEUROEMPIRICAL REMARK IC: "LOCATION" OF PHENOMENAL TIME

In contrast (and this is extremely important), these neuronal mechanisms are not sufficient by themselves and can therefore not be considered neural correlates of phenomenal time. For that, something additional is required, such as an extrinsic stimulus from either the body (an interoceptive stimulus), or the environment (an exteroceptive stimulus) to elicit sufficiently large changes in neural activity level of the resting state (see Chapter 29 in Part VIII). However, the mere occurrence of an extrinsic stimulus is not sufficient by itself. The extrinsic stimulus also needs to interact with the brain's intrinsic activity, its resting state, in a certain way, that is, in a nonlinear way, to allow the association of a phenomenal state, e.g., phenomenal time and space, to the purely neuronal stimulus-induced activity. Accordingly, nonlinearity during rest–stimulus interaction, rather than the extrinsic stimulus itself (or the brain's intrinsic activity), can be considered a sufficient neuronal condition of phenomenal time.

Where does this leave us with regard to the constitution of phenomenal time? Phenomenal time cannot be "located" in the brain itself and its intrinsic activity; nor can it be "located" in and exclusively associated with the extrinsic stimulus itself and its particular stimulus-induced activity. Instead, phenomenal time is constituted in the interaction between the brain's intrinsic activity and the environmental and bodily extrinsic stimuli. In short, phenomenal time (and space) is (are) constituted in the intrinsic–extrinsic interaction between brain and environment/body. Any "location" of time (and space) in either brain or environment/body must consequently fail.

NEUROEMPIRICAL REMARK ID: PHYSICAL TIME, "BIOPHYSICAL TIME," AND PHENOMENAL TIME

How does this characterization of phenomenal time stand in relation to physical time? Physical time is constituted within the world itself, which brain, body, and environment are part of. Metaphorically put, phenomenal time is constituted within the space of the physical time. Phenomenal time is the kind of time that biological organisms like humans (and other species) constitute on the basis of their respective biophysical equipment, their "biophysical-computational spectrum" (as I explicate in the second Introduction and especially in Chapters 20 and 21).

Due to this biological and, more specifically, biophysical context, the concept of phenomenal time (and space) may be complemented by the one "biophysical time (and space)." The concept of "biophysical time (and space)" describes the time (and space) of biological organisms in relation to their respective environments and their particular physical features. Most important, such a relationship between organism and environment does not yet imply any kind of consciousness. This distinguishes the concept of a "biophysical time (and space)" from that of phenomenal time, which describes the subjective experience and thus consciousness of time.

The relation between organism and environment is based on the degree of correspondence between the organism's biophysical features (of both his brain and body) and the physical features of his environment. This relationship, as I suggested earlier, is central for the constitution of "biophysical time (and space)" by the intrinsic–extrinsic interaction between the organism's brain, body, and environment.

How are all three concepts of time—physical time, biophysical time, and phenomenal time—related to each other? The "biophysical time (and space)" of biological organisms takes place within, and thus presupposes, the physical time (and space) of the purely physical world. In other words, physical time (and space) is (are) a necessary but not sufficient condition of possible "biophysical time (and space)." At the same time, "biophysical time (and space)" are necessary but not sufficient (by themselves) to constitute phenomenal time (and space). Accordingly, all three concepts of time (and space) are necessarily but not sufficiently dependent upon each other.

NEUROEMPIRICAL REMARK IIA: DISTINCTION BETWEEN NEURONAL, PREPHENOMENAL, AND PHENOMENAL ACCOUNTS OF TIME

I have so far provided the general framework for my neurophenomenal account of time. This let me distinguish between different concepts of time: physical time, biophysical time, and phenomenal time. These different concepts of time implied different concepts of the world—physical time references to the physical world, biophysical time to the biological world, and phenomenal world to the world as we experience it in consciousness, the conscious world (if one wants to say so).

This provides an overarching framework for time and how it stands in relation to the world. That is usually a matter of philosophical discussion and, more specifically, of a philosophy of time, which to discuss is far beyond the scope of this book. More important in the present context is the kind of time that is investigated empirically in current psychology and neuroscience. How does my neurophenomenal account of time and its concepts of biophysical and phenomenal time compare to approaches taken in current psychology and neuroscience?

As already illustrated earlier, the three concepts of time are not independent of each other. I demonstrated that *phenomenal* time necessarily presupposes *biophysical* time, which in turn is constituted and takes place within the space of the *physical* time. What we now need to understand is how the brain contributes to and makes possible the transformation of physical time into biophysical time and, ultimately, phenomenal time. That in turn is essential in order to understand how my neurophenomenal account of time differs from the accounts of time in current psychology and neuroscience.

The constitution of biophysical and phenomenal time was the subject of intense discussion in Chapters 13–15. There I discussed the neuronal processes underlying the constitution

of biophysical time as distinguished from physical time, and its conversion into phenomenal time in the "right" circumstances. Without repeating the various neuronal and neurophenomenal hypotheses postulated in these chapters, I now want shed a brief light on the kind of approaches and accounts I presupposed there in a rather implicit way. This is important for understanding how my neurophenomenal account of time compares with others that are discussed and put forward in current psychology and neuroscience. I first want to distinguish between different accounts of time and space: neuronal, prephenomenal, phenomenal, and postphenomenal. Let us start with the neuronal account.

NEUROEMPIRICAL REMARK IIB: FROM THE NEURONAL OVER THE PREPHENOMENAL TO THE PHENOMENAL ACCOUNT OF TIME

A neuronal account of time and space only considers how the brain processes and constitutes space and time for itself and its own intrinsic activity, regardless of whether the kind of space and time constituted is either physical or phenomenal. The neuronal account thus focuses on the neuronal mechanisms underlying what can be described as *spatialization and temporalization* of the brain's intrinsic activity. Thereby the brain's intrinsic activity constitutes a statistically based virtual spatiotemporal structure, as I discussed in Chapters 4–6 in Volume I. Most important, such a purely neuronal account remains completely independent of any phenomenal (or prephenomenal) considerations and hence of consciousness in general.

This changes, however, as soon as one investigates how the brain's resting-state activity makes possible and thus predisposes consciousness, including phenomenal time. The purely neuronal account of time is then transformed into what I describe as the prephenomenal rather than neuronal account. One now considers the neuronal mechanisms underlying the processing of temporal information with regard to how they predispose, that is, enable and make possible the experience of phenomenal time and thus "inner time consciousness."

Accordingly, the neuronal processes are now no longer considered within the purely neuronal context of the brain. Instead, they are now shifted into the phenomenal context of consciousness. I call such an approach the "prephenomenal account of time." Such a "prephenomenal account of time" can be regarded as a first step towards a neurophenomenal account of time that seeks those neuronal mechanisms that underlie the constitution of phenomenal time in consciousness.

Such a prephenomenal account of time and space must not only be distinguished from a purely neuronal account but also from phenomenal accounts. A phenomenal account of time and space focuses exclusively on how time and space are subjectively experienced in consciousness. This is, for instance, well reflected in the descriptions of inner time consciousness by Husserl (see chapter 14 here) and James (see earlier here). Here the context is purely phenomenal, thus focusing on consciousness independent of the brain and its neuronal mechanisms. And, even more important, experience itself; that is, consciousness, becomes the focus here. This distinguishes the phenomenal account of time from the prephenomenal account, where the brain's

neuronal processes are the prime target and how they relate to the features of phenomenal time (see Fig. A2-1).

NEUROEMPIRICAL REMARK
IIC: POSTPHENOMENAL VERSUS NEURONAL ACCOUNT OF TIME

Finally, one also needs to distinguish neuronal, prephenomenal, and phenomenal accounts from what I call "postphenomenal accounts" of time and space. Postphenomenal accounts of time and space presuppose phenomenal time, including their respectively underlying neuronal mechanisms. Post-phenomenal accounts of time therefore presuppose consciousness and focus on the functions, i.e., perception and cognition of time, that take place on the basis of and, metaphorically speaking, within the space of consciousness. Such a post-phenomenal account of time is presupposed in current psychology and neuroscience that investigate the neuronal and psychological mechanisms underlying the perception and cognition of time (see, for instance, Coull et al. 2011 for a review).

How is such a post-phenomenal account of time distinguished from the earlier-described

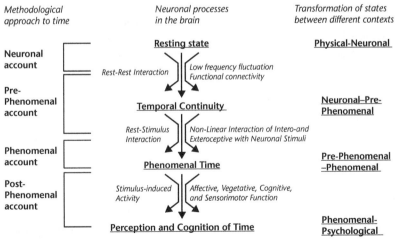

Figure A2-1 Different accounts of time. The figure shows the different approaches and accounts of time and their respective neuronal mechanisms. I distinguish between neuronal, prephenomenal, phenomenal, and postphenomenal accounts (*left*), which I suppose to be associated with distinct neuronal mechanisms (*middle*). The different accounts presuppose different contexts, physical, neuronal, phenomenal, and psychological, and their respective transformations between the different states (*right*).

neuronal, pre-phenomenal, and phenomenal accounts? The neuronal account focuses on the neuronal mechanisms by which the brain itself spatializes and temporalizes its intrinsic activity. This is to be distinguished from the neuronal mechanisms that are recruited during the perception and cognition of time.

Let us give a more concrete example. One neuronal mechanism of the brain for temporalizing its own intrinsic activity consisted of the constitution of low-frequency fluctuations (see Chapters 4–6 in Volume I). The neuronal account of time now investigates how these low-frequency fluctuations are constituted as for instance in terms of a statistically based temporal structure (see Chapters 4–6). This is to be distinguished from a postphenomenal account of time that investigates how the perception and cognition of time modulate and use these low-frequency fluctuations by, for instance, "slicing them up" into higher-frequency fluctuations (see Chapters 4–6 in Volume I and Chapters 13–15 in Volume II).

NEUROEMPIRICAL REMARK IID: POSTPHENOMENAL VERSUS PREPHENOMENAL AND PHENOMENAL ACCOUNTS OF TIME

How can the postphenomenal account be distinguished from a prephenomenal account of time? The prephenomenal account investigates how the neuronal mechanisms underlying the temporalization of the brain's intrinsic activity are related to the phenomenal features of consciousness. The prephenomenal account thus aims to directly link neuronal and phenomenal features, and can therefore also be characterized as a *neurophenomenal* account.

This is different in the *postphenomenal* account. Rather than linking neuronal and phenomenal features, as in the prephenomenal or neurophenomenal account, the postphenomenal account aims to link perceptual and cognitive features, i.e., the perception and cognition of time, to specific neuronal mechanisms. One may thus want to speak of *neuro-perceptual and neuro-cognitive* account of time as distinguished from a neurophenomenal account of time.

This is even more important considering that any kind of perception and cognition of time always presupposes consciousness of time and takes thus place, metaphorically speaking, within the "space" of consciousness. Hence, to confuse neuro-perceptual and neuro-cognitive accounts of time with a neurophenomenal account is to confuse furniture and floor, and thus to neglect that the furniture—the perception and cognition of time—always presupposes some kind of "floor," the consciousness of time.

Finally, the postphenomenal account of time must also be distinguished from the phenomenal account. The phenomenal account focuses only on the subjective-experiential features and how time is experienced from the first-person perspective in consciousness. This remains completely independent of any physical and neuronal features of time and is thus purely phenomenal. Putting the phenomenal features into a neuronal context allowed me then to target the underlying neuronal mechanisms in my neurophenomenal account.

The case is different in postphenomenal accounts of time, which do not care much about the subjective-experiential; that is, phenomenal, features of time. Instead, the postphenomenal account only cares about the perceptual and cognitive features of time as distinguished from the phenomenal features of consciousness itself. The postphenomenal account of time can therefore be described as a *perceptual-cognitive* account, which (very much like the phenomenal account) may be extended to the neuronal context of the brain and then resurface as a neuro-perceptual and neuro-cognitive account.

NEUROEMPIRICAL COMPARISON IA: NEURODYNAMICAL APPROACH TO TIME (VARELA)

After having distinguished among different concepts of time and different accounts of time, I now want to directly compare my neurophenomenal account to other approaches to time in recent neuroscience. Rather than discussing each position in full detail, I here focus on some of the main authors espousing a particular position and account of time at the border between neuronal and phenomenal accounts. Let me start with the neurodynamical approach to time by F. J. Varela, who explicitly refers to some of the phenomenal features of time I discussed in Chapters 14 and 15.

Varela (1999) hypothesizes that the three-fold temporal structure is related to the dynamic mechanisms of large-scale neuronal integration that is associated with perception-action, memory, and motivation. More specifically, he proposes specific cell assemblies for every particular cognitive act. These cell assemblies are selected through precise coincidence of the firing of cells; for example, synchronization. The synchronization is, however, dynamically unstable and will constantly give rise to new assemblies whereby the succeeding cell assemblies build upon or bifurcate from the previous one—these continuous jumps of the system can be called "trajectories."

Since each trajectory is the starting or bifurcation point for the next one to arise, there is a smooth transition between the various trajectories. The moments of transiently stable synchrony before the next trajectory arises may be linked to the "duration bloc" (see Chapters 13–15 in Volume II), or as Varela (1999) calls it, the "integration-relaxation processes (at the I-scale) are strict correlates of present-time consciousness." The threefold temporal structure may thus be traced back to neuronal synchronization and multistable or dynamical trajectories.

NEUROEMPIRICAL COMPARISON IB: NEURODYNAMICAL VERSUS NEUROPHENOMENAL APPROACH TO TIME

How does Varela's neurodynamical approach compare with my neurophenomenal account? The neurophenomenal account differs from Varela's neurodynamical approach in that it does not take a dynamical systems perspective. It is rather neuroanatomical and neurophysiological (and also neuropsychological) in that it hypothesizes that a particular kind of neural activity, that is, resting-state activity, in a particular set of regions, the default mode network (DMN), as well as a particular kind of coding, difference-based coding, are involved in constituting the duration bloc or the threefold temporal structure.

My approach is, at least in part, neurophysiological, in that it argues that the encoding of the changes in the continuously high resting-state neural activity, including its low- and high-frequency waves via difference-based coding may be crucial in providing temporal continuity. Though these features differ from Varela's neurodynamical approach, both approaches may nevertheless be compatible if not complementary with each other. The neural mechanisms I described here may eventually be well described with the tools of dynamic systems and neuronal synchronization sketched by Varela.

For instance, one could imagine that neuronal synchronization within the DMN may be established via their low-frequency fluctuations and functional/effective connectivity and thereby constitute transient temporal continuity and thus the duration bloc with the threefold temporal structure. As described in Part V, specific signal fluctuations have indeed been observed in the DMN, which may provide a starting point for investigation of neuronal synchronization. Hence, the present combination of neuroanatomical, neurophysiological, and neuropsychological perspectives may well be compatible with or even complementary to Varela's neurodynamical approach.[1] Both approaches may also be complementary in that my hypothesis of difference-based coding provides the kind of neural coding that is necessary to make possible the kind of neurodynamical mechanisms Varela postulates.

NEUROEMPIRICAL COMPARISON IC: AFFECT AND TIME

Finally, Varela (1999) links the third component of the threefold temporal structure, protention, with affect. Protention is supposed to be "always suffused with affect and emotional tone" because it concerns a nonpredictable openness that induces emotion. The very constitution of the threefold temporal structure and especially protention is thus ingrained by affect and emotion; this implies that time may open the door to study affect and emotional tonality and vice versa.

This is very compatible with my approach. I suppose that the anterior cortical midline structure (CMS) and their functional/effective connectivity to subcortical regions are central in constituting "protention"; that is, the anticipation of the future (see Chapters 13–15). Interestingly, the very same regions, the anterior CMS as well as subcortical midline regions like the amygdala, the nucleus accumbens, and the tectum have also been shown to be activated during emotion-processing and during subjective emotional experience (see Chapters 31 and 32 as well as Phan et al. 2002 for an overview; see also Grimm et al. 2006).

Such regional overlap in anterior CMS indeed suggests some kind of linkage between emotion/affect and protention, as postulated by Varela. This is further supported by the observation of both emotional and temporal abnormalities in depression, which shows abnormally high resting-state activity in precisely the anterior CMS (see Chapter 17 as well as Chapter 27). There is thus some empirical evidence, although indirect, for the affective and emotional nature of protention, which may complement Varela's approach. Future investigations are necessary, however, to demonstrate the inherently affective nature of protention like its coupling to especially positive emotions.

In contrast to his account of the affective nature of protention, Varela's assumption that retention is not inherently affective cannot be supported on empirical grounds. The posterior DMN like the posterior cingulate and the hippocampus that are supposed to implicate retention, that is, the past, have been observed to be also associated with emotions and affect (see Panksepp 1998; Phan et al. 2002); this makes it rather unlikely that retention is principally distinguished from protention with regard to emotional involvement.

Phenomenologically, this is supported by the fact that experience of the past becomes abnormally overloaded by negative affect in depression (see Chapters 17 and 27). This is not compatible with the assumption of an affect-free nature of retention postulated by Varela. Accordingly, the principal distinction between protention and retention with regard to the presence or absence of affect/emotion cannot be supported by the empirical data.

Instead of such a strict dichotomy, one might better propose a continuum between positive and negative affect/emotion that seems to be parallel those and be closely intertwined with the continuum between protention and retention. This is the lesson depressed patients seem to tell us, whose abnormal focus on the past (at the expense of the future) is associated with abnormally negative emotions (at the expense of positive emotions) (see also Northoff et al. 2011, see Chapter 17).

NEUROEMPIRICAL COMPARISON IIA: PRENOETIC ACCOUNT OF TIME (GALLAGHER AND POEPPEL)

Gallagher (1998, 135–7, 153, 182) proposes so-called *prenoetic* forces or factors that, on one hand, condition and constrain subjective temporal experience, while, on the other hand, they are not accessible by reflection and its act-object intentionality. In addition to superpersonal forces (linguistic, cultural, historical), he attributes the physiological body and social factors a crucial role in conditioning subjective temporal experience.

This is quite compatible with my approach and complements it on the conceptual level. What I call prephenomenal may more or less correspond to what Gallagher calls prenoetic. Similar to Gallagher's prenoetic factors, the here sketched neuronal processes underlying the constitution of temporal continuity are prephenomenal concepts and, to speak with Gallagher, cannot be accessed as such in phenomenal experience in terms of act-object intentionality. On the other hand, they condition, or better, enable and predispose, phenomenal states and thus subjective temporal experience. What I call *prephenomenal structures* may thus show some of the features Gallagher associates with his concept of *prenoetic factors,* which also mirrors what Poeppel (2009) calls "presemantic integration" (which may correspond more or less to what I here described as "temporal continuity" of neuronal activity).

Gallagher (1998, 161–163), relying on the work of Poeppel (as summarized in Poeppel 2009), proposes a relationship between neuronal and phenomenal time windows. Poeppel

(2009) suggests neuronal states of 30 ms as the "subpersonal quanta of primary consciousness." These 30 ms neuronal states may be integrated in successive order within temporal windows of 2–3 seconds which, on the phenomenal level of consciousness, may resurface in corresponding durations of an experienced specious present. There may, however, be neuronal states longer than 2–3 seconds that Poeppel associates with presemantic integration or content-independent retentional mechanisms. Gallagher (1998, 161–163) adheres to Poeppel's theory, since it helps "to make sense of many experiences" by explaining their "microgenesis in neuronal terms."

However, Gallagher critically remarks that Poeppel's theory "does not solve all problems." First, there are many events even on the 30 ms level that never enter consciousness and instead remain unconscious (and can therefore not even be considered as subpersonal). How and where are these events processed if the 30 ms windows account for primary consciousness of objects?

Second, the distinction between presemantic and semantic levels becomes blurred once one proposes, as Gallagher does, that semantic factors like historical, linguistic, and cultural forces condition and constrain subjective temporal experience. If this is true, semantic processes should already be at work on the microgenetic level and thus during the neuronal constitution of the 30 ms quanta (see Gallagher 1998, footnote 10 on p. 215). In other words, semantic factors are relevant from early on rather than appearing only late at the very end as the pinnacle of neuronal processing.

NEUROEMPIRICAL COMPARISON IIB: PRENOETIC VERSUS NEUROPHENOMENAL ACCOUNT OF TIME

Gallagher's account raises two questions for my hypothesis of the relationship between phenomenal time and difference-based coding. First, does neuronal processing within the dynamic temporal network (DTN) (see Chapter 13) constitute similar time windows? This question cannot be answered empirically at this point, since temporal investigations of this system using electroencephalography or magnetoencephalography have hardly been reported.

I hypothesize that the length and time span of possible time windows depends, at least in part, on the phases of the low-frequency fluctuations and on the speed of neural processing in functional connectivity within the DTN. This, however, is a rather speculative hypothesis that needs to be tested in studies that combine analysis of changes in resting-state connectivity within the DMN and reports about subjective temporal experience.

Second, Gallagher's account raises the question whether neural processing in terms of difference-based coding constitutes meaning and thus introduces the semantic dimension. I propose that by coding intero- and exteroceptive stimuli in difference to the brain's intrinsic activity, its resting-state activity, and vice versa, the semantic dimension and thus meaning is constituted. This would imply that the semantic dimension is present from early on in neural processing and that it determines what and how something is processed.

In other words, the semantic dimension may already be at work at the microgenetic level of difference-based coding and thus in rest–rest interaction; this is not only quite compatible with Gallagher's (1998, 162–163, footnote 10 on p. 215) criticism of both Poeppel and Varela, but also with the observation of meaningful semantic contents occurring already in the resting state itself, such as in mind wandering, daydreaming, and dreams (see Chapter 26).

NEUROEMPIRICAL COMPARISON IIIA: AFFECTIVE-VEGETATIVE ACCOUNT OF TIME (CRAIG AND WITTMANN)

One may now be inclined to raise the question how my prephenomenal account of time and space stands in relation to the postphenomenal accounts in current cognitive neuroscience. To address that question, we may need to go briefly into the current neuroscience about the perception and cognition of time.

Initially, the perception and cognition of time and space was considered to be mainly based on cognitive functions like working memory, attention, and executive functions (see later, for instance, Vogeley and Kupke 2007 and Coull et al. 2011). Such cognitive views of the perception and cognition of time, however, need to be complemented by affective and vegetative functions as it has been especially pointed out by Craig (2009, 2010a and b) and Wittmann (2009), who both propose a central role for the insula in the perception of time.

Based on his account of the insula, Craig (2009, 2010a and b) proposes this region to be central in constituting time, subjective time. The insula is central in generating emotions across time, a "finite series of emotional moments can provide an image of feelings across time." This is supposed to be based on the homeostatic, that is, interoceptive input from the body and possibly some endogenous activity in the insula at around 8 Hz. If now salient emotional moments occur, the subjective time may slow down with that emotional moment occupying a larger temporal space in the passage across time.

How can such a salient emotional moment and its relationship to the past and future moments be perceived and cognized? Craig (2010a and b, see figure 6 there) proposes what he calls a "comparative buffer": this allows for automatic and introspective comparison of the different emotional moments across time (which thereby provides the illusion of a self or subject). Since it is very much analogous to us watching a movie in a cinema, Craig calls his account a "cinemascopic model of awareness."

A 2011 account by Seth et al. (2011) associates the insula with time consciousness also, more specifically the subjective experience of presence (see also Chapters 13–15). They consider the insula to be a comparator that generates top-down predictions that are compared with bottom-up signals from vegetative afferences as triggered by interoceptive input. Such comparison is supposed to make possible the subjective experience of time and, more specifically, *presence*. This complements the assumption of Craig (2010a and b), who suggests the insula is central in the perception of time (see Appendix 2 for details).

Based on such an affective and interoceptive account of time, Wittmann et al. (2010, 2011) investigated the perception of time; more specifically, the perception of the duration of time. They demonstrated that the subjective perception of the duration of time was specifically encoded by neuronal activity in the posterior insula and was also dependent upon interoceptive awareness and the cardiac signals. This means that the perception of time is not a purely cognitive function but also an interoceptive, that is, vegetative, and affective (see also Wittmann 2009, 2011 as well as Wittmann et al. 2010a and b).

Both Craig and Wittmann focus on what happens prior to the recruitment of cognitive functions during the perception and cognition of time. They propose that affective and vegetative functions, and more specifically their perception by us, may be central in and predictive of how we perceive and cognize time (and space). Such a shift from cognitive to affective and vegetative functions is neuroanatomically accompanied by a shift from (for instance) the lateral prefrontal cortex and its essential role in higher order cognitive functions (see Vogeley and Kupke 2007) to the insula and its involvement in affective and vegetative processing.

Neuroempirical Comparison IIIB: Affective-Vegetative versus Neurophenomenal Account of Time

How is such a vegetative and affective approach to time related to my neurophenomenal account? Rather than focusing on the affective and vegetative functions and the insula's role in the perception and cognition of time, I go even one step further and focus on what must happen prior to both affective-vegetative and cognitive functions in order to make consciousness and subsequently perception and cognition of time possible.

In the same way Craig and Wittmann shift from cognitive functions to their very presuppositions in affective and vegetative function, I take the latter and go back to their very ground, that is, necessary conditions. More specifically, I go back to the brain's intrinsic activity, its resting-state activity, which occurs prior to any function, whether affective, vegetative, or cognitive. I just go one step further back than do Wittmann and Craig, which leads me from the affective and vegetative functions to the resting state and its purely neuronal functions.

For instance, recruitment of the insula during affective and vegetative functions presupposes a certain resting-state activity in the very same region and its modulation by especially the anterior cortical midline structures; that is, rest–rest interaction (see Wiebking et al. 2011, 2012; Duncan et al. 2011, 2013). Such rest–rest interaction between midline structures and insula may be central in constituting the degree of temporal continuity inherent in the resting state itself. That in turn may predispose the degree to which time can possibly be experienced within the context of affective and vegetative (and cognitive) functions during subsequent rest–stimulus interaction and stimulus-induced activity.

The here-proposed shift from affective and vegetative functions to the resting state and its purely neuronal function implies a shift from a postphenomenal account of time to a prephenomenal (and neurophenomenal) one (see earlier). This goes along with a shift from the sufficient neural conditions of the perception of time to the necessary, i.e., predisposing neural conditions of possible "inner time consciousness." Accordingly, unlike Craig and Wittmann, I thus focus on the neural predispositions of "inner time consciousness" rather than on the neural correlates of "inner time perception."

How can we now better link the neurophenomenal and the affective-vegetative accounts of time? Based on my neurophenomenal account and the assumption that perception presupposes consciousness, I hypothesize the following: The resting-state activity in the insula, and especially its temporal structure, including the phase durations of its low-frequency fluctuations, may predict the temporal range (or scope) within which one is able to experience and perceive the vegetative functions of one's own body, like one's own heartbeat. One could then propose that the deviation of the subjective heart beat perception from the objective heart beat rate, i.e., the accuracy of the heartbeat perception, may be predicted by the low-frequency fluctuations' phase durations and the timing of the heartbeat in relation to the low-frequency fluctuations' phase onsets as encoded in the resting-state activity of the insula: the more closely the low-frequency fluctuations' phase onsets align with the onset of the heartbeat, and the more closely the phase durations (in the resting-state activity of the insula) correspond to the durations between two different heartbeats, the more accurate is the subjective heartbeat perception (and thus the less deviation there is between objective heartbeat rate and subjective heartbeat perception).

NEUROEMPIRICAL COMPARISON IVA: COGNITIVE ACCOUNT OF RETENTION (FUSTER AND KELLEY)

Fuster (1997, 2003) proposes that the prefrontal cortex may be crucially involved in constituting the threefold temporal structure. The prefrontal cortex comprises the functions of working memory (past), interference control (present), and preparatory set (future) as basic functions of the prefrontal cortex; when combined, these functions provide temporal integration between past, present, and future, resulting in the threefold temporal structure.

Let us detail that. Working memory provides online maintenance of contents and may therefore be essential for providing online access to actual perceptions in the present moment. This allows working memory to hold items "online" across time, which makes linkage between the past and the present time dimensions and thus (see also Vogeley and Kupke 2007). Neuroanatomically, working memory has been associated with predominantly the lateral prefrontal cortical activity, including the ventrolateral and dorsolateral prefrontal cortex. Due to its integration of past and present, working memory and the lateral prefrontal cortical activity are proposed by Fuster to account for retention (see also Vogeley and Kupke 2007).

This assumption of the crucial involvement of working memory and the ventrolateral/dorsolateral prefrontal cortex in retention contrasts with my hypothesis in at least neuroanatomical terms. I hypothesize that retention corresponds to functional/effective connectivity between ventral and posterior CMS, whereas the lateral prefrontal cortex, including ventrolateral and dorsolateral prefrontal cortex, is rather associated with reflection than retention. Any kind of memory, even working memory, may be considered a cognitive process, if not a higher order cognitive process, which may correspond to what phenomenologically is described as reflection.

Reflection, however, mirrors a reflective and cognitive level rather than the prereflective and pre-cognitive level, as it is required to account for the phenomenal features of consciousness. One may subsequently suspect confusion between the prereflective/pre-cognitive and the reflective/cognitive levels in the characterization of retention by working memory and the lateral prefrontal cortex.

The cognitive proponents, however, may want to argue that working memory is just the wrong kind of memory. Instead, one may associate retention with a much more simple form of memory that does not yet require cognitive and thus reflective capacities and may therefore be closer to the prereflective and pre-cognitive level. One could, for instance, propose some form of iconic memory by means of which subjects can retain for short amounts of time a tachistocopically presented visual image and can read off some of its details after its actual occurrence (see, e.g., recent work by Ned Block). There may thus be some kind of short-term visual storage, an ultra-short-term memory, that allows us to link different discrete points in time, like those from past and present moments.

NEUROEMPIRICAL COMPARISON IVB: COGNITIVE VERSUS NEUROPHENOMENAL ACCOUNT OF RETENTION (FUSTER AND KELLEY)

However, following Kelley (2005), such iconic memory as short-term visual storage is not compatible with the subjects' phenomenological reports of moving objects. Subjects report that they experience moving objects as persistent in time rather than seeing and retaining after-images, as we would expect in the case of iconic memory as short-term visual storage. propose

I claim that the introduction of iconic memory as ultra-short-term memory does not solve the basic problem. Why? Because the assumption of some special short-term memory is simply incompatible with the phenomenology of retention. As Varela (1999) points out, the threefold temporal structure and thus retention presuppose

the original constitution of an object or event in time, which is constituted in the present moment and therefore phenomenally described as an impression or the "living present." Any kind of memory, including iconic memory, in contrast, presupposes an object or event already given to impression; the object or event is thus not originally constituted or presented, as in the case of retention, but rather modulated or re-presented.

Therefore, retention must be principally distinguished memory including iconic memory, working memory, autobiographical memory, and any other form of memory. Whatever the form of memory, it always presupposes some kind of perceptual and cognitive processing of particular objects, events, or persons. This signifies a memory-based approach to time as a postphenomenal approach. Neuronally, a memory-based approach targets the neuronal mechanisms underlying the perceptual and cognitive processing of the respective stimuli, thus focusing on stimulus-induced activity.

This is to be distinguished from a neurophenomenal account that focuses on the experience, that is consciousness, of time, rather than on the perception and cognition of time as in the memory-based approach. As such, the neurophenomenal approach is forced to target the brain's resting-state activity and its spatiotemporal structure rather the subsequent stimulus-induced activity.

NEUROEMPIRICAL COMPARISON IVC: COGNITIVE ACCOUNT OF PROTENTION (FUSTER AND KELLEY)

How can we explain protention? The goal-orientation and, more specifically, its preparatory set refers to the "preparation of action" (Fuster 1997, 2003) and includes therefore a prospective component with an orientation toward the future. The readiness potential may, for instance, be considered a neural mechanism that indicates planning, preparation, and anticipation of future actions,[2] which phenomenally may be associated with protention. These functions may be mediated by the medial and lateral premotor cortex as well as by the dorsolateral prefrontal cortex (see also Vogeley and Kupke 2007).

Similar to the case of retention, one can argue that preparation, planning, and anticipation constitute cognitive activities that may be linked to the reflective level rather than to the prereflective and pre-cognitive level and its threefold temporal structure. Developing, preparing, or anticipating motor activity is not the same as the original constitution of objects or events within and through the dynamic flow of time. Preparing, planning, and anticipating require higher order cognitive functions and thus reflection, for example, what can be described as "active synthesis" (Fuster 1997).

What is anticipated is already known or supposed to be known or imaginable, even though it has not yet actually occurred since otherwise it could not be predicted and thus anticipated. Anticipation presupposes determination of the future and thus of time in general. Protention, in contrast, dos not predetermine the future, implying that time remains open. Instead, the concept of *protention* constitutes (rather than predetermines) the future by opening a temporal horizon from past to future, which Husserl described as "passive synthesis" between past, present, and future (see Chapters 13–15).

NEUROEMPIRICAL COMPARISON
IVD: CONFUSION BETWEEN ANTICIPATION AND PROTENTION

Such "passive synthesis" and its temporal horizon, the openness toward the future, provide the basis for the anticipation of particular objects, events, or persons. Prior to the cognitive activity of anticipation, there must be thus some openness towards the future that first and foremost makes the former, anticipation, possible. To confuse protention and anticipation would thus be to neglect the fact that the window to the future must first be "opened," i.e., protention, before one can lean out of the window to anticipate how nice it would be to stand on the green lawn in the neighbor's garden, i.e., anticipation. Accordingly, anticipation presupposes protention.

One would suggest, based on these considerations, the following empirical hypotheses. One could hypothesize that the temporal scope of anticipation—the time window within which one can anticipate—may be predicted by the temporal constellations in both "inner time consciousness" and the brain's resting-state activity: the longer the phase durations of the resting state's low-frequency fluctuations, the more the subjective experience, that is, consciousness, can extend into the future, thus showing stronger degrees of protention. And the larger the extension of protention into the future, the wider the temporal range and scope within which anticipation can take place. Accordingly, the longer the phase durations in the resting state, the larger the extension of protention into the future, and the wider the temporal range and scope of anticipation.

However, as we all know, nothing is simple. Whether the longer phase durations of the resting state will really translate into wider temporal range and scope of anticipation depends also on the *timing* of the cognitive activity related to anticipation: If the onset of anticipation falls close to or is even identical to the phase onset of the resting state's low-frequency fluctuations, the anticipation may take more or less full advantage of the long phase durations. In that case, there may indeed be a good prediction of the temporal range and scope of anticipation by the resting state's phase durations. If, in contrast, the two onsets do not fall together, the prediction may decrease; the degree of deviation may then predict the probability of prediction with higher degrees of deviation (in onsets) leading to a lower probability of prediction.

Finally, on a more conceptual level, confusion between anticipation and protention means to confuse a cognitive (and more generally psychological) state, anticipation, with a phenomenal state, protention. As shown earlier, anticipation as a cognitive state necessarily presupposes consciousness in general and protention in particular. This means that phenomenal states like protention must precede psychological states like anticipation in very much the same way that the brain's intrinsic resting-state activity precedes its extrinsic stimulus-induced activity.

To confuse anticipation and protention would thus be to confuse not only psychological/cognitive and phenomenal states but also stimulus-induced and resting-state activity. This ultimately amounts to a confusion between pre-phenomenal and phenomenal accounts of protention on one hand, and postphenomenal accounts of anticipation on the other.

Notes

1. Another aspect that is missing in my account is the functional architecture within the DMN itself. Lloyd (2002) suggests that a recurrent network with an input layer, an output layer, a hidden layer, and an additional layer may be necessary to represent the predicted state (output layer), the current state (input layer), and the prior state (additional or hidden layer), and thus the threefold temporal structure of protention, presentation, and retention. Such a network model might be interesting to investigate in the specific case of the DMN.

2. Grush (2005) gives the timing of sensorimotor contingencies a central role in his emulator model of phenomenal time. This requires revealing the temporal order or movements and the temporal distance between the current, prior, and subsequent movements. He considers emulators to be process models in the brain, such as premotor cortex, that continuously anticipate, retain, and update sensorimotor feedback, which they can achieve by constantly timing their output in proportion possible to feedback from an actually ongoing process. Due to his focus on sensorimotor contingencies, he seems to avoid the slip to the reflective or cognitive level, as seems to be the case with Fuster. However, it remains unclear (1) how he bridges the gap from mere sensorimotor timing to subjective experience of a threefold temporal structure, and (2) how he links sensorimotor contingencies with prereflective self-awareness.

APPENDIX 3: BRAIN AND UNITY

The discussion of *unity* in the context of consciousness led us deeply into philosophical territory, as in the discussion of the concepts of unity and subjectivity. There is another point of convergence with philosophy, more specifically with the framework of German philosopher Immanuel Kant, whose transcendental approach I believe can be linked to the brain and neuroscience by advocating what I describe as a *neurotranscendental approach* (see also Northoff 2011, 2012a and c, 2013, for the linkage between Kant and neuroscience; as well as Churchland 2012, 1–5, 19). Interestingly, a connection of Kant's philosophy to neuroscience has also been observed by one of the main neuroscientists of visual consciousness, Semir Zeki. His consideration of Kant shall be discussed here and will be put into the current framework.

One concept centrally figuring in Kant's philosophy is that of transcendental unity, which he suggested is necessary for making consciousness possible. I here specify Kant's concept of transcendental unity by what I described earlier as the environment–brain unity that I suppose to occur prior to any subsequent unity; that is, prephenomenal unity and phenomenal unity. I also enrich Kant's concept of *synthesis* by postulating particular neuronal mechanisms that are supposedly involved in constituting the environment-brain unity as transcendental unity. I conclude the section with the charge of a possible category error; that is, the confusion between natural and logical levels of investigation.

NEUROEMPIRICAL REMARK IA: ZEKI'S THEORY OF "MICRO-CONSCIOUSNESS"

Semir Zeki (2003, 2008), based in London, has made major contributions to the understanding of the visual system. His neuroscientific (besides his aesthetic) work focuses mainly on the visual cortex and how it relates to visual consciousness, which he takes as a paradigmatic example of consciousness in general. Let us start with the visual cortex. The visual cortex contains neuroanatomically different systems for visual motion (V5) and color (V4) that have distinct anatomical inputs and are functionally segregated from each other. This is further supported by lesion studies. Patients with lesions in V5 show color blindness (achromatopsia), while they remain able to see and therefore conscious of visual motion. In contrast, lesions in V4 lead to motion blindness (akinetopsia), whereas the perception and thus consciousness of color is preserved. Since perception here is taken to be identical to consciousness, one cannot deny that these patients show consciousness, albeit limited to either visual motion or color with deficits in the respective other. Zeki speaks here of what he calls "micro-consciousness," which is "micro" because it is limited to certain contents like color or visual motion.

How is such micro-consciousness generated? Zeki (2003, 2008) conducted a series of imaging experiments where he presented either two identical or non-identical visual stimuli at the same time, for example, same or opposite faces and same or opposite houses. The same or identical faces/houses induced high activity in the visual cortex, for example, the face and house areas, and most important, were consciously perceived to 100%. In contrast, neither of the non-identical faces/houses were consciously perceived at all (0%) and went along with lower activity in the respective face and house regions. Interestingly, both regions, face and house regions, were also active when their respective stimulus type remained absent albeit to a much a lower degree.

From these results Zeki concludes that the difference between consciousness and non-consciousness does not lie in the presence or absence of neural activity in particular regions (as, for instance, the involvement of higher order regions like the prefrontal cortex). Instead of the involvement of a particular region, he proposes the degree of neuronal activity in the region processing a particular content (like faces or houses) to be central for inducing consciousness. The higher the activity in the region processing a particular content, the more likely it is that the content will become conscious. In contrast, lower activity levels in the same region will make consciousness of the particular content less likely, or even impossible.

Accordingly, the region's activity levels predict whether the respective contents will become conscious, entailing what Zeki calls "micro-consciousness." In addition to their spatial differences, that is, the regions associated with different conscious contents like color or visual motion, micro-consciousness must also be characterized in temporal terms. For instance, color is temporally perceived prior to visual motion, while locations are perceived earlier than color, which in turn precedes the perception of orientation. Different forms of micro-consciousness and their respective contents are thus not only distributed across space, that is, regions, but also across time. There is thus a certain temporal sequence in the occurrence of the different contents and their respective micro-consciousness.

Such intraregional temporal characterizations must be distinguished from interregional temporal synchronization, that is, binding, which must be assumed to occur later following the activation of a particular region at one particular point in time. Since it binds together different features or attributes of a stimulus into a whole, interregional binding and synchronization may be characterized by what Zeki (2003, 2008) calls "macro-consciousness" (and "unified consciousness"; see later), which must be assumed to temporally follow micro-consciousness.

NEUROEMPIRICAL REMARK IB: ZEKI'S THEORY OF "MICRO-CONSCIOUSNESS" AND KANT'S CONCEPT OF "TRANSCENDENTAL CONSCIOUSNESS"

Zeki proposes a clear temporal hierarchy with micro-consciousness occurring early and first, followed by macro-consciousness, and ultimately the overall and final "unified consciousness" (see below) as he calls it. What does Zeki mean by the concept of "unified consciousness"? "Unified consciousness" describes the final and ultimate stage that allows us to perceive ourselves as the perceiving person; it is *my* self (and no other person's self) that perceives the visual motion and the color, including their linkage in my perception. It is at this point where Zeki sees the similarity (or correspondence) to Kant, who, according to him, established the connection of micro- and macro-consciousness to the unified consciousness.

What Zeki describes as micro- and macro-consciousness corresponds to what Kant called "empirical consciousness," while Zeki considers his concept of "unified consciousness" as analogous to Kant's concept of "transcendental consciousness." Zeki (2008, 16) cites from Kant the following passage (without giving the exact location in *Critique of Pure Reason*):

> All representations have a necessary reference to possible empirical consciousness. For if they did not have this reference, and becoming conscious of them were entirely impossible, then this would be tantamount to saying that they do not exist at all. But all empirical consciousness has a necessary reference to a transcendental consciousness (a consciousness that precedes all particular experience), *viz.*, the consciousness of myself as original apperception.

What does Zeki think about what Kant described as "transcendental consciousness" and its relationship to empirical consciousness? Kant argues that any empirical consciousness can only occur on the basis of a prior transcendental consciousness, implying that the former is necessary related to the later. In contrast, Zeki disagrees with Kant in that any empirical consciousness, that is, micro- and macro-consciousness, must have a necessary relation to transcendental consciousness. This is so because there are cases where micro- and macro-consciousness can easily occur even without the consciousness of myself as the perceiving person that is, unified consciousness. In other words, empirical consciousness, i.e., micro- and macro-consciousness, can occur without and thus disassociated from unified consciousness. Therefore, these instances shed some empirical doubt on Kant's assumption of the necessary relation of micro- and macro-consciousness to transcendental consciousness.

In addition, Zeki also doubts Kant's assumption that any transcendental consciousness is prior to any experience, meaning that it precedes the occurrence of micro- and macro-consciousness. He, concedes however, that there must be special cortical programs in, for instance, the visual cortex that must indeed be present before any experience and thus visual consciousness can be acquired so that "all experience must therefore be read into them" (Zeki 2008, 16). The exact nature of the *a priori* cortical programs remains unclear, however. What is clear though, following Zeki, is that these *a priori* cortical programs must concern micro-consciousness and thus empirical consciousness, rather than unified consciousness, that is, transcendental consciousness:

> The cortical programs to construct visual attributes must also be present before any experience is acquired and all experience must therefore be read into them. It seems more likely that, ontogenetically, the micro-consciousness precedes the unified consciousness and that the programs for them are also present at birth. Hence, even though in adult life the unified consciousness is at the apex of the hierarchy of consciousness, ontogenetically, it is the micro-consciousness that occupies this position. (Zeki 2008, 16)

NEUROPHILOSOPHICAL REMARK IA: NONLINEAR INTERACTION AND CONSCIOUSNESS

There are two points where Zeki (2008) himself admits that he does not know the exact neuronal mechanisms. First, he admits that the neuronal mechanisms underlying the different levels of neural activity that are predictive and decide upon the presence or absence of consciousness remain unclear. Second, he does not give any indication of the exact neuronal nature of the *a priori* cortical programs that are necessary *a priori* for subsequent micro-consciousness to occur.

Let us start with the first point, the neuronal mechanisms that allow for the distinction between high and low levels of cortical activity and subsequently between conscious and unconscious perception. Zeki observes that even in the absence of a particular stimulus, for example, house or face, the respective region, that is, face or house region, still shows some degree of neuronal activity. Since the stimulus remains absent here, this neuronal activity must be characterized as what I have described as resting-state activity.

Most important, the level of activity in these regions during the resting state is apparently not sufficiently high enough to induce consciousness of, for instance, houses or faces during the resting state itself. For that, as I propose, a stimulus must interact with that region's resting-state activity, entailing (usually except in extreme cases of rest–rest interaction as in dreams; see Chapter 26) rest–stimulus interaction to change activity to a sufficient degree (see Chapter 29). But, as Zeki observes, only certain stimuli, that is, similar face or house stimuli, increase the respective regions' resting-state activity to such levels such that conscious perception of the stimulus becomes possible. In contrast, other stimuli, for example, different face or house stimuli, do increase the respective regions' resting-state activity, but not to a sufficiently high level as to induce conscious perception.

Why do only certain stimuli, the identical ones, induce consciousness? Neuronally, both cases, the conscious and the unconscious one, show rest–stimulus interaction. This suggests that, in both instances, the level of neural activity increases. However, the same neuronal mechanism, rest–stimulus interaction, leads to different levels of neural activity, which then seem to account for the difference between presence and absence of consciousness. There must therefore be some additional neuronal mechanisms at work during rest–stimulus interaction that accounts for the phenomenal difference.

I propose this additional neuronal mechanism to consist of the occurrence of non-linearity during rest-stimulus interaction which makes it possible to associate a phenomenal state, that is, consciousness, with the otherwise purely neuronal stimulus-induced activity (see Chapter 29). How does that stand to the earlier-described results by Zeki obtained during the presentation of similar or different house/face stimuli? I hypothesize that in Zeki's case of similar faces or houses, nonlinear interaction and consequently higher levels of neuronal activity are more likely to occur than in the case of different faces or houses. In the case of different stimuli, in contrast, rest–stimulus interaction may remain only linear, which makes the induction of sufficiently high changes in the levels of neuronal activity to associate consciousness with the stimuli impossible.

Taken all together, this amounts to the following neurophenomenal hypotheses. I hypothesize that the degree of nonlinear interaction during rest–stimulus interaction (see Volume I, Chapters 11 and 12) is directly related to the degree of neuronal activity in the respective regions and consequently to the degree of consciousness: The higher the degree of non-linearity during rest–stimulus interaction, the higher the degree of stimulus-induced activity, and the higher the likelihood that the resulting stimulus-induced activity will be associated with consciousness. This remains to be explicitly demonstrated in the future, however (see also Chapters 28 and 29).

We are now able to provide an answer to Zeki's first question, the one about the neuronal mechanisms that predict the high levels of neural activity and their association with consciousness. Based on the considerations discussed in this section, my answer to Zeki's first point is that the degree of nonlinearity during rest–stimulus interaction accounts for sufficiently high neural activity levels to subsequently associate consciousness with the stimulus and its purely neuronal stimulus-induced activity.

NEUROPHILOSOPHICAL REMARK IB: "CORTICAL PROGRAMS" AND DIFFERENCE-BASED CODING

The argument in the preceding section leads me to the second point. There must be some information encoded in the resting state that programs it to enable nonlinear rather than merely linear rest–stimulus interaction. I argue that this information is encoded in the resting state in the *gestalt* of the kind of neural code the brain's resting state applies to the processing of all changes in its activity levels (during either the resting state itself or during stimulus-induced activity).

Moreover, I propose this kind of neural coding to be difference-based coding, as detailed in Volume I, which I also suggest to predispose the occurrence of consciousness as discussed here in Volume II. I postulate that difference-based coding is central in allowing for nonlinear interaction, such as that between identical stimuli, as in Zeki's experiment with same or different houses and faces (see Chapter 29). Such nonlinear interaction in turn may allow the association of a phenomenal state, that is, consciousness, with the purely neuronal stimulus-induced activity as, for instance, related to the identical stimuli in Zeki's experiment.

Zeki's results of the neuronal and phenomenal difference between same and different face/house stimuli are nicely compatible with the assumption of difference-based coding and its nonlinear character in the presence of the "right," for example, identical stimuli. In both cases, same and different face/house stimuli, the stimulus material remains the same. Despite the presentation of the same stimulus material, there are differences in both regards—neuronally, i.e., in the degree or level of neural activity, and phenomenally, i.e., in the presence or absence of consciousness.

How can we account for these neuronal and phenomenal differences in the presence of the same stimulus material? If the stimuli were encoded by themselves, i.e., in isolation and thus independently of their respective combinations or constellations, there should be neither a neuronal nor a phenomenal difference. In other words, if stimulus-based coding were at work, there should be neither a neuronal nor a phenomenal difference between same and different face/house stimuli. This suggests that the constellation or combination between the stimuli as either the same or different is central for determining the neuronal and phenomenal differences. In other words, this suggests that difference-based coding is at work that allows the brain to encode the spatial and temporal differences between stimuli rather than the stimuli themselves into neural activity. Accordingly, Zeki's results speak in favor of difference-based coding rather than stimulus-based coding.

How does such difference-based coding relate to what Zeki described as the "cortical programs"? I propose that what Zeki calls "cortical programs" describe the programming of the brain's resting-state activity to apply a specific kind of encoding to its own activity changes; namely, difference-based coding rather than stimulus-based coding. In the same way the computer is programmed to apply the 0-1 code to its own processing of any incoming information, the brain and its resting-state activity apply difference- rather than stimulus-based coding to its own processing of any activity changes as induced either by the resting state itself or extrinsic stimuli. In short, I propose what Zeki calls a "cortical program" to consist of a particular neural code, difference-based coding.

NEUROPHILOSOPHICAL REMARK IIA: "CORTICAL PROGRAMS" AND "CONTENT- BASED CONCEPTS OF CONSCIOUSNESS"

How does all that relate to Kant? As discussed earlier, Zeki contests Kant's assumption of transcendental consciousness's being *a priori* and necessarily related to empirical consciousness. Why? Because, following him, micro- and macro-consciousness occur temporally prior to unified consciousness. He proposes this

because the perception and thus consciousness of attributes and features, e.g., micro- and macro-consciousness precede the consciousness of the self who perceives these attributes and features, e.g., unified consciousness.

However, Zeki does not contest Kant's assumption that there must be something occurring prior and thus *a priori* to micro- and macro-consciousness when he proposes specific cortical programs that make consciousness possible. Accordingly, Zeki does not deny the necessity that there must be something prior to empirical consciousness, e.g., micro- and macro-consciousness, in order for it to be possible. In contrast to Kant, Zeki does not associate this "something prior" with the concept of transcendental consciousness, but rather with what he describes as "cortical programs." This implies that the *a priori* cortical programs cannot be associated with the perception and consciousness of the perceiving self, the unified or transcendental consciousness. How can we clarify this conceptual puzzle? I argue that we need to distinguish different concepts of consciousness, which shall be detailed in the following.

Zeki presupposes a concept of consciousness that is based on contents. His concepts of micro- and macro-consciousness and unified consciousness are all based on different contents, features/attributes in micro-consciousness, objects and events in macro-consciousness, perceiving self in unified consciousness. This follows Kant's characterization of empirical consciousness and its determination by contents that are by their very nature empirical. I therefore speak of a "content-based concept of consciousness" (see Fig. A3-1).

NEUROPHILOSOPHICAL REMARK IIB: KANT'S TRANSCENDENTAL CONSCIOUSNESS AS A "MODE-BASED CONCEPT OF CONSCIOUSNESS"

How does Kant's concept of transcendental consciousness fit in? This is where the trouble starts. Kant seems to characterize consciousness as content based when he associates it with the "consciousness of myself as original apperception" (see above quote from Zeki). This corresponds well to Zeki's characterization of

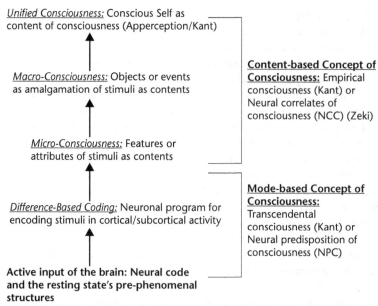

Figure A3-1 Content- versus mode-based concept of consciousness. The figure points out different concepts of consciousness, content-based and mode-based. Thereby both forms of consciousness are not mutually exclusive but rather build upon each other. I borrow the terms *micro-consciousness, macro-consciousness,* and *unified consciousness* from Zeki and associate them with my assumption of difference-based coding and the resting state's prephenomenal structures, which I consider both to be neural predispositions rather than neural correlates of consciousness. My view is quite compatible with Kant's view on the mode-based determination of transcendental consciousness, as well as with Zeki, who rather focuses on content-based consciousness. The concept of "content-based consciousness" describes the definition of consciousness by contents, such as by micro-contents or macro-contents, as Zeki seems to suppose; whereas the concept of *mode-based consciousness* pertains more to the form of consciousness that describes how the contents of consciousness are organized and structured. What Kant describes as *transcendental unity* provides such organization, which, I propose, is also predisposed by the resting state's spatiotemporal structures that are therefore prephenomenal rather than non-phenomenal.

unified consciousness as the consciousness of the perceiving self.

However, such a content-based determination of transcendental consciousness is incompatible with necessity of its occurring prior to empirical consciousness; that is, micro- and macro-consciousness. If transcendental consciousness is defined by the self that links, integrates, and thus unifies all preceding contents, including the ones associated with micro- and macro-consciousness, transcendental consciousness must *follow* rather than precede empirical consciousness. In short, a content-based determination of transcendental consciousness makes its characterization as

a priori impossible. If, however, transcendental consciousness is no longer characterized as *a priori*, empirical consciousness can no longer show necessary reference to it.

This is well observed by Zeki (2008, 16), who, as described earlier, denies Kant's assumption of necessity; that is, necessary reference. I propose the problem here to stem from an ambiguity in Kant himself in his determination of consciousness. When claiming for transcendental consciousness to be *a priori* and being the necessary reference for empirical consciousness, Kant does not presuppose a content-based determination anymore but rather a "mode-based concept of consciousness."

What do I mean by "mode-based concept of consciousness"?

The concept of mode refers here to the principally conscious mode as distinguished from the principally non-conscious mode thus referring to what, relying on Searle, I described in the introduction as "principal consciousness" as distinguished from "principal non-consciousness." Such mode-based concept of consciousness, that is, "principal consciousness," can well be characterized *a priori*, thereby signifying a specific "cortical program," as Zeki says, and a particular way of neural coding, difference-based coding as suggested earlier.

How can we characterize the concept of cortical programs in further detail on the basis of a mode-based concept of consciousness? I would propose that a particular coding strategy, that is, difference-based coding, to account for what Zeki calls "cortical programs" and what Kant describes as transcendental consciousness. Therefore, I consider that difference-based coding takes on the role of what may be called a transcendental (or better, neuro-transcendental) condition or, in my own terms, a *neural predisposition*, that is, necessary, non-sufficient condition, of possible consciousness, that is, mode-based consciousness (or Kant's transcendental consciousness, as determined in a mode-based way). This has important implications for the determination of Kant's concept of transcendental consciousness. Instead of implying a neural correlate and thus actual consciousness, that is content-based consciousness or, as Kant would say, empirical consciousness, transcendental consciousness must be characterized as mode-based (rather than content-based) and requires the search for neural predisposition (rather than neural correlate).

Neurophilosophical Remark
IIC: Mode-Based Concept
of Consciousness Requires
a Neurotranscendental Approach

I postulate that that difference-based coding is a transcendental (or neuro-transcendental) condition (or neural predisposition) of consciousness in a mode-based (rather than content-based) way. This however is not compatible with Kant's concept of transcendental consciousness when he presupposes it in a content-based way (as in the context of the "consciousness of myself as original apperception"). That means to confuse the mode of consciousness with its contents since being conscious of myself pertains to a content (one's own self) rather than a mode.

Such a content-based determination of transcendental consciousness in Kant, however, is to be distinguished from his assumption of a necessary and *a priori* role of transcendental consciousness for possible empirical consciousness. This pertains to what I said above: that there must be "something additional" besides empirical consciousness itself for it to be possible. This "something additional" is apparently what Kant refers to when he signifies transcendental consciousness as *a priori* and necessary for the possibility of empirical consciousness.

How can we characterize Kant's concept of transcendental consciousness and thus the "something additional" in further conceptual and empirical detail? I argue that what I described as mode-based consciousness signifies Kant's concept of transcendental consciousness, including its *a priori* and necessary character. Conceptually, the a priori and necessary character of Kant's concept of transcendental consciousness resurfaces in what I described in the second Introduction as "principal consciousness,".

What exactly does the concept of "principal consciousness" refer to? The concept of "principal consciousness refers to the principal possibility of the occurrence of a phenomenal state, that is, consciousness, independently of whether it is actually realized or not. Empirically, as stated earlier, the concept of transcendental consciousness and its conceptual analogue in my framework, "principal consciousness," are supposed to be related to a particular kind of neural coding, difference-based coding, that the brain and its resting-state activity apply to all changes in the brain's own activity.

Finally, another point of convergence with Kant shall be mentioned. Kant considered the mind as an active organ that provides an input that structures and organizes the stimuli from the environment such as that we can cognize them. This active input refers to the transcendental level and that is where he "located" the mode of consciousness and thus transcendental consciousness.

The same is true in the case of the brain. I characterize the brain as an active organ that provides an input, that is, its spatiotemporal structure of the resting state and its specific neural coding, that is, difference-based coding, that predispose the brain to process the stimuli from the environment in a certain way. This is what I here described as neural predisposition, which, taken from a Kantian perspective, may well be described as neurotranscendental (see also Northoff 2011, chapters 1 and 2 herein; Northoff 2012, 2013).

Kant's mode-based concept of consciousness, that is, transcendental consciousness, may consequently well be associated with the active input to the brain to its neural processing of stimuli from body and environment. This implies a neurotranscendental approach, which is here conceptualized as the search for the neural predispositions of consciousness. More specifically, this brain's active input may consists in its resting state's spatiotemporal structure and its specific way of neural coding, difference-based coding, which predisposes the brain to associate a phenomenal state, that is, consciousness, with its purely neuronal activity changes during either rest–rest or rest–stimulus interaction.

Philosophical Remark Ia: Concepts of Transcendental and Empirical Unity

So far, I have used the concept of the transcendental without going into further detail. I therefore will discuss the concept of the transcendental now in the subsequent sections.

The notion of the transcendental was introduced by Immanuel Kant. Roughly, Kant introduced the term "transcendental" to characterize all knowledge that focuses more on the *form* of our cognition and knowledge of ourselves and the world than on the *content* of our knowledge.[1] Since the form of our knowledge must also be "cognized" and known by us, Kant speaks here of a certain form of cognition or knowledge, *a priori* cognition, which remains independent of the specific contents: "I call all cognition transcendental that is occupied not so much with

objects but rather with our mode of cognition of objects insofar as this is to be possible *a priori*" (Kant 1998, A11–A12).

The concept of the "transcendental" must be distinguished from that of the "transcendent" that "goes beyond" or transcends any possible knowledge of humans into a world that lies beyond the world we inhabit. Let me rephrase this important distinction. The concept of "transcendental" concerns the possible knowledge of the objects within the world that we can possibly cognize. In contrast, the notion of "transcendent" goes beyond the objects we can possibly cognize by postulating some objects in a world that lies beyond our possible cognition and knowledge, for example, a transcendent world.

In sum, the notion of the "transcendental" concerns the mode in which we cognize objects in the world, whereas "transcendent" refers to objects in a non-natural world we cannot cognize at all (see also footnote 6 on p. 717 in the Introduction by P. Guyer and A. Wood in Kant 1998). In other words, the concept of "transcendence" has ontological-metaphysical implications, thus belonging to the ontological-metaphysical domain, while the concept of the transcendental remains (supposedly) purely epistemic.[2]

Philosophical Remark Ib: Transcendental Unity as Form or Structure

What exactly is meant by the "form" (or mode) of our knowledge? Kant refers here to a specific structure and organization that is inherent in our knowledge. One such central form that structures and organizes our knowledge is unity. Unity provides the most basic form or structure and organization of our cognition and knowledge of ourselves and the world.

In other words, unity is the basic form or structure and organization of consciousness:

> Every necessity (i.e., the necessity of connection) has a transcendental condition as its ground. A transcendental ground must therefore be found for the unity of consciousness in the synthesis of the manifold of all our intuitions, hence also the concepts of objects in general, consequently also of all objects of experience without which it would be impossible to think

of any objects for our intuitions; for the latter is nothing more than the something for which the concept expresses such a necessity of synthesis. Now this original and transcendental condition is nothing other than the transcendental apperception. (Kant 1998, A106–A107; see below for the determination of the terms "apperception"[3] and "synthesis")

The unity of consciousness reflects the most basic form or structure and organization, which as such must be distinguished from a more empirical unity, the unity we encounter in the contents of our perception, or *outer sense* as Kant would have said, and the contents in introspection, or *inner sense* in Kant's terms. Kant considered the more empirical unity of inner and outer sense, that is, perception and introspection, to be dependent upon the unity as basic form or structure and organization, i.e., a transcendental unity, as one might say. Without the unity as basic form or structure and organization, i.e., the transcendental unity, no unity, i.e., empirical unity, in either perception or introspection would be possible at all.[4]

Taking all this into consideration, the unity as basic form or structure and organization must be characterized as transcendental and thereby be distinguished from the unity in perception and introspection that is then empirical rather than transcendental. One may consequently distinguish between transcendental unity and empirical unity with the former providing the ground or necessary condition for the possibility of the latter.[5]

Philosophical Remark IC: Synthesis of Transcendental Unity

How is the transcendental unity of consciousness generated? Kant considers the transcendental unity to be the very basis of the empirical unity and, even more radical, of any other form or structure and organization in consciousness. He therefore proposes that the transcendental unity is *a priori* given.[6] Where, however, does the transcendental unity come from? Kant suggests some kind of process that generates the transcendental unity, and this process is described by the term "synthesis":

Only the spontaneity of our thought requires that this manifold first be gone through, taken up, and combined in a certain way in order for a cognition to be made out of it. I call this action synthesis. By synthesis in the most general sense, however, I understand the action of putting different representations together with each other and comprehending their manifold in one cognition. (Kant 1998, A77/B102–B103)

The concept of *synthesis* refers to a "putting together," "combination," "composition," and "nexus" (see footnote a in Kant 1998, A77/B103) of what Kant called the "manifold" resulting in unity: "But in addition to the concept of the manifold and of is synthesis, the concept of combination also carries with it the concept of the unity of the manifold. Combination is the representation of the synthetic unity of the manifold" (Kant 1998, B130–B131). This[7] entails that the transcendental unity is also a synthetic unity that (unlike an "analytical unity") underlies certain processes yielding its generation.[8] That is well reflected in the following quote where Kant speaks of a "synthetic unity of apperception":

This synthetic unity (of apperception), however, presupposes a synthesis, or includes it, and if the former is to be necessary *a priori* then the latter must also be a synthesis *a priori*. Thus the transcendental unity of apperception is related to the pure synthesis of the imagination.... Now we call the synthesis of the manifold in imagination transcendental if, without distinction of the intuitions, it concerns nothing but the connection of the manifold *a priori*, and the unity of this synthesis is called transcendental if it is represented as necessary *a priori* in relation to the original unity of apperception. (Kant 1998, A118; see also B135, where Kant speaks of the transcendental synthesis as the "faculty of combining *a priori*")

Neurophilosophical Remark IIIA: Environment–Brain Unity as Neurotranscendental Unity

How does Kant's concept of transcendental unity relate to the here-suggested "environment–brain unity"? Analogous to Kant's transcendental unity, the environment–brain unity is the most basic form or structure and organization upon which any kind of subsequent neuronal processing and ultimately consciousness depends and is built (see Chapters 20 and 21). The environment–brain unity is supposed to be based upon a statistically based spatiotemporal continuity between the environmental stimuli and the brain's resting-state activity. Such a statistically based spatiotemporal continuity leads, in an ideal case, to the constitution of a virtual spatiotemporal unity between environment and brain (see Chapter 21). This virtual spatiotemporal unity between environment and brain, the environment–brain unity, is supposed to bias and predispose the subsequent constitution of the phenomenal unity and thus consciousness during rest–stimulus interaction (see Chapters 18 and 29).

How is such biasing and predisposition of consciousness by the environment–brain unity possible? For instance, a rhythmic presentation of environmental stimuli may lead to a higher degree of a statistically and spatiotemporally based environment–brain unity than a non-rhythmic presentation of the same stimuli (see Chapter 20 for details). And the higher the degree of the environment–brain unity, the more likely it is that a phenomenal state, that is, consciousness, can be associated with the resulting change in the resting state's neural activity. This suggests that the environment–brain unity does indeed provide the basic form or structure and organization, that is, a particular temporal and spatial template, for the subsequent phenomenal unity as a hallmark of consciousness.

The dependence of the phenomenal unity on the preceding environment–brain unity is also reflected in the relationship between the different underlying neuronal mechanisms. More specifically, the phase of the resting state's low-frequency oscillation is adjusted in a specific way to the statistical structure of the environmental stimuli; as such, it biases and predisposes the phases and amplitudes of the more stimulus-related high-frequency oscillations, including their degree of entrainment by the low-frequency oscillations of the resting state.

How, then, is the relationship between low- and high-frequency oscillations related to the association of consciousness to the stimulus-induced activity? The degree of the

high- by low-frequency oscillation entrainment biases and predisposes how the actual stimulus, and its specific temporal (and spatial) discrete point in time (and space), will be processed during subsequent rest–stimulus interaction: The better the stimulus' discrete position in time and space corresponds to and matches with the phase durations of the ongoing high-by-low-frequency entrainment in the resting state, the higher the likelihood that consciousness will be associated with the stimulus and its respective stimulus-induced activity.

Taken together, this demonstrates that the phenomenal unity of consciousness can indeed be ultimately traced back to the virtual and statistically and spatiotemporally based environment–brain unity.. This means the environment–brain unity must be considered a necessary condition of possible consciousness. Moreover, the environment–brain unity must occur prior to the actual stimulus that is to be associated with consciousness. The environment–brain unity can consequently indeed be characterized as a transcendental unity in very much the same way Kant used this concept when presupposing it in a mode- rather than content-based way. Since it is based, at least in part, on the brain and its neuronal states, i.e., its intrinsic activity, one may want to characterize the environment–brain unity as *neurotranscendental* unity rather than merely as transcendental unity.

NEUROPHILOSOPHICAL REMARK IIIB: EMPIRICAL EVIDENCE FOR THE NEUROTRANSCENDENTAL ROLE OF THE ENVIRONMENT–BRAIN UNITY

Let me describe this striking analogy to Kant in slightly different terms. Both unities, Kant's transcendental unity and my environment–brain unity, are supposed to provide the base for any subsequent unity, be it the empirical unity of consciousness in Kant, or what I (and others) describe as phenomenal unity of consciousness (which for Kant would be subsumed under what he describes as empirical unity). I consequently propose that what Kant called transcendental unity (in a mode- rather than content-based way) may correspond more or less to the concept of environment–brain unity as posited here (see later for more detailed discussion of the suspicion of what philosophers call "category error"; as well as Northoff 2011, 2012, 2013; see also Fig. A3-2).

One may go even one step further. Kant associates the empirical unity with inner and outer sense, that is, perception and introspection. This is strikingly similar to what I here describe as phenomenal unity that can occur in either perception of the outer environment, that is, outer sense, or the perception of one's own self, that is, introspection or inner sense. Hence, I propose that what I here describe as phenomenal unity may more or less correspond to what Kant called empirical unity.

Most important, Kant claimed the empirical unity to be prevalent during perception and introspection, that is, inner and outer sense, and to depend on the preceding transcendental unity. I demonstrated here empirical support for the perception and thus outer sense to depend on the preceding environment–brain unity. This was, for instance, shown in the case of schizophrenia, where an abnormally altered environment–brain unity leads to bizarre perception of the environment and one's own self, thus including both inner and outer sense (see Chapters 22 and 27).

However, I did not show any data supporting that the perception of one's own self in introspection, that is, inner sense, is also dependent upon the prior environment–brain unity. I only showed that the environment–brain unity has an indirect impact via the resting state's self-specific organization upon the degree of self-specificity assigned to subsequent stimuli (see Chapters 23 and 24). In contrast, empirical support for the environment–brain unity's impact on the self (and self-consciousness) was only gathered indirectly, via the alteration of the self in schizophrenia (see Chapter 27). Hence, future research is warranted to demonstrate the dependence of our sense of self, i.e., self-consciousness, on the degree of the spatiotemporally and statistically based environment–brain unity.

In contrast to the here-presupposed characterization of the environment–brain unity as transcendental, Kitcher (1992) proposes higher-order cognitive functions like working memory and attention to be crucially involved in the generation of the transcendental unity. This, however, is challenged here by showing that what Kant called "transcendental unity" is very much synthesized by and based on a specific method of neural coding of stimuli at the interface between brain and environment. Hence, rather than going up to the highest logical functions as Kant did, or the highest cognitive functions as Kitcher does, I claim that we need to go down to the lowest

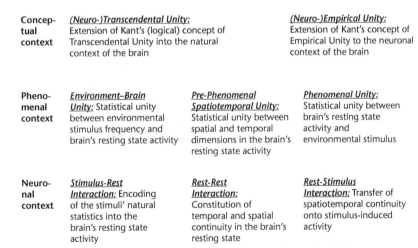

Conceptual context	*(Neuro-)Transcendental Unity:* Extension of Kant's (logical) concept of Transcendental Unity into the natural context of the brain		*(Neuro-)Empirical Unity:* Extension of Kant's concept of Empirical Unity to the neuronal context of the brain
Phenomenal context	*Environment–Brain Unity:* Statistical unity between environmental stimulus frequency and brain's resting state activity	*Pre-Phenomenal Spatiotemporal Unity:* Statistical unity between spatial and temporal dimensions in the brain's resting state activity	*Phenomenal Unity:* Statistical unity between brain's resting state activity and environmental stimulus
Neuronal context	*Stimulus-Rest Interaction:* Encoding of the stimuli' natural statistics into the brain's resting state activity	*Rest-Rest Interaction:* Constitution of temporal and spatial continuity in the brain's resting state	*Rest-Stimulus Interaction:* Transfer of spatiotemporal continuity onto stimulus-induced activity

Figure A3-2 Concept of unity in different contexts. The figure shows the different concepts of unity in the different contexts (neuronal, phenomenal, and conceptual) and how they correspond to each other. This provides a transition and complementarily between the concepts used here to describe neuronal and empirical mechanisms and Kant's concepts for describing the mind's input to cognition.

functions prior even to any sensorimotor and cognitive functions; namely, the kind of coding and subsequent neural activity the brain itself applies to its own neural processing of any stimuli from the environment. How can we express this difference in a more illustrative way? One may metaphorically say that I pull Kant from the lofty heights[9] of his head (being concerned only with logic as being devoid of any space and time) onto the very ground his feet stand on, where his environment–brain unity and its spatiotemporal template "locates" him as a biophysical subject in the midst of the physical world (see Chapter 21 for details about the concept of "biophysical subjectivity").

Neurophilosophical Remark
IIIC: Kant's Concept of "Synthesis" and the Constitution of the Nvironment–Brain Unity

So far, I have applied the conceptual framework of Kant to shed more light on the environment–brain unity using his concept of the transcendental unity to enrich and detail my own concept. However, the transfer may also go the reverse way, from my neuroscientifically based concepts to the more philosophical= ones of Kant. The neuroscientific data and findings may help to detail and further specify some of Kant's concepts like his concept of synthesis, as described earlier. Kant characterizes synthesis by "putting together," "combination," "composition," and "nexus" (see earlier). Though Kant distinguishes between distinct kinds of synthesis (mostly with regard to different material or content that is synthesized), the details of such "combination," "putting together," "composition," and "nexus" remain unclear (in either case of the different concepts of synthesis).

This is the point where I propose that the here suggested neuroscientifically based concepts and particularly their underlying neuronal mechanisms may contribute to fill the gap Kant left open in his concept of synthesis. Let me be more specific and detail the concept of synthesis by discussing each of its different features like "putting together," "combination," "composition," and "nexus" with regard to the environment–brain

unity (as transcendental unity). What exactly is "put together" in the synthesis of the environment–brain unity? Our empirical data provide a clear answer, as described in detail in Part VI). The environment and more specifically the occurrence of its stimuli across time (and space) are put together, integrated, and linked with the low-frequency oscillations in the brain. The phases of the resting state's low-frequency fluctuations are aligned to the onset of the stimuli from the environment as reflected in their statistical frequency distribution, i.e., their natural statistics.

This, in turn, makes possible the constitution of a statistically based virtual temporal (and spatial) continuity between the environment's stimuli and the brain's resting-state activity. Both brain and environment are thus directly linked together in a statistically based virtual temporal (and spatial) continuum, resulting in what I called "environment–brain unity." What Kant described as synthesis and "putting together" may thus be empirically specified by the resting state's neural alignment to the statistical frequency distribution of the environment stimuli, i.e., their natural statistics.

How are both stimuli and low-frequency oscillations "combined" in the synthesis of the environment–brain unity? They are combined by means of their statistical structures. More specifically, the statistical structure of the environmental stimuli's occurrence across time is "combined" with the phase of the low-frequency oscillations, that is, their cycling across time—hence, the statistical-based rather than physical-based nature of the environment–brain unity (see Chapter 20). Kant's concept of "combination" as hallmark feature of synthesis can consequently be empirically specified here by the matching processes between two different statistical frequency distributions, the one from the environmental stimuli and the one from the brain and its resting state's stimuli.

What kind of "composition" is going on in the synthesis of the environment–brain unity? The environment–brain unity is synthesized and thus composed by spatial and temporal differences between the different stimuli and their respective discrete points in time and space that are encoded into the brain's neural activity via difference-based coding. What is composed by the synthesis of the environment–brain unity is thus spatial and temporal differences, which is possible on the basis of difference-based coding. Hence, Kant's concept of "composition" can be specified by the difference-based (rather than stimulus-based) nature of the environment–brain unity.

Finally, based on its continuity-, statistical-, and difference-based nature, the environment–brain unity may well be described as "nexus" between environment and brain. A nexus is where two distinct set of properties or features overlap at a particular point in space and time while diverging in others. This is exactly what happens with regard to the resting state's low-frequency fluctuations, including their phases on one hand, and the rhythmic structure of the environmental stimuli on the other.

Let me be more specific. The phase onsets of the resting state's low-frequency fluctuations may align themselves to the onsets of the environmental stimuli and their rhythmic structures, thus accounting for the overlap between environment and brain. In contrast, it may be impossible for the resting state's low-frequency fluctuations to align their phase onsets to some other stimuli in the environment (simply because the former's phase onsets do not correspond to the latter and their rhythmic or non-rhythmic structure). Taken together, this means that the resting state's neuronal mechanisms of phase shift and neural alignment may empirically specify Kant's more metaphorical description of synthesis by the term "nexus."

Neurophilosophical Conclusion IA: Kant and the Brain—Nothing But a Category Error?

Leaving aside and neglecting most of the difficulties and controversies in interpreting Kant (this is left to the philosophers and especially the Kant specialists), I shall nevertheless briefly mention one central argument against my neurotranscendental interpretation (see Northoff 2011, 2012, 2013, for a more detailed neurotranscendental account of Kant). The traditional philosopher

and especially the Kant specialist may be very much puzzled by the fact that I propose correspondence between Kant's transcendental unity and the environment–brain unity.

Why may the traditional philosopher be puzzled? He may diagnose what is called a "category error" in philosophical circles. My assumption of a correspondence between Kant's transcendental unity and my concept of "environment–brain unity" is faulty in that it confuses logical and empirical categories: Kant used the term *transcendental unity* in a predominantly logical (and epistemic, I would claim) context, which is by definition devoid of any reference to empirical reality, including space and time.

Such a predominantly logical (and epistemic) domain excludes any empirical characterization. This means that the characterization by space and time, which are deemed to be empirical (or metaphysical-ontological), are also excluded: any concept that directly refers to time and space or at least indirectly presupposes them can only be characterized as empirical, not as transcendental. What does this imply for the characterization of my concept of the environment–brain unity? I characterized the concept of the "environment–brain unity" in strongly spatial and temporal terms; namely, by the spatial and temporal continuity between the environmental stimuli's statistical frequency distribution and that of the resting state's spatial and temporal neuronal measures. This even led me to describe the environment–brain unity as a spatiotemporal unity.

This, however, following the Kantian philosophers, designates the environment-brain unity as empirical rather than as transcendental. When characterizing the "environment–brain unity" as transcendental, or better, neurotranscendental, I thus confuse Kant's notion of the transcendental with the concept of the empirical: due to its reference to space and time, the concept of the "environment–brain unity" can at best be characterized as empirical but not as transcendental., I consequently commit what the philosophers call a "category error" that consists in the confusion between transcendental and empirical levels (and ultimately between logical and natural contexts).

NEUROPHILOSOPHICAL CONCLUSION IB: KANT AND THE BRAIN—IMMUNITY OF THE NEURAL PREDISPOSITIONS OF CONSCIOUSNESS AGAINST THE CATEGORY ERROR

Is the charge of a "category error" justified? Presupposing Kant's predominantly logical context, the charge of a category error is certainly justified. This, however, changes once one interprets Kant no longer in an exclusively logical context but rather in the natural context of embodiment and embeddedness (see, for instance, Svare 2006). The transcendental unity is then no longer supposed to be generated by "reason" and "understanding," as Kant himself proposed, but rather by the body and its integration within the environment. Most important, such a shift from a purely logical of reason to the more natural context of the body entails the reference to and inclusion of space and time. Space and time are then an integral part of the natural reality of the body, and, to put it even more strongly, they may *constitute* that natural reality by providing some kind of template or grid.

What does the shift from the logical to the natural context entail for the alleged "category error"? The terms "transcendental" and "empirical" do then need to be redefined in their relation to space and time. What in Kant's purely logical context would be deemed to be empirical, that is, the environment–brain unity, could then be designated as transcendental within a natural context, as I suggested earlier. This needs to be detailed.

My focus here is one our natural world rather than on the purely logical world as Kant presupposed it. This shift in context that is from the logical to the natural world entails a redesignation of the role of time and space as part of that very same natural world: If time and space necessarily precede consciousness in an *a priori* way, and do henceforth predispose possible consciousness (as distinguished from actual consciousness), space and time need to be characterized as transcendental. If, in contrast, time and space enable the manifestation of actual consciousness and thus correlates rather than predispositions, they must be characterized as merely empirical rather than transcendental.

I now claim that the spatiotemporal continuity that characterizes the environment–brain unity takes on exactly such transcendental, or better, neurotranscendental, role with regard to consciousness: The environment–brain unity precedes the occurrence of consciousness and is as such a necessary condition of its possibility, that is a predisposition (rather than a correlate). In other words, I propose the environment–brain unity that allows to constitute time and space to predispose possible consciousness and thus be a neural predisposition of consciousness (NPC). This clearly fulfills the criteria for a transcendental, or better, neurotranscendental, role of the environment–brain unity.

Does the environment-brain unity has a special and thus transcendental rather than merely empirical role? As NPC, the environment–brain unity must be distinguished from the neural conditions that are sufficient to induce actual consciousness, like nonlinear rest–stimulus interaction, which I consider the neural correlate of consciousness (NCC) (see Part VIII for details). In contrast to the NPC and their transcendental or neurotranscendental role, the NCC take on an empirical role. This means that the charge of a "category error" can well be directed toward the NCC, whereas it does not apply in the case of the NPC and particularly the environment–brain unity.

NEUROPHILOSOPHICAL CONCLUSION IC: KANT AND THE BRAIN—NATURAL VERSUS LOGICAL WORLDS

The traditional philosopher may now claim that all that sounds plausible. Yes, presupposing the framework of the natural context rather than the one of the logical context leads indeed to a re-definition of the transcendental and the empirical. And that in turn may indeed rule out the diagnosis of a category error in the case of the NPC and thus the environment–brain unity.

Kant, however, was not interested at all in the natural reality itself. Instead, he (and many other past and current philosophers) focus on the logical conditions, the transcendental conditions, that are necessarily presupposed by the natural, i.e., the empirical world. This, however, implies that the concept of the transcendental cannot be associated at all with the natural and thus the empirical world, but only with the logical domain. Since time and space are excluded by the logical domain, they cannot be associated at all with the concept of the transcendental and consequently with the environment–brain unity. That in turn means that the environment–brain unity can at best be characterized as empirical but not as transcendental. In other words, the diagnosis of a "category error" needs to be maintained as long as one follows Kant's original framework with its dichotomy between logical and natural domains.

How can we continue from here on? Now it all comes down to whether one accepts Kant's original framework with its dichotomy between natural and logical domains. Or whether, alternatively, one shifts Kant's logical (and epistemic) domain, including its transcendental conditions, into the natural world, thus presupposing what is described as "naturalization" in philosophy. This raises the question for what philosophers describe as 'naturalization'. I do not want to go into the philosophical debate here over whether one can "naturalize" Kant or not. I leave that to the philosophers and to the search for conceptually and logically plausible answers.

The only point I want to make here is a neurophilosophical one. From a neurophilosophical perspective, the question of the naturalization of Kant comes down to the question of empirical and more specifically neuronal plausibility. If such a naturalization of Kant and his concept of the transcendental is empirically plausible, i.e., in accordance with the empirical data of the brain, I can avoid the charge of a category error at least for claims that are limited to the natural world. My characterization of the environment–brain unity as transcendental or neurotranscendental is therefore at least valid in the natural world.

This however changes once one presupposes the logical world as the traditional philosophers do. My characterization of the environment–brain unity as transcendental is indeed a category error and may therefore not be valid in the purely logical world, which the philosophical traditionalists claim to hold in Kant. This has important implications.

Do I need to be concerned about the charge of a category error in the domain of the logical world? No, because as a neurophilosopher (and neuroscientist) I am primarily interested in the natural world, so that my work is done once I show that the naturalization of Kant's philosophy is empirically plausible. If so, I do not need to care much about the charge of a category error that applies only to the logical world because that world is simply not my primary concern as neurophilosopher. My aim is to explain how the brain and consciousness are related to each other in the natural world we live in, rather than in some merely logically possible world we do not actually live in.

Notes

1. Obviously, I will not be able to recount the details and the difficulties in interpreting Kant's stance here. I leave this to the philosophers to discuss.
2. This also makes it clear that the here-supposed concept of the "transcendental" does not refer to the possible cognition of objects outside the limits of our cognition and *a priori* cognition (see also McDowell 1994 for a more refined post-Kantian concept of the concept of the transcendental). Hence, there is nothing mysterious about the transcendental view of the mind's input to our cognition of objects and events of the world, while the search for transcendent objects is mysterious in its search for objects beyond and thus outside our (cognition of the) world.
3. It should, however, be noted that in his attempts at a deduction in between the A- and B-version (Prolegomena, Kant 1977); and after the B-version, Kant did not rely on apperception as a primary tool for the deduction. He does not even mention the term "apperception" in either the *Prolegomena to Any Future Metaphysics* or *Metaphysical Foundations of Natural Science*.
4. Within Kant's mainly logical and epistemic (and higher-order cognitive) framework (as I propose it to be), this requires the distinction of the transcendental unity of consciousness from the unity as one category within his list of categories, so that one may designate the former unity as extra categorical as distinguished from the categorical use of the term "unity" (see Caygill 1995, 407–409). This is also reflected in the following quote from Kant:

> This unity, which precedes all concepts of combination *a priori*, is not the former category of unity

(§10); for all categories are grounded on logical functions in judgements, but in these combination, thus the unity of given concepts, is already thought. The category therefore already presupposes combination. We must therefore seek this unity (as qualitative, §12) someplace higher, namely in that which itself contains the ground of the unity of different concepts in judgements, and hence of the possibility of the understanding, even in its logical use. (Kant 1998, B131).

5. Kant seems to describe the cognition of both transcendental and empirical unity by the term "apperception" (I deliberately say "seems" because the definition of the term "apperception" is highly controversial), where he correspondingly distinguishes between transcendental and empirical apperception. This is well reflected in the following quote that concerns the introspection, that is, the inner sense, of one's own self:

> Now this original and transcendental condition is nothing other than the transcendental apperception. The consciousness of oneself in accordance with the determinations of our state in internal perception is merely empirical forever variable; it can provide no standing or abiding self in this stream of inner appearances, and is customarily called inner sense or empirical apperception. (Kant 1998, A107; see also B132)

However, Allison (1983, 273–274) points out that the identification of empirical apperception and inner sense is problematic, because Kant thereby undermines the distinction between both kinds of apperception. Rather than treating both types of apperception as distinct activities or faculties, which is suggested by the identification of empirical apperception with inner sense, both shall rather be conceived as distinct ways in which apperception can be conceived. Allison suggests that empirical apperception may be regarded as the consciousness of its activity during cognition of objects (o), while transcendental apperception may be described as a thought about the same activity. This, however, is problematic, because then transcendental apperception must be characterized as an *analytical* unity, which, according to Kant, it is not; it is rather a *synthetic* unity (see later). Allison's characterization of transcendental apperception of the thought of synthesizing and cognizing activity, as distinguished from the consciousness during actual synthesis and cognition, opens the door for a purely logical account of transcendental apperception (see later). In this case, however, transcendental apperception could no longer be characterized as an epistemic function, as I propose was Kant's intention, but rather by a purely logical role.

6. I am aware that the notion of the "given" is by itself problematic and could include different meanings; this though is left for the philosophers to discuss.

7. I am well aware that this carries plenty of room for interpretation, which I leave to the Kant specialists.

8. Kant seems to speak here also of a "pure synthesis" that is pure because it neither concerns specific contents nor space and time, thus being beyond or "outside of space and time"; see later for further discussion of this point.

9. This is almost literally reflected in the following quote when Kant characterizes the transcendental unity as the highest point: "And thus the synthetic unity of apperception is the highest point to which one must affix all use of the understanding, even the whole of logic and, after it, transcendental philosophy; indeed this faculty is the understanding itself" (Kant 1998, B134*).

APPENDIX 4: BRAIN AND SELF

What is the self? So far, I have considered empirical results while neglecting more or less the concept of self. In this appendix, I want to give a brief account of the here presupposed concept of self. I contrast "content- and region/network-based concepts of self" with a more "process- and code-based concept of the self." This leads me finally to argue that what is often called "self-relatedness" within the phenomenal context corresponds well to what can be described as "brain-relatedness" within the neuronal context.

NEUROTHEORETICAL REMARK IA: DEFINITION OF THE SELF BY SENSORIMOTOR AND BODILY CONTENTS

The current neuroscientific and philosophical discussion about the concept of self is rather complex and cannot be recounted in full detail. I therefore focus only on some crucial concepts of the self that are relevant in the present context while leaving conceptual subtleties for subsequent philosophical discussion.

The question of the self has been one of the most salient problems throughout the history of philosophy and more recently also in psychology and neuroscience (H. L. Gallagher & Frith, 2003; I. I. Gallagher, 2000; Metzinger & Gallese, 2003; Northoff, 2004). For example, William James distinguished between a physical self, a mental self, and a spiritual self. These distinct selves are now related to distinct brain regions

(Churchland, 2002; Dalgleish, 2004; Damasio, 1999a and b, 2003a, 2003b; H. L. Gallagher & Frith, 2003; I. I. Gallagher, 2000; Keenan, Wheeler, Platek, Lardi, & Lassonde, 2003; Kelley et al., 2002; Kircher & David, 2003; Lambie & Marcel, 2002; LeDoux, 2002; Marcel & Lambie, 2004; Northoff & Bermpohl, 2004b; J. Panksepp, 1998a, 2003a and b; Stuss, Gallup, & Alexander, 2001; Turk et al., 2002; Turk, Heatherton, Macrae, Kelley, & Gazzaniga, 2003; Vogeley & Fink, 2003). Damasio (1999) and Panksepp (1998b, 2003) suggest a "protoself" that corresponds more or less to James's physical self. The protoself is supposed to outline one's body in affective and sensory-motor terms and is associated with subcortical regions like the periaqueductal gray, the colliculi, and the tectum (J. Panksepp, 2007a and b). Such bodily self-related sensorimotor contents strongly resemble William James's description of the physical self.

A variant of such sensorimotor-based self has recently been suggested by Legrand and Ruby (2009) (see Cristoff et al. 2011). Based on the phenomenological distinction between reflexive (e.g., cognitive) and prereflexive (e.g., precognitive self-awareness), they associate the latter with sensorimotor rather than cognitive contents. This emphasis on sensorimotor functions as the basis of the self goes well with their assumption of embodiment as being crucial for reflexive and thus cognitive functions (see Thompson 2007; Legrand 2007a and b). Following such a sensorimotor-based concept of self, they propose the neural structures underlying senso-rimotor functions, including sensorimotor feed-back loops, to be crucially involved in generating a sense of self (e.g., prereflexive self-awareness). However, this hypothesis remains to be tested experimentally.

NEUROTHEORETICAL REMARK IB: DEFINITION OF THE SELF BY MENTAL CONTENTS

Besides sensorimotor and bodily contents, mental contents are also regarded as specific for the self. What recently has been described as "minimal self"(H. L. Gallagher & Frith, 2003; I. I. Gallagher, 2000) or "core or mental self" with mental con-tents (Damasio, 1999a and b, 2010) might corre-spond more or less to James's concept of mental self. The core or mental self builds upon the proto-self in mental terms and is associated with regions like the thalamus and the ventromedial prefrontal cortex (see, for instance, Damasio, 1999a and b, 2003a). Instead of the sensorimotor and bodily contents that signify the protoself, the mental self is defined by mental content (e.g., the contents of our mental states) and their associated cognitive contents. For instance, one's own name may be considered such mental content that is specifically related to the self as mental self (see Chapters 23 and 24 for details).

Already this makes it clear that the mental self neither concerns parts of one's own body nor their underlying neural mechanisms. Instead, the men-tal self may concern stimuli from the outside of one's own body and person; the central feature is here thus not ownership as in the case of the body but rather the designation of certain stimuli either being self- or non-self-specific. Since the judge-ment of stimuli as either self- or non-self-specific is the guiding experimental paradigm in most current imaging studies, they seem to presuppose at least in part the concept of the mental self (see Chapters 23 and 24 as well as below for details).

NEUROTHEORETICAL REMARK IC: DEFINITION OF THE SELF BY AUTOBIOGRAPHICAL CONTENTS

Finally, a more extended concept of the self may be distinguished. This concept of self is no longer based on either sensorimotor or mental contents

as the "proto- and the mental self" but rather on autobiographical contents. Autobiographical contents concern those events and objects in the environment that were experienced as autobio-graphical in the history of that particular person.

The inclusion of autobiographical memories brings in the concept of time, more specifically the experience of time with its extension into past, present, and future. The concept of the autobiographical self strongly overlaps with the concept of personal identity that raises the ques-tion for temporal continuity. This is reflected in, for instance, Damasio's (1999a and b) con-cept of "autobiographical self" and Gallagher's (H. L. Gallagher & Frith, 2003; I. I. Gallagher, 2000) concept of "narrative self" that both strongly rely on linking past, present, and future events, thereby resembling James's concept of a spiritual self.

The "autobiographical or extended self" that allows one to reflect upon one's protoself and core or mental self is associated with cortical regions like the hippocampus and the cingulate cortex. Since the autobiographical dimension strongly impacts the ability to judge specific stimuli as either self- or non-self-specific, the current para-digms in brain imaging do also seem to presup-pose the "autobiographical self." The concept of self presupposed in imaging studies thus seems to amount to a mixture of mental and autobio-graphical self (see Chapters 23 and 24).

Taken together, the self is often defined on the basis of different contents. The protoself presupposes bodily contents, the ones of one's own body. The mental self is determined by spe-cific mental contents, one's own mental states as distinguished from the ones of other persons. Finally, the autobiographical self presupposes autobiographical contents and distinguishes them from heterobiographical contents. What does such content-based determination of the self imply in neuronal regard? Despite the recent multiplication of contents, the concept of self remains essentially determined by contents. These different contents provide the very basis for current neuroscience to "neuronalize" the self, and its aim to associate the different contents with different functions and regions/networks. The content-based approach to the self thus goes here hand in hand with what may be described as "region- or network-based approach."

NEUROTHEORETICAL REMARK
IIA: SELF-AWARENESS IN IMAGING STUDIES OF THE SELF

What remains unclear, however, is what unites the different content-based concepts of self, allowing us to speak of a self in all cases. One common denominator is that the stimuli are characterized often as self-referential, entailing self-referential processing that is considered common to the distinct concepts of self and its different contents. This has also been described as "self-related" or "self-relevant" processing. Let me go back briefly to the experimental paradigms used in the neuroscience of the self because they tell us a lot about the often rather implicit presupposition about the concept of the self.

Many of the subjects for these studies were presented with stimuli, that is, pictures, faces, words, or tones, and had to evaluate whether they were related to them. Faces, for instance, were presented from one's own person, relatives, family members, and other nonrelated famous and nonfamous persons. Subjects then had to decide upon the degree of the stimuli's closeness to one's own person and decide whether they have something to do with the subjects.

Another example is the way we perceive pictures of ourselves or close friends versus pictures of completely unknown people or pictures of our childhood houses versus pictures of unknown houses. Such comparisons are possible in different sensory modalities. Self-relatedness is here understood and presupposed in a rather cognitive sense. This implies self-awareness, meaning that one becomes aware of one's self once one sees the stimulus that is related to one's own self as distinguished from the stimuli that are not related to the self.

NEUROTHEORETICAL REMARK
IIB: SELF-REFERENTIAL PROCESSING AS COGNITIVE PROCESS

The experimental designs in current imaging studies focus most often on the judgement of specific contents, whether they are sensorimotor/bodily, mental, or autobiographical. Such judgement task implicates self-awareness or self-consciousness, the ability to become aware of that stimulus as high- or low self-specific. Imaging studies thus combine a content-based view of the self, e.g., bodily, mental, or autobiographical contents, with the recruitment of higher order cognitive functions required for self-awareness and reflection.

Legrand and Ruby (2009) criticized the latter, the requirement of a "general evaluation function" as they call it. They argue that the imaging results may be confounded by such general unspecific evaluation function and thus by the judgement task required in these imaging studies. At the same time they pertain to a content-based view of the self when characterizing it by sensorimotor rather than cognitive contents.

The strong focus on the judgement in the imaging studies entails that most of the aforementioned imaging studies implicitly presuppose a concept of self as self-consciousness or self-awareness. This is so because the various tasks applied in these studies require subjects to make explicit reference to some aspects of themselves and to consciously access and monitor representational content about one's self. Since subjects must reference to themselves relying on their self-consciousness or self-awareness in order to fulfil the task, one may speak of "self-*referential* processing" (see also Northoff 2007). Due to the fact that it requires self-consciousness or self-awareness, self-referential processing is supposed to involve higher order cognitive function, the "highest" and most advanced forms of cognitive processing, out of which the self emerges at the pinnacle of the psychological and neural hierarchy.

On the philosophical level, such a higher order view of self-referential processing may propose correspond to predominantly cognitive accounts of the self in, for instance, higher-order representational accounts suggested by current philosophers like Peter Carruthers and David Rosenthal, as well as some interpretations of Kant's concept of the self by mental unity and apperception (see for instance, Kitcher 1992,

2010; and Brooks 1994; see, though, Northoff 2011, 2012, and 2013, as well as Appendix 3 in this volume for a different reading of Kant).

NEUROTHEORETICAL
REMARK IIC: PROCESS-BASED
CONCEPT OF SELF-SPECIFICITY

What are the conceptual alternatives in the case of the definition of the self? We have to seek alternatives on both sides experimental and conceptual. Experimentally, we may need to replace the judgement by a less cognitive task, such as mere perception (without any judgement) of self-specific and non-self-specific stimuli. This strategy has been pursued by studies from our group (Qin et al. 2010; Schneider et al. 2008; Northoff et al. 2010, Qin and Northoff 2011). Subjects were instructed to either perceive emotional pictures (see Schneider et al. 2008; Northoff et al. 2009) or their own name (Qin et al. 2010) while not making any judgement.

This kind of experimental design no longer presupposes a judgement or general evaluation function. Interestingly, in these studies focusing on the perception rather than the judgement of self-specific stimuli, various cortical midline structures as well as subcortical midline regions were found to be active during the self-specific stimuli (see Chapters 23 and 24, as well as Northoff et al. 2009; Schneider et al. 2008; and Qin et al. 2010, 2011, for details). This indicates that the neural activity in these regions may not be related to the general evaluation function or judgement itself as suggested by Legrand and Ruby (2009). That was confirmed in a recent meta-analysis of ours where we again showed that the activity in the anterior midline regions is really to the degree of self-specificity of the stimuli rather than task-related effects (see Qin and Northoff 2011; see chapters 23 and 24 herein for details).

Another issue arising here is whether neural activity in the midline structures is necessary for phenomenal consciousness. Alternatively, neural activity in the cortical midline structure (CMS) may also remain independent of the consciousness of the self (e.g., self-consciousness). Qin et al. (2010) demonstrated neural activity in various cortical midline regions during perception of the subject's own name in vegetative patients who by definition are nonconscious (though this has been debated recently; see Chapters 28 and 29 for more details, as well as Huang et al. 2013, for confirmation and extension of such finding). These results indicate first that the self may be processed independent of consciousness, and second that the neural activity in the CMS may not be related to consciousness independently of whether such consciousness concerns one's own self or some other content.

Let us briefly rewind. Imaging results demonstrated that the neural activity in the CMS is not specific for self-specific stimuli (see also Chapters 23 and 24). Hence, distinction between self- and non-self-specific contents could not be mapped onto a corresponding anatomical distinction in the cortex. At the same time, however, neural activity in the CMS may not be associated with judgement/general evaluation function or consciousness either. This means that the neural activity in the CMS cannot be accounted for by a specific function, whether it is judgement/general evaluation or consciousness.

What though is the neural activity in the CMS specific for if neither for self-specific contents nor for a general evaluation function or consciousness? Rather than being specific for a specific content (bodily, mental, autobiographical) or a specific function (judgement/general evaluation, consciousness), neural activity in the CMS may be proposed to be specific for a specific process. Conceptually, this entails a shift from a content-based concept of self to a process-based view of the self. Neural activity in the CMS may then be determined by a specific process that is instantiated when being confronted with any kind of stimuli that by the nature of that very process are then determined as self-specific or not (see Fig. A4-1) (see also Chapters 22–24 for details).

NEUROTHEORETICAL REMARK IIIA: SELF-*RELATED* PROCESSING AS NON-COGNITIVE SIBLING OF THE MORE COGNITIVE SELF-*REFERENTIAL* PROCESSING

What could this specific process be? Let us briefly recall what exactly one needs to perceive

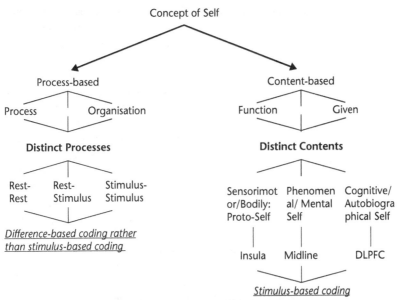

Figure A4-1 Content- versus process-based concept of the self. The figure shows idealized versions of different concepts of self as they are discussed and presupposed (often implicitly) in current neuroscience. (*Left*) This concerns the process-based self that is supposed to be based on various processes like rest–stimulus, stimulus–rest, and rest–rest interaction going on in the brain in its interaction with the environment. I propose that such interactions imply a specific way of neural coding of changes in neural activity. Rather than coding each stimulus by itself at its discrete point in time and space, the brain seems to code spatial and temporal differences between stimuli, resulting in difference-based coding as distinguished from stimulus-based coding. (*Right*) Here the alternative model of the self is shown that is more based on contents (taking them as a given) and associates them with different functions and regions in the brain. This presupposes ultimately stimulus-based coding rather than difference-based coding. DLPFC, dorsolateral prefrontal cortex.

or judge specific contents as either self- or non-self-specific. Before perceiving and judging them, these contents must be somehow related to the organism. If there is no relation at all of the contents to one's own organism, one is not able to subsequently perceive or judge them as such and hence as contents that are either self- or non-self-specific. This means that any stimuli, be they bodily, mental, or autobiographical, must first be related to the organism in order for the latter to be able to access the former as a specific content, be it self- or non-self-specific in subsequent perception or judgement. The constitution of any kind of content may thus be traced back to a specific relation between stimulus and organism, which by itself must be mediated by a specific process in order to yield content, whether it is bodily, mental, or autobiographical.

This process that establishes a relation between organism and stimulus may be called self-*related* processing. Self-*related* processing describes the relation between stimulus and organism that enables the constitution of any kind of content, be it bodily, mental, or autobiographical, including its associated continuum of different degrees of self-specificity. This distinguishes self-*related* processing from its cognitive counterpart, self-*referential* processing, which takes the contents, be they bodily, mental, or autobiographical, as given (and preexisting) and refers them to the self of the organism.

One may now want to argue that if self-related processing does not refer to specific contents, it refers to nothing, thus remaining empty. If, however, self-related processing does not refer to some specific content, we remain unable to investigate and reveal any corresponding neural contents. One may consequently criticize the concept of self-related processing as a mere conceptual figment that (refers to nothing and) does therefore not translate into any empirical and better neuronal relevance.

NEUROTHEORETICAL REMARK
IIIB: DIFFERENCE-BASED CODING MEDIATES SELF-*RELATED* PROCESSING

To counter this argument of the empirical and neuronal irrelevance of self-*related* processing, we need to address the issue of the possible neural realization of self-*related* processing. The neural mechanisms underlying the specific contents themselves, bodily, mental, or autobiographical, may not be viable candidates because they presuppose exactly that, e.g., the contents, which is supposed to be constituted by self-*related* processing.

How are the contents we perceive and judge as bodily, mental, or autobiographical constituted on the basis of our brain's neural processes? One may propose a specific form of neural coding by means of which the brain enables the various stimuli to be related to the organism and are thereby transformed into contents. Rather than presupposing the contents as a given and ready-made, that is, objects, events, and persons we perceive, we here focus on those neuronal mechanisms that are necessary and predispose the transformation of any stimuli into objects, events, persons; that is, contents.

The focus on those processes that transform stimuli into contents raises the question for the neural coding of the stimuli in the neural activity of the brain. Therefore, I focused in Volume I on the brain's neural code, which I supposed to be difference-based coding (rather than stimulus-based coding). This was complemented here in Volume II by showing how such neural code, difference-based coding, can account for the association of the contents and their respective stimulus-induced activity with phenomenal consciousness. Therefore, I hypothesized that difference-based coding is a necessary neuronal condition or predisposition for the possible constitution of contents out of stimuli in general;

this must be distinguished from the actual realization of specific contents and their underlying neural correlates (see Chapters 18 and 19). Most important, I propose such difference-based coding to go along with the characterization of the stimuli along a continuum of different degrees of self-specificity (see Chapters 23 and 24).

Self-related processing is thus supposed to be based on a particular way of neural coding, difference-based coding. This makes it impossible to associate it with a content- and region/network-based approach to the self. Instead, it is may be better compatible with what may be described as "process- and code-based approach" to the self. However, we have to be careful. The association of self-related processing with difference-based coding may strongly impact the definition of the former; this will be the focus of the next section here.

NEUROTHEORETICAL REMARK
IIIC: PHENOMENAL DETERMINATION OF SELF-RELATEDNESS

I here defined "self-related processing" in a purely operational sense, by the relationship between stimulus and organism. Such an operational definition must be distinguished from a more phenomenal definition of self-related processing, which I want to briefly describe as follows.

Presupposing a phenomenal context, self-related processing concerns stimuli that are experienced as strongly related to one's own person. Without going deeply into abstract philosophical considerations, I would like to give a brief theoretical description of what we mean by the terms "experience," "strongly related," and "to one's person." The concept of "experience" refers to phenomenal experience, such as, for example, the feeling of love, the smell of a rose, or the feeling of disgust. Thus, we focus on the subjective aspect of experience that is described as the "phenomenal aspect." The subjective aspect of experience as prereflective is often distinguished from its reflective or cognitive aspects.

Our definition of self-related processing by experience implies a focus on the implicit, subjective, and phenomenal aspects (to feel or experience self-referential stimuli)—what Kircher and David (2003) describe as "self-qualia" and Zahavi (2005) and others (Legrand 2007a and b; Legrand and Ruby 2009; see also Dainton 2008 for a phenomenal variant and Strawson 2011 for a metaphysical variant) as "prereflective." In contrast, our focus is less on associated cognitive and reflective functions, allowing to make it explicit (to know about or to be aware of stimuli as self-related). As such, I distinguish self-related processing also from what is commonly called "insight," which presupposes cognitive and reflective functions rather than being simply purely subjective and phenomenal.

NEUROTHEORETICAL REMARK
IIID: OPERATIONAL DETERMINATION OF SELF-RELATEDNESS

The term "strongly related" points out the process of associating and linking interoceptive and exteroceptive stimuli with a particular person. The main feature here is not the distinction between diverse sensory modalities but rather the linkage of the different stimuli to the individual person, that is, to its self. What unifies and categorizes stimuli in this regard is no longer their sensory origin but the strength of their relation to the self (this is what Kircher and David, 2003, call "ipseity"; see Chapter 30 for details about ipseity).

The more the respective stimulus is associated with the person's sense of belongingness, the more strongly it can be related to the self, and the stronger the degree of ipseity. The self-stimulus relationship results in the subjective experience of what has been called "mineness"; Lambie and Marcel (2002) speak of an "addition of the 'for me'" by means of which that particular stimulus becomes "mine," resulting in "mineness."

This definition of self-related processing is clearly phenomenal since it involves the explicit reference to experience, that is, consciousness when describing it by phenomenal features like ipseity and mineness. Finally, the phenomenal account of self-related processing presupposes some kind of self or specific person as a given since otherwise self-relatedness, including the phenomenal consciousness and

experience of that self-relatedness, would remain impossible.

Such a phenomenal approach is clearly different from my definition of self-relatedness. Though presupposing the same term, self-relatedness, the contexts are different in both cases, that is, phenomenal and nonphenomenal/operational, which leads to the difference in definition. Most important, my starting point is the relation between organism and stimulus, while in the phenomenal definition the starting point is the self itself and its experience independently of whether this "self" refers to a subjective self or objective self as, for instance, Legrand proposes (Legrand 2007a and b, 589).

The phenomenal approach takes the existence of a self as given, ready-made and granted; such a self is presupposed and serves then as starting point to explain how we can experience it, thus becoming phenomenally conscious of it. This is different from my starting point. My starting point is how what the phenomenal approach is taken as a given, ready-made and granted; that is, the self, is constituted on the basis of our brain and its neural coding and resting-state activity. My approach is thus code- and neuronally-based rather than phenomenally-based. As such, my approach must also be distinguished from Metzinger (2003), who takes a more functionalistic-representational approach and declares the self ultimately is an illusion.

CODA: "SELF-RELATEDNESS" VERSUS "BRAIN RELATEDNESS"

Why do I presuppose such an operational approach to the definition of self-related processing? This looks especially bizarre given my emphasis on prephenomenal features like self-specific organization. I do this in order to not confound the neuronal mechanisms by any phenomenal mechanisms or phenomenal projection. Hence, my first move is purely neuronal in order to avoid any confusion; my motivation is therefore primarily a methodological one. I want to avoid by all means that we project our own phenomenal features onto the brain and its neuronal features.

This is why I refrain from any (metaphysical or otherwise) concept of self for mainly methodological reasons. That does not prevent me, however, from using more operational terms in that context like "self-specific organization" as prephenomenal structure to characterize the resting state. And to use the concept of "self-specificity" to characterize larger activity changes as often observed during stimulus-induced activity (see Chapters 23 and 24).

One may nevertheless be confused about the term "self-related processing." If I do not presuppose any self, why then does the term self still appear in the concept of self-related processing? And why do I need the term "self" at all, for example, methodologically, if I aim to describe neuronal processes like stimulus–rest interaction, rest–rest, and rest–stimulus interaction. Stimulus–rest interaction is supposed to constitute the environment–brain unity (see Chapters 20 and 21), which is a neural predisposition for the constitution of self-specific organization during rest–rest interaction (see

Chapter 23). That, in turn, is a neural predisposition for the possible assignment of a high degree of self-specificity to stimuli (or larger neural activity changes in the resting state; see Chapter 24 and Fig. A4-2).

Why then do I still use the term "self" at all? Wouldn't it be better to replace it by the term "brain"? The terms "self-related processing" and "self-relatedness" would then be replaced by "brain-related processing" and "brain-relatedness" (see also Northoff 2011). Due to its active nature, as manifest in its neural code and its intrinsic activity, the brain can then relate the stimuli to itself along a continuum of different degrees; this may be called "brain-relatedness" and "brain-related processing." This is, for instance, well manifest when the resting state's low-frequency fluctuations and their phase onsets align themselves and thus relate to the stimuli in the environment (see Chapter 20).

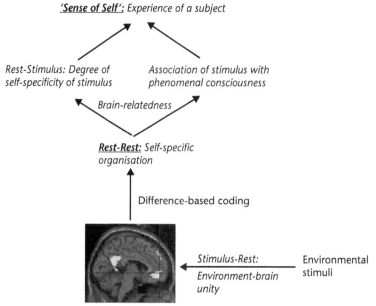

Figure A4-2 Self-relatedness and brain-relatedness. The figure shows the different kinds of processes that are proposed to be relevant in constituting a sense of self. Stimulus–rest, rest–rest, and rest–stimulus interaction and their associated prephenomenal features, environment–brain unity, and self-specific organization. If the interplay is right, they can all lead to the sense of self, the experience of a subject in phenomenal consciousness when associated with a stimulus that shows a high degree of self-specificity (see Chapters 23 and 24 for details).

Do we really still need the concept of self? Methodologically, probably not. While phenomenally the very concept, that is, brain relatedness, that replaces self-relatedness, makes possible the experience of a self, a sense of self in phenomenal consciousness. Such an experience of self is proposed to occur during specific constellations between intrinsic and extrinsic features, such as when the resting state shows a high degree of self-specific organization and encounters stimuli with high degrees of self-specificity (like one's own name).

Can we thus abandon the concept of self? No! Even if the researcher thinks that she does not need the concept of self anymore and declares it to be an illusion, it will nevertheless come back to her when she goes home and becomes phenomenally conscious and experiences a sense of self, i.e., of her own self. Most importantly, all that is possible only on the basis of her brain's very neuronal processes, resting-state activity and difference-based coding, which initially, in her working life, inclined her to reject the concept of self.

REFERENCES

Abraham, A., Schubotz, R. I., & von Cramon, D. Y. (2008). Thinking about the future versus the past in personal and non-personal contexts. *Brain Research*, *1233*, 106–19. doi:10.1016/j.brainres.2008.07.084

Addis, D. R., Moscovitch, M., & McAndrews, M. P. (2007). Consequences of hippocampal damage across the autobiographical memory network in left temporal lobe epilepsy. *Brain*, *130*(Pt 9), 2327–42. doi:10.1093/brain/awm166

Ahn, K., Gil, R., Seibyl, J., Sewell, R. A., & D'Souza, D. C. (2011). Probing GABA receptor function in schizophrenia with iomazenil. *Neuropsychopharmacology*, *36*(3), 677–83. doi:10.1038/npp.2010.198

Alcaro, A., Panksepp, J., Witczak, J., Hayes, D. J., & Northoff, G. (2010). Is subcortical-cortical midline activity in depression mediated by glutamate and GABA? A cross-species translational approach. *Neuroscience and Biobehavioral Reviews*, *34*(4), 592–605. doi:10.1016/j.neubiorev.2009.11.023

Ali, F., Rickards, H., & Cavanna, A. E. (2012). The assessment of consciousness during partial seizures. *Epilepsy and Behavior*, *23*(2), 98–102. doi:10.1016/j.yebeh.2011.11.021

Ali, F., Rickards, H., Bagary, M., Greenhill, L., McCorry, D., & Cavanna, A. E. (2010). Ictal consciousness in epilepsy and nonepileptic attack disorder. *Epilepsy and Behavior*, *19*(3), 522–5. doi:10.1016/j.yebeh.2010.08.014

Alkire, M. T. (2008). Probing the mind: anesthesia and neuroimaging. *Clinical Pharmacology and Therapeutics*, *84*(1), 149–52. doi:10.1038/clpt.2008.75

Alkire, M. T., Gruver, R., Miller, J., McReynolds, J. R., Hahn, E. L., & Cahill, L. (2008a). Neuroimaging analysis of an anesthetic gas that blocks human emotional memory. *Proceedings of the National Academy of Sciences USA*, *105*(5), 1722–27. doi:10.1073/pnas.0711651105

Alkire, M. T., Hudetz, A. G., & Tononi, G. (2008b). Consciousness and anesthesia. *Science*, *322*(5903), 876–80. doi:10.1126/science.1149213

Allen, P., Aleman, A., & McGuire, P. K. (2007a). Inner speech models of auditory verbal hallucinations: Evidence from behavioural and neuroimaging studies. *International Review of Psychiatry*, *19*(4), 407–15.

Allen, P., Amaro, E., Fu, C. H., Williams, S. C., Brammer, M. J., Johns, L. C., & McGuire, P. K. (2007b). Neural correlates of the misattribution of speech in psychosis. *British Journal of Psychiatry*, *190*, 162–69.

Allen, P., Laroi, F., McGuire, P. K., & Aleman, A. (2008). The hallucinating brain: a review of structural and functional neuroimaging studies of hallucinations. *Neuroscience and Biobehavioral Reviews*, *32*(1), 175–91.

Allison, H. E. (1983). *Kant's transcendental idealism: An interpretation and defense.* New Haven, CT: Yale University Press.

Anderson, B. (2011). There is no Such Thing as Attention. *Frontiers in Psychology*, *2*, 246. doi:10.3389/fpsyg.2011.00246

Andrews-Hanna, J. R. (2012). The brain's default network and its adaptive role in internal mentation. *Neuroscientist*, *18*(3), 251–70. doi:10.1177/1073858411403316

Andrews-Hanna, J. R., Reidler, J. S., Sepulcre, J., Poulin, R., & Buckner, R. L. (2010). Functional-anatomic fractionation of the brain's default network. *Neuron*, *65*(4), 550–62. doi:10.1016/j.neuron.2010.02.005

Aru, J., Bachmann, T., Singer, W., & Melloni, L. (2012). Distilling the neural correlates of consciousness. *Neuroscience and Biobehavioral Reviews*, 36(2), 737–46. doi:10.1016/j.neubiorev.2011.12.003

Augustenborg, C. C. (2010). The endogenous feedback network: A new approach to the comprehensive study of consciousness. *Consciousness and Cognition*, 19(2), 547–79. doi:10.1016/j.concog.2010.03.007

Baars, B. J. (2005). Global workspace theory of consciousness: toward a cognitive neuroscience of human experience. *Progress in Brain Research*, 150, 45–53. doi:10.1016/S0079-6123(05)50004-9

Baars, B. J. (2007). The global workspace theory of consciousness. In M. Velmans & S. Schneider (Eds.), *The Blackwell companion to consciousness* (pp. 236–47). Oxford, England: Blackwell Publishing.

Baars, B. J., & Franklin, S. (2007). An architectural model of conscious and unconscious brain functions: Global workspace theory and IDA. *Neural Networks*, 20(9), 955–61. doi:10.1016/j.neunet.2007.09.013

Baars, B. J., Ramsoy, T. Z., & Laureys, S. (2003). Brain, conscious experience and the observing self. *Trends in Neurosciences*, 26(12), 671–75.

Bagshaw, A. P., & Cavanna, A. E. (2012). Resting state networks in paroxysmal disorders of consciousness. *Epilepsy and Behavior*. doi:10.1016/j.yebeh.2012.09.020

Banasr, M., Chowdhury, G. M. I., Terwilliger, R., Newton, S. S., Duman, R. S., Behar, K. L., & Sanacora, G. (2010). Glial pathology in an animal model of depression: reversal of stress-induced cellular, metabolic and behavioral deficits by the glutamate-modulating drug riluzole. *Molecular Psychiatry*, 15(5), 501–11. doi:10.1038/mp.2008.106

Bartels A, & Zeki S. (2004) The chronoarchitecture of the human brain—natural viewing conditions reveal a time-based anatomy of the brain. *Neuroimage*, 22(1), 419–33.

Bartels, A., & Zeki, S. (2005). The chronoarchitecture of the cerebral cortex. *Philosophical Transactions of the Royal Society of London. Series B, Biological Sciences*, 360(1456), 733–50. doi:10.1098/rstb.2005.1627

Bayne, T. (2007). The unity of consciousness: A cartography. In M. Marraffa, M. de Caro, & F. Ferretti (Eds.), *Cartographies of the mind: Philosophy and psychology in intersection* (pp. 201–10). Dordrecht, The Netherlands: Kluwer.

Bayne, T. (2010). *The unity of consciousness*. Oxford, England: Oxford University Press.

Bayne, T., & Chalmers, D. (2003). What is the unity of consciousness? In A. Cleeremans (Ed.), *The unity of consciousness* (pp. 23–58). Oxford, England: Oxford University Press.

Beckmann, C. F., Jenkinson, M., Woolrich, M. W., Behrens, T. E., Flitney, D. E., Devlin, J. T., & Smith, S. M. (2006). Applying FSL to the FIAC data: Model-based and model-free analysis of voice and sentence repetition priming. *Human Brain Mapping*, 27(5), 380–91. doi:10.1002/hbm.20246

Benes, F. M. (2009). Neural circuitry models of schizophrenia: is it dopamine, GABA, glutamate, or something else? *Biological Psychiatry*, 65(12), 1003–5. doi:10.1016/j.biopsych.2009.04.006

Benes, F. M. (2010). Amygdalocortical circuitry in schizophrenia: from circuits to molecules. *Neuropsychopharmacology*, 35(1), 239–57. doi:10.1038/npp.2009.116

Bennett, M., & Hackler, P. (2003). *Philosophical foundation of neuroscience*. Oxford, England: Blackwell Pub. Retrieved from http://www.worldcat.org/title/philosophical-foundations-of-neuroscience/oclc/50410325&referer=brief_results

Bermpohl, F., Pascual-Leone, A., Amedi, A., Merabet, L. B., Fregni, F., Wrase, J., Schlagenhauf, F., et al. (2008). Novelty seeking modulates medial prefrontal activity during the anticipation of emotional stimuli. *Psychiatry Research*, 164(1), 81–5. doi:10.1016/j.pscychresns.2007.12.019

Bermpohl, F., Walter, M., Sajonz, B., Lücke, C., Hägele, C., Sterzer, P., Adli, M., et al. (2009). Attentional modulation of emotional stimulus processing in patients with major depression—alterations in prefrontal cortical regions. *Neuroscience Letters*, 463(2), 108–13. doi:10.1016/j.neulet.2009.07.061

Bernat, J. L. (2010). Current controversies in states of chronic unconsciousness. *Neurology*, 75(18 Suppl 1), S33–8.

Berze, J. (1914). *Die Primare insuffizienz der Psychischen aktivitat*. Leipzig, Germany: Franz Deuticke.

Besle, J., Schevon, C. A., Mehta, A. D., Lakatos, P., Goodman, R. R., McKhann, G. M., et al. (2011). Tuning of the human neocortex to the temporal dynamics of attended events. *Journal of Neuroscience*, 31(9), 3176–85. doi:10.1523/JNEUROSCI.4518-10.2011

Bin Kimura, B. (1997). "Cogito et le je." *L'Evolution Psychiatrique*, 62, 335–48.

Blanke, O. (2012). Multisensory brain mechanisms of bodily self-consciousness. *Nature Reviews Neuroscience*, *13*(8), 556–71. doi:10.1038/nrn3292

Blankenburg, W. (1969). Ansatze zu einer Psycholpathologie des "common sense". *Confinia Psychiatrica*, *12*, 144–63.

Bleuler, E. (1911). *Dementia praecox or the group of schizophrenias*. New York: International Universities Press.

Bleuler, E. (1916). *Lehrbuch der Psychiatrie*. (11. Aufl.). Berlin; Heidelberg; New York: Springer.

Block, N. (1995). How heritability misleads about race. *Cognition*, *56*(2), 99–128.

Block, N. (1996). How can we find the neural correlate of consciousness? *Trends in Neurosciences*, *19*(11), 456–59.

Block, N. (2005). Two neural correlates of consciousness. *Trends in Cognitive Sciences*, *9*(2), 46–52. doi:10.1016/j.tics.2004.12.006

Boeker, Heinz, Kleiser, M., Lehman, D., Jaenke, L., Bogerts, B., & Northoff, G. (n.d.). Executive dysfunction, self, and ego pathology in schizophrenia: an exploratory study of neuropsychology and personality. *Comprehensive Psychiatry*, *47*(1), 7–19. doi:10.1016/j.comppsych.2005.04.003

Boly, M., Balteau, E., Schnakers, C., Degueldre, C., Moonen, G., Luxen, A., et al. (2007a). Baseline brain activity fluctuations predict somatosensory perception in humans. *Proceedings of the National Academy of Sciences USA*, *104*(29), 12187–92. doi:10.1073/pnas.0611404104

Boly, M., Coleman, M. R., Davis, M. H., Hampshire, A., Bor, D., Moonen, G., et al. (2007b). When thoughts become action: An fMRI paradigm to study volitional brain activity in non-communicative brain injured patients. *NeuroImage*, *36*(3), 979–92. doi:10.1016/j.neuroimage.2007.02.047

Boly, M., Garrido, M. I., Gosseries, O., Bruno, M. A., Boveroux, P., Schnakers, C., et al. (2011). Preserved feed forward but impaired top-down processes in the vegetative state. *Science (New York)*, *332*(6031), 858–62. doi:10.1126/science.1202043

Boly, M., Phillips, C., Tshibanda, L., Vanhaudenhuyse, A., Schabus, M., Dang-Vu, T. T., Moonen, G., et al. (2008). Intrinsic brain activity in altered states of consciousness: how conscious is the default mode of brain function? *Annuals of the New York Academy of Sciences*, *1129*, 119–29. doi:10.1196/annals.1417.015

Boly, M., Tshibanda, L., Vanhaudenhuyse, A., Noirhomme, Q., Schnakers, C., Ledoux, D.,

et al. (2009). Functional connectivity in the default network during resting state is preserved in a vegetative but not in a brain dead patient. *Human Brain Mapping*, *30*(8), 2393–400. doi:10.1002/hbm.20672

Bonhomme, V., Boveroux, P., Vanhaudenhuyse, A., Hans, P., Brichant, J. F., Jaquet, O., et al. (2011). Linking sleep and general anesthesia mechanisms: This is no walkover. *Acta Anaesthesiologica Belgica*, *62*(3), 161–71.

Bossaerts, P. (2010). Risk and risk prediction error signals in anterior insula. *Brain Structure and Function*, *214*(5–6), 645–53. doi:10.1007/s00429-010-0253-1

Braboszcz, C., & Delorme, A. (2011). Lost in thoughts: Neural markers of low alertness during mind wandering. *NeuroImage*, *54*(4), 3040–7. doi:10.1016/j.neuroimage.2010.10.008

Brass, M., & Haggard, P. (2010). The hidden side of intentional action: The role of the anterior insular cortex. *Brain Structure and Function*, *214*(5–6), 603–10. doi:10.1007/s00429-010-0269-6

Brentano, F. (1874). *Psychologie vom empirischen Standpunkt [Psychology from an empirical Standpoint]* Meiner Publisher. Stuttgart

Brewer, J. A., Worhunsky, P. D., Gray, J. R., Tang, Y. Y., Weber, J., & Kober, H. (2011). Meditation experience is associated with differences in default mode network activity and connectivity. *Proceedings of the National Academy of Sciences USA*, *108*(50), 20254–9. doi:10.1073/pnas.1112029108

Britz, J., Landis, T., & Michel, C. M. (2009). Right parietal brain activity precedes perceptual alternation of bistable stimuli. *Cerebral Cortex*, *19*(1), 55–65. doi:10.1093/cercor/bhn056

Britz, J., Van De Ville, D., & Michel, C. M. (2010). BOLD correlates of EEG topography reveal rapid resting-state network dynamics. *NeuroImage*, *52*(4), 1162–70. doi:10.1016/j.neuroimage.2010.02.052

Brook A., & Raymont, P. (2006). The representational base of consciousness. *Psyche*, *12*(2–25).

Brook, A. (1994). *Kant and the mind*. Cambridge, England, and New York: Cambridge University Press.

Brook, A., & Raymont, P. (2006). *A unified theory of consciousness*. Cambridge, Mass.: MIT Press.

Brook, A., and Raymont, P., s.vv. "The unity of consciousness." *The Stanford Encyclopedia of Philosophy* (Spring 2013 Edition), Edward N. Zalta (ed.), URL = <http://plato.stanford.edu/archives/spr2013/entries/consciousness-unity/>.

Brown, E. N., Lydic, R., & Schiff, N. D. (2010). General anesthesia, sleep, and coma. *The New England Journal of Medicine, 363*(27), 2638–50. doi:10.1056/NEJMra0808281

Brown, G. G., & Thompson, W. K. (2010). Functional brain imaging in schizophrenia: Selected results and methods. *Current Topics in Behavioral Neurosciences, 4,* 181–214.

Brown, G. G., Mathalon, D. H., Stern, H., Ford, J., Mueller, B., Greve, D. N., et al. Function Biomedical Informatics Research Network. (2011). Multisite reliability of cognitive BOLD data. *NeuroImage, 54*(3), 2163–75. doi:10.1016/j.neuroimage.2010.09.076

Broyd, S. J., Demanuele, C., Debener, S., Helps, S. K., James, C. J., & Sonuga-Barke, E. J. (2009). Default-mode brain dysfunction in mental disorders: A systematic review. *Neuroscience and Biobehavioral Reviews, 33*(3), 279–96.

Buckner, R. L., & Carroll, D. C. (2007). Self-projection and the brain. *Trends in Cognitive Sciences, 11*(2), 49–57. doi:10.1016/j.tics.2006.11.004

Buckner, R. L., Andrews-Hanna, J. R., & Schacter, D. L. (2008). The brain's default network: Anatomy, function, and relevance to disease. *Annals of the New York Academy of Sciences, 1124,* 1–38.

Buzsaki, G. (2006). *Rhythms of the brain.* Oxford, England: Oxford University Press.

Buzsaki, G., & Draguhn, A. (2004). Neuronal oscillations in cortical networks. *Science, 304*(5679), 1926–9. doi:10.1126/science.1099745

Calhoun, V. D., Maciejewski, P. K., Pearlson, G. D., & Kiehl, K. A. (2008). Temporal lobe and "default" hemodynamic brain modes discriminate between schizophrenia and bipolar disorder. *Human Brain Mapping, 29*(11), 1265–75. doi:10.1002/hbm.20463

Callard, F., Smallwood, J., & Margulies, D. S. (2012). Default Positions: How Neuroscience's Historical Legacy has Hampered Investigation of the Resting Mind. *Frontiers in Psychology, 3,* 321. doi:10.3389/fpsyg.2012.00321

Canli, T., Sivers, H., Thomason, M. E., Whitfield-Gabrieli, S., Gabrieli, J. D. E., & Gotlib, I. H. (2004). Brain activation to emotional words in depressed vs healthy subjects. *Neuroreport, 15*(17), 2585–8. Retrieved from http://www.ncbi.nlm.nih.gov/pubmed/15570157

Canolty, R. T., & Knight, R. T. (2010). The functional role of cross-frequency coupling. *Trends in Cognitive Sciences, 14*(11), 506–15. doi:10.1016/j.tics.2010.09.001

Canolty, R. T., Cadieu, C. F., Koepsell, K., Ganguly, K., Knight, R. T., & Carmena, J. M. (2012). Detecting event-related changes of multivariate phase coupling in dynamic brain networks. *Journal of Neurophysiology, 107*(7), 2020–31. doi:10.1152/jn.00610.2011

Cauda, F., Micon, B. M., Sacco, K., Duca, S., D'Agata, F., Geminiani, G., & Canavero, S. (2009). Disrupted intrinsic functional connectivity in the vegetative state. *Journal of Neurology, Neurosurgery, and Psychiatry, 80*(4), 429–31. doi:10.1136/jnnp.2007.142349

Cavanna, A E, Mula, M., Servo, S., Strigaro, G., Tota, G., Barbagli, D., Collimedaglia, L., et al. (2008). Measuring the level and content of consciousness during epileptic seizures: the Ictal Consciousness Inventory. *Epilepsy and Behavior, 13*(1), 184–8. doi:10.1016/j.yebeh.2008.01.009

Cavanna, Andrea E, Shah, S., Eddy, C. M., Williams, A., & Rickards, H. (2011). Consciousness: a neurological perspective. *Behavioural Neurology, 24*(1), 107–16. doi:10.3233/BEN-2011-0322

Cavanna, Andrea Eugenio, & Monaco, F. (2009). Brain mechanisms of altered conscious states during epileptic seizures. *Nature Reviews. Neurology, 5*(5), 267–76. doi:10.1038/nrneurol.2009.38

Cavinato, M., Volpato, C., Silvoni, S., Sacchetto, M., Merico, A., & Piccione, F. (2011). Event-related brain potential modulation in patients with severe brain damage. *Clinical Neurophysiology, 122*(4), 719–24. doi:10.1016/j.clinph.2010.08.024

Caygill, H. (1995). *Kant dictionary.* Cambridge, MA: Blackwell.

Chalmers, D. (1996). *The conscious mind: In search of a fundamental theory.* New York: Oxford University Press.

Chalmers, D. (1998). On the search for the neural correlates of consciousness. In S. Hameroff, A. Kaszniak, & S. A. Scott (Eds.), *Toward a science of consciousness II: The second Tuscon discussions and debates* (pp. 34–54). Cambridge, MA: MIT Press.

Chalmers, D. (2002). *Philosophy of mind: Classical and contemporary readings.* New York: Oxford University Press. Retrieved from http://www.worldcat.org/title/philosophy-of-mind-classical-and-contemporary-readings/oclc/806407602&referer=brief_results

Chalmers, D. (2010). *The character of consciousness.* Oxford; New York: Oxford University Press. Retrieved from http://www.worldcat.org/title/character-of-consciousness/oclc/148750961&referer=brief_results

Chalmers, D. (2010). *The character of consciousness.* Oxford, England and New York: Oxford University Press.

Changeux, J. P., & Lou, H. C. (2011). Emergent pharmacology of conscious experience: New perspectives in substance addiction. *FASEB Journal, 25*(7), 2098–108. doi:10.1096/fj.11-0702ufm

Christoff, K. (2012). Undirected thought: neural determinants and correlates. *Brain Research, 1428,* 51–9. doi:10.1016/j.brainres.2011.09.060

Christoff, K., Cosmelli, D., Legrand, D., & Thompson, E. (2011). Specifying the self for cognitive neuroscience. *Trends in Cognitive Sciences, 15*(3), 104–12. doi:10.1016/j.tics.2011.01.001

Christoff, K., Gordon, A. M., Smallwood, J., Smith, R., & Schooler, J. W. (2009). Experience sampling during fMRI reveals default network and executive system contributions to mind wandering. *Proceedings of the National Academy of Sciences USA, 106*(21), 8719–24. doi:10.1073/pnas.0900234106

Christoff, K., Gordon, A. M., Smallwood, J., Smith, R., & Schooler, J. W. (2009). Experience sampling during fMRI reveals default network and executive system contributions to mind wandering. *Proceedings of the National Academy of Sciences USA, 106*(21), 8719–724.

Christoff, K., Ream, J. M., Geddes, L. P. T., & Gabrieli, J. D. E. (2003). Evaluating self-generated information: Anterior prefrontal contributions to human cognition. *Behavioral Neuroscience, 117*(6), 1161–8.

Churchland, P. (2012). *Plato's camera: how the physical brain captures a landscape of abstract universals.* Cambridge, MA: MIT Press. Retrieved from http://www.worldcat.org/title/platos-camera-how-the-physical-brain-captures-a-landscape-of-abstract-universals/oclc/727126736&referer=brief_results

Churchland, P. S. (2002). Self-representation in nervous systems. *Science, 296*(5566), 308–10.

Clauss, R. P. (2010). Neurotransmitters in coma, vegetative and minimally conscious states, pharmacological interventions. *Medical Hypotheses, 75*(3), 287–90. doi:10.1016/j.mehy.2010.03.005

Cole, M. W., Pathak, S., & Schneider, W. (2010). Identifying the brain's most globally connected regions. *NeuroImage, 49*(4), 3132–48.

Corlett, P. R., Frith, C. D., & Fletcher, P. C. (2009a). From drugs to deprivation: A Bayesian framework for understanding models of psychosis. *Psychopharmacology, 206*(4), 515–30. doi:10.1007/s00213-009-1561-0

Corlett, P. R., Krystal, J. H., Taylor, J. R., & Fletcher, P. C. (2009b). Why do delusions persist? *Frontiers in Human Neuroscience, 3,* 12. doi:10.3389/neuro.09.012.2009

Coull, J. T., Cheng, R. K., & Meck, W. H. (2011a). Neuroanatomical and neurochemical substrates of timing. *Neuropsychopharmacology, 36*(1), 3–25. doi:10.1038/npp.2010.113

Coull, J. T., Morgan, H., Cambridge, V. C., Moore, J. W., Giorlando, F., Adapa, R., et al. (2011b). Ketamine perturbs perception of the flow of time in healthy volunteers. *Psychopharmacology, 218*(3), 543–56. doi:10.1007/s00213-011-2346-9; 10.1007/s00213-011-2346-9

Craig, A. D. (2002). How do you feel? Interoception: The sense of the physiological condition of the body. *Nature Reviews. Neuroscience, 3*(8), 655–66. doi:10.1038/nrn894

Craig, A. D. (2003). Interoception: The sense of the physiological condition of the body. *Current Opinion in Neurobiology, 13*(4), 500–5.

Craig, A. D. (2004). Human feelings: Why are some more aware than others? *Trends in Cognitive Sciences, 8*(6), 239–41. doi:10.1016/j.tics.2004.04.004

Craig, A. D. (2009a). Emotional moments across time: A possible neural basis for time perception in the anterior insula. *Philosophical Transactions of the Royal Society of London Series B: Biological Sciences, 364*(1525), 1933–42. doi:10.1098/rstb.2009.0008

Craig, A. D. (2009b). How do you feel—now? The anterior insula and human awareness. *Nature Reviews Neuroscience, 10*(1), 59–70.

Craig, A. D. (2010a). Once an island, now the focus of attention. *Brain Structure and Function, 214*(5–6), 395–6. doi:10.1007/s00429-010-0270-0

Craig, A. D. (2010b). The sentient self. *Brain Structure and Function, 214*(5–6), 563–77. doi:10.1007/s00429-010-0248-y

Craig, A. D. (2010c). Why a soft touch can hurt. *The Journal of Physiology, 588*(Pt. 1), 13. doi:10.1113/jphysiol.2009.185116

Craig, A. D. (2011). Interoceptive cortex in the posterior insula: Comment on Garcia-Larrea et al. 2010 Brain 133, 2528. *Brain, 134*(Pt 4), e166; author reply e165. doi:10.1093/brain/awq308

Crick, F. (1994). *The astonishing hypothesis.* New York: Simon & Schuster.

Crick, F. (1995). *The astonishing hypothesis: The scientific search for the soul.* New York: Simon & Schuster. Retrieved from http://www.worldcat.org/oclc/32725569

Crick, F. C., & Koch, C. (2005). What is the function of the claustrum? *Philosophical Transactions of the Royal Society of London Series B: Biological Sciences*, *360*(1458), 1271–9. doi:10.1098/rstb.2005.1661

Crick, F., & Koch, C. (1998). Consciousness and neuroscience. *Cerebral Cortex*, *8*(2), 97–107.

Crick, F., & Koch, C. (2003). A framework for consciousness. *Nature Neuroscience*, *6*(2), 119–26. doi:10.1038/nn0203-119

Critchley, H. D. (2005). Neural mechanisms of autonomic, affective, and cognitive integration. *Journal of Comparative Neurology*, *493*(1), 154–66.

Critchley, H. D., Wiens, S., Rotshtein, P., Ohman, A., & Dolan, R. J. (2004). Neural systems supporting interoceptive awareness. *Nature Neuroscience*, *7*(2), 189–95. doi:10.1038/nn1176

Czisch, M., Wehrle, R., Kaufmann, C., Wetter, T. C., Holsboer, F., Pollmacher, T., & Auer, D. P. (2004). Functional MRI during sleep: BOLD signal decreases and their electrophysiological correlates. *European Journal of Neuroscience*, *20*(2), 566–74. doi:10.1111/j.1460-9568.2004.03518.x

D'Argembeau, A., Collette, F., Van der Linden, M., Laureys, S., Del Fiore, G., Degueldre, C., et al. (2005). Self-referential reflective activity and its relationship with rest: A PET study. *NeuroImage*, *25*(2), 616–24. doi:10.1016/j.neuroimage.2004.11.048

D'Argembeau, A., Feyers, D., Majerus, S., Collette, F., Van der Linden, M., Maquet, P., & Salmon, E. (2008a). Self-reflection across time: cortical midline structures differentiate between present and past selves. *Social Cognitive and Affective Neuroscience*, *3*(3), 244–52. doi:10.1093/scan/nsn020

D'Argembeau, A., Stawarczyk, D., Majerus, S., Collette, F., Van der Linden, M., Feyers, D., Maquet, P., et al. (2010). The neural basis of personal goal processing when envisioning future events. *Journal of Cognitive Neuroscience*, *22*(8), 1701–13. doi:10.1162/jocn.2009.21314

D'Argembeau, A., Stawarczyk, D., Majerus, S., Collette, F., Van der Linden, M., & Salmon, E. (2010). Modulation of medial prefrontal and inferior parietal cortices when thinking about past, present, and future selves. *Social Neuroscience*, *5*(2), 187–200. doi:10.1080/17470910903233562

D'Argembeau, A., Xue, G., Lu, Z. L., Van der Linden, M., & Bechara, A. (2008b). Neural correlates of envisioning emotional events in the near and far future. *NeuroImage*, *40*(1), 398–407. doi:10.1016/j.neuroimage.2007.11.025

Dainton, B. (2008). Sensing change. *Philosophical Issues*, *18*, 362–84.

Dainton, B. (2010). *Time and space*. Montreal, Quebec: McGill-Queen's University Press.

Dalgleish, T. (2004). The emotional brain. *Nature Reviews Neuroscience*, *5*(7), 583–9. doi:10.1038/nrn1432

Damasio, A. (1999a). *The feeling of what happens: Body and emotion in the making of consciousness*. New York: Harcourt Brace.

Damasio, A. (1999b). How the brain creates the mind. *Scientific American*, *281*(6), 112–17.

Damasio, A. (2003a). Feelings of emotion and the self. *Annals of the New York Academy of Sciences*, *1001*, 253–61.

Damasio, A. (2003b). Mental self: The person within. *Nature*, *423*(6937), 227.

Damasio, A. (2010). *Self comes to mind: Constructing the conscious brain*. New York: Harcourt Brace.

Damoiseaux, J. S., Rombouts, S. A. R. B., Barkhof, F., Scheltens, P., Stam, C. J., Smith, S. M., & Beckmann, C. F. (2006). Consistent resting-state networks across healthy subjects. *Proceedings of the National Academy of Sciences USA*, *103*(37), 13848–53. doi:10.1073/pnas.0601417103

Dang-Vu, T. T., Bonjean, M., Schabus, M., Boly, M., Darsaud, A., Desseilles, M., et al. (2011). Interplay between spontaneous and induced brain activity during human non-rapid eye movement sleep. *Proceedings of the National Academy of Sciences USA*, *108*(37), 15438–43. doi:10.1073/pnas.1112503108

Danielson, N. B., Guo, J. N., & Blumenfeld, H. (2011). The default mode network and altered consciousness in epilepsy. *Behavioural Neurology*, *24*(1), 55–65.

Danos, P., Schmidt, A., Baumann, B., Bernstein, H.-G., Northoff, G., Stauch, R., Krell, D., et al. (2005). Volume and neuron number of the mediodorsal thalamic nucleus in schizophrenia: a replication study. *Psychiatry Research*, *140*(3), 281–9. doi:10.1016/j.pscychresns.2005.09.005

Dastjerdi, M., Foster, B. L., Nasrullah, S., Rauschecker, A. M., Dougherty, R. F., Townsend, J. D., Chang, C., et al. (2011). Differential electrophysiological response during rest, self-referential, and non-self-referential tasks in human posteromedial cortex. *Proceedings of the National Academy of Sciences USA*, *108*(7), 3023–8. doi:10.1073/pnas.1017098108

Dawson, N., Morris, B. J., & Pratt, J. A. (2011). Subanaesthetic ketamine treatment alters prefrontal cortex connectivity with thalamus and ascending subcortical systems. *Schizophrenia Bulletin*. doi:10.1093/schbul/sbr144

De Graaf, T. A., Hsieh, P.-J., & Sack, A. T. (2012). The "correlates" in neural correlates of consciousness. *Neuroscience and Biobehavioral Reviews*, *36*(1), 191–7. doi:10.1016/j.neubiorev.2011.05.012

de Greck, M., Rotte, M., Paus, R., Moritz, D., Thiemann, R., Proesch, U., Bruer, U., et al. (2008a). Is our self based on reward? Self-relatedness recruits neural activity in the reward system. *NeuroImage*, *39*(4), 2066–75. doi:10.1016/j.neuroimage.2007.11.006

de Greck, M., Enzi, B., Prosch, U., Gantman, A., Tempelmann, C., & Northoff, G. (2010). Decreased neuronal activity in reward circuitry of pathological gamblers during processing of personal relevant stimuli. *Human Brain Mapping*, *31*(11), 1802–12. doi:10.1002/hbm.20981

de Greck, M., Rotte, M., Paus, R., Moritz, D., Thiemann, R., Proesch, U., et al. (2008b). Is our self based on reward? Self-relatedness recruits neural activity in the reward system. *NeuroImage*, *39*(4), 2066–75. doi:10.1016/j. neuroimage.2007.11.006

de Greck, M., Supady, A., Thiemann, R., Tempelmann, C., Bogerts, B., Forschner, L., et al. (2009). Decreased neural activity in reward circuitry during personal reference in abstinent alcoholics—a fMRI study. *Human Brain Mapping*, *30*(5), 1691–1704. doi:10.1002/hbm.20634

de Greck, Moritz, Enzi, B., Prösch, U., Gantman, A., Tempelmann, C., & Northoff, G. (2010). Decreased neuronal activity in reward circuitry of pathological gamblers during processing of personal relevant stimuli. *Human Brain Mapping*, *31*(11), 1802–12. doi:10.1002/hbm.20981

de Greck, Moritz, Scheidt, L., Bölter, A. F., Frommer, J., Ulrich, C., Stockum, E., Enzi, B., et al. (2011). Multimodal psychodynamic psychotherapy induces normalization of reward related activity in somatoform disorder. *World Journal of Biological Psychiatry*, *12*(4), 296–308. doi:10.31 09/15622975.2010.539269

de Greck, Moritz, Wang, G., Yang, X., Wang, X., Northoff, G., & Han, S. (2012). Neural substrates underlying intentional empathy. *Social Cognitive and Affective Neuroscience*, *7*(2), 135–44. doi:10.1093/scan/nsq093

De Vignemont, F. (2011). Embodiment, ownership and disownership. *Consciousness and Cognition*, *20*(1), 82–93. doi:10.1016/j.concog.2010.09.004

Dehaene, S., & Brannon, E. M. (2010). Space, time, and number: A Kantian research program. *Trends in Cognitive Sciences*, *14*(12), 517–9. doi:10.1016/j.tics.2010.09.009

Dehaene, S., & Changeux, J. P. (2005). Ongoing spontaneous activity controls access to consciousness: A neuronal model for inattentional blindness. *PLoS Biology*, *3*(5), e141. doi:10.1371/ journal.pbio.0030141

Dehaene, S., & Changeux, J. P. (2011). Experimental and theoretical approaches to conscious processing. *Neuron*, *70*(2), 200–27. doi:10.1016/j. neuron.2011.03.018

Dehaene, S., & Changeux, J.-P. (2005). Ongoing spontaneous activity controls access to consciousness: a neuronal model for inattentional blindness. *PLoS Biology*, *3*(5), e141. doi:10.1371/ journal.pbio.0030141

Dehaene, S., Changeux, J.-P., Naccache, L., Sackur, J., & Sergent, C. (2006). Conscious, preconscious, and subliminal processing: a testable taxonomy. *Trends in Cognitive Sciences*, *10*(5), 204–11. doi:10.1016/j.tics.2006.03.007

Del Cul, A., Baillet, S., & Dehaene, S. (2007). Brain dynamics underlying the nonlinear threshold for access to consciousness. *PLoS Biology*, *5*(10), e260. doi:10.1371/journal.pbio.0050260

Dennett, D. C. (1991). *Consciousness Explained*. Boston: Little, Brown and Company.

Dennett, D. C. (1992). The self as the center of narrative gravity". In F. Kessel, P. Cole, and D. L. Johnson, eds. *Self and Consciousness: Multiple Perspectives*. Hillsdale, NJ: Lawrence Erlbaum.

Dennett, D. (2001). Are we explaining consciousness yet? *Cognition*, *79*(1–2), 221–37.

Descartes, R. (1644/1911). *The Principles of Philosophy*. Translated by E. Haldane and G. Ross. Cambridge: Cambridge University Press.

Desseilles, M., Balteau, E., Sterpenich, V., Dang-Vu, T. T., Darsaud, A., Vandewalle, G., et al. (2009). Abnormal neural filtering of irrelevant visual information in depression. *Journal of Neuroscience*, *29*(5), 1395–1403. doi:10.1523/ JNEUROSCI.3341-08.2009

Di HB, Yu SM, Weng XC, Laureys S, Yu D, Li JQ, Qin PM, Zhu YH, Zhang SZ, Chen YZ. Cerebral response to patient's own name in the vegetative and minimally conscious states. *Neurology*. 2007 Mar 20;68(12):895–9.

Di Cristo, G. (2007). Development of cortical GABAergic circuits and its implications for neurodevelopmental disorders. *Clinical Genetics*, *72*(1), 1–8.

Di Cristo, G., Chattopadhyaya, B., Kuhlman, S. J., Fu, Y., Belanger, M. C., Wu, C. Z., et al. (2007).

Activity-dependent PSA expression regulates inhibitory maturation and onset of critical period plasticity. *Nature Neuroscience*, *10*(12), 1569–77. doi:10.1038/nn2008

Dias, E. C., Butler, P. D., Hoptman, M. J., & Javitt, D. C. (2011). Early sensory contributions to contextual encoding deficits in schizophrenia. *Archives of General Psychiatry*, *68*(7), 654–64. doi:10.1001/archgenpsychiatry.2011.17

Dierks, T., Linden, D. E., Jandl, M., Formisano, E., Goebel, R., Lanfermann, H., & Singer, W. (1999). Activation of Heschl's gyrus during auditory hallucinations. *Neuron*, *22*(3), 615–21.

Doege, K., Jansen, M., Mallikarjun, P., Liddle, E. B., & Liddle, P. F. (2010a). How much does phase resetting contribute to event-related EEG abnormalities in schizophrenia? *Neuroscience Letters*, *481*(1), 1–5. doi:10.1016/j.neulet.2010.06.008

Doege, K., Kumar, M., Bates, A. T., Das, D., Boks, M. P., & Liddle, P. F. (2010b). Time and frequency domain event-related electrical activity associated with response control in schizophrenia. *Clinical Neurophysiology*, *121*(10), 1760–71. doi:10.1016/j.clinph.2010.03.049

Doucet, G., Naveau, M., Petit, L., Zago, L., Crivello, F., Jobard, G., et al. (2012). Patterns of hemodynamic low-frequency oscillations in the brain are modulated by the nature of free thought during rest. *NeuroImage*, *59*(4), 3194–200. doi:10.1016/j.neuroimage.2011.11.059

Driesen, N. R., McCarthy, G., Bhagwagar, Z., Bloch, M., Calhoun, V., D'Souza, D. C., Gueorguieva, R., et al. (2013). Relationship of resting brain hyperconnectivity and schizophrenia-like symptoms produced by the NMDA receptor antagonist ketamine in humans. *Molecular Psychiatry*. doi:10.1038/mp.2012.194

Duncan, N. W., & Northoff, G. (2013). Overview of potential procedural and participant-related confounds for neuroimaging of the resting state. *Journal of Psychiatry and Neuroscience*, *38*(2), 84–96. doi:10.1503/jpn.120059

Duncan, N. W., Enzi, B., Wiebking, C., & Northoff, G. (2011). Involvement of glutamate in rest-stimulus interaction between perigenual and supragenual anterior cingulate cortex: A combined fMRI-MRS study. *Human Brain Mapping*, *32*(12), 2172–82. doi:10.1002/hbm.21179; 10.1002/hbm.21179

Duncan, N., Xian, J., Hayes, D., & Northoff, G. (2013). How is reward related to the resting state? A meta-analysis. In press, *Neuroimage*.

Edelman, D. B., & Seth, A. K. (2009). Animal consciousness: a synthetic approach. *Trends in Neurosciences*, *32*(9), 476–84. doi:10.1016/j.tins.2009.05.008

Edelman, D. B., Baars, B. J., & Seth, A. K. (2005). Identifying hallmarks of consciousness in non-mammalian species. *Consciousness and Cognition*, *14*(1), 169–87. doi:10.1016/j.concog.2004.09.001

Edelman, G. & Tononi, G. (2000). *A universe of consciousness: How matter becomes imagination.* New York; Basic books.

Edelman, G. (1993). Neural Darwinism: Selection and reentrant signaling in higher brain function. *Neuron*, *10*(2), 115–25.

Edelman, G. (2003). Naturalizing consciousness: a theoretical framework. *Proceedings of the National Academy of Sciences USA*, *100*(9), 5520–4. doi:10.1073/pnas.0931349100

Edelman, G. (2004). *Wider than the sky. The phenomenal gift of consciousness.* New Haven, CT: Yale University Press.

Eickhoff, S. B., Dafotakis, M., Grefkes, C., Stocker, T., Shah, N. J., Schnitzler, A., et al. (2008). fMRI reveals cognitive and emotional processing in a long-term comatose patient. *Experimental Neurology*, *214*(2), 240–46. doi:10.1016/j.expneurol.2008.08.007

Ellison-Wright, I., & Bullmore, E. (2009). Meta-analysis of diffusion tensor imaging studies in schizophrenia. *Schizophrenia Research*, *108*(1–3), 3–10. doi:10.1016/j.schres.2008.11.021

Engel, A. K., & Fries, P. (2010). Beta-band oscillations—signalling the status quo? *Current Opinion in Neurobiology*, *20*(2), 156–65. doi:10.1016/j.conb.2010.02.015

Enzi, B., Duncan, N. W., Kaufmann, J., Tempelmann, C., Wiebking, C., & Northoff, G. (2012). Glutamate modulates resting state activity in the perigenual anterior cingulate cortex—a combined fMRI-MRS study. *Neuroscience*, *227*, 102–9. doi:10.1016/j.neuroscience.2012.09.039

Enzi, B., de Greck, M., Prosch, U., Tempelmann, C., & Northoff, G. (2009). Is our self nothing but reward? Neuronal overlap and distinction between reward and personal relevance and its relation to human personality. *PloS One*, *4*(12), e8429. doi:10.1371/journal.pone.0008429

Enzi, Björn, De Greck, M., Prösch, U., Tempelmann, C., & Northoff, G. (2009). Is our self nothing but reward? Neuronal overlap and distinction between reward and personal relevance and its relation to human personality. *PloS One*, *4*(12), e8429. doi:10.1371/journal.pone.0008429

Ersner-Hershfield, H., Wimmer, G. E., & Knutson, B. (2009). Saving for the future self: Neural measures of future self-continuity predict temporal discounting. *Social Cognitive and Affective Neuroscience*, 4(1), 85–92. doi:10.1093/scan/nsn042

Esser, S. K., Hill, S., & Tononi, G. (2009). Breakdown of effective connectivity during slow wave sleep: Investigating the mechanism underlying a cortical gate using large-scale modeling. *Journal of Neurophysiology*, 102(4), 2096–111. doi:10.1152/jn.00059.2009

Esslen, M., Metzler, S., Pascual-Marqui, R., & Jancke, L. (2008). Pre-reflective and reflective self-reference: a spatiotemporal EEG analysis. *NeuroImage*, 42(1), 437–49. doi:10.1016/j.neuroimage.2008.01.060

Fan, Y., Wonneberger, C., Enzi, B., De Greck, M., Ulrich, C., Tempelmann, C., Bogerts, B., et al. (2011). The narcissistic self and its psychological and neural correlates: an exploratory fMRI study. *Psychological Medicine*, 41(8), 1641–50. doi:10.1017/S003329171000228X

Fan, Y., Duncan, N. W., de Greck, M., & Northoff, G. (2011a). Is there a core neural network in empathy? An fMRI based quantitative meta-analysis. *Neuroscience and Biobehavioral Reviews*, 35(3), 903–11. doi:10.1016/j.neubiorev.2010.10.009

Fan, Y., Wonneberger, C., Enzi, B., de Greck, M., Ulrich, C., Tempelmann, C., et al. (2011b). The narcissistic self and its psychological and neural correlates: An exploratory fMRI study. *Psychological Medicine*, 41(8), 1641–50. doi:10.1017/S003329171000228X

Farb, N. A. S., Segal, Z. V, & Anderson, A. K. (2013a). Attentional modulation of primary interoceptive and exteroceptive cortices. *Cerebral Cortex*, 23(1), 114–26. doi:10.1093/cercor/bhr385

Feinberg, T. E. (2009). *From axons to identity: Neurological explorations of the nature of the self.* New York: W. W. Norton.

Feinberg, T. E. (2011). Neuropathologies of the self: Clinical and anatomical features. *Consciousness and Cognition*, 20(1), 75–81. doi:10.1016/j.concog.2010.09.017

Feinberg, T. E. (2012). Neuroontology, neurobiological naturalism, and consciousness: A challenge to scientific reduction and a solution. *Physics of Life Reviews*, 9(1), 13–34. doi:10.1016/j.plrev.2011.10.019

Feinberg, T. E., Venneri, A., Simone, A. M., Fan, Y., & Northoff, G. (2010). The neuroanatomy of asomatognosia and somatoparaphrenia. *Journal of Neurology, Neurosurgery, and Psychiatry*, 81(3), 276–81. doi:10.1136/jnnp.2009.188946

Fell, J., & Axmacher, N. (2011). The role of phase synchronization in memory processes. *Nature Reviews Neuroscience*, 12(2), 105–18. doi:10.1038/nrn2979

Fell, J., Elger, C. E., & Kurthen, M. (2004). Do neural correlates of consciousness cause conscious states? *Medical Hypotheses*, 63(2), 367–9. doi:10.1016/j.mehy.2003.12.048

Fellinger, R., Klimesch, W., Schnakers, C., Perrin, F., Freunberger, R., Gruber, W., et al. (2011). Cognitive processes in disorders of consciousness as revealed by EEG time-frequency analyses. *Clinical Neurophysiology*, 122(11), 2177–84. doi:10.1016/j.clinph.2011.03.004

Ferrarelli, F., & Tononi, G. (2011). The thalamic reticular nucleus and schizophrenia. *Schizophrenia Bulletin*, 37(2), 306–15. doi:10.1093/schbul/sbq142

Ferrarelli, F., Massimini, M., Sarasso, S., Casali, A., Riedner, B. A., Angelini, G., et al. (2010). Breakdown in cortical effective connectivity during midazolam-induced loss of consciousness. *Proceedings of the National Academy of Sciences USA*, 107(6), 2681–6. doi:10.1073/pnas.0913008107

Ferrarelli, F., Sarasso, S., Guller, Y., Riedner, B. A., Peterson, M. J., Bellesi, M., Massimini, M., et al. (2012). Reduced natural oscillatory frequency of frontal thalamocortical circuits in schizophrenia. *Archives of General Psychiatry*, 69(8), 766–74. doi:10.1001/archgenpsychiatry.2012.147

Filevich, E., Kuhn, S., & Haggard, P. (2012). Intentional inhibition in human action: The power of 'no'. *Neuroscience and Biobehavioral Reviews*, 36(4), 1107–18. doi:10.1016/j.neubiorev.2012.01.006

Fingelkurts, A. A., Fingelkurts, A. A., & Kähkönen, S. (2005). Functional connectivity in the brain—is it an elusive concept? *Neuroscience and Biobehavioral Reviews*, 28(8), 827–36. doi:10.1016/j.neubiorev.2004.10.009

Fingelkurts, A. A., Fingelkurts, A. A., & Neves, C. F. (2010). Natural world physical, brain operational, and mind phenomenal space-time. *Physics of Life Reviews*, 7(2), 195–249. doi:10.1016/j.plrev.2010.04.001

Fingelkurts, A. A., Fingelkurts, A. A., Bagnato, S., Boccagni, C., & Galardi, G. (2011). Life or death: Prognostic value of a resting EEG with regards to survival in patients in vegetative and minimally conscious states. *PloS One*, 6(10), e25967. doi:10.1371/journal.pone.0025967

Fingelkurts, A. A., Fingelkurts, A. A., Kivisaari, R., Pekkonen, E., Ilmoniemi, R. J., & Kahkonen, S. (2004a). Enhancement of GABA-related signaling is associated with increase of functional connectivity in human cortex. *Human Brain Mapping*, *22*(1), 27–39. doi:10.1002/hbm.20014

Fingelkurts, A. A., Fingelkurts, A. A., Kivisaari, R., Pekkonen, E., Ilmoniemi, R. J., & Kahkonen, S. (2004b). Local and remote functional connectivity of neocortex under the inhibition influence. *NeuroImage*, *22*(3), 1390–406. doi:10.1016/j.neuroimage.2004.03.013

Fitzgerald, P. B., Oxley, T. J., Laird, A. R., Kulkarni, J., Egan, G. F., & Daskalakis, Z. J. (2006). An analysis of functional neuroimaging studies of dorsolateral prefrontal cortical activity in depression. *Psychiatry Research*, *148*(1), 33–45. doi:10.1016/j.pscychresns.2006.04.006

Fitzgerald, P. B., Sritharan, A., Daskalakis, Z. J., de Castella, A. R., Kulkarni, J., & Egan, G. (2007). A functional magnetic resonance imaging study of the effects of low frequency right prefrontal transcranial magnetic stimulation in depression. *Journal of Clinical Psychopharmacology*, *27*(5), 488–92. doi:10.1097/jcp.0b013e318151521c

Flohr, H. (1995). Sensations and brain processes. *Behavioral Brain Research*, *71*, 157–61.

Flohr, H. (2006). Unconsciousness. *Best Practice and Research. Clinical Anaesthesiology*, *20*(1), 11–22.

Flohr, H., Glade, U., & Motzko, D. (1998). The role of the NMDA synapse in general anesthesia. *Toxicology Letters*, *100–101*, 23–9.

Ford, J. M., Roach, B. J., Jorgensen, K. W., Turner, J. A., Brown, G. G., Notestine, R., et al. (2009). Tuning in to the voices: A multisite FMRI study of auditory hallucinations. *Schizophrenia Bulletin*, *35*(1), 58–66.

Fox, M. D., & Raichle, M. E. (2007). Spontaneous fluctuations in brain activity observed with functional magnetic resonance imaging. *Nature Reviews Neuroscience*, *8*(9), 700–11. doi:10.1038/nrn2201

Fox, M. D., Snyder, A. Z., Vincent, J. L., Corbetta, M., Van Essen, D. C., & Raichle, M. E. (2005). The human brain is intrinsically organized into dynamic, anticorrelated functional networks. *Proceedings of the National Academy of Sciences USA*, *102*(27), 9673–8. doi:10.1073/pnas.0504136102

Freeman, W. J. (2003). The wave packet: An action potential for the 21st century. *Journal of Integrative Neuroscience*, *2*(1), 3–30.

Freeman, W. J. (2007). Indirect biological measures of consciousness from field studies of brains as dynamical systems. *Neural Networks*, *20*(9), 1021–31. doi:10.1016/j.neunet.2007.09.004

Freeman, W. J. (2010). The use of codes to connect mental and material aspects of brain function: comment on: "Natural world physical, brain operational, and mind phenomenal space-time" by A. A. Fingelkurts, A. A. Fingelkurts and C. F. H. Neves. *Physics of Life Reviews*, *7*(2), 260–1. doi:10.1016/j.plrev.2010.04.010

Freeman, W. J. (2011a). The emergence of mind and emotion in the evolution of neocortex. *Rivista Di Psichiatria*, *46*(5–6), 281–7. doi:10.1708/1009.10972; 10.1708/1009.10972

Freeman, W. J. (2011b). Understanding perception through neural "codes." *IEEE Transactions on Bio-Medical Engineering*, *58*(7), 1884–90. doi:10.1109/TBME.2010.2095854

Fries, P., Reynolds, J. H., Rorie, A. E., & Desimone, R. (2001). Modulation of oscillatory neuronal synchronization by selective visual attention. *Science*, *291*(5508), 1560–3. doi:10.1126/science.291.5508.1560

Fries, P. (2005). A mechanism for cognitive dynamics: Neuronal communication through neuronal coherence. *Trends in Cognitive Sciences*, *9*(10), 474–80. doi:10.1016/j.tics.2005.08.011

Fries, P., Reynolds, J. H., Rorie, A. E., & Desimone, R. (2001). Modulation of oscillatory neuronal synchronization by selective visual attention. *Science*, *291*(5508), 1560–3. doi:10.1126/science.291.5508.1560

Fries, Pascal. (2005). A mechanism for cognitive dynamics: neuronal communication through neuronal coherence. *Trends in Cognitive Sciences*, *9*(10), 474–80. doi:10.1016/j.tics.2005.08.011

Friston, K. (2010). The free-energy principle: a unified brain theory? *Nature Reviews Neuroscience*, *11*(2), 127–38.

Friston, K. J. (1995). Neuronal transients. *Proceedings of the Royal Society of London Series B: Biological Sciences*, *261*(1362), 401–5. doi:10.1098/rspb.1995.0166

Frith, C., & Frith, U. (2008). Implicit and explicit processes in social cognition. *Neuron*, *60*(3), 503–10.

Frith, C., Perry, R., & Lumer, E. (1999). The neural correlates of conscious experience: an experimental framework. *Trends in Cognitive Sciences*, *3*(3), 105–14. Retrieved from http://www.ncbi.nlm.nih.gov/pubmed/10322462

Fu, C., & McGuire, P. K. (2003). *Hearing voices or hearing the self in disguise? Revealing the neural correlates of auditory hallucinations in schizophrenia. The self in neuroscience and psychiatry.* Cambridge University Press. Cambridge/UK

Fuchs, T. (2007a). *Das Gehirn—ein Beziehungsorgan. Eine Phänomenologisch-ökologische konzeption.* Kohlhammer Publisher in Stuttgart/Germany

Fuchs, T. (2011). *Das Relationale Gehirn—Ein Beziehungsorgan.* Stuttgart: Kohlhammer.

Fuchs, Thomas. (2007b). The temporal structure of intentionality and its disturbance in schizophrenia. *Psychopathology, 40*(4), 229–35. doi:10.1159/000101365

Fuster, J. M. (1997). *The prefrontal cortex: Anatomy, physiology, and neuropsychology of the frontal lobe.* Philadelphia, PA: Lippincott-Raven.

Fuster, J. M. (2003). *Cortex and mind: Unifying cognition.* Oxford, England: Oxford University Press.

Gadenne, V. (1996). *Bewusstsein, Kognition und Gehirn Erscheinungsjahr.* Bern, Switzerland: Huber.

Gallagher, H. L., & Frith, C. D. (2003). Functional imaging of "theory of mind." *Trends in Cognitive Science, 7*(2), 77–83.

Gallagher, I. I. (2000). Philosophical conceptions of the self: Implications for cognitive science. *Trends in Cognitive Science, 4*(1), 14–21.

Gallagher, S. (1998). *The inordinance of time.* Evanston, Ill.: Northwestern University Press.

Gallagher, S. (2007). Phenomenological approaches to consciousness. In M. Vemans & S. Schendier (Eds.), *Blackwell companion to consciousness* (pp. 134–56). Oxford, England: Blackwell.

Garrett, D. D., Kovacevic, N., McIntosh, A. R., & Grady, C. L. (2011). The importance of being variable. *Journal of Neuroscience, 31*(12), 4496–503. doi:10.1523/JNEUROSCI.5641-10.2011

Garrido, M. I., Friston, K. J., Kiebel, S. J., Stephan, K. E., Baldeweg, T., & Kilner, J. M. (2008). The functional anatomy of the MMN: a DCM study of the roving paradigm. *NeuroImage, 42*(2), 936–44. doi:10.1016/j.neuroimage.2008.05.018

Garrido, M. I., Kilner, J. M., Kiebel, S. J., & Friston, K. J. (2009a). Dynamic causal modeling of the response to frequency deviants. *Journal of Neurophysiology, 101*(5), 2620–31. doi:10.1152/jn.90291.2008

Garrido, M. I., Kilner, J. M., Kiebel, S. J., Stephan, K. E., Baldeweg, T., & Friston, K. J. (2009b). Repetition suppression and plasticity in the human brain. *NeuroImage, 48*(1), 269–79. doi:10.1016/j.neuroimage.2009.06.034

Garrido, M. I., Kilner, J. M., Stephan, K. E., & Friston, K. J. (2009). The mismatch

negativity: A review of underlying mechanisms. *Clinical Neurophysiology, 120*(3), 453–63.

Gillihan, S. J., & Farah, M. J. (2005). Is self special? A critical review of evidence from experimental psychology and cognitive neuroscience. *Psychology Bulletin, 131*(1), 76–97.

Goel, V., & Dolan, R. J. (2003). Explaining modulation of reasoning by belief. *Cognition, 87*(1), B11–22.

Goldberg, I. I., Harel, M., & Malach, R. (2006). When the brain loses its self: Prefrontal inactivation during sensorimotor processing. *Neuron, 50*(2), 329–39. doi:10.1016/j.neuron.2006.03.015

Golland, Y., Bentin, S., Gelbard, H., Benjamini, Y., Heller, R., Nir, Y., et al. (2007). Extrinsic and intrinsic systems in the posterior cortex of the human brain revealed during natural sensory stimulation. *Cerebral Cortex, 17*(4), 766–77. doi:10.1093/cercor/bhk030

Golomb, J. D., McDavitt, J. R., Ruf, B. M., Chen, J. I., Saricicek, A., Maloney, K. H., et al. (2009). Enhanced visual motion perception in major depressive disorder. *Journal of Neuroscience, 29*(28), 9072–77. doi:10.1523/JNEUROSCI.1003-09.2009

Gonzalez-Burgos, G., & Lewis, D. A. (2008). GABA neurons and the mechanisms of network oscillations: Implications for understanding cortical dysfunction in schizophrenia. *Schizophrenia Bulletin, 34*(5), 944–61. doi:10.1093/schbul/sbn070

Gonzalez-Burgos, G., & Lewis, D. A. (2012). NMDA receptor hypofunction, parvalbumin-positive neurons, and cortical gamma oscillations in schizophrenia. *Schizophrenia Bulletin, 38*(5), 950–7. doi:10.1093/schbul/sbs010

Gonzalez-Burgos, G., Fish, K. N., & Lewis, D. A. (2011). GABA neuron alterations, cortical circuit dysfunction and cognitive deficits in schizophrenia. *Neural Plasticity, 2011*, 723184. doi:10.1155/2011/723184

Graziano, M. S., & Kastner, S. (2011). Human consciousness and its relationship to social neuroscience: A novel hypothesis. *Cognitive Neuroscience, 2*(2), 98–113. doi:10.1080/17588928.2011.565121

Greicius, M. D., Flores, B. H., Menon, V., Glover, G. H., Solvason, H. B., Kenna, H., et al. (2007). Resting-state functional connectivity in major depression: Abnormally increased contributions from subgenual cingulate cortex and thalamus. *Biological Psychiatry, 62*(5), 429–37.

Greicius, M. D., Kiviniemi, V., Tervonen, O., Vainionpaa, V., Alahuhta, S., Reiss, A. L., &

Menon, V. (2008). Persistent default-mode network connectivity during light sedation. *Human Brain Mapping*, 29(7), 839–47. doi:10.1002/hbm.20537

Greicius, M. D., Supekar, K., Menon, V., & Dougherty, R. F. (2009). Resting-state functional connectivity reflects structural connectivity in the default mode network. *Cerebral Cortex*, 19(1), 72–8.

Grimm, S., Beck, J., Schuepbach, D., Hell, D., Boesiger, P., Bermpohl, F., Niehaus, L., et al. (2008). Imbalance between left and right dorsolateral prefrontal cortex in major depression is linked to negative emotional judgment: an fMRI study in severe major depressive disorder. *Biological Psychiatry*, 63(4), 369–76. doi:10.1016/j.biopsych.2007.05.033

Grimm, S., Boesiger, P., Beck, J., Schuepbach, D., Bermpohl, F., Walter, M., Ernst, J., et al. (2009). Altered negative BOLD responses in the default-mode network during emotion processing in depressed subjects. *Neuropsychopharmacology*, 34(4), 932–843. doi:10.1038/npp.2008.81

Grimm, S., Ernst, J., Boesiger, P., Schuepbach, D., Boeker, H., & Northoff, G. (2011). Reduced negative BOLD responses in the default-mode network and increased self-focus in depression. *World Journal of Biological Psychiatry*, 12(8), 627–637. doi:10.3109/15622975.2010.545145

Grimm, S., Ernst, J., Boesiger, P., Schuepbach, D., Hell, D., Boeker, H., & Northoff, G. (2009). Increased self-focus in major depressive disorder is related to neural abnormalities in subcortical-cortical midline structures. *Human Brain Mapping*, 30(8), 2617–27. doi:10.1002/hbm.20693

Grimm, S., Schmidt, C. F., Bermpohl, F., Heinzel, A., Dahlem, Y., Wyss, M., et al. (2006). Segregated neural representation of distinct emotion dimensions in the prefrontal cortex-an fMRI study. *NeuroImage*, 30(1), 325–40. doi:10.1016/j.neuroimage.2005.09.006

Gruberger, M., Ben-Simon, E., Levkovitz, Y., Zangen, A., & Hendler, T. (2011). Towards a neuroscience of mind-wandering. *Frontiers in Human Neuroscience*, 5, 56. doi:10.3389/fnhum.2011.00056

Grush, R. (2005). Internal models and the construction of time: Generalizing from state estimation to trajectory estimation to address temporal features of perception, including temporal illusions. *Journal of Neural Engineering*, 2(3), S209–18. doi:10.1088/1741-2560/2/3/S05

Guller, Y., Tononi, G., & Postle, B. R. (2012). Conserved functional connectivity but impaired effective connectivity of thalamocortical circuitry in schizophrenia. *Brain Connectivity*, 2(6), 311–9. doi:10.1089/brain.2012.0100

Gusnard, D. A., Akbudak, E., Shulman, G. L., & Raichle, M. E. (2001). Medial prefrontal cortex and self-referential mental activity: Relation to a default mode of brain function. *Proceedings of the National Academy of Sciences USA*, 98(7), 4259–64.

Haggard, P. (2008). Human volition: Towards a neuroscience of will. *Nature Reviews. Neuroscience*, 9(12), 934–46. doi:10.1038/nrn2497

Hamm, J. P., Gilmore, C. S., Picchetti, N. A., Sponheim, S. R., & Clementz, B. A. (2011). Abnormalities of neuronal oscillations and temporal integration to low- and high-frequency auditory stimulation in schizophrenia. *Biological Psychiatry*, 69(10), 989–96. doi:10.1016/j.biopsych.2010.11.021

Han, S., & Northoff, G. (2008). Culture-sensitive neural substrates of human cognition: a transcultural neuroimaging approach. *Nature Reviews Neuroscience*, 9(8), 646–54. doi:10.1038/nrn2456

Han, S., Northoff, G., Vogeley, K., Wexler, B. E., Kitayama, S., Varnum, M. E. (2013). A cultural neuroscience approach to the biosocial nature of the human brain. *Annual Review of Psychology*, 64, 335–59. doi: 10.1146/annurev-psych-071112-054629. Epub 2012 Sep 17. Review.

Hasler, G., & Northoff, G. (2011). Discovering imaging endophenotypes for major depression. *Molecular Psychiatry*, 16(6), 604–19. doi:10.1038/mp.2011.23

Hasler, Gregor, Van der Veen, J. W., Tumonis, T., Meyers, N., Shen, J., & Drevets, W. C. (2007). Reduced prefrontal glutamate/glutamine and gamma-aminobutyric acid levels in major depression determined using proton magnetic resonance spectroscopy. *Archives of General Psychiatry*, 64(2), 193–200. doi:10.1001/archpsyc.64.2.193

Hasson, U., Ghazanfar, A. A., Galantucci, B., Garrod, S., & Keysers, C. (2012). Brain-to-brain coupling: a mechanism for creating and sharing a social world. *Trends in Cognitive Sciences*, 16(2), 114–21. doi:10.1016/j.tics.2011.12.007

Hasson, U., Nir, Y., Levy, I., Fuhrmann, G., & Malach, R. (2004). Intersubject synchronization of cortical activity during natural vision.

Science, *303*(5664), 1634–40. doi:10.1126/science.1089506

Hayes, D. J., & Northoff, G. (2011). Identifying a network of brain regions involved in aversion-related processing: A cross-species translational investigation. *Frontiers in Integrative Neuroscience*, *5*, 49. doi:10.3389/fnint.2011.00049

Hayes, D. J., & Northoff, G. (2012). Common brain activations for painful and nonpainful aversive stimuli. *BMC Neuroscience*, *13*(1), 60. doi:10.1186/1471-2202-13-60

Haynes, J. D. (2009). Decoding visual consciousness from human brain signals. *Trends in Cognitive Sciences*, *13*(5), 194–202. doi:10.1016/j.tics.2009.02.004

Haynes, J. D. (2011). Decoding and predicting intentions. *Annals of the New York Academy of Sciences*, *1224*, 9–21. doi:10.1111/j.1749-6632.2011.05994.x; 10.1111/j.1749-6632.2011.05994.x

He, B. J., & Raichle, M. E. (2009). The fMRI signal, slow cortical potential and consciousness. *Trends in Cognitive Sciences*, *13*(7), 302–9. doi:10.1016/j.tics.2009.04.004

He, B. J., Snyder, A. Z., Zempel, J. M., Smyth, M. D., & Raichle, M. E. (2008). Electrophysiological correlates of the brain's intrinsic large-scale functional architecture. *Proceedings of the National Academy of Sciences USA*, *105*(41), 16039–44. doi:10.1073/pnas.0807010105

He, B. J., Zempel, J. M., Snyder, A. Z., & Raichle, M. E. (2010). The temporal structures and functional significance of scale-free brain activity. *Neuron*, *66*(3), 353–69. doi:10.1016/j.neuron.2010.04.020

Heinzel, A., & Northoff, G. (2009a). Emotional feeling and the orbitomedial prefrontal cortex: Theoretical and empirical considerations. *Philosophical Psychology*, *22*(4), 443–64.

Heinzel, A., Bermpohl, F., Niese, R., Pfennig, A., Pascual-Leone, A., Schlaug, G., & Northoff, G. (2005). How do we modulate our emotions? Parametric fMRI reveals cortical midline structures as regions specifically involved in the processing of emotional valences. *Brain Research. Cognitive Brain Research*, *25*(1), 348–58. doi:10.1016/j.cogbrainres.2005.06.009

Heinzel, A., Grimm, S., Beck, J., Schuepbach, D., Hell, D., Boesiger, P., et al. (2009). Segregated neural representation of psychological and somatic-vegetative symptoms in severe major depression. *Neuroscience Letters*, *456*(2), 49–53.

Heinzel, A., Steinke, R., Poeppel, T. D., Grosser, O., Bogerts, B., Otto, H., & Northoff, G. (2008). S-ketamine and GABA-A-receptor interaction in humans: an exploratory study with I-123-iomazenil SPECT. *Human Psychopharmacology*, *23*(7), 549–54. doi:10.1002/hup.960

Heiss, W.-D. (2012). PET in coma and in vegetative state. *European Journal of Neurology*, *19*(2), 207–11. doi:10.1111/j.1468-1331.2011.03489.x

Herbert, C., Herbert, B. M., Ethofer, T., & Pauli, P. (2011). His or mine? The time course of self-other discrimination in emotion processing. *Social Neuroscience*, *6*(3), 277–88. doi:10.1080/17470919.2010.523543

Hesselmann, G., Kell, C. A., & Kleinschmidt, A. (2008b). Ongoing activity fluctuations in hMT+ bias the perception of coherent visual motion. *Journal of Neuroscience*, *28*(53), 14481–5. doi:10.1523/JNEUROSCI.4398-08.2008

Hesselmann, G., Kell, C. A., Eger, E., & Kleinschmidt, A. (2008a). Spontaneous local variations in ongoing neural activity bias perceptual decisions. *Proceedings of the National Academy of Sciences USA*, *105*(31), 10984–9. doi:10.1073/pnas.0712043105

Hipp, J. F., Engel, A. K., & Siegel, M. (2011). Oscillatory synchronization in large-scale cortical networks predicts perception. *Neuron*, *69*(2), 387–96. doi:10.1016/j.neuron.2010.12.027

Hobson, J. A. (2009). REM sleep and dreaming: Towards a theory of protoconsciousness. *Nature Reviews Neuroscience*, *10*(11), 803–13. doi:10.1038/nrn2716

Hobson, J. A., & Friston, K. J. (2012). Waking and dreaming consciousness: neurobiological and functional considerations. *Progress in Neurobiology*, *98*(1), 82–98. doi:10.1016/j.pneurobio.2012.05.003

Hoffman, R. E. (2007). A social deafferentation hypothesis for induction of active schizophrenia. *Schizophrenia Bulletin*, *33*(5), 1066–70. doi:10.1093/schbul/sbm079

Hoffman, R. E. (2010). Revisiting Arieti's 'listening attitude' and hallucinated voices. *Schizophrenia Bulletin*, *36*(3), 440–2.

Hoffman, R. E., Anderson, A. W., Varanko, M., Gore, J. C., & Hampson, M. (2008). Time course of regional brain activation associated with onset of auditory/verbal hallucinations. *British Journal of Psychiatry*, *193*(5), 424–5.

Hoffman, R. E., Hampson, M., Wu, K., Anderson, A. W., Gore, J. C., Buchanan, R. J., et al. (2007).

Probing the pathophysiology of auditory/verbal hallucinations by combining functional magnetic resonance imaging and transcranial magnetic stimulation. *Cerebral Cortex 17*(11), 2733–43.

Hohwy, J. (2009). The neural correlates of consciousness: new experimental approaches needed? *Consciousness and Cognition, 18*(2), 428–38. doi:10.1016/j.concog.2009.02.006

Hohwy, J. (2012). Neural correlates and causal mechanisms. *Consciousness and Cognition, 21*(2), 691–2; author reply 693–4, doi:10.1016/j.concog.2011.06.006

Hohwy, J. (2012). Preserved aspects of consciousness in disorders of consciousness: A review and conceptual analysis. *Journal of Consciousness Studies, 19*(3–4), 87–120.

Holeckova, I., Fischer, C., Morlet, D., Delpuech, C., Costes, N., & Mauguière, F. (2008). Subject's own name as a novel in a MMN design: a combined ERP and PET study. *Brain Research, 1189*, 152–65. doi:10.1016/j.brainres.2007.10.091

Hoeller, Y., Kronbichler, M., Bergmann, J., Crone, J. S., Ladurner, G., & Golaszewski, S. (2011). EEG frequency analysis of responses to the own-name stimulus. *Clinical Neurophysiology, 122*(1), 99–106. doi:10.1016/j.clinph.2010.05.029

Hoeller, Y., Kronbichler, M., Bergmann, J., Crone, J. S., Schmid, E. V., Golaszewski, S., & Ladurner, G. (2011). Inter-individual variability of oscillatory responses to subject's own name. A single-subject analysis. *International Journal of Psychophysiology, 80*(3), 227–35. doi:10.1016/j.ijpsycho.2011.03.012

Holt, D. J., Cassidy, B. S., Andrews-Hanna, J. R., Lee, S. M., Coombs, G., Goff, D. C., Gabrieli, J. D., et al. (2011). An anterior-to-posterior shift in midline cortical activity in schizophrenia during self-reflection. *Biological Psychiatry, 69*(5), 415–23. doi:10.1016/j.biopsych.2010.10.003

Honey, C. J., Thesen, T., Donner, T. H., Silbert, L. J., Carlson, C. E., Devinsky, O., Doyle, W. K., et al. (2012). Slow cortical dynamics and the accumulation of information over long timescales. *Neuron, 76*(2), 423–34. doi:10.1016/j.neuron.2012.08.011

Hong, L. E., Summerfelt, A., Buchanan, R. W., O'Donnell, P., Thaker, G. K., Weiler, M. A., & Lahti, A. C. (2010). Gamma and delta neural oscillations and association with clinical symptoms under subanesthetic ketamine. *Neuropsychopharmacology, 35*(3), 632–40. doi:10.1038/npp.2009.168

Hoptman, M. J., Zuo, X. N., Butler, P. D., Javitt, D. C., D'Angelo, D., Mauro, C. J., & Milham, M. P. (2010). Amplitude of low-frequency oscillations in schizophrenia: A resting state fMRI study. *Schizophrenia Research, 117*(1), 13–20. doi:10.1016/j.schres.2009.09.030

Howard, M. F., & Poeppel, D. (2010). Discrimination of speech stimuli based on neuronal response phase patterns depends on acoustics but not comprehension. *Journal of Neurophysiology, 104*(5), 2500–11. doi:10.1152/jn.00251.2010

Hu, Z., Liu, H., Weng, X., & Northoff, G. (2012). Is there a valence-specific pattern in emotional conflict in major depressive disorder? An exploratory psychological study. *PloS One, 7*(2), e31983. doi:10.1371/journal.pone.0031983

Huang, Z., Wuhei, X., Weng X, Laureys S, Northoff, G. (2013). The self and its resting state in consciousness: An exploratory investigation in vegetative state. *Human Brain Mapping*, in press

Hume, D. (1739/1888). *A Treatise of Human Nature.* ed. L Selby-Bigge. Oxford: Oxford University Press.

Hunter, M. D., Eickhoff, S. B., Miller, T. W. R., Farrow, T. F. D., Wilkinson, I. D., & Woodruff, P. W. R. (2006). Neural activity in speech-sensitive auditory cortex during silence. *Proceedings of the National Academy of Sciences USA, 103*(1), 189–94. doi:10.1073/pnas.0506268103

Hurley, S. L. (1998). *Consciousness in action.* Cambridge, MA: Harvard University Press.

Husserl, E. (1929/1960). *Cartesian Meditations: an Introduction to Phenomenology.* Translated by Dorian Cairns. The Hague: M. Nijhoff.

Husserl, E. (1977). *Cartesian meditations: An introduction to phenomenology.* The Hague, The Netherlands: Nijhoff.

Husserl, E (1990) *On the Phenomenology of the Consciousness of Internal Time (1893–1917),* Translated by J. B. Brough, Dordrecht: Kluwer.

Hyder, F., Fulbright, R. K., Shulman, R. G., & Rothman, D. L. (2013). Glutamatergic function in the resting awake human brain is supported by uniformly high oxidative energy. *Journal of Cerebral Blood Flow and Metabolism.* doi:10.1038/jcbfm.2012.207

Hyder, F., Patel, A. B., Gjedde, A., Rothman, D. L., Behar, K. L., & Shulman, R. G. (2006). Neuronal-glial glucose oxidation and glutamatergic-GABAergic function. *Journal of Cerebral Blood Flow and Metabolism, 26*(7), 865–77. doi:10.1038/sj.jcbfm.9600263 1), 6–41.

Ingram, R. E. (1990). Self-focused attention in clinical disorders: Review and a conceptual model. *Psychology Bulletin, 107*(2), 156–76.

Ionta, S., Gassert, R., & Blanke, O. (2011a). Multi-sensory and sensorimotor foundation of bodily self-consciousness—an interdisciplinary approach. *Frontiers in Psychology, 2*, 383. doi:10.3389/fpsyg.2011.00383

Ionta, S., Heydrich, L., Lenggenhager, B., Mouthon, M., Fornari, E., Chapuis, D., et al. (2011b). Multisensory mechanisms in temporo-parietal cortex support self-location and first-person perspective. *Neuron, 70*(2), 363–74. doi:10.1016/j.neuron.2011.03.009

Jafri, M. J., Pearlson, G. D., Stevens, M., & Calhoun, V. D. (2008). A method for functional network connectivity among spatially independent resting-state components in schizophrenia. *Neuroimage, 39*(4), 1666–81.

James, W. (1890). *The Principles of Psychology* (Vols. 1–2). London: Macmillan.

Jaspers, K. (1963). *General Psychopathology.* Chicago, IL: University of Chicago Press.

Javitt, D. C. (2009a). Sensory processing in schizophrenia: neither simple nor intact. *Schizophrenia Bulletin, 35*(6), 1059–64. doi:10.1093/schbul/sbp110

Javitt, D. C. (2009b). When doors of perception close: Bottom-up models of disrupted cognition in psychosis. *Annual Review of Clinical Psychology, 5*, 249–75.

John, E. R. (2005). From synchronous neuronal discharges to subjective awareness? *Progress in Brain Research, 150*, 143–71. doi:10.1016/S0079-6123(05)50011-6

Kahan, T. L., & LaBerge, S. P. (2011). Dreaming and waking: Similarities and differences revisited. *Consciousness and Cognition, 20*(3), 494–514. doi:10.1016/j.concog.2010.09.002

Kant, I. (1787/1929). *Critique of Pure Reason.* Translated by N. Kemp Smith. New York: MacMillan.

Kant, I. (1998). *Critique of pure reason.* Translated by Guyer, P. & Wood, A. Cambridge, England: Cambridge University Press.

Kant, I. (1977). *Prolegomena to any future metaphysics that will Be able to Come forward as Science: The Paul Carus Translation.* Translated by Carus, P., & Ellington, J. W. Indianapolis, IN: Hackett.

Kaufmann, C., Wehrle, R., Wetter, T. C., Holsboer, F., Auer, D. P., Pollmacher, T., & Czisch, M. (2006). Brain activation and hypothalamic functional connectivity during human non-rapid eye movement sleep: An EEG/fMRI study. *Brain, 129*(Pt 3), 655–67. doi:10.1093/brain/awh686

Kay, B. P., Difrancesco, M. W., Privitera, M. D., Gotman, J., Holland, S. K., & Szaflarski, J. P. (2013). Reduced default mode network connectivity in treatment-resistant idiopathic generalized epilepsy. *Epilepsia.* doi:10.1111/epi.12057

Keedwell, P. A., Andrew, C., Williams, S. C., Brammer, M. J., & Phillips, M. L. (2005). The neural correlates of anhedonia in major depressive disorder. *Biological Psychiatry, 58*(11), 843–53.

Keedwell, P. A., Drapier, D., Surguladze, S., Giampietro, V., Brammer, M., & Phillips, M. (2010). Subgenual cingulate and visual cortex responses to sad faces predict clinical outcome during antidepressant treatment for depression. *Journal of Affective Disorders, 120*(1–3), 120–5. doi:10.1016/j.jad.2009.04.031

Keenan, J. P., Wheeler, M., Platek, S. M., Lardi, G., & Lassonde, M. (2003). Self-face processing in a callosotomy patient. *European Journal of Neuroscience, 18*(8), 2391–5.

Kelley, W. (2005). The puzzle of temporal experience. In A. Brook & K. Akins (Eds.), *Cognition and neuroscience* (pp. 156–75). Cambridge, England: Cambridge University Press.

Kelley, W. M., Macrae, C. N., Wyland, C. L., Caglar, S., Inati, S., & Heatherton, T. F. (2002). Finding the self? An event-related fMRI study. *Journal of Cognitive Neuroscience, 14*(5), 785–94.

Khader, P., Schicke, T., Röder, B., & Rösler, F. (2008). On the relationship between slow cortical potentials and BOLD signal changes in humans. *International Journal of Psychophysiology, 67*(3), 252–61. doi:10.1016/j.ijpsycho.2007.05.018

Khalsa, S. S., Rudrauf, D., Feinstein, J. S., & Tranel, D. (2009). The pathways of interoceptive awareness. *Nature Neuroscience, 12*(12), 1494–6. doi:10.1038/nn.2411

Kim, D. I., Manoach, D. S., Mathalon, D. H., Turner, J. A., Mannell, M., Brown, G. G., et al. (2009). Dysregulation of working memory and default-mode networks in schizophrenia using independent component analysis, an fBIRN and MCIC study. *Human Brain Mapping, 30*(11), 3795–811.

Kircher, T., & David, A. (2003). *The self in neuroscience and psychiatry.* Cambridge, England: Cambridge University Press.

Kirshner, L. A. (1991). The concept of the self in psychoanalytic theory and its philosophical foundations.

Journal of the American Psychoanalysis Association, 39(1), 157–82.

Kitcher, P. (1992). The naturalists return. *Philosophical Review, 101*(1), 53–114.

Kitcher, P. (2010) *Kant's Thinker*. Oxford: Oxford University Press.

Kjaer, T. W., Nowak, M., & Lou, H. C. (2002). Reflective self-awareness and conscious states: PET evidence for a common midline parietofrontal core. *NeuroImage, 17*(2), 1080–6. Retrieved from http://www.ncbi.nlm.nih.gov/pubmed/12377180

Klein, S. B. (2012). Self, memory, and the self-reference effect: An examination of conceptual and methodological issues. *Personality and Social Psychology Review, 16*(3), 283–300. doi:10.1177/1088868311434214

Klein, S. B., & Gangi, C. E. (2010). The multiplicity of self: Neuropsychological evidence and its implications for the self as a construct in psychological research. *Annals of the New York Academy of Sciences, 1191*, 1–15. doi:10.1111/j.1749–6632.2010.05441.x

Kleinschmidt, A. (2011). [Recovering the contents of consciousness in the noise of neuroimaging]. *Médecine Sciences: M/S, 27*(2), 199–203. doi:10.1051/medsci/2011272199

Kleinschmidt, A., Sterzer, P., & Rees, G. (2012). Variability of perceptual multistability: from brain state to individual trait. *Philosophical Transactions of the Royal Society of London. Series B, Biological Sciences, 367*(1591), 988–1000. doi:10.1098/rstb.2011.0367

Klimesch, W., Freunberger, R., & Sauseng, P. (2010). Oscillatory mechanisms of process binding in memory. *Neuroscience and Biobehavioral Reviews, 34*(7), 1002–14. doi:10.1016/j.neubiorev.2009.10.004

Koch, C. (2004). *The quest for consciousness: A neurobiological approach*. Engelwood, CO: Roberts.

Koch, C. (2009). The SCP is not specific enough to represent conscious content. *Trends in Cognitive Sciences, 13*(9), 367; author reply 368–9. doi:10.1016/j.tics.2009.07.002

Koch, C., & Tsuchiya, N. (2012). Attention and consciousness: Related yet different. *Trends in Cognitive Sciences, 16*(2), 103–5. doi:10.1016/j.tics.2011.11.012

Kokal, I., Engel, A., Kirschner, S., & Keysers, C. (2011). Synchronized drumming enhances activity in the caudate and facilitates prosocial commitment—if the rhythm comes easily. *PloS One, 6*(11), e27272. doi:10.1371/journal.pone.0027272

Kouider, S., & Dehaene, S. (2007). Levels of processing during non-conscious perception: a critical review of visual masking. *Philosophical Transactions of the Royal Society of London. Series B, Biological Sciences, 362*(1481), 857–75. doi:10.1098/rstb.2007.2093

Kouider, S., & Dehaene, S. (2009). Subliminal number priming within and across the visual and auditory modalities. *Experimental Psychology, 56*(6), 418–33. doi:10.1027/1618–3169.56.6.418

Kouider, S., De Gardelle, V., Sackur, J., & Dupoux, E. (2010). How rich is consciousness? The partial awareness hypothesis. *Trends in Cognitive Sciences, 14*(7), 301–7. doi:10.1016/j.tics.2010.04.006

Kraepelin, E. (1913). *Ein lehrbuch fur Studierende und arzte*. Leipzig, Germany: Barth.

Kühn, S., & Gallinat, J. (2013). Resting-State Brain Activity in Schizophrenia and Major Depression: A Quantitative Meta-Analysis. *Schizophrenia Bulletin, 39*(2), 358–65. doi: 10.1093/schbul/sbr151. Epub 2011 Nov 10.

Lakatos, P., Chen, C. M., O'Connell, M. N., Mills, A., & Schroeder, C. E. (2007). Neuronal oscillations and multisensory interaction in primary auditory cortex. *Neuron, 53*(2), 279–92. doi:10.1016/j.neuron.2006.12.011

Lakatos, P., Karmos, G., Mehta, A. D., Ulbert, I., & Schroeder, C. E. (2008). Entrainment of neuronal oscillations as a mechanism of attentional selection. *Science, 320*(5872), 110–3. doi:10.1126/science.1154735

Lakatos, P., O'Connell, M. N., Barczak, A., Mills, A., Javitt, D. C., & Schroeder, C. E. (2009). The leading sense: supramodal control of neurophysiological context by attention. *Neuron, 64*(3), 419–30. doi:10.1016/j.neuron.2009.10.014

Lakatos, P., Pincze, Z., Fu, K. M., Javitt, D. C., Karmos, G., & Schroeder, C. E. (2005a). Timing of pure tone and noise-evoked responses in macaque auditory cortex. *Neuroreport, 16*(9), 933–7.

Lakatos, P., Shah, A. S., Knuth, K. H., Ulbert, I., Karmos, G., & Schroeder, C. E. (2005b). An oscillatory hierarchy controlling neuronal excitability and stimulus processing in the auditory cortex. *Journal of Neurophysiology, 94*(3), 1904–11. doi:10.1152/jn.00263.2005

Lambie, J. A., & Marcel, A. J. (2002). Consciousness and the varieties of emotion experience: A theoretical framework. *Psychology Review, 109*(2), 219–59.

Lamm, C., & Singer, T. (2010). The role of anterior insular cortex in social emotions. *Brain*

Structure and Function, *214*(5–6), 579–91. doi:10.1007/s00429-010-0251-3

Lamme, V. A. (2006). Towards a true neural stance on consciousness. *Trends in Cognitive Sciences*, *10*(11), 494–501. doi:10.1016/j.tics.2006.09.001

Lamme, V. A., & Roelfsema, P. R. (2000). The distinct modes of vision offered by feedforward and recurrent processing. *Trends in Neurosciences*, *23*(11), 571–9.

Landsness, E., Bruno, M. A., Noirhomme, Q., Riedner, B., Gosseries, O., Schnakers, C., et al. Electrophysiological correlates of behavioural changes in vigilance in vegetative state and minimally conscious state. *Brain*, *134*(Pt. 8), 2222–32. doi:10.1093/brain/awr152

Lau, H., Rosenthal, D. (2012). Empirical support for higher-order theories of conscious awareness. *Trends in Cognitive Sciences*, *15*(8), 365–73. doi: 10.1016/j.tics.2011.05.009. Epub 2011 Jul 6. Review.

Långsjö, J. W., Alkire, M. T., Kaskinoro, K., Hayama, H., Maksimow, A., Kaisti, K. K., Aalto, S., et al. (2012). Returning from oblivion: imaging the neural core of consciousness. *The Journal of Neuroscience*, *32*(14), 4935–43. doi:10.1523/JNEUROSCI.4962-11.2012

Langston, R. F., Ainge, J. A., Couey, J. J., Canto, C. B., Bjerknes, T. L., Witter, M. P., et al. (2010). Development of the spatial representation system in the rat. *Science*, *328*(5985), 1576–80. doi:10.1126/science.1188210

Larson-Prior, L. J., Zempel, J. M., Nolan, T. S., Prior, F. W., Snyder, A. Z., & Raichle, M. E. (2009). Cortical network functional connectivity in the descent to sleep. *Proceedings of the National Academy of Sciences USA*, *106*(11), 4489–94. doi:10.1073/pnas.0900924106

Lau, H. C. (2008). A higher order Bayesian decision theory of consciousness. *Progress in Brain Research*, *168*, 35–48. doi:10.1016/S0079-6123(07)68004-2

Laureys, S., Perrin, F., Faymonville, M.-E., Schnakers, C., Boly, M., Bartsch, V., Majerus, S., et al. (2004). Cerebral processing in the minimally conscious state. *Neurology*, *63*(5), 916–8. Retrieved from http://www.ncbi.nlm.nih.gov/pubmed/15365150

Laureys, S., & Schiff, N. D. (2012). Coma and consciousness: Paradigms (re)framed by neuroimaging. *NeuroImage*, *61*(2), 478–91. doi:10.1016/j.neuroimage.2011.12.041

Laureys, S., Faymonville, M. E., De Tiege, X., Peigneux, P., Berre, J., Moonen, G., et al.

(2004a). Brain function in the vegetative state. *Advances in Experimental Medicine and Biology*, *550*, 229–38.

Laureys, S., Owen, A. M., & Schiff, N. D. (2004b). Brain function in coma, vegetative state, and related disorders. *Lancet Neurology*, *3*(9), 537–46. doi:10.1016/S1474-4422(04)00852-X

Laureys, S., Perrin, F., Faymonville, M. E., Schnakers, C., Boly, M., Bartsch, V., et al. (2004c). Cerebral processing in the minimally conscious state. *Neurology*, *63*(5), 916–8.

Laureys, S., Perrin, F., Schnakers, C., Boly, M., & Majerus, S. (2005). Residual cognitive function in comatose, vegetative and minimally conscious states. *Current Opinion in Neurology*, *18*(6), 726–33.

Laureys, Steven. (2005a). Science and society: death, unconsciousness and the brain. *Nature Reviews Neuroscience*, *6*(11), 899–909. doi:10.1038/nrn1789

Laureys, Steven. (2005b). The neural correlate of (un)awareness: lessons from the vegetative state. *Trends in Cognitive Sciences*, *9*(12), 556–9. doi:10.1016/j.tics.2005.10.010

Le Doux, J. (2002). *Synaptic self: How our brains become who we are*. New York: Viking.

Legrand, D. (2007a). Pre-reflective self-as-subject from experiential and empirical perspectives. *Consciousness and Cognition*, *16*(3), 583–99. doi:10.1016/j.concog.2007.04.002

Legrand, D. (2007b). Subjectivity and the body: Introducing basic forms of self-consciousness. *Consciousness and Cognition*, *16*(3), 577–82. doi:10.1016/j.concog.2007.06.011

Legrand, D., & Ruby, P. (2009). What is self-specific? Theoretical investigation and critical review of neuroimaging results. *Psychology Review*, *116*(1), 252–82.

Lehmann, D. (2010). Multimodal analysis of resting state cortical activity: What does fMRI add to our knowledge of microstates in resting state EEG activity? Commentary to the papers by Britz et al. and Musso et al. in the current issue of *NeuroImage*. *NeuroImage*, *52*(4), 1173–4. doi:10.1016/j.neuroimage.2010.05.033

Lehmann, D., & Michel, C. M. (2011). EEG-defined functional microstates as basic building blocks of mental processes. *Clinical Neurophysiology*, *122*(6), 1073–4. doi:10.1016/j.clinph.2010.11.003

Lehmann, D., Strik, W. K., Henggeler, B., Koenig, T., & Koukkou, M. (1998). Brain electric microstates and momentary conscious mind states as building blocks of spontaneous thinking: I. Visual imagery and abstract thoughts. *International Journal of Psychophysiology, 29*(1), 1–11.

Lemogne, C., Bergouignan, L., Piolino, P., Jouvent, R., Allilaire, J. F., & Fossati, P. (2009a). Cognitive avoidance of intrusive memories and autobiographical memory: Specificity, autonoetic consciousness, and self-perspective. *Memory (Hove, England), 17*(1), 1–7. doi:10.1080/09658210802438466

Lemogne, C., Delaveau, P., Freton, M., Guionnet, S., & Fossati, P. (2012). Medial prefrontal cortex and the self in major depression. *Journal of Affective Disorders, 136*(1–2), e1–11. doi:10.1016/j.jad.2010.11.034

Lemogne, C., le Bastard, G., Mayberg, H., Volle, E., Bergouignan, L., Lehericy, S., et al. (2009b). In search of the depressive self: Extended medial prefrontal network during self-referential processing in major depression. *Social Cognitive and Affective Neuroscience, 4*(3), 305–12. doi:10.1093/scan/nsp008

Lemogne, C., Mayberg, H., Bergouignan, L., Volle, E., Delaveau, P., Lehericy, S., et al. (2010). Self-referential processing and the prefrontal cortex over the course of depression: A pilot study. *Journal of Affective Disorders, 124*(1–2), 196–201. doi:10.1016/j.jad.2009.11.003

Lennox, B. R., Park, S. B., Jones, P. B., & Morris, P. G. (1999). Spatial and temporal mapping of neural activity associated with auditory hallucinations. *Lancet, 353*(9153), 644.

Leopold, D. A., & Logothetis, N. K. (1999). Multistable phenomena: Changing views in perception. *Trends in Cognitive Sciences, 3*(7), 254–64.

Levine, J. (1983), Materialism and qualia: The explanatory gap. *Pacific Philosophical Quarterly, 64*, 354–61.

Levine, J. (1993). On leaving out what it is like. In M. Davis & G. Humphreys (Eds.), *Consciousness: Psychological and philosophical issues* (pp. 34–56). Oxford, England: Blackwell.

Lewis, D. A. (2009a). Brain volume changes in schizophrenia: How do they arise? What do they mean? *Psychological Medicine, 39*(11), 1779–80. doi:10.1017/S003329170900573X

Lewis, D. A. (2009b). Neuroplasticity of excitatory and inhibitory cortical circuits in schizophrenia. *Dialogues in Clinical Neuroscience, 11*(3), 269–80.

Lewis, D. A., & Gonzalez-Burgos, G. (2008). Neuroplasticity of neocortical circuits in schizophrenia. *Neuropsychopharmacology, 33*(1), 141–65.

Lewis, D. A., & Levitt, P. (2002). Psychosis as a disorder of neurodevelopment. *Annual Review of Neuroscience, 25*, 409–32.

Lewis, D. A., & Levitt, P. (2002). Schizophrenia as a disorder of neurodevelopment. *Annual Review of Neuroscience, 25*, 409–32. doi:10.1146/annur

Lewis, D. A., Curley, A. A., Glausier, J. R., & Volk, D. W. (2012). Cortical parvalbumin interneurons and cognitive dysfunction in schizophrenia. *Trends in Neurosciences, 35*(1), 57–67. doi:10.1016/j.tins.2011.10.004

Lewis, D. A., Hashimoto, T., & Volk, D. W. (2005). Cortical inhibitory neurons and schizophrenia. *Nature Reviews Neuroscience, 6*(4), 312–24.

Libet, B. (2004). *Mind time: The temporal factor in consciousness.* Cambridge Mass.: Harvard University Press. Retrieved from http://www.worldcat.org/title/mind-time-the-temporal-factor-in-consciousness/oclc/53330937&referer=brief_results

Libet, B. (2006). Reflections on the interaction of the mind and brain. *Progress in Neurobiology, 78*(3–5), 322–26. doi:10.1016/j.pneurobio.2006.02.003

Lindenberger, U., Li, S.-C., Gruber, W., & Müller, V. (2009). Brains swinging in concert: cortical phase synchronization while playing guitar. *BMC Neuroscience, 10*, 22. doi:10.1186/1471-2202-10-22

Lindquist, K. A., & Barrett, L. F. (2012). A functional architecture of the human brain: emerging insights from the science of emotion. *Trends in Cognitive Sciences, 16*(11), 533–40. doi:10.1016/j.tics.2012.09.005

Lipska, B. K., & Weinberger, D. R. (2000). To model a psychiatric disorder in animals: Schizophrenia as a reality test. *Neuropsychopharmacology, 23*(3), 223–39. doi:10.1016/S0893-133X(00)00137-8

Lipsman, N., Nakao, T., Kuehn A,. Lozano A., Bajbouj M., Northoff, G. (2013). Neurophysiologic mechanisms of self-relevance in subcallosal cingulate cortex: Evidence from single-unit recording and local field potentials. *Cortex*, in press

Lisman, J. E., Coyle, J. T., Green, R. W., Javitt, D. C., Benes, F. M., Heckers, S., & Grace, A. A. (2008). Circuit-based framework for understanding neurotransmitter and risk gene interactions in psychosis. *Trends in Neuroscience, 31*(5), 234–42.

Llinas, R. (2002). *I of the vortex: From neurons to self.* Cambridge, MA: MIT Press.

Llinas, R., Ribary, U., Contreras, D., & Pedroarena, C. (1998). The neuronal basis for consciousness.

Philosophical Transactions of the Royal Society of London Series B: Biological Sciences, 353(1377), 1841–49.

Lloyd, D. (2002). Functional MRI and the study of human consciousness. *Journal of Cognitive Neuroscience, 14*(6), 818–31. doi:10.1162/089892902760191027

Lloyd, D. (2011). Neural correlates of temporality: Default mode variability and temporal awareness. *Consciousness and Cognition, 21*(2), 695–703. doi:10.1016/j.concog.2011.02.016

Lloyd, D. M. (2009). The space between us: a neurophilosophical framework for the investigation of human interpersonalspace. *Neuroscience and Biobehavioral Reviews, 33*(3), 297–304. doi: 10.1016/j.neubiorev.2008.09.007. Epub 2008 Sep 24. Review.

Logothetis, N. K., Murayama, Y., Augath, M., Steffen, T., Werner, J., & Oeltermann, A. (2009). How not to study spontaneous activity. *NeuroImage, 45*(4), 1080–9. doi:10.1016/j.neuroimage.2009.01.010

Longo, M. R., Azañón, E., & Haggard, P. (2010). More than skin deep: body representation beyond primary somatosensory cortex. *Neuropsychologia, 48*(3), 655–68. doi:10.1016/j.neuropsychologia.2009.08.022

Lorenz, K. (1977). *Behind the Mirror (Rückseite dyes Speigels)*. Translated by R. Taylor. New York: Harcourt Brace Jovanovich.

Lou, H C, Kjaer, T. W., Friberg, L., Wildschiodtz, G., Holm, S., & Nowak, M. (1999). A 15O-H2O PET study of meditation and the resting state of normal consciousness. *Human Brain Mapping, 7*(2), 98–105. Retrieved from http://www.ncbi.nlm.nih.gov/pubmed/9950067

Lou, H. C, Luber, B., Crupain, M., Keenan, J. P., Nowak, M., Kjaer, T. W., Sackeim, H. A., et al. (2004). Parietal cortex and representation of the mental Self. *Proceedings of the National Academy of Sciences USA, 101*(17), 6827–32. doi:10.1073/pnas.0400049101

Lou, H. C, Nowak, M., & Kjaer, T. W. (2005). The mental self. *Progress in Brain Research, 150*, 197–204. doi:10.1016/S0079-6123(05)50014-1

Lou, H. C., Gross, J., Biermann-Ruben, K., Kjaer, T. W., & Schnitzler, A. (2010a). Coherence in consciousness: Paralimbic gamma synchrony of self-reference links conscious experiences. *Human Brain Mapping, 31*(2), 185–92. doi:10.1002/hbm.20855

Lou, H. C., Luber, B., Stanford, A., & Lisanby, S. H. (2010b). Self-specific processing in the default network: A single-pulse TMS study. *Experimental Brain Research, 207*(1–2), 27–38. doi:10.1007/s00221-010-2425-x

Lou, H. C, Joensson, M., & Kringelbach, M. L. (2011a). Yoga lessons for consciousness research: a paralimbic network balancing brain resource allocation. *Frontiers in Psychology, 2*, 366. doi:10.3389/fpsyg.2011.00366

Lou, H. C, Joensson, M., Biermann-Ruben, K., Schnitzler, A., Østergaard, L., Kjaer, T. W., & Gross, J. (2011b). Recurrent activity in higher order, modality non-specific brain regions: a Granger causality analysis of autobiographic memory retrieval. *PloS One, 6*(7), e22286. doi:10.1371/journal.pone.0022286

Luber, B., Lou, H. C., Keenan, J. P., & Lisanby, S. H. (2012). Self-enhancement processing in the default network: a single-pulse TMS study. *Experimental Brain Research. Experimentelle Hirnforschung. Expérimentation Cérébrale, 223*(2), 177–87. doi:10.1007/s00221-012-3249-7

Lundervold, A. (2010). On consciousness, resting state fMRI, and neurodynamics. *Nonlinear Biomedical Physics, 4*(Suppl. 1), S9. doi:10.1186/1753-4631-4-S1-S9

Luo, Y., Zhang, Y., Feng, X., & Zhou, X. (2010). Electroencephalogram oscillations differentiate semantic and prosodic processes during sentence reading. *Neuroscience, 169*(2), 654–64. doi:10.1016/j.neuroscience.2010.05.032

Mancia, M. (2006). Implicit memory and early unrepressed unconscious: Their role in the therapeutic process (How the neurosciences can contribute to psychoanalysis). *International Journal of Psycho-Analysis, 87*(Pt. 1), 83–103.

Mancia, M. (2006). *Psychoanalysis and neuroscience*. Milan, Italy: Springer.

Mannell, M. V., Franco, A. R., Calhoun, V. D., Canive, J. M., Thoma, R. J., & Mayer, A. R. (2010). Resting state and task-induced deactivation: A methodological comparison in patients with schizophrenia and healthy controls. *Human Brain Mapping, 31*(3), 424–37. doi:10.1002/hbm.20876

Marsman, A., van den Heuvel, M. P., Klomp, D. W., Kahn, R. S., Luijten, P. R., & Hulshoff Pol, H. E. (2011). Glutamate in schizophrenia: A focused review and meta-analysis of 1H-MRS studies. *Schizophrenia Bulletin, 39*(1), 120–9. doi:10.1093/schbul/sbr069

Martinez, A., Hillyard, S. A., Dias, E. C., Hagler, D. J., Jr., Butler, P. D., Guilfoyle, D. N., et al.

(2008). Magnocellular pathway impairment in schizophrenia: Evidence from functional magnetic resonance imaging. *Journal of Neuroscience, 28*(30), 7492–500. doi:10.1523/JNEUROSCI.1852-08.2008

Martuzzi, R., Ramani, R., Qiu, M., Rajeevan, N., & Constable, R. T. (2010). Functional connectivity and alterations in baseline brain state in humans. *NeuroImage, 49*(1), 823–34. doi:10.1016/j.neuroimage.2009.07.028

Mascetti, L., Foret, A., Bourdiec, A. S., Muto, V., Kussé, C., Jaspar, M., Matarazzo, L., Dang-Vu, T., Schabus, M., Maquet, P. (2011) Spontaneous neural activity during human non-rapid eye movement sleep. *Prog Brain Res, 193*, 111–18. doi: 10.1016/B978-0-444-53839-0.00008-9. Review.

Mason, M. F., Norton, M. I., Van Horn, J. D., Wegner, D. M., Grafton, S. T., & Macrae, C. N. (2007). Wandering minds: The default network and stimulus-independent thought. *Science, 315*(5810), 393–5. doi:10.1126/science.1131295

Massimini, M., Ferrarelli, F., Sarasso, S., & Tononi, G. (2012). Cortical mechanisms of loss of consciousness: insight from TMS/EEG studies. *Archives Italiennes de Biologie, 150*(2–3), 44–55. Retrieved from http://www.ncbi.nlm.nih.gov/pubmed/23165870

Massimini, M., Boly, M., Casali, A., Rosanova, M., & Tononi, G. (2009). A perturbational approach for evaluating the brain's capacity for consciousness. *Progress in Brain Research, 177*, 201–14. doi:10.1016/S0079-6123(09)17714-2

Massimini, M., Ferrarelli, F., Murphy, M., Huber, R., Riedner, B., Casarotto, S., & Tononi, G. (2010). Cortical reactivity and effective connectivity during REM sleep in humans. *Cognitive Neuroscience, 1*(3), 176–83. doi:10.1080/17588921003731578

Mayberg, H. (2002). Depression, II—localization of pathophysiology. *American Journal of Psychiatry, 159*(12), 1979.

Mayberg, H. S. (2003a). Modulating dysfunctional limbic-cortical circuits in depression: Towards development of brain-based algorithms for diagnosis and optimised treatment. *British Medical Bulletin, 65*, 193–207.

Mayberg, H. S. (2003b). Positron emission tomography imaging in depression: A neural systems perspective. *Neuroimaging Clinics of North America, 13*(4), 805–15.

Mayberg, H. S. (2009). Targeted electrode-based modulation of neural circuits for depression. *Journal of Clinical Investigations, 119*(4), 717–25.

Mayberg, H. S., Liotti, M., Brannan, S. K., McGinnis, S., Mahurin, R. K., Jerabek, P. A., et al. (1999). Reciprocal limbic-cortical function and negative mood: Converging PET findings in depression and normal sadness. *American Journal of Psychiatry, 156*(5), 675–82.

McDonnell, M. D., & Ward, L. M. (2011). The benefits of noise in neural systems: Bridging theory and experiment. *Nature Reviews. Neuroscience, 12*(7), 415–26. doi:10.1038/nrn3061; 10.1038/nrn3061

McDowell, J. (1994). *Mind and World.* Camrbidge, MA: Harvard University Press.

McDowell, J. E., Brown, G. G., Paulus, M., Martinez, A., Stewart, S. E., Dubowitz, D. J., & Braff, D. L. (2002). Neural correlates of refixation saccades and antisaccades in normal and schizophrenia subjects. *Biological Psychiatry, 51*(3), 216–23.

McGinn, C. (1991). *The problem of consciousness: Essays towards a resolution.* Oxford, England: Blackwell. Retrieved from http://www.worldcat.org/title/problem-of-consciousness-essays-towards-a-resolution/oclc/21483291&referer=brief_results

McGlashan, T. H. (2009). Psychosis as a disorder of reduced cathectic capacity: Freud's analysis of the Schreber case revisited. *Schizophrenia Bulletin, 35*(3), 476–81. doi:10.1093/schbul/sbp019

McKiernan, K. A., D'Angelo, B. R., Kaufman, J. N., & Binder, J. R. (2006). Interrupting the ""stream of consciousness": An fMRI investigation. *NeuroImage, 29*(4), 1185–91.

Mechelli, A., Allen, P., Amaro, E. Jr., Fu, C. H., Williams, S. C., Brammer, M. J., et al. (2007). Misattribution of speech and impaired connectivity in patients with auditory verbal hallucinations. *Human Brain Mapping, 28*(11), 1213–22.

Medford, N., & Critchley, H. D. (2010). Conjoint activity of anterior insular and anterior cingulate cortex: Awareness and response. *Brain Structure and Function, 214*(5–6), 535–49. doi:10.1007/s00429-010-0265-x

Meissner, K., & Wittmann, M. (2011). Body signals, cardiac awareness, and the perception of time. *Biological Psychology, 86*(3), 289–97. doi:10.1016/j.biopsycho.2011.01.001

Melloni, L., Molina, C., Pena, M., Torres, D., Singer, W., & Rodriguez, E. (2007). Synchronization of neural activity across cortical areas correlates with conscious perception. *Journal of Neuroscience, 27*(11), 2858–65. doi:10.1523/JNEUROSCI.4623-06.2007

Melloni, L., Schwiedrzik, C. M., Muller, N., Rodriguez, E., & Singer, W. (2011). Expectations change the signatures and timing of electrophysiological correlates of perceptual awareness. *Journal of Neuroscience, 31*(4), 1386–96. doi:10.1523/JNEUROSCI.4570-10.2011

Menon, V. (2011). Large–scale brain networks and psychopathology: A unifying triple network model. *Trends in Cognitive Sciences, 15*(10), 483–506. doi:10.1016/j.tics.2011.08.003

Mentzos, S. (1982). *Neurotische Konfliktverarbeitung. Einführung in die Psychoanalytische Neurosenlehre unter Berücksichtigung neuer Perspektiven.* Munich, Germany: Kindler Verlag.

Mentzos, S. (1992.). *Psychose und Konflikt.* Goettingen, Germany: Vandenhoeck & Ruprecht).

Merker, B. (2005). The liabilities of mobility: A selection pressure for the transition to consciousness in animal evolution. *Consciousness and Cognition, 14*(1), 89–114. doi:10.1016/S1053-8100(03)00002-3

Merker, B. (2007). Consciousness without a cerebral cortex: A challenge for neuroscience and medicine. *Behavioral and Brain Sciences, 30*(1), 63–81; discussion 81–134. doi:10.1017/S0140525X07000891

Merker, B. H., Madison, G. S., & Eckerdal, P. (2009). On the role and origin of isochrony in human rhythmic entrainment. *Cortex, 45*(1), 4–17. doi:10.1016/j.cortex.2008.06.011

Merleau-Ponty, M. (1965). *Phanomenologie der Wahrnehmung.* Berlin, Germany: Walter de Gruyter.

Mesulam, M. (2008). Representation, inference, and transcendent encoding in neurocognitive networks of the human brain. *Annals of Neurology, 64*(4), 367–78. doi:10.1002/ana.21534

Metzinger, T. (1995). *Conscious experience.* Paderborn: Schöningh/Imprint Academic.

Metzinger, T. (2003). *Being no one.* Cambridge, MA: MIT Press.

Metzinger, T., & Gallese, V. (2003). the emergence of a shared action ontology: Building blocks for a theory. *Consciousness and Cognition, 12*(4), 549–71.

Mhuircheartaigh, R. N., Rosenorn-Lanng, D., Wise, R., Jbabdi, S., Rogers, R., & Tracey, I. (2010). Cortical and subcortical connectivity changes during decreasing levels of consciousness in humans: A functional magnetic resonance imaging study using propofol. *Journal of Neuroscience, 30*(27), 9095–102. doi:10.1523/JNEUROSCI.5516-09.2010

Molaee-Ardekani, B., Senhadji, L., Shamsollahi, M. B., Vosoughi-Vahdat, B., & Wodey, E. (2007). Brain activity modeling in general anesthesia: Enhancing local mean-field models using a slow adaptive firing rate. *Physical Review., 76*(4, Pt. 1), 041911.

Monaco, F., Mula, M., & Cavanna, A. E. (2005). Consciousness, epilepsy, and emotional qualia. *Epilepsy and Behavior, 7*(2), 150–60. doi:10.1016/j.yebeh.2005.05.018

Monti, M. M., Vanhaudenhuyse, A., Coleman, M. R., Boly, M., Pickard, J. D., Tshibanda, L., et al. (2010). Willful modulation of brain activity in disorders of consciousness. *New England Journal of Medicine, 362*(7), 579–89. doi:10.1056/NEJMoa0905370

Monto, S., Palva, S., Voipio, J., & Palva, J. M. (2008). Very slow EEG fluctuations predict the dynamics of stimulus detection and oscillation amplitudes in humans. *Journal of Neuroscience, 28*(33), 8268–72. doi:10.1523/JNEUROSCI.1910-08.2008

Moran, J. M., Macrae, C. N., Heatherton, T. F., Wyland, C. L., & Kelley, W. M. (2006). Neuroanatomical evidence for distinct cognitive and affective components of self. *Journal of Cognitive Neuroscience, 18*(9), 1586–94. doi:10.1162/jocn.2006.18.9.1586

Moran, L. V., & Hong, L. E. (2011). High vs low frequency neural oscillations in schizophrenia. *Schizophrenia Bulletin, 37*(4), 659–63. doi:10.1093/schbul/sbr056

Morgan, H. L., Turner, D. C., Corlett, P. R., Absalom, A. R., Adapa, R., Arana, F. S., et al. (2011). Exploring the impact of ketamine on the experience of illusory body ownership. *Biological Psychiatry, 69*(1), 35–41. doi:10.1016/j.biopsych.2010.07.032

Morgane, P. J., Galler, J. R., & Mokler, D. J. (2005). A review of systems and networks of the limbic forebrain/limbic midbrain. *Progress in Neurobiology, 75*(2), 143–60. doi:10.1016/j.pneurobio.2005.01.001

Mu, Y., & Han, S. (2010). Neural oscillations involved in self-referential processing. *NeuroImage, 53*(2), 757–68. doi:10.1016/j.neuroimage.2010.07.008

Mulert, C., Leicht, G., Hepp, P., Kirsch, V., Karch, S., Pogarell, O., et al. (2010). Single-trial coupling of the gamma-band response and the corresponding BOLD signal. *NeuroImage, 49*(3), 2238–47. doi:10.1016/j.neuroimage.2009.10.058

Naatanen, R., Paavilainen, P., Rinne, T., & Alho, K. (2007). The mismatch negativity (MMN) in basic research of central auditory processing: A review. *Clinical Neurophysiology, 118*(12), 2544–90. doi:10.1016/j.clinph.2007.04.026

Nachev, P., & Hacker, P. M. (2010). Covert cognition in the persistent vegetative state. *Progress in Neurobiology, 91*(1), 68–76. doi:10.1016/j.pneurobio.2010.01.009

Nagel, T. (1974). What is it like to be a bat? *Philosophical Review, 83*(4), 435–50.

Nagel, T. (2012). *Mind and cosmos. Why the materialist neo-Darwinian conception of nature is almost certainly false.* Oxford, New York: Oxford University Press.

Nakao, T., Bai, Y., Nashiwa, H., & Northoff, G. (2012a). Resting-state EEG power predicts conflict-related brain activity in internally guided but not in externally guided decision-making. *NeuroImage, 66C*, 9–21. doi:10.1016/j.neuroimage.2012.10.034

Nakao, T., Ohira, H., & Northoff, G. (2012b). Distinction between externally vs. internally guided decision-making: operational differences, meta-analytical comparisons and their theoretical implications. *Frontiers in Neuroscience, 6*, 31. doi:10.3389/fnins.2012.00031

Nakao, T., Osumi, T., Ohira, H., Kasuya, Y., Shinoda, J., Yamada, J., & Northoff, G. (2010). Medial prefrontal cortex-dorsal anterior cingulate cortex connectivity during behavior selection without an objective correct answer. *Neuroscience Letters, 482*(3), 220–4. doi:10.1016/j.neulet.2010.07.041

Nallasamy, N., & Tsao, D. Y. (2011). Functional connectivity in the brain: Effects of anesthesia. *Neuroscientist, 17*(1), 94–106. doi:10.1177/1073858410374126

Neisser, J. (2011a). Neural correlates of consciousness reconsidered. *Consciousness and Cognition, 21*(2), 681–90. doi:10.1016/j.concog.2011.03.012

Neisser, J. (2011b). Neural mechanisms and functional realization: A reply to Hohwy. *Consciousness and Cognition*, doi:10.1016/j.concog.2011.07.007

Niesters, M., Khalili-Mahani, N., Martini, C., Aarts, L., Van Gerven, J., Van Buchem, M. A., Dahan, A., et al. (2012). Effect of subanesthetic ketamine on intrinsic functional brain connectivity: a placebo-controlled functional magnetic resonance imaging study in healthy male volunteers. *Anesthesiology, 117*(4), 868–77. doi:10.1097/ALN.0b013e31826a0db3

Nikolov, S., Rahnev, D. A., & Lau, H. C. (2010). Probabilistic model of onset detection explains paradoxes in human time perception. *Frontiers in Psychology, 1*, 37. doi:10.3389/fpsyg.2010.00037

Nir, Y., & Tononi, G. (2010). Dreaming and the brain: from phenomenology to neurophysiology. *Trends in Cognitive Sciences, 14*(2), 88–100. doi:10.1016/j.tics.2009.12.001

Nir, Y., Staba, R. J., Andrillon, T., Vyazovskiy, V. V., Cirelli, C., Fried, I., & Tononi, G. (2011). Regional slow waves and spindles in human sleep. *Neuron, 70*(1), 153–69. doi:10.1016/j.neuron.2011.02.043

Noe, A. (2004). *Action and perception.* Cambridge, MA: MIT Press.

Northoff, G. (2003). Emotional qualia and ventromedial prefrontal cortex: A "neurophenomenological" hypothesis. *Journal of Consciousness Studies, 10*(8), 46–72.

Northoff, G. (2004a). *Philosophy of the brain.* Amsterdam/New York: John Benhamins Publisher.

Northoff, G. (2004b). What is neurophilosophy? A methodological account. *Journal of General Philosophy of Science, 35*(1), 91–127.

Northoff, G. (2004c). Why do we need a philosophy of the brain? *Trends in Cognitive Sciences, 8*(11), 484–5. doi:10.1016/j.tics.2004.09.003

Northoff, G. (2007). Psychopathology and pathophysiology of the self in depression—neuropsychiatric hypothesis. *Journal of Affective Disorders, 104*(1–3), 1–14.

Northoff, G. (2008a). Is appraisal embodied and embedded? A neurophilosophical investigation of emotions. *Journal of Consciousness Studies, 15*(5), 68–99.

Northoff, G. (2008b). What kind of neural coding and self does Hurely's shared circuit model presuppose? *Behavioral and Brain Sciences, 31*(1), 33–43.

Northoff, G. (2008c). Are our emotional feelings rational? A neurophilosophical investigation of the James-Lange theory. *Phenomenology and the Cognitive Sciences, 7*(4), 501–27.

Northoff, G. (2010a). Region-based approach versus mechanism-based approach to the brain. *Neuropsychoanalysis, 12*(2), 167–70.

Northoff, G. (2010b). Humans, brains, and their environment: marriage between neuroscience and anthropology? *Neuron, 65*(6), 748–51. doi:10.1016/j.neuron.2010.02.024

Northoff, G. (2011a). *Neuropsychoanalysis in practice: Brain, self, and objects.* New York: Oxford University Press.

Northoff, G. (2011b). Self and brain: what is self-related processing? *Trends in Cognitive Sciences*, 15(5), 186–7; author reply 187–8. doi:10.1016/j.tics.2011.03.001

Northoff, G. (2012a). Autoepistemic limitation and the brain's neural code: Comment on "Neuroontology, neurobiological naturalism, and consciousness: A challenge to scientific reduction and a solution" by Todd E. Feinberg. *Physics of Life Reviews*, 9(1), 38–39. doi:10.1016/j.plrev.2011.12.017

Northoff, G. (2012b). Psychoanalysis and the brain—why did Freud abandon neuroscience? *Frontiers in Psychology*, 3, 71. doi:10.3389/fpsyg.2012.00071

Northoff, G. (2012c). From emotions to consciousness—a neuro-phenomenal and neuro-relational approach. *Frontiers in Psychology*, 3, 303. doi:10.3389/fpsyg.2012.00303

Northoff, G. (2012d). *Das disziplinlose Gehirn— Was nun, Herr Kant?: Auf den Spuren unseres Bewusstseins mit der Neurophilosophie (Google eBook)*. Irisiana.

Northoff, G. (2012e). Immanuel Kant's mind and the brain's resting state. *Trends in Cognitive Sciences*, 16(7), 356–9. doi:10.1016/j.tics.2012.06.001

Northoff, G. (2013a). What the brain's intrinsic activity can tell us about consciousness? A tri-dimensional view. *Neuroscience and Biobehavioral Reviews*,. 37(4), 726–38. doi:10.1016/j.neubiorev.2012.12.004

Northoff, G. (2013b). Gene, brains, and environment-genetic neuroimaging of depression. *Current Opinion in Neurobiology*, 23(1), 133–42. doi:10.1016/j.conb.2012.08.004

Northoff, G., & Bermpohl, F. (2004a). Cortical midline structures and the self. *Trends in Cognitive Science*, 8(3), 102–07.

Northoff, G., & Hayes, D. J. (2011). Is our self nothing but reward? *Biological Psychiatry*, 69(11), 1019–25. doi:10.1016/j.biopsych.2010.12.014

Northoff, G., & Heinzel, A. (2003). The self in philosophy, neuroscience, and psychiatry. An epistemic approach. In T. Kircher & A. David (Eds.), *The self in neuroscience and psychiatry* (pp. 57–69). Cambridge, England: Cambridge University Press.

Northoff, G., & Panksepp, J. (2008). The trans-species concept of self and the subcortical-cortical midline system. *Trends in Cognitive Science*, 12(7), 259–64.

Northoff, G., & Qin, P. (2011). How can the brain's resting state activity generate hallucinations? A 'resting state hypothesis' of auditory verbal hallucinations. *Schizophrenia Research*, 127(1–3), 202–14. doi:10.1016/j.schres.2010.11.009

Northoff, G., Duncan, N. W., & Hayes, D. J. (2010). The brain and its resting state activity—experimental and methodological implications. *Progress in Neurobiology*, 92(4), 593–600. doi:10.1016/j.pneurobio.2010.09.002

Northoff, G., Grimm, S., Boeker, H., Schmidt, C., Bermpohl, F., Heinzel, A., Hell, D., et al. (2006). Affective judgment and beneficial decision making: ventromedial prefrontal activity correlates with performance in the Iowa Gambling Task. *Human Brain Mapping*, 27(7), 572–87. doi:10.1002/hbm.20202

Northoff, G., Heinzel, A., Bermpohl, F., Niese, R., Pfennig, A., Pascual-Leone, A., & Schlaug, G. (2004). Reciprocal modulation and attenuation in the prefrontal cortex: An fMRI study on emotional-cognitive interaction. *Human Brain Mapping*, 21(3), 202–12.

Northoff, G., Heinzel, A., de Greck, M., Bermpohl, F., Dobrowolny, H., & Panksepp, J. (2006). Self-referential processing in our brain—a meta-analysis of imaging studies on the self. *NeuroImage*, 31(1), 440–57. doi:10.1016/j.neuroimage.2005.12.002

Northoff, G., Kötter, R., Baumgart, F., Danos, P., Boeker, H., Kaulisch, T., Schlagenhauf, F., et al. (2004). Orbitofrontal cortical dysfunction in akinetic catatonia: a functional magnetic resonance imaging study during negative emotional stimulation. *Schizophrenia Bulletin*, 30(2), 405–27. Retrieved from http://www.ncbi.nlm.nih.gov/pubmed/15279056

Northoff, G., Qin, P., & Feinberg, T. E. (2011a). Brain imaging of the self—conceptual, anatomical and methodological issues. *Consciousness and Cognition*, 20(1), 52–63. doi:10.1016/j.concog.2010.09.011

Northoff, G., Qin, P., & Nakao, T. (2010). Rest-stimulus interaction in the brain: a review. *Trends in Neurosciences*, 33(6), 277–84. doi:10.1016/j.tins.2010.02.006

Northoff, G., Richter, A., Gessner, M., Schlagenhauf, F., Fell, J., Baumgart, F., et al. (2000). Functional dissociation between medial and lateral prefrontal cortical spatiotemporal activation in negative and positive emotions: A combined fMRI/MEG study. *Cerebral Cortex*, 10(1), 93–107.

Northoff, G., Richter, A., Wahl, C., Grimm, S., Boeker, H., Hell, D., Marquar, V., et al. (2005). NMDA-hypofunction in posterior cingulate as a model for schizophrenia: A Ketamine challenge study in fMRI. *Schizophrenia Research2*, *72*, 235–48.

Northoff, G., Schneider, F., Rotte, M., Matthiae, C., Tempelmann, C., Wiebking, C., Panksepp, J. (2009). Differential parametric modulation of self-relatedness and emotions in different brain regions. *Human Brain Mapping, 30*(2), 369–82.

Northoff, G., Walter, M., Schulte, R. F., Beck, J., Dydak, U., Henning, A., et al. (2007). GABA concentrations in the human anterior cingulate cortex predict negative BOLD responses in fMRI. *Nature Neuroscience, 10*, 1515–7.

Northoff, G., Wiebking, C., Feinberg, T., & Panksepp, J. (2011b). The 'resting-state hypothesis' of major depressive disorder-a translational subcortical-cortical framework for a system disorder. *Neuroscience and Biobehavioral Reviews, 35*(9), 1929–45. doi:10.1016/j.neubiorev.2010.12.007

Northoff, G., Witzel, T., Richter, A., Gessner, M., Schlagenhauf, F., Fell, J., Baumgart, F., et al. (2002). GABA-ergic modulation of prefrontal spatio-temporal activation pattern during emotional processing: a combined fMRI/MEG study with placebo and lorazepam. *Journal of Cognitive Neuroscience, 14*(3), 348–70. doi:10.1162/089892902317361895

Nunez, P. L., & Srinivasan, R. (2006). A theoretical basis for standing and traveling brain waves measured with human EEG with implications for an integrated consciousness. *Clinical Neurophysiology, 117*(11), 2424–35. Retrieved from http://www.pubmedcentral.nih.gov/articlerender.fcgi?artid=1991284&tool=pmcentrez&rendertype=abstract

Oestby, Y., Walhovd, K. B., Tamnes, C. K., Grydeland, H., Westlye, L. T., & Fjell, A. M. (2012). Mental time travel and default-mode network functional connectivity in the developing brain. *Proceedings of the National Academy of Sciences USA, 109*(42), 16800–4. doi:10.1073/pnas.1210627109

Oosterwijk, S., Lindquist, K. A., Anderson, E., Dautoff, R., Moriguchi, Y., & Barrett, L. F. (2012). States of mind: emotions, body feelings, and thoughts share distributed neural networks. *NeuroImage, 62*(3), 2110–28. doi:10.1016/j.neuroimage.2012.05.079

Orpwood, R D. (1994). A possible neural mechanism underlying consciousness based on the pattern processing capabilities of pyramidal neurons in the cerebral cortex. *Journal of Theoretical Biology, 169*(4), 403–18. doi:10.1006/jtbi.1994.1162

Orpwood, R. (2007). Neurobiological mechanisms underlying qualia. *Journal Of Integrative Neuroscience, 6*(4), 523–40. Retrieved from http://www.ncbi.nlm.nih.gov/pubmed/18181267

Orpwood, Roger D. (2010). Perceptual qualia and local network behavior in the cerebral cortex. *Journal of Integrative Neuroscience, 9*(2), 123–52. Retrieved from http://www.ncbi.nlm.nih.gov/pubmed/20589951

Overgaard, M., & Overgaard, R. (2010). Neural correlates of contents and levels of consciousness. *Frontiers in Psychology, 1*, 164. doi:10.3389/fpsyg.2010.00164

Owen, A. M., Coleman, M. R., Boly, M., Davis, M. H., Laureys, S., & Pickard, J. D. (2006). Detecting awareness in the vegetative state. *Science, 313*(5792), 1402. doi:10.1126/science.1130197

Palmer, L., & Lynch, G. (2010). Neuroscience. A Kantian view of space. *Science, 328*(5985), 1487–8. doi:10.1126/science.1191527

Panksepp, J. (1998a). *Affective neuroscience: The foundations of human and animal emotions.* New York: Oxford University Press.

Panksepp, J. (1998b). The pre-conscious substrates of consciousness: Affective states and the evolutionary origins of the SELF. *Journal of Consciousness Studies, 5*, 566–82.

Panksepp, J. (2003a). The neural nature of the core SELF: Implications for understanding schizophrenia. In T. Kircher & A. David (Eds.), *Schizophrenia and the self* (pp. 197–213). Oxford, England: Oxford University Press.

Panksepp, J. (2003b). At the interface of the affective, behavioral, and cognitive neurosciences: Decoding the emotional feelings of the brain. *Brain and Cognition, 52*(1), 4–14.

Panksepp, J. (2007a). Affective consciousness. In M. Velmans & S. Schneider (Eds.), *The Blackwell companion to consciousness* (pp. 114–30). Malden, MA: Blackwell.

Panksepp, J. (2007b). The neuroevolutionary and neuroaffective psychobiology of the prosocial brain. In R. I. M. Dunbar & L. Barrett (Eds.), *The Oxford handbook of evolutionary psychology* (pp. 145–62). Oxford, England: Oxford University Press.

Panksepp, J. (2011). Cross–species affective neuroscience decoding of the primal affective experiences of humans and related animals. *PloS One, 6*(9), e21236. doi:10.1371/journal.pone.0021236

Panksepp, J., & Northoff, G. (2009). The trans-species core self: The emergence of active cultural and neuro-ecological agents through self-related processing within subcortical-cortical midline networks. *Consciousness and Cognition, 18,* 193–215.

Panksepp, J., Fuchs, T., Garcia, V. A., & Lesiak, A. (2007). Does any aspect of mind survive brain damage that typically leads to a persistent vegetative state? Ethical considerations. *Philosophy, Ethics, and Humanities in Medicine, 2,* 32. doi:10.1186/1747-5341-2-32

Parfit, D. (1984). *Reasons and Persons.* Oxford University Press. New York, Oxford.

Park, I. H., Kim, J. J., Chun, J., Jung, Y. C., Seok, J. H., et al. (2009). Medial prefrontal default-mode hypoactivity affecting trait physical anhedonia in schizophrenia. *Psychiatry Research, 171*(3), 155–65.

Park, I. H., Kim, J. J., Chun, J., Jung, Y. C., Seok, J. H., Park, H. J., & Lee, J. D. (2009). Medial prefrontal default-mode hypoactivity affecting trait physical anhedonia in schizophrenia. *Psychiatry Research, 171*(3), 155–65. doi:10.1016/j.pscychresns.2008.03.010

Parnas, J., Handest, P., Saebye, D., & Jansson, L. (2003). Anomalies of subjective experience in schizophrenia and psychotic bipolar illness. *Acta Psychiatrica Scandinavica, 108*(2), 126–33. Retrieved from http://www.ncbi.nlm.nih.gov/pubmed/12823169

Parnas, J., Jansson, L., Sass, L., & Handest, P. (1998). Self-experience in the prodromal phases of schizophrenia: A pilot study of first-admissions. *Neurology, Psychiatry and Brain Research, 6,* 97–106.

Parnas, J., Vianin, P., Saebye, D., Jansson, L., Volmer-Larsen, A., & Bovet, P. (2001). Visual binding abilities in the initial and advanced stages of schizophrenia. *Acta Psychiatrica Scandinavica, 103*(3), 171–80. Retrieved from http://www.ncbi.nlm.nih.gov/pubmed/11240573

Parnas, J. (2003). Self and schizophrenia: A phenomenological perspective. In T. Kircher & A. David (Eds.), *The self in neuroscience and psychiatry* (pp. 45–67). Cambridge, England: Cambridge University Press.

Parvizi, J., & Damasio, A. (2001). Consciousness and the brainstem. *Cognition, 79*(1–2), 135–60.

Parvizi, Josef, & Damasio, A. R. (2003). Neuroanatomical correlates of brainstem coma. *Brain: A Journal of Neurology, 126*(Pt 7), 1524–36. doi:10.1093/brain/awg166

Pascal, B. (1966). *Pensées.* Harmondsworth, England: Penguin Books. Retrieved from http://www.worldcat.org/title/pensees/oclc/492612455&referer=brief_results

Pascal, B., & Krailsheimer, A. J. (1966). *Pascal's Pensées.* Harmondsworth, England: Penguin.

Perrin, F., Maquet, P., Peigneux, P., Ruby, P., Degueldre, C., Balteau, E., Del Fiore, G., et al. (2005). Neural mechanisms involved in the detection of our first name: a combined ERPs and PET study. *Neuropsychologia, 43*(1), 12–9. doi:10.1016/j.neuropsychologia.2004.07.002

Perrin, F., Schnakers, C., Schabus, M., Degueldre, C., Goldman, S., Brédart, S., Faymonville, M.-E., et al. (2006). Brain response to one's own name in vegetative state, minimally conscious state, and locked-in syndrome. *Archives of Neurology, 63*(4), 562–9. Retrieved from http://www.ncbi.nlm.nih.gov/pubmed/16606770

Pfeiffer, U. J., Timmermans, B., Vogeley, K., Frith, C. D., Schilbach, L. (2013) Towards a neuroscience of social interaction. *Front Hum Neurosci, 7,* 22. doi: 10.3389/fnhum.2013.00022. Epub 2013 Feb 1.

Phan, K. L., Wager, T., Taylor, S. F., & Liberzon, I. (2002). Functional neuroanatomy of emotion: A meta-analysis of emotion activation studies in PET and fMRI. *NeuroImage, 16*(2), 331–48. doi:10.1006/nimg.2002.1087

Phillips, M. L., Drevets, W. C., Rauch, S. L., & Lane, R. (2003). Neurobiology of emotion perception II: Implications for major psychiatric disorders. *Biological Psychiatry, 54*(5), 515–28.

Plum, F., & Posner, J. B. (1980). *The diagnosis of stupor and coma.* Philadelphia, PA: F. A. Davis.

Pöppel, E. (2009). Pre-semantically defined temporal windows for cognitive processing. *Philosophical Transactions of the Royal Society of London. Series B, Biological Sciences, 364*(1525), 1887–96. doi: 10.1098/rstb.2009.0015. Review.

Pollatos, O., Gramann, K., & Schandry, R. (2007a). Neural systems connecting interoceptive awareness and feelings. *Human Brain Mapping, 28*(1), 9–18. doi:10.1002/hbm.20258

Pollatos, O., Herbert, B. M., Matthias, E., & Schandry, R. (2007b). Heart rate response after emotional picture presentation is modulated by interoceptive awareness. *International Journal of Psychophysiology, 63*(1), 117–24. doi:10.1016/j.ijpsycho.2006.09.003

Pollatos, O., Kirsch, W., & Schandry, R. (2005a). Brain structures involved in interoceptive awareness and cardioafferent signal processing: A dipole source localization study. *Human Brain Mapping,* *26*(1), 54–64. doi:10.1002/hbm.20121

Pollatos, O., Kirsch, W., & Schandry, R. (2005b). On the relationship between interoceptive awareness, emotional experience, and brain processes. *Cognitive Brain Research, 25*(3), 948–62. doi:10.1016/j.cogbrainres.2005.09.019

Pollatos, O., Traut-Mattausch, E., Schroeder, H., & Schandry, R. (2007). Interoceptive awareness mediates the relationship between anxiety and the intensity of unpleasant feelings. *Journal of Anxiety Disorders, 21*(7), 931–43. doi:10.1016/j.janxdis.2006.12.004

Pomarol-Clotet, E., Honey, G. D., Murray, G. K., Corlett, P. R., Absalom, A. R., Lee, M., McKenna, P. J., et al. (2006). Psychological effects of ketamine in healthy volunteers. Phenomenological study. *British Journal of Psychiatry, 189,* 173–9. doi:10.1192/bjp.bp.105.015263

Pomarol-Clotet, E., Oh, T. M., Laws, K. R., & McKenna, P. J. (2008a). Semantic priming in schizophrenia: Systematic review and meta-analysis. *British Journal of Psychiatry, 192*(2), 92–7. doi:10.1192/bjp.bp.106.032102

Pomarol-Clotet, E., Salvador, R., Sarro, S., Gomar, J., Vila, F., Martinez, A., et al. (2008b). Failure to deactivate in the prefrontal cortex in schizophrenia: Dysfunction of the default mode network? *Psychological Medicine, 38*(8), 1185–93. doi:10.1017/S0033291708003565

Poppel, E. (2009). Pre-semantically defined temporal windows for cognitive processing. *Philosophical Transactions of the Royal Society of London, Series B: Biological Sciences, 364*(1525), 1887–96. doi:10.1098/rstb.2009.0015

Pred, R. (2005). *The dynamic flow of experience.* Cambridge, MA: MIT Press.

Price, J. L., & Drevets, W. C. (2010). Neurocircuitry of mood disorders. *Neuropsychopharmacology, 35*(1), 192–216. doi:10.1038/npp.2009.104

Price, J. L., & Drevets, W. C. (2012). Neural circuits underlying the pathophysiology of mood disorders. *Trends in Cognitive Sciences, 16*(1), 61–71. doi:10.1016/j.tics.2011.12.011

Prinz, J. (2012). *The conscious brain. How attention engenders experience.* New York: Oxford University Press.

Qin, P., & Northoff, G. (2011). How is our self related to midline regions and the default-mode network? *NeuroImage, 57*(3), 1221–33. doi:10.1016/j.neuroimage.2011.05.028

Qin, P., Di, H., Liu, Y., Yu, S., Gong, Q., Duncan, N., et al. (2010). Anterior cingulate activity and the self in disorders of consciousness. *Human Brain Mapping, 31*(12), 1993–2002. doi:10.1002/hbm.20989; 10.1002/hbm.20989

Qin, P., Di, H., Yan, X., Yu, S., Yu, D., Laureys, S., & Weng, X. (2008). Mismatch negativity to the patient's own name in chronic disorders of consciousness. *Neuroscience Letters, 448*(1), 24–8. doi:10.1016/j.neulet.2008.10.029

Qin, P., Duncan, N. W., Wiebking, C., Gravel, P., Lyttelton, O., Hayes, D. J., Verhaeghe, J., et al. (2012). GABA(A) receptors in visual and auditory cortex and neural activity changes during basic visual stimulation. *Frontiers in Human Neuroscience, 6,* 337. doi:10.3389/fnhum.2012.00337

Qin, P., Liu, Y., Shi, J. F., Wang, Y., Duncan, N., Gong, Q., et al. (2011). Dissociation between anterior and posterior cortical regions during self-specificity and familiarity to human brain mapping: A combined fMRI-meta-analytic study. *Human Brain Mapping, 33,* 154–64.

Raichle, M. E. (2009). A brief history of human brain mapping. *Trends in Neurosciences, 32*(2), 118–26. doi:10.1016/j.tins.2008.11.001

Raichle, M. E., MacLeod, A. M., Snyder, A. Z., Powers, W. J., Gusnard, D. A., & Shulman, G. L. (2001). A default mode of brain function. *Proceedings of the National Academy of Sciences USA, 98*(2), 676–82.

Revensuo, A. (2005). *Inner presence. Consciousness as biological phenomenon.* Cambridge, MA: MIT Press.

Revensuo, A. (2006). *Consciousness. The science of subjectivity.* Cambridge Mass.: MIT Press.

Richter, A., Grimm, S., & Northoff, G. (2010). Lorazepam modulates orbitofrontal signal changes during emotional processing in catatonia. *Human Psychopharmacology, 25*(1), 55–62. doi:10.1002/hup.1084

Riedner, B. A., Hulse, B. K., Murphy, M. J., Ferrarelli, F., & Tononi, G. (2011). Temporal dynamics of cortical sources underlying spontaneous and peripherally evoked slow waves. *Progress in Brain Research, 193,* 201–18. doi:10.1016/B978-0-444-53839-0.00013-2

Rosanova, M., Gosseries, O., Casarotto, S., Boly, M., Casali, A. G., Bruno, M. A., et al. (2012). Recovery of cortical effective connectivity and recovery of consciousness in vegetative patients. *Brain, 135*(Pt 4), 1308–20. doi:10.1093/brain/awr340

Rotarska-Jagiela, A., van de Ven, V., Oertel-Knochel, V., Uhlhaas, P. J., Vogeley, K., & Linden, D. E.

(2010). Resting-state functional network correlates of psychotic symptoms in schizophrenia. *Schizophrenia Research*, *117*(1), 21–30. doi:10.1016/j.schres.2010.01.001

Rowlands, M. (2010). *The new science of the mind: From extended mind to embodied phenomenology.* Cambridge, Mass.: MIT Press. Retrieved from http://www.worldcat.org/oclc/502393594

Roy, S., & Llinás, R. (2008). Dynamic geometry, brain function modeling, and consciousness. *Progress in Brain Research*, *168*, 133–44. doi:10.1016/S0079-6123(07)68011-X

Rudolf, J., Ghaemi, M., Haupt, W. F., Szelies, B., & Heiss, W. D. (1999). Cerebral glucose metabolism in acute and persistent vegetative state. *Journal of Neurosurgical Anesthesiology*, *11*(1), 17–24. Retrieved from http://www.ncbi.nlm.nih.gov/pubmed/9890381

Rudolf, J., Sobesky, J., Ghaemi, M., & Heiss, W. D. (2002). The correlation between cerebral glucose metabolism and benzodiazepine receptor density in the acute vegetative state. *European Journal of Neurology*, *9*(6), 671–7.

Rudolf, J., Sobesky, J., Grond, M., & Heiss, W. D. (2000). Identification by positron emission tomography of neuronal loss in acute vegetative state. *Lancet*, *355*(9198), 115–16.

Sadaghiani, S., Maier, J. X., & Noppeney, U. (2009). Natural, metaphoric, and linguistic auditory direction signals have distinct influences on visual motion processing. *Journal of Neuroscience*, *29*(20), 6490–9.

Sadaghiani, S., Scheeringa, R., Lehongre, K., Morillon, B., Giraud, A. L., & Kleinschmidt, A. (2010). Intrinsic connectivity networks, alpha oscillations, and tonic alertness: A simultaneous electroencephalography/functional magnetic resonance imaging study. *Journal of Neuroscience*, *30*(30), 10243–50. doi:10.1523/JNEUROSCI.1004-10.2010

Salvadore, G., Cornwell, B. R., Colon-Rosario, V., Coppola, R., Grillon, C., Zarate, C. A., & Manji, H. K. (2009). Increased anterior cingulate cortical activity in response to fearful faces: a neurophysiological biomarker that predicts rapid antidepressant response to ketamine. *Biological Psychiatry*, *65*(4), 289–95. doi:10.1016/j.biopsych.2008.08.014

Salvadore, G., Cornwell, B. R., Sambataro, F., Latov, D., Colon-Rosario, V., Carver, F., Holroyd, T., et al. (2010). Anterior cingulate desynchronization and functional connectivity with the amygdala during a working memory task predict rapid antidepressant response to ketamine. *Neuropsychopharmacology*, *35*(7), 1415–22. doi:10.1038/npp.2010.24

Salvadore, G., Van der Veen, J. W., Zhang, Y., Marenco, S., Machado-Vieira, R., Baumann, J., Ibrahim, L. A., et al. (2012). An investigation of amino-acid neurotransmitters as potential predictors of clinical improvement to ketamine in depression. *International Journal of Neuropsychopharmacology*, *15*(8), 1063–72. doi:10.1017/S1461145711001593

Sanacora, G. (2010). Cortical inhibition, gamma-aminobutyric acid, and major depression: there is plenty of smoke but is there fire? *Biological Psychiatry*, *67*(5), 397–8. doi:10.1016/j.biopsych.2010.01.003

Sanacora, G., Gueorguieva, R., Epperson, C. N., Wu, Y.-T., Appel, M., Rothman, D. L., Krystal, J. H., et al. (2004). Subtype-specific alterations of gamma-aminobutyric acid and glutamate in patients with major depression. *Archives of General Psychiatry*, *61*(7), 705–13. doi:10.1001/archpsyc.61.7.705

Sanacora, G., Treccani, G., & Popoli, M. (2012). Towards a glutamate hypothesis of depression: an emerging frontier of neuropsychopharmacology for mood disorders. *Neuropharmacology*, *62*(1), 63–77. doi:10.1016/j.neuropharm.2011.07.036

Saenger, J., Lindenberger, U., & Müller, V. (2011). Interactive brains, social minds. *Communicative and Integrative Biology*, *4*(6), 655–63. Retrieved from http://www.pubmedcentral.nih.gov/articlerender.fcgi?artid=3306325&tool=pmcentrez&rendertype=abstract

Saenger, J., Müller, V., & Lindenberger, U. (2012). Intra- and interbrain synchronization and network properties when playing guitar in duets. *Frontiers in Human Neuroscience*, *6*, 312. doi:10.3389/fnhum.2012.00312

Sass, L. (1996). The catastrophes of heaven': Modernism, primitivism, and the madness of Antonin Artaud. *Modernism/Modernity*, *3*, 73–92.

Sass, L. (2000). Schizophrenia, self-experience, and the so-called "negative symptoms." In J. Benjamins (Ed.), *Exploring the self: Philosophical and psychopathological perspectives on self-experience* (pp. 65–78). Amsterdam.

Sass, L. (2003). Self-disturbance in schizophrenia. In T. Kircher & A. David (Eds.), *The self in neuroscience and psychiatry* (pp. 89–105). Cambridge, England: Cambridge University Press.

Sass, L., & Parnas, J. (2001). Phenomenology of self disturbances in schizophrenia: some research findings and directions. *Philosophy, Psychiatry, Psychology, 8*, 347–56.

Sass, L., & Parnas, J. (2003). Schizophrenia, consciousness, and the self. *Schizophrenia Bulletin, 29*(3), 427–44. Retrieved from http://www.ncbi. nlm.nih.gov/pubmed/14609238

Sauseng, P., & Klimesch, W. (2008). What does phase information of oscillatory brain activity tell us about cognitive processes? *Neuroscience and Biobehavioral Reviews, 32*(5), 1001–13. doi:10.1016/j.neubiorev.2008.03.014

Savitz, J., & Drevets, W. C. (2009a). Bipolar and major depressive disorder: Neuroimaging the developmental-degenerative divide. *Neuroscience and Biobehavioral Reviews, 33*(5), 699–771. doi:10.1016/j.neubiorev.2009.01.004

Savitz, J., & Drevets, W. C. (2009b). Imaging phenotypes of major depressive disorder: Genetic correlates. *Neuroscience, 164*(1), 300–30. doi:10.1016/j.neuroscience.2009.03.082

Schacter, D. L., Addis, D. R., & Buckner, R. L. (2007). Remembering the past to imagine the future: The prospective brain. *Nature Reviews Neuroscience, 8*(9), 657–61. doi:10.1038/nrn2213

Scharfetter, C. (2003). The self in schizophrenia. In T. Kircher & A. David (Eds.), *The self in neuroscience and psychiatry 2*. Cambridge University Press.

Scharfetter, Christian. (1996). *The self-experience of schizophrenics: Empirical studies of the ego self in schizophrenia, borderline disorders and depression* (2nd ed.). Zurich, Switzerland: Private.

Scheidegger, M., Walter, M., Lehmann, M., Metzger, C., Grimm, S., Boeker, H., Boesiger, P., et al. (2012). Ketamine decreases resting state functional network connectivity in healthy subjects: implications for antidepressant drug action. *PloS One, 7*(9), e44799. doi:10.1371/ journal.pone.0044799

Schiff, N. D. (2009). Central thalamic deep-brain stimulation in the severely injured brain: Rationale and proposed mechanisms of action. *Annals of the New York Academy of Sciences, 1157*, 101–16. doi:10.1111/j.1749–6632.2008.04123.x

Schiff, N. D. (2010). Recovery of consciousness after severe brain injury: The role of arousal regulation mechanisms and some speculation on the heart-brain interface. *Cleveland Clinic Journal of Medicine, 77*(Suppl. 3), S27–33. doi:10.3949/ ccjm.77.s3.05

Schiff, N. D. (2012). Dissecting DBS dynamics through quantitative behavioral assessments and statistical modeling: A commentary on Cooper et al. 2011. *Experimental Neurology, 233*(2), 747–8. doi:10.1016/j. expneurol.2011.11.027

Schiff, N. D., Giacino, J. T., Kalmar, K., Victor, J. D., Baker, K., Gerber, M., Fritz, B., et al. (2007). Behavioural improvements with thalamic stimulation after severe traumatic brain injury. *Nature, 448*(7153), 600–3. doi:10.1038/ nature06041

Schilbach, L., Bzdok, D., Timmermans, B., Fox, P. T., Laird, A. R., Vogeley, K., Eickhoff, S. B. (2012). Introspective minds: using ALE meta-analyses to study commonalities in the neural correlates of emotional processing, social & unconstrained cognition. *PLoS One, 7*(2), e30920. doi: 10.1371/ journal.pone.0030920. Epub 2012 Feb 3.

Schilbach, L., Eickhoff, S. B., Schultze, T., Mojzisch, A., Vogeley, K. (2013). To you I am listening: perceived competence of advisors influences judgment and decision-making via recruitment of the amygdala. *Soc Neurosci, 8*(3), 189–202. doi: 10.1080/17470919.2013.775967. Epub 2013 Mar 13.

Schmitz, T. W., & Johnson, S. C. (2006). Self-appraisal decisions evoke dissociated dorsal-ventral aMPFC networks. *NeuroImage, 30*(3), 1050–8. doi:10.1016/j.neuroimage.2005.10.030

Schnakers, C., Perrin, F., Schabus, M., Majerus, S., Ledoux, D., Damas, P., et al. (2008). Voluntary brain processing in disorders of consciousness. *Neurology, 71*(20), 1614–20.

Schneider, F., Bermpohl, F., Heinzel, A., Rotte, M., Walter, M., Tempelmann, C., Wiebking, C., et al. (2008). The resting brain and our self: self-relatedness modulates resting state neural activity in cortical midline structures. *Neuroscience, 157*(1), 120–31. doi:10.1016/j. neuroscience.2008.08.014

Schooler, J. W., Smallwood, J., Christoff, K., Handy, T. C., Reichle, E. D., & Sayette, M. A. (2011). Meta-awareness, perceptual decoupling and the wandering mind. *Trends in Cognitive Sciences, 15*(7), 319–26. doi:10.1016/j.tics.2011.05.006

Schroeder, C. E., & Lakatos, P. (2009a). The gamma oscillation: Master or slave? *Brain Topography, 22*(1), 24–26. doi:10.1007/s10548-009-0080-y

Schroeder, C. E., & Lakatos, P. (2009b). Low-frequency neuronal oscillations as instruments of sensory selection. *Trends in Neurosciences, 32*(1), 9–18. doi:10.1016/j.tins.2008.09.012

Schroeder, C. E., & Lakatos, P. (2012). The signs of silence. *Neuron, 74*(5), 770–2. doi:10.1016/j. neuron.2012.05.012

Schroeder, C. E., Lakatos, P., Kajikawa, Y., Partan, S., & Puce, A. (2008). Neuronal oscillations and visual amplification of speech. *Trends in Cognitive Sciences, 12*(3), 106–13. doi:10.1016/j.tics.2008.01.002

Schroeder, C. E., Wilson, D. A., Radman, T., Scharfman, H., & Lakatos, P. (2010). Dynamics of Active Sensing and perceptual selection. *Current Opinion in Neurobiology, 20*(2), 172–6. doi:10.1016/j.conb.2010.02.010

Schrouff, J., Perlbarg, V., Boly, M., Marrelec, G., Boveroux, P., Vanhaudenhuyse, A., et al. (2011). Brain functional integration decreases during propofol-induced loss of consciousness. *NeuroImage, 57*(1), 198–205. doi:10.1016/j.neuroimage.2011.04.020

Searle, J. R. (1983). *Intentionality. An essay in the philosophy of mind*. Cambridge, England: Cambridge University Press.

Searle, J. (1992). *The Rediscovery of the Mind*. Cambridge, MA: MIT Press.

Searle, J. R. (1998). How to study consciousness scientifically. *Philosophical Transactions of the Royal Society of London, Series B: Biological Sciences, 353*(1377), 1935–42. doi:10.1098/rstb.1998.0346

Searle, J. R. (2000). Consciousness. *Annual Review of Neuroscience, 23*, 557–78.

Searle, J., R. (2004). *Mind. An introduction*. Oxford, England and New York: Oxford University Press.

Seger, C. A., Stone, M., & Keenan, J. P. (2004). Cortical activations during judgments about the self and an other person. *Neuropsychologia, 42*(9), 1168–77.

Sehatpour, P., Molholm, S., Schwartz, T. H., Mahoney, J. R., Mehta, A. D., Javitt, D. C., et al. (2008). A human intracranial study of long-range oscillatory coherence across a frontal-occipital-hippocampal brain network during visual object processing. *Proceedings of the National Academy of Sciences USA, 105*(11), 4399–404. doi:10.1073/pnas.0708418105

Sellars, W. (1963). *Science, perception, and reality*. New York: Humanities Press.

Seth, A. K., Baars, B. J., & Edelman, D. B. (2005). Criteria for consciousness in humans and other mammals. *Consciousness and Cognition, 14*(1), 119–39. doi:10.1016/j.concog.2004.08.006

Seth, A. K., Barrett, A. B., & Barnett, L. (2011). Causal density and integrated information as measures of conscious level. *Philosophical Transactions. Series A, Mathematical, Physical, and Engineering Sciences, 369*(1952), 3748–67. doi:10.1098/rsta.2011.0079

Seth, A. K., Dienes, Z., Cleeremans, A., Overgaard, M., & Pessoa, L. (2008). Measuring consciousness: relating behavioural and neurophysiological approaches. *Trends in Cognitive Sciences, 12*(8), 314–21. doi:10.1016/j.tics.2008.04.008

Seth, A. K., Izhikevich, E., Reeke, G. N., & Edelman, G. M. (2006). Theories and measures of consciousness: An extended framework. *Proceedings of the National Academy of Sciences USA, 103*(28), 10799–804. doi:10.1073/pnas.0604347103

Seth, A. K., Suzuki, K., & Critchley, H. D. (2011). An interoceptive predictive coding model of conscious presence. *Frontiers in Psychology, 2*, 395. doi:10.3389/fpsyg.2011.00395

Shapiro, L. A. (2011). *Embodied cognition*. New York: Routledge.

Shi, Z., Zhou, A., Han, W., & Liu, P. (2011). Effects of ownership expressed by the first-person possessive pronoun. *Consciousness and Cognition, 20*(3), 951–5. doi:10.1016/j.concog.2010.12.008

Shulman, R. G., Hyder, F., & Rothman, D. L. (2003). Cerebral metabolism and consciousness. *Comptes Rendus Biologies, 326*(3), 253–73.

Shulman. (2012). *Brain and consciousness*. Oxford, England and New York: Oxford University Press.

Siewert, Charles (2011). S.vv. "Consciousness and intentionality." *Stanford encyclopedia of philosophy* (Fall 2011 edition), Edward N. Zalta (ed.). URL = <http://plato.stanford.edu/archives/fall2011/ entries/consciousness-intentionality/>.). Stanford, CA:

Silberstein, M., & Chemero, A. (2012). Complexity and extended phenomenological-cognitive systems. *Topics in Cognitive Science, 4*(1), 35–50. doi:10.1111/j.1756-8765.2011.01168.x

Silva, S., Alacoque, X., Fourcade, O., Samii, K., Marque, P., Woods, R., et al., (2010). Wakefulness and loss of awareness: Brain and brainstem interaction in the vegetative state. *Neurology, 74*(4), 313–20. doi:10.1212/WNL.0b013e3181cbcd96

Singer, W. (1999). Neuronal synchrony: A versatile code for the definition of relations? *Neuron, 24*(1), 49–65, 111–25.

Singer, W. (2009). Distributed processing and temporal codes in neuronal networks. *Cognitive Neurodynamics, 3*(3), 189–96. doi:10.1007/s11571-009-9087-z

Slaby, J., & Stephan, A. (2008). Affective intentionality and self-consciousness. *Consciousness and Cognition, 17*(2), 506–13. doi:10.1016/j.concog.2008.03.007

Smallwood, J., & Schooler, J. W. (2006). The restless mind. *Psychological Bulletin, 132*(6), 946–58. doi:10.1037/0033-2909.132.6.946

Smallwood, J., Beach, E., Schooler, J. W., & Handy, T. C. (2008a). Going AWOL in the brain: Mind wandering reduces cortical analysis of external events. *Journal of Cognitive Neuroscience*, *20*(3), 458–69. doi:10.1162/jocn.2008.20037

Smallwood, J., McSpadden, M., Luus, B., & Schooler, J. (2008b). Segmenting the stream of consciousness: The psychological correlates of temporal structures in the time series data of a continuous performance task. *Brain and Cognition*, *66*(1), 50–6. doi:10.1016/j.bandc.2007.05.004

Solms, M. (1995). New findings on the neurological organization of dreaming: Implications for psychoanalysis. *Psychoanalytic Quarterly*, *64*(1), 43–67.

Solms, M. (1997). What is consciousness? *Journal of the American Psychoanalytic Association*, *45*(3), 681–703; discussion 704–78.

Solms, M. (2000). Dreaming and REM sleep are controlled by different brain mechanisms. *Behavioral and Brain Sciences*, *23*(6), 843–50; discussion 904–1121.

Soon, C. S., Brass, M., Heinze, H. J., & Haynes, J. D. (2008). Unconscious determinants of free decisions in the human brain. *Nature Neuroscience*, *11*(5), 543–5. doi:10.1038/nn.2112

Spencer, K. M. (2009). The functional consequences of cortical circuit abnormalities on gamma oscillations in schizophrenia: Insights from computational modeling. *Frontiers in Human Neuroscience*, *3*, 33. doi:10.3389/neuro.09.033.2009

Spencer, K. M., Nestor, P. G., Niznikiewicz, M. A., Salisbury, D. F., Shenton, M. E., & McCarley, R. W. (2003). Abnormal neural synchrony in schizophrenia. *Journal of Neuroscience*, *23*(19), 7407–11.

Spencer, K. M., Niznikiewicz, M. A., Nestor, P. G., Shenton, M. E., & McCarley, R. W. (2009). Left auditory cortex gamma synchronization and auditory hallucination symptoms in schizophrenia. *BMC Neuroscience*, *10*, 85. doi:10.1186/1471-2202-10-85

Spencer, K. M., Salisbury, D. F., Shenton, M. E., & McCarley, R. W. (2008). Gamma-band auditory steady-state responses are impaired in first episode psychosis. *Biological Psychiatry*, *64*(5), 369–75. doi:10.1016/j.biopsych.2008.02.021

Spreng, R. N., Mar, R. A., Kim, A. S. (2009). The common neural basis of autobiographical memory, prospection, navigation, theory of mind, and the default mode: a quantitative meta-analysis. *Journal of Cognitive Neuroscience*, *21*(3), 489–510. doi: 10.1162/jocn.2008.21029.

Spreng, R. N., Sepulcre, J., Turner, G. R., Stevens, W. D., Schacter, D. L. (2013) Intrinsic architecture underlying the relations among the default, dorsal attention, and frontoparietal control networks of the human brain. *Journal of Cognitive Neuroscience* *25*(1), 74–86. doi: 10.1162/jocn_a_00281. Epub 2012 Aug 20.

Sridharan, D., Levitin, D. J., & Menon, V. (2008). A critical role for the right fronto-insular cortex in switching between central-executive and default-mode networks. *Proceedings of the National Academy of Sciences USA*, *105*(34), 12569–74. doi:10.1073/pnas.0800005105

Stamatakis, E. A., Shafto, M. A., Williams, G., Tam, P., & Tyler, L. K. (2011). White matter changes and word finding failures with increasing age. *PloS One*, *6*(1), e14496. doi:10.1371/journal.pone.0014496

Stanghellini, G. (2009a). *Disembodied spirits and deanimated bodies: The psychopathology of common sense*. Oxford, England and New York: Oxford University Press.

Stanghellini, G. (2009b). Embodiment and schizophrenia. *World Psychiatry*, *8*(1), 56–9.

Stanghellini, G., & Ballerini, M. (2007). Criterion B (social dysfunction) in persons with schizophrenia: the puzzle. *Current Opinion in Psychiatry*, *20*(6), 582–7. doi:10.1097/YCO.0b013e3282f0d4e0

Stanghellini, G., & Ballerini, M. (2008). Qualitative analysis. Its use in psychopathological research. *Acta Psychiatrica Scandinavica*, *117*(3), 161–3. doi:10.1111/j.1600-0447.2007.01139.x

Stefanics, G., Haden, G. P., Sziller, I., Balazs, L., Beke, A., & Winkler, I. (2009). Newborn infants process pitch intervals. *Clinical Neurophysiology*, *120*(2), 304–8. doi:10.1016/j.clinph.2008.11.020

Stefanics, G., Hangya, B., Hernadi, I., Winkler, I., Lakatos, P., & Ulbert, I. (2010). Phase entrainment of human delta oscillations can mediate the effects of expectation on reaction speed. *Journal of Neuroscience*, *30*(41), 13578–85. doi:10.1523/JNEUROSCI.0703–10.2010

Stephan, K. E., Friston, K. J., & Frith, C. D. (2009). Dysconnection in schizophrenia: From abnormal synaptic plasticity to failures of self-monitoring. *Schizophrenia Bulletin*, *35*(3), 509–27. doi:10.1093/schbul/sbn176

Steriade, M., McCormick, D. A., & Sejnowski, T. J. (1993). Thalamocortical oscillations in the sleeping and aroused brain. *Science*, *262*(5134), 679–85.

Sterzer, P., Kleinschmidt, A., & Rees, G. (2009). The neural bases of multistable perception. *Trends in*

Cognitive Sciences, 13(7), 310–18. doi:10.1016/j. tics.2009.04.006

Strawson, G. (1994). *Mental reality*. Cambridge, MA: MIT Press.

Strawson, G. (2009). *Selves: An essay in revisionary metaphysics*. Oxford, England: Clarendon Press.

Sullivan, E. M., & O'Donnell, P. (2012). Inhibitory interneurons, oxidative stress, and schizophrenia. *Schizophrenia Bulletin, 38*(3), 373–6. doi:10.1093/schbul/sbs052

Svare, H. (2006). Body and practice in Kant. Doctoral dissertation, Oslo University Press, Oslo/Norway, 2006.

Szpunar, K. K., Watson, J. M., McDermott, K. B. (2007) Neural substrates of envisioning the future. *Proceedings of the National Academy of Sciences of the United States of America, 104*(2), 642–7. Epub 2007 Jan 3.

Taira, T. (2009). Intrathecal administration of GABA agonists in the vegetative state. *Progress in Brain Research, 177*, 317–28. doi:10.1016/ S0079-6123(09)17721-X

Tateuchi, T., Itoh, K., & Nakada, T. (2012). Neural mechanisms underlying the orienting response to subject's own name: an event-related potential study. *Psychophysiology, 49*(6), 786–91. doi:10.1111/j.1469-8986.2012.01363.x

Taylor, S. F., Welsh, R. C., Chen, A. C., Velander, A. J., & Liberzon, I. (2007). Medial frontal hyperactivity in reality distortion. *Biological Psychiatry, 61*(10), 1171–8. doi:10.1016/j. biopsych.2006.11.029

Tecchio, F., Salustri, C., Thaut, M. H., Pasqualetti, P., & Rossini, P. M. (2000). Conscious and preconscious adaptation to rhythmic auditory stimuli: A magnetoencephalographic study of human brain responses. *Experimental Brain Research, 135*(2), 222–30.

Thompson, E. (2007). *Mind in life: Biology, phenomenology, and the sciences of mind*. Cambridge, MA: Harvard University Press.

Tomasi, D., & Volkow, N. D. (2011). Functional connectivity hubs in the human brain. *NeuroImage, 57*(3), 908–17.

Tononi, G. (2004). An information integration theory of consciousness. *BMC Neuroscience, 5*, 42. doi:10.1186/1471-2202-5-42

Tononi, G. (2008). Consciousness as integrated information: A provisional manifesto. *The Biological Bulletin, 215*(3), 216–42.

Tononi, G. (2009). Slow wave homeostasis and synaptic plasticity. *Journal of Clinical Sleep Medicine, 5*(2 Suppl.), S16–19.

Tononi, G., Cirelli, C. (2003). Sleep and synaptic homeostasis: a hypothesis. *Brain Research Bulletin, 62*(2), 143–50.

Tononi, G., & Edelman, G. M. (2000). Schizophrenia and the mechanisms of conscious integration. *Brain Research Reviews, 31*(2–3), 391–400.

Tononi, G., & Koch, C. (2008). The neural correlates of consciousness: An update. *Annals of the New York Academy of Sciences, 1124*, 239–61. doi:10.1196/annals.1440.004

Turetsky, B. I., Calkins, M. E., Light, G. A., Olincy, A., Radant, A. D., & Swerdlow, N. R. (2007a). Neurophysiological endophenotypes of schizophrenia: The viability of selected candidate measures. *Schizophrenia Bulletin, 33*(1), 69–94. doi:10.1093/schbul/sbl060

Turetsky, B. I., Glass, C. A., Abbazia, J., Kohler, C. G., Gur, R. E., & Moberg, P. J. (2007b). Reduced posterior nasal cavity volume: A gender-specific neurodevelopmental abnormality in schizophrenia. *Schizophrenia Research, 93*(1–3), 237–44. doi:10.1016/j.schres.2007.02.014

Turetsky, B. I., Kohler, C. G., Indersmitten, T., Bhati, M. T., Charbonnier, D., & Gur, R. C. (2007c). Facial emotion recognition in schizophrenia: When and why does it go awry? *Schizophrenia Research, 94*(1–3), 253–63. doi:10.1016/j.schres.2007.05.001

Turk, D. J., Heatherton, T. F., Kelley, W. M., Funnell, M. G., Gazzaniga, M. S., & Macrae, C. N. (2002). Mike or me? Self-recognition in a split-brain patient. *Nature Neuroscience, 5*(9), 841–2.

Turk, D. J., Heatherton, T. F., Macrae, C. N., Kelley, W. M., & Gazzaniga, M. S. (2003). Out of contact, out of mind: The distributed nature of the self. *Annals of the New York Academy of Sciences, 1001*, 65–78.

Tye, M. (1995). *Ten Problems of Consciousness*. Cambridge, MA: Bradford/MIT Press.

Tye, M. (1999). *Ten Problems of Consciousness: A R epresentational theory of the Phenomenal mind*. Cambridge, MA: MIT Press.

Tye, M. (2003). *Consciousness and Persons: Unity and identity*. Cambridge, MA: MIT Press.

Tye, M. (2007). Philosophical problems of consciousness. In M. Velmans & S. Schneider (Eds.), *The Blackwell companion to consciousness* (pp. 23–37). Oxford, England: Blackwell.

Uddin, L. Q., Iacoboni, M., Lange, C., & Keenan, J. P. (2007). The self and social cognition: the role of cortical midline structures and mirror neurons. *Trends in Cognitive Science, 11*(4), 153–7.

Uhlhaas, P. J., & Singer, W. (2010). Abnormal neural oscillations and synchrony in schizophrenia.

Nature Reviews Neuroscience, 11(2), 100–13. doi:10.1038/nrn2774

Uhlhaas, P. J., Pipa, G., Lima, B., Melloni, L., Neuenschwander, S., Nikolic, D., & Singer, W. (2009a). Neural synchrony in cortical networks: History, concept and current status. *Frontiers in Integrative Neuroscience, 3*, 17. doi:10.3389/neuro.07.017.2009

Uhlhaas, P. J., Roux, F., Singer, W., Haenschel, C., Sireteanu, R., & Rodriguez, E. (2009b). The development of neural synchrony reflects late maturation and restructuring of functional networks in humans. *Proceedings of the National Academy of Sciences USA, 106*(24), 9866–71. doi:10.1073/pnas.0900390106

Uleman, J., S. (2005). Introduction. Becoming aware of the new unconscious. In R. Hassin, J. Uleman, & J. Bargh (Eds.), *The new unconscious* (pp. 1–10). Oxford, England: Oxford University Press.

van Boxtel, J. J., Tsuchiya, N., & Koch, C. (2010a). Opposing effects of attention and consciousness on afterimages. *Proceedings of the National Academy of Sciences USA, 107*(19), 8883–8. doi:10.1073/pnas.0913292107

van Boxtel, J. J., Tsuchiya, N., & Koch, C. (2010b). Consciousness and attention: On sufficiency and necessity. *Frontiers in Psychology, 1*, 217

Van Buuren, M., Gladwin, T. E., Zandbelt, B. B., Kahn, R. S., & Vink, M. (2010). Reduced functional coupling in the default-mode network during self-referential processing. *Human Brain Mapping, 31*(8), 1117–27. doi:10.1002/hbm.20920

Van de Ville, D., Britz, J., & Michel, C. M. (2010). EEG microstate sequences in healthy humans at rest reveal scale-free dynamics. *Proceedings of the National Academy of Sciences USA, 107*(42), 18179–84. doi:10.1073/pnas.1007841107

van der Meer, L., Costafreda, S., Aleman, A., & David, A. S. (2010). Self-reflection and the brain: A theoretical review and meta-analysis of neuroimaging studies with implications for schizophrenia. *Neuroscience and Biobehavioral Reviews, 34*(6), 935–46. doi:10.1016/j.neubiorev.2009.12.004

Van Dort, C. J., Baghdoyan, H. A., & Lydic, R. (2008). Neurochemical modulators of sleep and anesthetic states. *International Anesthesiology Clinics, 46*(3), 75–104. doi:10.1097/AIA.0b013e318181a8ca

van Eijsden, P., Hyder, F., Rothman, D. L., & Shulman, R. G. (2009). Neurophysiology of functional imaging. *NeuroImage, 45*(4), 1047–54. doi:10.1016/j.neuroimage.2008.08.026

van Gaal, S., & Lamme, V. A. (2012). Unconscious high-level information processing: Implication for neurobiological theories of consciousness. *Neuroscientist, 18*(3), 287–301. doi:10.1177/1073858411404079

Van Gulick, R. (2004). *Are there neural correlates of consciousness?* Exeter, England: Imprint Academic.

Van Gulick, R, (2011). Consciousness. In: Edward N. Zalta (ed.), *The Stanford Encyclopedia of Philosophy* (Summer 2011 Edition). URL http://plato.stanford.edu/archives/sum2011/entries/consciousness/.

van Loon, A. M., Scholte, H. S., van Gaal, S., van der Hoort, B. J., & Lamme, V. A. (2012). GABAA agonist reduces visual awareness: A masking-EEG experiment. *Journal of Cognitive Neuroscience, 24*(4), 965–74. doi:10.1162/jocn_a_00197

Van Someren, E. J., Van Der Werf, Y. D., Roelfsema, P. R., Mansvelder, H. D., & da Silva, F. H. (2011). Slow brain oscillations of sleep, resting state, and vigilance. *Progress in Brain Research, 193*, 3–15. doi:10.1016/B978-0-444-53839-0.00001-6

Van Wassenhove, V., Wittmann, M., Craig, A. D. B., & Paulus, M. P. (2011). Psychological and neural mechanisms of subjective time dilation. *Frontiers in Neuroscience, 5*, 56. doi:10.3389/fnins.2011.00056

Vandekerckhove, M., & Panksepp, J. (2009). The flow of anoetic to noetic and autonoetic consciousness: a vision of unknowing (anoetic) and knowing (noetic) consciousness in the remembrance of things past and imagined futures. *Consciousness and Cognition, 18*(4), 1018–28. doi:10.1016/j.concog.2009.08.002

Vanhaudenhuyse, A., Demertzi, A., Schabus, M., Noirhomme, Q., Bredart, S., Boly, M., et al. (2011). Two distinct neuronal networks mediate the awareness of environment and of self. *Journal of Cognitive Neuroscience, 23*(3), 570–8. doi:10.1162/jocn.2010.21488

Vanhaudenhuyse, A., Noirhomme, Q., Tshibanda, L. J., Bruno, M. A., Boveroux, P., Schnakers, C., et al. (2010). Default network connectivity reflects the level of consciousness in non-communicative brain-damaged patients. *Brain, 133*(Pt. 1), 161–71. doi:10.1093/brain/awp313

van Wassenhove, V., Wittmann, M., Craig, A. D., Paulus, M. P. (2011). Psychological and neural mechanisms of subjective time dilation. *Frontiers in Neurosciences, 5*, 56. doi: 10.3389/fnins.2011.00056.

Varela, F. J. (1997). Patterns of life: Intertwining identity and cognition. *Brain and Cognition, 34*(1), 72–87. doi:10.1006/brcg.1997.0907

Varela, F. J. (1999). Cognition without representations. *Rivista Di Biologia*, *92*(3), 511–12.

Varela, F., Lachaux, J-P., Rodriguez, E., & Martinerie, J. (2001). The brainweb: Phase synchronization and large-scale integration. *Nature Reviews Neuroscience*, *2*, 229–39.

Vincent, J. L., Patel, G. H., Fox, M. D., Snyder, A. Z., Baker, J. T., Van Essen, D. C., et al. (2007). Intrinsic functional architecture in the anaesthetized monkey brain. *Nature*, *447*(7140), 83–6.

Vogeley, K., & Fink, G. R. (2003). Neural correlates of the first-person-perspective. *Trends in Cognitive Science*, *7*(1), 38–42.

Vogeley, K., & Kupke, C. (2007). Disturbances of time consciousness from a phenomenological and a neuroscientific perspective. *Schizophrenia Bulletin*, *33*(1), 157–65. doi:10.1093/schbul/sbl056

Walker, M. P. (2009a). The role of sleep in cognition and emotion. *Annals of the New York Academy of Sciences*, *1156*, 168–97.

Walker, M. P. (2009b). The role of slow wave sleep in memory processing. *Journal of Clinical Sleep Medicine*, *5*(2 Suppl), S20–6.

Walla, P., Duregger, C., Greiner, K., Thurner, S., & Ehrenberger, K. (2008). Multiple aspects related to self-awareness and the awareness of others: An electroencephalography study. *Journal of Neural Transmission (Vienna, Austria: 1996)*, *115*(7), 983–92. doi:10.1007/s00702-008-0035-6

Walla, P., Greiner, K., Duregger, C., Deecke, L., & Thurner, S. (2007). Self-awareness and the subconscious effect of personal pronouns on word encoding: A magnetoencephalography (MEG) study. *Neuropsychologia*, *45*(4), 796–809. doi:10.1016/j.neuropsychologia.2006.08.017

Walter, M., Bermpohl, F., Mouras, H., Schiltz, K., Tempelmann, C., Rotte, M., Heinze, H. J., et al. (2008). Distinguishing specific sexual and general emotional effects in fMRI-subcortical and cortical arousal during erotic picture viewing. *NeuroImage*, *40*(4), 1482–94. doi:10.1016/j.neuroimage.2008.01.040

Walter, M., Henning, A., Grimm, S., Schulte, R. F., Beck, J., Dydak, U., Schnepf, B., et al. (2009a). The relationship between aberrant neuronal activation in the pregenual anterior cingulate, altered glutamatergic metabolism, and anhedonia in major depression. *Archives of General Psychiatry*, *66*(5), 478–86. doi:10.1001/archgenpsychiatry.2009.39

Walter, M., Matthiä, C., Wiebking, C., Rotte, M., Tempelmann, C., Bogerts, B., Heinze, H.-J., et al. (2009b). Preceding attention and the dorsomedial prefrontal cortex: process specificity versus domain dependence. *Human Brain Mapping*, *30*(1), 312–26. doi:10.1002/hbm.20506

Wehrle, R., Czisch, M., Kaufmann, C., Wetter, T. C., Holsboer, F., Auer, D. P., & Pollmacher, T. (2005). Rapid eye movement-related brain activation in human sleep: A functional magnetic resonance imaging study. *Neuroreport*, *16*(8), 853–7.

Wehrle, R., Kaufmann, C., Wetter, T. C., Holsboer, F., Auer, D. P., Pollmacher, T., & Czisch, M. (2007). Functional microstates within human REM sleep: First evidence from fMRI of a thalamocortical network specific for phasic REM periods. *European Journal of Neuroscience*, *25*(3), 863–71. doi:10.1111/j.1460-9568.2007.05314.x

Whitehead, A. (1978). *Process and reality: An essay in cosmology* (Corrected). New York: Free Press. Retrieved from http://www.worldcat.org/title/process-and-reality-an-essay-in-cosmology/oclc/3608752&referer=brief_results

Whitfield-Gabrieli, S., Moran, J. M., Nieto-Castañón, A., Triantafyllou, C., Saxe, R., & Gabrieli, J. D. E. (2011). Associations and dissociations between default and self-reference networks in the human brain. *NeuroImage*, *55*(1), 225–32. doi:10.1016/j.neuroimage.2010.11.048

Whitfield-Gabrieli, S., Thermenos, H. W., Milanovic, S., Tsuang, M. T., Faraone, S. V., McCarley, R. W., et al. (2009). Hyperactivity and hyperconnectivity of the default network in schizophrenia and in first-degree relatives of persons with schizophrenia. *Proceedings of the National Academy of Sciences USA*, *106*(4), 1279–84.

Wicker, B., Ruby, P., Royet, J. P., & Fonlupt, P. (2003). A relation between rest and the self in the brain? *Brain Research Brain Research Review*, *43*(2), 224–30.

Wiebking, C., Bauer, A., de Greck, M., Duncan, N. W., Tempelmann, C., & Northoff, G. (2010). Abnormal body perception and neural activity in the insula in depression: An fMRI study of the depressed "material me". *World Journal of Biological Psychiatry*, *11*(3), 538–49. doi:10.3109/15622970903563794

Wiebking, C., De Greck, M., Duncan, N. W., Heinzel, A., Tempelmann, C., & Northoff, G. (2011). Are emotions associated with activity during rest or interoception? An exploratory fMRI study in healthy subjects. *Neuroscience Letters*, *491*(1), 87–92. doi:10.1016/j.neulet.2011.01.012

Wiebking, C., Duncan, N. W., Qin, P., Hayes, D. J., Lyttelton, O., Gravel, P., Verhaeghe, J., et al. (2012). External awareness and GABA-A multimodal imaging study combining fMRI and [(18) F]flumazenil-PET. *Human Brain Mapping*. Sep 21, doi:10.1002/hbm.22166

Wiebking, C., Duncan, N. W., Tiret, B., Hayes, D. J., Marjańska, M., Doyon, J., Bajbouj, M., Northoff, G. (2013) GABA in the insula—a predictor of the neural response to interoceptive awareness. *Neuroimage,* Apr 22. doi: pii: S1053-8119(13)00 389-3. 10.1016/j.neuroimage.2013.04.042 [Epub ahead of print].

Williamson, P. (2007). Are anticorrelated networks in the brain relevant to schizophrenia?. *Schizophrenia Bulletin, 33*(4), 994–1003.

Wills, T. J., Cacucci, F., Burgess, N., & O'Keefe, J. (2010). Development of the hippocampal cognitive map in pre-weanling rats. *Science, 328*(5985), 1573–6. doi:10.1126/science.1188224

Wittgenstein, L. (1921/1961). *Tractatus Logico-Philosophicus.* Translated by Pears, D. & McGuinness, B. London: Routledge and Kegan Paul.

Wittmann, M. (2009). The inner experience of time. *Philosophical Transactions of the Royal Society of London. Series B: Biological Sciences, 364*(1525), 1955–67. doi:10.1098/rstb.2009.0003

Wittmann, M. (2011). Moments in time. *Frontiers in Integrative Neuroscience,* 5, 66. doi:10.3389/fnint.2011.00066

Wittmann, M., & Paulus, M. P. (2008). Decision making, impulsivity and time perception. *Trends in Cognitive Sciences, 12*(1), 7–12. doi:10.1016/j.tics.2007.10.004

Wittmann, M., & Van Wassenhove, V. (2009). The experience of time: neural mechanisms and the interplay of emotion, cognition and embodiment. *Philosophical Transactions of the Royal Society of London. Series B, Biological Sciences, 364*(1525), 1809–13. doi:10.1098/rstb.2009.0025

Wittmann, M., Simmons, A. N., Aron, J. L., & Paulus, M. P. (2010). Accumulation of neural activity in the posterior insula encodes the passage of time. *Neuropsychologia, 48*(10), 3110–20. doi:10.1016/j.neuropsychologia.2010.06.023

Wittmann, M., Simmons, A. N., Flagan, T., Lane, S. D., Wackermann, J., & Paulus, M. P. (2011). Neural substrates of time perception and impulsivity. *Brain Research, 1406,* 43–58. doi:10.1016/j.brainres.2011.06.048

Wittmann, M., van Wassenhove, V., Craig, A. D., & Paulus, M. P. (2010). The neural substrates of subjective time dilation. *Frontiers in Human Neuroscience,* 4, 2. doi:10.3389/neuro.09.002.2010

Yan, C., Liu, D., He, Y., Zou, Q., Zhu, C., Zuo, X., Long, X., et al. (2009). Spontaneous brain activity in the default mode network is sensitive to different resting-state conditions with limited cognitive load. *PloS One, 4*(5), e5743. doi:10.1371/journal.pone.0005743

Yaoi, K., Osaka, N., & Osaka, M. (2009). Is the self special in the dorsomedial prefrontal cortex? An fMRI study. *Social Neuroscience, 4,* 455–63.

Yoon, J. H., Maddock, R. J., Rokem, A., Silver, M. A., Minzenberg, M. J., Ragland, J. D., & Carter, C. S. (2010). GABA concentration is reduced in visual cortex in schizophrenia and correlates with orientation-specific surround suppression. *Journal of Neuroscience, 30*(10), 3777–81.

Zahavi, D. (2005). Subjectivity and selfhood investigating the first-person perspective. Cambridge, Mass.: MIT Press

Zeki, S. (2008). The disunity of consciousness. *Progress in Brain Research, 168,* 11–18. doi:10.1016/S0079-6123(07)68002-9

Zhao, K., Wu, Q., Zimmer, H. D., & Fu, X. (2011). Electrophysiological correlates of visually processing subject's own name. *Neuroscience Letters, 491*(2), 143–7. doi:10.1016/j.neulet.2011.01.025

Zhou, A., Shi, Z., Zhang, P., Liu, P., Han, W., Wu, H., Li, Q., et al. (2010). An ERP study on the effect of self-relevant possessive pronoun. *Neuroscience Letters, 480*(2), 162–6. doi:10.1016/j.neulet.2010.06.033

Zhou, J., Liu, X., Song, W., Yang, Y., Zhao, Z., Ling, F., et al. (2011). Specific and nonspecific thalamocortical functional connectivity in normal and vegetative states. *Consciousness and Cognition, 20*(2), 257–68.

Zhu, J., Wu, X., Gao, L., Mao, Y., Zhong, P., Tang, W., & Zhou, L. (2009). Cortical activity after emotional visual stimulation in minimally conscious state patients. *Journal of Neurotrauma, 26*(5), 677–88. doi:10.1089/neu.2008.0691

Zhu, Y., Zhang, L., Fan, J., & Han, S. (2007). Neural basis of cultural influence on self-representation. *Neuroimage, 34*(3), 1310–16.

Zmigrod, S., & Hommel, B. (2011). The relationship between feature binding and consciousness: Evidence from asynchronous multi-modal stimuli. *Consciousness and Cognition, 20*(3), 586–93. doi:10.1016/j.concog.2011.01.011

INDEX

aboutness, 329

aboutness of mental states, 329

absolute amplitude of low-frequency fluctuations (ALFF), 232

access consciousness, *lxii*, 153–154

access unity, 154, 155–157

active synthesis, 561

activity time curves (ACTs), 49

actual consciousness, *lviii*, *lvi–lvii*, *lxiv*

affect
    consciousness, 487
    qualia and, 506
    subcortical regions, 495–496
    vegetative state, 492–495

affective functions, self-specificity, 279, 290, 291–292*f*

Affective Neuroscience, Panksepp, 495

affective qualia, 503–504
    subcortical regions mediating, 496

affective-vegetative account of time, 557–558
    vs. neurophenomenal account, 558–559

affordance, 220

Alzheimer's disease, 257

amalgamated mind *vs.* amalgamated brain, 546–547

amantadine, 456

amplification hypothesis, 75

amygdala, 284–285*f*

anatomical rings, self-specificity, 254–256

anatomical structure, 10

anesthesia, *xli*
    dissociation between width of point and dimension bloc, 85
    effective *vs.* ineffective connectivity, 74–75
    functional connectivity in, 78–79
    glutamatergic transmission, 95
    neurophenomenal *vs.* neurocognitive account of, 102–103

anoetic consciousness, 503–504

ANOVA (analysis of variance), 125

anterior cortical midline structures (aCMS), schizophrenia, 393

anterior midline regions, resting-state activity and self-specificity, 257–258, 259*f*

apperception, 571, 577*n*.3, 578*n*.5

a priori cortical programs, 565

arousal, 45

ascending reticular activating system (ARAS), vegetative state, 79

aspectual shapes, 359

attend auditory (AA), ideal and worst phases in resting-state activity, 131, 133–134*f*

attend visual (AV), ideal and worst phases in resting-state activity, 131, 133–134*f*

attention, 151, 280

attention, mind wandering and, 383–384

attunement deficits, schizophrenia, 236–237

auditory-evoked potentials (ssAEPs), steady-state, 231

auditory hallucinations, external contents in resting state, 349

auditory oddball paradigm, 384

auditory processing, schizophrenia, 230

auditory stimuli, mind wandering, 384

autobiographical memory, 257

autobiographical self, 580–581

automatic nonconscious processors, 151

automatic processing, schizophrenia, 231

availability thesis, dependence of unity on subjectivity, 222–223

awake state, *xxiii–xxiv*
    carryover and transfer of resting state's structures to consciousness, 372–373
    constitution of perceptions in, and dreaming state, 376*f*
    intentionality, 379
    rest-rest interaction and resemblance of dreams and, 378–379
    stimulus-rest interaction encoding resting-state activity, 377–378

awareness, 104
    internal and external, in resting state, 332–334
    relationship between midline and lateral networks, 337–338*f*